Nonpharmacological Therapy of Arrhythmias for the 21st Century
The State of the Art

Editors:

Igor Singer, MBBS, FRACP, FACP, FACC, FACA
Professor of Medicine
Director, Cardiac Electrophysiology and Pacing
Chief, Arrhythmia Service
University of Louisville
Louisville, Kentucky

S. Serge Barold, MD, FRACP, FACP, FACC, FESC
Chief, Arrhythmia Service
Cardiology Division
Mt. Sinai Medical Center
Cleveland, Ohio

A. John Camm, MD, FRCP, FESC, FACC
Professor of Clinical Cardiology
St. George's Hospital Medical School
London, England

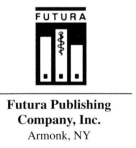

Futura Publishing Company, Inc.
Armonk, NY

Library of Congress Cataloging-in-Publication Data

Nonpharmacological therapy of arrhythmias for the 21st century. The
   state of the art / editor, Igor Singer; associate editors, S. Serge
   Barold, A. John Camm.
       p.   cm.
   Includes bibliographical references and index.
   ISBN 0-87993-690-8 (alk. paper)
    1. Arrhythmia—Treatment.   2. Catheter ablation.   3. Implantable
cardioverter-defibrillators.   I. Singer, Igor.   II. Barold, S.
Serge.   III. Camm, A. John.
    [DNLM: 1. Arrhythmia—therapy.   WG 330 N8139   1998]
   RC685.A65N65   1998
   616.1′2806—dc21
   DNLM/DLC
   for Library of Congress   98-4105
                                                   CIP

Copyright 1998
Futura Publishing Company, Inc.
135 Bedford Road
Armonk, New York 10504-0418
LC#: 98-4105
ISBN: 0-87993-6908

Printed in the United States of America.

This book is printed on acid-free paper.

*This book is dedicated to my children
Justin Joseph, Jessica Sarah, and Christina Rebecca,
my wife Sylvia Ann, and to my mother and father.
I hope that this book may provide further inspiration to scientists
and scholars who strive to better mankind
and help their fellow man.*
—Igor Singer

---

*To Helen S. Barold, MD,
who made us proud.*
— S. Serge Barold

To Joy and the kids.
—A. John Camm

Contributors

Ayman S. Al-Khadra, MD
Clinical Associate Staff, Department of Cardiology, Section of Electrophysiology, Cleveland Clinic, Cleveland, Ohio

Etienne Aliot, MD
Hôpital Central, Cardiology Department, Nancy, France

Boaz Avitall, MD, PhD
Associate Professor and Director, Clinical and Research Cardiac Electrophysiology Laboratories, Division of Cardiology, University of Chicago, Chicago, Illinois

Gust H. Bardy, MD
Professor of Medicine, University of Washington, Department of Medicine, Division of Cardiology, Seattle, Washington

S. Serge Barold, MD, FRACP, FACP, FACC, FESC
Chief, Arrhythmia Service, Cardiology Division, Mt. Sinai Medical Center, Cleveland, Ohio

J. Thomas Bigger Jr, MD
Professor of Medicine and Pharmacology, College of Physicians and Surgeons of Columbia University, New York, New York

Peter H. Belott, MD, FACC
Clinical Instructor, University of California at San Diego, School of Medicine, Director, Pacemaker Center, El Cajon, California

David G. Benditt, MD
Professor of Medicine, Co-Director Cardiac Arrhythmia Center, University of Minnesota, Minneapolis, Minnesota

Alfred E. Buxton, MD
Professor of Medicine, Temple University School of Medicine, Philadelphia, Pennsylvania

Hugh Calkins, MD
Associate Professor of Medicine, Director of Electrophysiology, Johns Hopkins Hospital, Baltimore, Maryland

A. John Camm, MD, FRCP, FESC, FACC
Professor of Clinical Cardiology, St. George's Hospital Medical School, London, England

Jacques Clémenty, MD
Professor of Medicine and Head Cardiac Electrophysiology and Pacing Department, Centre Hospitalier Universitaire de Bordeaux, Hôpital Cardiologique du Haut-Lévêque, Bordeaux-Pessac, France

Randolph A.S. Cooper, MD
Assistant Professor, Division of Cardiovascular Disease of the School of Medicine, University of Alabama at Birmingham, Birmingham, Alabama

David A. Danford, MD
Joint Division of Pediatric Cardiology, University of Nebraska Medical Center/Creighton College of Medicine, Children's Hospital, Omaha, Nebraska

C. de Chillou, MD
Hôpital Central, Cardiology Department, Nancy, France

Edwin G. Duffin, PhD
Bakken Fellow, Medtronic, Inc., Minneapolis, Minnesota

Kenneth A. Ellenbogen, MD
Director, Clinical Electrophysiology Laboratory, Division of Cardiology, Department of Medicine, Medical College of Virginia and the McGuire VA Medical Center, Richmond, Virginia

N.A. Mark Estes III, MD
Professor of Medicine, Tufts University School of Medicine, Chief, Divison of Cardiovascular Medicine, New England Medical Center, Boston, Massachusetts

Gerard Fahy, MD
Assistant Professor of Medicine, Director, ECG Laboratory, University of Minnesota, Minneapolis, Minnesota

Gary Felix, BS
Joint Division of Pediatric Cardiology, University of Nebraska Medical Center/Creighton College of Medicine, Children's Hospital, Omaha, Nebraska

T. Bruce Ferguson Jr. MD
Roper HeartCare, Roper CareAlliance, Charleston, South Carolina

Ross D. Fletcher, MD
Chief, Cardiology, VA Medical Center; Professor of Medicine, Georgetown University, Cardiology Section, Washington, DC

Stéphane Garrigue, MD
Centre Hospitalier Universitaire de Bordeaux, Hôpital Cardiologique du Haut-Lévêque, Bordeaux-Pessac, France

Colette M. Guiraudon, MD
Professor of Pathology, Director of Transplant Pathology, University of Western Ontario, London, Ontario, Canada

Gerard M. Guiraudon, MD
Chairman, Department of Thoracic and Cardiovascular Surgery, Professor of Surgery, Associate Chief, Division of Cardiothoracic Surgery, State University of New York, Buffalo, New York

Gopal Gupta, BS
Research Specialist, Clinical and Research Cardiac Electrophysiology Laboratories, Division of Cardiology, University of Chicago, Chicago, Illinois

Michel Haïssaguerre, MD
Professor of Medicine, Centre Hospitalier Universitaire de Bordeaux, Hôpital Cardiologique du Haut-Lévêque, Bordeaux-Pessac, France

David L. Hayes, MD
Consultant, Division of Cardiovascular Diseases and Internal Medicine, Director, Cardiac Pacing Services, Mayo Clinic and Mayo Foundation, Rochester, Minnesota

Ray Helms, BSE
Research Specialist, Clinical Research Cardiac Electrophysiology Laboratories, Division of Cardiology, University of Chicago, Chicago, Illinois

Mélèze Hocini, MD
Centre Hospitalier Universitaire de Bordeaux, Hôpital Cardiologique du Haut-Lévêque, Bordeaux-Pessac, France

Kris Houston, RN, BSN, MA
Joint Division of Pediatric Cardiology, University of Nebraska Medical Center/Creighton College of Medicine, Children's Hospital, Omaha, Nebraska

Henry H. Hsia, MD
Cardiology Section, Department of Medicine, Temple University School of Medicine and Temple University Hospital, Philadelphia, Pennsylvania

Jian Huang, MD
Fellow, Department of Medicine, Division of Cardiovascular Disease, University of Alabama-Birmingham, Birmingham, Alabama

Raymond E. Ideker, MD, PhD
Professor of Physiology, Medicine, and Biomedical Engineering, Division of Cardiovascular Disease, University of Alabama-Birmingham, Birmingham, Alabama

Demosthenes Iskos, MD
Fellow in Clinical Cardiac Electrophysiology, University of Minnesota, Minneapolis, Minnesota

Pierre Jaïs, MD
Staff Cardiologist, Centre Hospitalier Universitaire de Bordeaux, Hôpital Cardiologique du Haut-Lévêque, Bordeaux-Pessac, France

Gregory K. Jones, MD
The Department of Medicine, Division of Cardiology, University of Washington, Seattle, Washington

Werner Jung, MD, FESC
Department of Medicine and Cardiology, University of Bonn, Bonn, Germany

Pamela Karasik, MD
Associate Director, Electrophysiology, VA Medical Center; Assistant Professor of Medicine, Georgetown University, Cardiology Section, Washington, DC

Bruce H. KenKnight, PhD
Department of Therapy Research, Guidant/CPI, St. Paul, Minnesota

George J. Klein, MD, FRCPC, FACC
Professor of Medicine, Director, Arrhythmia Service, University of Western Ontario, Faculty of Medicine, London, Ontario, Canada

Helmut U. Klein, MD
Department of Cardiology, University Hospital of the Otto-von-Guericke University, Magdeburg, Germany

John D. Kugler, MD
Professor of Pediatrics, Joint Division of Pediatric Cardiology, University of Nebraska Medical Center/Creighton College of Medicine, Children's Hospital, Omaha, Nebraska

Douglas J. Lang, PhD
Department of Therapy Research, Guidant/CPI, St. Paul, Minnesota

T. Lavergne, MD
Cardiology Department, Hôpital Broussai, Paris, France

Paul A. Levine, MD
Clinical Professor of Medicine, Loma Linda University Medical Center, Loma Linda; Clinical Associate Professor of Medicine, University of California, Los Angeles, California; St. Jude Medical, Sylmar, California

M. Limousin, PhD
ELA Recherche, La Boursidière, Le Plessis Robinson, France

Berndt Lüderitz, MD, FESC, FACC
Professor of Medicine, Head, Department of Medicine and Cardiology, University of Bonn, Bonn, Germany

Keith G. Lurie, MD
Associate Professor of Medicine, Co-Director Cardiac Arrhythmia Center, University of Minnesota, Minneapolis, Minnesota

Bruce M. McManus, MD, PhD, FRCPC, FACC
Professor and Head, Department of Pathology and Laboratory Medicine, University of British Columbia; Director, Cardiovascular Research Laboratory, St. Paul's Hospital, Vancouver, B.C., Canada

William Miles, MD
Professor of Medicine, Krannert Institute of Cardiology, Department of Medicine, Indiana University School of Medicine, Indianapolis, Indiana

Scott Millard, BSE
Research Assistant, Clinical and Research Cardiac Electrophysiology Laboratories, Division of Cardiology, University of Chicago, Chicago, Illinois

John M. Miller, MD
Professor of Medicine, Krannert Institute of Cardiology, Department of Medicine, Indiana University School of Medicine, Indianapolis, Indiana

L. Brent Mitchell, MD, FRCPC
Professor and Head, Divison of Cardiology, Calgary Regional Health Authority/University of Calgary, Calgary, Alberta, Canada

Harry G. Mond, MD
Department of Cardiology, The Royal Melbourne Hospital, Victoria, Australia

Fred Morady, MD
Professor of Internal Medicine, Director, Clinical Electrophysiology Laboratory, University of Michigan Medical Center, Ann Arbor, Michigan

Seah Nisam
Director Medical Sciences, CPI/Guidant, Zaventem, Belgium

R. Nitzsche, PhD
Ela Recherch, La Boursidière, Le Plessis Robinson, France

Jeffrey E. Olgin, MD
Assistant Professor of Medicine, Krannert Institute of Cardiology, Department of Medicine, Indiana University School of Medicine, Indianapolis, Indiana

Walter H. Olson, PhD
Senior Research Fellow, Bakken Foundation, Tachyarrhythmia Research, Medtronic, Minneapolis, Minnesota

Ramakota K. Reddy, MD
The Department of Medicine, Division of Cardiology, University of Washington, Seattle, Washington

Sven Reek, MD
Department of Cardiology, University Hospital of the Otto-von-Guericke University, Magdeburg, Germany

Steven A. Rothman, MD
Cardiology Section, Department of Medicine, Temple University School of Medicine and Temple University Hospital, Philadelphia, Pennsylvania

N. Sadoul, MD
Hôpital Central, Cardiology Department, Nancy, France

Scott Sakaguchi, MD
Assistant Professor of Medicine, Fellowship Coordinator, Clinical Cardiac Electrophysiology, University of Minnesota, Minneapolis, Minnesota

Nadir Saoudi, MD
Cardiology Department, Centre Hospitalier Universitaire, Rouen, France

Avram Scheiner, PhD
Department of Therapy Research, Guidant/CPI, St. Paul, Minnesota

Dipen C. Shah, MD
Centre Hospitalier Universitaire de Bordeaux, Hôpital Cardiologique du Haut-Lévêque, Bordeaux-Pessac, France

Michael J. Silka, MD
Joint Division of Pediatric Cardiology, University of Nebraska Medical Center/Creighton College of Medicine, Children's Hospital, Omaha, Nebraska

Igor Singer, MBBS, FRACP, FACP, FACC, FACA
Professor of Medicine, Director, Cardiac Electrophysiology and Pacing, Chief, Arrhythmia Service, University of Louisville, Louisville, Kentucky

William M. Smith, PhD
Departments of Medicine, Physiology, and Biomedical Engineering, The University of Alabama at Birmingham, Birmingham, Alabama

S. Mark Sopher, MRCP
Department of Cardiological Sciences, St. George's Hospital Medical School, London, England

Donald Switzer, MD
Millard Fillmore Health System and State University of New York at Buffalo, School of Medicine, Department of Thoracic Surgery, Department of Medicine, Division of Cardiology, Buffalo, New York

Atsushi Takahashi, MD
Centre Hospitalier Universitaire de Bordeaux, Hôpital Cardiologique du Haut-Lévêque, Bordeaux-Pessac, France

Gregory P. Walcott, MD
Assistant Professor, Department of Medicine, The University of Alabama at Birmingham, Birmingham, Alabama

Paul J. Wang, MD
Associate Professor of Medicine, Tufts University School of Medicine, Director, Cardiac Arrhythmia Service, New England Medical Center, Boston, Massachusetts

Bruce L. Wilkoff, MD
Director, Cardiac Pacing and Tachyarrhythmia Devices, The Cleveland Clinic Foundation, Department of Cardiology, Cleveland, Ohio

Mark A. Wood, MD
Electrophysiology Section, Division of Cardiology, Department of Medicine, Medical College of Virginia and the McGuire VA Medical Center, Richmond, Virginia

Shelley M. Wood, BA
Assistant Coordinator, Cardiovascular Research Laboratory, St. Paul's Hospital, Vancouver, B.C., Canada

Raymond Yee, MD, FRCP(C), FACC
Associate Professor of Medicine, Director, Arrhythmia Monitoring Unit, The University of Western Ontario Faculty of Medicine, London, Ontario, Canada

Xiaohong Zhou, MD
Assistant Professor, Department of Medicine, Division of Cardiovascular Disease, University of Alabama-Birmingham, Birmingham, Alabama

Dennis W.X. Zhu, MD
Assistant Professor of Medicine, Director, Clinical Cardiac Electrophysiology, Baylor College of Medicine, Houston, Texas

Preface

Interventional electrophysiology has emerged as a major subspecialty of clinical electrophysiology. It continues to evolve with breathtaking speed. Technological developments, scientific advances, and computerization have made possible today what pioneers of this dynamic specialty could only dream of only two decades ago. It was only 18 years since the implantable defibrillator (ICD) debuted at the Johns Hopkins Hospital in Baltimore under the pioneering genius of Michel Mirowski, and barely 30 years since His bundle recordings were first introduced into clinical practice. In the last decade the advances in catheter technologies, mapping systems, and microcircuits have made possible therapies that were once considered unthinkable. The ICD, once considered by some as a bizarre and unethical invention, has now become commonplace. The ICD has not only been demonstrated to be superior to all other therapies for lethal ventricular arrhythmias, but is now being tested for primary prevention of sudden cardiac death. Parallel developments in pacing and defibrillation have led to the marriage of antitachycardia devices, dual chamber pacemakers, and defibrillators. Development of small caliber transvenous electrodes and small devices have made it possible for ICDs to be implanted in the electrophysiology laboratory by trained electrophysiologists. Similarly, evolution of steerable catheters and percutaneous multi-electrode mapping systems has provided electrophysiologists with tools to ablate most reentrant tachycardias, with few notable exceptions. Boundaries of interventional electrophysiology are continuously challenged by new discoveries, refinements in technology, and imaginative procedures.

It is with this backdrop in mind that this book was conceived. We are at the threshold of the new century. Consequently, we have chosen as the title for this book *Nonpharmacological Therapy of Arrhythmias for the 21st Century: The State of the Art* to reflect our current knowledge. This is a carefully integrated book covering most relevant subjects of interest to interventional electrophysiologists. It was our intention at the outset that this should be up to date, as difficult and elusive as this goal might seem, be practically oriented, and especially geared to the interventionists and others interested in this rapidly growing field: general cardiologists, cardiothoracic surgeons, cardiology fellows, engineers, nurses, and technicians.

The book is divided into four sections:

Section I deals with advances in catheter ablation techniques and covers specific procedures for accessory pathways, AV node reentrant tachycardia, atrial flutter, atrial fibrillation, and ventricular tachycardia. Scientific and anatomic basis for ablation therapies are extensively discussed. A chapter is also devoted to new catheter designs for interventional electrophysiology.

Section II describes the current knowledge base of ICD therapy, indications, and implantation techniques, including new developments in dual chamber and atrial defibrillators. The recently completed and published randomized multicenter trials of ICD therapy and trials for prophylaxis of sudden cardiac death are presented. Implications for current and future use of ICDs are discussed, as well as the role of pharmacological therapy.

Section III is devoted to arrhythmia surgery and mapping technologies. Although indications for operative intervention for arrhythmias are narrowing due to astonishing progress in percutaneous ablation, surgical techniques remain an essential therapeutic component for arrhythmias. Operative mapping, surgical techniques for supraventricular and ventricular arrhythmias, and atrial fibrillation are discussed.

Section IV is devoted to advances in pacing. A review of implantation techniques for pacemakers, with emphasis on the new, and methods for lead extraction, an increasingly important subject, are discussed at length. This section also contains extensive discussions of new indications for pacing, including vasodepressor syncope, the latest developments in rate-adaptive pacing, and clinical application of mode-switching and pacemaker automation.

It is our hope that this book will be useful to interventional electrophysiologists, general cardiologists, cardiovascular surgeons, and all others dealing with complex cardiac arrhythmias. We would like to thank the many talented authors and scientists as well as the staff at Futura Publishing Company, especially Ms. Linda Shaw, who have all made this book possible.

Igor Singer, MBBS, FRACP, FACP, FACC, FACA

S. Serge Barold, MD, FRACP, FACP, FACC, FESC

A. John Camm, MD, FRCP, FESC, FACC

Contents

SECTION I. Advances in Catheter Ablation
Section Editor: A. John Camm

SECTION II. Implantable Cardioverter-Defibrillators
Section Editor: Igor Singer

SECTION III. Surgical Alternatives for Arrhythmia Management
Section Editor: Igor Singer

SECTION IV. Advances in Cardiac Pacing
Section Editor: S. Serge Barold

Section I

Advances in Catheter Ablation

Section Editor: A. John Camm

Chapter 1

Physics and Biology of Catheter Ablation

Paul J. Wang, N. A. Mark Estes III

Introduction

Catheter ablation has become an important therapeutic tool in the treatment of many cardiac arrhythmias. The various techniques of catheter ablation share a common basis in the selective destruction of myocardial tissue responsible for the genesis or perpetuation of the cardiac arrhythmias. The conventional energy source used for nearly all clinical catheter ablations being performed is radiofrequency energy.[1–30] Alternative methods for catheter ablation include microwave,[31–57] laser,[58–94] cryoablation,[95–107] ultrasound,[108–116] and chemical ablation.[117–133]

Radiofrequency Ablation

Biophysics of Radiofrequency Ablation

Radiofrequency (RF) energy has been used as a clinical tool for the catheter ablation of numerous cardiac arrhythmias.[1–30] Radiofrequency energy spans a wide range of frequencies, exhibiting a varying combination of resistive and dielectric properties. At the lower frequencies, 300 to 900 kHz, representing the range of clinically used RF energy, the resistive properties predomi-

nate while at higher frequencies such as 915 MHz to 3 GHz, the range of medical microwave energies, the dielectric properties are mainly observed.

The resistive properties of RF energy result in the creation of heat within the myocardial tissue as energy passes from the electrode into the tissue. The amount of energy dissipated decreases rapidly over distance, approximately as a fourth power function.[7] Only a small volume of myocardial tissue is heated directly by the RF energy with the remaining tissue heating via conduction.

Haines and Watson developed a thermodynamic model that predicts the RF ablation lesion size.[7] The basic equation used in this analysis was $r_i/r = (t - T)/(t_o - T)$ where r is the distance from the electrode center, r_i is the radius of the thin rim of volume heated tissue, t is the tissue temperature at distance r, T is the basal temperature, and t_o is the temperature at the electrode-tissue interface. Using a model of an isolated perfused right ventricular tissue, the thermodynamic model was compared to the temperature measurements during ablation. The time-temperature rise exhibited a monoexponential relationship (Figure 1). The temperature at depth decreased rapidly, approximated by a hyperbolic relationship

From Singer I, Barold SS, Camm AJ (eds): *Nonpharmacological Therapy of Arrhythmias for the 21st Century: The State of the Art.* Futura Publishing Co, Inc., Armonk, NY, © 1998.

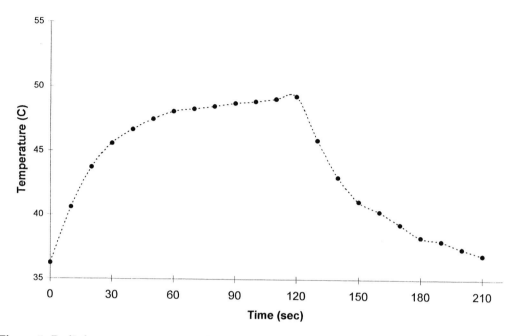

Figure 1. Radiofrequency energy was delivered to isolated perfused and superfused canine right ventricular free wall. The tissue temperature (°C) was measured using a thermistor at a distance 2.5 ± 0.2 mm from the RF electrode during and after the 120 sec of radiofrequency energy delivery. The electrode tip temperature was 80°C. Adapted with permission from Haines DE, et al.[7]

(Figure 2). Lesion depth was 4.4 ± 0.5 mm under these conditions at a mean power of 1.51 ± 0.15 watts, resulting in a volume of 96 ± 29 mm³. Temperature of the electrode was the best predictor of lesion size.

An ablation system for the delivery of energy to myocardial tissue consists of an electrode at the end of a catheter, a ground, and a radiofrequency energy source. Radiofrequency energy current passes between the indifferent ground plate and the electrode tip. The position of the ground plate does not significantly alter the lesion size. However, by increasing the ground plate surface area, the impedance may decline and the current may increase, leading to higher electrode temperatures.[8]

Effects of Radiofrequency Ablation

Radiofrequency ablation results in cell injury mediated primarily via thermal mecha-

nisms. Increased temperature of myocardial tissue has a number of effects electrophysiologically. In an isolated guinea pig papillary muscle preparation, there may be an increase in the dV/dt_{max} during heating to 38°C to 45°C for 1 minute. In contrast, heating to 45°C to 50°C may result in a decrease in dV/dt_{max}. The increase in dV/dt_{max} may be caused by a thermally mediated increase in sodium channel function while the decrease in dV/dt_{max} may be caused by voltage-dependent sodium channel inactivation. Abnormal automaticity was observed at temperatures above 45°C. Reversible changes in excitability were seen above 50°C.

Thermally mediated cell death appears to depend on both time and temperature. Prolonged heating may cause cell death at temperatures as low as 45°C while irreversible myocardial cell death during conventional ablation likely occurs between 52°C and

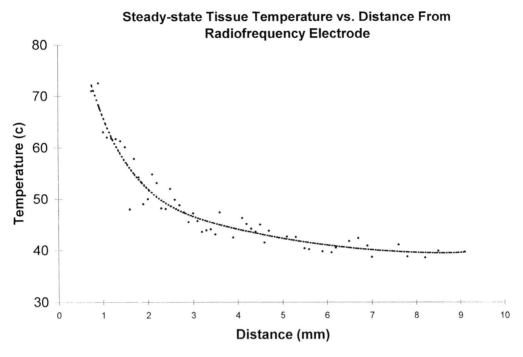

Figure 2. Radiofrequency energy was delivered to isolated perfused and superfused canine right ventricular free wall. The tissue temperature (°C) was measured using a thermistor. The steady-state temperature as a function of distance is shown. Adapted with permission from Haines DE, et al.[7]

55°C. Denaturation of membrane proteins and tissue dessication are important steps leading to cell death.

Myocyte heating by RF ablation may result in damage to the cell membrane, the sarcoplasmic reticulum, and mitochondria. Temperature-sensitive changes in membrane proteins involved in transport processes may be important in the electrophysiological changes observed. As the ablation continues, the tissue surrounding the electrode retracts. If temperatures rapidly increase, liquids under the electrode may boil and form vapor. Release of this vapor may lead to a "pop," which is likely associated with tissue destruction.[1]

In addition to thermal injury, there may be some direct effects of electrical energy on the integrity of the myocyte membrane. Studies examining the effects of high-energy fields on isolated chick myocytes have demonstrated that cellular depolarization

may occur. High-intensity RF fields have been shown to result in breakdown of the membrane lipid bilayer. However, there are few studies that examine membrane effects using the energies used during clinical radiofrequency ablation.

As RF ablation occurs, the impedance frequently decreases, reflecting changes in the electrical properties of myocardial tissue from the ablation. At excessively high temperatures, in excess of 90°C or 100°C, coagulation of tissue and blood occurs at the electrode-myocardial tissue interface. The impedance markedly rises due to these changes in tissue property, effectively stopping current flow.

A number of mathematical models have been developed to describe the biophysical changes that occur during RF ablation. Theoretical models must consider factors such as electrode configuration, materials, and size, blood flow, myocardial tissue properties, and the geometric relationship of the electrode and the myocardium.

Models such as that proposed by Labonte[3] consider heat transfer using the bioheat equation, in which the temperature distribution is simplified by ignoring metabolic heat generation and myocardial perfusion. The cooling effects of circulating blood are also considered. The electrical conductivity of heart tissue is approximated to be 0.6 Sm^{-1} at 1 MHz. Electrical conductivity varies by $2\%/^\circ\text{C}^{-1}$. The extent of thermal damage is predicted by a standard chemical rate process equation. A finite element analysis may be applied because of the complex geometries involved in radiofrequency ablation. A phantom consisting of tissue-equivalent material was used for experimental validation of the mathematical model (Figure 3). The theoretical model was quite accurate in predicting temperatures at 3 mm or greater depths. At depths less than 3 mm the predicted temperature was less than the observed temperature. There are several possible reasons given for this discrepancy. The phantom is cooled due to convection loss and evaporation. In addition, the thermographic method of measuring temperatures experimentally may have important spatial limitations.

Other models have used three-dimensional finite element analysis in order to analyze the effects of electrode geometry, electrode-tissue angle, and circulating blood flow on the lesion size and temperature distribution. In such a study by Panescu et al.,

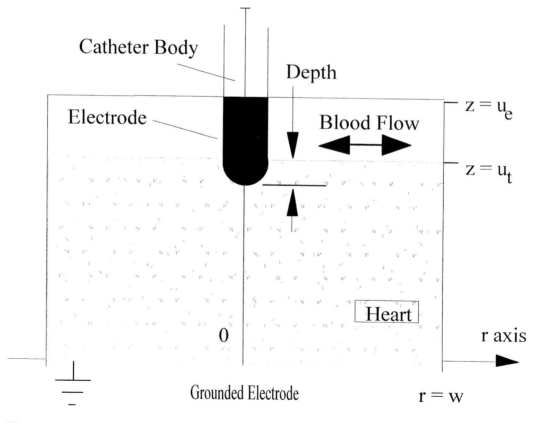

Figure 3. A common theoretical model for the radiofrequency ablation of the endocardium is shown. The electrode is placed perpendicular to the endocardium. The tissue is considered to be homogeneous. A grounded electrode is present on the opposite side of the heart tissue. Blood flows around the ablation electrode. Adapted with permission from Labonte S, et al.[3]

the maximal temperature was observed a fraction of a millimeter from the electrode surface. The greatest power to reach target temperature was at 45° angle, which also resulted in the largest lesions.[2]

The volume of heating predicted theoretically agrees with the experimentally observed temperature profile. In a study by Wonnell et al., the radial distance to 50% of the maximal temperature change was 1.11 ± 0.21 mm and volume representing greater than 25% of the change in maximal temperature was 150 ± 40 mm³.[32]

Factors Affecting Radiofrequency Ablation

Because the ultimate biological effect of RF energy is thermal injury, the temperature of the myocardial tissue is an important determinant of lesion size. The lesion size is affected by the electrode configuration and size, the power, and myocardial tissue properties.

Electrode Design

As outlined by mathematical models and experimental and clinical evidence, the lesion size and effectiveness of RF ablation are greatly affected by the electrode configuration and design. The conventional electrode is a dome-shaped tip electrode. This design has been used mainly because of its ease and safety of delivery. Other designs may result in increased lesion size. An elongated electrode in the shape of a peanut or dumbbell exhibits a current distribution which extends over a longer distance (Figure 4). Blouin and Marcus[21] have investigated a large number of electrode designs and their effects on lesion dimensions. They found that designs such as a needle electrode may yield the largest lesion size. However, these designs are not as practical for clinical use because of concerns of safety and catheter delivery. Blouin and Marcus demonstrated that power densities greater

than 0.6 W/mm² increase the incidence of impedance rises.

The thermal properties of the electrode may also be important. Effective heat transfer from the electrode to the myocardium may be an important determinant of lesion size. The use of thermally conductive materials such as gold has been shown to result in improved energy transfer.[15]

The surface area of the electrode may be augmented by increasing its dimensions and also by increasing its porosity.[16] Numerous small beads connected together provide an increased surface area, improving heat transfer and increasing the effective surface area for energy delivery.

Electrode Size

Electrode size has been shown to be an important determinant of RF ablation lesion size. As the electrode size increases, for a given power, the current density decreases. However, by increasing the power, the current density may be maintained, resulting in tissue heating over the entire electrode surface. The larger surface area increases the lesion size. For practical purposes, as long as the electrode surface area maintains contact with the endocardial surface and the power is used to maintain the current density, the lesion size will increase as a function of electrode size. Temperature monitoring has been used to determine whether adequate power is used to maintain desirable electrode-myocardial tissue interface temperatures over a large range of clinical conditions in which the degree of contact and geometry of the electrode and endocardium may vary considerably. Increasing the electrode size at some point may decrease the lesion size when a significant proportion of the electrode is not in contact with the myocardium. In such a case, some energy is dissipated into the blood pool when the electrode surface is not entirely in contact with the endocardium. In addition, if one part of the electrode is in better contact than another part of the electrode, uneven heating of the myocardial tissue may occur.

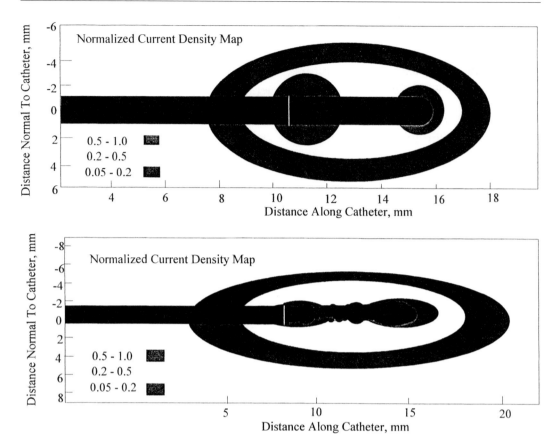

Figure 4. Schematic diagram of the normalized current density for an 8F 5-mm tip electrode (top panel) and an 8F 8-mm hourglass electrode (bottom panel). Adapted with permission from Panescu D, et al.[2]

Studies have demonstrated that 4-mm tip electrodes double the lesion size compared to 2-mm tip electrodes. Similarly, Langberg et al.[12,13] demonstrated that lesion size increases from 4 mm to 8 mm tip electrode sizes but that the lesion size decreases using larger electrode sizes. In addition significant char and coagulation formation was observed with electrode size greater than 8 mm. Despite tip temperature monitoring, the more proximal parts of the electrode may have better contact depending on the electrode-myocardial geometry resulting in increased current density at these sites and excessive heating. The current density also falls, resulting in decreased lesion size since it may be difficult to estimate the increased power required because it must be distributed over the entire electrode surface area.

Myocardial Tissue Properties

Myocardial tissue properties are important determinants of lesion size. Different regions of the normal heart have different geometries and tissue characteristics that may affect the heating properties during RF ablation. Myocardium that may have increased fibrosis or scarring will have significant different thermal and electrical properties. Radiofrequency ablation performed on diseased myocardial tissue results in significantly smaller lesions compared to normal myocardial tissue.

Power

As the power delivered increases, the current density at the myocardial interface and the resultant myocardial temperature increase. The overall lesion size increases up to the point that excessive temperatures occur, resulting in a decrease in lesion size at increased powers. Wittkampf et al. demonstrated that 6 W of power exhibited a greater lesion size compared to 4 W.[4]

Duration

As the duration of RF ablation increases, the lesion size increases up to a point. Whayne et al. have shown in vitro that RF ablation lesion size increases within the first 30 seconds but then begins to plateau.[34] Using a 2-mm tip electrode, Wittkampf et al. demonstrated that lesion length increased over the first 20 seconds of ablation with only small changes subsequently.[4]

Pulsing of RF energy has been hypothesized to result in cooling at the endocardial surface. This might permit one to deliver a larger amount of energy, creating an increased lesion size. However, limited in vitro studies did not demonstrate an increase in lesion size during pulsing.[20]

Temperature

Since RF ablation is thermally mediated, lesion size increases as the temperature increases. However, as discussed above, when the temperatures become excessive, the incidence of coagulation formation increases, significantly impairing the ability to increase lesion size.

Contact and Pressure

Improved contact of the electrode with the endocardium will maximize the surface area of the electrode-myocardial tissue interface, increasing lesion size. Increasing contact pressure similarly increases lesion size. Instability of the catheter electrode will result in fluctuating temperatures, convective losses of energy during ablation, and poor tissue heating. At extreme degrees

of instability, the likelihood of clinically successful ablation decreases substantially.

Temperature Measurement During Radiofrequency Ablation

A number of clinically available RF ablation systems use temperature monitoring during ablation. A thermocouple in contact with the tip of the electrode or the body of the electrode may be used (Figure 5). Also, a thermistor may be placed at the catheter tip for temperature measurement.

These techniques of temperature measurement approximate the temperature at the electrode-myocardial tissue interface during ablation. Temperature monitoring usually prevents excessive temperatures from occurring. Clinical use of temperature monitoring has been shown to result in a decreased incidence of coagulum formation during ablation. Calkins et al. showed that there was a 0.8% incidence of coagulum formation with the temperature control mode compared to 2.2% incidence with the power control mode.[6]

However, there are a number of limitations that may result in discrepancies between the recorded temperature and the true electrode-myocardial tissue temperature. The catheter electrode may not be in

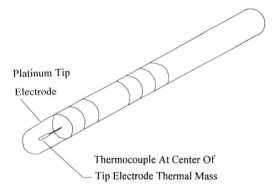

Platinum Tip
Electrode

Thermocouple At Center Of
Tip Electrode Thermal Mass

Figure 5. Schematic diagram of an RF ablation catheter with a thermocouple for temperature measurement. The thermocouple is placed in the center of a platinum tip electrode. Adapted with permission from Calkins H, et al.[6]

intimate contact with the myocardium at the site of the thermistor or thermocouple or at all parts of the electrode. Therefore any conventional temperature monitoring design may underestimate the myocardial interface temperature. This is particularly true at locations in which the catheter electrode may be parallel rather than perpendicular to the endocardial surface. Clinically, during accessory pathway ablation via the transseptal approach, the ablation electrode may be almost parallel to the mitral annulus, resulting in temperatures recorded from the electrode as low as 40°C while clinically effective ablation occurs, supporting this concept of underestimation of the peak temperature.

Recording of the temperature using a thermocouple against the catheter electrode but not directly at the surface also may result in an underestimation of the peak temperature. Such a design may provide an estimate of the overall temperature of the electrode rather than the peak temperature seen at the distal tip. However, the electrode mass that must be heated may result in a recorded temperature that is lower than the electrode-myocardial tissue temperature.

The tip temperature may be continuously monitored during ablation in order to assess the degree of contact. Marked variations in tip temperature typically represent catheter instability, often seen with the respiratory or cardiac cycle.

Recently, in addition to temperature monitoring, many clinically available ablation systems use feedback closed loop temperature control system. The RF generator regulates the power in order to maintain the set target temperature, usually between 60°C and 80°C. Changes in catheter contact may also result in marked variations in delivered power as well as sometimes in temperature as the power rapidly adjusts.

Temperature monitoring is particularly difficult as electrode size increases or the electrode geometry changes. As discussed above, as the electrode size increases, the maximal temperature may be greatly underestimated by the tip temperature. In order to perform linear catheter ablation lesions in the atrium for atrial fibrillation and flutter, longer electrode designs are being used. Temperature monitoring using a single point thermocouple is difficult since the side of the electrode in contact with the endocardium may be unpredictable. In addition, electrodes for the linear lesions may be longer, magnifying differences in the temperature over the electrode surface. Temperatures at the edges (so-called "edge effect") may exceed the temperature in the electrode body. Therefore, measuring temperatures in the midpoint will underestimate the peak temperature.

Cooled Radiofrequency Ablation

Since the electrode-myocardial interface temperature is an important factor that limits the power delivery during radiofrequency, saline cooling of the interface permits a higher power to be delivered, increasing lesion size while avoiding an impedance rise.[23–30] In vivo and in vitro experimental studies have supported this concept. Cooling during RF ablation may result in a higher temperature just below the surface of the endocardium. The maximal temperature is typically just under the endocardial surface and is less than or equal to 1 mm in depth. Even the temperature at the electrode-myocardial interface may be close to maximal temperature.[27,28] Therefore, improved methods of measuring temperature at the interface might be found that are superior to recording by the electrode temperature cooled by the saline flow.

The cooling permitted delivery of a higher mean power 22.0 ± 4.5 W compared to 6.1 ± 2.5 W without cooling. This resulted in a larger lesion volume of $1,247.8 \pm 520.5$ mm^3 compared to 436.1 ± 177.0 mm^3.[30]

Cooled RF ablation catheters may have a closed cooling design in which saline is recirculated or an open design in which saline is sprayed via small holes in the electrode. Cooling using either design interferes

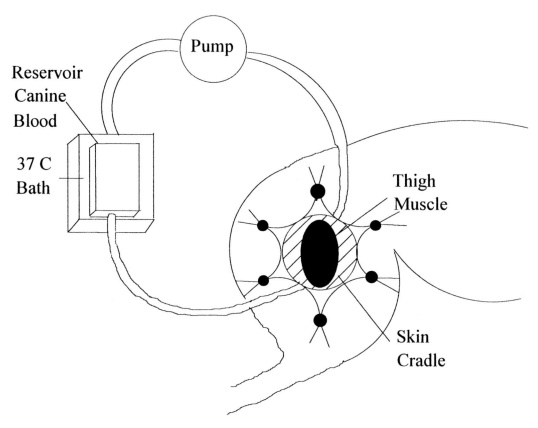

Figure 6. Schematic drawing of the thigh muscle model. The skin and superficial muscle were dissected, exposing underlying facial layer. A skin cradle was formed and was filled with heparinized canine blood at 36°C to 37°C at a flow rate of 20 mL/min. Adapted with permission from Nakagawa H, et al.[26]

with accurate temperature measurement since the electrode temperature will greatly underestimate the interface temperature.

Nakagawa et al., using a perfused canine thigh muscle model shown in Figure 6, demonstrated that saline-irrigated electrode ablation lesions were ellipsoid below the surface with a maximal lesion diameter at a depth of 4.1 ± 0.7 mm from the surface. At constant voltage, the mean lesion depth with saline irrigation was 9.9 ± 1.1 mm compared to 4.7 ± 0.6 mm without. This yielded total volumes of 700 ± 217 mm^3 and 135 ± 33 mm^3 for the irrigated and non-irrigated lesions, respectively. Similar results have been obtained with a closed-system saline-cooled RF ablation system.[26]

Microwave Ablation

Microwave ablation acts via dielectric heating of the myocardium.[31–57] The microwave energy results in oscillation of the water molecule dipoles within the myocardium, resulting in heating due to molecular interaction or friction. The microwave antenna placed at the end of a catheter radiates electromagnetic energy. Therefore, contact with the myocardium is not required in order to heat myocardial tissue.[1]

The microwave ablation system consists of a microwave generator and a microwave antenna incorporated into the ablation catheter. Microwave generators operate at either 915 MHz or 2,450 MHz frequencies.

Microwave ablation antennas may have one of a number of designs. A helical coil design is most commonly used. This design consists of a coaxial cable that terminates in an inner conductor extending beyond the coaxial cable and attached to a helical coil. Other designs include a monopolar antenna consisting of an inner conductor extending beyond the outer conductor and an O-applicator (Figure 7).

Several measurements are used to characterize microwave systems for myocardial ablation. A three-dimensional profile of the antenna's energy pattern is assessed. Most commonly, the specific absorption rate (SAR) is measured systematically in three dimensions. A brief energy pulse is given and the temperature rise at each point is measured. Since the temperature rise is nearly instantaneous, it is assumed that the SAR reflects almost entirely radiative properties of the ablation system rather than its conductive properties. The SAR pattern provides a three-dimensional picture of the electromagnetic field created during microwave ablation. Most commonly, the SAR measurements are performed in a medium with dielectric properties similar to myocardial tissue. Normal saline solution is often used because of its convenience although more precise measurements may be made using a medium containing substances that more precisely mimic the dielectric properties of myocardium. These so-called "phantom" solutions may contain, for example, water, sodium chloride, polyethylene, and a solidifying agent.

Other tests of the ablation system reflect the efficiency with which energy is deposited into the tissue. The ability of the energy source to deliver energy to the medium is considered "matching" of the antenna to

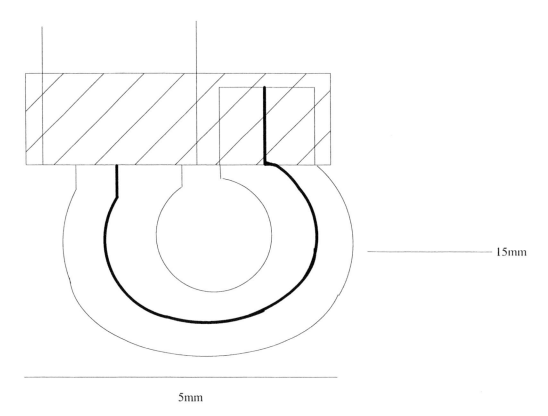

15mm

5mm

Figure 7. An O-applicator design for a microwave energy delivery. The radiation properties of this small loop antenna depend on the area of the loop. Adapted with permission from Shetty S, et al.[41]

the dielectric properties of the medium. An instrument called a systems analyzer is used to rapidly deliver energy over a large range of microwave frequencies and to measure at each frequency the amount of energy that is deposited into the tissue. One selects an antenna that exhibits the greatest efficiency at the frequency to be delivered. Another index of the "matching" of the energy to the myocardium is the ratio of reflected power to power delivered. During microwave energy delivery, some amount of the energy is reflected or returned back to the microwave generator from the myocardium. When the antenna and tissue are optimally matched, very little power is reflected. While most ablation systems are optimized for a specific load or impedance, some ablation systems have the capacity to vary the impedance of the system, compensating for differences in myocardial tissue properties.

Most commonly, the two frequencies (915 MHz and 2450 MHz) are used because they are permitted by the Federal Communications Commission and generators are available in these frequencies. Theoretically for myocardial tissue, 915 MHz results in a deeper degree of penetration but this is highly dependent on the antenna characteristics and efficiency. The 915 MHz frequency has the practical advantage of resulting in a lower amount of loss in the coaxial cable that connects the generator to the antenna compared with 2,450 MHz. Coaxial cable heating may become a particularly challenging problem when high forward powers are used for ablation. The coaxial cable may become too hot to handle and exceed the temperature safety limits that have been established.

The heating pattern and efficiency of microwave ablation systems are dependent on the antenna design. An antenna such as a helical coil creates a circumferential heating pattern, making placement parallel to the endocardial surface optimal. Other designs such as some dipole antennas may project the ablation energy forward. Selection of the appropriate antenna design will depend on the specific arrhythmia targeted. Helical coil antennas that result in circumferential heating may be suited to making long linear lesions such as for atrial fibrillation ablation, while a forward-projecting antenna might be ideal for accessory pathway ablation using a retrograde approach.

Comparisons have been made of microwave ablation and RF ablation. Wonnell et al. observed that there was a greater temperature rise during microwave ablation as a function of depth compared to RF ablation using an in vitro phantom model. The radial distance for a 50% change in temperature was 2.67 ± 0.28 mm for microwave ablation compared to 1.11 ± 0.21 mm for RF ablation[32] (Figure 8).

In an isolated perfused porcine right ventricular tissue model, Whayne et al.[34] demonstrated that microwave lesion size using a 915 MHz monopolar antenna system continued to increase over 300 seconds of ablation. At 300 seconds, a comparable lesion depth was obtained but at significantly lower antenna-tissue interface temperatures $70.4 \pm 13.5°C$ and $83.6 \pm 7.9°C$ for microwave and RF lesions, respectively ($p = 0.004$). This suggests that although microwave heating is considerably slower, if a greater amount of energy were used to achieve comparable surface temperatures, deeper lesions would be created (Figure 9). Pires et al. demonstrated that using a split-tip microwave antenna and 30 W for 20 seconds, the lesion depth was 3.8 ± 0.7 mm and 2.6 ± 0.7 mm for microwave and RF lesions in an excised bovine heart model ($p < 0.0001$).[33]

Pathologically, microwave lesions are comparable to RF lesions. Acutely, they demonstrate considerable hemorrhage; but chronically, they become a dense fibrous scar and are well-circumscribed (Figure 10). Microwave ablation has been performed in the right and left ventricles, the atria, the AV junction, the coronary sinus, and the mitral annulus.

Langberg[68] used a helical antenna ablation catheter to create AV block chronically using microwave energy at 2,450 MHz

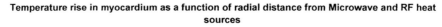

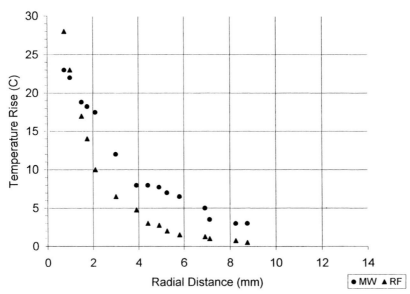

Figure 8. At each radial distance, there is a higher average temperature as function of distance, during microwave ablation using a helical antenna design. Adapted with permission from Wonnell et al.[32]

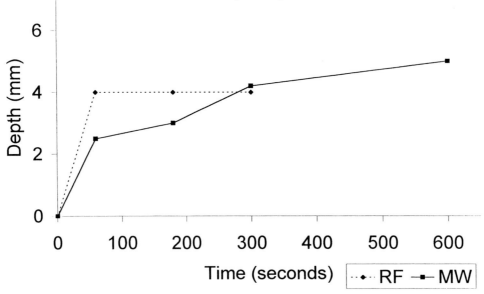

Figure 9. Comparison of lesion depth between microwave and RF ablation. Although microwave heating is considerably slower, if more energy is used, deeper lesions are created.

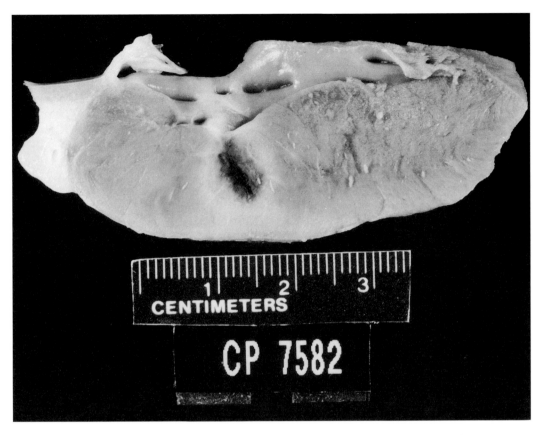

Figure 10. A microwave dense, fibrous, and well circumscribed microwave lesion.

(Figure 11). Lesions were 4.7 ± 2.1 mm in length, 2.8 ± 1.3 mm in width, and 0.9 ± 0.25 mm in depth. In the 6 animals, AV block was permanent. The mean escape rate was 44 ± 10 beats per minute at 6 weeks. The mean QRS duration was 87 ± 12 ms.

Microwave ablation also may be used for ventricular myocardial ablation at either 2,450 MHz or 915 MHz. As the power and duration of microwave energy delivery are increased, the lesion size also increases.[48,64–66] However, with high power, excessive temperatures resulting in thrombus formation have been observed.[58] Microwave energy, unlike RF energy, may be delivered despite tissue coagulation. Therefore, particular caution is required in order to prevent excessive heating. There is likely an important role of temperature monitoring during microwave ablation. A

feedback control microwave ablation system has been developed.[59]

Microwave ablation has also been used to ablate atrial myocardial tissue.[71] Microwave energy successfully ablated aconitine-induced atrial tachycardia.

Laser Ablation

Laser energy may use a wide range of wavelengths, from 250 nm to 10,600 nm.[58–94] The tissue response to ablation varies according to the wavelength delivered. Laser myocardial ablation is predominantly thermal in mechanism. Wavelengths in the infrared region such as Nd:YAG (neodynium-yttrium-aluminum-garnet) result in scattering of photons causing tissue destruction via photocoagulation without va-

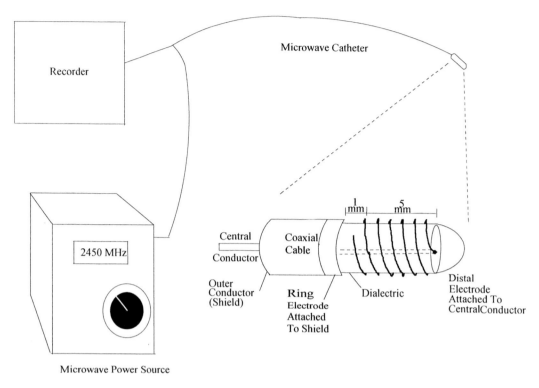

Figure 11. Schematic diagram of a microwave ablation system for myocardial ablation. The catheter is capable of electrical recordings and delivery of microwave energy via an antenna. Adapted with permission from Langberg JJ, et al.[46]

porization. This results in deeper lesions and has been extensively applied to the intraoperative ablation of ventricular tachycardia. In contrast, the CO_2 laser produces predominantly absorption compared to scatter, resulting in tissue evaporation and cutting. Ultraviolet radiation such as xenon fluoride excimer produces vaporization of tissue caused by absorption of energy concentrated in a thin layer.[1,58]

The laser ablation system includes a laser energy source and a transmission fiberoptic cable. Some forms of energy are not suitable for transmission via optic fibers. There are a number of design issues that are important in catheter-based laser ablation. There are a number of different designs that have been developed for energy delivery (Figure 12). Frequently, a considerable amount of heat is generated at the ablation site. Use of saline for cooling has been important to

limit the heating at this site. Saline also acts to clear the blood in front of the catheter tip.

Increased energy may be required to create a comparable lesion in diseased ventricular tissue compared to normal ventricular tissue. Pulsing of laser energy at low repetition rates has been investigated to decrease the degree of tissue charring. Cooling of the endocardial surface using saline irrigation also may decrease excessive heating. Flexibility and steerability of the catheter-based system is also important for a clinical ablation system. Temperature-monitoring also may be important to prevent excessive heating of the tissue. Lesion size increases with greater energy. However, laser ablation in situ results in lesions that are considerably larger than in vitro ($p < 0.005$) (Figure 13).[60]

Laser lesions exhibit coagulation necrosis, vacuolization, and crater formation. A central vaporized crater may be produced

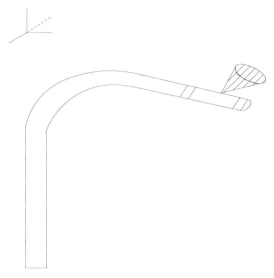

Figure 12. Schematic drawing of a laser-electrode catheter. A 300 μ silica fiber projects a Nd: YAG laser light at 1.06 μ perpendicular to the long axis of the catheter. The beam expands into a conical shape with a half-angle of 21°. Adapted with permission from Curtis AB, et al.[72]

surrounded by a rim of necrotic tissue. Chronically the lesions are healed with a homogeneous region of fibrosis comparable to cryoablative lesions. Byproducts of laser ablation have included primarily water soluble gaseous substances. These byproducts are small, in the range of 3 μm in size. Perforation is a potential risk of laser ablation.

Electrophysiologically, laser ablation results in reduction in resting membrane potential, action potential amplitude, and upstroke velocity, extending to a border zone 2 to 3 mm from the edge of the necrotic myocardium.[61]

Laser ablation has been successfully used to create permanent AV block. An argon laser using a 200 nm fiber was used to create prolongation of AV conduction and complete AV block.[116,117] A Nd:YAG laser has also been used to create complete AV block.[118]

Laser energy has been applied to supraventricular arrhythmias. Nd:YAG transcatheter ablation has been used to successfully treat 9 patients with AV nodal

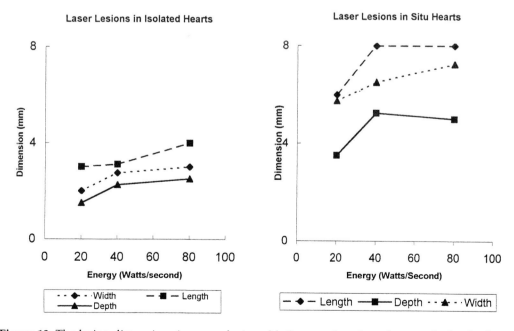

Figure 13. The lesion dimensions increase during ablation as a function of energy is clearly shown. The in vitro results are shown in the left panel. The results for in situ studies demonstrate larger lesion dimensions (right panel) compared to in vitro. Adapted with permission from Lee BI, et al.[60]

reentrant tachycardia using fast pathway ablation.[122]

Laser ablation has been extensively used intraoperatively to treat ventricular tachycardia. In a study of 57 patients, a Nd:YAG laser system was used to treat ventricular tachycardia. The operative mortality was 14% and of the 49 survivors three patients remained inducible for ventricular tachycardia.[127]

A steerable laser ablation catheter is currently being developed and has begun initial clinical studies for the treatment of ventricular tachycardia. Additional studies are needed to determine the efficacy of catheter-based laser therapy.

Cryoablation

Cryoablation has been used extensively intraoperatively for the creation of AV block or the ablation of atrial and ventricular tachycardias. Application of a cryosurgical probe to the AV junction is extremely effective in creating AV block.[100,101] Monomorphic ventricular tachycardia has been successfully treated using intraoperative cryoablation as the sole therapy.[104]

Catheter-based techniques for the cryoablation of arrhythmias are capable of freezing myocardial tissue.[95–107] Cryoablation of myocardial tissue is usually accomplished by achieving temperatures of $-60°C$ for 2 or more minutes. Several designs have been employed to achieve cryoablation using a catheter-based system. Some designs are based on the Joule Thompson effect, in which a pressure drop results in significant cooling or freezing. Gases such as nitrous oxide have been used in such systems. Cooling by employing a phase change has also been incorporated into a catheter design. Other designs have used the Peltier effect, in which a semiconductor is used to establish a temperature differential. Such systems may have multiple stages that permit the heat to be moved away in steps from the distal tip at the end of the catheter.

The size of the cryoablative lesion is de-pendent on factors such as the temperature, duration, surface area of the cooling probe, and the number of applications. The size of cryoablative lesion is limited greatly by the volume of heating provided by the circulating blood flow in the ventricles.[96]

Pathologically and electrophysiologically, the chronic cryoablative lesion consists of dense scar without electrical activity. There is a sharp demarcation between living and nonliving tissue. Acutely after cryoablation, frequent ventricular ectopic beats occur, particularly within the first 24 hours. In one study, five of six animals undergoing epicardial cryoablation exhibited ventricular tachycardia in the first 1 to 4 days. However, ventricular tachycardia was never observed 1 week or more after cryoablation. These acute arrhythmias are felt most likely to be due to enhanced automaticity. As expected, isolated cryoablative lesions do not affect epicardial activation. At 1 week after cryoablation, a circular hemorrhagic lesion was present. In some examples, an endocardial thrombus was present.

Cooling rather than ablation of myocardial tissue provides one of the most powerful tools for arrhythmia mapping.[95] Cryothermal mapping using a cooling source may permit one to accurately identify the critical zones in a tachycardia circuit. The application of sterile ice cubes was used to locate the site of cryotermination. In five of seven patients in one series, the cryotermination site differed from the site of earliest electrical recording by 3.0 to 7.5 cm.

The epicardial application of a 0°C cooling source resulted in a decrease of surface temperature by $-18 \pm 3.1°C$ at 0 mm, $-17.5 \pm 2.1°C$ in infarcted tissue, and $-4.2 \pm 2.3°C$ at 2–3 mm subepicardially, and $-1.3 \pm 1.3°C$ at 5 to 7 mm depths.[99] Preliminary results suggest that reversible mapping may be possible with a cryoablation catheter.[95]

Experimental studies have demonstrated that cryoablative catheter techniques are capable of creating permanent AV block.[105,106] In a study of eight pigs, complete AV block was created in five animals. Chronic lesions

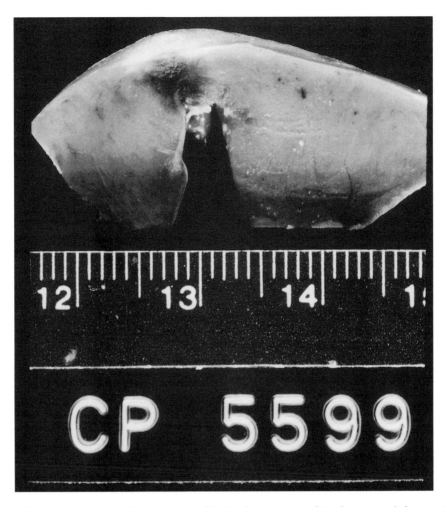

Figure 14. Gross appearance of chronic cryoablation lesion created in the canine left ventricle. The lesion is well demarcated. The lesion was produced using a cryoablation catheter utilizing nitrous oxide to freeze myocardial tissue based on the Joule-Thomson effect.

were small and well-circumscribed[106] (Figure 14). Lesions may also be created under the mitral annulus using a cryoablation catheter.[107] Clinical studies using a transvenous cryoablation catheter have yet to be performed.

Ultrasound Ablation

Ultrasound ablation has been investigated as a potential method of catheter ablation. Ultrasound energy at greater than 18,000 cycles per second causes propagation of a pressure wave. The energy is converted into heat within the myocardium. Recent studies have demonstrated the feasibility of ultrasound energy delivery for myocardial ablation.[108–113] The ultrasound system consists of ultrasound transducers and an energy source (Figure 15). Ultrasound ablation lesions are well circumscribed with evidence of myocyte cell death. The lesion size produced by ultrasound increase with duration and power. Lesions as deep as 7.6 mm were reported using cylindrical transducers of 2.3 mm at 9 MHz. In one study, lesions had a mean depth of 8.7 ± 2.9 mm in the left ventricle.[113]

Design issues include development of a

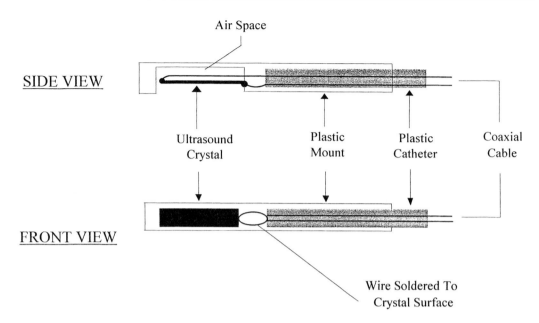

Figure 15. Schematic diagram of ultrasound transducer for myocardial ablation. The rectangle-shaped transducer of 12 mm long and 5 mm wide delivers ultrasound energy at a frequency of 5 MHz. Adapted with permission from He DS, et al.[113]

forward-projecting transducer rather than a side-projecting transducer. Further studies may explore the potential to focus multiple ultrasound energy transducers in order to increase the depth of penetration. Theoretically it may be possible to combine ultrasound ablation with ultrasound imaging.[114–116]

Chemical Ablation

The delivery of ablative agents via the coronary circulation has been shown to be effective in destroying myocardial tissue responsible for various cardiac arrhythmias.[117–133] Branches of the coronary circulation are selectively cannulated using angioplasty techniques. Cytotoxic agents such as ethanol may be delivered via an infusion catheter into these small branches. These ablative agents act nearly instantaneously to destroy the myocytes supplied by the coronary artery branch. Experimental and clinical cardiac arrhythmias such as

ventricular and atrial tachycardias have been treated using these techniques.

Clinically, ventricular tachycardia has been successfully ablated using chemical ablation. In a clinical study of 23 patients with sustained monomorphic ventricular tachycardia, ventricular tachycardia terminated after injection of contrast or saline into a coronary arterial branch in 10 patients. In nine of these 10 patients, acutely ventricular tachycardia could no longer be induced after injection of 2 cc of 96% ethanol into the termination vessel. However, ventricular arrhythmias developed in two patients at 5 to 7 days.[127]

In addition, the AV junction has been ablated by selective delivery of ethanol into the AV nodal artery. Ethanol has been injected as a bolus of 0.3 cc to 3 cc of 96% ethanol[110] or has been delivered as a continuous infusion of 2 cc or 96% ethanol over 2 minutes,[111] or 0.5 to 1.0 cc/minute of 25% to 50% ethanol for 10 to 40 minutes.[108]

Delivery of cytotoxic agents has also been achieved using selective catheterization of the cardiac venous system.[122,123] The delivery of agents via the cardiac venous system may have the advantage that unlike coronary arteries the cardiac veins are rarely stenosed.

Agents that occlude the arterial blood supply have been also used to treat cardiac arrhythmias. Agents such as glutaraldehyde cross-linked collagen and detachable coils[117,130] have been selectively delivered into small arterial branches to occlude the blood supply and irreversibly damage the myocytes which the vessels supply.

Issues in chemical ablation center predominantly on methods of controlling the size of myocardial necrosis. Injection of contrast prior to delivery of the cytotoxic agent may be used to estimate the region of necrosis. Preventing reflux of the cytotoxic agents into adjacent branches has also been the focus of efforts to improve these techniques. Recently, a flexible balloon proximal to the infusion port at the distal end of the catheter has been developed in order to prevent reflux during delivery of the cytotoxic agents. Improved catheters permit delivery into very small and distal coronary or cardiac venous branches.

Summary

A range of catheter ablation techniques have been developed for the selective destruction of myocardial cells for the abolition of cardiac arrhythmias. The energy sources of radiofrequency, microwave, laser, and ultrasound destroy myocardial cells through absorption of energy or heat. Cryoablation is unique in that freezing of cells results in myocyte death. Chemical ablation acts via the selective delivery of agents that result in cell death through ischemia or cytotoxicity. Future studies are needed to determine the relative utility of these various techniques.

Acknowledgment: The authors thank Brian Vander Brink, BS, for his assistance in preparation of the figures.

References

1. Avitall B, Khan M, Krum D, et al. Physics and engineering of transcatheter cardiac tissue ablation. J Am Coll Cardiol 1993;22:932.
2. Panescu D, Whayne JG, Fleischman, et al. Three dimensional finite element analysis of current density and temperature distributions during radiofrequency ablation. IEEE Trans Biomed Eng 1995;42:879–889.
3. Labonte S. Numerical model for radiofrequency ablation of the endocardium and its experimental validation. IEEE Trans Biomed Eng 1994;108–114.
4. Wittkampf FHM, Hauer RNW, Robles de Medina EO. Control of radiofrequency lesion size by power regulation. Circulation 1989;80:962–968.
5. Franklin JO, Langberg JJ, Oeff M, et al. Catheter ablation of canine myocardium with radiofrequency energy. PACE 1989;12:170–176.
6. Calkins H, Prystowsky E, Carlson M, et al. Temperature monitoring during radiofrequency catheter ablation procedures using closed loop control. Circulation 1994;90:1279–1286.
7. Haines DE, Watson DD. Tissue heating during radiofrequency catheter ablations: a thermodynamic model and observations in isolated perfused and superfused canine right ventricular free wall. PACE 1989;12:962–976.
8. Nath S, DiMarco JP, Gallop RG, et al. Effects of dispersive electrode position and surface area on electrical parameters and temperature during radiofrequency catheter ablation. Am J Cardiol 1996;77:765–767.
9. Oeff M, Langberg JJ, Chim ML, et al. Ablation of ventricular tachycardia using multiple sequential trans-catheter applications of radiofrequency energy. PACE 1992;15:1167–1176.
10. Swartz JF, Pellersels G, Silvers J, et al. A catheter-based curative approach to atrial fibrillation in human [Abstract]. Circulation 1994;90(4 Pt 2):I–335.
11. Baal T, Chen X, Kottkamp H, Borggrefe M. Radiofrequency catheter ablation: improving lesion size achieved with conventional catheters [Abstract]. Circulation 1994;90(4 Pt 2):I–272.
12. Langberg JJ, Gallagher M, Strickberger SA, et al. Temperature-guided radiofrequency

catheter ablation with very large distal electrodes. Circulation 1993;88:245–249.

13. Langberg JJ, Lee Michael A, Chin MC, et al. Radiofrequency catheter ablation: the effect of electrode size on lesion volume in vivo. PACE 1990;13:1242–1248.

14. Satake S, Ohira H, Okishige K et al. Temperature-guided radiofrequency ablation using a new catheter electrode of 12 F gold tip [Abstract]. Circulation 1993;88:I–62.

15. Simmons WN, Mackey SC, He DS, et al. Comparison of maximum myocardial lesion depth using radio-frequency energy delivered with a gold or platinum electrode [Abstract]. Circulation 1994;90(4 Pt 2): I–270.

16. Bergau D, Brucker GG, Saul JP. Porous metal tipped catheter produces larger radiofrequency lesions through tip cooling [Abstract]. Circulation 1993;88:I–164.

17. Wang PJ, Groeneveld PW, Gadhoke A, et al. Electrode panels: a new design for radiofrequency ablation catheters [Abstract]. J Am Coll Cardiol 1993;21:265A.

18. Groeneveld PW, Haugh C, Estes NAM, et al. Panel electrode "pigtail" catheter using flexible electrically conductive material: a new design for increasing radiofrequency ablation lesion size [Abstract]. PACE 1993; 16:923.

19. Satake S, Ohira H, Okishige K, et al. Temperature guided radiofrequency ablation of ventricular tachycardia using 12 F sphere tip electrode [Abstract]. Circulation 1994; 90(4 Pt 2):I–271.

20. Nath S, Whayne JG, Haines DE. Does pulsed radiofrequency delivery result in greater tissue heating and lesion size from catheter ablation [Abstract]. PACE 1993; 16(Pt II):947.

21. Blouin LT, Marcus FI. The effect of electrode design on the efficiency of delivery of radiofrequency energy to cardiac tissue in vitro. Pacing Clin Electrophysiol 1989;12(Pt 2):136–43.

22. Nath S, Lynch C 3d, Whayne JG, et al. Cellular electrophysiological effects of hyperthermia on isolated guinea pig papillary muscle: implications for catheter ablation. Circulation 1993;88:1826–1831.

23. Sykes C, Riley R, Pomeranz M, et al. Cooled tip ablation results in increased radiofrequency power delivery and lesion size [Abstract]. PACE 1994;17(4 Pt II):782.

24. Skrumeda LL, Maguire MA, Mehra R. Effect of delivering saline at a low flow rate on FT lesion size in the left ventricle [Abstract]. PACE 1995;18(4 Pt II):921.

25. Mittleman RS, Huang SKS, DeGuzman WT, et al. Use of the saline infusion electrode

catheter for improved energy delivery and increased lesion size in radiofrequency catheter ablation. PACE 1995;18(5 Pt 1): 1022–1027.

26. Nakagawa H, Yamanashi WS, Pitha JV, et al. Comparison of in vivo tissue temperature profile and lesion geometry for radiofrequency ablation with a saline-irrigated electrode versus temperature control in a canine thigh muscle preparation. Circulation 1995;91:2264–2273.

27. Panescu D, Fleishman SD, Whayne JG, et al. Effects of cooled-electrode ablation on maximum tissue temperature. PACE 1997; 20:1205.

28. Demazumder D, Kallash HL, Schwartzman D. Myocardial heating patterns during radiofrequency energy delivery via an irrigated electrode. PACE 1997;20:1203.

29. Arruda M, Nakagawa H, Khastgir T, et al. Facilitation of accessory pathway ablation from the middle cardiac vein by a saline irrigated catheter electrode [Abstract]. PACE 1995;18(4 Pt II):832.

30. Ruffy R, Imran MA, Santel DJ, et al. Radiofrequency delivery through a cooled catheter tip allows the creation of larger endomyocardial lesions in the ovine heart. J Cardiovasc Electrophysiol 1995;6:12: 1089–1096.

31. Stauffer PR, Suen SA, Satoh T, et al. Comparative thermal dosimetry of interstitial microwave and radiofrequency-LCF hyperthermia. Int J Hyperthermia 1989;5(3): 307–318.

32. Wonnell TL, Stauffer PR, Langberg JJ. Evaluation of microwave and radiofrequency catheter ablation in a myocardium-equivalent phantom model. IEEE Trans Biomed Eng 1992;39:1086–1095.

33. Pires LA, Huang SKS, Lin JC, et al. Comparison of radiofrequency (RF) versus microwave (MW) energy catheter ablation of the bovine ventricular myocardium. PACE 1994;17(4 Pt II):782.

34. Whayne JG, Nath S, Haines DE. Microwave catheter ablation of myocardium in vitro: assessment of the characteristics of tissue heating and injury. Circulation 1994;89: 2390–2395.

35. Whayne JG, Haines DE. Comparison of thermal profiles produced by new antenna designs for microwave catheter ablation [Abstract]. PACE 1992;15:580.

36. Whayne JG, Haines DE. Computer modeling of microwave antenna designs using the finite element analysis method [Abstract]. PACE 1993;16(4 Pt II):921.

37. Whayne JG, Nath S, Haines DE. The effect of antenna design and microwave fre-

quency on tissue temperature profiles during microwave catheter ablation in vitro [Abstract]. Circulation 1992;86:I–192.

38. Ahmad A, Estes NAM, Manolis AS, et al. Does microwave heating in saline predict the 3-dimensional heating pattern in myocardium [Abstract]. J Am Coll Cardiol 1994; 35A.

39. Huang SKS, Lin JC, Mazzola F, et al. Percutaneous microwave ablation of the ventricular myocardium using a 4-mm split-tip antenna electrode: a novel method for potential ablation of ventricular tachycardia [Abstract]. J Am Coll Cardiol 1994;34A.

40. Liem LB, Mead RH, Shenasa M, et al. In vitro and in vivo results of transcatheter microwave ablation using foreward-firing tip antenna design. PACE 1996;11:2004–2008.

41. Shetty S, Ishii TK, Krum DP et al. Microwave applicator design for cardiac tissue ablations. J Microwave Power Electromag Energy 1996;31:59–66.

42. Haines DE, Whayne JG. What is the radial temperature profile achieved during microwave catheter ablation with a helical cord antenna in canine myocardium? J Am Coll Cardiol 1992;19:99A.

43. Haugh C, Davidson E, Estes NAM, et al. Pulsing microwave energy: a method to create more uniform temperature gradients. J Int Cardiac Electrophys 1997;1: 57–65.

44. Wang PJ, Haugh CJ, Schoen FJ, et al. Left ventricular thrombus formation after high power microwave ablation: implications for temperature and power regulation [Abstract]. Circulation 1993;88(4 Pt 2):I–354.

45. Wang PJ, Ahmad A, Lenihan T, et al. Developing and testing a feedback control system for microwave ablation: in vitro and in vivo results [Abstract]. PACE 1994;17(4 Pt II): 782.

46. Langberg JJ, Wonnell T, Chin MC, et al. Catheter ablation of the atrioventricular junction using a helical microwave antenna: a novel means of coupling energy to the endocardium. PACE 1991;14:2105–2113.

47. Yang X, Watanabe I, Kojima T, et al. Microwave ablation of the atrioventricular junction in vivo and ventricular myocardium in vitro and in vivo. Jpn Heart J 1994;34: 175–191.

48. Lin JC, Wang Y, Hariman RJ. Microwave catheter ablation of the canine atrioventricular junction [Abstract]. J Am Coll Cardiol 1993;16:357A.

49. Beckman KJ, Lin JC, Wang Y, et al. Production of reversible and irreversible atrioventricular block by microwave energy [Abstract]. Circulation 1987;76:IV–405.

50. Coggins D, Chin M, Wonnell T, et al. Efficacy of microwave energy for ventricular ablation [Abstract]. PACE 1991;14:703.

51. Ruder M, Mead RH, Baron K, et al. Microwave ablation: in vivo data. PACE 1994; 17(4 Pt II):781.

52. Cohen TJ, Coggins D, Chin MC, et al. Microwave ablation of ventricular myocardium: the effects of varying duration on lesion volume [Abstract]. Circulation 1991;II–711.

53. Ikeda T, Sugi K, Emjoji E, et al. Relation between the size of lesions and arrhythmias produced by microwave catheter ablation with a special electrode device. Jpn Circ J 1994;58:214–221.

54. Wang PJ, Schoen FJ, Aronovitz M, et al. Microwave catheter ablation under the mitral annulus: a new method of accessory pathway ablation [Abstract]. PACE 1993;16(4 Pt II):866.

55. Wang PJ, Gadhoke A, Schoen FJ, et al. Microwave catheter ablation via the coronary sinus: the need for power and temperature regulation [Abstract]. PACE 1994;17(4 Pt II):813.

56. Cohen TJ, Coggins DL, Chin MC, et al. Microwave ablation of atrial myocardium: the effects of varying duration on lesion volume [Abstract]. Circulation 1992;86(4): I–784.

57. Rho TH, Ito M, Pride HP, et al. Microwave ablation of canine atrial tachycardia induced by aconitine. Am Heart J 1995;129(5): 1021–1025.

58. Saksena S. Catheter ablation of tachycardia with laser energy: issues and answers. PACE 1989;12:196–203.

59. Isner JM, Donaldson RF, Deckelbaum LI, et al. The excimer laser: gross, light microscopic and ultrastructural analysis of potential advantages for use in laser therapy of cardiovascular disease. J Am Coll Cardiol 1985;6:1102.

60. Lee BI, Gottdiener JS, Fletcher RD, et al. Transcatheter ablation: comparison between laser photoablation and electrode shock ablation in the dog. Circulation 1985; 71:579–586.

61. Levine JH, Merillat JC, Stern M, et al. The cellular electrophysiologic changes induced by ablation: comparison between argon laser photoablation and high-energy electrical ablation. Circulation 1987;76: 217–225.

62. Svenson RH, Littmann L, Splinter R, et al. Application of lasers for arrhythmia ablation. In: Zipes DP, Jalife J, eds. Cardiac Electrophysiology: From Cell to Bedside. Philadelphia: WB Saunders, 1990.

63. Svenson RH, Marroum MC, Frank F, et al.

Successful Nd:YAG laser photocoagulation of arrhythmogenic myocardium: potential limitations of current optical delivery systems. Proc SPIE 1986;713:74.

64. Svenson RH, Hessel S, Selle JG, et al. Nd:YAG laser photocoagulation of drug resistant ventricular tachycardia: results in 27 consecutive cases and operative factors influencing surgical outcome. Presented at International Society for Laser Surgery and Medicine, Munich, Germany, June 1987.

65. Enders S, Weber HP, Heinze A, et al. Laser and radiofrequency catheter ablation of ventricular myocardium in dogs: a comparative test [Abstract]. PACE 1994;17(4 Pt II): 782.

66. Weber H, Enders S, Keiditisch E. Percutaneous Nd:YAG laser coagulation of ventricular myocardium in dogs using a special electrode laser catheter. PACE 1989;12: 899–910.

67. Littmann L, Svenson RH, Brucker G, et al. Percutaneous neodymium:YAG laser photoablation of ventricular tachycardia [Abstract]. Circulation 1992;86(4):I–192.

68. Oeff M, Hug B, Stormer U, et al. Fluorescence spectroscopy for identification of the AV node prior to laser ablation. Circulation 1991;84:11–13.

69. Bartorelli AL, Leon MB, Almagor Y, et al. In vivo human atherosclerotic plaque recognition by laser-excited fluorescence spectroscopy. J Am Coll Cardiol 1991;17: 160B–168B.

70. Rosenthal E, Montarello JK, Bucknall CA, et al. His bundle ablation with the laser thermal probe ("hot tip"): a feasibility study. PACE 1989;12:812–822.

71. Haines DE. Thermal ablation of perfused porcine left ventricle in vitro with the neodymium-YAG laser hot tip catheter system. PACE 1992;15:979–985.

72. Curtis AB, Mansour M, Friedl SE, et al. Modification of atrioventricular conduction using a combined laser-electrode catheter. PACE 1994;17(3 Pt I):337–348.

73. Weber HP, Heinze A, Enders, et al. Catheter-directed laser coagulation of atrial myocardium in dogs. Eur Heart J 1994;15: 971–980.

74. Hirao K, Yamamoto N, Ishihara N, et al. Catheter ablation of canine ventricle using transballoon Nd:YAG laser irradiation technique under direct vision [Abstract]. Circulation 1994;90(4):I–486.

75. Zheng SM, Kloner RA, Whittaker P. Ablation and coagulation of myocardial tissue by means of a pulsed holmium:YAG laser. Am Heart J 1993;126:1474–1477.

76. Curtis AB, Abela GS, Griffin JC, et al. Trans-vascular argon laser ablation of atrioventricular conduction in dogs: feasibility and morphological results. PACE 1989;12(2): 347–357.

77. Ohtake H, Misaki T, Watanade G, et al. Myocardial coagulation by intraoperative Nd:YAG laser ablation and its dependence on blood perfusion. PACE 1994;17(10): 1627–1631.

78. Oeff M, Hug B, Muller G. Transcatheter laser photocoagulation for treatment of cardiac arrhythmias. Lasers Med Sci 1991;6: 355–361.

79. Narula OS, Bharati S, Chan MC, et al. Microtransection of the His bundle with laser radiation through a pervenous catheter: correlation of histologic and electrophysiologic data. Am J Cardiol 1984;54:186–192.

80. Narula OS, Boveja BK, Cohen DM, et al. Laser catheter-induced atrioventricular nodal delays and atrioventricular block in dogs: acute and chronic observations. J Am Coll Cardiol 1985;5:259–267.

81. Weber HP, Heinze A, Enders S, et al. Modification of atrioventricular node transmission properties by transcatheter endocardial laser irradiation in dogs [Abstract]. PACE 1994;17(4 Pt II):832.

82. Schuger CD, McMath L, Abrams G, et al. Long-term effects of percutaneous laser balloon ablation from the canine coronary sinus. Circulation 1992;86:947–954.

83. Obelienius V, Knepa A, Ambartzumian R, et al. Transvenous ablation of the atrioventricular conduction system by laser irradiation under endoscopic control. Lasers Surg Med 1985;5:469–474.

84. Saksena S, Gielchinsky I. Argon laser ablation of modification of the atrioventricular conduction system in refractory supraventricular tachycardia. Am J Cardiol 1990;66: 767–770.

85. Weber HP, Kaltenbrunner W, Heinze A, et al. Laser catheter ablation for patients with atrioventricular nodal reentrant tachycardia [Abstract]. PACE 1994;17(4 Pt II):815.

86. Weber HP, Heinze A. Laser catheter ablation of atrial flutter and of atrioventricular nodal reentrant tachycardia in a single session. Eur Heart J 1994;15:1147–1149.

87. Mehta D, Bharati S, Lev M, et al. Histopathological changes following laser ablation of a left-sided accessory pathway in a human. PACE 1994;17(4 Pt II):672–677.

88. Littmann L, Svenson RH, Brucker G, et al. Comparative study on the efficacy and safety of transcatheter radiofrequency ablation and contact neodymium-YAG laser photoablation of the left ventricular endo-

cardium in dogs [Abstract]. PACE 1993;16(4 Pt II):859.

89. Enders S, Weber HP, Heinze A, et al. Laser and radiofrequency catheter ablation of ventricular myocardium in dogs: a comparative test [Abstract]. PACE 1994;17(4 Pt II): 782.

90. Svenson RH, Littmann L, Splinter R, et al. Current status of lasers for arrhythmia ablation. J Cardiovasc Electrophysiol 1992;3: 345–353.

91. Weber HP, Heinze A, Enders S, et al. Catheter-directed laser coagulation of ventricular myocardium in dogs [Abstract]. PACE 1994;17(4 Pt II):832.

92. Vincent GM, Fox J, Knowlton K, et al. Catheter-directed neodymium:YAG laser injury of the left ventricle for arrhythmia ablation: dosimetry and hemodynamic, hematologic, and electrophysiologic effects. Lasers Surg Med 1989;9:446–453.

93. Weber H, Enders S, Coppenrath K, et al. Effects of Nd:YAG laser coagulation of myocardium on coronary vessels. Lasers Surg Med 1990;10:133–139.

94. Fram DB, Berns E, Aretz T, et al. Feasibility of radiofrequency powered, thermal balloon ablation of atrioventricular bypass tracts via the coronary sinus: in vivo canine studies. PACE 1995;18:1518–1530.

95. Dubuc M, Friedman PL, Roy D, et al. Reversible electrophysiologic effects using ice mapping with a cryoablation catheter. PACE 1997;20:1203.

96. Imai S, Nakagawa H, Ymanashi W, et al. Cryo-catheter ablation: effect of blood flow on lesion formation. PACE 1997;20:1204.

97. Okishige K, Stanhope W, Couper G, et al. Feasibility of catheter cryoablation of epicardial ventricular tachycardia [Abstract]. PACE 1993;16(4 Pt II):923.

98. Wood DL, Hammill SC, Porter CJ, et al. Cryosurgical modification of atrioventricular conduction for treatment of atrioventricular node reentrant tachycardia. Mayo Clin Proc 1988;63:988–992.

99. Gessman LJ, Agarwal JB, Endo T, et al. Localization and mechanism of ventricular tachycardia by ice mapping 1 week after the onset of myocardial infarction in dogs. Circulation 1983;68:657–666.

100. Harrison L, Gallagher JJ, Kasell J, et al. Cryosurgical ablation of the AV node. Circulation 1977;55:463–470.

101. Gallagher LA, Selay WC, Anderson W, et al. Cryo-surgical ablation of accessory atrioventricular connections: a method for correction of the pre-excitation syndrome. Circulation 1977;55:471–478.

102. Hollman WL, Hakel DB, Lease JG, et al.

Cryo-surgical ablation of the atrioventricular nodal reentry: histologic localization of the proximal common pathway. Circulation 1988;77:1356–1363.

103. Ott DA, Garson A, Cooley DA, et al. Cryoablative techniques in the treatment of cardiac tachyarrhythmias. Ann Thorac Surg 1987;26:438–441.

104. Caceres J, Werner P, Jazayeri M, et al. Efficacy of cryosurgery alone for refractory monomorphic sustained ventricular tachycardia due to inferior wall infarction. J Am Coll Cardiol 1988;11:1254.

105. Gillette PC, Swindle MM, Thompson RP, et al. Transvenous cryoablation of the bundle of His. PACE 1991;14:504–510.

106. Fujino H, Thompson RP, Germroth PG, et al. Histologic study of chronic catheter cryoablation of the atrioventricular conduction in swine. Am Heart J 1993;125:1632–1637.

107. Wang PJ, Aronovitz M, Schoen FJ, et al. Catheter cryoablation under the mitral annulus: a new method of accessory pathway ablation [Abstract]. J Am Coll Cardiol 1993; 21(2):357A.

108. He D, Zimmer JE, Hynynen KH, et al. Application of ultrasound energy for intracardiac ablation of arrhythmias [Abstract]. Circulation 1992;86(4):I–783.

109. He DS, Zimmer J, Hynynen K, et al. The effect of acoustic power, sonication time and transducer temperature on myocardial lesion size in vitro [Abstract]. Circulation 1993;88(4):I–399.

110. He DS, Simmons WN, Zimmer JE, et al. Comparison of several ultrasonic frequencies for cardiac ablation [Abstract]. Circulation 1994;90(4):I–271.

111. He DS, Marcus FL, Hynynen K, et al. In vivo studies of ultrasound energy for intracardiac ablation of arrhythmias [Abstract]. PACE 1995;18(4 Pt II):800.

112. Zimmer JE, Hynynen K, He DS, et al. The feasibility of using ultrasound for cardiac ablation. IEEE Trans Biomed Eng 1995;42: 9:891–897.

113. He DS, Zimmer JE, Hynynen K, et al. Preliminary results using ultrasound energy for ablation of the ventricular myocardium in dogs. Am J Cardiol 1994;73:1029–1031.

114. Chan RC, Johnson SB, Seward JB, et al. Initial experience with left ventricular endocardial catheter manipulation guided by intracardiac ultrasound visualization: improved accuracy over fluoroscopy imaging [Abstract]. J Am Coll Cardiol 1995;41A.

115. Packer DL, Chan R, Johnson SB, et al. Ultrasound cardioscopy: initial experience with a new high resolution combined intracar-

diac ultrasound/ablation system. PACE 1994;17(Pt II):863.

116. Packer DL, Seward JB, Chan RC, et al. The utility of a new integrated high resolution intracardiac ultrasound/ablation system in a canine model [Abstract]. J Am Coll Cardiol 1995;353A.

117. Hsia TY, Billingham M, Sung RJ. Intracoronary arterial occlusion: a novel technique potentially useful for ablation of cardiac arrhythmias. J Int Cardiac Electrophys 1997; 1:7–14.

118. Chilson DA, Peigh PS, Mahomed Y, et al. Chemical ablation of ventricular tachycardia in the dog. Am Heart J 1986;111: 113–118.

119. Inoue H, Waller BF, Zipes DP. Intracoronary ethyl alcohol or phenol injection ablates aconitine-induced ventricular tachycardia in dogs. J Am Coll Cardiol 1987; 10(6):1342–1349.

120. Brugada P, DeSwart H, Smeets JLRM, et al. Termination of tachycardias by interrupting blood flow to the arrhythmogenic area. Am J Cardiol 1988;62:387–392.

121. Friedman PL, Selwyn AP, Edelman E, et al. Effect of selective intracoronary antiarrhythmic drug administration in sustained ventricular tachycardia. Am J Cardiol 1989; 64:475–479.

122. Kay GN, Epstein AE, Bubien RS et al. Intracoronary ethanol ablation for recurrent sustained ventricular tachycardia. J Am Coll Cardiol 1992;19:159–168.

123. Strickberger SA, Foster PR, Wang PJ, et al. Intracoronary infusion of dilute ethanol for control of ventricular rate in patients with atrial fibrillation. PACE 1993;16(10): 1984–1993.

124. Brugada P, DeSwart H, Smeets JLRM, et al. Transcoronary chemical ablation of ventricular tachycardia. Circulation 1989;79: 475–482.

125. DeMaio SJ, Walter PF, Douglas JS. Treatment of ventricular tachycardia induced cardiogenic shock by percoronary chemical ablation. Cathet Cardiovasc Diagn 1990;21: 170–176.

126. Okishige K, Andrews TC, Friedman PL. Suppression of incessant polymorphic ventricular tachycardia by selective intracoronary ethanol infusion. PACE 1991;14: 188–185.

127. Sneddon JF, Ward DE, Simpson IA, et al. Alcohol ablation of atrioventricular conduction. Br Heart J 1991;65:143–147.

128. Brugada P, DeSwart H, Smeets J, et al. Transcoronary chemical ablation of atrioventricular conduction. Circulation 1990; 81:757–761.

129. Kay GN, Bubien R, Dailey S, et al. A prospective evaluation of intracoronary ethanol ablation of the atrioventricular conduction system. J Am Coll Cardiol 1991;17: 1634–1640.

130. Wang P, Schoen F, Reagan K, et al. Modification of atrioventricular conduction by selective AV nodal artery catheterization. PACE 1990;13:88–102.

131. Wang P, Schoen FJ, Aronovitz M, et al. Myocardial ablation using selective cardiac venous catheterization and ethanol injection [Abstract]. Circulation 1990;82:III–719.

132. Gadhoke A, Schoen F, Zebede J, et al. Acute and chronic effects of myocardial ablation using selective cardiac venous system catheterization and ethanol injection [Abstract]. J Am Coll Cardiol 1992;19(3):99A.

133. Lu C, Liu X, Jia G. Experimental ventricular tachycardia treated by transcatheter intramyocardial chemical ablation [Abstract]. PACE 1994;17(4 Pt II):861.

Chapter 2

Morphological Features of Normal and Abnormal Conduction System:
Essentials for Electrophysiologists

Bruce M. McManus, Shelley M. Wood

Introduction

In 1845, Purkinje first identified prominent ventricular fibers involved in the heart's "apparatus of motion." Since then, our understanding of the complex electrophysiological properties and processes of the cardiovascular system has grown immensely. Within 50 years of Purkinje's discovery, Kent had described the atrioventricular functional area, His the penetrating bundle, and Tawara the atrioventricular node. In 1907, Keith and Flack discovered the sinus node. Thorel, in 1909, suggested the presence of specialized conduction pathways linking the sinus and atrioventricular nodes. Today, almost a century later, the combined expertise of cardiologists, basic electrophysiologists, and pathologists has produced an elaborate picture of the cardiac conduction system, the heart's normal physiological and electrical function, and the pathobiology underlying rhythm disturbances and aberrant conduction.

An understanding of the normal development of cardiac structures in the fetus and

infant helps us appreciate how conduction abnormalities arise, particularly in the context of well-documented congenital anomalies or syndromes.[1–3] A more comprehensive discussion of embryological changes pertaining to the conduction system is available elsewhere.[4] Briefly, the primordium of the sinus node can be seen in the position it will assume postnatally after cardiac looping has occurred. Following cardiac chamber septation, the embryonic ring forms, composed of outer sulcus tissue, inner cushion tissue, and interposed ring tissue. Initially, in the developing human fetus, the atrial and ventricular myocardium are not anatomically separated. Sulcus tissue must grow into the atrioventricular junction, isolating atria from ventricles. Prior to this development, however, the atrioventricular junction appears to produce a slight delay between atrial and ventricular depolarizations, thereby modulating cardiac rhythm during the development of the heart chambers. The penetrating bundle and bundle branches are separated from the ventricular myocardium by an extended sheath of sulcus tissue. With time, the conductive pri-

From Singer I, Barold SS, Camm AJ (eds): Nonpharmacological Therapy of Arrhythmias for the 21st Century: The State of the Art. Futura Publishing Co., Armonk, NY, © 1998.

mordium, overlying the septal surfaces of the ventricles, extends forming the distal bundle and Purkinje system. With the continuity of the atrioventricular axis established, a remnant of the sulcus tissue normally adopts an insulating, protective role for the remainder of postnatal life.

Ectopic atrioventricular connections are commonly found in fetal hearts and are usually severed during development of the central fibrous body and valve annuli. Persistence of these ectopic fibers beyond infancy can form the basis for preexcitation in adult hearts.

Major Components of Cardiac Conduction System: Normal Anatomy

Sinus Node

The sinus node (the sinoatrial node) in the adult heart is usually described as an "upside-down teardrop" measuring up to 1.5 cm in length and 0.5 × 0.3 cm transversally, located in the epicardial groove of the sulcus terminalis at the junction of the superior vena cava and the right atrium[5] (Figure

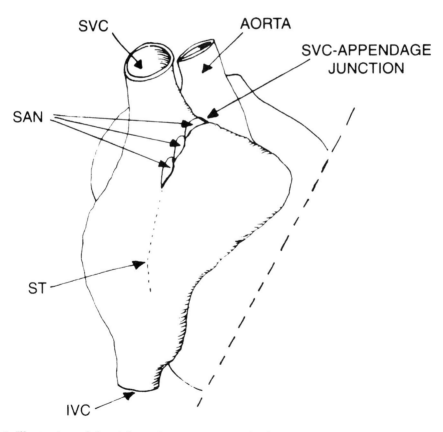

Figure 1. Illustration of the right atrium portraying the location of the sinus node in the sulcus terminalis at the superior vena cava–right atrial appendage junction. The node is typically quite constant in its position in an anatomically normal heart, overlapping the roof-peak of the right atrial appendage in certain hearts. SAN = sinus node; ST = sulcus terminalis; IVC = inferior vena cava; SVC = superior vena cava. Reproduced with permission from Singer I, ed., p 135.[126]

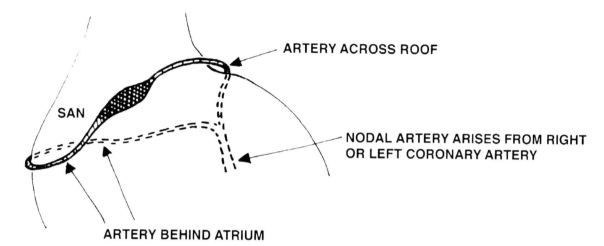

Figure 2. Illustration of the typical anterior-posterior and posterior-anterior course of the sinus node artery running through the long axis of the node. SAN = sinoatrial [sinus] node. Reproduced with permission from Singer I, ed., p 136.[126]

1). The specificity of this description, however, can be misleading since the shape and position of the node appear to vary according to the shape of the sulcus terminalis and, to some degree, to the variable positioning and extent of its arterial supply (Figure 2). In infants, the node may extend toward the inferior vena cava.[6] Appreciation of the sinus node as a *region* of pacemaker cells reduces the potential for accidental damage during surgery. Proposed approaches to determining the exact location of the node include the cavo-auricular incision described by Calmat Par et al,[7] identification of the curved sinoatrial notch reported by He et al.,[6] and localization of the antrum atria dextri. Postganglionic parasympathetic nerve fibers in the epicardium surround and innervate the node. Histological examination of the node reveals whorled, interwoven muscle fascicles, and collagenous connective tissue elements (Figure 3). In the sinus node, the interlacing myofibers are small and pale, interspersed with matrix. Light microscopy permits differentiation of apparent pacemaking cells, transitional cells, and atrial working muscle cells.

Atrioventricular Nodal Axis

The atrioventricular node (AV node) can be considered as three related regions: the compact node, the transitional zone, and the penetrating bundle (Figure 4). The compact atrioventricular node (AV node) is shaped like a half oval and, fully formed, measures approximately $1 \times 3 \times 5$ mm. Arterial supply normally originates as a branch of the right coronary artery at the crux of the heart, constituting the atrioventricular nodal artery; however, in certain hearts, the left circumflex artery may serve this function. The AV node is located epicardially, just underlying the right atrial epicardium posteriorly, anterior to the nodal artery and between the coronary sinus and the medial tricuspid valve leaflet, posterosuperior to the membranous septum. Koch's triangle is a useful anatomical landmark for identifying the compact node, delineated leftward by the intersection of the eustachian valve and the tricuspid valve annulus, with the ostium of the coronary sinus forming the rightward base of the triangle (Figure 5). The node is located at the apex of Koch's

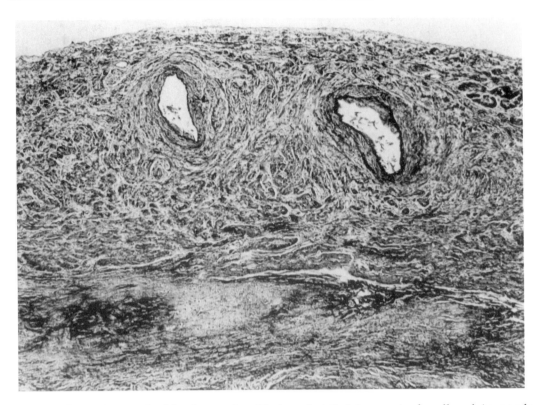

Figure 3. Photomicrograph of the sinus node with characteristic interweaving bundles of sinus node cardiocytes and connective tissue, both of which surround branches of the sinus node artery. The epicardial surface of the right atrium is located to the top of the photograph, illustrating the close proximity of the node to the epicardium. A similar degree of proximity exists with regard to the endocardium in the antrum atria dextri. Reproduced with permission from Singer I, ed., p 137.[126]

triangle, abutted by the annulus fibrosis and Todaro's tendon (Figure 6). The latter reflects the condensation of connective tissue in the thebesian and eustachian valves, in essence a lengthy, slender commissure. The AV node projects leftward into the His bundle at the apex of Koch's triangle and merges this conductive axis with ventricular tissue below the intersection of Todaro's tendon and the central fibrous body.

The notion of a compact AV node refers to the most easily distinguishable tissue (histologically) within a continuous axis of specialized tissue. It is made up of interconnecting fasciculi of small cells, morphologically comparable to the interlacing myofibers of the sinus node. Small archipelagos of these nodal cells frequently extend from the compact node into the central fibrous body.

From the compact body of the node, two extensions made up of identical cells run posteriorly from the node and branch to approach the mitral and tricuspid annuli.

Transitional cells comprising a well-defined layer surround the compact node and inferior (posterior) extensions. The transitional zone is further differentiated by the three main approaches to the compact node that are designated as *superficial transitional cells* which run anteriorly and inferiorly to the compact node, *posterior transitional cells* which approach the node from the coronary sinus area, and *deep transitional cells* which link the left atrium to the compact node. The transitional zone may be implicated in the dual atrioventricular nodal conduction seen in patients with atrioventricular junctional reentrant tachycardia (see below).

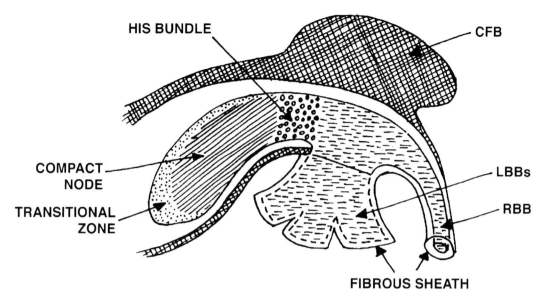

Figure 4. Illustration of the atrioventricular node, His bundle, and proximal left and right bundle branches. Of note, the central fibrous body (CFB) is adjacent to the AV nodal complex, and, in continuity with the rest of the fibrous skeleton, it provides a protective sheath to insulate the upper reaches of the transitional and compact node from the distal ventricular contact points of the bundle branches. LBB = left bundle branch; RBB = right bundle branch. Reproduced with permission from Singer I, ed., p 138.[126]

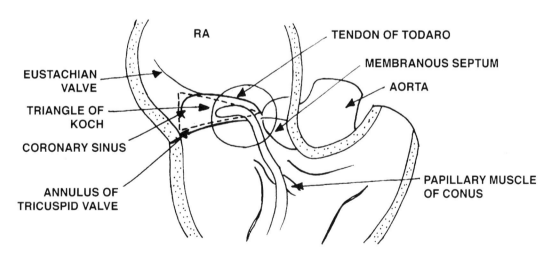

Figure 5. Illustration of cutaway view of right-sided, cardiac chambers displaying the essential anatomic landmarks of the atrioventricular node and His bundle system. The triangle of Koch is denoted with the atrioventricular node situated at its apex; the His bundle courses through the fibrous skeleton giving rise to the proximal bundle branches and inferior to the membranous septum. RA = right atrium.

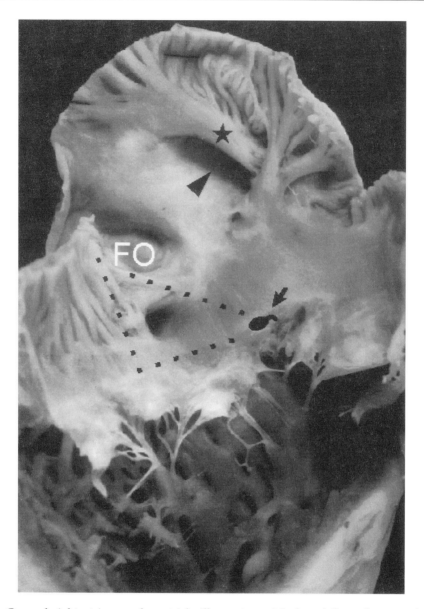

Figure 6. Opened right atrium and ventricle illustrating with dotted lines the triangle of Koch including the typical location of the atrioventricular node and proximal His bundle at its apex (arrow). Other relevant landmarks in this picture include the tendon of Todaro as a confluence of the eustachian and thebesian valves, the coronary sinus within the triangle of Koch, the fossa ovale (FO) region, the entry site of the superior vena cava (arrow head), and the crista terminalis (star). The posterior leaflet of the tricuspid valve defines the lower margin of the triangle of Koch by its point of attachment.

The junction between the compact AV node and the penetrating atrioventricular bundle is designated as the point at which the axis of nodal cells penetrate the annulus fibrosis. Whereas the nodal cells of the com- pact AV node are in contact with the atrial myocardium (through the transitional cells), the cells of the atrioventricular bun- dle, while histologically similar to those of the compact node, are separated from the atrial myocardium by the annulus fibrosis. Tongues of tissue extending from the compact AV node into the central fibrous body connecting the bundle axis to the ventricular septum, or from the initial part of the bundle branches to the septal crest, have been implicated as potential substrates for preexcitation and circus rhythm circuits.

His Bundle, Bundle Branches, and Purkinje Fibers

The penetrating bundle, or His bundle, is defined histologically as a continuation of the compact AV node where it projects through the central fibrous body (Figure 4) and descends along the posterior border of the membranous ventricular septum. The bundle itself is approximately 2 mm long and divided into three anatomical components. The proximal or nonpenetrating tract is located distal to the AV node. The middle or penetrating tract is embedded within the central fibrous body. The distal tract branches into the right and left bundle branches at the crest of the ventricular septum with the right bundle branch continuing as an extension of the main bundle, sometimes running deep into the endomyocardium. Upon exiting the central fibrous body, the left bundle branch divides, forming additional multifasciculi. The Purkinje fibers which act as extensions of the bundle branches typically run in fine trabeculae within the immediate subendocardium of both ventricles. Purkinje fibers are only slightly larger than working myofibers. They are readily observed in papillary muscles.

Cardiac Skeleton and Membranous Septum

The primary components of the cardiac conduction system and, indeed, of the basic musculature of the heart are largely supported by the sturdy fibrocollagenous tissue that comprises the cardiac skeleton. The central fibrous body provides connective tissue continuity between the aortic, mitral, and tricuspid valves (Figure 7). Extending posteroinferiorly and anteriorly from the central fibrous body is the left fibrous trigone comprised of firm bundles of connective tissue. The mitral and tricuspid valve annuli are essentially fibroelastic extensions of the left and right fibrous trigones, respectively. The membranous septum acts as an extension of the cardiac skeleton at the base of the ventricular septum. In forming a segment of the medial right atrial wall, the membranous septum acts as the primary supporting structure for the right aortic valve cusp. After the atrioventricular nodal tissue has penetrated the central fibrous body as the His bundle, the inferior margin of the membranous septum marks the course of the His bundle between the right and noncoronary aortic valve cusps.

Age-Related Changes Affecting the Cardiac Conduction System

Replacement of cell populations by fat and fibrous tissue occurs throughout the conduction system as part of the normal aging process. In the sinus node, myocardial cells are replaced by fibrous tissue with nodal cells persisting in the collagen and thicker elastic cells developing around nodal myocytes. Aging in the atrioventricular node is characterized by fatty infiltration, an increase in nodal collagen and elastic tissue, with slight infiltration of mononuclear cells and degeneration of nodal myocytes. Atria dilatation, myocyte atrophy, lipofuschin accumulation, and interstitial fibrosis in all four chambers of the heart may participate in arrhythmogenesis and are not unique to, or even preferential to, the conduction system.

Abnormal Anatomy of the Conduction System

Atresia

Atresia of the sinoatrial node is rare, normally seen when the predominant pace-

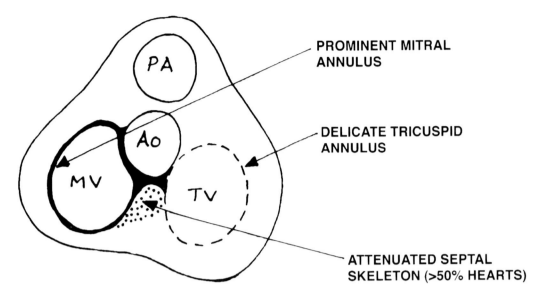

Figure 7. Illustration of transversely sectioned atrioventricular junctional region of a heart illustrating the relative completeness of the fibrous skeleton toward the left side of the heart and the relative delicacy of the corresponding right-sided skeleton. Typically, there is attenuation of the skeleton in the region of the posterior septal space. The latter may be of practical relevance since a number of bypass tracts are detected by electrophysiological mapping of this region. A greater number of bypass tracts, however, are located in the left lateral location, perhaps a surprising finding considering that the fibrous skeleton is more fully developed in this region than anywhere in the heart. Reproduced with permission from Singer I, ed., p 142.[126]

maker is at the level of the atrioventricular or ventricular tissue. Interruption of conduction between the atria and ventricles is attributed to differing origins of tissue in the crucial interface between conduction fibers of the His bundle, central fibrous body, and endocardial cushion tissue.

Displacement

Complex congenital cardiac malformations can affect the developmental positioning of the sinus node. In particular, atrioventricular canal defects, transposition of the great arteries, and ventricular septal defects may all lead to displacement of the sinus node. Normally located along the sulcus terminalis anteriorly and over the rooftop junction of the right atrial appendage and the superior vena cava, the sinus node may be congenitally displaced, thus, it may be out of the sulcus terminalis and more to-

ward the left side of the right atrial appendage.

Duplication

Duplication of the sinus node can occur in situs ambiguous (also known as atrial isomerism) of the heart. The anatomy of the heart with normal atria is usually classified as situs solitus, in which the morphological right atrium is found on the right side of the body and the left on the left, and situs inversus, in which the atria is arranged in an opposite fashion, in effect 'mirroring' the arrangement seen in situs solitus. The abdominal viscera are also mirror-image versus normal in situs inversus. Situs ambiguous describes a heart in which the atrial features fall neither into solitus nor inversus categories. Right isomerism describes a heart with duplication of right-sided structures; left isomerism describes a heart with duplication of left-sided structures. Thus, duplication of the sinus node can occur in right isomerism,[8] creating alternative or competing pacemakers capable of producing a range of conduction disturbances. A comprehensive review of the cardiac conduction system in situs ambiguous is available elsewhere.[9]

Infection and Inflammation

Conduction disturbances can arise from a range of infections and other inflammatory conditions, either secondary to specific microbial or postinfectious processes or due to an immune response. Lyme disease, Chagas' disease, and diphtheria are three of the most common infections that exhibit a tropism for the heart, while cardiac sarcoidosis

and Wegener's granulomatosis are well documented to produce arrhythmogenic sequelae.

Infarction

The nature and degree of conduction system disturbances in the setting of a myocardial infarction depends on the location of the infarct and the extent of scarring and related fibroelastosis[5] (Figure 8). S-T segment depression (denoting ischemia), premature contractions, ventricular tachycardia, fibrillation, and/or standstill are common arrhythmias secondary to myocardial injury including acute, subacute, and chronic myocardial injury and the healing process.

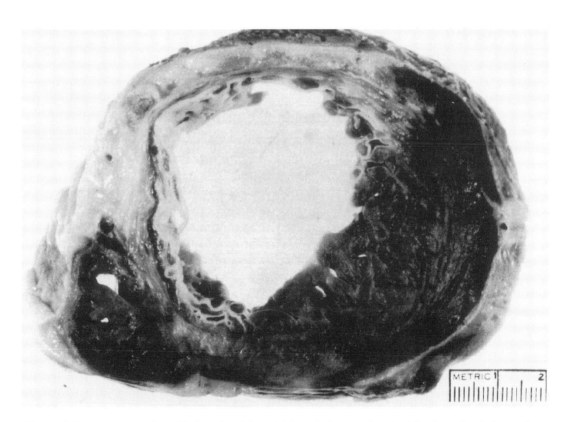

Figure 8. Transverse section of left and right ventricles of a human heart with a large healed anteriorseptal myocardial infarct. A lesion of this size, associated with left ventricular chamber dilatation and variable islands of viable but potentially ischemic myocardium, may provide sites for local reentry circuits and arrhythmogenesis. Reproduced with permission from Singer I, ed., p 149.[126]

Infiltration

Deposits of eosinophilic, amorphous amyloid protein typically produce atrial fibrillation and heart block and, less commonly, ventricular arrhythmias. Amyloidosis is common in aged human hearts and can also contribute to arrhythmogenesis at earlier ages in association with chronic inflammatory conditions and multiple myeloma or neoplasms. Primary tumors, including rhabdomyomata (Purkinje cell tumors) and mesotheliomas (endotheliomas) are believed to produce heart block through tumor enlargement. Rhabdomyomata, also associated with paroxysmal arrhythmias, may be congenital in origin and are seen predominantly in children. Mesotheliomas normally affect the AV node, interrupting the conduction axis and resulting in block or atrial fibrillation. Exogenous or endogenous hemochromatosis can lead to atrial flutter and/or fibrillation, sinus tachycardia, heart block, and syncope. Iron deposits and associated fibrosis are more common in the subepicardial region and in the atrioventricular node, and less so in the subendocardial region and sinus node. Finally, fibrosis occurring secondary to injury and necrosis or as part of the normal aging process can act as a substrate for arrhythmogenesis.

Congenital Cardiac Malformations Associated with Arrhythmogenesis Both Preoperatively and Postoperatively

Accessory pathways are frequently found in otherwise normal hearts and are also associated with a number of grossly evident cardiovascular malformations. Moreover, an underlying, sometimes asymptomatic congenital malformation of the heart can itself represent an important risk factor for arrhythmogenesis and sudden death. Several well-defined congenital conditions involve a fundamental malalignment of the principal conduction components which,

not surprisingly, affects the electrical activation patterns of the heart. For the electrophysiologist, a knowledge of common congenital abnormalities is important not only because of the conduction patterns related to the malformations themselves, but also because of the conduction disturbances that can arise *after* the patient has undergone corrective surgery.

Congenital Complete Atrioventricular Block

Impairment of conduction through the atrioventricular junction tissues can be present at birth or result from a number of acquired diseases. True congenital block, resulting from a developmental anomaly that is intrinsic to the atrioventricular node or branches, must be distinguished from congenital conditions in which block is secondary to well-defined structural malformations. The latter include congenitally corrected transposition, in which a malalignment of the atrial and ventricular septa can produce atrioventricular conduction disturbances, or atrioventricular septal defects and double inlet left ventricle wherein a deficiency or absence of the right ventricle results in block.

Accessory Pathways

The existence of accessory or anomalous pathways that "short circuit" the normal conduction pathway from the sinus node through to the ventricular myocardium can produce preexcitation. In the human fetus, accessory atrioventricular connections are common, rarely producing disturbances that are clinically apparent, and normally severed during postnatal development. When accessory pathways crossing the atrioventricular ring tissue persist beyond the normal developmental period, the delay-producing activity of the compact AV node is bypassed and additional and/or conflicting wavefronts of activation are produced. Preexcitation, and arrhythmias such as atrial fibrillation or ventricular fibrillation may result. It is important to note that accessory pathways, while associated with a number of gross, congenital abnormalities, are also common in otherwise "normal" hearts.

Classification of Accessory Pathways

Researchers have studied aberrant electrical links between the atrial and the ventricular myocardium for more than a century. In 1983, Davies et al.[4] summarized the observations gleaned from their own work and that of their predecessors and defined five types of anomalous connections capable of producing preexcitation (Figure 9). The most common of these are accessory atrioventricular connections, which exist outside the specialized atrioventricular junctional tissues, spanning from atria to ventricles. Two other categories link the atrioventricular node/His bundle to the ventricular septal musculature and these

are denoted as nodoventricular or fasciculoventricular connections. Differentiation of the latter pathways is made on the basis of their starting points, with the former originating in the compact node and the latter originating in the bundle or proximal bundle branches. The fourth possibility for an accessory tract is an atriofascicular pathway comprised of atrial fibers that connect with the His bundle or branches, penetrating the collagenous insulation provided by the central fibrous body. Finally, intranodal bypass tracts, which also take their point of departure from within the atria, circumvent the main delay-producing region by joining the atrioventricular junctional tissues distal to the compact node but *before* the bundle penetrates the central fibrous body.

Recent reviews have focused on the course and location of accessory pathways.[10] Cain et al.[11,12] have documented the regional distribution of accessory pathways, noting that 58% are found in the left free wall, 24% in the posterior septal site,

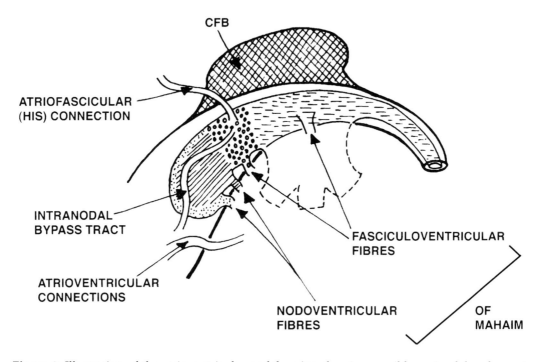

Figure 9. Illustration of the atrioventricular nodal region showing possible perinodal and remote atrioventricular bypass tracts. These tracts are described in more detail within the text. It is of note that, in recent years, fibers of Mahaim have been localized more remotely from the node-His axis then depicted in this diagram. Reproduced with permission from Singer I, ed., p 145.[126]

13% in the right free wall, and 5% in the anterior septal site. The importance of differentiating between the different sites and insertion points of bypass tracts has been underscored in numerous investigations and clinical observations.

Left free wall pathways are usually ablated at the point of ventricular insertion which is believed to be the "weak link" in left-sided pathways.[13] The ablation catheter may be advanced into the left ventricle across the aortic valve in a retrograde direction (Figure 10). The catheter tip is then wedged beneath the mitral valve annulus, affording a stable position. When ablation of the region of ventricular insertion region fails to interrupt aberrant conduction, an atrial approach is used wherein the ablation catheter is advanced across the mitral valve into the left atrium. A third approach, tar-

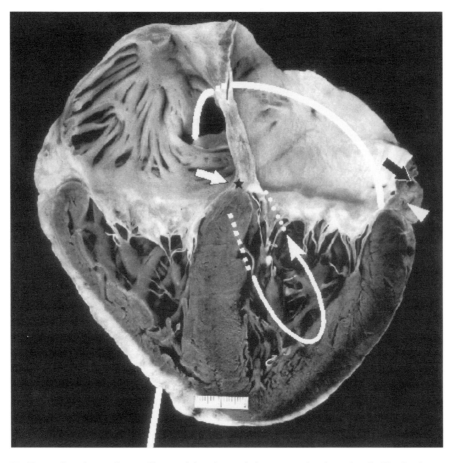

Figure 10. Four-chamber echocardiographic view of the posterior-interior half of a human heart illustrating two routes for ablation catheters to reach atrioventricular bypass tracts in the left side of the heart. The passage of a catheter retrograde from the aorta and up underneath the medial posterior mitral leaflet may provide access to certain pathways adjacent to the posterior septal space. Other more lateral pathways may be reached using a transseptal atrial approach, introducing the catheter by way of the inferior vena cava. The site of the atrioventricular node is designated (white arrow), and the left circumflex coronary artery is denoted (arrowhead) in close adjacency, the coronary vein (black arrow). The relevance of the latter structures relates to their potential damage when radiofrequency energy is delivered to the site of a bypass tract. It is now known that the size of ablation lesions is generally larger than originally anticipated, and neighboring structures must be kept squarely in mind.

geting the interface between the left atrium and the anomalous pathway, is to access the left atrium via a transseptal approach (Figure 10). Ablation delivered from within the coronary sinus can be used in the rare occurrence of a subepicardial left free wall pathway.[13] Ablation of right free wall pathways is approached from the atrial aspect of the tricuspid valve, targeting the weak atrial insertion point. The difficulty in achieving a stable catheter position is cited as the primary reason for failed ablation of right-sided pathways, frequently necessitating repeat sessions.[13]

Experience with surgical and ablation procedures for septal pathways in general, and posterior septal pathways in particular, emphasizes the complexity of the surrounding architecture[14–16] (Figure 11) and the specificity required for isolating an aberrant pathway.[17–20] Posterior septal pathways are typically located between the insertion of the atrial extension of the membranous septum into the right fibrous trigone anteriorly and the epicardium overlying the crux of the heart posteriorly. Laterally, posteroseptal pathways are bound by the walls of the left and right atria. This pyramidal space contains Todaro's tendon, the AV nodal artery, epicardial fat, and the proximal portion of the coronary sinus, and is immediately adjacent to the triangle of Koch.[11] The majority of posteroseptal pathways appear to course in a right atrial–left ventricle direction. Nearby, certain bypass pathways map to diverticula in the deep coronary sinus, at the connecting site for the posterior coronary vein (Figure 12). Anterior septal pathways are much less common than posterior septal pathways. They are normally located just anterior to the AV node, anterosuperior to the bundle of His. They pass through the fat pad separating the atrioventricular insertion of the right coronary artery and the right and left fibrous trigone of the cardiac skeleton.[11,13] Ablation is usually conducted via the right atrium using a jugular venous approach. Over the past 10 years, a number of groups have reported an additional intermediate septal pathway, which

differs from an anterior septal pathway that inserts in the anteromedial right atrium and activates the ventricular septum anteriorly, and from a posterior septal pathway that inserts near the ostium of the coronary sinus and activates the right and left ventricles more posteriorly.[20,21]

Acquired cardiac malformations including areas of scarring, aneurysm formation, or hypertrophy can also act as anatomically discreet, electrical pathways between the atria and ventricles or related conduction tissue, producing rhythm disturbances.

The Wolff-Parkinson-White Syndrome and Variants

Accessory pathways are well-documented as being the underlying cause of the Wolff-Parkinson-White (WPW) syndrome. Described in the early 20th century[22] and in more detail by the investigators for whom the syndrome is named.[23] WPW is an electrophysiological condition characterized by a normal electrocardiogram and short P-R intervals with preexcitation. Paroxysmal tachycardia and/or paroxysmal atrial fibrillation or flutter are the common arrhythmic manifestations. The WPW syndrome is often observed in normal hearts, but may also be associated with specific congenital malformations including Ebstein's anomaly, mitral valve prolapse, or cardiomyopathy.

Investigators have defined several variants of the WPW syndrome that are also related to the presence of one or more accessory pathways. The most common of these is the so-called "silent" WPW syndrome or concealed bypass tract wherein the pathway(s) is only capable of retrograde conduction and cannot therefore be identified by a surface ECG, nor be mapped to the ventricular insertion point by conventional methods. Permanent junctional reciprocating tachycardia (PJRT) has also been identified as a subset of the WPW syndrome. In this condition, an accessory pathway, frequently located in the posterior septal area,

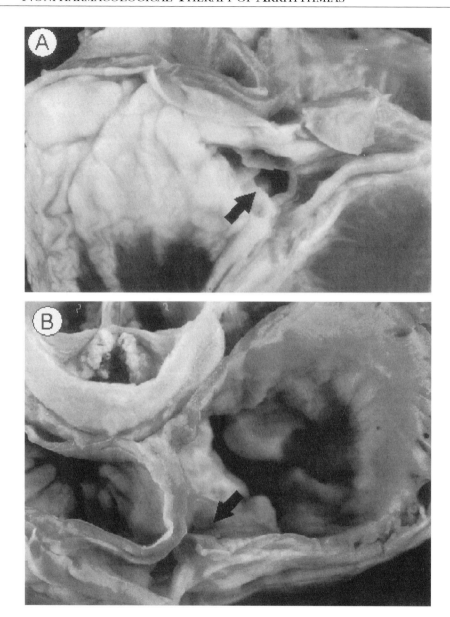

Figure 11. The posterior septal space, viewed from directly posterior (panel **A**) and superior (panel **B**). In **A**, the site of penetration of the atrioventricular nodal artery into the posterior septal space is denoted (arrow). In **B**, the mouth of the coronary sinus is designated and the juxtaposition of the coronary sinus, posterior-medial right atrial cavity, posterior-medial left atrial cavity, and the confluence of the two atrial walls is quite apparent. A substantial number of bypass tracts are located in this region.

conducts in a retrograde direction and is conspicuous for its unusually slow conduction and atrial insertion at the coronary sinus ostium. The AV junctional region including the compact node and His bundle

acts as the anterograde limb. A major clue to the presence of accessory pathway PJRT is incessant supraventricular tachycardia with a long R-P interval, narrow QRS complex, and inverted P waves in inferior

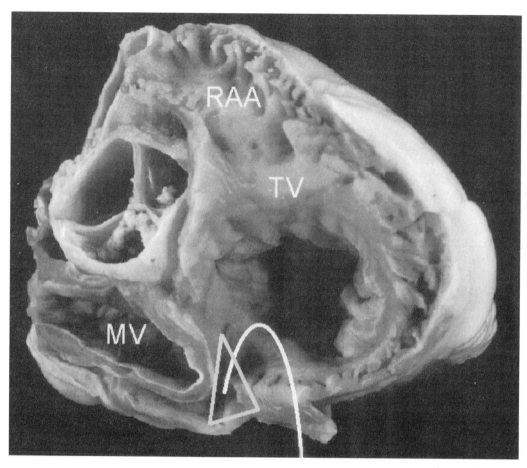

Figure 12. Superior view of heart with atria unroofed illustrating the approximate location of the posterior septal space and the approximate position of a catheter entering the ostium of the coronary sinus and projecting to a site of a potential coronary sinus diverticulum. Such diverticula are deemed to be the site of uncommon bypass tracts. RAA = right atrial appendage; TV = tricuspid valve annulus; MV = mitral valve.

leads.[24] Caution must be exercised in ablating such a posterior septal accessory pathway because of its proximity to the AV junctional region.[24]

Recently, Plumb[25] highlighted some of the important anatomical landmarks and mapping procedures used for catheter ablation for the WPW syndrome. He emphasizes the results obtained by electrophysiological mapping and the different accessory pathways and insertion points with which these results are frequently associated. Percutaneous, vascular, multipolar electrode catheters are used to record the pacing of the atria and ventricles, and to confirm the number and location of accessory pathways. The advent of large-tip deflectable electrode catheters has enabled ablationists to map the aberrant pathway and deliver the radiofrequency current within the same session.[26]

Lown-Ganong-Levine Syndrome

Accessory bypass tracts linking the bundle of His directly to the atrium or linking the atrial septum directly to the ventricular septum are speculated to produce the arrhythmias seen in the Lown-Ganong-Levine syndrome. Earlier investigations of this condition have not been comprehensively expanded in recent years.[27,28]

Postoperative Issues in Radiofrequency Ablation

In the three decades that have passed since the first surgical ablation for an accessory pathway associated with WPW syndrome, nonsurgical, catheter-based ablation techniques have revolutionized the treatment and cure of patients with a wide range of conduction disturbances. Direct current (DC) ablation has been largely supplanted by radiofrequency (RF) ablation, which is now widely used to target accessory pathways, the AV nodal junction, and AV node. RF ablation is, however, a relatively new technique and the risk factors associated with the procedures and the late, postoperative sequelae are only gradually emerging.

Much of the literature discussing successes and failures of RF ablation emphasizes the recurrence of conduction disturbances following RF ablation for WPW syndrome, Mahaim fibers (nodoventricular fibers), or other preexcitation syndromes.[29-38] The incidence of recurring arrhythmias following ablation has been estimated to be as much as 12%,[39] often returning in less than 24 hours. In most instances, recurrent conduction along an previously ablated pathway is manifest within 2 months,[31] and a second ablation session usually succeeds in permanently interrupting the recalcitrant bypass tract. One study reported that initial recurrence of aberrant conduction within 24 hours of ablation may cease spontaneously over ensuing weeks.[40]

Investigators in major electrophysiology and pacing centers have attempted to pinpoint issues that may account for or contribute to failed interruption of an accessory pathway.[13,25,29,31,39-43] In general, post-ablation arrhythmias appear to be more common in younger patients, in patients with multiple accessory pathways, or in patients whose initial ablation session is particularly

long and complex.[39] Right free wall and septal pathways fall under this category and carry a higher risk of post-ablation recurrence.[31,39] Langberg et al.[39] reported that 14 patients out of 200 receiving RF ablation for an accessory pathway experienced conduction recurrence along the accessory pathway. They also noted a trend, substantiating a previous claim by Twidale and colleagues,[31] of increased conduction recurrence along an accessory pathway in regions where the ablation electrode failed to record accessory pathway potentials during the initial catheter probing. Yet other investigators have corroborated this finding.[29] A second predictor of recurrent accessory pathway conduction appears to be an absence of recorded antegrade conduction.[29,31]

Langberg et al.[39] proposed that the disproportionately higher incidence of recurrence in right-sided and septal pathways may be due in part to the specific positioning of the catheter as dictated by the ablation site. Since left-sided accessory pathways are often ablated by "wedging" the catheter tip between the mitral valve annulus and the left ventricle, the RF current can be delivered with a high degree of stability and accuracy. By contrast, catheters placed against the tricuspid annulus cannot achieve the same contact pressure and stability, in part because of endocardial shifting due to the normal cardiac or respiratory motion.[39]

A number of recent papers have focussed on electrode temperature and tissue heating in relation to recurrent conduction.[39,44,45] Several groups have proposed that lower electrode temperatures may result in insufficient or transient interruption of conduction along an aberrant pathway. A recent study by Calkins and associates[39] found no difference in electrode temperatures at successful ablation sites versus sites of recurrent conduction. They suggested, however, that imprecise positioning of the catheter for a particular pathway, or an ablation target located in a mid-myocardial or epicardial region, can lead to inaccurate assumptions about the exact temperature reaching the intended lesion site. With increased distance from the exact point of electrode contact, tissue temperature drops significantly; thus, the correlation between a higher recurrence of conduction and specific accessory pathway locations may be linked to inadequate heating of the intended target. Greater accuracy in accessing or pinpointing anomalous conduction locales will stem from an ever-increasing understanding of conduction system anatomy and ongoing refinements to present-day ablation technology.

Equally important to electrophysiologists is the issue of catheter-induced mechanical trauma and the impact of both the catheter itself and the lesions it induces on future electrical and hemodynamic activity. Most investigators agree that arrhythmias post-ablation are usually due to an unsuccessful first ablation attempt and are not secondary to the procedure. Lev and Bharati,[46] however, have postulated that inflammatory changes resulting from RF ablation may provide a "nidus" for future arrhythmic events. Others have suggested that small, homogenous, catheter-induced lesions in the adjacent myocardium may lead to late contractility and conduction disturbances.[25] The possibility that other forms of catheter-induced damage could form the substrate for conduction disturbances has not been comprehensively explored. Chiang et al.,[47] in a review of 666 patients, documented 17 with catheter-induced mechanical trauma. They suggested that the traumatized tissues may be either temporarily or permanently damaged by either the electrode tip or shaft; revival of traumatized tissues may account for the recurrence of conduction along an accessory pathway. King et al.[48] reviewed the incidence of atrioventricular nodal block (AVNB) secondary to catheter positioning in 613 patients undergoing radiofrequency ablation for atrioventricular nodal reentrant tachycardia or atrioventricular reentrant tachycardia. They reported that AVNB due to mechanical trauma occurred in 10 patients (1.6%) during positioning of

a stiff large-tip steerable catheter in the junctional area but, in all cases, resolved after repositioning of the catheter. To date, mechanical trauma, coronary artery blockage, myocardial perforation, pericardial bleeding, and thromboembolism have been reported secondary to RF ablation catheters[25,26,47,49–51]; however, these complications are reasonably rare.

A recent study by Friedman et al.[52] addressed the effects of RF ablation on the autonomic nervous system. They proposed that transient AV block and sinus bradycardia during application of RF current, and inappropriate sinus tachycardia, following ablation for AV node modification or an accessory pathway, may be due to a loss of parasympathetic influence on the sinus node. Previous reports[53,54] addressing this issue also support the claims put forward by Friedman's group. Denervation of the ventricular myocardium has not yet been reported; however, as the authors suggest,[52] newer, more powerful ablation techniques, including saline-irrigated ablation and cryoablation, capable of producing transmural ventricular lesions, may in turn lead to denervation supersensitivity and arrhythmogenesis.

Ebstein's Anomaly

In Ebstein's anomaly, the septal and posterior (inferior) tricuspid valve leaflets are displaced caudally with the point of maximum displacement located in the commissure between the two leaflets, found at the posterior border of the ventricular septum. The anterior leaflet is usually enlarged and attaches posteroinferiorly to the bridge between the trabecular and inlet portions of the right ventricle. The orifice of the valve is displaced apically into the right ventricle near the junction of the inlet and trabecular regions. In congenitally corrected transposition of the great arteries, Ebstein's anomaly can affect the left atrioventricular valve (essentially the displaced tricuspid valve). Dilatation of the right atrium and enlargement of the right atrioventricular junction results in a prominent eustachian valve.

The downward displacement of the valve effectively divides the ventricle into an atrialized posterior ventricle which acts as an inlet and the trabecular and outlet portions which operate as the functional ventricle. Additional congenital abnormalities commonly associated with Ebstein's anomaly of the tricuspid valve include atrial septal defect, patent foramen ovale, right atrial enlargement, and myocardial abnormalities.

Preexcitation is common in patients with Ebstein's anomaly and is usually caused by the existence of one or more accessory pathways. A recent study claims that as many as 15% of patients with Ebstein's anomaly experience supraventricular tachycardia most frequently associated with WPW syndrome.[55,56] Enhanced atrioventricular nodal conduction and dual atrioventricular nodal physiology have also been reported.[57]

Cappato et al.[58] have explored the role of RF catheter ablation for accessory pathways associated with Ebstein's anomaly. They observed that the abnormal morphology, including the atrialized right ventricle, and associated conduction irregularities complicate electrophysiological mapping and ablation. The higher incidence of failed accessory pathway ablation is likely due to the structural complexity of the disease.

Septal Defects

Malformations involving the atrioventricular septal junction fall under the category of atrial septal defects (ASDs). These include isolated atrial septal defects which are in some way characterized by an opening between the left and right atria, and atrioventricular canal defects (or endocardial cushion defects) which result from incomplete embryological partitioning of the atrioventricular canal. The most common arrhythmias associated with unoperated ASDs are atrial fibrillation and flutter, although supraventricular tachycardia has also been reported.[59–62] Incomplete development of the endocardial primordia is suspected to be the cause of most electrophysiologically problematic ASDs; the majority involve incomplete or abnormal development of the lower portion of the atrial septum, the inflow portion of the ventricular septum and/or the atrioventricular valves. The two principal ASDs of relevance to this discussion are ostium primum defects (or partial atrioventricular canal) and complete atrial septal defects (or common orifice/common atrioventricular canal). The former refers to a septal malformation that extends to the atrioventricular valves and normally involves a cleft mitral valve with leaflets that are fused to a deficient ventricular septum preventing communication at that level. The latter type arises from a lack of fusion between the anterior and posterior leaflets on the septal crest, resulting in failed differentiation of the primitive canal into two discrete atrioventricular apertures. The atrioventricular node can be hypoplastic or displaced as a result of a deficient atrial septum. Backward displacement of the compact node and associated tissues can result in early posterior activation. Ventricular septal defects (VSDs) may be as common as ASDs, but do not carry the same potential for arrhythmogenesis.

Postoperative arrhythmias following repair of an atrial septal defect can occur immediately following surgery or late postoperatively and vary depending on the age of the patient. In children, junctional escape rhythms, atrioventricular dissociation, and ectopic atrial rhythm (sick sinus syndrome) are common in the early postoperative period, whereas adults, by contrast, typically present with atrial flutter. Late postoperatively, tachyarrhythmias are reasonably common in both adults and children. Atrioventricular block has occasionally been observed in adults both early and late, postoperatively. The most common conduction system disturbance seen following repair of an ASD is right bundle branch block. AV node and His-Purkinje conduction delays are also common early postsurgery. Up to one-third of all patients undergoing repair of an ASD experience complete heart block. Surgery for VSDs in the region of the membranous septum frequently result in right bundle branch block, with reports in the past citing an incidence of up to 100%.[63-66] Ventricular tachycardia, atrial flutter, atrial fibrillation, paroxysmal supraventricular tachycardia, and junctional tachycardia have also been reported.[67-69]

Tetralogy of Fallot

An anterior malalignment of the infundibular septum is responsible for the four co-existent congenital malformations that comprise the tetralogy of Fallot, namely a ventricular septal defect, infundibular pulmonary stenosis, overriding of the ventricular septum by the aortic valve, and right ventricular hypertrophy.[70] The ventricular septal defect in tetralogy of Fallot can be an infundibular perimembranous defect or infundibular muscular in type. The former is more common. Depending on the nature of the septal defect, the conduction system is normally unaffected although right bundle branch block has been reported. Postoperatively, however, repaired tetralogy of Fallot can be associated with a number of conduction disturbances including right bundle branch, sinus node dysfunction, ventricular arrhythmias, and complete heart block.[71-79]

Hemorrhage, necrosis, and/or inflammatory changes secondary to surgery are believed to be responsible for most conduction problems in patients undergoing surgical repair[64]; however, the multifactorial nature of both the malformation and the surgical steps required for its repair make it difficult to pinpoint the precise conditions responsible for arrhythmogenesis. As Ross[74] has pointed out, no classification system exists for determining the severity of a given malformation nor for cataloging the anatomic variability that exists between patients. Nevertheless, a growing number of clinical reports and experimental models have identified issues that appear to be impor-

tant. For example, several studies have indicated that age at the time of surgery is an important factor in determining the risk of sudden death, although the cause of death is a subject of ongoing debate. Postoperative sudden death in children and adolescents may be due to heart block[80,81] or to ventricular arrhythmias and tachyarrhythmias.[78,80-85] A recent study of adults (age 18 years and older) with previous corrective surgery suggested that conduction defects and rhythm disturbances were rare, potentially due to careful monitoring and correction of hemodynamic changes following surgery. Several authors have proposed that ventricular arrhythmias are more prevalent in patients who undergo repair later, either as adolescents or young adults.[73,79,82,86-88] Different surgical approaches are also believed to carry different degrees of arrhythmic risk. Dietl et al.[71] reported that the incidence of postoperative ventricular arrhythmias in adults was significantly higher when a right ventricular approach was used and lower with a right atrial procedure. In particular, their study and others[80,82,84,85] indicate that scarring in the right ventricle may serve as the site of origin for a reentrant mechanism resulting in ventricular tachycardia, and/or may affect normal contractility and function of the right ventricle. Additional studies have qualitatively assessed aspects of different repair procedures and have highlighted issues that may increase the risk of postoperative arrhythmias or hemodynamics.[76,89,90]

Univentricular Hearts

Univentricular hearts, lacking a ventricular septum between the right and left ventricular inlet structures, are categorized as left and right according to the morphological orientation of the single, operative ventricle. Hearts with a single, morphologically right ventricle and rudimentary left ventricular chamber normally do not suffer from conduction disturbances, since the His bundle and node are able to develop normally.

In single left ventricular hearts, however, the posterior AV node is typically hypoplastic and detached from the ventricular musculature. An anterior atrioventricular pathway forms in lieu of the His bundle (which would ordinarily connect with the posterior AV node). Prolonged P-R interval, potentially culminating in complete heart block, is observed in left-sided univentricular hearts with a rudimentary right-sided chamber.

Transposition of the Great Arteries

Congenitally corrected transposition of the great arteries (CCTGA) embodies a physiological "correction" of a malalignment of the atrial and ventricular septa. The morphological left ventricle is situated on the right and vice versa, while the L-transposed aorta connects to the morphological right ventricle on the left side and the pulmonary trunk connects to the left ventricle on the right side. In CCTGA, the atrioventricular node is separated from the inlet septum, normally as a result of an expansive membranous septum or a ventricular septal defect. Typically, a second atrioventricular bundle forms, descending anteriorly to reach the trabecular septum. This nonbranching bundle from the anomalous AV node can become fibrotic with aging, leading to atrioventricular block. Additional accessory pathways are often associated with CCTGA and can lead to preexcitation syndromes. Additional conduction disturbances have been reported, including premature atrial depolarization, junctional escape rhythms, sinoatrial block, and sinus bradycardia.

A procedure aimed at rechanneling the pulmonary and systemic venous drainage in hearts with complete transposition of the great arteries was developed by Mustard[91] in 1964. After undergoing decades of modification, the preferred method for reconstructing a heart with complete TGA is an arterial switch operation.[92] While postsurgical arrhythmias are still reported, refinement of surgical techniques has greatly reduced the number of postoperative conduction disturbances.[64] Physiological alterations implicated in arrhythmogenesis postsurgery include intraoperative damage to the sinus node, sinus node artery, or atrioventricular nodal tissue. Supraventricular arrhythmias, such as premature atrial complexes, atrial flutter, atrial fibrillation, ectopic atrial rhythms, slow junctional rhythms, junctional ectopic tachycardia, sick sinus syndrome, and, less commonly, atrioventricular block have been reported[64,93,94] after atrial switch operations.

Emerging Issues in Conduction System Morphology

Slow/Fast Pathways of the Atrioventricular Node: Implications for the Treatment of Atrioventricular Node Reentry Tachycardia

The observations by Scherf and Shookhoff in 1926 of returning atrial impulses in animal models has fueled more than seven decades of research into the reentrant tachycardias of the AV nodal region. The concept of dual nodal pathways within the AV junction, explored by Moe and colleagues throughout the 1950s and 1960s, has grown increasingly complex. Over ensuing years, investigators put forth the concept of a functional dissociation of the AV node into slow and fast pathways. These pathways form the basis for atrioventricular node reentrant tachycardia (AVNRT) with one pathway acting as the retrograde reentry route for conduction impulses to reactive the atria. In the most common form of AVNRT, antegrade conduction occurs over the slow AV nodal pathway, while the fast pathway provides the route for retrograde conduction. This form is generally referred to as *slow/fast* AVNRT. Less common is *fast/slow* AVNRT in which antegrade conduction occurs over the fast pathway with the retrograde return via the slow pathway. A third, very rare form of AVNRT has also been identified involving two slow pathways, one of which provides the antegrade route and the other the retrograde route. More recently, several groups[95,96] have proposed that AVNRT involves multiple intranodal and perinodal tissues that operate as functional slow and fast routes.

The application of intracardiac mapping and catheter ablation techniques in the diagnosis and treatment of AVNRT, the latter through AV node modification, has permitted electrophysiologists to gain a clearer understanding of reentry circuits and potential routes for slow and fast/anterograde and retrograde conduction. The anatomic delimitations of the reentrant circuits, however, continue to be a major point of contention in AVNRT research and patient care. The perinodal atrium, compact AV node and proximal His bundle may be involved electrophysiologically.

For several years, investigators have debated whether functional dissociation of the atrioventricular nodal conduction into fast and slow pathways has any anatomic correlate.[97–100] The possibility that reentry circuits involve tissues *outside* of the compact node has been explored by a number of groups and continues to be a major research focus. Kadish and Goldberg[97] have argued that the approaches to the AV node, identified as being part of reentry circuits, are anatomically distinct with different conduction system components. Thus, several investigators have suggested that the functional fast and slow pathways may be located anatomically within the differentiated tissues of the transitional zone surrounding the compact node, with the superficial transitional cells forming part of the fast pathway and the posterior zone constituting part of the slow pathway.[99,101] Success of ablation sessions that have targeted the approach to the AV node seems to uphold these claims.[102–105] An earlier study[106] reported that patients with dual AV node conduction demonstrated distinct atrial insertion points for slow and fast pathways during retrograde conduction. Using intra-

cardiac mapping, Sung et al.[106] located the retrograde atrial exit of the fast AV node pathway at the low septal region of the right atrium near the His bundle recording site. The retrograde atrial exit of the slow AV node pathway was localized in or near the coronary sinus ostium, inferior and posterior to the exit of the fast AV node pathway (Figure 13). A broad tissue region is postulated to be the upper point of connection between the fast and slow pathways.[106] Tondo et al.[107] have also explored the atrial component of the AV nodal reentrant circuit, focusing primarily on the coronary sinus as an ablation target. They reported that the atrial muscle within the coronary sinus or adjacent myocardium may form part of the reentry route in certain patients.[107] Additional reports have corroborated these observations.[108,109] Likewise, observations that reentrant tachycardias of the AV region can persist despite 2:1 conduction block superior to the His bundle[110–112] support the hypothesis that the lower turnaround point where the two pathways converge may be located within or close to the His bundle.

Radiofrequency Catheter Ablation for Atrial Fibrillation and Atrial Flutter

Surgical strategies for atrial fibrillation, including the corridor and maze procedures, revolve around the creation of nonconductive boundaries which prevent reentry of wavelet circulation by anatomically limiting the contiguous tissue area required by reentrant circuits. Today, the maze procedure, having undergone a number of refinements, affords high success rates and long-term cure. The procedure restores the synchrony of the atria and ventricles and reestablishes sinus node control of ventricular rate by serial partitioning of both atria. The major shortcomings of the maze procedure as an open heart surgery are its cost and associated risks. Currently, attempts to design catheter-based methods to achieve the same linear, nonconductive barriers to

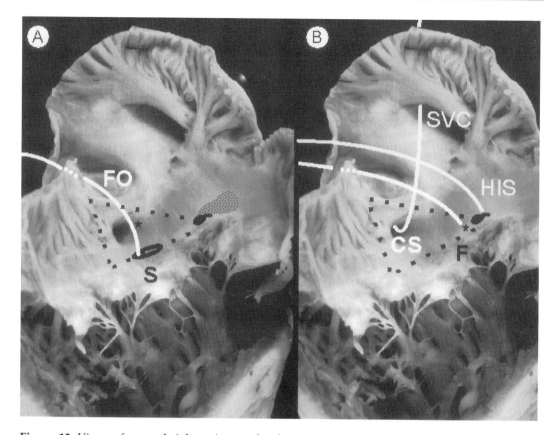

Figure 13. Views of opened right atrium and right ventricle in which the slow (panel **A**) and fast (panel **B**) pathways for atrioventricular reentrant tachycardia are depicted as sites for possible ablation. In panel **A**, the oblong region for the slow pathway may be a site for ablation, as well as at the anterior margin of the coronary sinus (designated with a star). Koch's triangle is outlined with the atrioventricular node adjacent to the septal leaflet of the tricuspid valve and inferior/posterior to the membranous septum (shaded region). The fossa ovale (FO) is also noted. In panel **B**, with precisely the same photograph, representation is provided of an ablation catheter for the fast (F) pathway (star), a His recording catheter, and a catheter in the ostium of the coronary sinus. The coronary sinus catheter enters through the superior vena cava (SVC).

intra-atrial reentry are being explored. For example, Avitall et al.[113] reported successful interruption of atrial fibrillation in dogs using radiofrequency-induced lesions to "compartmentalize" the right atrium. Likewise, Haissaguerre et al.[41] reported successful ablation of atrial fibrillation through the creation of serial, vertical lesions along the posterior wall of the right atrium, a second series along the lateral wall of the right atrium, and, finally, a third series along the anterior wall of the right atrium.

In recent years, the His bundle region has

been the anatomical focus of RF ablation for atrial fibrillation associated with rapid ventricular rates. Radiofrequency current can be used to modify AV conduction and reduce the maximum ventricular rate during atrial tachyarrhythmias, while maintaining normal AV conduction.[114,115] Baker et al.[116] have reviewed additional nonpharmacological approaches used in the management of atrial arrhythmias and new avenues of therapy currently being explored.

Lesh et al.[117] have summarized many of the observations made by investigators over the past 80 years regarding the anatomical delineation of reentrant circuits implicated in atrial flutter (Figure 14). They note that macroscopic anatomical regions play a key role in determining circuit boundaries.

Olgin et al.[118] have recently demonstrated that the entire crista terminalis and its continuation as the eustachian ridge form the posterior barrier in atrial flutter, while the tricuspid annulus acts as the anterior bar-

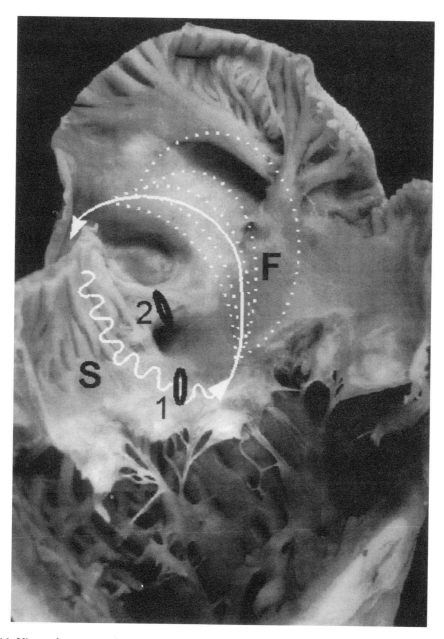

Figure 14. View of an opened right atrium and right ventricle illustrating potential routes of slow (S) and fast (F) pathways in atrial flutter. At #1 and #2, respectively, the preferred sites for successful ablation of atrial flutter pathway are denoted.

rier.[119] In a different series, Guiraudon et al.[120] have identified the narrow isthmus of tissue found between the inferior vena cava and the tricuspid annulus as the region of slow conduction.

Pathology of Ablation Lesions: Radiofrequency and Alternative Energy Sources

Our current understanding of tissue destruction in RF ablation is based on a number of animal models and clinical observations[44,121,122] that indicate the injury process is thermally mediated. In one study, guinea pig papillary muscle subjected to temperatures greater than or equal to 45°C demonstrated increased resting tension and, at temperatures greater than or equal to 50°C, showed signs of irreversible myocardial contracture.[123] One group[123] has postulated that hyperthermally mediated injury damages plasma membranes permitting influx of extracellular sodium and calcium, which results in depolarization and increased myocardial resting tension, respectively. Intracellular buffering systems are also affected by excessive heat; activity of adenosine triphophatase in the sarcoplasmic reticulum is suppressed at temperatures in excess of 50°C.[124]

Studies of myocardial macrovasculature in animals indicate that cellular damage induced through tissue heating is linked to compromised vessel function and perfusion. Histological examination reveals microvascular swelling and disruption, intravascular thrombosis, and neutrophil adherence to vessel walls. As recently proposed,[123] early and late changes in tissue conductivity may be due to recovery and reperfusion of an area following ablation or, in contrast, loss of aberrant conduction in an initially resilient pathway may be a late effect of impaired vascular function. Of note, vascular preservation appears to be greater following direct current ablation than radiofrequency ablation, providing one reason for a higher incidence of conduc-

tion interruption when radiofrequency energy is used.[125]

In their recent, comprehensive review, Nath and Haines[123] have characterized the gross and pathological features of lesions produced by RF ablation, and have compared the pathophysiological effects and efficacy of alternative methods of ablation. Very briefly, the endocardium following RF ablation may be slightly deformed and pale in color, although hemorrhage is not uncommon (Figure 15). Charring can occur if ablation temperatures exceed 100°C or following a swift increase in electrical impedence.[123] Early microscopic study reveals distinct pale, necrotic lesions surrounded by hemorrhagic tissue (Figure 16). After 5 days, this peripheral hemorrhaging is accompanied by inflammatory infiltrates encircling a well-differentiated nidus of coagulation necrosis. Within 2 months following ablation, lesions are considerably smaller and made up of granulation and fibrous tissue, fat cells, cartilagenous tissue, and a chronic inflammatory infiltrate.[123]

In electrophysiology centers today, radiofrequency, replacing high- and low-energy direct current technology, has become the modality of choice for catheter ablation. Despite ongoing research into other energy sources—including laser energy, microwave ablation, ultrasound, and cryoablation—no alternative forms of energy delivery have surpassed existing RF ablation techniques. Although a comprehensive examination of alternative ablation methods is beyond the scope of this chapter, it is important to emphasize that RF ablation, while highly successful and relatively inexpensive, does have its drawbacks. In particular, the small lesions that radiofrequency produces are implicated in the failure of ablation to effectively or lastingly block conduction. New developments in catheter design, aimed at improving maneuverability and stability, may help to optimize radiofrequency lesion size and placement. Both microwave and ultrasound carry the potential to produce larger, discrete lesions; these too, however, are limited by existing methods of

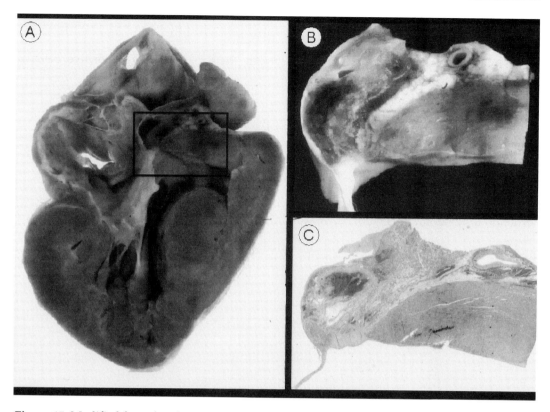

Figure 15. Modified four-chamber section of a heart with complex congenital heart disease (dextroversion, double inlet left ventricle, rudimentary right ventricle, ventricular inversion, Wolff-Parkinson-White syndrome, attenuated His bundle). In panel **A,** the boxed region includes an area where attempted ablation of a bypass tract was undertaken. At higher power, a section from that region depicts gross **(B)** and microscopic **(C)** areas of hemorrhage (dark discoloration) that permeate the tissue adjacent to the myocardium including adipose tissue. There is hemorrhage adjacent to the sectioned epicardial coronary artery.

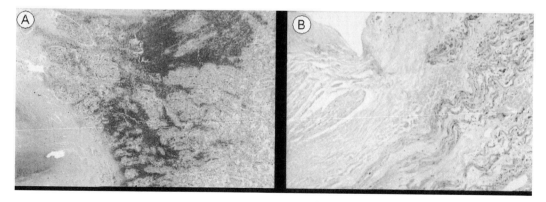

Figure 16. Photomicrographs of region in Figure 15 wherein hemorrhage and necrosis were induced by radiofrequency ablation. In panel **A** there are areas of coagulative necrosis adjacent to large areas of hemorrhage (darker staining). The areas of necrosis can be highlighted using an antibody to muscle-specific actin (MSA, panel **B**) wherein no immunoreactivity is present in injured tissue adjacent to deeply staining viable myocytes ($\times 25$, both panels; H&E [A], MSA [B]).

safe and effective energy delivery. It seems likely that, with time and technological refinements, different energy sources might be used in different anatomic settings or conditions.

Post-Script

Management of patients with automaticity and conduction abnormalities has markedly improved over the last two decades. An understanding of the technology, the anatomy, the potential sequelae, and the opportunities for innovation will continue to advance the field. Closer interaction between electrophysiologists and pathologists will help to clarify remaining structure-function conundrums that underlie arrhythmogenesis.

Acknowledgments: The authors wish to express their gratitude to Dr. John Yeung for the suggestions and guidance he provided regarding electrophysiology "essentials." We are also grateful to Drs. Kugler, Kerr, and Singer for their feedback and advice. Thank you also to Stuart Greene, Janet Wilson, and Jennifer Hards for their artistic and photographic expertise.

References

1. Rajadurai VS, Menahem S. Fetal arrhythmias: a 3-year experience. Aust NZ J Obstet Gynaecol 1992;32:28.
2. Reed KL. Fetal arrhythmias: etiology, diagnosis, pathophysiology, and treatment. Semin Perinat 1989;13:294.
3. Colvin EV. Cardiac Embryology. In: Garson Jr A, Bricker JT, McNamara, DG, eds. The Science and Practice of Pediatric Cardiology. Lea and Febiger, Philadelphia, 1990, p 71.
4. Davies MJ, Anderson RH, Becker AE. The Conduction System of the Heart. London, Butterworths, 1983.
5. McManus BM, Wood SM. Key morphological features of the normal and abnormal, modified and unmodified conduction system. In: Singer I, ed., Interventional Electrophysiology. Williams and Wilkins, Baltimore, 1997, p 133.
6. He BM, Tan YX, Cheng M, et al. The surgical anatomy of the sinoatrial node. Surg Radiol Anat 1991;13:123.
7. Calmat Par A, Hammou J-C, Chomette G, et al. Localization precise du noeud sino-auriculaire. Arch Mal Coeur 1973;66:855.
8. Van Mierop LHS, Wiglesworth FW. Isomerism of the cardiac atria in asplenia syndrome. Lab Invest 1962;11:1303.
9. Dickinson DF, Wilkinson MB, Anderson KR, et al. The cardiac conduction system in situs ambiguus. Circulation 1979;59:879.
10. Tai YT, Lau CP. Patterns of radiofrequency catheter ablation of left free-wall accessory pathways: implications for accessory pathway anatomy. Clin Cardiol 1993;16:644.
11. Cain ME, Luke RA, Lindsay BD. Diagnosis and localization of accessory pathways. PACE 1992;15:801.
12. Cain ME, Cox JL. Surgical treatment of supraventricular arrhythmias. In Platia E, ed. Management of Cardiac Arrhythmias: The Non-Pharmalogic Approach. JB Lippincott, Philadelphia, 1987, p 304.
13. Schluter M, Kuck KH. Radiofrequency current therapy of supraventricular tachycardia: accessory atrioventricular pathways. PACE 1993;16:643.
14. Edwards FH, Weston L. Surgical management of posteroseptal accessory atrioventricular pathways. Ann Thorac Surg 1992;53:321.
15. Davis LM, Byth K, Ellis P, et al. Dimensions of the human posterior septal space and coronary sinus. Am J Cardiol 1991;68:621.
16. Cox JL. Anatomy of the posterior septal space. Am J Cardiol 1991;68:675.
17. Wen MS, Yeh SJ, Wang CC, et al. Radiofrequency ablation therapy of the posteroseptal accessory pathway. Am Heart J 1996;132:612.
18. Dhala AA, Deshpande SS, Bremner S, et al. Transcatheter ablation of posteroseptal accessory pathways using a venous approach and radiofrequency energy. Circulation 1994;90:1799.
19. Sealy WC, Mikat EM. Anatomical problems with identification and interruption of posterior septal Kent bundles. Ann Thorac Surg 1983;36:584.
20. Sealy WC, Gallagher JJ. The surgical approach to the septal area of the heart based on experiences with 45 patients with Kent bundles. J Thorac Cardiovasc Surg 1980;79:542.
21. Epstein AE, Kirklin JK, Holman WL, et al. Intermediate septal accessory pathways: electrocardiographic characteristics, electrophysiologic observations and their surgical implications. J Am Coll Cardiol 1991;17:1570.

22. Cohn AE, Fraser FR. Paroxysmal stimulation of the vagus nerves by pressure. Heart 1913–1914;4:93.

23. Wolff L, Parkinson J, White PD. Bundle-branch block with short P-R interval in healthy young people prone to paroxysmal tachycardia. Am Heart J 1930;5:685.

24. Shih HT, Miles WM, Klein LS, et al. Multiple accessory pathways in the permanent form of junctional reciprocating tachycardia. Am J Cardiol 1994;73:361.

25. Plumb VJ. Catheter ablation of the accessory pathways of the Wolff-Parkinson-White syndrome and its variants. Prog Cardiovasc Dis 1995;37:295.

26. Kay GN, Epstein AE, Dailey SM, et al. Role of radiofrequency ablation in the management of supraventricular arrhythmias: experience in 760 consecutive patients. J Cardiovasc Electrophysiol 1993;4:372.

27. James TN. Morphology of the human atrioventricular node, with remarks pertinent to its electrophysiology. Am Heart J 1961;62:756.

28. Douglas JE, Mandel WJ, Danzig R, et al. Lown-Ganong-Levine syndrome. Circulation 1972;45:1143.

29. Chen SA, Chiang CE, Tsang WP, et al. Recurrent conduction in accessory pathway and possible new arrhythmias after radiofrequency catheter ablation. Am Heart J 1993;125:381.

30. Gursoy S, Schluter M, Kuck KH. Radiofrequency current catheter ablation for control of supraventricular arrhythmias. J Cardiovasc Electrophysiol 1993;4:194.

31. Twidale N, Wang XZ, Beckman KJ, et al. Factors associated with recurrence of accessory pathway conduction after radiofrequency catheter ablation. PACE 1991;14:2042.

32. Klein GJ, Bashore TM, Sellers TD, et al. Ventricular fibrillation in the Wolff-Parkinson-White syndrome. N Engl J Med 1979;301:1080.

33. Bockeria LA, Chigogidze NA, Golukhova EZ, et al. Diagnosis and surgical treatment of tachycardias in patients with nodoventricular fibers. PACE 1991;14:2004.

34. Ellenbogen KA, Ramirez NM, Packer DL, et al. Accessory nodoventricular (Mahaim) fibers: a clinical review. PACE 1986;9:868.

35. Moss AJ. Clinical significance of ventricular arrhythmias in patients with and without coronary artery disease. Prog Cardiovasc Dis 1980;23:33.

36. Gallagher JJ, Pritchett EL, Sealy WC, et al. The preexcitation syndromes. Prog Cardiovasc Dis 1978;20:285.

37. Short DS. The syndrome of alternating bradycardia and tachycardia. Br Heart J 1954;16:208.

38. MacWilliam JA. Some applications of physiology to medicine. II. Ventricular fibrillation and sudden death. Br Heart J 1923;2:215.

39. Langberg JJ, Calkins H, Kim YN, et al. Recurrence of conduction in accessory atrioventricular connections after initially successful radiofrequency catheter ablation. J Am Coll Cardiol 1992;19:1588.

40. Wagshal AB, Pires LA, Mittleman RS, et al. Early recurrence of accessory pathways after radiofrequency catheter ablation does not preclude long-term cure. Am J Cardiol 1993;72:843.

41. Haissaguerre M, Fischer B, Labbe T, et al. Frequency of recurrent atrial fibrillation after catheter ablation of overt accessory pathways. Am J Cardiol 1992;69:493.

42. Morady F, Strickberger A, Man C, et al. Reasons for prolonged or failed attempts at radiofrequency catheter ablation of accessory pathways. J Am Coll Cardiol 1996;27:683.

43. Huang JL, Chen SA, Tai CT, et al. Long-term results of radiofrequency catheter ablation in patients with multiple accessory pathways. Am J Cardiol 1996;78:1375.

44. Nath S, Lynch C 3rd, Whayne JG, et al. Cellular electrophysiological effects of hyperthermia on isolated guinea pig papillary muscle. Implications for catheter ablation. Circulation 1993;88:1826.

45. Hirao K, Sato T, Otomo K, et al. The response of atrioventricular junctional tissue to temperature. Jpn Circ J 1994;58:351.

46. Bharati S, Lev M. The Cardiac Conduction System in Unexplained Sudden Death. Futura Publishing Co, Mount Kisco, NY, 1990.

47. Chiang CE, Chen SA, Wu TJ, et al. Incidence, significance, and pharmacological responses of catheter-induced mechanical trauma in patients receiving radiofrequency ablation for supraventricular tachycardia. Circulation 1994;90:1847.

48. King A, Wen MS, Yeh SJ, et al. Catheter-induced atrioventricular nodal block during radiofrequency ablation. Am Heart J 1996;132:979.

49. Willems S, Shenasa M, Borggrefe M, et al. Unexpected emergence of manifest preexcitation following transcatheter ablation of concealed accessory pathways. J Cardiovasc Electrophysiol 1993;4:467.

50. Jackman WM, Wang XZ, Friday KJ, et al. Catheter ablation of accessory atrioventricular pathways (Wolff-Parkinson-White syndrome) by radiofrequency current. N Engl J Med 1991;324:1605.

51. Epstein MR, Knapp LD, Martindill M, et al.

Embolic complications associated with radiofrequency catheter ablation. Am J Cardiol 1996;77:655.

52. Friedman PL, Stevenson WG, Kokovic DZ. Autonomic dysfunction after catheter ablation. J Cardiovasc Electrophysiol 1996;7:450.

53. Ehlert FA, Goldberger JJ, Brooks R, et al. Persistent inappropriate sinus tachycardia after radiofrequency current catheter modification of the atrioventricular node. Am J Cardiol 1992;69:1092.

54. Kokovic DZ, Harada T, Shea JB, et al. Alterations of heart rate and heart rate variability after radiofrequency catheter ablation of supraventricular tachycardia. Circulation 1993;88:1671.

55. Kocheril AG, Rosenfeld LE. Radiofrequency ablation of an accessory pathway in a patient with corrected Ebstein's anomaly. PACE 1994;17:986.

56. Mair DD. Ebstein's anomaly: natural history and management. J Am Coll Cardiol 1992;19:1047.

57. Porter CJ. Ebstein's anomaly of the tricuspid valve. In: Garson A, Bricker JT, McNamara DG, eds. The Science and Practice of Pediatric Cardiology. 2. Lea and Febiger, Philadelphia, 1990, p 1134.

58. Cappato R, Schluter M, Weib C, et al. Radiofrequency current catheter ablation of accessory atrioventricular pathways in Ebstein's anomaly. Circulation 1996;94:376.

59. Dave KS, Parkrashi BC, Wooler GH, et al. Atrial septal defects in adults. Am J Cardiol 1973;31:7.

60. Gault JH, Morrow AG, Gay WA, et al. Atrial septal defect in patients over the age of 40 years. Circulation 1968;37:261.

61. Kuzman WJ, Yuskis AS. Atrial septal defects in the older patient simulating acquired valvular heart disease. Am J Cardiol 1965;15:303.

62. Saksena FB, Aldridge HE. Atrial septal defect in the older patient. Circulation 1970;42:1009.

63. Kulbertus HE, Coyne JJ, Hallidie-Smith KA. Conduction disturbances before and after surgical closure of ventricular septal defect. Am Heart J 1969;77:123.

64. Vetter VL, Horowitz LN. Electrophysiological residua and sequelae of surgery for congenital heart defects. In Engle MA, Perloff JK, eds. Congenital Heart Disease After Surgery: Benefits, Residua, Sequelae. Yorke Medical Books, New York, 1983, p 261.

65. Dickens I, Maranhao V, Goldbert H. Right bundle branch block: a vectorcardiographic and electrocardiographic study of ventricular septal defect following open heart surgery. Circulation 1959;20:201.

66. Okoroma EO, Guller B, Maloney JD, et al. Etiology of right bundle branch block pattern after surgical closure of ventricular septal defects. Am Heart J 1975;90:14.

67. Perloff JK. The Clinical Recognition of Congenital Heart Disease. W.B. Saunders, Philadelphia, 1987.

68. Clark DS, Hirsch HD, Tamer DM, et al. Electrocardiographic changes following surgical treatment of congenital cardiac malformations. Prog Cardiovasc Dis 1975;17:451.

69. Sasaki R, Theilen EO, January LE, et al. Cardiac arrhythmias associated with the repair of atrial and ventricular septal defects. Circulation 1958;18:909.

70. Anderson RH, Becker AE. Pathology of Congenital Heart Disease. Butterworths, London, 1981.

71. Dietl CA, Cazzaniga ME, Dubner SJ, et al. Life-threatening arrhythmias and RV dysfunction after surgical repair of tetralogy of Fallot: comparison between transventricular and transatrial approaches. Circulation 1994;90:II7.

72. Cullen S, Celermajer DS, Franklin RC, et al. Prognostic significance of ventricular arrhythmia after repair of tetralogy of Fallot: a 12-year prospective study. J Am Coll Cardiol 1994;23:1151.

73. Joffe H, Georgakopoulos D, Celermajer DS, et al. Late ventricular arrhythmia is rare after early repair of tetralogy of Fallot [see comments]. J Am Coll Cardiol 1994;23:1146.

74. Ross BA. From the bedside to the basic science laboratory: arrhythmias in Fallot's tetralogy. J Am Coll Cardiol 1993;21:1738.

75. Dreyer WJ, Paridon SM, Fisher DJ, et al. Rapid ventricular pacing in dogs with right ventricular outflow tract obstruction: insights into a mechanism of sudden death in postoperative tetralogy of Fallot. J Am Coll Cardiol 1993;21:1731.

76. Murphy JG, Gersh BJ, Mair DD, et al. Long-term outcome in patients undergoing surgical repair of tetralogy of Fallot. N Engl J Med 1993;329:593.

77. Rosenthal A. Adults with tetralogy of Fallot: repaired, yes; cured, no. N Engl J Med 1993;329:655.

78. Waien SA, Liu PP, Ross BL, et al. Serial follow-up of adults with repaired tetralogy of Fallot. J Am Coll Cardiol 1992;20:295.

79. Chandar JS, Wolff GS, Garson A Jr, et al. Ventricular arrhythmias in postoperative tetralogy of Fallot. Am J Cardiol 1990;65:655.

80. Deanfield JE, Ho SY, Anderson RH, et al.

Late sudden death after repair of tetralogy of Fallot: a clinicopathologic study. Circulation 1983;67:626.

81. James FW, Kaplan S, Chou T. Unexpected cardiac arrest in patients after surgical correction of tetralogy of Fallot. Circulation 1975;52:691.

82. Kobayashi J, Hirose H, Nakano S, et al. Ambulatory electrocardiographic study of the frequency and cause of ventricular arrhythmia after correction of tetralogy of Fallot. Am J Cardiol 1984;54:1310.

83. Gillette PC, Yeoman MA, Mullins CE, et al. Sudden death after repair of tetralogy of Fallot. Circulation 1977;56:566.

84. Kavey RE, Blackman MS, Sondheimer HM. Incidence and severity of chronic ventricular dysrhythmias after repair of tetralogy of Fallot. Am Heart J 1982;103:342.

85. Horowitz LN, Vetter VL, Harken AH, et al. Electrophysiologic characteristics of sustained ventricular tachycardia occurring after repair of tetralogy of Fallot. Am J Cardiol 1980;46:446.

86. Garson A Jr, Gillette PC, Gutgesell HP, et al. Stress-induced ventricular arrhythmia after repair of tetralogy of Fallot. Am J Cardiol 1980;46:1006.

87. Deanfield JE, McKenna WJ, Presbitero P, et al. Ventricular arrhythmia in unrepaired and repaired tetralogy of Fallot: relation to age, timing of repair, and haemodynamic status. Br Heart J 1984;57:77.

88. Marie PY, Marcon F, Brunotte F, et al. Right ventricular overload and induced sustained ventricular tachycardia in operatively "repaired" tetralogy of Fallot. Am J Cardiol 1992;69:785.

89. Katz NM, Blackstone EH, Kirklin JW, et al. Late survival and symptoms after repair of tetralogy of Fallot. Circulation 1982;65:403.

90. Fuster V, McGoon DC, Kennedy MA, et al. Long-term evaluation (12 to 22 years) of open heart surgery for tetralogy of Fallot. Am J Cardiol 1980;46:635.

91. Mustard WT. Successful two-stage correction of transposition of the great vessels. Surgery 1964;55:469.

92. Webb GD, McLaughlin PR, Gow RM, et al. Transposition complexes. Cardiol Clin 1993;11:651.

93. Braunstein PW Jr, Sade RM, Gillette PC. Life-threatening postoperative junctional ectopic tachycardia Ann Thorac Surg 1992; 53:726.

94. Mair DD, Danielson GK, Wallace RB, et al. Long-term follow-up of Mustard operation survivors. Circulation 1974;49(Suppl II):11.

95. Shakespeare CF, Anderson M, Camm AJ. Pathophysiology of supraventricular tachycardia. Eur Heart J 1993;14 (Suppl E):2.

96. Swiryn S, Bauernfeind RA, Palileo EA, et al. Electrophysiologic study demonstrating triple antegrade AV nodal pathways in patients with spontaneous and/or induced supraventricular tachycardia. Am Heart J 1982;103:168.

97. Kadish A, Goldberg J. Ablative therapy for atrioventricular nodal reentry arrhythmias. Prog Cardiovasc Dis 1996;37:273.

98. Shah DC, Jais P, Gencel L, et al. Radiofrequency catheter ablation for AV nodal reentrant tachycardias (AVNRT). Ind. Heart J 1996;48:231.

99. Sung RJ, Lauer MR, Chun H. Atrioventricular node reentry: current concepts and new perspectives. PACE 1994;17:1413.

100. McGuire MA, Janse MJ. New insights on anatomical location of components of the reentrant circuit and ablation therapy for atrioventricular junctional reentrant tachycardia [Review]. Curr Opinion Cardiol 1995;10:3.

101. Racker DK. Atrioventricular node and input pathways: A correlated gross anatomical and histological study of the canine atrioventricular junctional region. Anat Rec 1989;224:336.

102. Wu D, Yeh SJ, Wang CC, et al. Double loop figure-of-8 reentry as the mechanism of multiple atrioventricular node reentry tachycardias. Am Heart J 1994;127:83.

103. Spach MS, Josephson ME. Initiating reentry: the role of nonuniform anisotropy in small circuits [Review]. J Cardiovasc Electrophysiol 1994;5:182.

104. Akhtar M, Jazayeri MR, Sra J, et al. Atrioventricular nodal reentry. Clinical, electrophysiological, and therapeutic considerations. Circulation 1993;88:282.

105. Fromer M, Shenasa M. Ultrarapid subthreshold stimulation for termination of atrioventricular node reentrant tachycardia. J Am Coll Cardiol 1992;20:879.

106. Sung RJ, Waxman HL, Saksena S, et al. Sequence of retrograde atrial activation in patients with dual atrioventricular nodal pathways. Circulation 1981;64:1059.

107. Tondo C, Beckman KJ, McClelland JH, et al. Response to radiofrequency catheter ablation suggests that the coronary sinus forms part of the reentrant circuit in some patients with atrioventricular nodal reentrant tachycardia. Circulation 1996;94 (Suppl 1):2220A.

108. Keim S, Werner P, Jazayeri M, et al. Localization of the fast and slow pathways in atrioventricular nodal reentrant tachycar-

dia by intraoperative ice mapping. Circulation 1992;86:919.

109. Ross DL, Johnson DC, Denniss AR, et al. Curative surgery for atrioventricular junctional ("AV nodal") reentrant tachycardia. J Am Coll Cardiol 1985;6:1383.

110. Chaoui R, Bollmann R, Hoffmann H, et al. [Fetal echocardiography: Part III. Fetal arrhythmia] [Review] [German]. Zentralblatt fur Gynakologie 1991;113:1335.

111. Meinertz T, Hofmann T, Zehender M. Can we predict sudden cardiac death? [Review]. Drugs 1991;41 Suppl 2:9.

112. Larsen L, Markham J, Haffajee CI. Sudden death in idiopathic dilated cardiomyopathy: role of ventricular arrhythmias [Review]. PACE 1993;16:1051.

113. Avitall B, Hare J, Mughal K, et al. Ablation of atrial fibrillation in a dog model. J Am Coll Cardiol 1994;484:276A.

114. Williamson BD, Man KC, Daoud E, et al. Radiofrequency catheter modification of atrioventricular conduction to control the ventricular rate during atrial fibrillation. J Am Coll Cardiol 1994;331:910.

115. Kunze KP, Schluter M, Geiger M, et al. Modulation of atrioventricular nodal conduction using radiofrequency current. Am J Cardiol 1988;61:657.

116. Baker BM, Smith JM, Cain ME. Nonpharmacologic approaches to the treatment of atrial fibrillation and atrial flutter. J Cardiovasc Electrophysiol 1995;6:972.

117. Lesh MD, Van Hare G, Kao AK, et al. Radiofrequency catheter ablation for Wolff-Parkinson-White syndrome associated with a coronary sinus diverticulum. PACE 1991; 14:1479.

118. Olgin JE, Kalman JM, Fitzpatrick AP, et al. Role of right atrial endocardial structures as barriers to conduction during human type I atrial flutter: activation and entrainment mapping guided by intracardiac echocardiography. Circulation 1995;92:1839.

119. Kalman J, Olgin J, Lee R, et al. The anterior barrier in human atrial flutter: Role of the tricuspid annulus. Circulation 1995;92:406.

120. Guiraudon GM, Klein GJ, van Hemel N, et al. Atrial flutter: lessons from surgical interventions (musing on atrial flutter mechanism). PACE 1996;19:1933.

121. Whayne JG, Nath S, Haines DE. Microwave catheter ablation of myocardium in vitro: assessment of the characteristics of tissue heating and injury. Circulation 1994;89: 2390.

122. Langberg JJ, Calkins H, el-Atassi R, et al. Temperature monitoring during radiofrequency catheter ablation of accessory pathways. Circulation 1992;86:1469.

123. Nath S, Haines DE. Biophysics and pathology of catheter energy delivery systems [Review]. Prog Cardiovasc Dis 1995;37:185.

124. Inesi G, Millman M, Eletr S. Temperature-induced transitions of function and structure in sarcoplasmic reticulum membranes. J Mol Biol 1973;81:483.

125. Idikio HA, Humen DP. Fine structural alterations in radiofrequency energy-induced lesions in dog hearts: possible basis for reduced arrhythmic complications. Can J Cardiol 1991;7:270.

126. Singer I, ed. Interventional Electrophysiology. Williams and Wilkins, Baltimore, 1997.

Chapter 3

A Conceptual Approach to Radiofrequency Catheter Ablation of Accessory Pathways Focusing on Electrogram Criteria

Michel Haïssaguerre, Pierre Jaïs, Dipen C. Shah, A. Takahashi, S. Serge Barold, Jacques Clémenty

Introduction

The curative treatment of patients with tachycardia related to an accessory pathway (AP) is now regularly performed by transcutaneous catheter ablation. The first catheter fulguration of an AP was performed by Weber and Schmitz in 1983.[1] In 1984, Morady and Scheinman described a technique for ablation of posteroseptal AP[2] in which DC shocks were delivered at the site of an anatomic landmark—the coronary sinus ostium. In 1986, Warin et al demonstrated the ability to map along both atrioventricular (AV) rings using endocardial ventricular electrograms and AP potentials, thus making it possible to ablate consistently in any location.[3-7] Finally, Jackman, Kuck, et al. showed that radiofrequency (RF) energy could reproduce the high efficacy of DC energy with little risk thus opening wide the door for catheter ablation as the treatment of choice for AP ablation.[8-35]

Catheter ablation techniques are now routinely performed for arrhythmias caused by APs. The majority of AP can be ablated with minimal aggression, i.e., one RF application, provided that enough attention is paid to electrophysiological recordings without losing any time. This chapter will describe an overall approach based on electrogram criteria to minimize the number of RF applications and attendant risks. The techniques specific to various AP locations are described in other chapters.

Technical Considerations

There is a near perfect match between the anatomic size of the AP (0.5–7 mm, mean 1.3 mm)[14,15] and lesions created by RF current with 4-mm tip electrode. The most commonly used RF ablation catheter is a 7F, steerable catheter with a platinum tip electrode 4 mm in length, and RF energy is delivered through different generators as a 400–750 kHz sine wave current. Although impedance monitoring can be used during RF delivery, the automatic monitoring of electrode tip temperature has significant advantages. The energy is modulated in order to achieve a preset distal temperature with the highest power that does not cause an

From Singer I, Barold SS, Camm AJ (eds): Nonpharmacological Therapy of Arrhythmias for the 21st Century: The State of the Art. Futura Publishing Co, Inc., Armonk, NY, © 1998.

impedance rise. However, because the tip temperature sensor is not always optimally placed in relation to the electrode-tissue configuration, the optimal preset temperature varies between 60°C and 80°C. This suppresses or minimizes the coagulum formation that can occur either progressively or suddenly (and may therefore be unavoidable during manual power titration). The temperature controlled mode of RF delivery has been associated with a lower incidence of recurrent AP conduction (3% vs. 8%) in our experience compared to power mode delivery.

The total duration of energy delivery varies from 30 to 120 seconds when AP conduction is interrupted or commonly 10 seconds when there is no change in the electrical signals. In view of some instances of successful abolition of accessory pathway conduction noted after longer delivery of RF energy, we extend the duration of energy delivery to 20–30 seconds, when the electrogram criteria are favorable (see below).

Energy delivery must be stopped immediately if an impedance rise occurs or the catheter is displaced, or if there is any indication of complications. In general, the electrocardiogram is continuously monitored while the catheter position on the fluoroscopic screen is periodically checked during energy delivery. The ablating catheter must have a stable position during sinus rhythm, ventricular pacing, or tachycardia.

"Safety" pulses are not necessary unless there is difficulty achieving a stable catheter position such as in right lateral sites, or when AP conduction has not been eliminated soon (<7 sec) after the onset of energy. A longer duration or an increased power/temperature of the successful pulse are more efficient than the use of a "bonus" pulse.[33]

Heparin is usually given during and after the procedure. In our laboratory, we administer IV heparin immediately *after* the procedure and this approach is associated with a very low incidence of complications, in particular only one case of tamponade and a 0.5% incidence of minor cerebral embolic

phenomenon. We use a bolus of 1 mg/kg of IV heparin for left-sided ablations and half of this dose for right-sided ablations followed by 20–40 mg/day of subcutaneous enoxaparine for 5 days. For left-sided AP, aspirin (250 mg) is also given for a few weeks after the procedure by others. Routine post-ablation echocardiography is performed in most centers.

Determination of the Optimal Ablation Site

A plethora of different ECG algorithms to localize preexcitation have been published.[34] The most important information is to recognize midseptal APs with their attendant higher risk of AV block or the epicardial AP which requires ablation in the coronary sinus.

An initial electrophysiological study is required to identify the mechanism of the clinical tachycardia and to ascertain that the AP is a part of the circuit since occasionally AV nodal reentrant tachycardia or atrial tachycardia can be the primary cause of the clinical tachycardia associated with a preexcitation. Two catheters, including one deflectable catheter, are generally enough to effect ablation of manifest AP and assess antegrade and retrograde AP properties. The use of oblique fluoroscopic views is helpful although more often a matter of operator preference.

Atrial or Ventricular Approach?

The AP may be ablated either from the atrium (above the AV valve leaflet) or from the ventricle (below the leaflet), the latter being more stable because the electrode is wedged between the leaflet base and the ventricular aspect of the annulus. These "atrial or ventricular" approaches are equally successful provided that the ablating catheter is in close proximity to the AP. Both anatomic and technical considerations determine the direction of catheters on one or the other side of the annulus. Generally, a retrograde aortic approach for a left-sided AP easily allows a ventricular catheter position, whereas a transseptal approach allows full exploration of the atrial aspect of the mitral annulus.[6] However, an atrial position can be reached retrogradely after manipulating and pulling back a fully curved catheter in the posterior region of the left ventricle. On the right side of the heart, most APs are ablated from the atrium by catheters introduced from the inferior vena cava, but some APs, located at sites where the catheter position is particularly unstable, can occasionally be ablated only with the catheter inserted beneath the leaflet to reach the ventricular side of the tricuspid annulus. Therefore, the A/V electrogram ratio at the ablation site does not help in predicting a successful outcome. Ratio values varying from 0.05 to 6 have been found at successful ablation sites.

Concealed Versus Manifest APs

Fewer criteria are available for targeting concealed APs than for manifest APs, chiefly the shortest ventriculoatrial (VA) interval. The effects of subthreshold stimulation on AP conduction as a pretest for successful ablation has been proposed, but this technique unfortunately has the potential of inducing atrial fibrillation. Also, most concealed APs have a left lateral location and the common retrograde approach below the mitral annulus obscures the AP and atrial potentials within the ventricular electrograms unless pacing techniques are used to differentiate them. These data explain why more RF applications are usually required in ablation of concealed AP (median: 3 in our center) compared to manifest AP (median: 1 in patients without any prior attempts).

Electrogram Parameters

Given that most APs are tiny pathways,[36,37] they should be ablated with one or two RF applications. However, two conditions are concomitantly required for successful ablation: adequate mapping and interpretation of local electrograms, and sufficiently stable firm catheter contact to reach a tissue temperature >55°C and produce irreversible tissue injury. Catheter stability is better assessed by stable electrograms than by the degree of catheter excursion on fluoroscopy. Needless to say, interpretation of electrograms is facilitated by the strict use of identical filters and gain settings in a given laboratory. Therefore, an unsuccessful RF application can be due to an unstable catheter position (even at an adequate site with good electrograms) or to a site with suboptimal electrograms. The failures in right-sided APs are mainly due to unstable catheter positions whereas failures in left-sided APs are due mainly to inadequate mapping and/or electrogram interpretation.

Several parameters can be used to determine the optimal target site.

Recording the AP Potential

Direct recording of the AP potential should be the gold standard of criteria used to localize the site for effective ablation.[3,4,7,9] Unfortunately, since the AP origin of such potentials is accepted usually on probability grounds, this decreases its specificity because most AP potentials are not appropriately validated by excluding both an atrial and a ventricular origin. The maneuvers for validation induce conduction block that occurs consistently at the same interface, usually between the atrial electrogram and the suspected potential in our experience. This implies that this potential could be separated from both the atrial and the ventricular activity in only a minority of patients (Figure 1). Therefore, the AP potential is usually referred to as "possible" or "probable," and it is not surprising that the use of this criterion by itself has a relatively low predictive value for successful ablation in some studies.[18,19]

In our experience, validated AP poten-

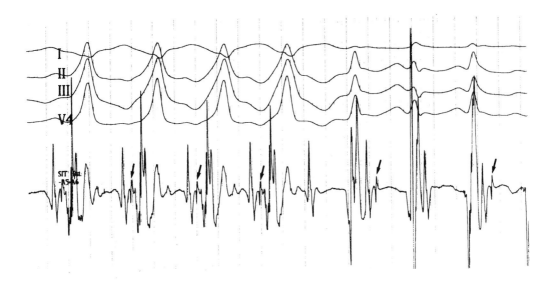

Figure 1. A bipolar endocardial recording from a patient with a left lateral accessory pathway during atrial pacing. Transient loss of preexcitation (5th–7th complex from the left) is associated with alternating block at the atrial and ventricular sites. K potential (arrow) interfaces with resultant alternating disappearance of this sharp potential. This is proof that the K potential is neither atrial nor ventricular. Note that the local AV interval is longer than usual.

tials are usually very sharp (His bundle like) and have a very low bipolar "amplitude," most between 0.03 and 0.07 mV, so that they require high gain amplification in the range of 50–100 mm/mV to be evidenced (Figures 2, 3). However, a large AP potential measuring 0.1 to 0.2 mV can be sometimes recorded notably in anteroseptal or epicardial intracoronary sinus locations. In unipolar unfiltered recordings, the AP potentials have a much lower amplitude so that they can be recognized as a tiny notch or potential only by comparison with the timing of the simultaneous bipolar recording. However, such unipolar AP potentials are usually inscribed *before* the timing of the ventricular waveform deflection, thus indicating that they are not of ventricular origin. If atrial pacing then elicits a block between the atrial electrogram and the AP potential, this is a strong argument that the potential really originates from the AP.

AV Interval

The shortest AV conduction time during preexcitation is widely used initially to identify the approximate site of AP insertion. This can be ascertained by observing the oscilloscope screen as the catheter position is changed. Importantly, the AV interval is actually the time from the local atrial tissue which is independent of AP activation to the local ventricular tissue activated through the AP. A very short AV time should be the rule if APs are always short straight bypasses crossing the annulus. For the AP that is long, oblique, tortuous, or with multiple insertion points, the AV time can be a misleading criterion if interpreted in isolation, i.e., short at unsuccessful sites or long at successful ablation sites. However, in practice, long AV intervals ($\geq$50 ms from peak to peak) are nearly always predictive of ablation failures except in some posteroseptal AP or in patients who previously had ineffective surgical or catheter ablation procedures (Figure 4).

Localizing the Ventricular Insertion Site

This is indicated by the site with the earliest ventricular electrogram relative to the

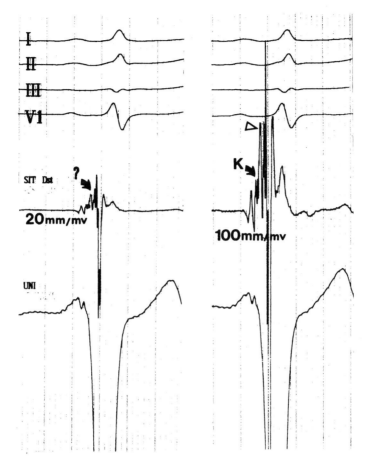

Figure 2. High gains are required to correctly identify a K potential. On the left panel, with a gain of 20 mm/mV the curved arrow marked (?) identifies a presumptive sharp K potential; however, with a higher gain (100 mm/mV on right panel) correlation with the unfiltered unipolar tracing identifies a much lower amplitude sharper transient potential (K, dark arrow) as occurring between the unipolar A and V electrograms. Note that the previously identified potential (arrowhead) occurs in fact after the onset of ventricular depolarization on the unipolar electrogram.

onset of the delta wave. It is expressed as the V-delta interval. The exact onset of the delta wave is difficult to identify and probably not reproducible at subsequent manual measurements. For right free wall AP, the earliest delta wave is recorded in V_1-V_3 leads which must be used as the reference. For other AP locations, there is no significant difference between limb and chest leads. The maximum peak of the bipolar electrogram rather than its onset is to be preferred for estimating activation because there is a better correlation of the maximal

peak with the local activation time, and because it is a powerful independent predictor of successful sites.[35] Therefore, interpretation of bipolar mapping electrograms is straightforward when the initial ventricular potential is large and sharp but ambiguous in other situations. In the presence of polyphasic signals, it is difficult to determine the true local activation timing using large recording electrodes such as the 4-mm tip electrode that is commonly used. The local activation time should be more reliably defined by using either the unipolar intrinsic deflection or closely spaced bipolar electrograms (requiring specially designed catheters). The degree of prematurity of ventricular electrograms (maximum peak or dv/dt) depends on AP location[35] and varies from patient to patient. Its value for an individual patient cannot be predicted. The earliest timings are observed in right lateral and anteroseptal AP (-18 ± 11 ms), or in right posteroseptal AP (-13 ± 9 ms). The ventricular potentials relative to delta wave onset are not as early in left posteroseptal (-2 ± 5 ms) and left lateral AP (0 ± 5 ms) (Figure 2). Therefore, a precocity of -10 or -15 ms is often insufficient in right free wall AP whereas 0 ms is adequate in most left-sided APs. Because the left ventricular wall is relatively thick, some APs can have a relatively deep insertion with regard to the endocardial electrode inserted below the mitral leaflet. These ''epicardial'' APs can be suspected when all the endocardial ventricular potentials scanning the region of interest show initial low frequency (distant with a low dv/dt) vectors in unipolar and bipolar recordings instead of a large sharp potential (Figure 5). Pacing the ventricular aspect of the annulus (pacemapping) can be used to reproduce QRS complexes similar or identical to fully preexcited QRS complexes recorded in the 12-lead ECG. This technique can be used as

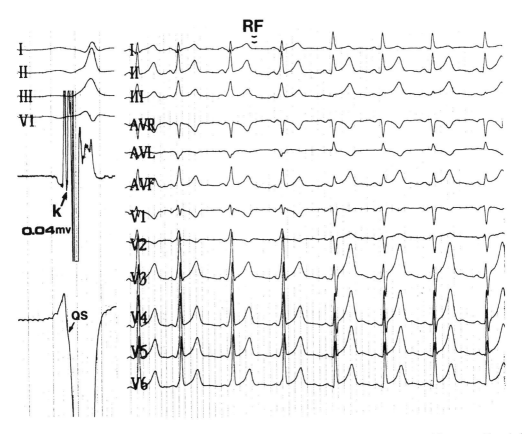

Figure 3. A typical micro-K potential recorded at the ablation site in a patient with a manifest left lateral accessory AV connection. On the left, the local bipolar and unfiltered unipolar electrograms at the site of ablation show the PQS morphology of the latter and the sharp low amplitude (0.04 mV) K potential (indicated by the arrow) on the bipolar electrograms. Preexcitation disappears within one beat after application of RF current at this site.

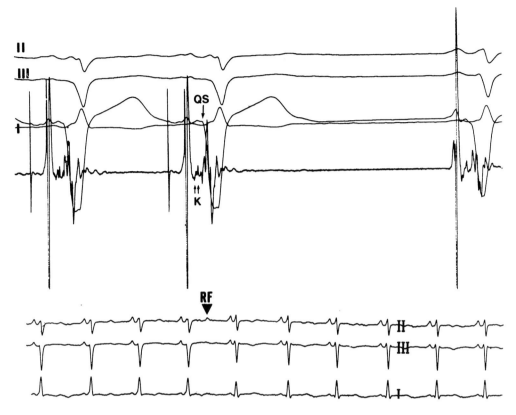

Figure 4. Ablation site for a patient with a manifest posteroseptal accessory AV connection who had undergone (unsuccessfully) a previous catheter ablation procedure elsewhere. Below the surface ECGs (leads II, III, and I) are shown the local unfiltered unipolar and bipolar electrograms during atrial pacing (first two complexes) and sinus rhythm. Note the long local AV interval and small arrows indicating presumptive K potentials, both being the probable sequelae of previous ablation. The unfiltered unipolar electrogram has a QS morphology. RF application at this site promptly abolished preexcitation.

an additional criterion for identifying the ventricular insertion site but with a limited resolution estimated to be around 5 mm.

Unfiltered Distal Unipolar Recordings

Some series in the literature report a rather high median number of RF applications (i.e., >5) for ablating manifest APs and we are of the opinion that this is simply because the authors managed without unipolar recordings. The unfiltered unipolar recording is extremely reliable in the selection of AP ablation sites in order to minimize the

number of unnecessary RF pulses. Recordings are obtained from the distal electrode of the ablation catheter which then serves to deliver ablative energy, whereas a bipolar recording might show an apparent optimal pattern due to the contribution of the proximal electrode. Furthermore, the unipolar intrinsic deflection provides more precise local activation timing than bipolar recordings, notably when multicomponent electrograms are recorded (as in Ebstein's disease). The intrinsic deflection can disclose a local late ventricular activation despite an apparently favorable bipolar electrogram or vice-versa. The most important information

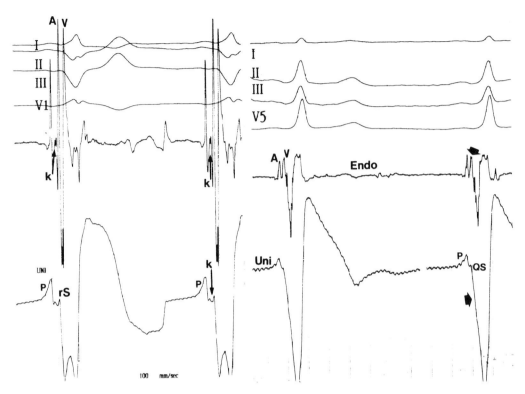

Figure 5. The right-hand panel depicts the "best" local endocardial electrograms from a patient with a left free wall epicardial accessory AV connection. The bipolar electrogram shows a relatively low amplitude ventricular electrogram (arrow); and the intrinsic deflection of the unipolar ventricular electrogram has a low dv/dt (arrow), indicating a relatively remote origin. Such electrograms should prompt epicardial mapping. The left-hand panel also depicts local endocardial bipolar and unipolar electrograms in a patient with a manifest posteroseptal accessory AV connection. Though in general a unipolar rS configuration (as shown here) is not desirable at a probable ablation site, the association with an accessory pathway potential on the bipolar electrogram (K, arrow) indicates catheter proximity to the pathway as opposed to the ventricular insertion and can be an effective ablation site as for the case shown here.

is provided by the morphology of the "unfiltered" (0.05–500 Hz) ventricular depolarization which gives *direct* information on the proximity of the catheter to the origin of the ventricular activation[20,25,26] and this can be ascertained at a glance on the recorder screen. The presence of a clear initial positive deflection in the unipolar ventricular waveform indicates that there is intervening excitable myocardial tissue between the recording electrode and the origin of ventricular excitation. The higher and wider the r wave, the further the origin of ventricular excitation and correspondingly a lower likelihood of successful ablation at the site.

Unnecessary energy applications must be avoided when such electrograms are recorded. The only exception is when the rS ventricular pattern is preceded by a spike AP potential on the simultaneous bipolar recordings, which indicates a long or oblique AP, a situation observed in about 10%–20% of left lateral AP (Figure 5).

A purely negative ventricular pattern (i.e., a QS wave) indicates proximity of the ventricular activation origin (Figures 2–4). It is a highly sensitive marker for successful ablation but it is not highly specific because such a pattern can be recorded about 5 mm from the earliest ventricular activation site.

Its specificity increases when the initial intrinsic deflection is both sharp and early. These conditions are best obtained with a ventricular position of the catheter (below the leaflet) than with an atrial position (or in the coronary sinus) where the intrinsic deflection is often smooth and the maximal dv/dt difficult to determine.

Finally, the presence of marked ST segment elevation on unipolar waveforms[35] indicates either excessive catheter contact with the myocardium, which can frequently result in an impedance rise using power mode RF delivery) or the effect of a previous RF burn.

Localizing the Atrial Insertion Site by the VA Interval

The shortest VA time is the main marker for successful ablation at the atrial insertion site: typically for a concealed AP. In a study by Smeets et al.[38] using high-density intraoperative computerized mapping, the atrial insertion site could cover a broad zone measuring 2 cm in contrast with histological studies showing AP widths ranging from 1 to 3 mm in size. In left lateral concealed AP using a retrograde aortic approach for mapping below the leaflet, retrograde continuous electrical activity is frequent, thus making the determination of the optimal site imprecise, unless pacing techniques are used to differentiate the ventricular potentials from the superimposed retrograde AP atrial potential. It is common to see the disappearance of the atrial potential during tachycardia because of temporal superimposition. A transseptal approach providing more vivid atrial potentials greatly facilitates mapping as shown by Fischer and Swartz. Atrial electrogram polarity reversal can also be used for left-sided AP: the AP insertion is modeled as a discrete point source from which activation spreads directly anterior and posterior along the mitral annulus.[32] A recording bipole, if placed parallel to the mitral annulus, will record a negative electrogram posterior to the AP

insertion site, then a fractionated and isoelectric electrogram at the site of the AP atrial insertion and the polarity reversal will be completed with further anterior movement of the catheter. Similar information could be expected using the morphology of unfiltered unipolar retrograde atrial electrograms provided that the electrogram onset can be distinguished.

In practice, the ablation site for manifest AP can be approached by finding the area of the shortest AV interval. Then the earliest ventricular potential relative to delta wave onset must be looked for, in combination with unipolar electrograms to exclude sites with an rS pattern. A main ventricular potential synchronous with onset of the delta wave is acceptable as a target site in left-sided preexcitations, while earlier timings are necessary to locate the optimal ablation site for right-sided preexcitations. Then "fine" tuning must be performed to disclose a tiny spike preceding the ventricular potential which dramatically enhances the probability of success for an RF application provided that the catheter position is sufficiently stable. This strategy allows ablation of most AP with one RF application.

Management of "Resistant" AP

The AP may be resistant to ablation attempts due to inability to stabilize the catheter on the target site or because of inadequate electrograms. Sometimes the AP is anatomically deep but rarely it may be broad.

Inadequate Tissue Contact/Stability of the Ablation Catheter

The problems related to stability of tissue contact are much more common with AP located on the right side due to the smooth and contractile nature of the atrial aspect of the tricuspid annulus. A catheter introduced from the superior vena cava may allow the tip to be looped in the right ventricle and positioned beneath the tricuspid leaflet. Such a ventricular approach can also be performed from an inferior vein with a large curved catheter resting against the septum. Also the use of different ablation catheters with varying distal configurations or long intravascular guiding sheaths can be very helpful. For a left-sided AP, switching from a transseptal to a retrograde aortic approach should be tried.

Inadequate Electrograms

In some patients, the electrograms are obviously inadequate or misinterpreted: the ventricular electrogram is not the earliest (since there is a unipolar r wave) or has a slow initial slope or no AP potential has been recorded. In others, ablation is unsuccessful in spite of apparently favorable electrograms, catheter stability, and adequate monitored temperature. This means that the AP or its targeted insertion is wide or deep. A change in the anatomic site or the mapping criterion can be helpful simply because the electrode will face a narrower or shallower aspect of the AP.

The following should be kept in mind when a "resistant" AP is encountered:

1. Target the other side of the annulus.

In left-sided APs that cannot be ablated retrogradely from beneath the leaflet, the catheter may be advanced into the left atrium and then progressively withdrawn to ablate the atrial side of the mitral annulus with the same antegrade parameters. Otherwise, a transseptal approach must be considered, particularly to reach the anterior most left AP. In posteroseptal APs, changing to sites with a higher or lower A/V ratio can be helpful. Also switching to the other side of the septum must be envisaged early in resistant posteroseptal APs. A positive preexcitation in lead V_1 can often be reached from the right side but occasionally an AP with a negative preexcitation in V_1 can be ablated only from the left posterior septum. In right-sided AP, the ventricular approach is often useful from either the superior or the inferior vena cava as described above.

2. Changing the mapping criterion.

Switching from the earliest antegrade to the earliest retrograde activation site is useful in posteroseptal or left lateral AP, where an oblique course has been encountered relatively frequently. In some posteroseptal APs ablated in the proximal coronary sinus or afferent branches, the local retrograde VA time can be very short despite a relatively long AV time during preexcitation. It should be emphasized that the mere anatomic positioning of the ablation catheter at the atrial or ventricular side of the annulus (as reflected by a high or low A/V electrogram ratio) is to be distinguished from mapping of the atrial or ventricular insertion of the AP.

3. Seeking an AP potential.

High amplification is frequently required to record a tiny sharp potential preceding the first ventricular activity. The AP potential must be searched for, particularly when previous multiple RF applications guided by atrial or ventricular insertion mapping have been unsuccessful. The AP potential can be present between atrial and ventricular potentials that are separated more than usual (Figure 4), suggesting that previous ablations have altered a part of the AP insertion.

4. Deeply or epicardially located AP.

Such epicardial AP can be suspected when all the endocardial ventricular electrograms have an initial low amplitude and slope as well as a late intrinsic deflection. In 21 of 104 consecutive "right or left" posteroseptal AP, ablation was required in the proximal coronary sinus or afferent vessels (posterior or middle cardiac veins). Such APs had distinctive ECG patterns (Figure 6), notably a steep positive delta wave in

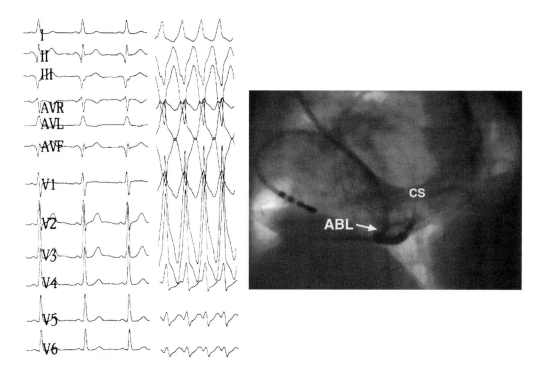

Figure 6. Typical surface ECG patterns in a patient with a manifest posteroseptal accessory AV pathway successfully ablated within a small posterior cardiac vein arising from the proximal coronary sinus (right panel). Note the steep positive delta wave in lead aVR and the distinct large S waves in V_5 and V_6 (during rapid atrial pacing in the panel on the right).

aVR and R<S in V_5/V_6 during rapid atrial pacing.[39] Some posteroseptal AP can be associated with a coronary sinus diverticulum or aneurysm that can be visualized by echocardiography or direct angiography.[29,40]

In about 5% of our left lateral AP, the AP could not be ablated endocardially including on the atrial aspect of the annulus. Ablation inside the mid/distal coronary sinus is legitimate, particularly if the coronary sinus electrograms are more favorable than the endocardial ones.[40,41] The target temperature used in the coronary sinus is preset to a lower value (50–60°C) than usual to minimize the risks of venous thrombi or perforation or catheter adherence.

Exceptionally, the AP can be situated in the area of mitral-aortic continuity. We have seen a single case with the optimal electrograms inside the proximal left anterior descending coronary artery (Figure 7) that was naturally not ablated.

Use of Different Modes of Higher Energy Delivery

Limiting unsuccessful pulse duration to 10 sec may miss a successful site that would require longer energy delivery. This applies to posteroseptal AP (possibly deep) and also to presumed wide AP for which the use of short pulses, although at appropriate sites, would not create significant confluent lesions for effective ablation. Such a wide AP should be identified a priori by a mapping bracketing the AP insertion and showing along several millimeters identical electrograms *including AP potentials*. A longer

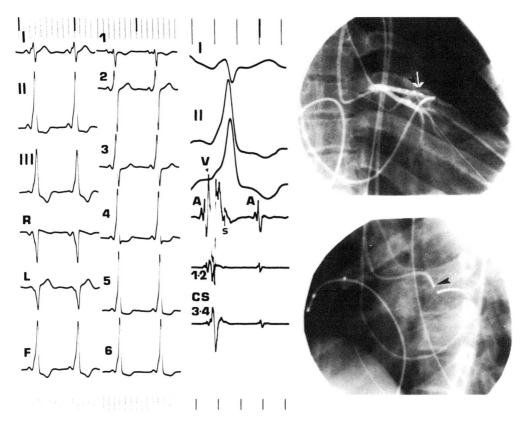

Figure 7. An exceptional instance of a manifest accessory AV connection located in the area of mitral aortic fibrous continuity. The surface ECGs indicate preexcitation of the QRS during sinus rhythm with an inferior frontal plane axis (left panel). Inadvertent positioning of a catheter inside the proximal LAD revealed optimal electrograms (better than those recorded during both endocardial and epicardial mapping) and the x-ray pictures (right panel) document the location of this catheter (arrows) verified by coronary angiography (arrow). No ablation was attempted at this site.

interval and later timing in the local electrograms after ablation (with or without change in the preexcitation pattern) is probably the best indication that a part of the AP has been ablated, and a confirmation that the AP is anatomically wide. In one extreme case, we found AP potential and optimal electrograms along 6 cm. The AP corresponded to the insertion of a giant right atrial appendage diverticulum onto the anterior right ventricle, which was successfully ablated by sequential contiguous RF applications (Figure 8).

Bipolar transseptal RF pulses have been proposed to ablate posteroseptal APs[30] that could not be ablated by unipolar pulses applied on either side of the septum. This technique was effective in two of our patients.

During sequential applications of RF energy to cover a wider area, the final "successful" sites can show less favorable electrograms than "unsuccessful" sites because previous applications guided by the shortest AV conduction times may have altered a part of AP insertions, leaving some fibers with longer conduction times that will be ablated with additional applications. Finally, we have observed that scar tissue due to previous prior RF application limits heat transmission and effectiveness of subsequent RF pulses. If RF ablation applied through the usual catheters is ineffective,

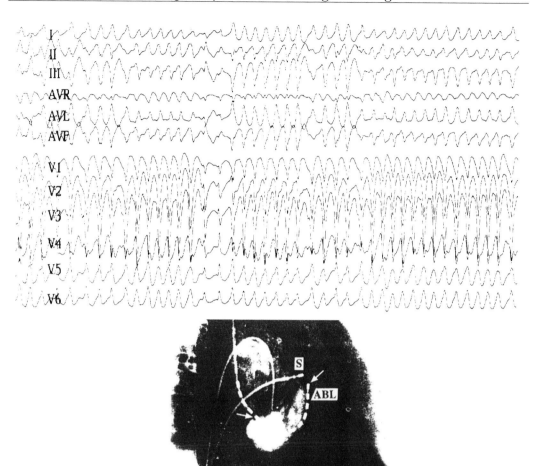

Figure 8. A rare case with a wide and giant right atrial appendage inserting onto the anterior right ventricle and functioning as a broad and manifest accessory AV connection. The 12-lead ECG during continuing atrial fibrillation exhibits almost exclusively preexcited QRS complexes with a stereotypic morphology in the chest leads but a changing frontal plane QRS indicative of a shifting vector of preexcitation. The x-ray picture depicts an angiogram of the diverticulum with a 14-pole electrode catheter placed inside it. Sequential ablation was performed from each electrode with a progressive disappearance of the preexcitation.

the use of more powerful energies or RF energy through new types of electrodes, particularly including an irrigated tip, can be envisaged as shown by Jackman et al.

Conclusion

Successful ablation of AP can be achieved in most patients with one or few RF applications, based on precise electrogram criteria. Electrograms can also be used to identify wide or deep AP which will require a different strategy. If ablation is unsuccessful, the next step is to target another part of either the AP or the AV annulus. As a last resort, the use of more penetrating energies will ablate the most recalcitrant AP.

References

1. Weber H, Schmitz L. Catheter technique for closed-chest ablation of an accessory pathway. N Engl J Med 1983;308:654.
2. Morady F, Scheinman MM. Transvenous catheter ablation of a posteroseptal accessory pathway in a patient with the Wolff-Parkinson-White syndrome. N Engl J Med 1984; 310:705–707.
3. Jackman WM, Friday KJ, Scherlag BJ, et al. Direct endocardial recording from an atrioventricular pathway: localization of the site of block effect of antiarrhythmic drugs and attempt at nonsurgical ablation. Circulation 1983;5:906–916.
4. Haissaguerre M, Warin JF, Regaudie JJ, et al. Fulguration après enregistrement électrique direct de la voie de Kent. Arch Mal Coeur 1986;79:1072–1081.
5. Warin JF, Haissaguerre M, Le Metayer Ph, et al. Catheter ablation of accessory pathways with a direct approach. Circulation 1988;78: 800–815.
6. Haissaguerre M, Warin JF. Closed-chest ablation of left lateral atrioventricular accessory pathways. Eur Heart J 1989;10:602–610.
7. Warin JF, Haissaguerre M, d'Ivernois Ch, et al. Catheter ablation of accessory pathways: technique and results in 248 patients. PACE 1990;13:1609–1614.
8. Jackman WM, Kuck KH, Naccarelli GV, et al. Radiofrequency current directed across the mitral annulus with a bipolar epicardial-endocardial catheter electrode configuration in dogs. Circulation 1988;78:1288–1298.
9. Jackman WM, Friday KJ, Yeung-Lai-Wah JA, et al. New catheter technique for recording left free wall accessory atrioventricular pathway activation: identification of pathway fiber orientation. Circulation 1988;78: 598–611.
10. Marcus FI. The use of radiofrequency energy for intracardiac ablation: historical perspective and results of experiments in animals. In Breithardt G, Borggrefe M, Zipes DP, eds. Nonpharmacological Therapy of Tachyarrhythmias. Futura Publishing Co, Mount Kisco, NY, 1987, pp 213–219.
11. Borggrefe M, Budde T, Podczeck A, et al. High frequency alternating current ablation of an accessory pathway in humans. J Am Coll Cardiol 1987;10:576–582.
12. Jackman WM, Wang W, Friday KJ, et al. Catheter ablation of accessory atrioventricular pathways (Wolff-Parkinson-White syndrome) by radiofrequency current. N Engl J Med 1991;324:1605–1611.
13. Kuck KH, Schluter M. Single-catheter approach to radiofrequency ablation of left-side accessory pathways in patients with Wolff Parkinson White syndrome. Circulation 1991;84:2366–2375.
14. Schluter M, Geiger M, Siebles J, et al. Catheter ablation using radiofrequency current to cure symptomatic patients with tachyarrhythmias related to an accessory atrioventricular pathway. Circulation 1991;84: 1644–1661.
15. Huang SKS. Radiofrequency catheter ablation of cardiac arrhythmias: appraisal of an evolving therapeutic modality. Am Heart J 1989;118:1317–1323.
16. Calkins H, Souza J, El-Atassi R, et al. Diagnosis and cure of the Wolff-Parkinson-White syndrome of paroxysmal supraventricular tachycardias during a single electrophysiologic test. N Engl J Med 1991;324:1612–1618.
17. Lesh MD, Van Hare GF, Schamp DJ, et al. Curative percutaneous catheter ablation using radiofrequency energy for accessory pathways in all locations: results in 100 consecutive patients. Am J Cardiol 1992;19: 1303–1309.
18. Calkins H, Kim Y, Schmaltz S, et al. Electrogram criteria for identification of appropriate target sites for radiofrequency catheter ablation of accessory pathways. Circulation 1992;85:565–573.
19. Silka MJ, Kron J, Halperin BD, et al. Analysis of local electrogram characteristics correlates with successful radiofrequency ablation of accessory pathways. PACE 1992;15: 1000–1007.
20. Haissaguerre M, Fischer B, Warin JF, et al. Electrogram patterns predictive of successful radiofrequency catheter ablation of accessory pathways. PACE 1992;15(II):2138–2145.
21. Natale A, Wathen M, Yee R, et al. Atrial and ventricular approaches for radiofrequency catheter ablation of left-sided accessory pathways. Am J Cardiol 1992;70:114–116.
22. Chen XU, Borggrefe M, Hindricks G, et al. Radiofrequency ablation of accessory pathways: characteristics of transiently and permanently effective pulses. PACE 1992;15: 1122–1130.
23. Swartz JF, Tracy CM, Fletcher RD. Radiofrequency endocardial catheter ablation of accessory atrioventricular pathway atrial insertion sites. Circulation 1993;87:487–499.
24. Chen SA, Chiang CE, Tsang WP, et al. Recurrent conduction in accessory pathway and possible new arrhythmias after radiofrequency catheter ablation. Am Heart J 1993; 125:381–387.

25. Simmers TA, Hauer RN, Wittkampf FH, et al. Radiofrequency catheter ablation of accessory pathways: prediction of ablation outcome by unipolar electrogram characteristics. PACE 1993;16(II):866.

26. Grimm W, Miller J, Josephson ME. Successful and unsuccessful sites of radiofrequency catheter ablation of accessory atrioventricular connections. Am Heart J 1994;128:77–87.

27. Damle RS, Choe W, Kanaan NM, et al. Atrial and accessory pathway activation direction in patients with orthodromic supraventricular tachycardia: insights from vector mapping. J Am Coll Cardiol 1994;23:684–692.

28. Dhala AA, Deshpande SS, Bremner S, et al. Transcatheter ablation of posteroseptal accessory pathways using a venous approach and radiofrequency energy. Circulation 1994;90:1799–1810.

29. Arruda MS, Beckman KJ, McClelland JH, et al. Coronary sinus anatomy and anomalies in patients with posteroseptal accessory pathway requiring ablation within a venous branch of the coronary sinus [abstract]. J Am Coll Cardiol 1994;23:224A.

30. Bashir Y, Heald SC, O'Nunain S, et al. Radiofrequency current delivery by way of a bipolar tricuspid annulus-mitral annulus electrode configuration for ablation of posteroseptal accessory pathways. J Am Coll Cardiol 1993;21:550–556.

31. Wen MS, Yeh SJ, Wand CC, et al. Radiofrequency ablation therapy of the posteroseptal accessory pathway. Am Heart J 1996;132: 612–620.

32. Fisher WG, Swartz JF. Three dimensional electrogram mapping improves ablation of left-sided AP. PACE 1992;15:2344–2356.

33. Wittkampf FHM, Simmers TA, Hauer RNW. Repeated radiofrequency catheter ablation: effect of a bonus pulse on myocardial temperature. [Abstract] Eur Heart J 1994;14:256.

34. Fitzpatrick AP. The ECG in Wolff-Parkinson-White syndrome. PACE 1995;18:1469–1473.

35. Haïssaguerre M, Dartigues JF, Warin JF, et al. Electrogram patterns predictive of successful catheter ablation of accessory pathways. Value of unipolar recording mode. Circulation 1991;84:188–202.

36. Becker AE, Anderson RH, Durrer D, et al. The anatomic substrates of Wolff Parkinson White: a clinicopathologic correlation in seven patients. Circulation 1978;57:870–879.

37. Frank R, Brechenmacher C, Fontaine G. Apport de l'histologie dans l'étude des syndromes de préexcitation ventriculaire. Coeur Med Int 1976;15:337–343.

38. Smeets J, Allessie M; Kirchlof CH, et al. High resolution mapping of ventriculoatrial conduction over the accessory pathway in patients with the Wolff Parkinson White syndrome [abstract]. Eur Heart J 1990;11:1.

39. Takahashi A, Shah DC, Jaïs P, et al. Electrocardiographic features predicting a coronary sinus ablation site for posteroseptal accessory pathways. Cardiovasc Electrophysiol (in press).

40. Guiraudon GM, Guiraudon CM, Klein GJ, et al. The coronary sinus diverticulum: a pathologic entity associated with the Wolff Parkinson White syndrome. Am J Cardiol 1988;62: 733–755.

41. Haïssaguerre M, Gaïta F, Fischer B, et al. Radiofrequency catheter ablation of left lateral accessory pathways via the coronary sinus. Circulation 1992;86:1464–1468.

42. Langberg JJ, Man KC, Vorperian VR, et al. Recognition and catheter ablation of subepicardial accessory pathways. J Am Coll Cardiol 1993;22:1100–1104.

Ablation of Left-Sided Accessory Pathways:
Transatrial, Retrograde, or Coronary Sinus Approach?

John D. Kugler, David A. Danford, Michael J. Silka, Kris Houston, Gary Felix, and the other participating members* of the Pediatric Electrophysiology Society

Introduction

The procedural approach during radiofrequency (RF) catheter ablation for patients with left-sided accessory atrioventricular (AV) pathways (APs) has been a subject of debate among electrophysiologists since RF catheter ablation was introduced as an alternative (to surgery) curative technique.

When the first RF catheter ablation large series of both pediatric and adult patients were reported in 1991–1992, authors described using the "retrograde approach" for most patients with left-sided AP.[1-7] This technique requires an arterial sheath in the femoral artery for the ablation catheter to be manipulated under fluoroscopic guidance superiorly to the aortic arch, then inferiorly in the ascending aorta across the aortic valve (Figures 1, 2). After the catheter is in the ventricle (left ventricle except for those with congenital heart defects such as ventricular inversion, single ventricle, etc.), the tip is manipulated under the mitral valve leaflets in an effort to locate, then ablate, the ventricular insertion of the AP along the annulus from the left anteriolateral to the posterior septal area. When the atrial insertion is sought, the catheter tip is manipulated toward the left atrium and can be directed on the annulus or on the atrial side of the annulus.

In the early reports, the "transatrial" route was mentioned as an alternative when the catheter tip could not be manipulated to the desired site during the retrograde approach.[1,7] However, during the following few years, the transseptal or atrial approach was reported by some investigators as a primary choice in both pediatric and adult patients.[8-13] The transseptal technique, like the retrograde, was adapted for RF catheter ablation from methods already in use for hemodynamic and angiographic catheterization. Using either the transseptal sheath technique (e.g., Mullins sheath with needle puncture of the atrial septum),[14] or the patent foramen ovale when present, the cathe-

---

* See Appendix I for listing of other participating members of the Pediatric Radiofrequency Catheter Ablation Registry.

From Singer I, Barold SS, Camm AJ (eds): Nonpharmacological Therapy of Arrhythmias for the 21st Century: The State of the Art. Futura Publishing Co, Inc., Armonk, NY, © 1998.

RAO

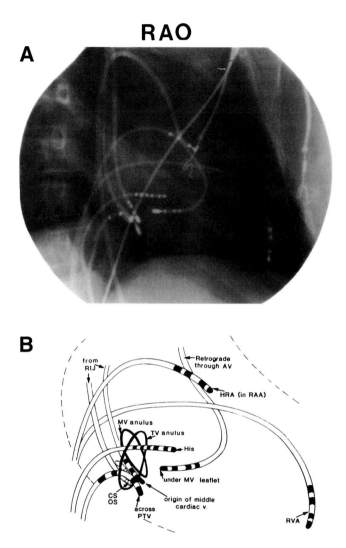

Figure 1. Right anterior oblique (RAO) projection of a cinecardiographic frame **(A)** with illustration **(B)** demonstrating the courses of seven catheters required for successful ablation of a posterior septal accessory pathway in a 12-year-old girl. Two catheter approaches were required for successful radiofrequency catheter (RF) ablation: (1) coronary sinus, and (2) retrograde. Five catheters were initially used: right ventricular apex (RVA), high right atrium (HRA), in the right atrial appendage (RAA), His bundle (HIS), coronary sinus (CS), from the right internal jugular (RIJ) approach, and the 4-mm tip ablation catheter across the posterior tricuspid valve (PTV) area. RF ablation current was initially applied near the CS os (advanced from femoral vein), where a prominent accessory pathway potential was recorded. Although the accessory pathway potential was eliminated, the tachycardia continued. Next, a second, 4-mm tip ablation catheter was advanced through a second sheath placed in the RIJ vein and positioned in the origin of the middle cardiac vein, where another accessory pathway potential was recorded. Although the tachycardia terminated 5 sec after RF current was applied at the site, the tachycardia recurred. After several further attempts, similar results revealed only temporary termination of the tachycardia. Finally, a third 4-mm tip ablation catheter was advanced retrogradly via a right femoral artery sheath, across the aortic valve (AV), and positioned under the mitral valve (MV) leaflet in the posterior septal area. Final success was achieved at this left posterior septal site, which was approximately 2 cm from the initial application near the CS os. Reproduced with permission in part from Kugler JD.[43]

LAO

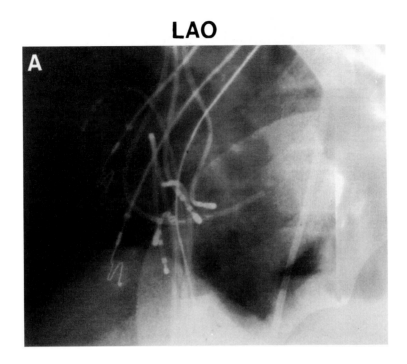

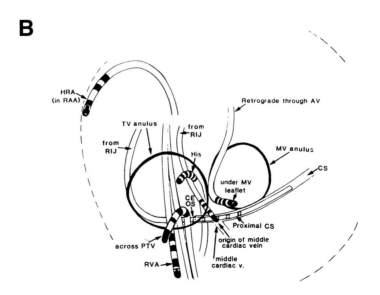

Figure 2. Left anterior oblique (LAO) view of the same catheter courses as described in Figure 1. Reproduced with permission in part from Kugler JD.[43]

RAO   LAO

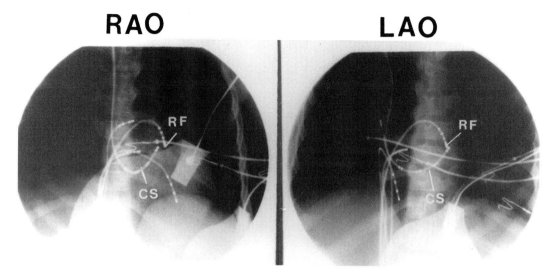

Figure 3. Labeled radiographs in a 7-year-old girl with a left lateral free wall accessory pathway in which the transseptal technique (Mullins sheath) was used. With the application of radiofrequency energy during ventricular paced rhythm, conduction was eliminated within a few seconds. At the end of the procedure, only normal retrograde conduction was demonstrated. CS = coronary sinus catheter; LAO = left anterior oblique; RAO = right anterior oblique; RF = radiofrequency catheter.

ter is advanced to the left atrium from the right atrium (Figure 3). In most patients, the tip is manipulated directly on the mitral annulus or on the atrial side of the annulus to map and then ablate the AP atrial insertion. Sites ranging from the anterior free wall to the posterior septum and sometimes even the mid-anterior septal area are accessible using this method. For patients in whom ablation of the atrial insertion is unsuccessful, it is possible to advance and manipulate the catheter into the left ventricle so that the tip can be directed back under the mitral valve annulus to ablate the AP ventricular insertion.

Historically, the utilization of the coronary sinus (CS) has been interesting. In the first case reports of RF catheter ablation and for the early patients in the first large RF catheter ablation series, a second large-tipped catheter in the CS was utilized.[1,15] Radiofrequency energy current flowed from the retrograde catheter in contact with the left ventricular insertion site to the CS electrode nearby. This technique of using a catheter in the CS was abandoned soon thereafter in favor of using a skin pad. Even

before the advent of RF catheter ablation, ablation of APs using direct current energy was carried out through catheters in the CS.[16–19] Moreover, after RF had become the energy source of choice by most electrophysiologists, "low-dose" direct current was still advocated by some investigators.[20,21] Even in the early RF catheter ablation reports, using the ablation catheter in the CS was essential to ablate left posterior septal AP, especially in difficult sites approachable only by advancing the catheter tip into CS diverticulae and branches (Figures 1,2) such as the middle cardiac vein.[1,22–25] Based on ongoing reports of success, some investigators have recently returned to using the CS approach to gain access to difficult left free wall presumed "epicardial" AP sites.[26–28] Regardless of the site within the length of the CS or of its diverticulae and/or venous branching vessels, angiography is advocated by most experienced investigators.[29–31] The angiography is carried out predominantly by direct CS angiography, but some have found coronary artery angiography helpful because it provides coronary artery anatomic information in addition to the levophase venous anatomy.

In this chapter, the first section provides data from the Pediatric Electrophysiology Society's Pediatric Radiofrequency Catheter Ablation Registry. Next, the published work of others from both adult and pediatric patients that have involved approaches to left-sided pathways are summarized, compared, and discussed in the context of the Pediatric Registry data. Last, based on these data, conclusions are drawn that focus on how the electrophysiologist can maximize success while minimizing complications for patients with left-sided APs.

Pediatric Radiofrequency Catheter Ablation Registry Data

The Pediatric Radiofrequency Catheter Ablation Registry was started in 1991. The major aim of this voluntary Registry was to establish a database of pediatric patients (upper age limit 21 years) who underwent RF catheter ablation. The database allows the study of factors that influence outcomes such as RF catheter ablation immediate success/failure, recurrence rates, complication rates, specific complications (e.g., AV block), and procedural issues (e.g., fluoroscopy and procedure times). The accumulation of a very large pediatric RF catheter ablation database has promoted outcome-based research into many controversial and clinically relevant aspects of the procedure. One such project addresses issues associated with the catheter approach to left-sided pathways.

Enrollment of patients in the Registry is done by reporting clinical variables and the procedural outcomes listed above on a case-by-case basis. One of the clinical variables reported is whether a transatrial procedure was done. The database is compiled and analyzed biannually, looking for association of clinical variables with outcomes as described in the initial Registry results reported in 1994.[32] As with other clinical variables, the transatrial approach was investigated first by univariate analysis of the factor transatrial approach on outcome measures of complications, success/failure, fluoroscopy and procedure times, then, if significant ($P<0.10$), multivariate analysis was performed to determine whether there is a significant association independent of the other variables ($P<0.05$). However, the regular Registry data form does not include questions pertaining to all ablation catheter approaches used and which failed or succeeded. The regular Registry asks only whether an ablation catheter was advanced across the atrial septum and whether an ablation catheter was advanced into the CS because at the onset of the Registry these data were considered to be potential risk factors for complications but were not considered factors related to success/failure. Therefore, it was clear that further data were required to address questions that were not attainable in the Registry database.

The method by which further data and answers were sought was investigated by creating and sending two questionnaires. First, a questionnaire containing 13 questions was mailed to all 57 pediatric electrophysiologists in the Registry. The questionnaire did not include questions related to specific data from procedures. Instead, it addressed issues such as whether the electrophysiologist used only the retrograde approach or only the transseptal approach, or if both were used, which approach was tried first and which criteria were then followed to make the decision to crossover to another approach.

Second, a list was generated of each center's patients with left-sided pathways who had previously been submitted to the Registry. Specific questions were added to the list that related to each patient's RF catheter ablation procedure as to the approach or approaches used (transseptal, patent foramen ovale, retrograde, CS) as well as to the corresponding success or failure. The list of each center's patients and procedure with the specific questions addressing the catheter approach were then sent to the respective center to be completed and returned to the coordinating center (University of Nebraska).

Initial Transatrial Analysis Derived from Standard Registry Data

There was no association between the transatrial technique and the incidence of major complications (defined in the Registry as death or any complication that required treatment or follow-up). Similarly, there were no associations between transatrial technique and AV block or non-AV block major complications.

There was a univariate association between transatrial approach and success or failure of the RF catheter ablation ($P < 0.05$), but this disappeared on the multivariate analysis when the effect of AP site, presence of underlying structural heart disease, and previous experience were taken into account. Because the Registry analysis consistently has shown that experience is significantly associated with a higher success rate,[32-34] it was considered possible that more experience leads to greater use of the transseptal approach, which meets with greater success because it is used by more experienced operators. This was further investigated by performing chi square analysis comparing the proportions of total procedures that used the approach for each of six levels of experience. As listed in Table 1,

more experienced operators in the Registry use the transseptal approach more frequently ($P < 0.001$). It may be reasonable to conclude that the univariate relationship between transseptal approach and success is an epiphenomenon of the relationship between experience and success.

Both procedural outcome measures of fluoroscopy time and procedure time had significant univariate and multivariate correlations of longer times with the transatrial approach. On average, the transseptal approach was associated with an additional 14.5 minutes of fluoroscopy time and 31.2 minutes of procedural time to the RF catheter ablation procedure. The additional time could be attributable to persistence with an unsuccessful nontransatrial approach before crossing over, or to the transseptal approach itself, or to both.

Operator Preference

Of 57 questionnaires sent to the Registry members, 36 (63%) were returned. Of the 36 respondents, 35 had performed more than 30 total RF catheter ablation procedures, 33 more than 40 procedures, and 29 more than 50 procedures. All but two respondents were involved as the primary operator, and for them, the RF catheter ablation procedure was performed by a pediatric interventionalist colleague. For specifically performing the transseptal technique during the RF

Table 1
Catheter Approaches for Radiofrequency Ablation of Left Accessory Pathways

Number of Transatrial Procedures/ Left Accessory Pathways*	vs.	Previous Experience: Number of Procedures
92/216, 44%		<10
102/177, 58%		10–19
73/144, 51%		20–29
136/261, 52%		30–49
287/468, 61%		50–99
486/680, 71%		100+

*p < 0.001.
See text for description.

catheter ablation, 34 use it for some or all of the procedures and, if used, another cardiologist performs the transseptal technique for 9 of these 34. Of those 34 who use the transseptal technique, including those who previously learned the technique but do not perform it now, 25 learned the transseptal technique during fellowship training. The RF catheter ablation procedures are performed in both single plane (n = 11) and biplane (n = 25) laboratories.

Neither retrograde nor transseptal was strongly favored as the initial approach. Transseptal generally is used first by 18/36 (50%) compared to 11/36 (31%) for the retrograde approach. Although not specifically documented by the respondents, seven therefore appear not to systematically favor one method over the other as an initial approach. Of the 11 who use the retrograde approach first, all 11 usually cross over to the transseptal approach if success is not obtained. Of the 18 who use the transseptal approach first, seven seldom and five never cross over to retrograde. Regardless of which route is favored first, the two most common indications for those who cross over to the other approach are the same: fluoroscopy/procedure time and number of applications. Of the six respondents who listed specific thresholds for crossovers, a wide range was found. The range of unsuccessful RF energy applications before considering crossing over to the other technique was 5 to 20 and the range of fluoroscopy time was 60–90 minutes.

Data Generated from Second Questionnaire of Previously Entered Registry Patients with Left-Sided Accessory Pathways

Data for all patients and procedures from the 46 pediatric centers entered into the Registry from January 1, 1991, through September 15, 1996, included a total of 4,135 patients who underwent 4,651 procedures, of which 3,509 involved APs. Of the AP procedures, 1,940 were left-sided pathways which included 277 left septal (sites 7,8 on Figure 4) and 1,663 left free wall (sites 9,10,11 on Figure 4) pathways. Twenty-nine centers returned data for further analysis from patients who had a total of 1,391 left-sided APs.

Demographic data from those left-sided AP procedures returned for further analysis revealed a mean/median age of 12.3/13.1 years (range, 0.1–20.9; 10th percentile 5.2, 90th percentile 17.5); mean/median weight of 49.5/50 kg (range, 1.9–139; 10th percentile 19.3, 90th percentile 75.0). Most patients had an otherwise normal heart (no structural or hemodynamic heart disease: 1,072/1,153, 93%).

Of the 1,391 APs analyzed, at some time during the procedure the transatrial approach was used 966 times (transseptal technique, 790; PFO, 176), the retrograde approach 462, and the CS approach 105.

One of the three approaches used without crossover to one or two of the other approaches:

1. Transatrial Approach

Crossover to another approach was not carried out from the transatrial approach in 845 (transseptal, 696; PFO, 149) of the 966 procedures in which it was used. Of the 845 procedures in which only the transatrial approach was used, success was found in 804, 95.1% (transseptal, 665/696, 95.5%; PFO, 139/149, 93.3%). In 41/845, 4.9% (transseptal, 31/696, 4.5%; PFO, 10/149, 6.7%), further efforts were abandoned during the procedure to try another approach when failure was encountered with the transatrial approach. These data overstate success associated with the transatrial approach in general because many patients whose initial method was a failed transatrial approach are not included here, but reported in the crossover statistics below.

2. Retrograde

The retrograde arterial technique was used as the only approach in 364 procedures

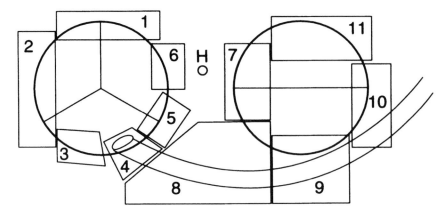

Figure 4. Illustration of the Pediatric Radiofrequency Catheter Ablation diagram, from which participating members select the number corresponding to the accessory pathway location. Sites 1, 2, and 3 depict right free wall accessory pathways along the tricuspid valve; sites 4, 5, and 6 depict right septal pathways; sites 7 and 8 depict left septal accessory pathways; sites 9, 10, and 11 depict left free wall accessory pathways. In this LAO view, the coronary sinus starts in site 4 and runs to the right through sites 8, 9 and 10. H = His bundle.

of the 462 in which it was used. Success was accomplished in 336/364 (92.3%). Therefore, in 28/364 (7.7%) crossover to another approach was not chosen despite failure with the retrograde approach alone. Exclusion of failed retrograde attempts that resulted in crossover to other approaches artificially inflates the success rate over that which would be expected if retrograde was the only available method.

3. Coronary Sinus

The coronary sinus was utilized as the only approach in 49 procedures of the 105 in which it was used. Success was achieved in 43/49 (87.8%) so efforts were abandoned in 6/49 (12.2%) without proceeding on to other approaches during the procedure. Again, the exclusion of failed CS attempts that resulted in crossover to other approaches skews these success rates upward.

Two of the three approaches used (one approach failed and crossover to only one other approach):

1. Transatrial and Retrograde

There were 77 APs in which this combination of approaches was utilized. Success was achieved in 61/77, 79%. The CS approach was not used for the 16 failures. Ret-

rograde was the successful approach in 41 and transatrial in 20.

2. Transatrial and CS

This combination was used for 35 APs with 33 successes (94%). Further crossover to the retrograde approach was not used for the two failures. There were 19 transatrial and 14 CS successes in this group.

3. Retrograde and CS

Of the 12 APs in which this combination was used, success was found for 10 (83%). In the two failures, the atrial approach was not utilized. Four of the successes were retrograde and six were CS.

All three approaches used:

Of the nine cases in which all three approaches were used, there were three successes by CS, two by transatrial, three by retrograde, and one failure.

In summary, the above data in which the multiple combinations were used (or not used) is revealing. Although the quantification of the success rates for each approach was not possible in this analysis because we do not know the number of times each approach was in fact the first one used, it is not surprising that all three approaches have many successes as the primary route to ablation. Moreover, all approaches have a record of success after failure of one or more of the other two approaches. Again, because it is unknown in the database the number of times each approach was applied as the second choice (as opposed to the primary or even the third choice), it is not possible to quantitate the success rates. However, it seems reasonable to conclude that when the first choice fails, and a second and/or third approach is tried, success usually is achieved (112/133, 84.2%). It then follows that, as Natale et al. and Lesh et al. have recognized, greater success may have been achieved had all three approaches been used in the 92 failures in which only one approach was tried and in the 40 failures in which only two approaches were attempted.[8,11] However, caution with this conclusion is needed because it is unknown whether one or more of the approaches had been tried during a previous procedure. With this caveat aside, the question arises: why are there cases where the operator tries only one approach and if it fails, another approach is not attempted?

Correlation of Factors with One Attempt

To better understand possible reasons why there were failed RF catheter ablations in which only one approach was tried, univariate and multivariate analysis was used to identify features that may correlate with the one-failed-approach procedure.

The following were analyzed: age (very young, ≤2 yr.; young, ≤4 yr.; continuous variable); weight (light, ≤15 kg; heavy, ≥80 kg; continuous variable); underlying structural or hemodynamic heart disease; operator experience (expert, ≥20 procedures; previous procedures as continuous variable); major complications; location of AP (Posterior septal; posterior free wall; lateral free wall; anteriolateral free wall). Initially, uni-

variate analysis was performed and, for all factors, those with univariate association with a one-failed-approach procedure were then subjected to multivariate analysis to test for the independence of those associations.

Multivariate analysis revealed that one-failed-approach procedures had independently positive association with only two factors: underlying heart disease ($P < 0.001$) and major procedural complication ($P < 0.001$). Underlying heart disease may discourage secondary approaches because of concern that a longer procedure may be poorly tolerated. Perhaps the anatomy in some patients is not conducive to other approaches (e.g., anomalous coronary sinus).[35] It seems reasonable to speculate that when a major complication occurred, operators were appropriately reluctant to proceed on with any further attempt at different approach.

One-failed-approach procedures had independent negative association with three variables: lateral free wall AP location ($P = 0.002$), experience as "expert" operator ($P < 0.001$), as well as the continuous variable experience as defined as previous cases ($P = 0.011$). Therefore, experienced operators were more likely to proceed on to try another approach, whereas, conversely, inexperienced operators were more likely to give up after only one approach. The AP site was unlikely to be left lateral when the operator gave up after one failed approach. The most likely explanation relates to the high success rate found with this AP location so it follows that there are probably a low number of failures after trying only one approach for left lateral AP.

Correlation of factors with AP ablation success/failure: uni- and multivariate analysis was carried out to identify factors with independent associations with procedural success or failure. Age, weight, heart disease, pathway location, operator experience, atrial approach attempted, retrograde approach attempted, and CS approach attempted were analyzed for possible independent associations with success or failure. As has been found for all tachyarrhythmias and for paroxysmal supraventricular tachycardias (AP together with AV node reentry) in past Registry analyses, success was associated with experience (expert, $P<0.001$; continuous variable, p = 0.034), and with left lateral location ($P<0.001$).[32–34] The presence of structural heart disease ($P<0.001$) and the posterior septal AP site ($P<0.001$) were features that made success less likely. No demonstrable independent correlation was found between success and having tried one particular approach over another.

Correlation of Success for All Cases Whenever One of the Three Approaches Was Tried

To further evaluate the outcome of success for each specific approach, the next analysis was limited to all of those cases when the transseptal technique was tried (at any time during the procedure). Among the cases in which transseptal was attempted, experience (the continuous variable) correlated ($P< 0.001$) with success, but structural heart disease ($P<0.005$) and posterior septal AP location ($P<0.001$) both correlated with failure. These results were similar to those in which the success/failure outcome was analyzed for all approaches together.

The other atrial approach, PFO, was examined separately in the same manner. Experience ($P<0.001$) again correlated with success, as did an additional variable, the very young ($P<0.001$). The latter (those children ≤2 years old) perhaps could be explained by enhanced catheter maneuverability in a smaller heart via the PFO compared with transseptal technique. Another possibility could relate to some centers foregoing transseptal approach in small children, thereby the PFO atrial approach in some centers may be the only one used in this age group.

For the analysis that was limited to those cases in which the retrograde approach was tried, experience did not correlate with success as it did for other approaches. However, similar to the transseptal technique, the posterior septal AP location correlated with failure ($P = 0.002$). An additional factor, weight (continuous variable) correlated with failure ($P<0.001$). It is difficult to explain the reason for this correlation.

The inquiry revealed interesting correlations for the cases in which the CS was attempted in addition to the experience factor correlation with success ($P<0.001$). Contrary to the data for the retrograde approach and both atrial approaches, CS success correlated with the posterior septal AP location ($P<0.001$). Moreover, failure correlated with the left lateral AP site ($P = 0.02$).

From the investigations involved with AP location, it seems reasonable to conclude that the CS approach should be used more frequently for AP sites in the posterior septal area and a strong point could be made that this approach should be attempted first for AP in this area. For the left lateral AP site, both transseptal and retrograde approaches are correlated with success so it does not seem to matter which is used first. However, the CS should probably not be used for AP at this left lateral area unless both of the other approaches have been tried.

Correlation with Fluoroscopy Time

The duration of fluoroscopy time is a procedural matter that has been a concern, and therefore a subject of study, since the advent of the procedure and thereby the Registry. When fluoroscopy time was analyzed as an outcome, the following variables correlated with a greater chance of longer fluoroscopy time: presence of structural heart disease ($P<0.001$); weight as a continuous variable ($P = 0.02$); posterior septal AP location ($P = 0.02$); attempt using CS approach ($P = 0.04$); attempt using transseptal technique ($P<0.001$). A shorter fluoroscopy time correlated with experience when analyzed both as an expert ($P<0.001$) and as a continuous variable ($P<0.001$).

It can be concluded that experience reduces fluoroscopy time in a nonlinear fashion, with a demonstrable threshold effect at 20 cases and a continuous benefit from further cases. It seems logical, and moreover it is supported by data from previous reports of learning curves and experience, that experience is beneficial in limiting fluoroscopy and procedure time.[36–38]

Fluoroscopy time increases with increasing patient weight. This adverse association with weight is not a threshold phenomenon associated only with very heavy patients, but is a continuous association across all patient weights. The explanation for this correlation is unknown, but one that has been consistent with virtually all Registry investigations.[32–34] Moreover, in the multicenter Atakr study, a longer fluoroscopy time correlated with age, a finding that also probably relates to weight.[39] It is no surprise to experienced ablation electrophysiologists that, independent of the approaches used, a longer fluoroscopy time is expected when an AP is within the difficult anatomic area of the posterior septum.

The retrograde approach did not add fluoroscopy time. When either the transseptal approach or the CS approach was tried, more fluoroscopy time was spent (mean 10.32 and 9.2 minutes, respectively). It is likely that some of the additional time is unrelated to placement of the transseptal or CS catheter, because time may have been spent trying other approaches before deciding to use either the transseptal or the CS approach.

The finding that the transseptal technique adds time is directly contrary to that reported by Dick et al.[40] These investigators found in their center that the transseptal technique was associated with significantly less fluoroscopy time compared to the retrograde approach. One explanation may be related to the issue of a single center versus multiple centers, thereby the single center expertise in the transseptal technique may be considerable compared with many of those from the Registry. The era in which the respective techniques were predomi-

nantly used may also be important. The initial experience of most operators who began performing RF catheter ablation in the early era (late 1980s, early 1990s) was with the retrograde approach whereas the transseptal technique has become more prevalent recently.[1–13] With experience (independent from the technique used), fluoroscopy time shortens, so the data and conclusion of Dick et al. may be biased from the experience factor rather than due to the technique itself. Failure to control for the confounding influence of operator experience may account for the contradictory findings of Dick et al.

Correlation with Complications

Major complications are less likely with greater experience ($P = 0.003$) and more likely in younger (continuous variable) patients ($P = 0.008$). There was no independent correlation between major complication and any one particular approach. The five most frequent complications were analyzed. There was no difference ($P > 0.05$) between specific complication rates for each catheter approach when each of the five most frequent complications were analyzed separately (2x2 chi square). For perforation, effusion, or hemothorax: TA, n = 14, rate = 0.014; retrograde, n = 4, rate = 0.008; CS, n = 0. For brachial plexus: TA, n = 9, rate 0.009; retrograde, n = 1, rate 0.002, CS, n = 0. For emboli: TA, n = 4, rate 0.004; retrograde, n = 2, rate 0.004, CS = 0. For valve regurgitation: TA, n = 2, rate = 0.002; retrograde, n = 3, rate = 0.006; CS, n = 1, n = 0.01. For AV block: TA, n = 1, rate = 0.001, retrograde, n = 3, rate = 0.006; CS, n = 0. Lau and associates compared their lower incidence of aortic and mitral valve regurgitation in children using the transseptal approach to an earlier report by Minich et al. in which the retrograde approach was used.[41,42] However, Lau and colleagues did not compare the technique within their own center as did Dick and associates who found no difference in complication rate between the two approaches.[40–42]

Conclusions

The three issues appear to be success rate, complications, and fluoroscopy time. As has been consistently found with all previously reported Registry data, experience at the pediatric center was a highly significant factor that correlated with ablation success.[32–34] Although a high success rate is demonstrated individually for all approaches, it appears prudent to conclude, as have Natale et al. and Lesh et al., that an even higher success rate can be achieved when more than one approach is tried after failure is found using the initial approach (whatever it may be).[8,11] The specific correlation of higher success for posterior septal APs when the CS approach is tried suggests that this route should be tried first in these patients. Enhanced success within the CS would be expected when a diverticulum is demonstrated by CS angiography.[21–25] Moreover, the CS approach should be reserved for last (after both other approaches fail) in patients with lateral free wall APs.

As others have reported, the complication rate is not different for a specific catheter approach.[8,11,40] However, again, experience correlated with a low complication rate. A higher complication rate should be expected when RF ablation is carried out in young children.

The importance of experience is again demonstrated with fluoroscopy time: shorter fluoroscopy time is associated with experience. Longer fluoroscopy times should be expected in heavier patients and in those who have underlying structural or hemodynamic heart disease or a posterior septal AP. For members of the Pediatric Radiofrequency Catheter Ablation Registry, the transseptal technique was associated with longer fluoroscopy time, although this finding conflicts with those from other reports.[8,11] The CS approach was also an independent variable associated with a longer fluoroscopy time.

By applying these data, patients with left-sided APs will probably enjoy higher success rates, lower complication rates, and shorter fluoroscopy times.

Acknowledgment: We wish to thank Louise Larsen for assisting in the preparation of this chapter.

Appendix I
Members of the Pediatric Electrophysiology Society who Participated in the Transatrial, Retrograde, and Coronary Sinus Catheter Approach Project

Arkansas Children's Hospital
Arrhythmia Associates, Fairfax, VA
Atlanta Children's Heart Center

Boston Children's Hospital

Children's Hospital of Philadelphia

Children's Hospital of Pittsburgh, M.D.
Children's Hospital of San Diego
Children's Hospital of Seattle
Cook Children's Medical Center - Fort Worth

Denver Children's Hospital

Christopher Erickson, M.D.
Margaret Schenck, M.D.
Robert Campbell, M.D.
Edward Hulse, M.D.
Edward Walsh, M.D.
J. Philip Saul, M.D.
Victoria Vetter, M.D.
Larry Rhodes, M.D.
Lee Beerman, M.D.
James Perry, M.D.
Frank Cecchin, M.D.
Paul Gillette, M.D.
Christopher Case, M.D.
Michael Schaffer, M.D.

(continued)

Duke University Medical Center	*Ronald Kanter, M.D.*
Geisinger Medical Center	*Mark Cohen, M.D.*
Loma Linda University	*Jorge McCormack, M.D.*
Mayo Clinic	*Co-burn Porter, M.D.*
Miami University School of Medicine	*Grace Wolff, M.D.*
	Ming-Lon Young, M.D.
Mount Sinai Medical Center	*Steve Fishberger, M.D.*
Oregon Health Science University	*Michael Silka, M.D.*
Primary Children's Medical Center	*Victoria Judd, M.D.*
	Susan Etheridge, M.D.
Rainbow Babies & Children's Hospital	*George Van Hare, M.D.*
South Carolina Children's Heart Center	*Christopher Case, M.D.*
	Paul Gillette, M.D.
Stanford University	*Anne Dubin, M.D.*
SUNY Health Science Center	*Craig Byrum, M.D.*
Tampa General	*Jorge McCormack, M.D.*
Texas Children's Hospital	*Rich Friedman, M.D.*
	Arnold Fenrich, M.D.
Toronto Hospital for Sick Children	*Robert Gow, M.D.*
	Robert Hamilton, M.D.
University of California, Davis	*Jeanny Park, M.D.*
University of California, San Francisco	*George Van Hare, M.D.*
University of Nebraska Medical Center	*John Kugler, M.D.*
Vanderbilt University	*Frank Fish, M.D.*

References

1. Jackman WM, Xunzhang W, Friday KJ, et al. Catheter ablation of accessory atrioventricular pathways (Wolff-Parkinson-White syndrome) by radiofrequency current. N Engl J Med 1991;324:1605–1611.
2. Calkins H, Sousa J, El-Atassi R, et al. Diagnosis and cure of the Wolff-Parkinson-White syndrome or paroxysmal supraventricular tachycardias during a single electrophysiologic test. N Engl J Med 1991;324:1612–1618.
3. Van Hare GF, Lesh MD, Scheinman M, et al. Percutaneous radiofrequency catheter ablation for supraventricular arrhythmias in children. J Am Coll Cardiol 1991;17:1613–1620.
4. Schluter M, Geiger M, Siebels J, et al. Catheter ablation using radiofrequency current to cure symptomatic patients with tachyarrhythmias related to an accessory atrioventricular pathway. Circulation 1991;84:1644–1661.
5. Kuck K-H, Schluter M. Single-catheter approach to radiofrequency current ablation of left-sided accessory pathways in patients with Wolff-Parkinson-White syndrome. Circulation 1991;84:2366–2375.
6. Dick M II, O'Connor BK, Serwer GA, et al. Use of radiofrequency current to ablate accessory connections in children. Circulation 1991;84:2318–2324.
7. Lesh MD, Van Hare GF, Schamp DJ, et al. Curative percutaneous catheter ablation using radiofrequency energy for accessory pathways in all locations: results in 100 consecutive patients. J Am Coll Cardiol 1992; 19:1303–1909.
8. Natale A, Wathen M, Yee R, et al. Atrial and ventricular approaches for radiofrequency catheter ablation of left-sided accessory pathways. Am J Cardiol 1992;70:114–116.
9. Case CL, Gillette PC, Oslizlok PC, et al. Radiofrequency catheter ablation of incessant, medically resistant supraventricular tachycardia in infants and small children. J Am Coll Cardiol 1992;20:1405–1410.
10. Swartz JF, Tracy CM, Fletcher RD. Radiofrequency endocardial catheter ablation of

accessory atrioventricular pathway atrial insertion sites. Circulation 1993;87:487–499.

11. Lesh MD, Van Hare GF, Scheinman MM, et al. Comparison of the retrograde and transseptal methods for ablation of left free wall accessory pathways. J Am Coll Cardiol 1993;22:542–549.

12. Saul JP, Hulse E, De W, et al. Catheter ablation of accessory atrioventricular pathways in young patients: use of long vascular sheaths, the transseptal approach and a retrograde left posterior parallel approach. J Am Coll Cardiol 1993;21:571–583.

13. Manolis AS, Wang PJ, Estes NAM II. Radiofrequency ablation of left-sided accessory pathways: transaortic versus transseptal approach. Am Heart J 1994;128:896–902.

14. Mullins CE. Transseptal left heart catheterization: experience with a new technique in 520 pediatric and adult patients. Pediatr Cardiol 1983;4:239–245.

15. Kuck K-H, Kunze K-P, Schluter M, et al. Modification of a left-sided accessory atrioventricular pathway by radiofrequency current using a bipolar epicaridal-endocardial electrode configuration. Eur Heart J 1988;9:927–932.

16. Fisher JD, Brodman R, Kim SG, et al. Attempted nonsurgical electrical ablation of accessory pathways via the coronary sinus in the Wolff-Parkinson-White syndrome. J Am Coll Cardiol 1984;4:685–694.

17. Morady F, Scheinman MM. Transvenous catheter ablation of a posteroseptal accessory pathway in a patient with the Wolff-Parkinson-White syndrome. N Engl J Med 1984;310:705–707.

18. Morady F, Scheinman MM, Winston ST, et al. Efficacy and safety of transcatheter ablation of posteroseptal accessory pathways. Circulation 1985;72:170–177.

19. Smith RT Jr, Gillette PC, Massumi A, et al. Transcatheter ablative techniques for treatment of the permanent form of junctional reciprocating tachycardia in young patients. J Am Coll Cardiol 1986;8:385–390.

20. Lemery R, Leung TK, Lavallee E, et al. In vitro and in vivo effects within the coronary sinus of nonarcing and arcing shocks using a new system of low-energy DC ablation. Circulation 1991;83:279–293.

21. Connelly DT, Rowland E, Ahsan AJ, et al. Low energy catheter ablation of a posteroseptal accessory pathway associated with a diverticulum of the coronary sinus. PACE 1991;14:1217–1221.

22. Lesh MD, Van Hare G, Kao AK, et al. Radiofrequency catheter ablation for Wolff-Parkinson-White syndrome associated with a coronary sinus diverticulum. PACE 1991; 14:1479–1484.

23. Pedersen AK, Benetis R, Thomsen PEB. A posteroseptal accessory pathway located in a coronary sinus aneurysm: diagnosis and radiofrequency catheter ablation. Br Heart J 1992;68:414–416.

24. Arruda MS, Beckman KJ, McClelland JH. Coronary sinus anatomy and anomalies in patients with posteroseptal accessory pathway requiring ablation within a venous branch of the coronary sinus [Abstract]. J Am Coll Cardiol 1994;1A–484A, 224A.

25. Doig JC, Saito J, Harris L, et al. Coronary sinus morphology in patients with atrioventricular junctional reentry tachycardia and other supraventricular tachyarrhythmias. Circulation 1995;92:436–441.

26. Haissaguerre M, Gaita F, Fischer B, et al. Radiofrequency catheter ablation of left lateral accessory pathways via the coronary sinus. Circulation 1992;86:1464–1468.

27. Giorgberidze I, Saksena S, Krol RB, et al. Efficacy and safety of radiofrequency catheter ablation of left-sided accessory pathways through the coronary sinus. Am J Cardiol 1995;76:359–365.

28. Nakagawa H, Yamanashi WS, Pitha JV, et al. Effective delivery of radiofrequency energy through the coronary sinus without impedance rise using a saline irrigated electrode [Abstract]. J Am Coll Cardiol 1995; 293A.

29. Tebbenjohanns J, Pfeiffer D, Schumacher B, et al. Prospective angiography of the coronary sinus: impact for posteroseptal accessory pathway ablation. PACE 1994;17:741.

30. Arruda M, Otomo K, Tondo C, et al. Coronary sinus angiography using an "occlusion" technique as an aid to RF ablation of epicardial accessory pathways. PACE 1995; 18:833.

31. Tebbenjohanns J, Pfeiffer D, Schumacher B, et al. Direct angiography of the coronary sinus: impact on left posteroseptal accessory pathway ablation. PACE 1996;19: 1075–1081.

32. Kugler JD, Danford DA, Deal B, et al. Radiofrequency catheter ablation in children and adolescents. N Engl J Med 1994;330: 1481–1487.

33. Kugler JD, Houston K, and other participating members of the Pediatric EP Society. Pediatric radiofrequency catheter ablation (RFCA) Registry: update of immediate results [Abstract]. PACE 1995;18(II):814.

34. Kugler J, Danford D, Houston K, et al. Pediatric Radiofrequency Catheter Ablation Registry: update of immediate results. In Imai Y, Momma K, eds. Proceedings of the

2nd World Congress of Pediatric Cardiology and Cardiac Surgery. Armonk, NY, Futura Publishing Co, Inc. 1998.

35. Levine JC, Walsh EP, Saul JP. Radiofrequency ablation of accessory pathways associated with congenital heart disease including heterotaxy syndrome. Am J Cardiol 1993;72:689–693.

36. Leather RA, Leitch JW, Klein GJ, et al. Radiofrequency catheter ablation of accessory pathways: a learning experience. Am J Cardiol 1991;68:1651–1655.

37. Calkins H, El-Atassi R, Kalbfleisch SJ, et al. Effect of operator experience on outcome of radiofrequency catheter ablation of accessory pathways. Am J Cardiol 1993;71:1104–1105.

38. Danford DA, Kugler JD, Deal B, et al. The learning curve for radiofrequency ablation of tachyarrhythmias in pediatric patients. Am J Cardiol 1995;75:587–590.

39. Rosenthal LS, Klein LS, Prystowsky, et al. The relationship between age, fluoroscopy duration, and arrhythmia target: a multicenter study [Abstract]. PACE 1997;20(II);1088.

40. Dick M II, Serwer GS, Armstrong B, et al. Access to left-sided accessory pathways in young patients: transseptal vs. retrograde aortic routes [Abstract]. Circulation 1996;94:I–120.

41. Lau YR, Case CL, Gillette PC, et al. Frequency of atrioventricular valve dysfunction after radiofrequency catheter ablation via the atrial approach in children. Am J Cardiol 1994;74:617–618.

42. Minich LL, Snider AR, Dick M II. Doppler detection of valvular regurgitation after radiofrequency ablation of accessory connections. Am J Cardiol 1992;70:116–117.

43. Kugler JD. Cardiac ablation in pediatric patients. In Zipes D, Jalife J, eds. Cardiac Electrophysiology: From Cell to Bedside. WB Saunders Co, Philadelphia, 1995, pp 1524–1537.

Chapter 5

Ablation of Right Free Wall and Mahaim Accessory Pathways

Dennis W.X. Zhu

Introduction

Radiofrequency (RF) catheter ablation has revolutionized management of patients with paroxysmal supraventricular tachycardia, including those involving an atrioventricular (AV) accessory pathway (AP). The success rate at most centers exceeds 90%. The incidence of complications and rate of recurrence are low. Right free wall APs represent an important subset of APs, accounting for about 14% of all patients in published series.[1-10] In spite of their relatively low occurrence, right free wall APs are at times the most technically challenging ones to be treated successfully with catheter ablation.

The purpose of this chapter is to review the anatomic features related to the right free wall APs, to characterize the electrocardiographic manifestations of the preexcitation, and to discuss the techniques of catheter mapping and ablation of APs located in this region. Patients with Mahaim APs form a distinct subgroup of the preexcitation syndrome. Because of its unique anatomic and electrophysiological characteristics, the mapping and ablation of Mahaim APs will be described in a separate section of this chapter.

Right Free Wall Accessory Pathways

Anatomic Considerations

Right free wall APs are located along the tricuspid annulus except the septal region. Overall, mapping and ablation of the right free wall pathways are more challenging than left free wall pathways for the following reasons: (1) the circumference of the tricuspid annulus is about 2 cm longer than that of the mitral annulus,[11] therefore, longer circumferential distance needs to be covered during mapping the right free wall pathways; (2) the tricuspid valve attaches to the annulus at a much more acute angle than that of the mitral valve, hindering catheter manipulation from mapping the ventricular insertion of the right free wall APs;[12] (3) while left free wall APs can easily be localized by a multielectrode catheter positioned in the coronary sinus, an equivalent venous structure is absent for inserting a catheter to localize right free wall APs. Although the right coronary artery has been used for this purpose in difficult cases, complications can occur, and its value in clinical practice is limited;[12] (4) multiple APs are more commonly located along the tricuspid

From Singer I, Barold SS, Camm AJ (eds): *Nonpharmacological Therapy of Arrhythmias for the 21st Century: The State of the Art.* Futura Publishing Co, Inc., Armonk, NY, © 1998.

annulus than the mitral annulus; and (5) Ebstein's anomaly occurs in about 10% of patients with right-sided APs.[13–15] In Ebstein's anomaly, the tricuspid valve is deformed and the attachments of the tricuspid septal and posterior leaflets are displaced away from the anatomic annulus and extended into the right ventricle.[16,17] The AP, however, bridges the anatomic annulus regardless of where the valve itself is attached.[18] Abnormal endocardial electrograms are often present on the dysplastic tricuspid annulus and interfere with the mapping procedure.[19]

Because of these anatomic features and the likelihood of association with congenital abnormalities, the success rate of catheter ablation of APs in the right free wall is lower and the recurrence rates are higher than those of APs in the left free wall. An echocardiogram is usually recommended prior to the procedure to exclude or establish the diagnosis of Ebstein's anomaly. Since right free wall APs are located distant from the normal AV conduction system, there should be no risk of inadvertent AV block if energy is delivered at the proper location.

Electrocardiographic Features

When ventricular preexcitation is present, the delta wave patterns on the 12-lead electrocardiogram (ECG) have traditionally been used for estimating the ventricular insertion site of the AP. These localization criteria were developed previously by using the relatively coarse intraoperative mapping as the "gold standard."[20–22] Several new ECG criteria for AP localization have been developed recently based on the site of successful catheter ablation as a new "gold standard."[23–27]

Since right free wall APs can be located anywhere along the tricuspid annulus except the septal region, some variations of the surface ECG pattern of preexcitation are expected (Figure 1). Generally (1) the main deflection of the frontal QRS is directed leftward ($15°$ to $-60°$); (2) the main QRS deflec-

tion in leads V_1 to V_3 is predominantly negative resulting in a left bundle branch block-like pattern; (3) the frontal plane delta wave axis is directed toward about $-30°$ ($0°$ to $-60°$) such that negative or biphasic delta waves may be present in leads III and aVF, and positive delta waves are seen in leads I and aVL; and (4) Ebstein's anomaly is sometimes associated with preexcitation from right free wall pathways (Figure 2). It should be pointed out that significant overlapping of preexcitation patterns is present among patients with right anterior free wall, anteroseptal and midseptal pathways and that the differences in the surface ECG are sometimes insufficient enough to distinguish these locations.[26,27] As a result, electrophysiological study and mapping are necessary for the definitive localization.

Electrophysiological Evaluation

A diagnostic electrophysiological study is required to identify the mechanism of clinical tachycardia and to ascertain that the AP is part of the circuit. It is usually performed during a single session followed by mapping and ablation. Ideally, all antiarrhythmic drugs should be discontinued for at least five half-lives prior to the procedure for an accurate assessment of the conduction properties of the normal and abnormal AV connections and to facilitate tachycardia induction. The patient is brought to the cardiac electrophysiology laboratory in the fasting state. After local anesthesia, 6F quadripolar catheters are introduced into the femoral vein using the Seldinger technique and advanced into the right ventricular apex, right atrial appendage, and across the tricuspid valve for recording His bundle potentials.

A coronary sinus electrogram is important in identifying and localizing a left-sided AP that may occasionally coexist with right free wall APs. Usually this is accomplished by introducing a 6F or 7F orthogonal decapolar catheter into the right subclavian or internal jugular vein and position-

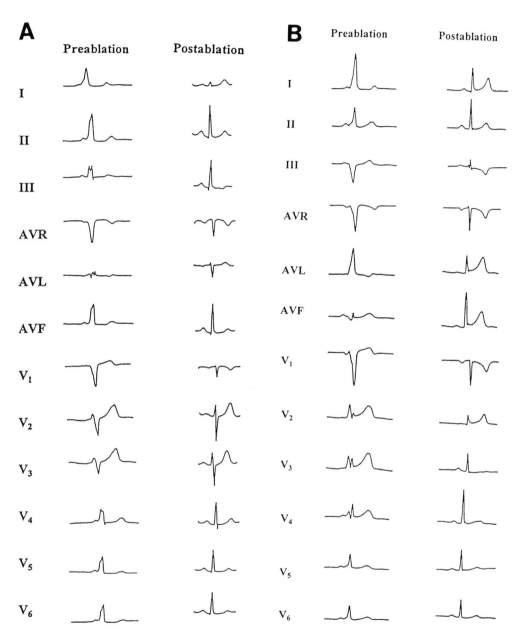

Figure 1. Twelve-lead ECG during sinus rhythm from two patients with a manifest right lateral AP. **(A)** The main deflection of QRS complex is negative in V_1-V_3 and the transition occurs in V_4, giving rise to a left bundle branch block pattern. **(B)** The transition of QRS complex occurs in V_2, mimicking a midseptal pathway. After ablation, the preexcitation is no longer present in either patient.

Preablation   Postablation

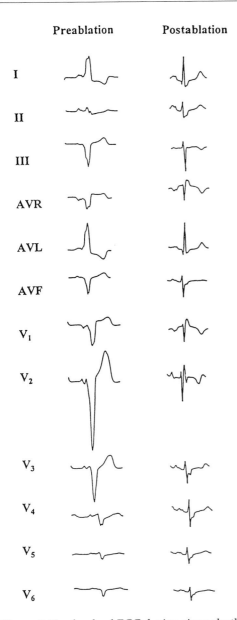

Figure 2. Twelve-lead ECG during sinus rhythm from a patient with a manifest right free wall AP and Ebstein's anomaly. Before ablation, the main QRS deflection in precordial leads is negative throughout. After ablation, an underlying right bundle branch block is shown.

the mapping catheter usually also serves as the ablation catheter, it should have a distal electrode of 4 mm and a deflectable segment. A 7F quadripolar catheter with an interelectrode distance of 2 mm and spacing of 5 mm between the proximal and distal pair of electrodes has been most commonly used. The mapping catheter is usually inserted into the right femoral vein. The venous access sheath should generally be one French size larger than the mapping catheter to allow for easy manipulation. A variety of preformed intravascular long sheaths may be used to stabilize the catheter for optimal mapping. At the preference of the operator, the mapping catheter can also be inserted into the right subclavian or internal jugular vein to facilitate mapping and ablation.

After the catheters are in place, the ventricle is stimulated to study the retrograde conduction property of the AP. Incremental ventricular pacing and single ventricular extrastimulation are performed to assess the pattern of atrial activation, the conduction time of the retrograde impulse, and the retrograde effective refractory period of the AP. Pacing is then performed from the high right atrium. Incremental atrial pacing and single atrial extrastimulation are used to assess the antegrade conduction property of the AP and the patterns of preexcitation.

For the majority of patients with a right free wall AP, reentrant tachycardia is induced during ventricular or atrial pacing. Whenever the reentrant tachycardia is induced, the protocol is interrupted so that the characteristics of the arrhythmia may be studied. The most common tachycardia is orthodromic reciprocating tachycardia. The reentrant circuit uses the AV node and His-Purkinje system as the antegrade limb and the AP as the retrograde limb. Portions of the atrial and ventricular myocardia provide the upper and lower connections, respectively. The retrograde sequence of atrial activation during orthodromic reciprocating tachycardia is useful in identifying the location of the AP. Usually, orthodromic reciprocating tachycardia presents as a nar-

ing it in the coronary sinus so that the proximal pair of electrodes are in the vicinity of the ostium. No heparin is administered routinely unless the patient has recognized risk for thromboembolic complications. Because row QRS complex tachycardia and can be differentiated from AV nodal reentrant tachycardia and atrial tachycardia by resetting the atrial activation with a single premature ventricular stimulus delivered during tachycardia when the His bundle is still refractory from its prior antegrade conduction.[28] Termination of the tachycardia by a single premature ventricular stimulus at a time of His bundle refractoriness without activating the atrium is also indicative of orthodromic reciprocating tachycardia. The occurrence of functional right bundle branch block during orthodromic reciprocating tachycardia will result in VA interval prolongation of 35 sec or greater.[29] If there is minimal prolongation of VA interval with functional right bundle branch block during induced orthodromic reciprocating tachycardia, the AP is likely to be septal rather than in the right free wall.[29] The occurrence of functional left bundle branch block during tachycardia should not affect the VA interval.

When an AP participates in the antegrade conduction during the reentrant tachycardia, the resultant tachycardia is antidromic reciprocating tachycardia. During antidromic reciprocating tachycardia, the QRS complex shows a full degree of preexcitation.[30] Atrial fibrillation, atrial flutter, atrial tachycardia, and AV nodal reentrant tachycardia may occur in patients with a right free wall AP. In this setting, the AP may participate in AV conduction as a bystander. Antidromic reciprocating tachycardia should be distinguished from atrial tachycardia or AV nodal reentrant tachycardia with bystander AP conduction. It is most readily accomplished by introduction of a single premature atrial stimulus near the atrial insertion site of the AP during tachycardia. Such an atrial stimulus introduced at a time when the atrium near the AV node is refractory preexcites the ventricle with a similar QRS morphology, indicating the presence of an AP conducting in the antegrade direction. More importantly, if that preexcited QRS complex is followed by advancement of the next retrograde His

bundle potential and the next atrial activation, antidromic reciprocating tachycardia is confirmed.[31]

Mapping Techniques

General Considerations

The most common fluoroscopic view used for mapping and ablation of the right free wall AP is the left anterior oblique view (LAO) at 40°–60° assisted by the right anterior oblique view (RAO) at 15°–30° (Figure 3). Usually a monoplane fluoroscopy is adequate. Biplane fluoroscopy shortens the transition time from one view to the other but also adds to the cost and the mass of equipment beside the patient. In the LAO projection, the tricuspid annulus is viewed as a clockface, with the His bundle potential recorded at 2:00 and the coronary sinus ostium at 5:00. The mapping catheter is manipulated with clockwise or counterclockwise rotation to move along the tricuspid annulus. The right anterior AP is at the most superior aspect (12:00), the right lateral pathway located at the most lateral aspect (9:00); whereas, the right posterior pathway is at the most inferior aspect (6:00) of the tricuspid annulus.

In our practice, the APs in the right posterior, posterolateral, and lateral regions are initially mapped from the femoral venous approach (Figure 4). The right anterior and anterolateral regions can also be mapped using the femoral venous approach, but alternatively a catheter introduced from the right subclavian vein sometimes may obtain a better tissue contact in these regions (Figure 5). The majority of the right free wall APs can be mapped and ablated by positioning the catheter on the atrial side of the tricuspid annulus. Occasionally, a right free wall AP may be better approached by placing the catheter underneath the tricuspid annulus. To accomplish this, the catheter is introduced across the tricuspid annulus and looped back up in the right ventricle underneath the tricuspid annulus until a small atrial potential and a large ventricular po-

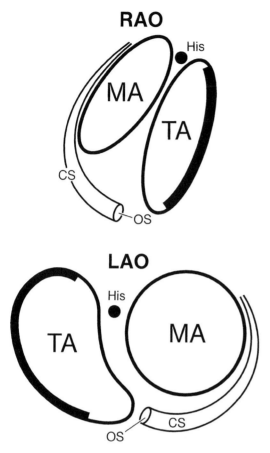

Figure 3. Diagrams of fluoroscopic views commonly used for mapping right free wall APs. In the RAO view, the tricuspid annulus is foreshortened, and the atrioventricular groove is in profile. In the LAO view, the tricuspid annulus is viewed as a clockface, with the His bundle potential recorded at 2:00 and the coronary sinus ostium at 5:00. LAO = left anterior oblique view; RAO = right anterior oblique view; MA = mitral annulus; TA = tricuspid annulus; CS = coronary sinus; OS = ostium.

tential are recorded, confirming its proximity to the ventricular aspect of the tricuspid annulus.

Several parameters have been used to determine the optimal target site for ablation:[32]

1. Earliest Site of Ventricular Activation.

In patients with manifest preexcitation, the site that records the earliest ventricular

activation should be identified. If the QRS complex shows only a minimal delta wave during sinus rhythm, atrial pacing may be used to increase the degree of ventricular preexcitation. A surface ECG lead that clearly shows the delta wave onset can be used as the reference. While a local ventricular activation which coincides with the onset of delta wave is usually acceptable for a target site in left-sided pathways, earlier values are to be found for right free wall APs.

2. Earliest Site of Atrial Activation.

The earliest site of retrograde atrial activation could be identified during orthodromic reciprocating tachycardia or ventricular pacing at a rate associated with exclusive or predominant conduction over the AP. In a patient with an AP that conducts in both directions, the earliest site of retrograde atrial activation usually shows a concordance to the site of earliest ventricular activation. Right-sided pathways are not consistently oblique as they cross the AV groove, as are left-sided pathways.

3. Accessory Pathway Potentials.

Accessory pathway potentials have been characterized as discrete, high-frequency potentials that can arise anywhere along the course of the AP, from the atrial end to the ventricular insertion site, during both antegrade and retrograde activation. AP potentials should precede the onset of the delta wave during antegrade conduction (Figure 6) and precede the onset of atrial activation during retrograde conduction. It may be more easily identified when the bipolar recording is obtained from closely spaced bipoles perpendicular to the annulus and parallel to the course of the AP. Lower amplification may attenuate overlapping atrial and ventricular potentials thus facilitating the recognition of AP potentials. Different pacing maneuvers have been developed to demonstrate that AP potentials are essential for intact AP conduction and can be dissociated from those local atrial and ventricular electrograms.[33]

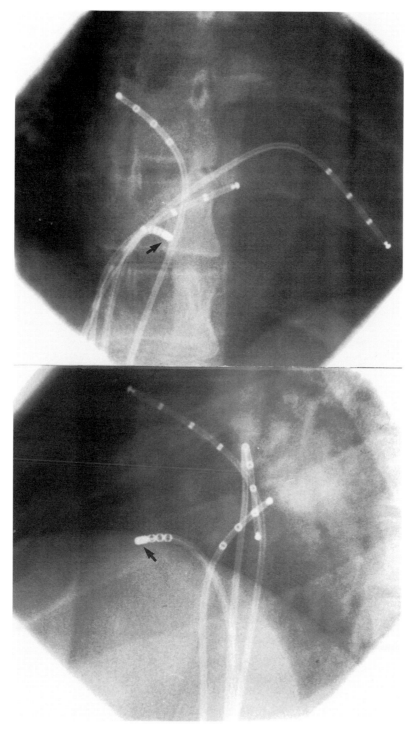

Figure 4. Radiographs of catheter ablation of a right free wall AP. The RAO (upper panel) and LAO (lower panel) views of the intracardiac catheters are illustrated. The mapping/ablation catheter (arrow) is inserted into the right femoral vein and placed at the atrial aspect of the tricuspid annulus.

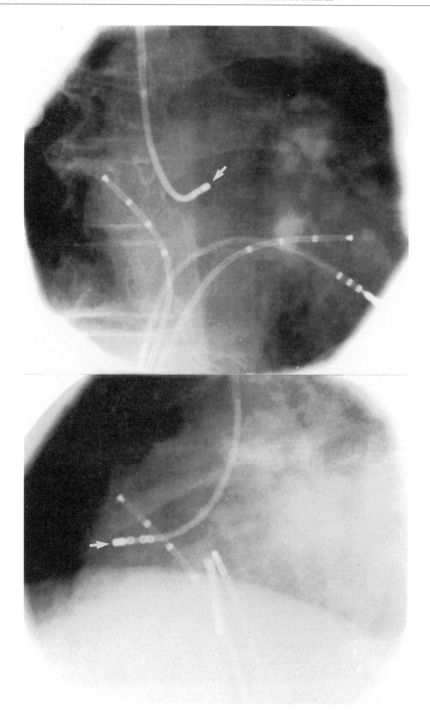

Figure 5. Radiographs of catheter ablation of a right free wall AP with the mapping/ablation catheter (arrow) introduced from the right subclavian vein and positioned at the atrial aspect of the tricuspid annulus. The upper panel is in the RAO view. The lower panel is in the LAO view.

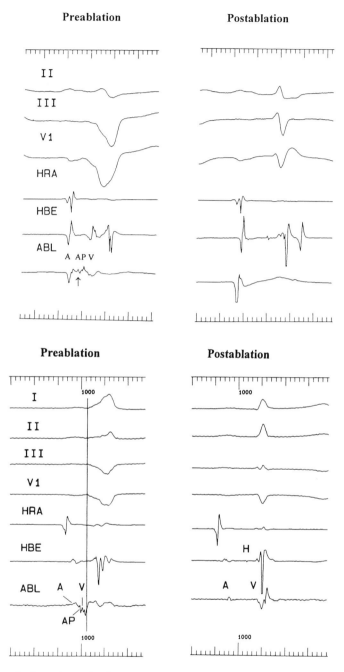

Figure 6. Mapping during sinus rhythm in two patients with a manifest right free wall AP. In the upper left panel (preablation), a large atrial deflection (A), an AP potential (AP), and a small ventricular potential (V) are recorded on the ablation catheter (ABL) positioned at the atrial aspect of the tricuspid annulus. In the lower left panel (preablation), a small atrial deflection (A), an AP potential (AP), and a large ventricular potential (V) are recorded as the ablation catheter (ABL) positioned at the ventricular aspect of the tricuspid annulus. Surface ECG (I, II, III, V_1) and intracardiac electrograms after successful ablation are shown in the right panels. HRA = high right atrium; HBE = His bundle electrogram.

4. Shortest Interval between Local Atrial and Ventricular Electrograms.

At the site where the APs are located, the local AV interval during preexcited sinus rhythm or atrial pacing, and the VA interval during orthodromic reciprocating tachycardia or ventricular pacing are usually less than 60 ms.[34] Frequently, a continuous electrical activity of multiphasic potential is recorded between the local atrial and ventricular electrograms at the site of earliest activation. These potentials may be generated by the AP or by the fusion of the terminal and initial portions of the local atrial and ventricular electrograms.

5. Stability of Local Electrograms.

Stability is considered to be present when AV ratio variation of the local electrograms is less than 10% regardless of the degree of catheter excursion on fluoroscopy. Local electrogram stability implies that the catheter tip is securely positioned against the annular myocardial tissue. A stable local electrogram will increase the likelihood of a successful ablation.

Special Techniques

If positioning and stabilizing the catheter along the tricuspid annulus is difficult, specially designed long sheaths are available to facilitate the catheter manipulation at the different parts of the annulus. A circular "halo" 20-electrode catheter is also available which can be positioned along the tricuspid annulus to expedite endocardial mapping of the right free wall APs.

The right coronary artery has a relatively constant relationship to the anatomic tricuspid annulus along the epicardium and has been used for right free wall AP localization in selected patients.[12] Several investigational mapping catheters have been developed. These catheters have a size of 2F to 3F. Some of the catheters have a central lumen, allowing placement over a standard angioplasty guidewire. An initial coronary angiogram is performed to ensure that the right coronary artery is dominant and that there

are no abnormalities. After full heparization, the mapping catheter is introduced into the right coronary artery and advanced to the crux of the heart and then slowly withdrawn in 0.5- to 1.0-cm increments. Bipolar recordings and measurements are made at each site. Localization of the AP is based on the shortest local AV interval during preexcited sinus rhythm and the shortest VA interval during orthodromic reciprocating tachycardia or ventricular pacing. Once the mapping has been completed, the ablation catheter is manipulated to the endocardial surface of the tricuspid annulus using the radiopaque electrodes on the coronary artery mapping catheter as the marker to direct the placement of the ablation catheter (Figure 7). Intracoronary artery mapping is generally well tolerated. However, serious complications such as inducing coronary artery spasm or ventricular fibrillation have been reported.[12] Thus, this technique should be used only by experienced operators with great caution when conventional mapping attempts have failed. Radiofrequency energy should never be delivered to the mapping catheter in the coronary artery. A follow-up coronary angiogram is mandatory to ascertain that there has been no damage to the artery.

Radiofrequency Ablation

The ablation itself starts once the AP has been precisely localized and a stable catheter position has been achieved. Radiofrequency current is delivered between the catheter tip electrode and an adhesive electrode-surgical dispersive pad applied to the right posterior chest. Temperature-controlled energy delivery is preferred. Studies have shown that ablation catheter temperature monitoring provides important information about the adequacy of tissue heating. Reversible loss of tissue excitability occurs at an average temperature of 43°C. Irreversible tissue injury occurs at a temperature of 50°C.[35] When the temperature at electrode-tissue injuries exceeds 100°C, tissue and plasma protein immediately adja-

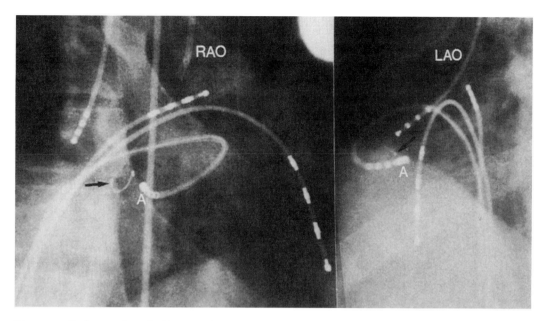

Figure 7. Radiographs of ablation of a right free wall AP guided by a mapping catheter (black arrow) in the right coronary artery. The ablation catheter (A) is advanced into the right ventricle and placed underneath the tricuspid valve for ablating the ventricular insertion of the pathway. RAO = right anterior oblique view; LAO = left anterior oblique view. Reproduced with permission from Lesh MD.[12]

cent to the electrode desiccates to form a coagulum. Inadequate tissue heating is often due to catheter instability. Closed-loop temperature-controlled energy delivery can significantly reduce the incidence of coagulum formation, allowing for application of maximal energy to a given site thus maximizing the lesion size. During current delivery, it is necessary to monitor fluoroscopically the stability of the catheter position. The time required for the temperature to approach the stable state has been estimated to be 2.2 ± 3 sec.[36] We typically preset the temperature at 65°C. In those with preexcitation, RF energy is usually delivered during sinus rhythm or atrial pacing (Figure 8). In patients with APs that conduct bidirectionally or in the retrograde direction only, ablation could be performed during orthodromic reciprocating tachycardia or ventricular pacing at a rate associated with exclusive or predominant conduction over the AP. Radiofrequency energy application is typically interrupted if AP conduction is

not blocked or if tachycardia does not terminate within 15 sec. Radiofrequency delivery should be continued for 30 to 60 sec when the AP block has occurred early during the energy application.

Transient interruption of right free wall AP conduction during RF application is common with subsequent reappearance of conduction seconds to minutes after the energy delivery is terminated. Therefore, the patient should be observed in the electrophysiology laboratory for at least 30 min to make sure that there is no return of AP conduction and that additional applications of RF energy are not needed. Early prediction that RF delivery would be painless was inaccurate, and the discomfort developed in some patients as well as the need to lay still for a prolonged period of time have prompted us to use additional intravenous sedatives and analgesics prior to the beginning of RF application. It is routine for patients to be ambulatory after 4 hours, discharged the same day or after overnight observation,

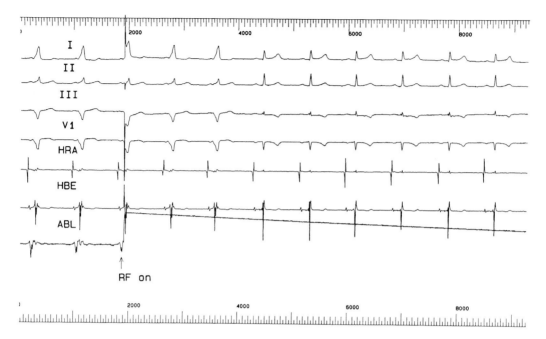

Figure 8. Surface ECG (I, II, III, V_1) showing a sudden loss of preexcitation with radiofrequency application (RF) during sinus rhythm in a patient with a right free wall AP. HRA = high right atrium; HBE = His bundle electrogram; ABL = ablation catheter.

and to return to their usual activities the next day.

Results

The outcome of catheter ablation of right free wall APs in several clinical series are summarized in Table 1. The success rate for catheter ablation of right free wall APs averages 91%. It is lower than those achieved for left free wall pathways (99%), and similar to those for septal pathways (90%). These differences reflect the technical difficulties associated with catheter ablation of right

Table 1
Outcome of Radiofrequency Catheter Ablation of Accessory Pathways at Right Free Wall and Other Locations

Study	Date	Initial Success			Recurrence		
		RFW	Septal	LFW	RFW	Septal	LFW
Jackman et al. (1)	1991	15/15	53/56	106/106	2/15	8/56	5/105
Leather et al. (2)	1991	8/16	10/18	45/47	8/16	8/18	12/47
Lesh et al. (3)	1992	17/21	36/43	44/45	2/17	4/36	2/44
Chen et al. (4)	1993	25/27	40/43	63/69	2/27	3/43	6/69
Kay et al. (5)	1993	57/62	114/123	186/187	5/57	10/125	4/186
Wang et al. (6)	1994	41/41	34/34	164/164	7/41	2/34	6/164
Iesaka et al. (7)	1994	30/30	15/17	88/88	1/30	0/15	0/88
Total		193/212 (91%)	302/334 (90%)	696/706 (99%)	27/203 (13%)	35/327 (11%)	35/703 (5%)

RFW = right free wall; LFW = left free wall

free wall APs. On the other hand, major complications associated with right free wall AP ablation are rare, similar to a routine diagnostic electrophysiological study. Recurrence of right free wall AP conduction after successful catheter ablation is relatively high, ranging from 3% to 50% with a mean recurrence rate of 13%. In our experience pathways that were difficult to ablate initially tended to have a higher recurrence rate. Pathways requiring a longer time for ablation of conduction during RF energy delivery were found to have a higher recurrence. Repeated attempts of ablation will result in successful elimination of AP conduction in most of these patients, although, the incidence of further recurrences tends to be higher. The reason for the lower success and higher recurrence rate in these individuals is not clear. Generally, it is more difficult to maintain the ablation catheter in a stable position along the tricuspid annulus to allow for adequate tissue contact in these patients. As with other procedures, a greater operator experience correlates with higher success rate, shorter ablation time, and fewer complications.

Ebsteins' Anomaly

Ebstein's anomaly is the most common congenital heart abnormality associated with Wolff-Parkinson-White syndrome.[13] Approximately 30% of patients with Ebstein's anomaly have APs.[14] The pathway is usually located around the tricuspid

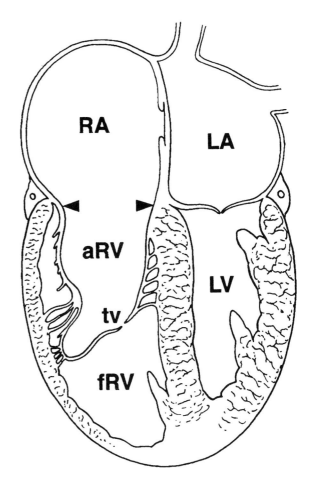

Figure 9. Diagram of Ebstein's anomaly in which abnormally developed tricuspid valve attaches abnormally to an enlarged tricuspid annulus and right ventricle. The attachments of the septal and posterior leaflets are displaced from anatomic tricuspid annulus (black arrows) and tethered toward the right ventricular apex. RA = right atrium; LA = left atrium; LV = left ventricle; RV = right ventricle; tv = tricuspid valve; fRV = functional right ventricle; aRV = atrialized right ventricle.

annulus, and multiple APs are frequently present.[19] Ebstein's anomaly consists of abnormally developed tricuspid valve that is attached abnormally to an enlarged tricuspid annulus and right ventricle. The attachments of the septal and posterior leaflets are displaced from the anatomic tricuspid annulus toward the right ventricular apex (Figure 9).[16–18] The abnormal attachment of the tricuspid valve leaflets produces anatomic separation of the proximal portion of the right ventricular inlet (atrialized portion of the right ventricle) from the right ventric-

ular body. When the catheter tip is positioned in the atrialized portion of the right ventricle, the pressure tracing is atrial but the electrical tracing is ventricular (Figure 10). The AP, however, bridges the anatomic annulus regardless of where the valve itself is attached. Fragmented endocardial electrograms are often present on the dysplastic tricuspid annulus and prevent the clear distinction of local atrial and ventricular electrograms as well as AP potentials during the mapping procedure (Figure 11).[19] Atrial septal defects and other congenital abnor-

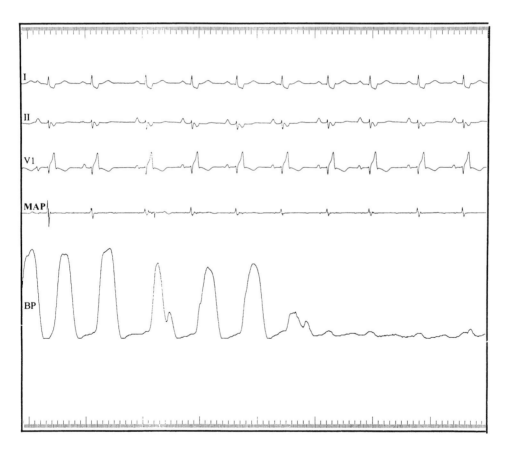

Figure 10. A bipolar catheter with a central lumen for blood pressure recording is initially placed at the right ventricular apex, and then slowly pulled back toward the right atrium. Simultaneous recordings of the intracavitary pressure (BP) and electrograms (MAP) are shown. Although ventricular electrograms are recorded constantly by the catheter during the pullback, the intracavitary pressure changed from right ventricular pressure to right atrial pressure indicating that the catheter has crossed the deformed tricuspid valve and entered the atrialized right ventricle.

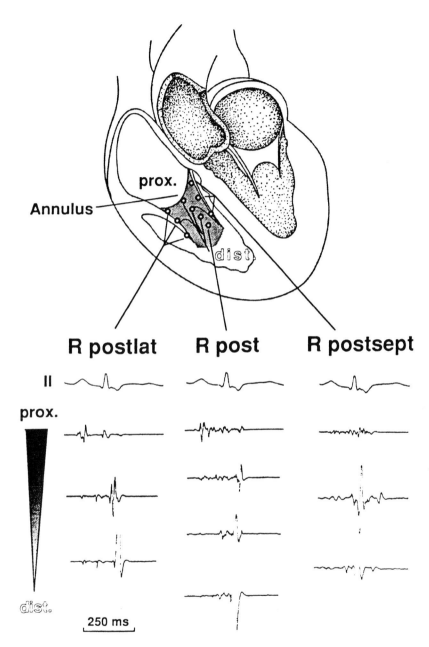

Figure 11. Local electrograms recorded from the dysplastic tricuspid valve area during sinus rhythm in a patient with Ebstein's anomaly and a right-sided AP. Recordings are made from three to four sites between the annulus (prox.) and the attachment of the displaced tricuspid valve (dist.) in the posterolateral (R postlat.), posterior (R post.), and posteroseptal (R postsept) regions. The electrograms at the annulus exhibit continuous fragmentation of local potentials at the posteroseptal and posterior regions but tend to normalize at the posterolateral region. The fragmentation of the electrograms decreases as the catheter is placed more apically (from prox. to dist.) in each region. Reproduced with permission from Cappato R, et al.[51]

malities are commonly associated with Ebstein's anomaly.[17] Pressley et al. reported surgical ablation of 38 patients with Wolff-Parkinson-White syndrome and Ebstein's anomaly.[37] Right-sided APs were present in the majority of the patients. Fifty percent of the patients had multiple APs.

Recently, Cappato and colleagues reported catheter ablation of APs in 21 patients with Ebstein's anomaly and supraventricular tachycardia.[19] Thirty-four right-sided APs were found to be located along the atrialized right ventricle (Figure 12). Eleven of the 21 patients had multiple APs. Local electrograms were normal in 10 patients and fragmented in 11 patients. Atrial extrastimulation during orthodromic tachycardia appeared helpful in dissociating atrial electrograms from ventricular fragmented potentials recorded by the mapping catheter. Right coronary artery mapping was useful in patients in whom APs could not be localized by endocardial mapping. Twenty-

six APs were successfully ablated in 10 patients with normal local electrograms and in 6 of 11 patients with fragmented electrograms. Of the eight APs in the remaining five patients with abnormal electrograms, only two APs could be ablated. During a mean follow-up period of 22 months, five patients who had undergone successful ablation developed clinical recurrences. Factors likely to account for ablation failure included: location of APs along the atrialized right ventricle, and the fragmented endocardial electrograms. Some of these patients also had fragmented epicardial atrial and ventricular electrograms recorded during right coronary artery mapping.

Mahaim Pathways

Evolving Anatomic and Physiological Correlations

In 1938, Mahaim and colleagues described anatomic connections between the

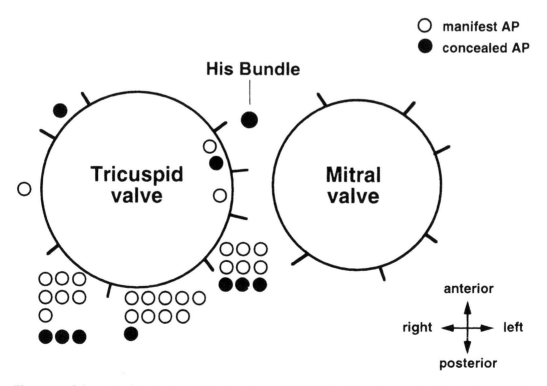

Figure 12. Schematic distribution of the locations of 34 APs in 21 patients with Ebstein's anomaly. Eleven of the 21 patients had multiple pathways. Reproduced with permission from Cappato R, et al.[51]

AV node and the ventricles as well as discrete connections from the fascicles to the ventricles.[38,39] Patients with Mahaim pathways form a special type of the preexcitation syndrome. They have minimal preexcitation during sinus rhythm. Full preexcitation develops during tachycardia which has a left bundle branch block morphology. At electrophysiological study, an AP is identified which exhibits slow and decremental antegrade conduction. Retrograde conduction over the pathway is usually absent. Because of these characteristics, Wellens invoked the concept of a nodoventricular fiber to explain this phenomenon.[40] It was assumed that these aytpical pathways derived their unusual characteristics by virtue of originating from the normal AV node.[41,42]

A classification of Mahaim pathways, based on anatomic insertion sites, was subsequently proposed with nodoventricular pathways linking AV node to the ventricle, nodofascicular pathways connecting AV node to the fascicle and fasciculoventricular pathways joining the distal conduction system to the ventricle.[43]

These concepts remained largely unchallenged until the era of surgical intervention. Gillette and colleagues, in 1982, described a group of patients who were clinically diagnosed to have a nodoventricular pathway but were actually related to an AP ablated surgically at the tricuspid annulus in the free wall region.[44] This observation was confirmed intraoperatively by Klein and others, i.e., that patients with clinical features thought to be nodoventricular Mahaim pathways usually had atriofascicular pathways connecting the right free wall at the tricuspid annulus to the distal fascicular system of the right ventricle or less frequently AV pathways inserted into the right ventricular free wall at the tricuspid annulus with decremental properties.[45,46] Later, high-energy DC shocks were applied through the catheter to ablate the AV node in patients with Mahaim pathway-mediated tachycardia.[47,48] After the AV node has been destroyed, the preexcited tachycardia was

eliminated. However, patients developed fully preexcited QRS complex with a long and decremental AV conduction. This interesting finding suggested that the AV node and Mahaim pathways were anatomically distant from each other. Recently, an increasing number of patients with Mahaim pathways underwent successful RF catheter ablation.[49–53] It is now clear that most pathways exhibiting Mahaim properties are located at the tricuspid annulus along the right free wall. The majority of these pathways have a long anatomic course. The atrial end is located close to the lateral tricuspid annulus. The ventricular end either inserts into the apical region of the right ventricular free wall close to the distal right bundle branch or may link directly with the distal right bundle branch at the right ventricular free wall (Figure 13). A smaller number of Mahaim pathways insert into the right ventricle close to the tricuspid annulus.

Electrophysiological Features

Atriofascicular pathways are associated with unique electrophysiological features. During sinus rhythm, preexcitation on the routine 12-lead ECG is usually minimal or absent. The preexcited QRS complex during atrial pacing has a left bundle branch block morphology and leftward axis and is identical to those seen during spontaneous tachycardia (Figure 14). More preexcitation and a shorter stimulus to QRS interval are seen during pacing from the high right atrium than pacing from the distal coronary sinus at similar cycle lengths. In contrast to the typical AP which has a relatively short conduction time and exhibits all or no conduction when stressed by progressive premature stimulus or rapid rates, the antegrade conduction of a Mahaim pathway is slow and decremental. With incremental atrial pacing, a rate-dependent prolongation of the A to delta interval is demonstrated (Figure 15). Retrograde conduction over the AP

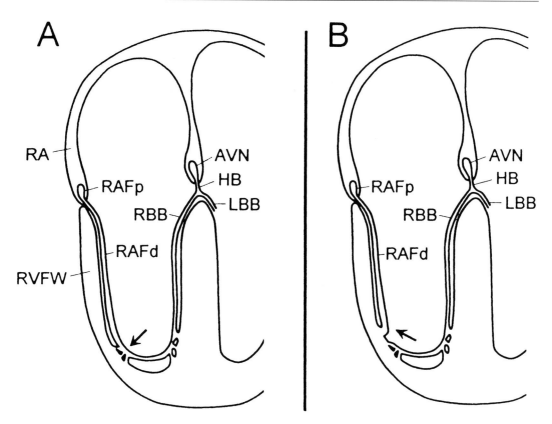

Figure 13. Schematic representation of a right atriofascicular AP consisting of proximal portion (RAFp) which is responsible for the conduction delay and decremental conduction properties, and a long distal segment (RAFd) located along the endocardial surface of the right ventricular free wall which has electrophysiological properties similar to the right bundle branch. The distal end of the right atriofascicular AP might insert into the apical region of the right ventricular free wall close to the distal components of the right bundle branch (arrow, panel **A**), or might fuse with the distal components of the right bundle branch (arrow, panel **B**). AVN = AV node; HB = His bundle; LBB = left bundle branch; RBB = right bundle branch; RVFW = right ventricular free wall; RA = right atrial free wall. Reproduced with permission from Jackman WM, et al.[54]

is usually absent. Unlike typical APs, atriofascicular pathway conduction is usually blocked by adenosine administration. During catheter mapping, the earliest site of ventricular activation during preexcitation is recorded near the right ventricular apex with local activation at or before the onset of the QRS complex on the surface ECG. Antidromic reciprocating tachycardia using the atriofascicular pathway as the antegrade limb and the normal AV conduction system as the retrograde limb is the most commonly observed tachycardia in these patients (Figure 16).[54] A second AP is utilized for retrograde conduction in about

10% of the patients. Patients with Mahaim pathways often have other APs as well as dual AV nodal physiology and AV nodal reentrant tachycardia.

Atrioventricular pathways with decremental conduction resemble atriofascicular pathways electrophysiologically. The two can be differentiated by identifying the earliest site of ventricular activation. During preexcited tachycardia or atrial pacing, the earliest ventricular activation is recorded adjacent to the tricuspid annulus in patients with right atrioventricular APs. Right ventricular apex activation and retrograde His bundle activation occur well after the onset of QRS complex on the surface ECG. In patients with atriofascicular APs, earliest activation occurs close to the apex of the right ventricle and is preceded by a distinct potential representing activation of a distal

segment of the right bundle branch. Catheter-induced right bundle branch block does not effect the antegrade conduction of the AP suggesting that the atriofascicular pathway connects only to the distal components

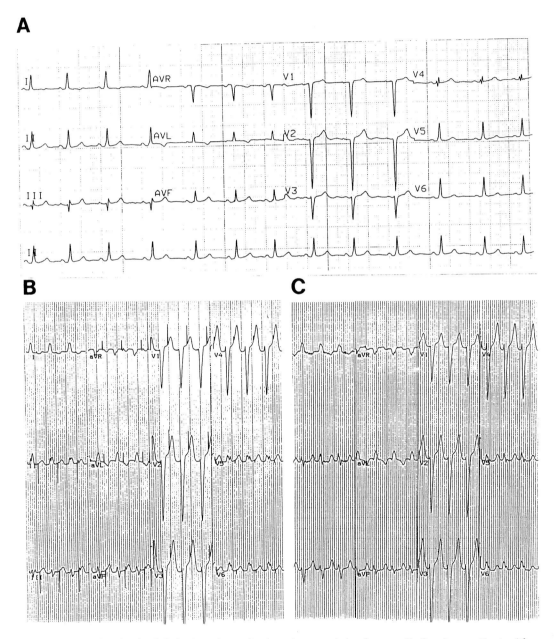

Figure 14. Twelve-lead ECG during sinus rhythm shows minimal preexcitation in a patient with a right atriofascicular pathway **(A)**. The preexcited QRS complex during atrial pacing has a left bundle branch block morphology and leftward axis **(B)**, and is identical to those during spontaneous tachycardia using the atriofascicular pathway **(C)**. Continued.

D

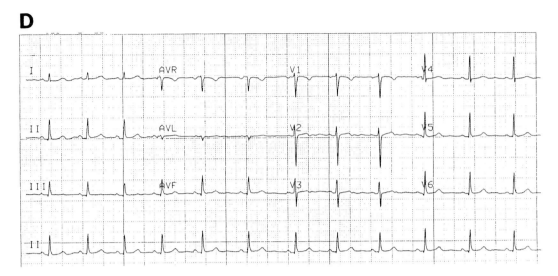

Figure 14. (D) Twelve-lead ECG during sinus rhythm after ablation of the right atriofascicular AP.

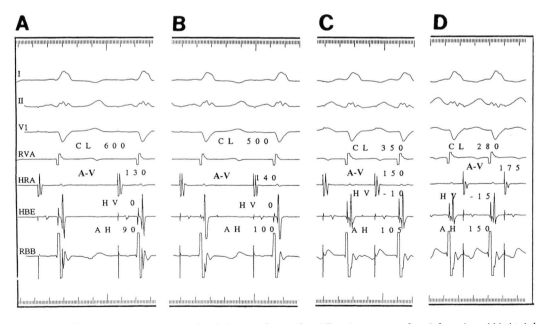

Figure 15. Decremental response of a right atriofascicular AP to incremental atrial pacing. **(A)** Atrial pacing at a cycle length of 600 ms results in an A-V interval of 130 ms, A-H interval of 90 ms, and HV interval of 0 ms. **(B)** Atrial pacing at a cycle length of 500 ms results in an A-V interval of 140 ms, A-H interval of 100 ms, and HV interval of 0 ms. **(C)** Atrial pacing at a cycle length of 350 ms results in an A-V interval of 150 ms, A-H interval of 105 ms, and HV interval of −10 ms. **(D)** Atrial pacing at a cycle length of 280 ms results in an A-V interval of 175 ms, A-H interval of 150 ms, and HV interval of −15 ms. HRA = high right atrium; HBE = His bundle electrogram; RBB = right bundle branch potential; RVA = right ventricular apex.

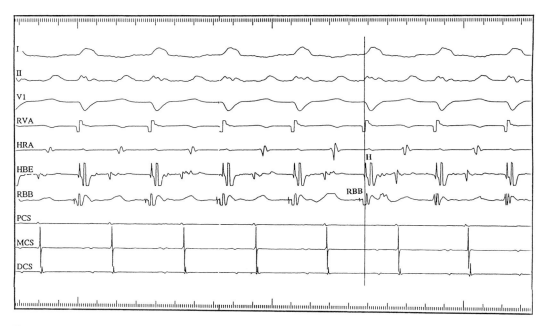

Figure 16. Antidromic reciprocating tachycardia using a right atriofascicular AP for antegrade conduction. Retrograde conduction occurs over the right bundle branch (RBB), His bundle (H), and AV node. The characteristics features of this tachycardia include a left bundle branch block pattern, early ventricular activation at the right ventricular apex, early retrograde activation of the right bundle branch (RBB) and His bundle (H), and a long AV interval resulting from the long antegrade conduction time over the right atriofascicular pathway. Vertical line indicates onset of the QRS complex. HRA = high right atrium; HBE = His bundle electrogram; RBB = right bundle branch; RVA = right ventricular apex; PCS = proximal coronary sinus; MCS = middle coronary sinus; DCS = distal coronary sinus.

of the right bundle branch. Right bundle branch block, however, will increase the tachycardia cycle length and the VA interval since right bundle branch forms part of the retrograde limb of the reentrant circuit of the tachycardia.

During antidromic reciprocating tachycardia, a late extrastimulus can be delivered to the right atrium to differentiate right atriofascicular APs from nodofascicular pathways. The latter, if ever present, is extremely rare. A right atrial extrastimulus should be delivered late enough so that the activation timing at the atrial septum is not advanced and the AV node is not penetrated. Such a right atrial extrastimulus should advance the timing of the next QRS complex without a change in the ventricular activation sequence or the mor-

phology of the QRS complex in a tachycardia utilizing a right atriofascicular AP (Figure 17). When a nodofascicular AP is involved in tachycardia, a late right atrial extrastimulus should not advance the timing of the next QRS complex since the atrium is not part of the reentrant circuit and the atrial extrastimulus does not penetrate the AV node.

Mapping and Ablation

The distinct anatomic and electrophysiological features of atriofascicular pathways make them more difficult to be localized by the conventional techniques used in mapping typical AV APs. Usually, the mapping catheter is introduced either through the right femoral vein or sub-

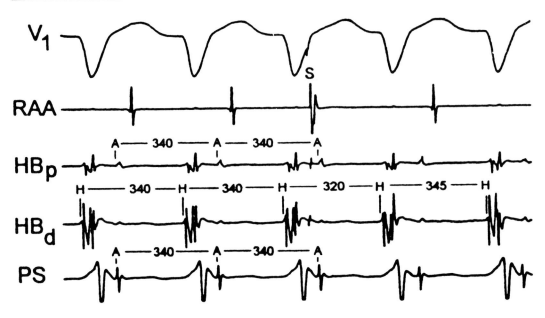

Figure 17. Verification of a right atriofascicular AP participating antidromic reciprocating tachycardia by delivering a late atrial extrastimulus which did not advance the timing of atrial activation in the His bundle electrogram (HBp) (A-A = 340 ms) or in the posterior septum (PS) (A-A = 340 ms) indicating the atrial extrastimulus did not penetrate the AV node. However, the atrial extrastimulus advanced the next ventricular activation by 20 ms (H-H shortened to 320 ms), indicating the presence of an AP with a right atrial connection. Reproduced with permission from Jackman WM, et al.[54]

clavian vein and positioned either above or below the tricuspid valve. Since retrograde conduction over the pathway is usually absent, the mapping is targeted at the antegrade conduction of the pathway and is usually performed during atrial pacing. Because the distal insertion site of the atriofascicular pathway is not at the tricuspid annulus, a search for the earliest ventricular activation along the tricuspid annulus during preexcitation is not useful. Atrial pacemapping at the tricuspid annulus searching for a site providing the shortest A to delta interval was relatively imprecise and technically challenging.[54] Induction of late atrial extrastimulus along the tricuspid annulus during antidromic reciprocating tachycardia to localize the site that results in the greatest advance of the timing of the subsequent QRS complex theoretically corresponds to the atrial insertion of the pathway. Practically, this approach is difficult

and time-consuming.[49] Localization of the atrial insertion of the right atriofascicular pathway by mapping the AP potential has proven to be useful and more precise. In the majority of patients with atriofascicular APs, mapping along the lateral and anterolateral tricuspid annulus during sinus rhythm may record a distinct AP potential which appears similar to a His bundle potential.[50] There are atrial APs and ventricular potentials with relatively long isoelectric intervals between them (Figure 18). It has been shown that the increase in AP conduction time during atrial incremental pacing or atrial extrastimulation occurs between the atrial and AP potentials and is similar to the normal AV conduction system with an AV node, His bundle, and right bundle branch. This has led to the speculation that atriofascicular pathways may represent a secondary or congenitally displaced AV node and His-Purkinje-like conduction system.[41] The AP potential is confirmed by showing a fixed relationship between the potential and the following QRS complex and by demonstrating the loss of the potential during decremental atrial pacing or adenosine administration with the conduction block over the AP.

Cappato and colleagues presented a unique technique of mapping in which a deliberate attempt was made to interrupt conduction of the pathway by catheter manipulation. Radiofrequency energy was delivered at the site of mechanical block after resumption of preexcitation.[51] This technique needs further verification since most electrophysiologists try to avoid bumping the pathway during mapping so that the target for ablation will not be missing for a prolonged period.

We generally use the atrial pacemapping on the tricuspid annulus searching for the site providing the shortest stimulus to delta wave interval. From that site, further detailed mapping is performed to record a Mahaim pathway potential. Theoretically, a right atriofascicular AP can be ablated at any site recording the Mahaim pathway potential from the tricuspid annulus to the apical region of the right ventricular free wall. Targeting the AP ventricular insertion site near the apex is not recommended, since several activation potentials may be present at that region and may be difficult to determine which potential represents the Mahaim pathway potential instead of potentials originating from the distal right bundle branch. Damage producing distal right bundle branch block may be proarrhythmic since retrograde right bundle branch block will increase the VA interval during antidromic reciprocating tachycardia, thus

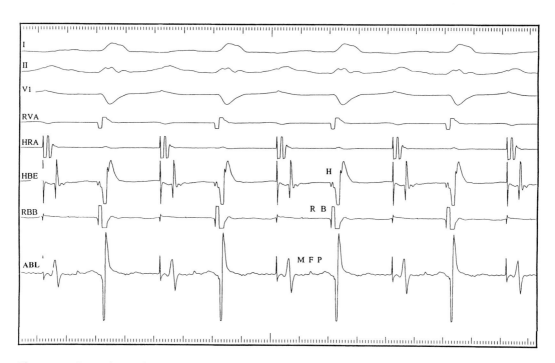

Figure 18. Recording of Mahaim fiber potential (MFP), a right atriofascicular AP potential, at the lateral tricuspid annulus by the ablation catheter (ABL) during atrial pacing. The discrete atrial, AP, and ventricular potentials with relatively long isoelectric intervals between them produce an electrogram appearing similar to the His bundle. Radiofrequency energy delivery at this site successfully eliminate the AP conduction. HBE = His bundle potential; RBB = right bundle branch potential; HRA = high right atrium; RVA = right ventricular apex.

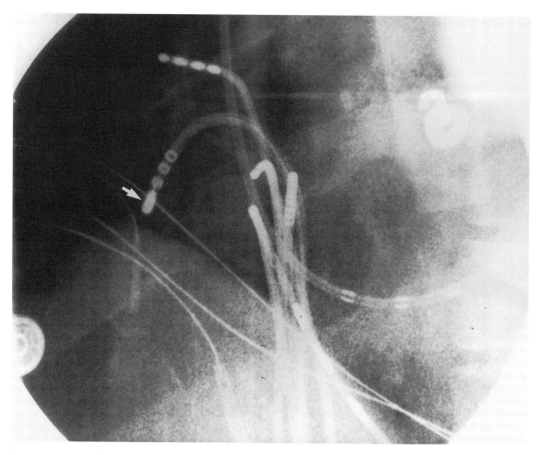

Figure 19. Radiogram in the left anterior oblique view during the successful ablation of a right atriofascicular AP via the femoral approach. The ablation catheter (arrow) is positioned at the atrial aspect of the lateral tricuspid annulus.

making the tachycardia more easy to start and sustain. Therefore, RF catheter ablation of right atriofascicular APs should be performed at the tricuspid annulus guided by a pathway potential (Figure 19). When the AP is traumatized by catheter manipulation, it is associated with loss of the Mahaim potential at the block site and at the site distal to the block site. The Mahaim potential can usually still be recorded at the tricuspid annulus and along the AP proximal to the site of block. If AP conduction does not return, ablation may be performed at sites recording the Mahaim potential proximal to the block site.[54] Radiofrequency energy delivery is usually applied either during right atrial pacing or during antidromic recipro-

cating tachycardia to detect loss of pathway conduction (Figure 20).

Results

Table 2 summarizes the results of catheter ablation of the Mahaim pathways using a variety of techniques. The overall success rate is 94%. Ninety-five percent of the APs are located in the right free wall regardless of whether they are atriofascicular or atrioventricular. No significant complications occurred. Recurrence of AP conduction occurred in two patients but the conduction was successfully eliminated during subsequent procedures.

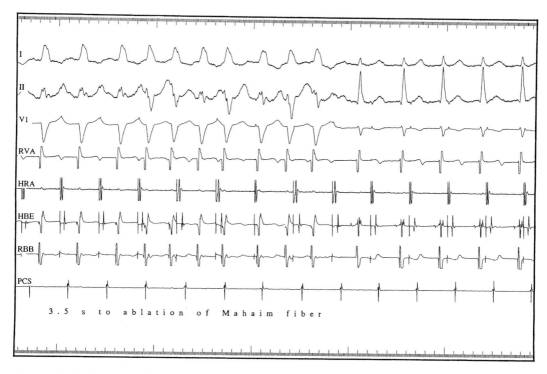

Figure 20. Catheter ablation of a right atriofascicular AP during atrial pacing. Pathway conduction block occurred 3.5 sec after the onset of energy delivery.

Summary

Successful catheter ablation of right free wall APs can at times challenge even an experienced interventional electrophysiologist. Certain anatomic features, the presence of multiple pathways, and the likelihood of associated congenital abnormalities such as Ebstein's anomaly can all increase the technical difficulties, thus giving a lower success rate and a higher recurrence rate. Adequate training, careful preparation, and appropriate use of special catheters and techniques should improve the outcome of the procedure. The majority of Mahaim APs (antegrade conduction only, long conduc-

Table 2
Outcome of Radiofrequency Catheter Ablation of Mahaim Accessory Pathways

Study	Date	Patient (n)	AF	AV	Success (%)	Compli-cations	Recurrence (%)	Mapping Techniques
Klein et al. (49)	1993	4	3	1	4 (100%)	0	0	Stim to Δ interval
McClelland et al. (50)	1994	26	23	3	26 (100%)	0	0	Mahaim potentials
Grogin et al. (52)	1994	6	4	2	6 (100%)	0	0	Mahaim potentials
Cappato et al. (51)	1994	11	11	—	9 (82%)	0	1 (10%)	Mechanical block
Heald et al. (53)	1995	20	16	4	18 (90%)	0	1 (5%)	Mahaim potentials
Total		67	57	10	63 (94%)	0	2 (3%)	

— = unspecified; AF = atriofascicular pathways; AV = atrioventricular pathways; Stim = stimulus.

tion time, and decremental properties) are located along the right free wall. Most of these pathways connect the lateral right atrium to the distal components of the right bundle branch and may represent a duplication of the AV conduction system. Successful ablation is usually guided by a distinct Mahaim pathway potential.

Acknowledgments: The author wishes to thank Dr. Huabin Sun for his contribution in preparing the figures for this manuscript and to Marianne Anderson for her excellent secretarial assistance.

References

1. Jackman WM, Wang XZ, Friday KJ, et al. Catheter ablation of accessory atrioventricular pathways (Wolff-Parkinson-White syndrome) by radiofrequency current. N Engl J Med 1991;324:1605–1611.
2. Leather RA, Leitch JW, Klein GJ, et al. Radiofrequency catheter ablation of accessory pathways: a learning experience. Am J Cardiol 1991;68:1651–1655.
3. Lesh MD, Van Hare GF, Schamp DJ, et al. Curative percutaneous catheter ablation using radiofrequency energy for accessory pathways in all locations: results in 100 consecutive patients. J Am Coll Cardiol 1992;19:1303–1309.
4. Chen SA, Chiang CE, Chiou CW, et al. Serial electrophysiological studies in the late outcome of radiofrequency ablation for accessory atrioventricular-mediated tachyarrhythmias. Eur Heart J 1993;14:734–743.
5. Kay GN, Epstein AE, Dailey SM, et al. Role of radiofrequency ablation in the management of supraventricular arrhythmias: experience in 760 consecutive patients. J Cardiovasc Electrophysiol 1993;4:371–389.
6. Wang L, Hu D, Ding Y, et al. Predictors of early and late recurrence of atrioventricular accessory pathway conduction after apparently successful radiofrequency catheter ablation. Int J Cardiol 1994;46:61–65.
7. Iesaka Y, Takahashi A, Chun Y, et al. Radiofrequency catheter ablation of atrioventricular accessory pathways in Wolff-Parkinson-White syndrome with drug-refractory and symptomatic supraventricular tachycardia—its high effectiveness irrespective of accessory pathway location and properties. Jpn Circ J 1994;58:767–777.
8. Calkins H, Langberg J, Sousa J, et al. Radiofrequency catheter ablation of accessory atrioventricular connections in 250 patients: abbreviated therapeutic approach to Wolff-Parkinson-White syndrome. Circulation 1992;85:1337–1346.
9. Swartz JF, Tracy CM, Fletcher RD. Radiofrequency endocardial catheter ablation of accessory atrioventricular pathway atrial insertion sites. Circulation 1993;87:487–499.
10. Haissaguerre M, Gaita F, Marcus FI, et al. Radiofrequency catheter ablation of accessory pathways: a contemporary review. J Cardiovasc Electrophysiol 1994;5:532–552.
11. Sunderman F. Normal Values in Clinical Medicine. WB Saunders, Philadelphia, PA, 1950.
12. Lesh MD. Ablation of right free wall atrioventricular accessory pathways. In Huang SKS, ed. Radiofrequency Catheter Ablation of Cardiac Arrhythmias: Basic Concepts and Clinical Applications. Futura Publishing Company Co, Armonk, New York, 1995, pp 311–334.
13. Kastor JA, Goldreyer BN, Josephson ME, et al. Electrophysiologic characteristics of Ebstein's anomaly of the tricuspid valve. Circulation 1975;52:987–995.
14. Smith WM, Gallagher JJ, Kerr CR, et al. The electrophysiologic basis and management of symptomatic recurrent tachycardia in patients with Ebstein's anomaly of the tricuspid valve. Am J Cardiol 1982;49:1223–1234.
15. Colavita PG, Packer DL, Pressley JC, et al. Frequency, diagnosis and clinical characteristics of patients with multiple accessory atrioventricular pathways. Am J Cardiol 1987;59:601–606.
16. Ebstein W. Über einen sehr seltenen Fall von Insuffizienz der Valvula tricuspidalis, bedingt durch eine angeborene hochgradige Missbildung derselben. Arch Anat Physiol Wissensch Med 1866;238–254.
17. Giuliani ER, Fuster V, Brandenburg RO, et al. Ebstein's anomaly: the clinical features and natural history of Ebstein's anomaly of the tricuspid valve. Mayo Clinic Proc 1979;54:163–173.
18. Becker AE, Anderson RH, Durrer D, et al. The anatomical substrates of the Wolff-Parkinson-White syndrome: a clinicopathologic correlation in seven patients. Circulation 1978;57:870–879.
19. Cappato R, Schlüter M, Weiss C, et al. Radiofrequency current catheter ablation of accessory atrioventricular pathways in Ebstein's anomaly. Circulation 1996;94:376–383.
20. Tonkin AM, Wagner GS, Gallagher JJ, et al.

Initial forces of ventricular depolarization in the Wolff-Parkinson-White syndrome: analysis based upon localization of the accessory pathway by epicardial mapping. Circulation 1975;52:1030–1036.

21. Milstein S, Sharma AD, Guiraudon GM, et al. An algorithm for the electrocardiographic localization of accessory pathways in the Wolff-Parkinson-White syndrome. PACE 1987;10:555–563.

22. Reddy GV, Schamroth L. The localization of bypass tracts in the Wolff-Parkinson-White syndrome from the surface electrocardiogram. Am Heart J 1987;113:984–993.

23. Fitzpatrick AP, Gonzales RP, Lesh MD, et al. New algorithm for the localization of accessory atrioventricular connections using a baseline electrocardiogram. J Am Coll Cardiol 1994;23:107–116.

24. Arruda M, Wang X, McClelland J, et al. ECG algorithm for predicting radiofrequency ablation site in posteroseptal accessory pathways [Abstract]. PACE 1992;15:535.

25. Xie B, Heald SC, Bashir Y, et al. Localization of accessory pathways from the 12-lead electrocardiogram using a new algorithm. Am J Cardiol 1994;74:161–165.

26. Scheinman MM, Wang YS, Van Hare GF, et al. Electrocardiographic and electrophysiologic characteristics of anterior, midseptal and right anterior free wall accessory pathways. J Am Coll Cardiol 1992;20:1220–1229.

27. Chiang CE, Chen SA, Teo WS, et al. An accurate stepwise electrocardiographic algorithm for localization of accessory pathways in patients with Wolff-Parkinson-White syndrome from a comprehensive analysis of delta waves and R/S ratio during sinus rhythm. Am J Cardiol 1995;76:40–46.

28. Zhu DWX, Maloney JD. Radiofrequency catheter ablative therapy for atrioventricular nodal reentrant tachycardia. In Singer I, ed. Interventional Electrophysiology. Williams & Wilkins, Baltimore, 1996, pp 275–316.

29. Kerr CR, Gallagher JJ, German LD. Changes in ventriculoatrial intervals with bundle branch block aberration during reciprocating tachycardia in patients with accessory atrioventricular pathways. Circulation 1982; 66:196–201.

30. Brady GH, Packer DL, German LD, et al. Pre-excited reciprocating tachycardia in patients with Wolff-Parkinson-White syndrome: incidence and mechanism. Circulation 1984;70: 377–391.

31. Packer DL, Prystowsky EN. Anatomical and physiological substrate for antidromic reciprocating tachycardia. In DP Zipes, Jalife J, eds. Cardiac Electrophysiology: From Cell to Bedside. Philadelphia, WB Saunders Company, 1990, pp 655–666.

32. Zhu DWX. Radiofrequency catheter ablative therapy for anteroseptal and midseptal accessory atrioventricular pathways. In Singer I, ed. Interventional Electrophysiology. Williams & Wilkins, Baltimore, 1996, pp 253–273.

33. Jackman WM, Kuck KH, Friday KJ, et al. Catheter recordings of accessory atrioventricular pathway activation. In DP Zipes, Jalife J, eds. Cardiac Electrophysiology: From Cell to Bedside. WB Saunders, Philadelphia, 1990, pp 491–502.

34. Haissaguerre M, Clémenty J, Warin JF. Catheter ablation of atrioventricular reentrant tachycardias. In DP Zipes, Jalife J, eds. Cardiac Electrophysiology: From Cell to Bedside, WB Saunders, Philadelphia, 1995, pp 1487–1499.

35. Nath S, Lynch C, Whayne JG, et al. Cellular electrophysiological effects of hyperthermia on isolated guinea pig papillary muscle: implications for catheter ablation. Circulation 1993;88:1826–1831.

36. Langberg JJ, Calkins H, El-Atassi R, et al. Temperature monitoring during radiofrequency catheter ablation of accessory pathways. Circulation 1992;86:1469–1474.

37. Pressley JC, Wharton JM, Tang AS, et al. Effect of Ebstein's anomaly on short- and long-term outcome of surgically treated patients with Wolff-Parkinson-White syndrome. Circulation 1992;86:1147–1155.

38. Mahaim I, Benatt A. Nouvelles recherches sur les connexions superieures de la branche gauche du fasiceau de His-Tawara avec cloison interventriculaire. Cardiologia 1938;1: 61–76.

39. Mahaim I, Winston MR. Recherches d'pranatomie comparée et de pathologie experimentale sur les connexions hautes du faisceau de His-Tawara. Cardiologia 1941;5:189–260.

40. Wellens HJJ. Tachycardias related to the pre-excitation syndrome. In: Electrical Stimulation of the Heart in the Study and Treatment of Tachycardias. University Park Press, Baltimore, 1971, pp 97–109.

41. Gallagher JJ, Smith WM, Kasel JH, et al. Role of Mahaim fibers in cardiac arrhythmias in man. Circulation 1981;64:176–189.

42. Lerman BB, Waxman HL, Proclemer A, et al. Supraventricular tachycardia associated with nodoventricular and concealed atrioventricular bypass tracts. Am Heart J 1982; 104:1097–1102.

43. Anderson RH, Becker AE, Brechenmacher C, et al. Ventricular preexcitation: a proposed nomenclature for its substrates. Eur J Cardiol 1975;3:27–36.

44. Gillette PC, Garson A Jr, Cooley DA, et al. Prolonged and decremental antegrade conduction properties in right anterior accessory connections: Wide QRS antidromic tachycardia of left bundle branch block pattern without Wolff-Parkinson-White configuration in sinus rhythm. Am Heart J 1982;103:66–74.

45. Klein GJ, Guiraudon GM, Kerr CR, et al. "Nodoventricular" accessory pathway: evidence for a distinct accessory atrioventricular pathway with atrioventricular node-like properties. J Am Coll Cardiol 1988;11: 1035–1040.

46. Tchou P, Lehmann MH, Jazayeri M, et al. Atriofascicular connection or a nodoventricular Mahaim fiber? Electrophysiologic elucidation of the pathway and associated reentrant circuit. Circulation 1988;77:837–848.

47. Bhandari A, Morady F, Shen EN, et al. Catheter-induced His bundle ablation in a patient with reentrant tachycardia associated with a nodoventricular tract. J Am Coll Cardiol 1984;4:611–616.

48. Ellenbogen KA, O'Callaghan WG, Colavita PG, et al. Catheter atrioventricular junction ablation for recurrent supraventricular tachycardia with nodoventricular fibers. Am J Cardiol 1985;55:1227–1229.

49. Klein LS, Hackett FK, Zipes DP, et al. Radiofrequency catheter ablation of Mahaim fibers at the tricuspid annulus. Circulation 1993;87: 738–747.

50. McClelland JH, Wang X, Beckman KJ, et al. Radiofrequency catheter ablation of right atriofascicular (Mahaim) accessory pathways guided by accessory pathway activation potentials. Circulation 1994;89: 2655–2666.

51. Cappato R, Schluter M, Weiss C, et al. Catheter-induced mechanical conduction block of right-sided accessory fibers with Mahaim-type preexcitation to guide radiofrequency ablation. Circulation 1994;90:282–290.

52. Grogin HR, Lee RJ, Kwasman M, et al. Radiofrequency catheter ablation of atriofascicular and nodoventricular Mahaim tracts. Circulation 1994;90:272–281.

53. Heald SC, Davies DW, Ward DE, et al. Radiofrequency catheter ablation of Mahaim tachycardia by targeting Mahaim potentials at the tricuspid annulus. Br Heart J 1995;73: 250–257.

54. Jackman WM, McClelland JH, Nakagawa H, et al. Ablation of right atriofascicular (Mahaim) accessory pathways. In Zipes DP, ed. Catheter Ablation of Arrhythmias. Futura Publishing Co., Armonk, NY, 1994, pp 187–210.

Chapter 6

Catheter Ablation of Anteroseptal and Midseptal Accessory Pathways

Hugh Calkins

Introduction

Since the first introduction of catheter ablation as a therapeutic tool for use in the treatment of cardiac arrhythmias in 1982[1,2] and the first report of successful catheter ablation of an accessory pathway (AP) using direct current energy in 1983,[3] radiofrequency (RF) catheter ablation has emerged as a first-line therapy for the treatment of many cardiac arrhythmias including the Wolff-Parkinson-White syndrome and paroxysmal supraventricular tachycardia involving an AP. Accessory pathways can be classified according to their location, direction of conduction (manifest or concealed), and rate of conduction (decremental or nondecremental, rapid or slow conduction). The purpose of this chapter is to review the technique, results, and complications associated with RF catheter ablation of anteroseptal and midseptal APs. Anteroseptal and midseptal APs are uncommon, accounting for less than 10% of APs among 11 published ablation series[4-15] (Tables 1, 2). Their importance rests primarily on the increased risk of developing AV block as a complication of catheter ablation as a result of the close proximity of these APs to the specialized conduction system. Because of this, particular attention will be focused on reviewing the anatomy of the anteroseptal and midseptal space and also discussing potential techniques for reducing the risk of AV block.

Anatomic Considerations

The location of APs have historically been subdivided into four regions of the heart: right free wall, left free wall, anteroseptal, and posteroseptal.[16,17] Although these descriptions were adequate in the era of surgical ablation, the era of RF catheter ablation has brought about a renewed interest in the localization of APs to more precise regions of the heart. Perhaps the most commonly used approach today is to divide the myocardial regions surrounding the tricuspid and mitral annuli into 13 regions, as would be visualized using the left anterior oblique (LAO) fluoroscopic projection of the heart (Figure 1). APs can be located anywhere along the tricuspid or mitral annulus with the exception of the area along the anterior leaflet of the mitral valve which lies in direct continuity with the aortic valve (thus no ventricular myocardium is present in this area). According to this schema, midseptal

From Singer I, Barold SS, Camm AJ (eds): Nonpharmacological Therapy of Arrhythmias for the 21st Century: The State of the Art. Futura Publishing Co, Inc., Armonk, NY, © 1998.

Table 1
Catheter Ablation of Anteroseptal Accessory Pathways

Study	No. of Pts.	Incidence	Approach (IVC/SVC)	Approach (A/V)	Success n (%)	AV Block n	Other AV Block n	RBBB n	Recurrence n (%)
Jackman (5)	13	8%	SVC	V	13 (100%)	0	0	5	2 (15%)
Lesh (6)	7	6%	IVC	V	7 (100%)	0	0	3	0 (0%)
Calkins (4)	10	4%	IVC		8 (80%)	2	0	0	
Swartz (7)	10	8%	IVC	A	9 (90%)	0	0		0
Kay (8)	19	5%	IVC or SVC	V	19 (100%)	0	0		0
Yeh (14)	11	4%	IVC		9 (82%)	0	3	4	
Haissaguerre (9)	8	1%	IVC or SVC	V	8 (100%)	0	0	1	0
Satake (10)	10		IVC	V	10 (100%)	0	0	0	0
Xie (11)	6		IVC		5 (83%)	0	0	0	
Schluter (13)	12	8%	SVC	A	12 (100%)	0	0	2	1 (10%)
Total	106				100 (94%)	2 (2%)	3 (3%)	15 (15%)	3 (3%)

See text for abbreviations.

APs are defined as those which lie anterior to the coronary sinus os and posterior to a catheter positioned to record a His bundle potential. Anteroseptal APs are defined as those which lie in close proximity to or immediately anterior to the His bundle. It is generally accepted that the term *anteroseptal accessory pathways* should be reserved for the subset of APs that have a His potential associated with the atrial or ventricular insertion of the AP (as evidenced by the presence of an AP potential or earliest activation) (Figure 2). Haissaguerre and colleagues have proposed that the term *para-Hisian accessory pathway* be reserved for the small subset of anteroseptal APs whose atrial and ventricular insertions are associated with a large His bundle (>0.1 mV) with virtually no distance between the tip electrode of the ablation catheter and the His bundle catheter in any fluoroscopic view.[9]

While this simplified scheme for AP localization has gained widespread acceptance among the community of interventional electrophysiologists, a potential risk of this simplified approach is that it does not draw

Table 2
Catheter Ablation of Midseptal Accessory Pathways

Study	No. of Pts.	Incidence	Approach (IVC/SVC)	Approach (A/V)	Success n (%)	AV Block n	Other AV Block n	RBBB n	Recurrence n (%)
Lesh (6)	6	6%	IVC	V	6 (100%)	0	0	0	2 (33%)
Calkins (4)	5	2%	IVC		5 (100%)	0	0	0	0
Swartz (7)	11	9%	IVC	A	11 (100%)	1		0	
Kay (8)	12	3%	IVC or SVC	V	11 (92%)	0	1	np	
Yeh (14)	3	1%	IVC		1 (33%)	1	1	0	
Satake (10)	7		IVC	V	7 (100%)	0	0	0	0
Xie (11)	20		IVC		17 (85%)	2	0	0	
Kuck (15)	6	4%	SVC	A	6 (100%)	0	0	0	1 (17%)
Lorga (12)	15		IVC		15 (100%)	0	0	0	3 (20%)
Total	85				79 (84%)	4 (5%)	2 (3%)		6 (8%)

See text for abbreviations.

His Bundle

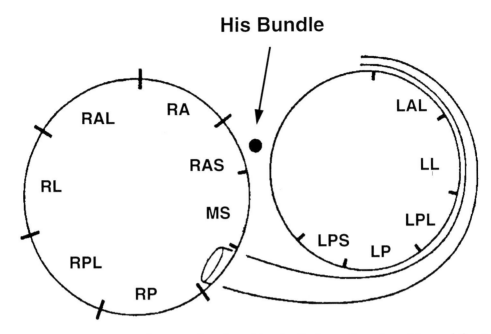

Figure 1. Schematic drawing depicting the tricuspid and mitral annuli as viewed from a left anterior oblique projection. The standard classification of the location of APs into 13 distinct anatomic regions is shown.

attention to the anatomic complexity of the midseptal and anteroseptal space.[18,19] Shown in Figure 3 is a series of dissections created by removing the segment of the heart where the atrial musculature inserts into the ventricular mass. It can be appreciated that the aortic valve is in effect wedged between the mitral and the tricuspid valves and interposes between the tricuspid and the pulmonary orifices. The leaflets of the mitral and aortic valves are in fibrous continuity, with the fibrous tissue at each end thickened to form the right and left fibrous trigones. The central fibrous body is formed from right fibrous trigone plus the membranous septum. It can be appreciated that APs cannot lie in the region of the fibrous connection between the mitral and aortic valves because there is no potential continuity between the atrium and ventricle in this region. Because the septal leaflet of the tricuspid valve inserts more apically than the septal attachments of the mitral valve, a muscular atrioventricular (AV) septum exists between the right atrium and the left

ventricle. Anterior to this muscular AV septum is a fibrous AV septum, which is part of the membranous septum and together with the right fibrous trigone forms the central fibrous body, which is the keystone of the cardiac fibrous skeleton. It is the regions anterior and posterior to these AV septal components that have been referred to as anteroseptal and posteroseptal, respectively.

The term AV junction refers to the AV myocardial continuity that allows atrial impulses to be transmitted to the ventricular myocardium via the normal AV node and His bundle system. The compact AV node lies at the apex of the triangle of Koch and rests on the atrial aspect of the central fibrous body. The triangle of Koch is bordered superiorly by the tendon of Todaro and inferiorly by the annular extent of the septal tricuspid leaflet; it contains the ostium of the coronary sinus in its posterior part (Figure 4). The tendon of Todaro merges with the central fibrous body at the anterior tip of Koch's triangle. In humans it has been estimated that the compact AV

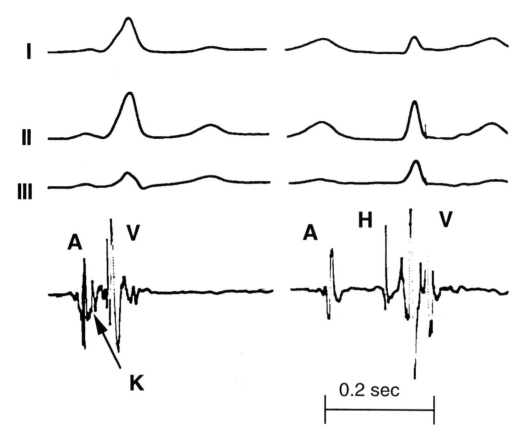

Figure 2. Local electrogram recorded at the successful ablation site of an anteroseptal AP. Note the presence of an AP potential during preexcited rhythm as well as a large His potential which can be observed following spontaneous block in the AP. Whenever possible the size of the His potential should be <0.1 mV at sites of RF energy delivery.

node is between 1.7 and 3 mm in length.[19] More anteriorly, the conduction axis becomes surrounded by a fibrous collar as it penetrates the central fibrous body to become the bundle of His, which is between 1 and 1.5 cm in length. The penetrating bundle then branches as it arrives at the summit of the ventricular septum. The proximal portions of the ventricular bundle branches are encased by a thin sheath of fibrous tissue. The Wolff-Parkinson-White syndrome is associated with myocardial AV connections distinct from the normal AV node-His bundle system, which allows the atrial or ventricular impulses to bypass the normal AV junction.

When considered from this anatomic perspective, it can be appreciated that the mid-septum is in reality the only true area of muscular septal contiguity in the AV junction and represents the area between the offset attachments of the leaflets of the mitral and tricuspid valves. This area can therefore also be identified as the muscular AV septum. The triangle of Koch lies on its atrial surface and contains the compact portion of the AV node and the zone of transitional fibers. The bundle of His, which penetrates the AV membranous septum to reach the crest of the muscular ventricular septum, lies at its apex. The anteroseptal and posteroseptal areas could be more accurately described as the areas anterior and posterior to the true septum.

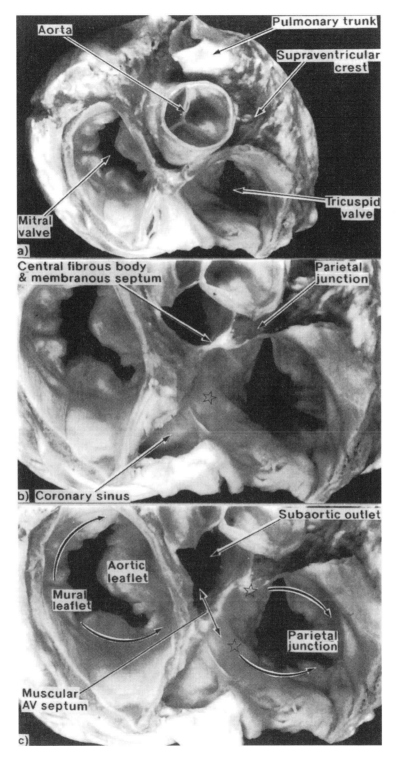

Figure 3. Series of dissections created by removing the segment of the heart where the atrial musculature inserts into the ventricular mass. Used with permission from Dean JW, et al.[18]

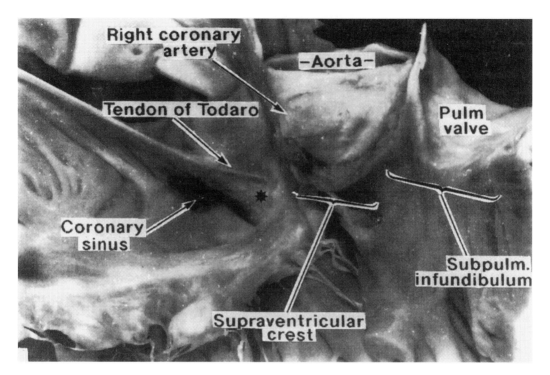

Figure 4. Dissection showing relation of the triangle of Koch to the anterior area of the septum. The position of the AV node is marked by an asterisk. Used with permission from Dean JW, et al.[18]

Identification of Anteroseptal and Midseptal Accessory Pathways Based on ECG Characteristics

The characteristics of the 12-lead electrocardiogram can be useful in the localization of manifest APs. This method of evaluation is of particular value among patients with midseptal and anteroseptal APs. If the 12-lead ECG suggests the presence of an AP in this location, discussions regarding the potential risk of complete heart block can be initiated with the patient and their family prior to proceeding with electrophysiology testing and catheter ablation.

The normal sequence of ventricular depolarization begins with activation of the midportion of the interventricular septum. This occurs in a left-to-right direction on the surface ECG, resulting in septal q waves in ECG leads I and V_5-V_6 and r waves in leads V_1-V_2. In contrast, in the presence of an

antegrade conducting AP, atrioventricular conduction occurs not only via the specialized His-Purkinje system, but also via the AP, resulting in preexcitation of the portion of the right ventricle at the site where insertion of the AP occurs. The morphology of the resultant fused QRS complex depends not only on the AP location, but also on the degree of preexcitation.

With manifest anteroseptal and midseptal APs, premature activation of the summit of the right ventricle, with relatively unopposed left free wall forces, results in a left bundle branch block (LBBB) pattern (Figures 5, 6). Fitzpatrick and colleagues[20] studied the 12-lead ECG tracings recorded from 93 patients with manifest APs and developed an algorithm for predicting the location of manifest APs based on the results of a maximally preexcited ECG (Figure 7). Right-sided septal APs (anteroseptal, midseptal, and posteroseptal) could be distinguished from right free wall APs based on the presence of a QRS transition (from nega-

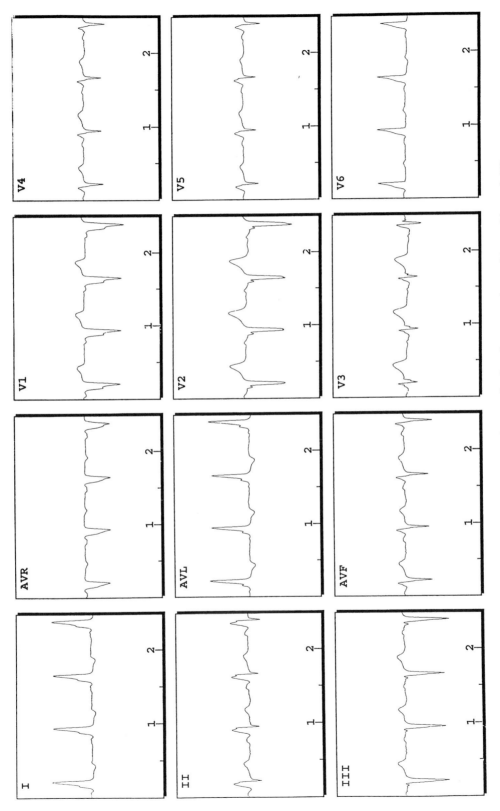

Figure 5. Twelve-lead ECG during normal sinus rhythm from a patient with a midseptal AP.

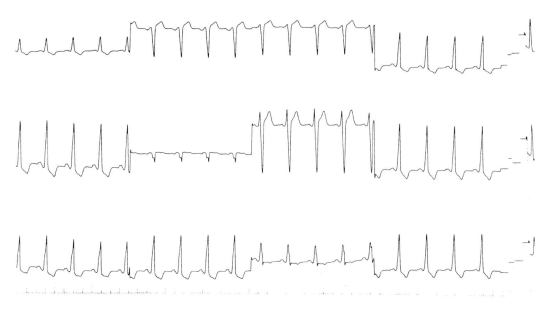

Figure 6. Twelve-lead ECG during normal sinus rhythm from a patient with an anteroseptal AP.

tive to positive) at or before lead V_3 or a QRS transition in V_4 combined with a delta wave in lead II ≥1.0 mV. The sum of the delta wave polarities in the inferior leads II, III, and aVF was the most important variable for distinguishing among APs located in the septal area. If this sum was greater than +1, the AP was anteroseptal. If the sum was less than −1 it was posteroseptal and if it was −1, 0, or +1 it was midseptal. Shown in Figures 5 and 6 are 12-lead ECGs obtained from two patients with a midseptal and an anteroseptal AP, respectively. An alternative algorithm, based on the polarity and morphology of QRS complexes rather than delta waves, has also been proposed (referred to as the St. George's algorithm[21]) (Figure 8). This algorithm was evaluated prospectively and found to correctly identify the location of 85% of APs.

Several others studies have been published that have focused on the ECG characteristics of specific subsets of anteroseptal and midseptal APs. Lorga and colleagues subdivided the location of midseptal APs into three zones spanning the region between the His bundle catheter and the coronary sinus os (zones 1–3 with zone 1 being

most anterior).[12] Each patient had a positive delta wave in leads I, II, aVL, and V_3-V_6, and a negative delta wave in lead III and aVR. The delta wave polarity in aVF was the only ECG parameter that predicted the AP location. Six of eight ablated in zone 3 had a negative delta wave in aVF while six of seven ablated in zones 1 and 2 had positive or isoelectric delta waves in aVF. Haissaguerre et al. analyzed the ECG patterns from eight patients with what was termed a "para-Hisian AP."[9] This subset of anteroseptal APs were defined as present when its atrial and ventricular insertions were associated with a large His bundle of >0.1 mV with virtually no distance between tip electrode of the ablation catheter and the His bundle catheter in any fluoroscopic view. The ECG characteristics of para-Hisian APs are similar to anteroseptal APs including positive delta waves in leads I, II, and aVF. However, they can be differentiated from anteroseptal APs by the presence of negative delta waves in V_1 and V_2 with a positive and negative predictive accuracy of 86% and 93%, respectively.

In summary, the results of these studies suggest that in the presence of significant

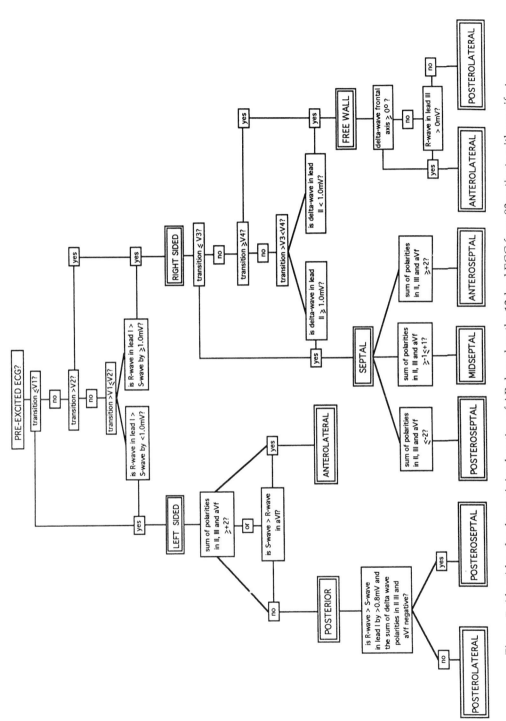

Figure 7. Algorithm for determining location of APs based on the 12-lead ECG from 93 patients with manifest pathways. Used with permission from Fitzpatrick AP, et al.[20]

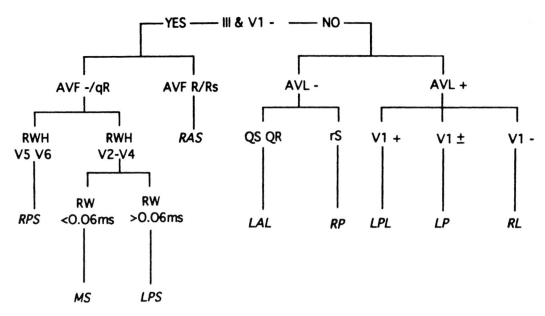

Figure 8. Algorithm for determining location of APs based on polarity and morphology of QRS complexes from patients with manifest pathways. Used with permission from Xie B, et al.[21]

preexcitation, physicians should be alert to the presence of an anteroseptal or midseptal AP in a patient who presents with a 12-lead ECG characterized by a left bundle pattern in lead V_1, a QRS transition at or before lead III, and positive delta wave polarities in one or more of leads II, III, and aVF. Because of the importance of the degree of preexcitation in the accuracy of these algorithms, attempts to bring out preexcitation using adenosine, exercise, or transesophageal pacing should be considered, particularly if the decision of whether to proceed with electrophysiology testing rests on the likelihood of an anteroseptal or midseptal AP.

Catheter Ablation Technique

A diagnostic electrophysiology study is performed prior to, or in conjunction with, the catheter ablation procedure. The diagnostic electrophysiology study serves to confirm the presence of an AP and to determine the number and conduction characteristics of the APs, as well as define the role of the AP in the patient's clinical tachycardia. Standard quadripolar electrode catheters

are introduced via the inferior vena cava and positioned in the high right atrium, the His bundle position, and at the apex of the right ventricle. Typically, a multielectrode catheter is also positioned in the coronary sinus via either the superior vena cava or the inferior vena cava. Atrial and ventricular pacing and programmed stimulation are then performed using standard techniques. Orthodromic AV reciprocating tachycardia (AVRT) is the most commonly induced sustained arrhythmia. This can be distinguished from AVNRT and atrial tachycardia by resetting atrial activation with a single premature ventricular stimulus during tachycardia at a time when the His bundle is refractory. For anteroseptal APs, the preexcitation index is usually <25 ms.[22] Termination of the tachycardia with a premature ventricular stimulus at a time when the His bundle is refractory without exciting the atrium is also indicative of an AP. When functional left or right BBB occurs spontaneously during orthodromic AVRT involving a midseptal or anteroseptal AP, the VA interval either does not change or lengthens by less than 30 ms.[23] The development of ipsilateral functional BBB during orthodromic AVRT will result in VA interval prolongation of 35 ms or greater in the presence of a free wall AP.[24] When an AP participates in the antegrade direction during the reentrant tachycardia, the resulting tachycardia is termed antidromic AVRT. Antidromic AVRT occurs rarely in the presence of a single midseptal or anteroseptal AP.[25] The administration of intravenous adenosine to selectively block retrograde AV node conduction can be very helpful in mapping and ablating anteroseptal and midseptal APs. Demonstration of VA conduction block with adenosine following but not prior to catheter ablation can also provide a useful endpoint for catheter ablation.[26,27]

Once the diagnostic electrophysiology study has been performed, confirming the indication for catheter ablation, efforts are focused on localization of the AP. In patients with a manifest AP, regional localization is accomplished with analysis of a maximally preexcited ECG as described above. In patients with a concealed AP, localization of the AP is performed by mapping the sequence of retrograde atrial activation either during orthodromic AVRT or during ventricular pacing. Whenever possible, mapping of the retrograde activation sequence should be performed during orthodromic AVRT because this eliminates the confounding factor of fusion of atrial activation due to retrograde VA conduction across both the AP and the AV node.

Electrode mapping of right-sided APs (including midseptal and anteroseptal APs) can be performed by determining the activation sequence of the right ventricle (for antegrade conducting APs) or the retrograde activation sequence of the right atrium (for retrograde conducting APs) or both. In either case, a steerable quadripolar electrode catheter, with a 4-mm distal electrode is initially positioned in the right ventricle and withdrawn to position the electrode pairs along the tricuspid annulus. Bipolar intracardiac electrograms (2- or 5-mm interelectrode spacing) from the distal and proximal

electrode pairs are recorded. In this manner, one can establish a prominent ventricular signal distally and a smaller atrial signal proximally along the ablation catheter. The electrograms are recorded using a bandpass filter of 50 to 500 Hz, amplified at a low gain (20 mm/mV), and recorded at paper speeds of 100 or 200/sec. Mapping of APs, including anteroseptal and midseptal APs, is most readily accomplished by viewing the position of the intracardiac electrode catheters in the LAO and RAO projections. Use of the LAO projection allows the tricuspid annulus to be viewed as a clockface, with His bundle position at 1:00 and the coronary sinus os at 5:00. In the LAO fluoroscopic projection, the catheter can be manipulated with clockwise or counterclockwise rotation and moved along the tricuspid annulus. In the RAO view, the position of the tricuspid valve can be identified as a relative lucency due to the presence of the fat pad located along the AV groove.

Localization of APs can be determined by evaluating the antegrade (manifest APs) or the retrograde (manifest or concealed APs) activation sequence. Earliest activation occurs at the site of insertion of the AP into the atrium or ventricle. Accurate localization requires that the AP be "bracketed" with later activation times demonstrated on either side of the AP insertion site. Once the AP has been localized to a precise region of the tricuspid annulus, the ablation catheter is manipulated until the local electrogram recorded from the distal electrode pair demonstrates "optimal" electrogram characteristics for ablation. Particular attention should be focused on identifying a deflection consistent with an AP potential. Once electrogram stability has been established, RF energy is delivered. Generally, between 30 and 50 W of RF energy is delivered for 30 to 60 sec. In the past several years, temperature-controlled catheter ablation with target electrode temperatures of 60°C to 70°C has been increasingly used.[28,29] If no effect is observed after 10 to 15 sec, the application of RF energy is generally aborted and the catheter repositioned. Because of the increased risk of conduction block occurring as a complication of catheter ablation in the midseptal or anteroseptal region, a more cautious approach to energy delivery should be used in this region. In general, catheter ablation should be performed using a low power output (i.e., 10 W), which can gradually be increased while carefully monitoring for the development of a junctional rhythm or AV block. If temperature-controlled RF ablation is used, the initial target temperature should be set to 50°C and progressively increased if necessary. Applications of energy should be interrupted if AP block does not occur within 10 sec or if a sustained junctional rhythm of more than five consecutive beats develops. During current delivery, the catheter position should be continuously monitored fluoroscopically in the LAO projection to verify catheter position stability. Following a successful application of RF energy, the patient is monitored for 30 minutes for recurrence. Electrophysiology testing and administration of adenosine is performed prior to withdrawal of the electrode catheters to confirm the absence of early recurrence.

At the conclusion of the ablation procedure, the sheaths are removed and the patient is monitored for a minimum of 3 hours. Although recent studies have demonstrated that catheter ablation can be safely accomplished on an outpatient basis,[30] post-procedure hospitalization for 24 hours should be considered particularly among patients in whom RF energy was delivered in close proximity to the His bundle. If transient AV block occurs during the ablation procedure, monitoring for at least 24 hours following the procedure is strongly recommended as late recurrence of AV block may occur. Although the benefit of aspirin has not been proven, particularly among those patients undergoing catheter ablation on the right side of the heart, we recommend that patients take aspirin for 4 weeks following the ablation procedure. Follow-up electrophysiology studies are generally no longer performed on a routine basis following catheter

ablation procedures unless symptoms recur.[31,32]

Identification of Optimal Target Site

Criteria have been developed to identify appropriate target sites for RF ablation of APs, which can generally be applied during catheter ablation of APs in all locations. Calkins et al.[33] have identified electrogram characteristics at successful and unsuccessful sites during the delivery of RF energy during the ablation of manifest and concealed APs. During the ablation of manifest APs, multivariate analysis identified three electrogram characteristics that were independent predictors of a successful outcome: electrogram stability, the interval between activation of the ventricular component of the local ventricular electrogram and the onset of the delta wave, and the presence of a probable or possible AP potential. Electrograms were classified as unstable if there was more than a 10% change in the A:V ratio, or if there was an appearance or a disappearance of a major deflection in the local electrogram. Accessory pathway potentials were identified only on a morphological basis. A probable AP potential was identified as a deflection in the local electrogram pathway potential that proceeded the onset of the QRS complex and was distinct from the atrial and ventricular components of the local electrogram. A possible AP potential was defined as a deflection that preceded the onset of the QRS complex and merged with the atrial or ventricular components of the local electrogram. The predicted probabilities of success based on the presence or absence of these electrogram characteristics are shown in Table 3. The probability of success was 57% at sites demonstrating electrogram stability, an AP potential, and an activation of the local ventricular electrogram before the delta wave. In contrast, the probability of success was only 3% if all of these characteristics were absent.

During the ablation of concealed APs, multivariate analysis identified three electrogram characteristics that were independent predictors of a successful outcome: electrogram stability, the presence of retrograde continuous electrical activity, and the presence of a probable or possible AP potential. The predicted probabilities of success based on the presence or absence of these electrogram characteristics are shown in Table 4. The probability of success was 82% at sites demonstrating electrical stability, an AP potential, and retrograde continuous electrical activity. In contrast, the probability of success was only 5% if these three characteristics were absent.

Particular caution should be used in avoiding use of a short AV interval as a criterion for identification of an appropriate site for ablation. As pointed out by Haissaguerre and colleagues,[34] this approach may not be the best predictor of successful ablation sites, especially with right anteroseptal and right lateral APs. The atrial signal is independent of AP activation and cannot be used by itself to locate successful ablation sites.

Table 3
Predicted Probability of Success During Ablation of Manifest Accessory AV Connections

Stability	K Potential	VaQRS >/= 0 msec	Probability of Success (%)
y	y	y	57 ± 6
y	y	n	36 ± 4
y	n	y	28 ± 6
n	y	y	18 ± 8
y	n	n	14 ± 3
n	y	n	9 ± 4
n	n	y	6 ± 3
n	n	n	3 ± 1

Stability indicates no major change in the morphology or amplitude of the local egm before delivery of RF energy, K potential indicates the presence of an AP potential, VAQRS > 0 msec indicates the activation of the V component of the egm begins before onset of the QRS. y = yes; n = no.
Reproduced with permission from Calkins H, et al.[133]

Table 4
Predicted Probability of Success During Ablation of Concealed Accessory AV Connections

Stability	K Potential	CEA	Probability of Success (%)
y	y	y	82 ± 8
y	n	y	64 ± 10
y	y	n	51 ± 9
n	y	y	38 ± 14
y	n	n	30 ± 9
n	n	y	20 ± 10
n	n	n	5 ± 4

Stability indicates no major change in the morphology or amplitude of the local egm before delivery of RF energy, K potential indicates the presence of an AP potential, CEA indicates retrograde continuous activity.
Reproduced with permission from Calkins et al (33)
y = yes; n = no.

The Role of Temperature During Ablation Procedures

Thermal injury is the principal mechanism of tissue destruction during RF catheter ablation procedures. Elevation of tissue temperature results in the denaturation of proteins, evaporation of fluids with subsequent destruction of tissue, and coagulation of tissue and blood.[35] Temperature-dependent depolarization of myocardial tissue and loss of excitability occur at temperatures greater than 43°C.[36] Reversible loss of excitability occurs at a temperature of approximately 48°C (range 43°C to 51°C). Irreversible tissue injury occurs at temperatures of approximately 50°C. During RF catheter ablation procedures, the temperature at the border between viable and nonviable tissue has been estimated to be approximately 48°C.[37] When the temperature at the electrode-tissue interface exceeds 100°C, tissue immediately adjacent to the electrode desiccates and plasma proteins denature to form a coagulum. The development of a coagulum results in a rapid increase in the measured lead impedance. If sudden boiling occurs, an audible popping may be heard.

This abrupt increase in impedance leads to a dramatic decrease in current density, effectively limiting the possibility of further lesion growth. Thus, as a result of the 100°C temperature ceiling for tissue heating during RF catheter ablation procedures, a theoretical maximum lesion size exists for a given electrode.[38] Because of the critical importance of temperature during RF catheter ablation procedures, temperature monitoring and closed loop temperature control have been developed as tools to facilitate catheter ablation procedures.[28]

Recent studies have provided important information regarding the potential role of temperature monitoring during RF catheter ablation procedures.[28,39] Langberg et al.[39] reported a minimal temperature of 48°C and mean electrode temperatures of 62°C ± 15°C at successful ablation site. Similarly, Calkins et al.[28] reported a minimal temperature of 44°C and a mean temperature of 64°C ± 12°C at successful ablation sites. However, no difference was reported between the mean electrode temperature obtained during successful and unsuccessful applications of RF energy (64°C ± 12°C versus 65°C ± 13°C, p = 0.8). Furthermore, no difference was found between the mean electrode temperature obtained at sites associated with and without late recurrence of conduction following an initially successful ablation procedure.[32] The absence of a temperature difference between successful versus failed sites and between sites with and without a recurrence likely reflects the fact that successful catheter ablation requires both tissue heating and accurate mapping. Calkins et al.[28] further evaluated the potential benefit of closed loop temperature control in reducing the incidence of coagulum development. The likelihood of developing a coagulum or impedance rise was greater in the power control mode than in the temperature control mode. In the temperature control mode, a coagulum was never observed when the target temperature was 70°C, whereas a coagulum was noted for 7% of applications with a target temperature of 85°C.

Prior studies evaluating electrode temperature during RF catheter ablation procedures have reported the presence of significant target-dependent differences in electrode temperature. Langberg et al.[29] reported that ablation of right-sided and posteroseptal APs on the atrial side of the tricuspid annulus resulted in lower electrode temperatures than applications on the ventricular side of the mitral annulus used during ablation of left free wall APs (48°C ± 7°C versus 60°C ± 16°C). A similar relationship was reported by Calkins et al.[28] Electrode temperatures were highest during ablation of left free wall and posteroseptal APs (66°C ± 13°C and 65°C ± 11°C) and lowest during ablation of right free wall and septal APs (58°C ± 10°C and 57°C ± 9°C).

These target-dependent differences may reflect important differences in electrode-tissue contact, catheter stability, and/or convective heat loss to the blood pool during catheter ablation at these anatomic sites. Catheter positions used during ablation of posteroseptal and left free wall APs generally result in more stable catheter contact with less exposure to high velocity blood flow compared with those used for right free wall APs.

Thus, temperature monitoring and temperature control are valuable tools during RF catheter ablation procedures. First, electrode temperature provides important information about adequacy of tissue heating. Failure of an application of RF energy associated with tissue temperatures less than 50°C may likely be due to inadequate heating, often due to catheter instability, rather than inaccurate mapping. Second, closed loop temperature control can markedly decrease the incidence of coagulum development. And third, closed loop temperature control allows for application of maximal power to a given site, thereby maximizing lesion size.

Special Considerations During Catheter Ablation of Midseptal and Anteroseptal Accessory Pathways

The increased risk of complete heart block associated with RF catheter ablation of anteroseptal APs was first brought to attention in 1992.[4] In this study, complete heart block occurred during catheter ablation in 3 of 250 patients undergoing catheter ablation of one or more APs (1%). Two of 10 patients who underwent catheter ablation of an anteroseptal AP developed complete heart block (20%). These findings have subsequently been confirmed by others. Chen and colleagues reported two instances of complete heart block among 191 patients undergoing catheter ablation of an AP.[40] Both patients who developed complete heart block were undergoing catheter ablation of an "anteromidseptal" AP. Yeh and colleagues reported a 33% incidence of complete heart block among patients undergoing catheter ablation of a midseptal AP.[14] Similarly, the Pediatric Catheter Ablation Registry recently reported the development of second or third degree AV block among 11 of 106 children (10%) who underwent catheter ablation of a midseptal AP (with four children developing complete heart block) and in 3 of 111 children (3%)

undergoing catheter ablation of an anteroseptal AP (with two children developing complete heart block)[41] (Figure 9). Thus, convincing evidence exists to demonstrate the importance of this complication during catheter ablation of midseptal and anteroseptal APs.

Several techniques have been proposed to minimize the risk of complete heart block in this area. The first involves the use of low power output, low temperatures, and short applications of RF energy. We will typically perform catheter ablation in this region using a low power output (i.e., 10 W), which can gradually be increased while carefully monitoring for the development of a junctional rhythm or AV block. If temperature-controlled RF ablation is used, we set the initial target temperature to 50°C. Applications of energy are interrupted if AP block does not occur within 10 sec or if a sustained junctional rhythm of more than five consecutive beats develops. During current delivery, the catheter position should be continuously monitored fluoroscopically in the

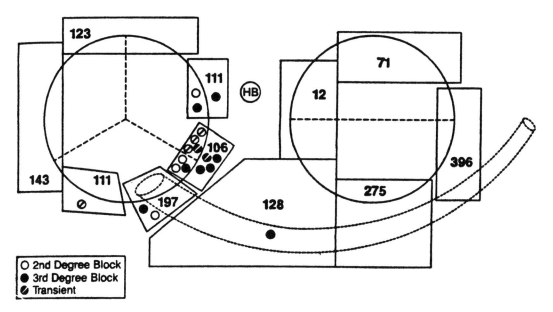

Figure 9. Schematic drawing showing the sites of AV block that occurred during catheter ablation in children based on the Pediatric Radiofrequency Ablation Registry. The increased risk of AV block during ablation in the anteroseptal and especially the midseptal area can be appreciated. Used with permission from Schaffer MS, et al.[41]

LAO projection to verify catheter position stability. The second technique involves maximizing the distance between the ablation catheter and the catheter positioned to record the His bundle. If possible, catheter ablation should be performed at sites at which either no His bundle potential is present or if necessary a site at which the His potential is <0.1 mV. The third technique concerns the selective delivery of RF energy on either the atrial or ventricular side of the annulus. Advocates of delivering RF energy on the ventricular side of the annulus claim that the fibrous tissue that surrounds the penetrating His bundle, combined with its location deep to the endocardium, renders it less susceptible to thermal injury.[5,6,8–10] Others have advocated that delivering energy on the atrial side of the annulus reduces the risk of AV block.[7,13,15] These authors propose that the

atrial approach is preferable based on the observation that conduction block typically occurs between the atrial electrogram and the AP potential during RF catheter ablation procedures.[42] Furthermore, Warin and colleagues reported no instances of complete heart block among 25 patients who underwent catheter ablation of an anteroseptal AP using DC energy delivered on the atrial side of the annulus just anterior to the His bundle.[43] Thus, advocates of both the atrial and ventricular approach exist. It remains unlikely that a prospective study will ever be performed to determined which approach is associated with a lower risk of complete heart block.

At Johns Hopkins we prefer approaching anteroseptal and midseptal APs using an inferior vena cava approach and delivering RF energy at sites with an AV ratio <1. When catheter stability is a problem we rap-

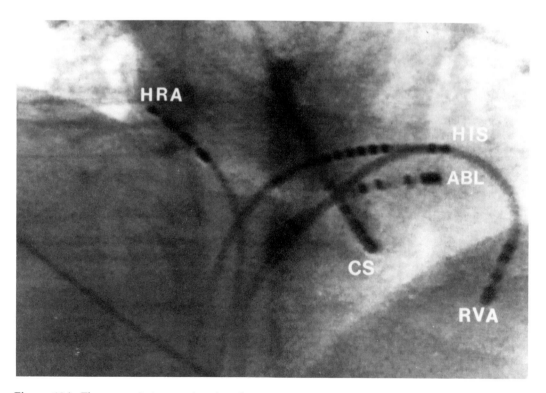

Figure 10A. Fluoroscopic image showing the position of catheters during ablation of a midseptal AP as viewed in the RAO projection. A long sheath has been used to help stabilize the ablation catheter.

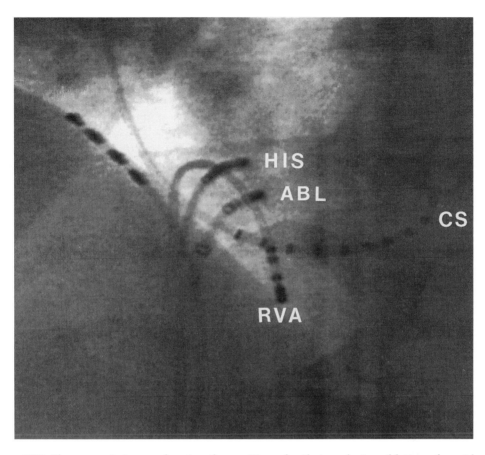

Figure 10B. Fluoroscopic image showing the position of catheters during ablation of a midseptal AP as viewed in the LAO projection. A long sheath has been used to help stabilize the ablation catheter.

idly move to using a long sheath to stabilize the ablation catheter (Figure 10 A, B). Regardless of which strategies are used, the risk of AV block will remain. For this reason it is critical for the electrophysiologist to evaluate the risks of AV block in light of the severity and potential risks of the AP which is being ablated. Whereas a 3% risk of complete AV block may be very acceptable in a highly symptomatic patient who has failed conventional medical therapy or a patient who presented with atrial fibrillation with a rapid ventricular response, the risk of AV block would clearly not be acceptable in an asymptomatic or minimally symptomatic patient in whom the AP refractory period is long.

Catheter ablation of an anteroseptal or midseptal AP may initially fail due to inaccurate mapping, inadequate tissue heating, or rarely the presence of a left midseptal AP. When initial attempts at catheter ablation fail, it is important to consider each of these three factors. In our experience, the most common reasons for failure is inadequate tissue heating, often due to catheter instability. Awareness of this problem is readily apparent when temperature monitoring is used. Approaches to remedy this problem include the use of different ablation catheters with different handling characteristics, an alternative approach to ablation (superior vena cava versus inferior vena cava), or the use of intravascular sheaths. Less common causes for failure are inaccurate mapping or the presence of a left-sided midseptal AP.[21]

Results: Anteroseptal Accessory Pathways

Despite the challenges associated with catheter ablation of anteroseptal APs, RF catheter ablation can be accomplished with a high success rate, approaching that of APs in other locations, and with only a small risk of complete AV block. The overall results of catheter ablation of APs in all locations that have been reported in large series are summarized in Table 5. The overall success rate for ablation of APs in all locations ranged from 89% to 99%. Overall, catheter ablation was successful in 1,334 of 1,401 patients (95%). Recurrence of conduction occurred in 10% of patients.

The technique and results of catheter ablation of anteroseptal APs that have been reported in 10 published series are summarized in Table 1. Among a total of 106 APs, catheter ablation was successful in 100 (94%). Complications included complete AV block in two patients (2%), transient or second degree AV block in an additional three patients (3%), and a new RBBB in 15 patients (15%). Recurrence of AP conduc-

tion occurred in three patients. Among 420 patients who have undergone RF catheter ablation of an AP at Johns Hopkins Hospital over the past 5 years, an anteroseptal AP was present in 10. Among these patients, nine were sufficiently symptomatic to justify the potential risk of complete AV block. The IVC approach was used in each with delivery of RF energy at sites with an AV ratio <1. Catheter ablation was successful in eight of these nine patients. Catheter ablation was prematurely terminated in the final patient, with a para-Hisian AP who developed transient complete heart block with RF energy delivery.

Results: Midseptal Accessory Pathways

The technique and results of catheter ablation of midseptal APs which have reported in nine published series are summarized in Table 2. Among a total of 85 APs, catheter ablation was successful in 79 (84%). Complications included complete AV block in four patients (5%) and transient or second degree AV block in two patients. Recurrence of conduction occurring in two patients. Among 420 patients who have undergone RF catheter ablation of an AP at Johns Hopkins Hospital over the past 5

Table 5
Review of Catheter Ablation Series

Author	No. of Pts.	No. of APs	AP Location					Success (%)
			LFW	PS	MS	AS	RFW	
Calkins (4)	250	267	161	44	5	10	47	94
Jackman (5)	166	177	106	43	0	13	15	99
Lesh (6)	100	109	45	30	6	7	21	89
Swartz (7)	114	122	76	13	11	10	12	95
Haissaguerre (39)	408	436	286	77	0	41	32	97
Kay (18)	363	384	187	92	12	19	62	96
Total	1401	1495	861	299	34	100	189	1334/1401 (95%)

See text for abbreviations.

years, seven underwent catheter ablation of a midseptal AP. The IVC approach was used in each with delivery of RF energy at sites with an AV ratio <1. Catheter ablation was successfully accomplished in each patient.

Summary

In summary, APs located in the anteroseptal and midseptal region represent an important subset of APs due to an increased risk of AV block that is associated with delivery of RF energy in this region. Catheter ablation of APs located in this region can be successfully accomplished in greater than 85% of patients with a risk of complete heart block of approximately 2%. Because of this increased risk of AV block, catheter ablation of APs in this region must be approached cautiously and particular attention should be focused on analyzing the risk benefit ratio of proceeding with catheter ablation when an AP localized to this region has been identified.

References

1. Gallagher JJ, Svenson RH, Kasell JH, et al. Catheter technique for closed-chest ablation of the atrioventricular conduction system: a therapeutic alternative for the treatment of refractory supraventricular tachycardia. N Engl J Med 1982;306:194–200.
2. Scheinman MM, Morady F, Hess DS, et al. Catheter-induced ablation of the atrioventricular junction to control supraventricular arrhythmias. JAMA 1982;851–855.
3. Weber H, Schmidt L. Catheter technique for closed-chest ablation of an accessory pathway. N Engl J Med 1983;308:653–654.
4. Calkins H, Langberg J, Sousa J, et al. Radiofrequency catheter ablation of accessory atrioventricular connections in 250 patients. Circulation 1992;85:1337–1346.
5. Jackman WM, Xunzhang W, Friday KJ, et al. Catheter ablation of accessory atrioventricular pathways (Wolff-Parkinson-White syndrome) by radiofrequency current. N Engl J Med 1991;324:1605–1611.
6. Lesh MD, Van Hare GF, Schamp DJ, et al. Curative percutaneous catheter ablation using radiofrequency energy for accessory pathways in all locations: results in 100 consecutive patients. J Am Coll Cardiol 1992;19: 1303–1309.
7. Swartz JF, Tracy CM, Fletcher RD. Radiofrequency endocardial catheter ablation of accessory atrioventricular pathway atrial insertion sites. Circulation 1993;87:487–499.
8. Kay GN, Epstein AE, Dailey SM, et al. Role of radiofrequency ablation in the management of supraventricular arrhythmias: experience in 760 consecutive patients. J Cardiovasc Electrophysiol 1993;4:371–389.
9. Haissaguerre M, Marcus F, Poquet F, et al. Electrocardiographic characteristics and catheter ablation of para-Hisian accessory pathways. Circulation 1994;90:1124–1128.
10. Satake S, Okishige K, Azegami K, et al. Radiofrequency ablation for WPW syndrome with monitoring the local electrogram at the ablation site. Jpn Heart J 1996;37:741–750.
11. Xie B, Herald SC, Bashir Y, et al. Localization of accessory pathways from the 12-lead electrocardiogram using a new algorithm. Am J Cardiol 1994;74:161–165.
12. Lorga FA, Sosa E, Scanavacca M, et al. Electrocardiographic identification of midseptal accessory pathways in close proximity to the atrioventricular conduction system. PACE 1996;10(Pt II):1984–1987.
13. Schluter M, Kuck KH. Catheter ablation from right atrium of anteroseptal accessory pathways using radiofrequency current. J Am Coll Cardiol 1992;19:663–670.
14. Yeh SJ, Wang CC, Wen MS, et al. Characteristics and radiofrequency ablation therapy of intermediate septal accessory pathway. Am J Cardiol 1994;73:50–56.
15. Kuck KH, Schluter M, Gursoy S. Preservation of atrioventricular nodal conduction during radiofrequency current catheter ablation of midseptal accessory pathways. Circulation 1992;86:1743–1752.
16. Sealy WC, Gallagher JJ. The surgical approach to the septal area of the heart based on experiences with 45 patients with Kent bundles. J Thorac Cardiovasc Surg 1980;79: 542–551.
17. Sealy WC. Kent bundles in the anterior septal space. Ann Thorac Surg 1983;36:2.
18. Dean JW, Ho SY, Rowland E, et al. Clinical anatomy of the atrioventricular junctions. J Am Coll Cardiol 1994;24:1725–1731.

19. Ho SY, Kilpatrick L, Kanai T, et al. The architecture of the atrioventricular conduction axis in dog compared to man: its significance to ablation of the atrioventricular nodal approaches. J Cardiovasc Electrophysiol 1995; 6:26–39.

20. Fitzpatrick AP, Gonzales RP, Lesh MD, et al. New algorithm for the localization of accessory atrioventricular connections using a baseline electrocardiogram. J Am Coll Cardiol 1994;23:107–116.

21. Xie B, Heald SC, Bashir Y, et al. Localization of accessory pathways from the 12-lead using a new algorithm. Am J Cardiol 1986; 74:161–165.

22. Miles WM, Yee R, Klein G, et al. The preexcitation index: an aid in determining the mechanism of supraventricular tachycardia and localizing accessory pathways of atrioventricular nodal conduction during radiofrequency current catheter ablation. Circulation 1990;74(3)494–500.

23. Scheinman MM, Wang YS, Van Hare GF, et al. Electrocardiographic and electrophysiologic characteristics of anterior, midseptal and right anterior free wall accessory pathways. J Am Coll Cardiol 1992;20:1220–1229.

24. Kerr CR, Gallagher JJ, German LD. Changes in ventriculoatrial intervals with bundle branch block aberration during reciprocating tachycardia in patients with accessory atrioventricular pathways. Circulation 1982; 66:197.

25. Bardy GH, Packer DL, German LD, et al. Preexcited reciprocating tachycardia in patients with Wolff-Parkinson-White syndrome incidence and mechanism. Circulation 1984;70: 377–391.

26. Keim S, Curtis AB, Belardinelli L, et al. Adenosine-induced atrioventricular block: a rapid and reliable method to assess surgical and radiofrequency catheter ablation of accessory atrioventricular pathways. J Am Coll Cardiol 1992;19:1005–1012.

27. Engelstein ED, Wilber D, Wadas M, et al. Limitations of adenosine in assessing the efficacy of radiofrequency catheter ablation of accessory pathways. Am J Cardiol 1994;73: 774–779.

28. Calkins H, Prystowsky E, Carlson M, et al. and the Atakar Multicenter Investigators Group. Temperature monitoring during radiofrequency catheter ablation procedures using closed loop control. Circulation 1994; 90:1279–1286.

29. Dinerman JL, Berger RD, Calkins H. Temperature monitoring during radiofrequency ablation. J Cardiovasc Electrophysiol 1996;7: 163–173.

30. Kalbfleisch SJ, El-Atassi R, Calkins H, et al. Safety, feasibility and cost of outpatient radiofrequency catheter ablation of accessory atrioventricular connections. J Am Coll Cardiol 1993;21:567–570.

31. Chen SA, Chiang CE, Yang CJ, et al. Usefulness of serial follow-up electrophysiologic studies in predicting late outcome of radiofrequency ablation for accessory pathways and atrioventricular nodal reentrant tachycardia. Am Heart J 1993;126:619–625.

32. Calkins H, Prystowsky E, Berger RD, et al. and the Atakar Multicenter Investigators Group. Recurrence of Conduction following radiofrequency catheter ablation procedures: relationship to ablation target and electrode temperature. J Cardiovasc Electrophysiol 1996;7:704–712.

33. Calkins H, Kim YN, Schmaltz S, et al. Electrogram criteria for identification of appropriate target sites for radiofrequency catheter ablation of accessory atrioventricular connections. Circulation 1992;85:565–573.

34. Haissaguerre M, Gaita F, Marcus FI, et al. Radiofrequency catheter ablation of accessory pathways: a contemporary review. J Cardiovasc Electrophysiol 1994;5:532–552.

35. Frez A, Shitzer A. Controlled destruction and temperature distributions in biological tissues subjected to monoactive electrocoagulation. J Biochem Engineering 1980;102: 42–49.

36. Nath S, Lynch C, Whayne JG, et al. Cellular electrophysiological effects of hyperthermia on isolated guinea pig papillary muscle: implications for catheter ablation. Circulation 1993;88(Pt 1):1826–1831.

37. Haines DE, Watson DD. Tissue heating during radiofrequency catheter ablation: a thermodynamic model and observations in isolated perfused and superfused canine right ventricular free wall. PACE 1989;12:962–976.

38. Haines DE, Verow AF. Observations on electrode-tissue interface temperature and effect on electrical impedance during radiofrequency ablation of ventricular myocardium. Circulation 1990;82:1034–1038.

39. Langberg JJ, Calkins H, El-Atassi R, et al. Temperature monitoring during radiofrequency catheter ablation of accessory pathways. Circulation 1992;86:1469–1474.

40. Chen SA, Chiang CE, Tai CT, et al. Complications of diagnostic electrophysiologic studies and radiofrequency catheter ablation in patients with tachyarrhythmias: an eight-year survey of 3,996 consecutive procedures in a tertiary referral center. Am J Cardiol 1996; 77:41–46.

41. Schaffer MS, Silka MJ, Ross BA, et al. Inadvertent atrioventricular block during radio-

frequency catheter ablation: results of the Pediatric Radiofrequency Ablation Registry. Circulation 1996;94:3214–3220.

42. Calkins H, Mann C, Kalbfleisch S, et al. Site of accessory pathway block after radiofrequency catheter ablation in patients with the Wolff-Parkinson-White syndrome. J Cardiovasc Electrophysiol 1994;5:20–27.

43. Warin J, Haissaguerre M, Divernois C, et al. Catheter ablation of accessory pathways: technique and results in 248 patients. PACE 1990;3:1609–1614.

Catheter Ablation of Posteroseptal Accessory Pathways

Fred Morady

Introduction

It has now been 14 years since the publication of the first report of successful catheter ablation of an accessory pathway (AP).[1] The AP was posteroseptal in location and was ablated using a direct current shock delivered near the ostium of the coronary sinus. A subsequent series of 48 patients demonstrated that direct current ablation of posteroseptal APs had a success rate of approximately 70% and was associated with a small risk of cardiac tamponade and atrioventricular block.[2] Because of the potential for complications related to barotrauma, direct current ablation of posteroseptal APs generally was limited to patients with severe symptoms who could not be adequately managed with pharmacological therapy.

With the advent of radiofrequency (RF) catheter ablation several years ago, the efficacy and safety of catheter ablation of APs dramatically improved, to the point that catheter ablation of APs quickly became first-line therapy for patients symptomatic from arrhythmias involving an AP. The purpose of this chapter is to review the current body of knowledge having to do with various aspects of RF catheter ablation of posteroseptal APs.

Anatomy of the Posteroseptal Space

An understanding of the anatomy of the posteroseptal space is important for electrophysiologists who perform catheter ablation procedures. Based on his experience as a pioneer in the development of techniques for the surgical interruption of APs, Dr. Will Sealy elucidated the surgical anatomy of the posteroseptal space, where posteroseptal AP are located.[3] This space has a configuration similar to that of a trihedral pyramid with unequal faces that is lying on its side (Figure 1). The base of the pyramid is the epicardium of the crux, and the apex is the right fibrous trigone, which is the junction of the mitral and tricuspid annuli, the aortic annulus, the membranous septum, and the atrial septum. The right side of the pyramid is the septal portion of the right atrium, the left side is the left atrium, and the third side, which also is the floor, consists of the posterior superior process of the left ventricle and the muscular ventricular septum. The ostium of the coronary sinus is located at the

From Singer I, Barold SS, Camm AJ (eds): Nonpharmacological Therapy of Arrhythmias for the 21st Century: The State of the Art. Futura Publishing Co., Inc., Armonk, NY, © 1998.

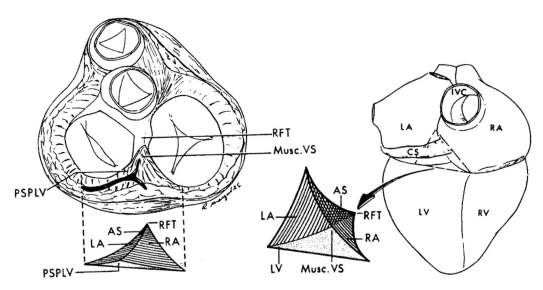

Figure 1. Schematic representation of the posteroseptal space. AS = anterior septum; CS = coronary sinus; IVC = inferior vena cava; LA = left atrium; LV = left ventricle; Musc. VS = muscular ventricular septum; PSPLV = posteroseptal process of the left ventricle; RA = right atrium; RFT = right fibrous trigone; RV = right ventricle. Reproduced from Sealy WC, et al. with permission from the Journal of Thoracic and Cardiovascular Surgery.[3]

posterior superior aspect of the right face of the pyramid. The pyramidal space contains adipose tissue, the atrioventricular node artery, and in its superior portion, the anterior part of the coronary sinus.

In the electrophysiology laboratory, the ostium of the coronary sinus provides a convenient landmark for identification of the posteroseptal region and of APs that result in earliest antegrade or retrograde activation in the vicinity of the ostium. If the earliest antegrade or retrograde activation occurs inside the coronary sinus, the question arises as to how far leftward the posteroseptal space extends from the ostium. In conventional practice, APs that are localized to within 1–2 cm of the ostium have been considered to be posteroseptal, and APs that are localized to areas beyond 1–2 cm from the ostium have been considered to be left free wall in location. This practice was questioned by a study that measured the dimensions of the posteroseptal space in 48 human cadaver hearts.[4] The mean distance from the coronary sinus ostium to the left border

of the posteroseptal space was 2.3 ± 0.4 cm (± standard deviation). The proximal 1.5 cm of the coronary sinus was found to be almost always within the posteroseptal space, and the junction of the posterior septum and the left free wall was located more than 1.75 cm to the left of the coronary sinus ostium in all adults with a body weight of 60 kg or more.[4] These data suggest that some APs that are categorized as being in the left free wall, based on localization within the coronary sinus more than 1 cm from the ostium, may actually be posteroseptal APs. However, because the dimensions of the cadaver heart may not accurately reflect the in vivo dimensions, the best criterion for delineation of the left margin of the posteroseptal space is not entirely clear. While the use of the 1 cm criterion likely results in an underestimate of the true frequency of posteroseptal APs, this probably has little or no clinical impact in the electrophysiology laboratory. In practice, when APs are localized within the coronary sinus beyond 1 cm from the os, a left-sided endocardial approach is almost always effective, regardless of whether the AP is in the left free wall or actually within the posterior septum.

Anatomic and Surgical Delineation of Posteroseptal Accessory Pathways

There are only three anatomic descriptions of posteroseptal AP based on postmortem examination of the human heart.[5–7] In these reports, the APs were found to connect the right atrium[5,7] or left atrium[6] with the top of the interventricular septum.

In their initial experience with surgical interruption of posteroseptal APs in 31 patients, Sealy and Gallagher found that approximately 40% of the APs were located between the right fibrous trigone and the coronary sinus, approximately 20% coursed with the bundle of His, and another 20% were located underneath the coronary sinus at the crux of the heart.[3] In one of the 31 patients, the AP coursed from the left atrium to the posterior superior process of the left ventricle. The posteroseptal APs were found to usually run from the atrium to the ventricle through the fat within the pyramidal space, at some distance from the cardiac walls. In some patients, the posteroseptal APs seemed to arise in the atrial muscle surrounding the coronary sinus. The successful surgical interruption of these APs was accomplished most commonly through a right atriotomy, and often required both a left and right atriotomy. In a small number of patients, a left atriotomy by itself was used, and in a single patient, cryoablation applied using an epicardial approach was effective. In subsequent reports involving larger numbers of patients, posteroseptal APs were often found to connect the right atrium and the left ventricle.[8,9]

In 1988 Guiraudon and coworkers reported an important intraoperative observation about posteroseptal APs.[10] Among 65 patients, six were found in the operating room to have a coronary sinus diverticulum in the posteroseptal region. The coronary sinus diverticula consisted of a venous pouch 2–5 cm in diameter within the left ventricular wall, proximal to the midcardiac vein, with a 5–10 mm neck opening into the coronary sinus (Figure 2). Successful interruption of the AP in these six patients required separation of the neck of the coronary sinus diverticulum from the left ventricle. Therefore, this report indicated that in some patients, posteroseptal APs are located within a coronary sinus diverticulum that serves as a bridge between the left ventricle and right or left atrium.

The surgical experience with interruption of posteroseptal APs explains why some posteroseptal APs can be ablated with a right-sided approach and delivery of RF en-

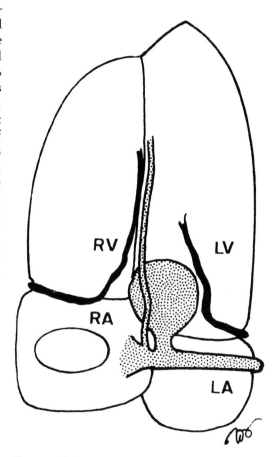

Figure 2. Schematic representation of a coronary sinus diverticulum. Abbreviations as in Figure 1. Reproduced from Guiraudon GM, et al. with permission from the American Journal of Cardiology.[10]

ergy at or near the ostium of the coronary sinus, some require a left-sided approach, and some can be ablated only from within the body of the coronary sinus, one of its branches, or a coronary sinus diverticulum.

Electrocardiographic Manifestations of Posteroseptal Accessory Pathways

Manifest posteroseptal APs are typically associated with negative delta waves in the inferior leads, often mimicking the Q waves of an inferior infarction (Figure 3). While a negative delta wave is always present in lead III, the prevalence of a negative delta wave is 90% in aVF, and 50% in lead II.[11] The delta waves in leads I and aVL are positive, there is an R/S ratio greater than 1 in V_2, and tall R waves in V_2 through V_6 (Figure 3).[11] The QRS frontal plane axis is be-

tween $+30°$ and $-60°$. The configuration of the delta wave and QRS complex in V_1 is variable. Right posteroseptal APs are usually associated with a negative or isoelectric delta wave in V_1 (Figure 3), and left posteroseptal APs are usually associated with a positive delta wave and R/S ratio greater than 1 in V_1 (Figure 4). While the configuration of the delta wave and QRS complex in lead V_1 are often helpful in distinguishing right and left posteroseptal APs, exceptions are not uncommon, and the accurate differentiation of right and left posteroseptal APs is not always possible based on the electrocardiogram.

Identification of Posteroseptal Accessory Pathways in the Electrophysiology Laboratory

Mapping of manifest posteroseptal APs usually demonstrates the site of earliest

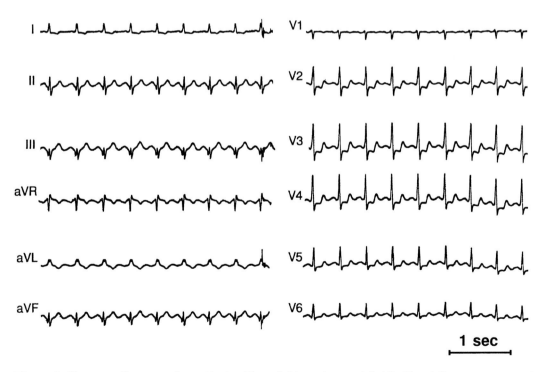

Figure 3. Electrocardiogram of a patient with a right posteroseptal AP. The delta waves are not prominent, because of fusion between conduction through the AP and the atrioventricular node. In the Emergency Department, the negative delta waves in the inferior leads were misinterpreted as pathologic Q waves indicative of an inferior myocardial infarction.

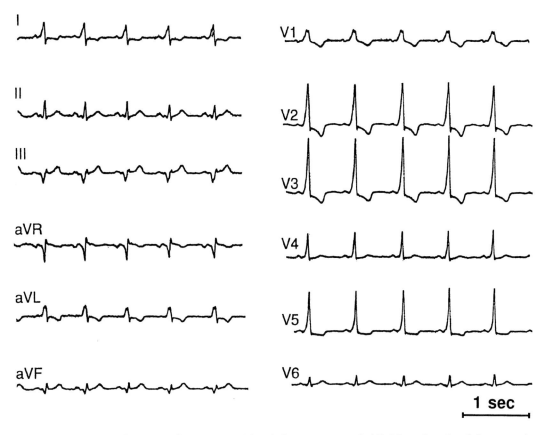

Figure 4. Electrocardiogram of a patient with a left posteroseptal AP. Note that the delta wave in V_1 is positive, and that the QRS complex in V_1 has a monophasic R wave configuration. This pattern is typical of left posteroseptal APs. In contrast, right posteroseptal APs usually are associated with a negative or isoelectric delta wave and an R/S ratio less than 1 in V_1.

ventricular activation to be at the ostium of the coronary sinus, or inside the coronary sinus, within 1–2 cm of the ostium. Mapping of retrograde atrial activation, best performed during orthodromic reciprocating tachycardia to avoid the confounding effects of retrograde atrioventricular nodal conduction, demonstrates earliest atrial activation at these same areas. Because of the oblique course of some APs, the site of earliest ventricular activation in manifest APs may not correspond with the site of earliest atrial activation during retrograde conduction.

In some patients with a posteroseptal AP, extensive mapping of antegrade and retrograde activation with a right-sided approach and a left ventricular approach fails to reveal a specific site that is earlier than its neighboring sites. This may be an indication that the AP is epicardial, with earliest activation within the coronary sinus, one of its branches, or within a coronary sinus diverticulum.

During orthodromic reciprocating tachycardia utilizing a posteroseptal AP, a ventricular depolarization introduced during His bundle refractoriness will advance the atrial electrograms by at least 15–20 ms. At times, ventricular depolarizations introduced at the right ventricular apex are unable to preexcite the atrium during His bundle refractoriness, in which case introduction of the premature stimulus near the ventricular septum is helpful (Figure 5).[12]

In orthodromic reciprocating tachycardia utilizing a posteroseptal AP, functional right bundle branch block has no effect on

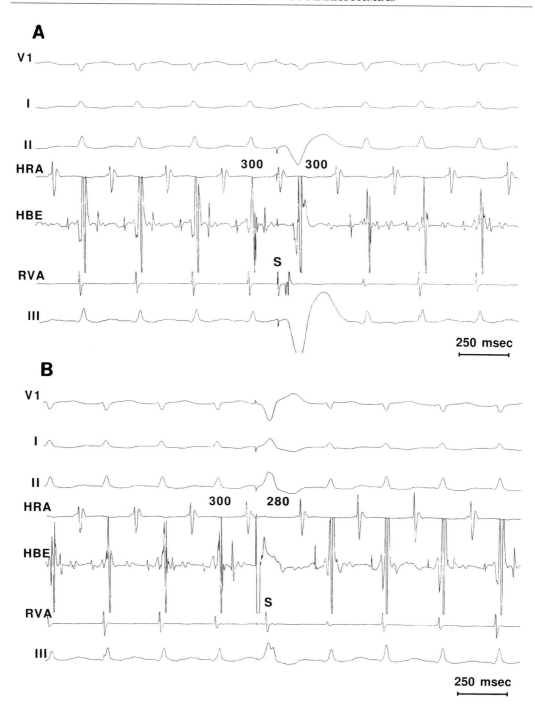

Figure 5. Orthodromic reciprocating tachycardia utilizing a conceal posteroseptal AP. **A.** A ventricular premature depolarization introduced at the right ventricular apex during His bundle refractoriness does not affect the atrial electrograms. As indicated, the atrial cycle length remains constant at 300 ms. **B**. A ventricular premature depolarization introduced at the summit of the right ventricular septum during His bundle refractoriness advances the atrial electrogram by 20 ms, as shown. HBE = His bundle electrogram; HRA = high right atrium; RVA = right ventricular apex; S = stimulus.

the ventriculoatrial interval, and functional left bundle branch block typically prolongs the ventriculoatrial interval by less than 25 ms.[13] This is helpful in distinguishing posteroseptal APs from left free wall APs, which are associated with prolongation of the ventriculoatrial interval by 30 ms or more during left bundle branch block aberration.[13] An increase in the ventriculoatrial interval during a left bundle branch block suggests that a posteroseptal AP inserts into the left side of the ventricular septum. However, because many posteroseptal APs course from the right atrium to the left ventricle, catheter ablation of an AP that is "left-sided" in regard to its ventricular insertion may often be feasible using a right-sided approach.[14]

At times, electrophysiological testing may demonstrate rapid, nondecremental ventriculoatrial conduction and earliest atrial activation near the ostium of the coronary sinus, compatible with a posteroseptal AP, but tachycardia may not be inducible. The absence of inducible tachycardia precludes the usual diagnostic maneuvers that are helpful in distinguishing a concealed posteroseptal AP from retrograde conduction over an atrioventricular nodal pathway, including introduction of a ventricular depolarization during His bundle refractoriness, the response to a functional bundle branch block, and comparison of the His-atrial intervals during tachycardia and ventricular pacing.[15] In this type of situation, a comparison of ventriculoatrial intervals during ventricular pacing at the right ventricular apex and at a posterobasal right ventricular site may be helpful in distinguishing a concealed posteroseptal AP from a retrograde atrioventricular nodal pathway.[16] If a posteroseptal AP is present, the ventriculoatrial interval during right ventricular pacing at a basal site is shorter than when pacing at the apex; if retrograde conduction occurs through the atrioventricular node-His-Purkinje axis, the converse will occur. Accordingly, Martinez-Alday et al. reported that the difference between the ventriculoatrial interval measured during apical pacing and posterobasal pacing ranged from +10 to +70 ms in the presence of a posteroseptal AP, compared to values of −50 to +5 ms when retrograde conduction was through the atrioventricular node.[16] Therefore, if the ventriculoatrial interval measured during ventricular pacing at a posterobasal site ≥10 ms shorter than during apical pacing, this is strong evidence that a posteroseptal AP is present, even if tachycardia is not inducible.[16]

Right- vs. Left-sided Target Sites for Ablation of Posteroseptal Accessory Pathways

Based on the configuration of the QRS complex in lead V_1, the site of earliest ventricular activation (if the AP is manifest), and the response to a functional left bundle branch block during orthodromic tachycardia, posteroseptal APs can be categorized as being right-sided or left-sided. However, this categorization of posteroseptal APs does not necessarily predict whether an effective target site for ablation of the AP will be right-sided or left-sided. In a study of 50 consecutive patients with a posteroseptal AP, Dhala et al. found that 10 patients had a positive delta wave in V_1 and ventriculoatrial interval prolongation of 10 to 30 ms in association with a functional left bundle branch block during orthodromic tachycardia.[14] Although these findings indicated that the APs inserted into the left side of the ventricular septum, successful RF ablation required a left-sided approach in only one of the 10 patients. In the other nine patients with a left-sided posteroseptal AP, the successful target sites for ablation were at the coronary sinus ostium or within the first 1 cm of the coronary sinus in five patients, at the posteroseptal aspect of the tricuspid annulus in two patients, and at the inferomedial right atrium posterior to the coronary sinus ostium in two patients. Among the 40 other patients with a posteroseptal AP, the AP was successfully ablated using a venous approach in 39. Therefore, the results of this study suggested that the majority of posteroseptal APs can be ablated at or near the coronary sinus ostium, regardless of whether the AP is classified as right- or left-sided based on electrocardiographic and electrophysiological criteria.

Although it is appropriate to first attempt ablation of a posteroseptal AP from the right side, it must be kept in mind that a left-sided approach may be necessary, even when the AP does not have the typical electrocardiographic pattern of a left-sided posteroseptal AP. In a series of patients in whom lengthy or multiple procedures were needed before successful ablation was achieved, several patients had a posteroseptal AP that was thought to be right-sided based on the absence of a positive delta wave in V_1, the presence of an R/S ratio <1 in V_1, and also because right-sided applications often resulted in transient AP block.[17] After multiple ineffective applications of RF energy at or near the ostium of the coronary sinus, successful ablation was achieved by delivery of RF energy at the posteroseptal aspect of the mitral annulus. Therefore, a left ventricular or left atrial approach should be considered if several right-sided applications of RF energy are ineffective in ablating a posteroseptal AP.

The configuration of the delta wave in lead II may be helpful in identifying posteroseptal APs that can be ablated using a right-sided approach. Two studies have demonstrated that the successful ablation site is in the right posteroseptal region in 80–82% of patients who have a positive or biphasic delta wave in lead II.[14,18]

It also may be possible to predict whether a right- or left-sided approach is necessary based on analysis of atrial activation during orthodromic tachycardia. In a study of 89 consecutive patients with a concealed posteroseptal AP, 36 patients (39%) required a left atrial or left ventricular endocardial approach for ablation.[19] The ΔVA (the ventriculoatrial interval recorded during orthodromic tachycardia or ventricular pacing by the His bundle catheter minus the shortest

ventriculoatrial interval recorded within the proximal coronary sinus) was found to be predictive of the location of successful ablation.[19] When the ΔVA was 25 ms or more, a left endocardial approach was necessary, and when the ΔVA was less than 25 ms, successful ablation usually was achieved by delivery of RF energy on the right side, at or near the ostium of the coronary sinus (Figure 6). This study demonstrated that the use of a left ventricular endocardial approach early in the procedure when the ΔVA is 25 ms or more is associated with a significant reduction in procedure duration, radiation exposure, and number of RF energy applications.

Ablation of Posteroseptal Accessory Pathways from Within the Coronary Sinus

Because some posteroseptal APs are epicardial or located in close proximity to the coronary sinus or one of its branches, or within a coronary sinus anomaly, an endocardial approach to ablation is not always effective, and delivery of RF energy within the coronary sinus or one of its branches is sometimes necessary. An electrocardiographic finding that may be useful in predicting the need for delivery of energy within the coronary sinus is the presence of a steeply negative delta wave in lead II (Figure 7). In a preliminary report, among 15 patients with a posteroseptal AP who had a steeply negative delta wave in lead II, eight patients (53%) were found to require ablation from within a venous branch of the coronary sinus.[18] In an expanded study of 166 consecutive patients with a posteroseptal AP, Arruda et al. found that 23 patients required ablation from within a venous branch of the coronary sinus (Arruda MS, personal communication); the sensitivity of a markedly negative delta wave in lead II for predicting the need for ablation from within a branch or diverticulum of the coronary sinus was 78%, while the specificity of this finding was 99%. The positive and

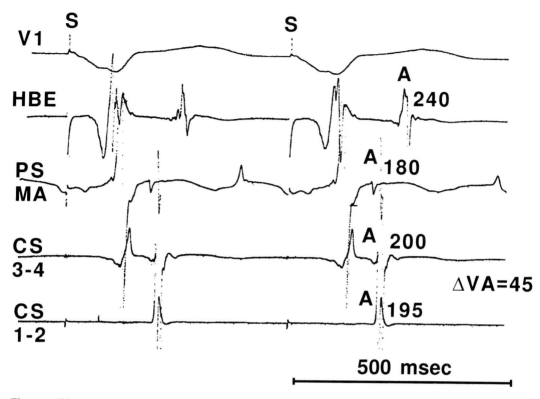

Figure 6. Ventricular pacing in a patient with a concealed left posteroseptal AP. From top to bottom are lead V_1, the His bundle electrogram (HBE), an electrogram recorded in the left ventricle at the posteroseptal mitral annulus (PS MA), and coronary sinus electrograms recorded at the ostium (CS 3–4) and in the proximal coronary sinus (CS 1–2), which was the site of the shortest ventriculoatrial interval within the coronary sinus. The ventriculoatrial conduction intervals in milliseconds are indicated adjacent to the corresponding atrial electrograms (A). The difference between the ventriculoatrial interval measured by the His bundle catheter and the shortest ventriculoatrial interval recorded within the coronary sinus (ΔVA) was 45 ms. When the ΔVA is less than 25 ms, successful ablation of a posteroseptal AP usually is achieved using a right-sided approach.[19] In contrast, when the ΔVA is 25 ms or more, a left endocardial approach usually is necessary, as was the case in this patient. The AP was ablated at the posteroseptal mitral annulus, where the ventriculoatrial interval was 180 ms.

negative predictive values of a deeply inverted delta wave in lead II for predicting the need for ablation from within a venous branch of the coronary sinus were 95% and 97%, respectively.

During mapping, the characteristic features of posteroseptal APs that require ablation from within the coronary sinus include: the absence of a clear-cut earliest site of endocardial activation during antegrade and/or retrograde AP conduction; a diminutive or absent endocardial AP potential; an AP potential within the coronary sinus or

one of its branches that is larger than the largest amplitude AP potential that can be found at the endocardial surface; a presumed AP potential recorded within the coronary sinus that is larger in amplitude than the atrial and ventricular electrograms (Figure 8).[20]

If the electrocardiogram and results of initial endocardial and coronary sinus mapping suggest the presence of a posteroseptal AP that will require ablation from within the coronary sinus, it is often helpful to visualize the coronary sinus by injection of

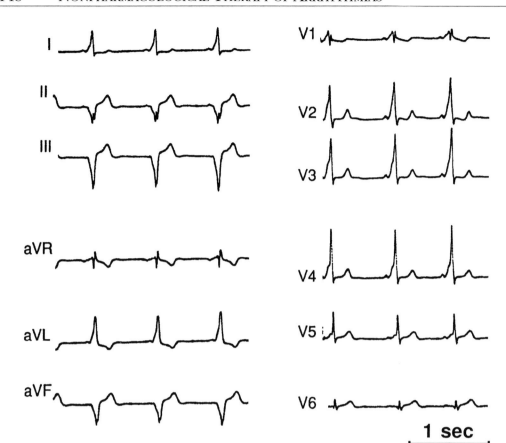

Figure 7. Electrocardiogram of a patient with a posteroseptal AP that was ablated by delivery of RF energy in a middle cardiac vein of the coronary sinus. Note that the delta wave in lead II is steeply negative. Approximately 50% of patients with a posteroseptal AP who have this type of delta wave in lead II will require ablation from within the coronary sinus or middle cardiac vein.[18]

contrast, to determine the location and size of branches of the coronary sinus, and to look for venous anomalies such as a diverticulum.[21]

It has been suggested that a transesophageal echocardiogram prior to the electrophysiology procedure is useful in patients with posteroseptal APs, because it allows visualization of the middle cardiac vein and coronary sinus diverticula. In a study of 18 consecutive patients with a posteroseptal AP who underwent both a transesophageal echocardiogram and a coronary sinus angiogram, five of five coronary sinus diverticula and 22 of 22 middle cardiac veins were correctly identified with the transesophageal echocardiogram.[22] In the five patients

who had a coronary sinus diverticulum, the AP was successfully ablated in each by delivery of RF energy at the neck of the diverticulum.[22] Therefore, whether by transesophageal echocardiography before the ablation procedure, or coronary sinus angiography during the procedure, it may be very helpful to directly visualize the coronary sinus.

The results of experimental and clinical studies have suggested that the application of RF energy within the coronary sinus is generally safe. A mean of approximately 25 W of RF energy delivered inside the coronary sinus in closed-chest dogs resulted in well-circumscribed areas of necrosis and fibrosis in the fat of the atrioventricular sul-

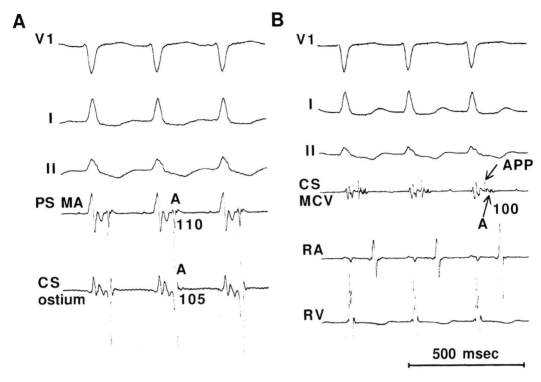

Figure 8. Mapping of a posteroseptal AP during orthodromic reciprocating tachycardia. **A.** The shortest ventriculoatrial intervals recorded during orthodromic reciprocating tachycardia at the posteroseptal mitral annulus (PS MA) and coronary sinus (CS) ostium were 110 and 105 ms, respectively. The AP could not be ablated by delivery of RF energy at either site. **B.** The shortest ventriculoatrial interval of 100 ms was recorded in the middle cardiac vein of the coronary sinus (CS MCV), where a presumed AP potential (APP) was present. As is typical of posteroseptal APs that require ablation from within the coronary sinus or one of its branches, a distinct AP potential could not be recorded endocardially, and the AP potential recorded within the coronary sinus was larger in amplitude than the ventricular and atrial electrograms. A = atrial electrogram; RA = right atrial electrogram; RV = right ventricular electrogram.

cus, with no involvement of the circumflex coronary artery and no instances of coronary sinus perforation.[23]

In a clinical study, 5–30 W of RF energy were delivered for 5–30 sec inside the coronary sinus in nine patients who had a left posteroseptal AP.[24] The criterion used to select patients for this approach was the presence of a prominent presumed AP potential within the proximal coronary sinus. Seven of the nine APs (78%) were successfully ablated, and in five of these patients, the ablation site was within the middle cardiac vein or a venous anomaly. The only complication was transient coronary sinus spasm, but this had no clinical sequelae. Therefore,

this study demonstrated that successful ablation of posteroseptal APs within the coronary sinus or one of its branches can be accomplished safely. However, it is important to keep in mind that energy levels greater than 30 W and applications within small branches of the coronary sinus where the vessel lumen was occluded by the ablation catheter were avoided.[24] In another study, hemopericardium and cardiac tamponade occurred when RF energy was delivered within a small venous branch of the coronary sinus,[25] emphasizing the importance of exercising great care when attempting ablation of an AP from within the coronary sinus.

Electrogram Criteria for Selection of Target Sites

The electrogram criteria that are used to select sites for ablation of posteroseptal APs are the same as for APs in other locations. When the AP is manifest, the highest probability of success occurs at sites that have stable electrograms, a presumed AP potential (Figure 9), and where local ventricular activation occurs before the onset of the delta wave.[26] When the AP is concealed, the best predictors of successful ablation are electrogram stability, a presumed retrograde AP potential, and retrograde continuous electrical activity during ventricular pacing or orthodromic tachycardia (Figure 10).[26]

Methods of Power Delivery

When posteroseptal APs are ablated using a right- or left-sided endocardial approach, an electrode-tissue interface temperature of at least 60°C should be attained, to minimize the possibility of a recurrence of AP conduction.[27] Temperatures greater

than 90°C should be avoided, to prevent coagulum formation.[27]

Two techniques are available for titrating power to achieve the optimal temperature at the electrode–tissue interface. Ablation catheters that have a thermistor embedded in the distal electrode are widely available, and these catheters allow either manual or automatic titration of power to maintain an electrode–tissue interface temperature between 60°C and 80°C. If a thermistor catheter is not available, impedance monitoring can be substituted. With this technique, the application of RF energy is initiated at a low power setting (10–12 W) and the initial impedance is noted. The power is then titrated upward until the impedance falls by 5–10 ohms, which correlates well with an electrode–tissue interface temperature of 60°C.[28] In a randomized study, temperature and impedance monitoring were found to be equally effective in optimizing the results of AP ablation.[28]

A more cautious approach is warranted when ablating posteroseptal APs that are within the coronary sinus, one of its branches, or a venous anomaly. To mini-

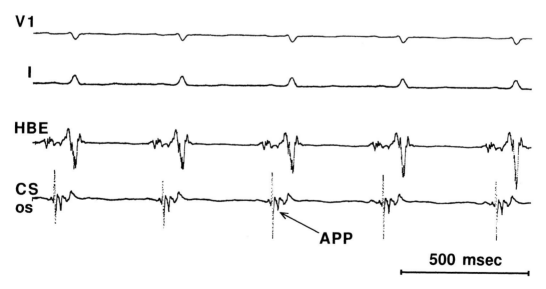

Figure 9. An effective target site for ablation of a right posteroseptal AP. A presumed accessory pathway potential (APP) is present at the coronary sinus ostium, sandwiched between a large atrial depolarization and a small ventricular depolarization. The APP is simultaneous with the His bundle depolarization in the His bundle electrogram (HBE).

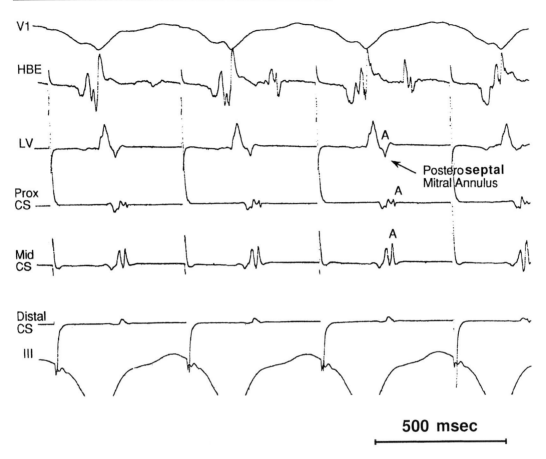

Figure 10. Mapping of a concealed left posteroseptal AP during ventricular pacing. Shown are V_1, the His bundle electrogram, a left ventricular recording (LV) obtained with the ablation catheter positioned at the posteroseptal aspect of the mitral annulus, recordings at the proximal (prox), mid, and distal coronary sinus (CS), and lead III. Continuity of the atrial electrogram (A) with the ventricular electrogram, as seen in this case in the left ventricular recording, is a predictor of successful ablation. Delivery of RF energy at this site was effective in ablating the AP.

mize the possibility of perforation and cardiac tamponade, pericarditis, and injury to a coronary artery, temperature monitoring should be performed with the goal of identifying the lowest effective temperature. In contrast to endocardial ablation sites, an electrode–tissue interface temperature of 60°C is not necessary, and may be dangerous. A target temperature of 45°C is initially used, with gradual titration upward until AP conduction is eliminated. The application is then continued for 20–30 sec at the temperature that first resulted in AP block. It should be emphasized that if the ablation

catheter appears to be occluding the vein, an attempt at ablation may not be advisable.

Efficacy of Catheter Ablation of Posteroseptal Accessory Pathways

In the first part of the 1990s, several large series of patients undergoing RF ablation of APs were published, and in the subgroup of patients with posteroseptal APs, the success rates ranged from 81% to 98%.[25,30–33] Some investigators noted that the success rate for ablation of posteroseptal APs was somewhat lower than for left free wall APs[32] and that a larger number of RF applications were necessary than for APs in other locations.[30] In these initial studies, the recurrence rate of AP conduction ranged from 7% to 10%, with no indication that posteroseptal APs were associated with a higher recurrence rate than were APs in other locations.[25,31–33]

In more recent studies focusing specifically on RF ablation of posteroseptal APs, refinements in mapping and ablation techniques have been reflected in higher success rates of 97%–100%,[14,19] and a recurrence rate as low as zero.[14]

The overall experience with RF ablation of posteroseptal APs at the University of Michigan from 1990 through 1996 now encompasses 173 pathways, of which 165 (95%) were successfully ablated (unpublished data). The recurrence rate after an initially successful procedure was 3%, with all but one patient having a successful long-term outcome after a repeat procedure.

Distribution of Effective Target Sites for Ablation

In a study of 74 consecutive patients with a posteroseptal AP at the University of Oklahoma, the distribution of successful ablation sites was as follows: right-sided in 51 patients (69%); left-sided in 15 patients (20%); and within the coronary sinus or a middle cardiac vein in 8 patients (11%).[34]

At the University of Michigan Medical Center, 173 of 970 accessory pathways (18%) in 919 patients who underwent catheter ablation of an AP were found to be posteroseptal (unpublished data). Among the 165 posteroseptal APs that were successfully ablated, 116 (70%) were ablated with a right-sided approach and delivery of RF energy at or near the ostium of the coronary sinus, 43 (26%) were ablated using a left ventricular approach and delivery of RF energy at the posteroseptal aspect of the mitral annulus, and the remaining 6 (4%) were ab-

lated by delivery of RF energy inside the coronary sinus, either within the middle cardiac vein or a diverticulum (unpublished data). The higher prevalence of APs requiring ablation within a venous branch or anomaly of the coronary sinus at the University of Oklahoma may reflect the fact that a large proportion of patients are referred to this center after a failed ablation attempt elsewhere. Therefore, the 4% prevalence in the University of Michigan series may be more representative of a random sample of posteroseptal APs.

While experience at the Universities of Oklahoma and Michigan has suggested that 20%–26% of posteroseptal APs require a left ventricular approach for ablation, the results from other centers have been widely divergent, with the percentage of posteroseptal APs requiring a left ventricular approach varying from only 4%[14] to as high as 39%.[19] It is likely that this marked variability in the need for a left ventricular approach is largely attributable to a difference in the criteria used to identify posteroseptal APs. For example, Dhala et al.[14] considered an AP to be posteroseptal when the earliest site of atrial or ventricular activation was within the proximal 1 cm of the coronary sinus, whereas Chiang et al.[19] used a 2-cm criterion. The use of a 1-cm criterion would be expected to exclude posteroseptal APs most likely to require a left ventricular approach, explaining why only 4% of pathways were ablated from the left side in the study of Dhala et al. compared to 39% when the 2-cm criterion was used. It also is possible that some posteroseptal APs can be ablated from either side of the septum, depending on how persistently a given approach is attempted.

Bipolar Tricuspid Annulus–Mitral Annulus Configuration

Delivery of RF energy between the distal electrodes of two catheters positioned against the posteroseptal aspects of the tricuspid and mitral annuli at times may be effective in ablating a posteroseptal AP when conventional unipolar applications at these locations individually have been ineffective. In one study, right- and left-sided unipolar applications of RF energy at sites where local ventricular activation occurred 0–20 ms prior to the delta wave were unsuccessful in ablating a posteroseptal AP in five patients; energy delivery simultaneously at the same sites in a bipolar configuration resulted in a successful outcome.[35] It was postulated that the bipolar applications resulted in necrosis extending from one electrode tip to the other, thereby interrupting an AP deep within the septum.[35] Although the bipolar technique of RF energy delivery was helpful in this small series of patients, it is also possible that these APs could have been ablated by more precise delivery of unipolar applications of energy. In addition, energy applications were delivered at a fixed power setting, without either impedance or temperature monitoring, and it is possible that the unipolar applications did not result in adequate tissue heating. Nevertheless, the bipolar technique of energy delivery should be kept in mind as a possible alternative to unipolar ablation in patients with posteroseptal APs that are difficult to ablate.

Complications

Aside from the complications that may result from any electrophysiological procedure, such as thrombophlebitis, damage to the femoral artery, or right ventricular perforation, the only complication that has been associated with the endocardial approach to RF ablation of posteroseptal APs has been high-degree AV block. One patient in each of two studies developed AV block as a complication of posteroseptal AP ablation, resulting in an incidence of approximately 2%.[25,31] However, one of these patients had corrected transposition of the great vessels and a baseline abnormality in AV nodal conduction.[25] The single patient

with AV block in the other study remains the only patient with this complication in the updated University of Michigan series of 173 patients who have undergone RF ablation of a posteroseptal AP (unpublished data). Therefore, the actual risk of AV block as a complication of posteroseptal AP ablation in patients normal AV nodal conduction in the baseline state appears to be less than 1%.

Additional types of complications have been reported in associated with ablation of posteroseptal APs from within the coronary sinus or one of its branches. These include pericarditis,[25] pericardial effusion,[14] cardiac tamponade,[25] coronary artery spasm,[33] and coronary sinus spasm.[24] It is likely that the risk of these types of complications can be minimized by the avoidance of energy delivery within small branches of the coronary sinus that are completely occluded by the ablation electrode.

Conclusions

Because of the complexity of the posteroseptal space, posteroseptal APs may be more challenging to ablate than are free wall APs. However, a high success rate is achievable if mapping is approached in a systematic fashion. When there is manifest preexcitation, the configuration of delta waves can provide helpful clues for determining whether a right-sided, left-sided, or coronary sinus approach is needed for ablation. The ΔVA during orthodromic tachycardia also may provide information helpful in determining whether a right- or left-sided approach is needed. Based on these clues and on the results of preliminary mapping within the coronary sinus, detailed mapping can then be commenced using the approach deemed to be most likely to succeed. For example, if the delta wave is positive in lead II and the ΔVA during orthodromic tachycardia is less than 25 ms, detailed right-sided mapping in the region around the coronary sinus ostium and in the first centimeter of the coronary sinus is warranted. On the other hand, if coronary sinus mapping demonstrates the earliest site of atrial and/or ventricular activation to be 2 cm from the os, and the ΔVA during orthodromic tachycardia is greater than 25 ms, a left-sided endocardial approach is appropriate, utilizing either transseptal catheterization or retrograde aortic entry into the left ventricle. If there is a markedly negative delta wave in lead II, the possibility of an epicardial AP must be kept in mind, and the coronary sinus and its branches should be thoroughly mapped if right- and left-sided endocardial mapping fail to reveal a successful target site for ablation.

When clues as to the location of an effective target site are not available, are contradictory, or prove to be incorrect, the following stepwise approach may be appropriate:

1. Delivery of RF energy at the right-sided site of earliest atrial or ventricular activation through the AP or at sites where a presumed AP potential is recorded.
2. Delivery of RF energy at the left-sided site of earliest atrial or ventricular activation through the AP,

or at sites where a presumed AP potential is recorded.

3. Injection of contrast into the coronary sinus to determine the location and caliber of the middle cardiac vein or veins and to look for a coronary sinus diverticulum, followed by detailed mapping within the coronary sinus and its branches. Careful delivery of RF energy within the coronary sinus, middle cardiac vein, or coronary sinus diverticulum may be appropriate if mapping demonstrates a site that is more attractive than the right- and left-sided endocardial sites, and if the ablation catheter does not appear to be completely occluding the venous structure.

4. Delivery of RF energy in bipolar fashion between electrodes positioned at the most attractive right- and left-sided endocardial sites.

Although this stepwise approach to ablation of posteroseptal APs requires prospective validation, the results of published studies suggest that its use will allow a success rate approaching 100%.

References

1. Morady F, Scheinman MM. Transvenous catheter ablation of a posteroseptal accessory pathway in a patient with the Wolff-Parkinson-White syndrome. N Engl J Med 1984; 310:705–707.
2. Morady F, Scheinman MM, Kou WH, et al. Long-term results of catheter ablation of a posteroseptal accessory atrioventricular connection in 48 patients. Circulation 1989;79:1160–1170.
3. Sealy WC, Gallagher JJ. The surgical approach to the septal area of the heart based on experiences with 45 patients with Kent bundles. J Thorac Cardiovasc Surg 1980;79:542–551.
4. Davies LM, Byth K, Ellis P, et al. Dimensions of the posterior septal space and coronary sinus. Am J Cardiol 1991;68:621–625.
5. Truex RC, Bishof JK, Downing DF. Accessory atrioventricular muscle bundles. II. Cardiac conduction system in a human speci-

men with Wolff-Parkinson-White syndrome. Anat Rec 1960;137:417–435.
6. Dreifus LS, Wellens HJ, Watanabe Y, et al. Sinus bradycardia and atrial fibrillation associated with the Wolff-Parkinson-White syndrome. Am J Cardiol 1976;38:149–156.
7. Becker AE, Anderson RH, Durrer D, et al. The anatomical substrates of Wolff-Parkinson-White syndrome: a clinicopathologic correlation in seven patients. Circulation 1978;57:870–879.
8. Sealy WC, Mikat EM. Anatomical problems with identification and interruption of posterior septal Kent bundles. Ann Thorac Surg 1983;36:584–595.
9. Guiraudon GM, Klein GJ, Sharma AD, et al. Surgical ablation of posterior septal accessory pathways in the Wolff-Parkinson-White syndrome by a closed heart circuit. J Thorac Cardiovasc Surg 1986;92:406–413.
10. Guiraudon GM, Guiraudon CM, Klein GJ, et

al. The coronary sinus diverticulum: a pathologic entity associated with the Wolff-Parkinson-White syndrome. Am J Cardiol 1988;
62:733–735.

11. Rodriguez LM, Smeets JL, de Chillou C, et al.
The 12-lead electrocardiogram in midseptal,
anteroseptal, posteroseptal and right free
wall accessory pathways. Am J Cardiol 1993;
72:1274–1280.

12. Goldberger J, Wang Y, Scheinman M. Stimulation of the summit of the right ventricular
aspect of the ventricular septum during orthodromic atrioventricular reentrant tachycardia. Am J Cardiol 1992;70:78–85.

13. Kerr CR, Gallagher JJ, German LD. Changes
in ventriculoatrial intervals with bundle
branch block aberration during reciprocating tachycardia in patients with accessory
atrioventricular pathways. Circulation 1982;
66:196–201.

14. Dhala AA, Deshpande SS, Bremner S, et al.
Transcatheter ablation of posteroseptal accessory pathways using a venous approach
and radiofrequency energy. Circulation
1994;90:1799–1810.

15. Miller JM, Rosenthal ME, Gottlieb CD, et al.
Usefulness of the delta HA interval to accurately distinguish atrioventricular nodal
reentry from orthodromic septal bypass tract
tachycardias. Am J Cardiol 1991;68:
1037–1044.

16. Martinez-Alday JD, Almendral J, Arenal A,
et al. Identification of concealed posteroseptal Kent pathways by comparison of ventriculoatrial intervals from apical and posterobasal right ventricular sites. Circulation
1994;89:1060–1067.

17. Morady F, Strickberger SA, Man KC, et al.
Reasons for prolonged or failed attempts at
radiofrequency catheter ablation of accessory pathways. J Am Coll Cardiol 1996;27:
683–689.

18. Arruda M, Wang X, McClelland J, et al. ECG
algorithm for predicting radiofrequency ablation site in posteroseptal accessory pathways [abstract]. PACE 1992;15:535.

19. Chiang CE, Chen SA, Tai CT, et al. Prediction
of successful ablation site of concealed posteroseptal accessory pathways by a novel algorithm using baseline electrophysiologic
parameters: Implication for an abbreviated
ablation procedure. Circulation 1996;93:
982–991.

20. Langberg JJ, Man KC, Vorperian VR, et al.
Recognition and catheter ablation of subepicardial accessory pathways. J Am Coll Cardiol 1993;22:1100–1104.

21. Lesh MD, Van Hare G, Kao AK, Scheinman
MM. Radiofrequency catheter ablation for

Wolff-Parkinson-White syndrome associated with a coronary sinus diverticulum.
PACE 1991;1410:1479–1484.

22. Omran H, Pfeiffer, Tebbenjohanns J, et al.
Echocardiographic imaging of coronary
sinus diverticula and middle cardiac veins
in patients with preexcitation syndrome: impact on radiofrequency catheter ablation of
posteroseptal accessory pathways. PACE
1995;18:1236–1243.

23. Langberg J, Griffin JC, Herre JM, et al. Catheter ablation of accessory pathways using radiofrequency energy in the canine coronary sinus. J Am Coll Cardiol 1989;13:491–
496.

24. Giorgberidze I, Saksena S, Krol RB, et al. Efficacy and safety of radiofrequency catheter
ablation of left-sided accessory pathways
through the coronary sinus. Am J Cardiol
1995;76:359–365.

25. Jackman WM, Wang X, Friday KJ, et al. Catheter ablation of accessory atrioventricular
pathways (Wolff-Parkinson-White syndrome) by radiofrequency current. N Engl J
Med 1991;324:1605–1611.

26. Calkins H, Kim YN, Schmaltz S, et al. Electrogram criteria for identification of appropriate target sites for radiofrequency catheter ablation of accessory atrioventricular
connections. Circulation 1992;85:565–573.

27. Langberg JJ, Calkins H, Atassi R, et al. Temperature monitoring during radiofrequency
catheter ablation of accessory pathways. Circulation 1992;86:1469–1474.

28. Strickberger SA, Ravi S, Daoud E, et al. Relation between impedance and temperature
during radiofrequency ablation of accessory
pathways. Am Heart J 1995;130:1026–
1030.

29. Strickberger SA, Weiss R, Knight BP, et al.
Randomized comparison of two techniques
for titrating power during radiofrequency
ablation of accessory pathways. J Cardiovasc
Electrophysiol 1996;7:795–801.

30. Schluter M, Geiger M, Siebels J, et al. Catheter ablation using radiofrequency current to
cure symptomatic patients with tachyarrhythmias related to an accessory atrioventricular pathway. Circulation 1991;84:
1644–1661.

31. Calkins H, Langberg J, Sousa J, et al. Radiofrequency catheter ablation of accessory
atrioventricular connections in 250 patients:
abbreviated therapeutic approach to Wolff-
Parkinson-White syndrome. Circulation
1992;85:1337–1346.

32. Lesh MD, Van Hare GF, Schamp DJ, et al.
Curative percutaneous catheter ablation
using radiofrequency energy for accessory
pathways in all locations: results in 100 con-

secutive patients. J Am Coll Cardiol 1992;19:1303–1309.

33. Swartz JF, Tracy CM, Fletcher RD. Radiofrequency endocardial catheter ablation of accessory atrioventricular pathway atrial insertion sites. Circulation 1993;87:487–499.

34. Wang X, Jackman WM, McClelland J, et al. Sites of successful radiofrequency ablation of posteroseptal accessory pathways [abstract]. PACE 1992;15:535.

35. Bashir Y, Heald SC, O'Nunain S, et al. Radiofrequency current delivery by way of a bipolar tricuspid annulus-mitral annulus electrode configuration for ablation of posteroseptal accessory pathways. J Am Coll Cardiol 1993;22:550–556.

Chapter 8

Modification of Atrioventricular Node for Management of Atrioventricular Nodal Reentrant Tachycardia

Dennis W.X. Zhu

Introduction

The most common form of paroxysmal supraventricular tachycardia in adults is atrioventricular nodal reentrant tachycardia (AVNRT).[1–3] It accounts for approximately 60%–70% of patients with paroxysmal supraventricular tachycardia at referral centers. In the past, pharmacological therapy was the principal modality of management. In spite of its effectiveness in reducing the frequency and severity of recurrence, chronic drug treatment was limited by side effects, risk of proarrhythmia, expense, and patient compliance. Although surgical modification of atrioventricular (AV) node provided potentially curative results, the procedure was limited by operative morbidity and prolonged hospital stay.[4–7] Thus, it was reserved only for severely symptomatic and drug-refractory patients.

During the last decade, the development of the radiofrequency (RF) catheter modification technique has revolutionized the management of AVNRT.[8–26] It not only has been highly efficacious, but has also proven to be low risk. In addition, it is the most cost-effective form of therapy for the long term.[27,28] As a result, catheter modification has obviated the need for chronic antiarrhythmic therapy, and has virtually eliminated surgical procedures for AVNRT.

Evolving Anatomic and Physiological Concepts of Atrioventricular Node

The advent of catheter modification not only has provided a curative therapy for AVNRT, but has also rekindled research interest in the anatomy and physiology of the AV node. In spite of extensive investigation for nearly a century, the understanding of the anatomic structure of the AV node as well as the reentrant circuit for AVNRT continues to evolve.

In the normal heart, the AV node provides the only electrical connection between the atria and the ventricles. The classic description of the AV node is accredited to Tawara, who identified a spindle-shaped compact network of cells known as "knoten," which was located anteriorly at the base of the interatrial septum.[29] The ana-

From Singer I, Barold SS, Camm AJ (eds): Nonpharmacological Therapy of Arrhythmias for the 21st Century: The State of the Art. Futura Publishing Co, Inc., Armonk, NY, © 1998.

tomic boundary of the AV node was defined by Koch as a triangular region confined by the tendon of Todaro superiorly, the coronary sinus ostium posteriorly, and the attachment of tricuspid septal leaflet inferiorly.[30] The compact AV node is situated in the apex of this triangle anteriorly at the membranous septum, where it penetrates the central fibrous body to become the His bundle. Histologically, three different areas of specialized tissues have been observed connecting the working atrial and ventricular myocardia: (1) a transitional cell zone located between the atrial myocardium and the compact AV node, (2) the compact AV node, and (3) the bundle traveling through the membranous septum.[31]

To explore the anatomic substrate of the atrial connections of the compact AV node, Truex and Smythe performed detailed morphometric reconstruction of the AV junction in the human heart. They divided the AV junction into three parts: the anterior-superior approach, located in the anterosuperior atrial septum; the posterior approach, extending toward the coronary sinus ostium; and the compact AV node.[32] James described two principal groups of fibers projecting from the interatrial septum and entering the compact AV node.[33] Becker and Anderson grouped the atrial–AV nodal transitional cells into three zones: superficial, deep, and posterior.[34] The superficial zone was continuous with the anterior and superior aspect of the compact node, the posterior zone joined the inferior and posterior aspect of the compact node, and the deep zone connected the left atrium to the deep portion of the compact node. Racker investigated the anatomic and functional substrates of atrial–AV nodal connections in the dog heart.[35,36] She described discrete atrionodal bundles: superior, medial, and lateral, with the latter two converging to form a proximal AV bundle that in turn is continuous with the compact AV node. She demonstrated that the superior atrionodal bundle and the proximal AV bundle possessed functional properties of specialized conducting tissue distinctly different

from those of working atrial myocardium. The superior atrionodal bundle might form a part of the fast pathway, whereas the posterior and medial atrionodal bundles and proximal AV bundle might constitute a major portion of the slow pathway. Despite these basic investigations, most clinical electrophysiologists in the 1970s and 1980s embraced the simple concept of complete intranodal confinement of the AV nodal pathways to explain the anatomic substrate of AVNRT.[37,38] To support the concept of an entirely intranodal location of the reentrant circuit for AVNRT, it has been proposed that there are upper and lower common pathways that connect the slow and the fast pathways. There is evidence to support the concept of a lower common pathway, with the point of turnaround located above the His bundle recording site. In support of this, it has been shown that transient block can occur below the His bundle during AVNRT without changing the cycle length of the tachycardia. The H-Ae interval is shorter during tachycardia than the HA interval during ventricular pacing. Finally, the introduction of premature ventricular extrastimuli that penetrate the His bundle does not effect the cycle length of the tachycardia. The evidence for an upper common pathway is more controversial and certainly not considered definitive at the present time. More recently, the data accumulated from the intraoperative mapping and catheter modification have changed our compact circular paradigm of the AV node to the participation of the paranodal atrial myocardium within the reentrant circuit.[39]

Perhaps the most common observation put forth at the present time is the fact that catheter ablation of the slow or fast pathway is successful at sites that are distinct from the compact AV node (Figure 1).[40] However, it is not yet clear whether patients with AVNRT have any specific anatomic differences from normal individuals, or whether the propensity for developing AVNRT relates more to functional differences in the conduction characteristics of the two pathways.

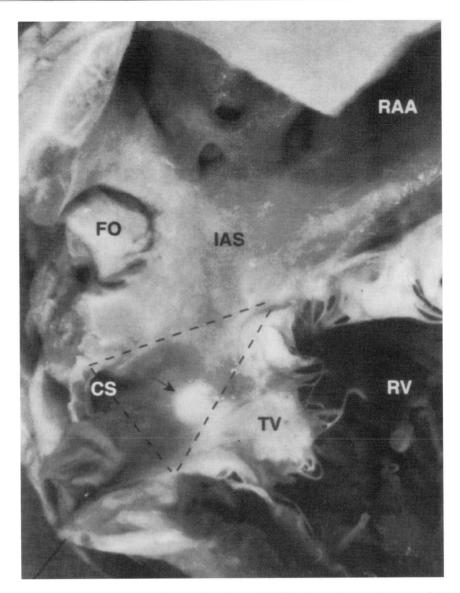

Figure 1. Heart specimen from a patient with typical AVNRT who underwent a successful AV nodal slow pathway modification with a single RF application 5 months earlier. Koch's triangle is marked with dashed lines. The lesion is seen as a pale circular area (arrow) adjacent to the tricuspid annulus, just anterior to the coronary sinus (CS) ostium, and lies 11.5 mm from the apex of the triangle where the compact AV node is located. FO = fossa ovalis; IAS = intra-atrial septum; RAA = right atrial appendage; RV = right ventricle; TV = tricuspid valve. Reproduced with permission from Olgin JE, et al.[43]

Anatomic studies on the AV junction in patients with dual AV nodal physiology and AVNRT are limited. In 10 patients with dual AV nodal physiology who underwent heart transplantation, no obvious histological difference was noted in the explanted hearts.[41] The morphology of the proximal coronary sinus in patients with AVNRT has been studied by angiography. The ostium was larger and appeared like a windsock in patients with AVNRT but was tubular in the individuals without AVNRT.[42,43] Since the posterior transitional cell zone of the AV junction is located in the proximity of the coronary sinus ostium, the anatomic difference may be implicated in the arrhythmogenesis of AVNRT.

It is important to know the dimensions of the AV junction in the human heart in order to achieve an optimal outcome for catheter modification of AVNRT. In adults, the compact AV node has a length of 5–7 mm and a width of 2–5 mm.[44] The size of Koch's triangle has been measured during intraoperative mapping and postmortem examination.[45] The mean length of this triangle (from the nearest edge of the coronary sinus to the central fibrous body) was 17 ± 3 mm and mean height was 13 ± 3 mm. Certain variability in AV junction dimensions has been reported.[46] The dimensions of Koch's triangle were also measured fluoroscopically in 218 patients during catheter modification of AVNRT.[47] In the right anterior oblique view, the distance between the proximal His bundle area and the base of the coronary sinus ostium was 25.9 ± 7.9 mm, whereas the site of successful slow pathway modification was consistently located at about 13 mm from the site recording the proximal His bundle deflection.

Clinical Presentation

Most frequently, AVNRT presents in young to middle-aged adults. However, it is not uncommon to have the initial manifestation of AVNRT starting at age 70 or even 80. It seems to be more common in women. At Baylor College of Medicine, the mean age of patients with AVNRT undergoing catheter modification was 49 ± 14 years (range 14–92); 73% of them were female. Atrioventricular nodal reentrant tachycardia could also occur in the transplanted heart.[48] Depending on age at presentation, concomitant structural heart disease may or may not be present. The literature does not suggest any particular relation to a specific form of organic heart disease. After initial presentation, recurrent

episodes vary in frequency and duration, and usually persist for years. A causal relationship of posture or exercise to initiation of tachycardia is noticed by some patients. Typically, the onset and termination of the tachycardia occur abruptly. In some patients, however, termination of tachycardia is frequently perceived as gradual, perhaps due to the presence of sinus tachycardia after sudden termination of AVNRT. Palpitations or the feeling of a rapid heart beat is the most common symptom. This can be accompanied by the sensation of rapid, regular pounding in the neck, dyspnea, chest tightness, and dizziness. Syncope may occur and may be related more to impaired vasomotor adaptation to tachycardia than to rapid heart rate itself.[49] Occasionally, syncope may be the presenting symptom with the patient not having any awareness of a rapid heart beat. The signs are not specific, with most patients presenting with a rapid and diminished pulse. In the absence of concomitant heart disease, the prognosis is usually excellent.

Electrocardiographic Manifestations

During sinus rhythm, ECG manifestations compatible with dual AV nodal physiology are relatively uncommon but include: (1) sudden and persistent prolongation of PR interval (Figure 2); (2) PR alternans; and (3) dual ventricular responses to a single supraventricular impulse conducted simultaneously along the fast and slow pathways.[50] During AVNRT, a regular, narrow QRS complex tachycardia is observed with rates usually ranging from 140 to 240 bpm. The rate of tachycardia may vary greatly from episode to episode, and even within the same long episode. This variation reflects the dynamic influence of the autonomic nervous system on both antegrade and retrograde conductions of the AV node reentrant circuit. With rapid tachycardia, alternans of QRS amplitude may be present. In typical

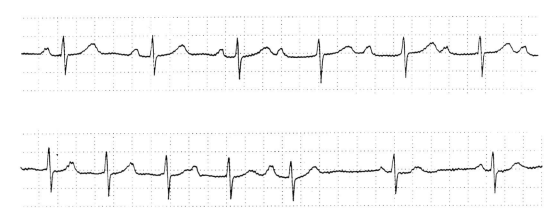

Figure 2. A continuous rhythm strip from a patient with dual AV nodal physiology and typical AVNRT. In the top tracing, abrupt prolongation of the fourth PR interval from 190 to 400 ms followed an atrial premature complex. In the bottom tracing, the long PR interval normalized as with slowing of atrial rate. The change in PP intervals probably alters the conduction of the fast pathway, shifting conduction to the slow pathway. Perpetuation of slow pathway conduction is more likely due to repetitive concealment of conduction from the slow pathway to the fast pathway, thus blocking conduction in the latter.

AVNRT, which is seen in the majority of patients, the P wave is seen in close proximity to the QRS complex (Figure 3). Commonly, the P wave is obscured by the QRS complex or may be seen slightly before or after the QRS complex. The presence of a pseudo-r wave in lead V_1, or a pseudo-s wave in leads II, III, and aVF is highly suggestive of typical AVNRT (Figure 4). In the atypical form of AVNRT, the RP interval is greater than the PR interval (Figure 5). The P wave is inverted in leads II, III, AVF, positive in V_1, V_2, aVL, and isoelectric or biphasic in lead I. ST-T change of considerable magnitude is often observed and is a nonspecific phenomenon

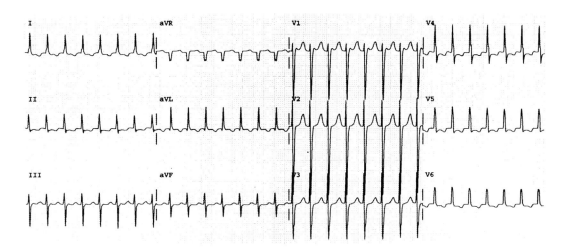

Figure 3. Typical AVNRT. No P wave is identifiable in any of the leads. Non-specific ST-T changes are present. Reproduced with permission from Singer I, ed., p 281.[110]

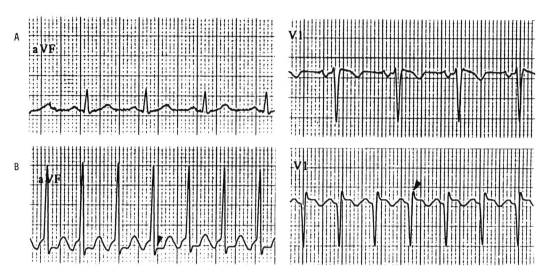

Figure 4. Electrocardiographic clues to typical AVNRT. Panel A shows sinus rhythm in leads AVF and V_1. During typical AVNRT (panel B), the retrograde P waves are observed at the terminal portion of the QRS complex in lead AVF, mimicking terminal delay (arrowhead), and as a pseudo r' wave (arrowhead) in lead V_1. Reproduced with permission from Zhu DWX, et al.[42]

generally unrelated to structural heart disease. Functional bundle branch block may develop, thus rendering a wide QRS complex tachycardia. However, functional bundle branch block should not affect the rate of tachycardia. since the bundle branches are not part of the reentrant circuit (Figure 6). The onset of tachycardia is commonly preceded by a premature atrial beat which results in a sudden prolongation of the PR interval. When spontaneous termination is observed and the P wave can be identified, the last QRS of the tachycardia is frequently associated with a P

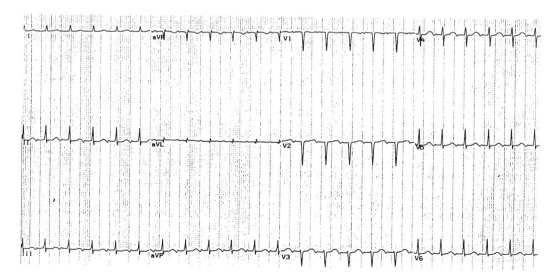

Figure 5. Atypical AVNRT. The P wave is recognizable and is inverted in leads II, III, and AVF. Also, note that the P wave is immediately following the T wave with a RP interval longer than PR interval. Reproduced with permission from Zhu DWX, et al.[42]

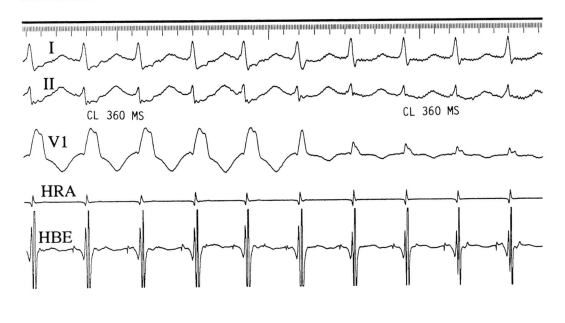

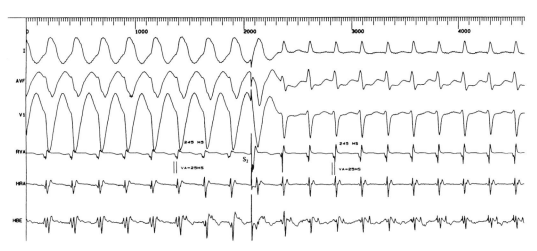

Figure 6. Surface electrocardiogram (I, II, aVF, and V_1) and intracardiac recordings during typical AVNRT. In the upper panel, the right bundle branch block aberration spontaneously resolves. In the lower panel, the left bundle branch block aberration resolves with the introduction of a single ventricular extra stimulus (S_2). Note that the functional right or left bundle branch block does not affect the rate or the VA interval of the tachycardia since the bundle branches are not part of the reentrant circuit. RVA = right ventricular apex; HRA = high right atrium; HBE = His bundle electrogram. Reproduced with permission from Zhu DWX, et al.[42]

wave since AVNRT usually stops by blocking in the antegrade limb of the reentrant circuit. Because these electrocardiographic manifestations may also be seen occasionally in other forms of supraventricular tachycardia, electrophysiological study is necessary for differential diagnosis.

Electrophysiological Features

Dual AV Nodal Physiology

Moe and colleagues demonstrated the presence of two functionally distinct AV nodal pathways in an animal model and hy-

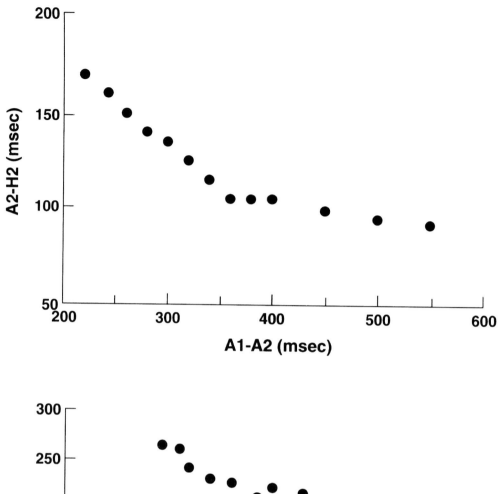

Figure 7. Antegrade AV nodal conduction curves (A_2-H_2 vs. A_1-A_2) showing the "normal" pattern (upper panel) and dual AV nodal physiology (lower panel). Reproduced with permission from Zhu DWX, et al.[42]

pothesized that such conduction patterns may be the basis of AV nodal reentry.[51] Similar AV nodal conduction patterns were described later in humans.[52] The "normal" AV nodal conduction curve is shown in Figure 7, upper panel. With increasing prematurity of the atrial extrastimulus, there is a gradual and progressive conduction delay in the AV node. A discontinuous AV nodal conduction curve is shown in Figure 7, lower panel. At a critical atrial coupling interval, a 10-ms decrement in A_1-A_2 results in a marked prolongation (>50 ms) in A_2-H_2. This sudden increase in conduction time (jump) has been called dual AV nodal physiology. Further 10-ms decrements in A_1-A_2 result in relatively smaller additional prolongations (<50 ms) in A_2-H_2. Dual AV nodal physiology is probably due to two anatomically or functionally dissociated conduction pathways in the AV node; the fast pathway has a shorter conduction time and a longer refractory period, and the slow pathway has a longer conduction time (by at least 50 ms) and a shorter refractory period. The abrupt rise in AV nodal conduction time is believed to represent a switch in conduction from the fast pathway to the slow pathway. Using a single atrial extrastimulus, dual AV nodal physiology has been identified in 50%-90% of patients with documented AVNRT.[39] On the other hand, dual AV nodal physiology has also been demonstrated with a single atrial extrastimulus in 5%-10% of subjects without a history of AVNRT.[53] Rosen and colleagues extended Moe's concept of dual AV nodal physiology to clinical AVNRT. They suggested that unidirectional block in one of the pathways with conduction over the alternate route leading to retrograde conduction over the previous blocked pathway allowed for reentry.[54,55] This fundamental concept is well established and is no longer a subject of controversy, although the specific anatomic correlates underlying the physiological phenomenon remain less clear.[37–40,56–59] In some patients, multiple jumps are demonstrated in the antegrade AV nodal conduction curve (Figure 8). This may represent the presence of multiple

antegrade slow pathways and probably more complex reentrant tissue mass.[60]

Dual AV nodal physiology has also been demonstrated in the retrograde AV nodal conduction. It is defined by a discontinuous V_1-V_2 versus A_1-A_2 curve. With increasing prematurity of the ventricular extrastimulus, there is a gradual and progressive retrograde conduction delay in the AV node or the His-Purkinje system. At a certain coupling interval of the ventricular extrastimulus, the ventriculoatrial (VA) interval abruptly lengthens. This pattern of retrograde conduction was first described by Wu and colleagues in a patient with atypical AVNRT.[61] In 1981, Sung and colleagues studied the pattern of retrograde AV nodal conduction and noted that the sequence of retrograde atrial activation changed when conduction switched from the fast pathway to the slow pathway.[62] When retrograde conduction proceeds over the fast pathway, the earliest atrial activation occurs near the His potential recording site; in contrast, the retrograde slow pathway conduction first activates the atrium near the coronary sinus ostium. High-resolution intraoperative mapping studies have confirmed that earliest activation of the atrium during retrograde fast pathway conduction occurs near the apex of the triangle of Koch[63] and that retrograde conduction over the slow pathway resulted in earliest atrial activation near the coronary sinus ostium.[64] A posterior exit site near the coronary sinus ostium during retrograde slow pathway conduction may be demonstrated in nearly one-half of patients with spontaneous AVNRT.[17]

Atrioventricular Nodal Reentrant Tachycardia

Typical (Slow/Fast) Atrioventricular Nodal Reentrant Tachycardia

This is by far the most prevalent type and it accounts for approximately 90% of AVNRT cases. When an atrial premature beat blocks in the fast pathway and proceeds down slowly along the slow pathway, the fast pathway has enough time to recover from its refractoriness. This allows the impulse to activate the fast pathway retrogradely and return to the atrium, giving rise to an AV nodal reentrant echo beat. The impulse then travels down along the slow pathway again. The continuation of this process leads to the develop-

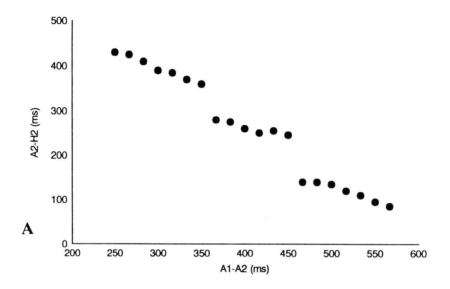

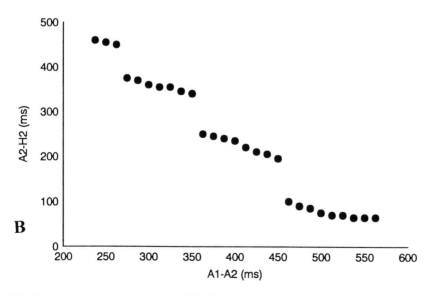

Figure 8. Multiple jumps are demonstrated in the antegrade AV nodal conduction curves in two patients with AVNRT, suggesting the presence of multiple slow pathways. (**A**) In patient A, the A_2-H_2 interval prolongs markedly (jump) at A_1-A_2 coupling intervals of 460 and 360 ms. (**B**) In patient B, the jumps occurred at A_1-A_2 coupling intervals of 460, 360, and 280 ms.

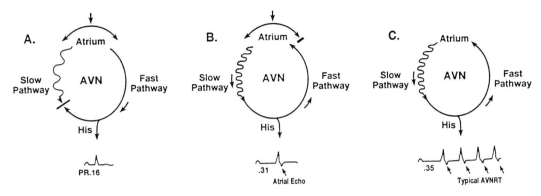

Figure 9. The diagrams illustrating the mechanism of typical (slow/fast) AVNRT. (**A**) During sinus rhythm, the impulse antegradely penetrates both the fast and slow pathways simultaneously. Because the impulse reaches the His bundle via the fast pathway, the PR interval is normal. The impulse conducting down the distal fast pathway may continue to activate the slow pathway retrogradely and collide with the incoming antegrade impulse in the slow pathway. (**B**) Because the effective refractory period of the fast pathway is longer than the slow pathway, an atrial premature beat may block in the fast pathway and conduct down the slow pathway to activate the His bundle. Therefore, PR interval is prolonged. Because the antegrade conduction along the slow pathway is slow, the fast pathway has enough time to regain its excitability. The impulse that has reached distal slow pathway may continue to activate the fast pathway retrogradely and return to the atrium, giving rise to a typical AV nodal reentrant echo beat (arrow). The impulse continues to conduct down the slow pathway, but the latter has not recovered from its refractoriness yet. Thus, the impulse blocks in the slow pathway antegradely. (**C**) An even earlier atrial premature beat blocks in the fast pathway and conducts down the slow pathway more slowly. This provides more time not only for the fast pathway to recover from its refractoriness and giving rise to a single reentrant echo, but also allows the slow pathway to recover to have repetitive antegrade reentrance. The continuation of this process leads to the development of typical AVNRT. Reproduced with permission from Zhu DWX, et al.[42]

ment of typical AVNRT (Figure 9). The essential features of typical AVNRT are as follows:

1. Dual AV nodal physiology is present in more than two-thirds of the patients. At a critical coupling interval, a 10-ms decrement in A_1-A_2 blocks the fast pathway. The impulse proceeds down the slow pathway and results in a marked increase (>50 ms) in A_2-H_2. This abrupt rise in AV nodal conduction time is often associated with the initiation of AV nodal reentrant echo beat or AVNRT (Figure 10).

2. Because the retrograde AV conduction is through the fast pathway, the retrograde atrial activation sequence during tachycardia is concentric, with the earliest atrial activation recorded at His bundle site.

3. The VA interval during tachycardia is usually less than 60 ms if atrial activation is measured at the His potential recording site, and is usually less than 90 ms if measured at high right atrium.[65]

4. Premature ventricular stimulation during tachycardia should not preexcite the atrium when delivered at a time that the His bundle is refractory. When an earlier coupled premature ventricular stimulation advances the timing of the His bundle activation, the timing of atrial activation may also be advanced.[39] However, the atrial activation sequence should remain unaltered. There is almost invariably a 1:1 AV relationship. However, this is not obligatory and AVNRT may continue in the presence of intermittent 2:1 or Wenckebach AV block probably due to functional infrahisian block (Figure 11).[66]

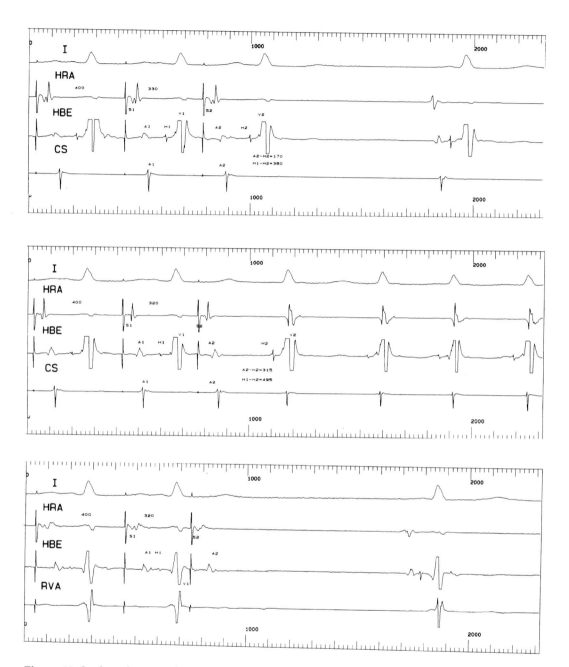

Figure 10. Surface electrocardiogram and intracardiac recordings during single atrial extrastimulus at a drive cycle length of 400 ms. (Top) When a single atrial extrastimulus (S_2) is introduced at a coupling interval of 330 ms, the AH interval (A_2-H_2) is 170 ms. (Middle) When the coupling interval of the atrial extra stimulus (S_2) is decreased by 10 ms to 320 ms, the AH interval (A_2-H_2) is markedly lengthened to 315 ms (jump), demonstrating dual AV nodal physiology. Typical AVNRT is initiated in association with the jump in AV nodal conduction time. (Bottom) After ablation of the slow pathway, there is no antegrade slow pathway conduction or AVNRT induction when a single atrial extrastimuli (S_2) is introduced at the same coupling interval (320 ms). HRA = high right atrium; HBE = His bundle electrogram; CS = coronary sinus electrogram; RVA = right ventricular apex.

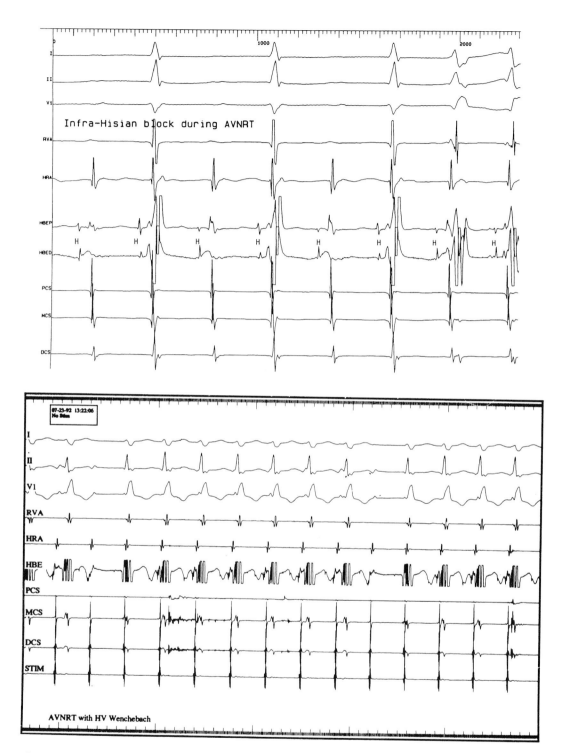

Figure 11. Surface electrocardiogram (I, II, V$_1$) and intracardiac recordings demonstrating typical AVNRT with intermittent 2:1 infrahisian block and a 1:1 AV conduction with functional right bundle branch block aberration during the last two beats (top panel). Wenckebach infra-Hisian block and right bundle branch block during typical AVNRT are shown in the bottom panel. RVA = right ventricular apex; HRA = high right atrium; HBE = His bundle electrogram; CS = coronary sinus electrogram.

Atypical (Fast/Slow and Slow/Slow) Atrioventricular Nodal Reentry Tachycardia

Atypical AVNRT is observed in approximately 10% of patients presenting with AVNRT.[39,67,68] Because the retrograde conduction occurs over the slow pathway, it is characterized by a long RP interval (RP>PR or RP=PR). The diagnosis of atypical AV nodal reentry can be confirmed by the following features:

1. Retrograde dual AV nodal conduction curve is present in some patients.

2. Tachycardia induction depends on a critical VA or His–atrial interval during retrograde slow pathway conduction.

3. The retrograde atrial activation sequence during the tachycardia is concentric with the earliest atrial activation recorded at/or near the ostium of the coronary sinus (Figure 12).

4. VA interval during tachycardia is greater than 60 ms if atrial activation is measured at the His potential site and is usually greater than 90 ms if measured at high right atrium.

5. Premature ventricular stimulation during tachycardia should not reset the atrium when delivered at a time that the His bundle is refractory. When an earlier coupled premature ventricular stimulation advances the timing of the His bundle activation, the timing of atrial activation may also be advanced. However, the atrial activation sequence should remain unchanged.[39]

Slow/slow AVNRT theoretically requires the presence of two or more slow pathways with different conduction properties and refractory periods. In slow/slow AVNRT, one slow pathway is used for antegrade conduction and another slow pathway for retrograde conduction.[39,69,70] During tachycardia, the earliest retrograde atrial activation is recorded posteroinferiorly and the retrograde conduction time is similar to the antegrade conduction time.

Diagnostic Electrophysiological Study

The typical diagnostic electrophysiological study and catheter ablation procedure are usually performed during a single session. Ideally, all antiarrhythmic drugs should be discontinued for at least five half-lives prior to the procedure to facilitate tachycardia induction and accurate assessment of conduction properties. The patient

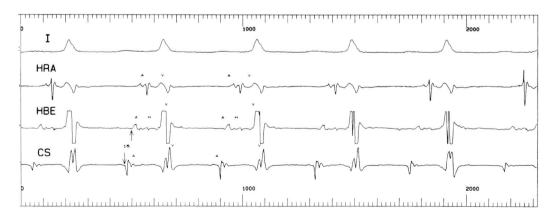

Figure 12. Surface electrogram (1) and intracardiac recordings during atypical AVNRT. The earliest retrograde atrial activation is recorded at the ostium of the coronary sinus (CS) and is about 16 ms earlier than the atrial activation recorded on the His catheter (HBE). HRA = high right atrium.

is brought to the electrophysiology laboratory in the fasting state. After sedation with benzodiazapine (midazolam or diazapine), and an intravenous narcotic (meperidine, morphine, fentanyl, or propofol), local anesthesia is applied with 1%–2% lidocaine. Six French quadripolar catheters are routinely introduced into the femoral vein using the Seldinger technique and advanced into the right ventricle, right atrial appendage, and across the tricuspid valve for recording the His bundle potential. Although coronary sinus recording is not critical for the diagnosis of typical AVNRT, the placement of the coronary sinus catheter is helpful in the diagnosis of atypical AVNRT and in identifying the mechanism of other superventricular tachycardias that may coexist with AVNRT. It is also useful to aid in anatomic recognition of the ostium of the coronary sinus (where the coronary sinus catheter makes a sharp angulation) as a marker for slow pathway modification. This is usually accomplished by introducing a 6F or 7F hexapolar or decapolar catheter into the internal jugular, subclavian, or femoral vein and positioning it in the coronary sinus so that the proximal pair of the electrodes are in the vicinity of the ostium. We commonly insert a 7F quadripolar deflectable ablation catheter (2-5-2 mm with a 4- or 5-mm tip) into the right femoral vein and position it in the coronary sinus. If there is no evidence of accessory pathway present and there is no other types of supraventricular tachycardias inducible during the diagnostic electrophysiological study, the same catheter may be withdrawn and used for modification of AVNRT. No heparin is given routinely unless the patient has recognized risk for thromboembolic complications.

When the basic intervals are measured, it is important to note that preexisting prolonged PR interval may indicate an abnormal or absent fast pathway in the antegrade direction. Although there is concern about AV block when the antegrade slow pathway modification is contemplated, slow pathway ablation is usually safely accomplished in these patients.[71]

Decremental right ventricular pacing is usually performed first to evaluate the sequence of retrograde atrial activation, the VA, and His-atrial intervals. It is started at a cycle length slightly shorter than that of the sinus rhythm and decreased gradually (by 10 or 20 ms) until a VA conduction block is observed. Four patterns of response may be observed.[72] The usual response seen in patients with typical AVNRT is a rapid VA conduction via the fast pathway. Usually no incremental conduction is noted, down to the cycle length of VA block. The other pattern of response is VA conduction occurring predominantly via the fast pathway at relatively long cycle lengths and a sudden shift of conduction to the slow pathway associated with abrupt VA conduction prolongation at a critical cycle length. Once this shift occurs, further VA conduction prolongation may occur with pacing cycle length shortening until retrograde conduction block occurs. In some patients, the retrograde conduction is predominantly over the slow pathway. These patients are prone to atypical AVNRT and may manifest typical AVNRT only after improvement of the retrograde fast pathway conduction with isoproterenol infusion. Occasionally, VA conduction may be absent in the baseline and only present during isoproterenol infusion.

Programmed ventricular stimulation is performed using an eight-beat drive train followed by the introduction of single ventricular extrastimulus decremented by 10 or 20 ms. The cycle length of the drive train is slightly shorter than that of the sinus rhythm. With progressive shortening of the V_1-V_2 coupling interval, a gradual VA prolongation is seen in some individuals, primarily due to His-Purkinje system or AV nodal retrograde conduction delay. In other patients, a sudden VA prolongation develops at a critical coupling interval, either due to shift of retrograde conduction from the fast to slow AV nodal pathway, or due to shift of the retrograde His bundle activation route from the right bundle–His axis to the left bundle–His axis. In the latter, the sudden prolongation of VA interval usually is less than 50 ms.

Decremental atrial pacing is usually performed from the right atrial appendage starting at a cycle length slightly shorter than that of the sinus rhythm and shortened gradually (by 10 or 20 ms) until an AV conduction block is observed. In the majority of patients, the gradual increase in AH interval is followed by an abrupt and marked AH prolongation (more than 50 ms), frequently resulting in the initiation of AV nodal reentrant echo beats or AVNRT. For the remaining patients, a gradual and smooth AH interval prolongation is seen until antegrade block occurs.

Programmed atrial stimulation is performed using an eight-beat drive train followed by the introduction of a single atrial extrastimulus decremented by 10 or 20 ms. The cycle length of the drive train is slightly shorter than that of the sinus rhythm. Dual AV nodal physiology associated with initiation of an AV nodal reentrant echo beat or AVNRT occurs in 70% of patients. Failure to demonstrate dual pathways may occur if conduction times over the slow and fast pathways are similar, if the refractory period of the fast pathway is similar to that of the slow pathway, or if the refractory period of the fast pathway is not obtainable due to atrial refractoriness or if either pathway exhibits unidirectional conduction, i.e., antegrade conduction occurs exclusively over the slow pathway and retrograde conduction exclusively over the fast pathway. Multiple jumps are demonstrable in some patients. These patients may have multiple slow pathways and a more complex reentrant tissue mass. The other type of response is a continuous curve with initiation of AVNRT at a critical A_1-A_2 coupling interval.[73] This occurs when conduction times of the two pathways are not markedly different, yet the effective refractory period of the fast pathway is longer than the slow pathway. Addition of a second drive train and/or a second extrastimulus may alter the refractory periods in such a way as to allow the dual AV nodal physiology to become manifest and AVNRT to be initiated.

Induction of AVNRT is essential prior to catheter modification. Typical AVNRT is usually induced when a critical degree of AV nodal conduction delay is achieved, either with decremental atrial pacing and/or delivery of critically timed atrial premature stimulation. Retrograde His–Purkinje system conduction delay during ventricular premature stimulation prevents significant delay or block in the AV nodal region; therefore, the initiation of typical AVNRT is uncommon with this approach. Atypical AVNRT can be initiated with either atrial or ventricular stimulation. Sometimes, both typical and atypical AVNRT may be induced in the same patient. Isoproterenol may be required for initiation of AVNRT in about 50% of the patients. Isoproterenol infusion is usually started at 1 mcg/min and should be titrated to increase the sinus rate by 20%–30%. This will improve antegrade slow pathway conduction and/or retrograde fast pathway conduction, thus facilitating the induction of AVNRT. Administration of atropine or beta blockers may also be helpful for induction of AVNRT on occasion.

Differentiating typical AVNRT from other forms of supraventricular tachycardias is usually not difficult. AV reciprocating tachycardia using a concealed septal accessory pathway as the retrograde limb can be ruled out if atrial activation during tachycardia occurs before or simultaneously with ventricular activation (VA interval $\leq$50 ms) and premature ventricular stimulation delivered during tachycardia when the His bundle is refractory fails to preexcite the atrium (not very specific). Atrial reentrant tachycardia is unlikely if there is an identical sequence of retrograde atrial activation during both tachycardia and ventricular pacing. Premature ventricular stimulation that retrogradely advances the timing of His bundle activation by 30 ms or more will advance the timing of atrial activation in typical AVNRT or produce VA block and terminate the tachycardia, but

Table 1
Differential Diagnosis of Atypical Atrioventricular Nodal Reciprocating Tachycardia

	Atrial Tachycardia	Atypical AVNRT	AVRT (Posteroseptal Pathway)
Earliest site of atrial activation	Right or left atrium	Coronary sinus ostium	Proximal coronary sinus
PVC delivered during tachycardia when His bundle is refractory	No preexcitation	No preexcitation	Preexcitation
Induction of tachycardia with ventricular pacing	Rare	Common	Common
Termination of tachycardia with PVC that does not preexcite atrium	No	Yes	Yes
Functional BBB during tachycardia	No change in cycle length or VA interval	No change in cycle length or VA interval	Small increase in cycle length and VA interval with BBB ipsilateral to pathway
AV block during tachycardia	May occur	2:1 AV block below His bundle occasionally seen	No

AVNRT = Atrioventricular reciprocating nodal tachycardia; BBB = bundle branch block; PVC = premature ventricular stimulus.

should not usually affect the timing of atrial activation in atrial reentrant tachycardia. It is more difficult to distinguish AV reciprocating tachycardia utilizing a slow conducting accessory pathway in the retrograde direction or atrial tachycardia from atypical AVNRT (Table 1). Orthodromic AV reciprocating tachycardia can be excluded by the failure to advance the timing of atrial activation by a premature ventricular stimulation that results in a 30 ms or greater advance in the timing of local ventricular activation close to the site of earliest atrial activation. The difference between the VA interval during ventricular pacing at the right ventricular apex and base may also be helpful. It has been shown that the VA interval shortens when the ventricular stimulus is moved from the apex to the base in the presence of a posteroseptal pathway, whereas the VA interval tends to lengthen in patients with normal conduction or AVNRT. Para-Hisian pacing during sinus rhythm with intermittent His bundle capture can be used to differentiate retrograde conduction over a posteroseptal accessory pathway from retrograde conduction over the AV node.[74] Entrainment of the tachycardia by ventricular pacing at a cycle length 15 to 20 ms shorter than the tachycardia cycle length, with an identical atrial activation sequence distinguishes AVNRT from atrial tachycardia. Termination of the tachycardia by a premature ventricular stimulation that did not conduct to the atrium definitely excludes atrial tachycardia. When an accessory pathway does coexist with AVNRT, the former should be targeted first before proceeding to selective modification of the AV node.

In spite of extensive efforts, tachycardia occasionally cannot be induced in some patients with dual AV nodal physiology and documented spontaneous supraventricular tachycardia which has the electrocardiographic features of AVNRT. Such incidence of noninducibility appears to be around 2%.[75] The American College of Cardiology/ American Heart Association Committee on Clinical Intracardiac Electrophysiology and Catheter Ablation Procedures considered slow pathway modification in such patients to be a class II indication, reflecting the uncertainty and divided opinion on this issue.[76] Due to the lack of a valid endpoint, we previously did not perform catheter modification of the AV node in three such patients. Two of them returned after additional episodes of spontaneous tachycardia. Typical AVNRT was induced and ablated in both patients during the subsequent procedure. Recently, the outcome of slow pathway modification was reported in seven patients with dual AV nodal physiology and supraventricular tachycardia but who did not have inducible tachycardia in the electrophysiology laboratory.[75] Dual AV nodal physiology was eliminated in six patients and remained present in one. During a follow-up period of 15 ± 10 months, no patient had recurrence of symptomatic tachycardia. Since then, we have modified the slow pathway in three such patients; all of them remained free of symptoms at follow-up.

Catheter Modification of the AV Node

In the last decade, catheter ablation has evolved rapidly from AV junction ablation to selective modification of the AV node. The early application of catheter modification of the AV node involved the use of direct current shocks.[77,78] The introduction of radiofrequency (RF) catheter modification has revolutionized the treatment for AVNRT.[8-26] The lesions generated by RF current are small, discrete, and more homogenous than those produced by direct current shocks. Radiofrequency ablation avoids complications from barotrauma associated with intracardiac direct current shocks and eliminates the need for general anesthesia. The energy output of the RF current can be either temperature controlled or manually titrated to achieve the desired effects.[79] Although newer energy sources and tools are emerging,[80] RF catheter ablation

is superior to any other currently available technique.

The ablation catheter should have a distal electrode of 4 or 5 mm in length and a deflectable distal segment. The length of the deflectable segment of the catheter that has proved most effective for modification of AVNRT ranges from 2.5 to 3.0 inches. A 7F quadripolar catheter with an interelectrode distance of 2 mm and a spacing of 5 mm between the proximal and distal pairs has been most commonly used. Six or 8 French ablation catheters are also commercially available. The ablation catheter is usually inserted into the right femoral vein. The venous access sheath should generally be one French size bigger than the ablation catheter to allow for convenient manipulation. The RF energy generator is typically able to produce an unmodulated bipolar output at 300–750 kHz, which is delivered between the catheter tip electrode and an adhesive electrosurgical dispersive pad applied to the right posterior chest. Temperature-controlled energy delivery is generally preferred. Temperature, impedance, voltage, and current should be continuously monitored.[81] The fluoroscopic right anterior oblique view (RAO) at 15°–30° and the left anterior oblique view (LAO) at 40°–60° are usually used for mapping and ablation. Usually monoplane fluoroscopy is adequate. Biplane fluoroscopy shortens the RAO–LAO transition time but adds the cost and the mass of equipment beside the patient. The position of the tip electrode of the ablation catheter is closely monitored during RF energy delivery to detect displacement. Energy is usually applied for 30–60 sec during sinus rhythm. Occasionally, current may be applied during ventricular pacing, atrial pacing, or tachycardia. Energy delivery is immediately terminated at first sight of a nonconducted P wave and in the event of an impedance rise or displacement of the catheter tip. Inducibility of AVNRT is tested following each likely successful energy application to determine whether the endpoint of the procedure has been achieved. It is safe and feasible to perform catheter modification of the slow pathway on an outpatient basis.[28] At our center, over 95% of the patients were discharged home on the same day of the procedure. For patients after fast pathway modification, continuous ambulatory electrocardiographic monitoring as an inpatient for 1 or 2 days is appropriate due to the likelihood of delayed onset of AV block.[82]

Selective Modification of the Fast Pathway

Technique

The retrograde fast pathway of AVNRT is usually located near the anterosuperior tricuspid annulus along the atrial septum, just proximal to where the maximal His potential is recorded.[63] The ablation catheter is initially positioned at the AV junction in a routine fashion to record the maximal amplitude of the bipolar His potential from the distal pair of the electrodes. The catheter is then slowly withdrawn for several millimeters and manipulated slightly superiorly from the site where the maximal His potential is recorded. A gentle clockwise torque is applied to direct the catheter tip toward the atrial septum. While the RAO view is generally utilized for placement of the ablation catheter, the LAO view is sometimes utilized to confirm the position of the ablation catheter tip on the tricuspid annulus (Figure 13).

The electrograms at target sites (Figure 14) are characterized by the following: (1) the amplitude of the local atrial potential is usually at least twice as high as the local ventricular potential; and (2) the His potential is proximal and small (less than 0.1 mV). Additionally, electrograms at the ablation site may be evaluated for retrograde atrial activation via the fast pathway during either ventricular pacing or AVNRT to ensure that it occurs earlier than or simultaneously with that recorded by the His catheter.

Usually, RF energy is delivered during sinus rhythm. The ablation catheter is held steadily with a gentle clockwise torque applied to maintain close contact to the atrial septum. The surface electrocardiogram is continuously monitored for PR prolongation and/or occurrence of AV block. Radiofrequency application at an effective site invariably results in the occurrence of an accelerated junctional rhythm. However, accelerated junctional rhythm is a nonspecific finding that may also occur during 25% of RF applications at ineffective sites.[83] Ventriculoatrial dissociation is expected to be present during the accelerated junctional rhythm that occurs during modification of the AV nodal fast pathway. When accelerated junctional rhythm develops, it is advisable to pace the atrium at a faster rate to allow for continuous monitoring of the integrity of antegrade AV conduction.

The RF current is initially applied at a power output of 10 W for 15 sec, and then increased by 5 W every 10 sec up to a maximum of 30 W.[12] During temperature-controlled energy application, the temperature should be preselected at 50°C initially and then upgraded in 5°C steps every 10 sec up to a maximum of 80°C.[15] When the accelerated junctional rhythm or prolongation of PR interval (≤50%) occurs, energy delivery or temperature setting should be held constant for an additional 20–30 sec. Radiofrequency current application is immediately terminated if the PR interval increases by more than 50% or if a nonconducted P wave is noted. The endpoints of the procedure are: (1) a PR interval prolongation by about 50% over baseline and/or the elimination or marked attenuation of retrograde fast pathway conduction, and (2) noninducibility of AVNRT before and during isoproterenol infusion. If AVNRT remains inducible or retrograde fast pathway conduction persists, the ablation catheter is moved stepwise slightly inferiorly toward the midseptum, and energy is applied again until the endpoints are met. The gradual titration of energy or temperature during each RF application may reduce the risk of AV block.

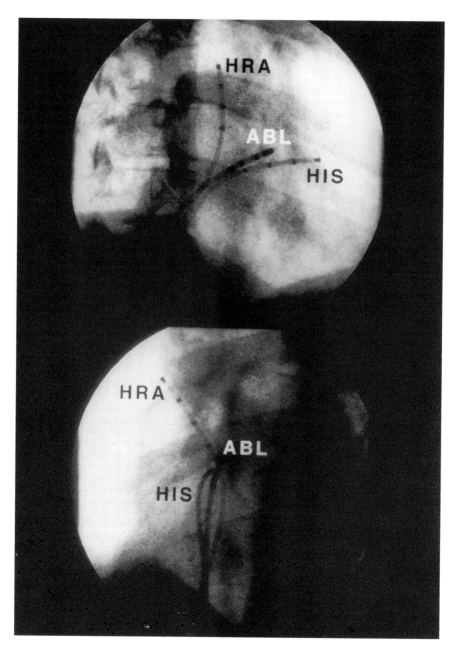

Figure 13. Fast pathway ablation site in the fluoroscopic RAO view (upper panel). A quadripolar catheter is in the His potential recording site (HIS). The distal electrode of the ablation catheter (ABL) is at the site of successful ablation. The target site of fast pathway ablation usually is located proximally and superiorly to the site where the maximal His potential is recorded. HRA = catheter positioned at high right atrium. The lower panel shows the catheter positions in the LAO view. Reproduced with permission from Zhu DWX, et al.[42]

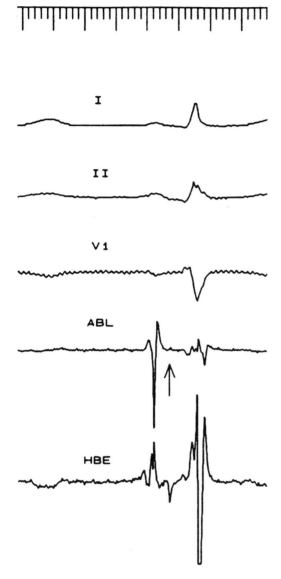

Figure 14. The surface electrocardiogram (I, II, V₁) and typical intracardiac electrogram recorded from the distal pair electrodes of the ablation catheter (ABL) at the successful site of fast pathway ablation. The amplitude of the local atrial electrogram is more than twice as the local ventricular electrogram. The recorded His potential is small and proximal. HBE = His bundle electrogram. Reproduced with permission from Zhu DWX, et al.[42]

Electrophysiological Changes after Fast Pathway Modification

Electrophysiological testing is repeated following successful energy application. The major electrophysiological findings after fast pathway modification are as follows: (1) prolongation of the AH interval and elimination of dual AV nodal physiology (Figure 15); (2) elimination or significant attenuation of retrograde fast pathway conduction; and (3) insignificant changes in the AV block cycle length and AV nodal effective refractory period. Following fast pathway modification, the average increase in the AH interval was about 50%. Complete elimination of retrograde fast pathway conduction occurred in 40%–72% of the patients, and the remainder had a marked increase in the VA block cycle length.[10,12,15] Dual AV nodal physiology was eliminated in 85%–100% of the patients in whom it was present before the ablation. Because the slow pathway of the AV node usually has a shorter antegrade block cycle length and effective refractory period than does the fast pathway, the change in shortest 1:1 AV conduction cycle length and AV nodal effective refractory period after the fast pathway ablation is minimal.

After successful modification of the fast pathway and elimination of typical AVNRT, about 10% of patients may have inducible atypical AVNRT that was not apparent before modification.[84] This arrhythmia usually does not occur spontaneously at follow-up, and therefore, additional modification efforts may not be necessary. Occasionally, patients who underwent fast pathway modification had only the retrograde fast pathway modified. This resulted in elimination of retrograde fast pathway conduction without a change in the AH interval or antegrade dual AV nodal physiology. This observation implies that, at least in some patients, the antegrade and retrograde fast pathways may be anatomically separate. In the majority of patients, however, fast pathway modification results in elimination or attenuation of both antegrade and retrograde fast pathway conduction.

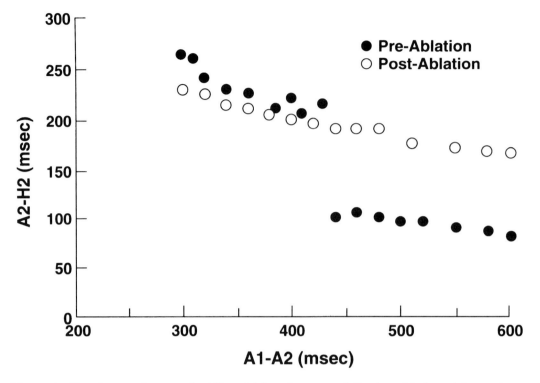

Figure 15. The change of antegrade AV nodal function curve following ablation of fast pathway. Before ablation, dual AV nodal physiology is present. The marked prolongation in the A_2-H_2 interval occurs when the A_1-A_2 coupling interval shortens by 10 ms from 440 ms to 430 ms. Following fast pathway ablation, all antegrade conduction is proceeded through the slow pathway and the dual AV nodal physiology is eliminated. Reproduced with permission from Zhu DWX, et al.[42]

Results

Early attempts of catheter modification of AV node for management of AVNRT targeted the fast pathway. The results of published series of selective fast pathway modi-fication are summarized in Table 2.[8–15] A clear learning curve was present. The later series achieved a success rate of up to 96%.[15]

The tachycardia recurrence rate after fast pathway modification is approximately 3%–10%.[9–12,14,15] The majority of recur-

Table 2
Outcome of Radiofrequency Catheter Modification of AV Nodal Fast Pathway

Study	Date	Patients (n)	Success Rate (%)	Heart Block (%)	Recurrence (%)
Goy et al.[8]	1990	8	5 (63%)	0	1 (13%)
Lee et al.[9]	1991	39	33 (85%)	3 (8%)	2 (5%)
Calkins et al.[10]	1991	44	42 (95%)	1 (2%)	5 (11%)
Jazayeri et al.[11]	1992	19	15 (78%)	4 (21%)	0
Langberg et al.[12]	1993	127	10 (76%)	9 (8%)	0
Mitrani et al.[13]	1993	13	113 (87%)	3 (23%)	4 (30%)
Chen et al.[14]	1993	32	30 (93%)	2 (5%)	1 (3%)
Kottkamp et al.[15]	1995	53	51 (96%)	0	3 (5%)

rences occur within the first 3 months. Repeat modification for recurrent tachycardia has been as safe and efficacious as the initial modification procedure.[8-15]

Complications

The most significant complication associated with modification of fast pathway is the development of inadvertent complete heart block necessitating permanent pacemaker implantation. According to early series of selective fast pathway modification, the incidence of complete heart block was substantial, ranging from 2% to 21%. The difference may reflect the operators' technique and experience.[9-12,14] In a recent study by Kottkamp and colleagues, no complete AV block occurred in 53 consecutive patients who underwent selective modification of the fast pathway.[15]

Careful attention to the details of the technique may decrease the incidence of AV block. First, atrial pacing at whatever rate is necessary to override the accelerated junctional rhythm so that the AV conduction can be closely monitored throughout the duration of energy application. Second, energy should be delivered in a titrated fashion, and temperature-controlled energy delivery is preferred. If inadvertent complete AV block occurs, it is usually apparent during the procedure.[9-11] Patients who have recovered from transient complete AV block should be followed closely because development of late complete AV block has been reported and may occur days or weeks after the procedure.[11-13] Other complications of fast pathway modification are rare and are similar to the complications associated with any invasive electrophysiological study including vascular damage, deep venous thrombosis, pulmonary emboli, and cardiac tamponade.

Selective Modification of the Slow Pathway

Basic Considerations

Two principal approaches for modifying the slow pathway of AVNRT have been used extensively. In the first approach, the intracardiac atrial electrogram configuration is used to identify the target site for modification.[16,17] In the second approach, target sites are localized primarily on fluoroscopically based anatomic landmarks.[11,18-20] Several other approaches have also been described.

Regardless of the approach, RF energy is applied in the same manner. When an appropriate target site for slow pathway modification is identified, RF energy is usually delivered at a preselected temperature of 60°C[85,86] or a power output of 20–30 W for up to 60 sec. If the target site is close to where the His potential is recorded, it is prudent to start with a lower temperature or energy output and to titrate upward using the onset of accelerated junctional rhythm as the endpoint. Successful modification of AV nodal slow pathway is usually achieved at an electrode–tissue interface temperature of about 50°C (range 42°C to 56°C).[85] Accelerated junctional rhythm during RF energy application occurs in nearly 100% of effective sites. However, it also occurs in up to 65% of ineffective applications.[83] On the other hand, the absence of junctional rhythm usually predicts inefficacy of the application, and the RF energy delivery should not be continued for more than 15 sec at the same site. Intact VA conduction is expected during the accelerated junctional rhythm that accompanies slow pathway ablation, even when there is poor VA conduction during baseline ventricular pacing (Figure 16). The appearance of VA block during accelerated junctional rhythm may herald the onset of AV block and the energy application should be discontinued immediately.[83,87] On the other hand, it has been noted that patients with unrecognized VA block during accelerated junctional rhythm during slow pathway modification often did not have impairment of AV conduction afterward.[88]

Electrogram-Guided Approach

The RAO view is initially used for catheter placement because it best displays

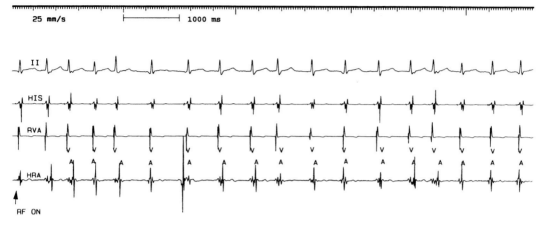

Figure 16. Accelerated junctional rhythm during RF ablation of the AV nodal slow pathway. The electrograms recorded in the right ventricular apex (RVA) and high right atrium (HRA) are labeled as "V" and "A," respectively. There is a 1:1 VA conduction with a short VA conduction time during accelerated junctional rhythm. This is the desired response during RF application for ablation of the slow pathway. The appearance of VA block during accelerated junctional rhythm may herald the development of AV block and the RF application should be discontinued immediately. His = His bundle electrogram. Reproduced with permission from Zhu DWX, et al.[42]

Koch's triangle in profile. Positioning of the ablation catheter is best performed during sinus rhythm because the atrial and ventricular electrograms on the tricuspid valve are more easily distinguishable. After the ablation catheter has been manipulated to cross the tricuspid valve and recording the His bundle potential, an inferoposterior deflection of the distal segment is made, and the catheter is slowly withdrawn with gentle clockwise torque applied so that the tip of the catheter lies along the tricuspid annulus near the ostium of the coronary sinus (but not in or posterior to the coronary sinus ostium). During sinus rhythm, the area along the posteromedial tricuspid annulus in proximity to the coronary sinus ostium is carefully mapped with bipolar recordings from the distal pair of electrodes of the ablation catheter. The electrogram criteria used to identify the target site are an atrial-to-ventricular electrogram ratio of <1.0 and the presence of a probable slow pathway potential (Figure 17).[16,17] Two types of slow pathway potentials have been identified: a sharp, discrete, high-frequency potential following the initial atrial electrogram[17] (Figure 18, upper panel) and a multicompo-

nent atrial electrogram[16] (Figure 18, lower panel). Usually, the slow pathway potentials are recorded at the mid or posterior right atrial septum near tricuspid annulus, anterior to the coronary sinus ostium.[16] Occasionally, slow pathway potentials have been recorded posterior to or within the ostium of coronary sinus. If the characteristic electrograms are recorded from multiple sites, the site with the largest, sharpest, and latest slow pathway potential should be attempted first. Using slow pathway potentials in the posteroseptal right atrium to guide ablation, Jackman and colleagues[39] reported that only a single application of RF energy was required to eliminate AVNRT in 90 of 173 patients (52%). The inducibility of AVNRT is assessed after each likely successful application of RF energy. The endpoint for successful modification of the slow pathway is the inability to induce AVNRT both before and during isoproterenol infusion that is sufficient to increase sinus rate to 120–130 bpm.

Recently, it has been reported that the characteristic atrial electrograms useful in identifying ablation sites in patients with AVNRT are equally prevalent in patients

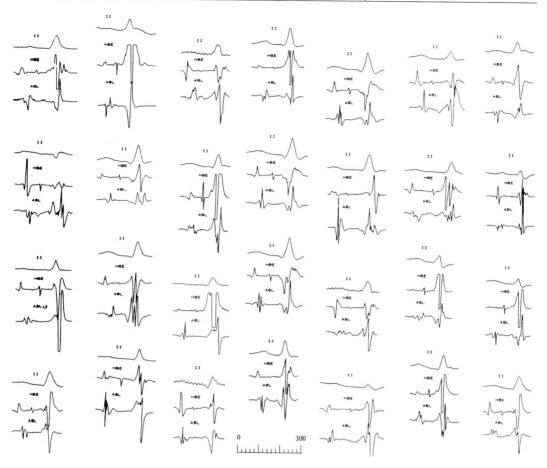

Figure 17. Electrograms recorded from the distal pair of electrodes of the ablation catheter at the successful sites of slow pathway ablation in 28 consecutive patients with AVNRT. At each of the successful site, the atrial to ventricular electrogram ratio is <1.0, and the atrial electrogram shows probable slow pathway potentials. Tracings from lead II and His bundle are also shown.

without AVNRT.[89] This finding suggests that the anatomic and electrophysiological components of the AV node such as the slow pathway are probably present in all individuals. Dual AV nodal physiology and AVNRT may occur as a result of difference in the electrophysiological properties of these components.

Anatomic Approach

In the anatomic approach, target sites are selected mainly based on fluoroscopic landmarks. The only electrogram criteria used was an atrial-to-ventricular electrogram ratio of less than 0.5–1.0. No effort is made in particular to search for a slow pathway potential to guide catheter modification.

Jazayeri and colleagues reported the initial series of patients who underwent slow pathway modification guided by an anatomic approach.[11] The posteromedial tricuspid annulus between the level of the coronary sinus ostium and the His potential recording site was divided into three (posterior, medial, and anterior) anatomic areas. The RAO view was used to visualize the position of the ablation catheter. Serial RF energy applications were delivered along the tricuspid annulus in each area starting at the most posterior site, at the level of the

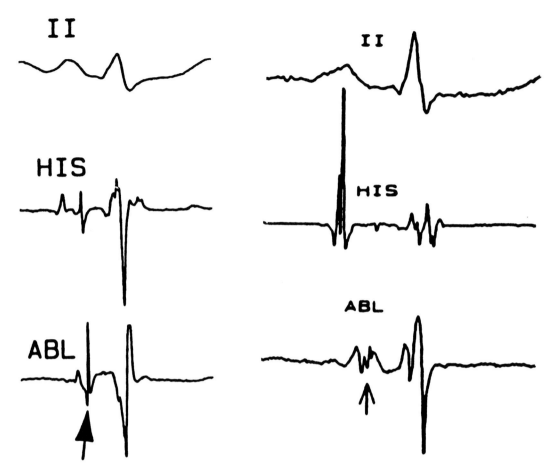

Figure 18. Two types of probable slow pathway potentials identified at successful sites of ablation. A discrete, sharp, high-frequency deflection resembling His potential occurring 10–40 ms following the local atrial electrogram is shown in the left panel. An atrial electrogram with multiple low amplitude components is shown in the right panel. Reproduced with permission from Zhu DWX, et al.[42]

floor of the coronary sinus ostium, and progressing to the most anterior site, just inferior to the His potential recording site. The inducibility of AVNRT was assessed after each likely successful application of RF energy. If the tachycardia was still inducible after one RF energy application had been delivered at each of the anatomic positions, the process was repeated. With this approach, the slow pathway was successfully ablated in 188 of 193 (97%) patients.[22] No patient developed AV block.

Wathen and colleagues[18] reported a method in which the ablation catheter tip was positioned inferiorly on the tricuspid annulus at 6:00 plane in the LAO view. The RF energy was initially applied toward the ventricular side as suggested by a large ventricular and a much smaller atrial electrogram. As the catheter was then withdrawn gradually in a stepwise fashion along the 6:00 plane, the atrial electrogram progressively increased in size relative to the ventricular electrogram. Two to four RF energy applications were made during the pullback sequence. If AVNRT remained inducible, the process was repeated along a more anterior line (in the 5:30, 5:00, 4:30,

4:00 plane directions) on the tricuspid annulus until the slow pathway conduction was eliminated.

Moulton and colleagues[19] described a catheter migratory transection technique. Instead of using a series of RF energy applications to generate a linear lesion in the corridor between the tricuspid annulus and the ostium of the coronary sinus, a linear lesion was created by inscribing an arc with the catheter tip through the inferior half of Koch's triangle during continuous RF energy delivery and fluoroscopic image monitoring in the RAO view. The most anterior limit of the ablation catheter tip within the triangle was a position midway between the His bundle catheter and the coronary sinus ostium. During this migratory application of RF energy, the first episode of accelerated junctional rhythm was usually observed when the ablation catheter tip was withdrawn 2–3 mm from its initial position on the posteromedial tricuspid annulus where small atrial and large ventricular electrograms were recorded. Bursts of accelerated junctional rhythm might subside after several seconds, but when the catheter tip was moved to an adjacent position, accelerated junctional rhythm often reemerged. If bursts of junctional ectopy persisted at any one tip location, further withdrawal was avoided until the arrhythmia subsided. In their series of 46 patients, inscribing 1–3 linear lesions perpendicular to the slow pathway near its midpoint in the atrial septum was able to block slow pathway conduction in 89% of patients and eliminate AVNRT in 100% of patients.

Wu and colleagues[20] reported a simplified midseptal technique in 189 consecutive patients. In the RAO view, the ablation catheter was initially manipulated to record the largest His potential. The catheter tip was then slowly curved down in a clockwise fashion until the His potential was no longer visible and the ratio of atrial to ventricular electrogram was less than 1. At this point, the catheter tip was usually sited at the midseptal area, somewhere between the recording site of the maximal His potential and the ostium of the coronary sinus. The immediate success rate was 97.9%. High-grade AV block occurred in two patients.

The Integrated Approach

In our practice, an integrated approach has been developed for slow pathway ablation. The right atrium near tricuspid annulus between the coronary sinus ostium and the His potential recording site is divided into posterior (P), medial (M), and anterior (A) zones. The electrogram-guided approach is used initially to identify the target sites where an atrial to ventricular electrogram ratio is less than 0.5 and a probable slow pathway potential is present. The mapping is started in the P and M zones and proceeded into the A zone. If the characteristic atrial electrogram is not identified in the above regions, the area posterior to or within the coronary sinus ostium will be mapped (Figure 19). The mapping is usually perform in the RAO view, and the ablation catheter tip position is confirmed in the LAO view (Figure 20).

Under continuous electrocardiographic monitoring, the RF energy is delivered during sinus rhythm. Bursts of accelerated junctional rhythm should develop and then subside after several seconds. The ablation catheter tip may be slowly withdrawn 2–3 mm from its initial site until accelerated junctional rhythm reemerges. When bursts of junctional rhythm persist at one catheter tip location, further pullback should be held until the junctional rhythm subsides. Guided by the electrograms, several such linear lesions may be generated if necessary within the triangle of Koch to interrupt slow pathway conduction.

Using this approach in 78 consecutive patients with AVNRT, we have achieved a success rate of 100%.[42] One patient experienced transient AV block for 5 sec but completely recovered. Atrioventricular nodal reentrant tachycardia recurred in one pa-

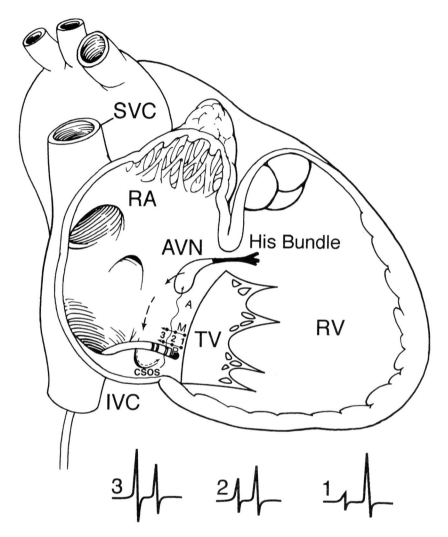

Figure 19. Schematic representation of catheter position in AV nodal slow pathway ablation using the integrated approach in the RAO view. The tricuspid annulus between the coronary sinus ostium and the His potential recording site is divided into posterior (P), midial (M), and anterior (A) zones. The mapping is started in the M and P zones and proceeded to the A zone to search for the possible slow pathway potentials. If the characteristic atrial electrogram is not identifiable in the above areas, the areas posterior to or within the coronary sinus ostium should be mapped. Positions 1, 2, and 3 on the right atrium represent three consecutive sites during a single ablation catheter pullback with continuous RF energy delivery. The corresponding electrograms of positions 1, 2, and 3 demonstrate the increasing size of the atrial electrogram relative to the ventricular electrogram. Position 1 is identified on the basis of the atrial electrogram to ventricular electrogram ratio of <0.5 and the presence of a probable slow pathway potential. Additional such linear lesions may be created until the AVNRT is eliminated. AVN = compact AV node; CSOS = coronary sinus ostium; TV = septal leaflet of tricuspid valve; RA = right atrium; RV = right ventricle; IVC = inferior vena cava; SVC = superior vena cava.

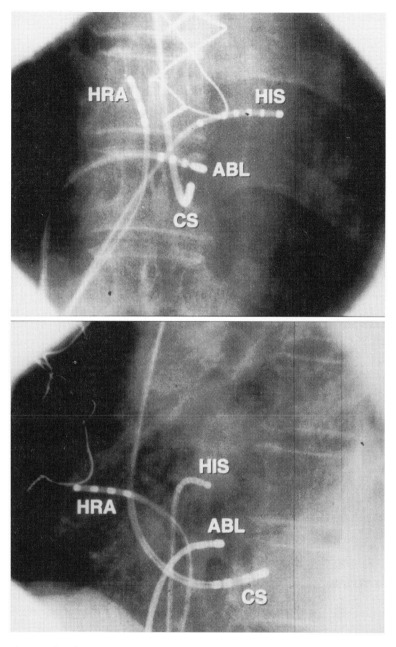

Figure 20. Radiograph of successful site of catheter ablation of slow pathway in a patient with typical AVNRT. The upper panel was in RAO view. The lower panel was in LAO view. The ablation catheter (ABL) was positioned at right atrial septum near the posteromedial tricuspid annulus, between the coronary sinus ostium (where the coronary sinus catheter (CS) makes a sharp angulation on the RAO) and the His potential recording site. A slow pathway potential was recorded on the distal pair of electrodes. The application of RF energy led to the development of accelerated junctional rhythm. Slow pathway conduction and AVNRT were eliminated. HIS = the catheter recording the maximal His potential; HRA = the catheter positioned at high right atrium. Reproduced with permission from Zhu DWX, et al.[42]

tient 3 months later and was successfully eliminated during a second procedure. Distribution of successful sites for slow pathway ablation in these patients is shown in Figure 21. The majority of the successful sites are near the tricuspid annulus either at the level of, or superior to the coronary sinus ostium. Occasionally, the target sites have been identified posterior to, or within the coronary sinus ostium. The slow pathway was also successfully modified in a patient with typical AVNRT in the transplanted heart.[48] Interestingly, no accelerated junctional rhythm was initiated during the ablation in this patient. Among

our patients, typical dual AV nodal physiology was demonstrable in 57% of the individuals. Eighteen percent of the patients had a smooth AV nodal conduction curve. Multiple jumps in the AV nodal conduction curve were present in 25% of the patients. When comparing the number of RF energy applications required to eliminate AVNRT, it became obvious that more energy applications were needed in patients with multiple jumps than in those with no jump or only a single jump in the AV nodal conduction curve.[60] The former group required a total of 10 ± 9 applications, while the latter group had a total of 4 ± 3 applications (p

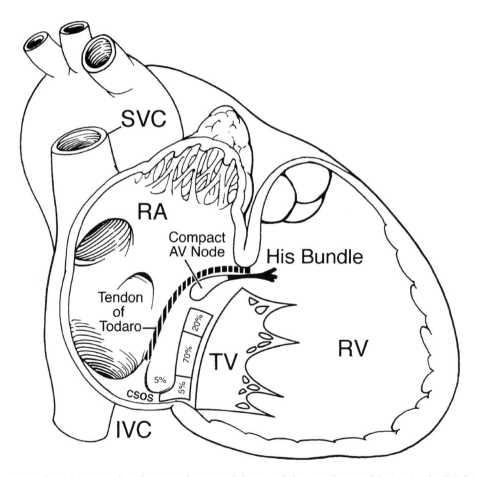

Figure 21. The schematic distribution of successful sites of slow pathway ablation in the RAO view. The majority of the sites are located near the tricuspid annulus either at the level of or superior to the coronary sinus ostium. The remaining 5% sites are located posterior to or within the coronary sinus ostium. CSOS = coronary sinus ostium; TV = septal leaflet of tricuspid valve; RA = right atrium; RV = right ventricle; IVC = inferior vena cava; SVC = superior vena cava.

< 0.0001). If only those energy deliveries that initiated accelerated junctional rhythm were counted, the former group needed 5 ± 4 and the latter group required only 2 ± 1 applications (p < 0.0001). These findings suggest that multiple jumps in the antegrade AV nodal conduction curve may represent the presence of multiple slow pathways and reflect a more complex reentrant tissue mass. Thus, more energy deliveries are necessary to eliminate AVNRT in these patients.

Other Approaches

Retrograde conduction of slow pathway may be demonstrated in 23%–41% of patients with AVNRT.[11,17] The target site is identified on the basis of earliest atrial activation recorded during retrograde slow pathway conduction, and an AV ratio <1.0 during sinus rhythm. Radiofrequency energy is delivered either during atypical AVNRT or ventricular pacing. The endpoints are noninducibility of AVNRT and/or selective loss of retrograde slow pathway conduction. Sometimes it is not possible to maintain constant retrograde conduction of the slow pathway, making this method less practical.

The response of typical AVNRT to subthreshold stimulation or to a single atrial extrastimulus delivered from the ablation catheter distal pair electrodes has been used to identify a target site for slow pathway modification.[90,91] The majority of AVNRT can be terminated in the antegrade direction by the subthreshold stimulation or a single extrastimulus delivered along the posteroseptal right atrium near tricuspid annulus. The RF energy should be applied to the site where termination of tachycardia in the antegrade direction occurred with the application of subthreshold stimulation or delivery of a single extrastimulus with the longest coupling interval. This approach may minimize the applications of RF energy delivery. However, multiple episodes of AVNRT may need to be induced and the

procedure can be time-consuming. Comparison of this approach to the others are not available currently.

Electrophysiological Changes Following Slow Pathway Modification

The major electrophysiological effects of complete slow pathway ablation are as follows: (1) prolongation of AV block cycle length; (2) prolongation of the antegrade AV nodal effective refractory period; (3) loss of previously demonstrable critical delay in A_2-H_2 interval during atrial extrastimulation that resulted in the initiation of AVNRT.[16–24,42] The above changes can be explained by the fact that slow pathway usually has a shorter antegrade AV block cycle length as well as effective refractory period than the fast pathway (Figure 22). Although the antegrade AV nodal effective refractory period may not change after successful slow pathway modification in patients with AVNRT and a smooth AV nodal conduction curve, the maximal AH interval usually shortens significantly after slow pathway modification in these individuals.[92]

Studies have reported that slow pathway modification may affect fast pathway function.[93,94] The fast pathway effective refractory period may shorten following slow pathway modification, and this shortening may not be due to a change in autonomic tone.[94]

The endpoint for slow pathway modification is the elimination of AVNRT inducibility before and during infusion of isoproterenol. Although it remains controversial whether the risk of recurrent AVNRT is higher when residual slow pathway function persists after successful elimination of AVNRT,[95–103] the presence of dual AV nodal physiology with or without single AV nodal reentrant echo beats is generally considered acceptable and is usually not an indicator for continuing attempts at ablation. When there is persistence of residual slow pathway conduction after successful modi-

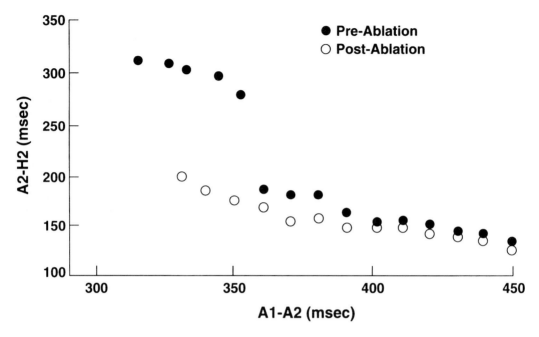

Figure 22. AV nodal conduction curves before and after ablation of slow pathway. Before ablation, dual AV nodal physiology is present. A marked prolongation in the A_2-H_2 interval occurs when the A_1-A_2 coupling interval shortens by 10 ms from 360 ms to 350 ms. After ablation of the slow pathway, all antegrade conduction is through the fast pathway. Dual AV nodal physiology is eliminated. The AV nodal effective refractory period has increased from 300 ms preablation to 320 ms postablation. Reproduced with permission from Zhu DWX, et al.[42]

Table 3
Outcome of Radiofrequency Catheter Modification of AV Nodal Slow Pathway

Study	Date	Patients (n)	Success Rate (%)	Heart Block (%)	Recurrence (%)	Technique
Haissaguerre et al.[16]	1992	64	64 (100%)	0	0	Potentials
Jackman et al.[17]	1992	80	79 (99%)	1 (1%)	0	Potentials
Epstein et al.[24]	1995	60	59 (98%)	1 (1.6%)	4 (6%)	Anatomic-midseptal
Wathen et al.[18]	1992	25	24 (96%)	0	1 (4%)	Anatomic
Chen et al.[14]	1993	68	68 (100%)	0	1 (1%)	Potential
Mitrani et al.[13]	1993	29	28 (97%)	1 (3%)	0	Potentials
Moulton et al.[19]	1993	30	30 (100%)	0	2 (6%)	Anatomic-migratory
Wu et al.[20]	1993	100	97 (97%)	3 (3%)	1 (1%)	Anatomic-midseptal
Kay et al.[21]	1993	242	239 (98%)	3 (1%)	16 (6%)	Anatomic
Akhtar et al.[22]	1993	193	188 (97%)	2 (1%)	0	Anatomic
Trohman et al.[23]	1994	93	91 (98%)	0	3 (3%)	Anatomic
Zhu et al.[42]	1996	78	78 (100%)	0	1 (1%)	Integrated

fication, the patient may not have changes in the AV block cycle length as well as AV nodal effective refractory period.

It has been reported that RF energy ablation directed posteriorly in an attempt to modify the slow pathway may occasionally result in fast pathway ablation.[104] In one study using a posterior approach aimed at the slow pathway, unintentional ablation of the fast pathway occurred in 14% of cases.[105] The retrograde fast pathway may be present posteriorly near the coronary sinus ostium in some patients as shown in the intraoperative mappings.[63] It is therefore essential to precisely map and localize not only the pathway targeted for modification but also the reciprocal pathway, because both pathways may course in close proximity to each other.

Results

Table 3 summarizes the results of RF catheter modification of the slow pathway using a variety of techniques. Overall, primary success rates ranged from 96% to 100%, and the incidence of inadvertent complete AV block was less than 3%. Other complications of slow pathway ablation are rare and are similar to the complications associated with any invasive electrophysiology study including vascular damage, deep venous thrombosis, pulmonary emboli, and cardiac tamponade.

Recurrence

The late recurrence rate after slow pathway modification, ranges from 1% to 8%. The predictors of recurrence of AVNRT after successful slow pathway modification have been studied. Several reports[95–97,101] showed that the recurrence rate was significantly higher in patients with residual slow pathway conduction than in those without slow pathway conduction. The recurrence rate was 13%–55% in patients with residual slow pathway conduction with or without inducible single echo beats, and was only 3%–4% in those without residual slow pathway conduction. In contrast, other studies

found that after successful elimination of AVNRT, residual slow pathway conduction with or without inducible single echo beats does not correlate with clinical tachycardia recurrence.[98–100,102,103] Since evidence of residual slow pathway conduction may still be present in approximately 40% of patients after successful elimination of AVNRT,[16,17,21,22] it is not a specific predictor for recurrence. The risk of causing complete AV block may increase substantially by continuing ablation attempts to eliminate the residual slow pathway conduction. On the other hand, the outcome of repeat modification for recurrent tachycardia has been excellent just as the initial procedure. Therefore, the persistence of residual dual AV nodal physiology and inducible single AV nodal reentrant echo beats should not be considered as an indication for continuing the modification effort as long as isoproterenol infusion is administered and AVNRT is no longer inducible.

Comparison of the Electrogram-Guided and Anatomic Approaches

Several large series[13,14,16,17] using the electrogram-guided approach for slow pathway modification have achieved a success rate greater than 97%. Those who used the anatomic approach have reported a success rate of 88%–96%.[18–24] The incidence of complete AV block by either approach[13,14,16–24] has been less than 2%. Kalbfleisch and colleagues[106] reported a prospective randomized comparison of the anatomic and electrogram-guided approaches for modification of slow pathway. The anatomic approach was effective in 21 of 25 patients (84%), and the electrogram-guided approach was effective in all 25 (100%) patients. The four patients for whom the anatomic approach was ineffective had a successful outcome with the electrogram-guided approach. There was no significant difference with respect to the time required for modification, duration of fluoroscopic exposure, or mean number of RF energy applications. It was interesting to note that the atrial electrogram duration and number of spikes were significantly greater at successful target sites, regardless of whether the anatomic or the electrogram-guided approach was used. Although both methods are comparable in efficacy and duration for modification of the slow pathway, the target sites may be outside the region of the anatomic approach in some patients, and the electrogram-guided approach may be required.

Catheter Modification of Atypical AVNRT

It has been shown that the slow pathway is the preferred target for modification in patients with atypical AVNRT.[17,26] Guided by a distinct slow pathway potential, Jackman and colleagues[17] successfully modified the slow pathway in four patients with atypical AVNRT and in seven patients with both atypical and typical AVNRT. Strickberger and colleagues[26] reported their experience in 10 consecutive patients with atypical AVNRT undergoing successful slow pathway modification. In four patients, target sites were identified during sinus rhythm by mapping for slow pathway potentials. In the other six patients, target sites were identified by mapping earliest retrograde atrial activation during atypical AVNRT or ventricular pacing.

Comparison of Fast and Slow Pathway Modification

Early experience with selective catheter AV nodal modification principally targeted the fast pathway. However, variable success rates and inadvertent AV block led to the development of selective slow pathway modification as an alternate method. In the earlier experience of Jazayeri and colleagues,[11] modification of fast pathway had a 100% success rate, but 21% of the patients developed complete heart block. In addition, 13% of the cases developed atypical AVNRT after successful modification of the fast pathway, and might require a slow path-

way modification. The slow pathway modification success rate was 97%, and no patient developed complete AV block. Mitrani and colleagues[13] reported a success rate of 69% for selective fast pathway modification and a 97% success rate for selective slow pathway modification. The incidence of complete AV block was 23% with fast pathway modification and 3% with slow pathway ablation. Three hundred ninety three patients with AVNRT underwent RF catheter modification of the AV node at the University of Michigan.[107] One hundred sixty patients had fast pathway modification and 223 underwent slow pathway modification. The overall success rate was 87% for the fast pathway approach and 98% for the slow pathway approach. The incidence of complete AV block was 4% with the fast pathway approach and 0.4% with the slow pathway approach. Both differences reached statistical significance. The 1992 NASPE survey[108] included 3,052 patients who had slow pathway modification and 255 patients who had fast pathway modification. The success rate was 96% for slow pathway approach and 90% for fast pathway approach. In the Multicenter European Radiofrequency Survey (MERFS), which included 880 patients who had undergone AV nodal modification for AVNRT, the incidence of complete AV block was significantly higher for fast pathway modification (5.3%) than for slow pathway modification (2.0%).[109] Accordingly, selective slow pathway modification is recommended as the preferred approach even in those institutions that originally developed the fast pathway ablation method.[15] Langberg and colleagues performed a randomized prospective study to compare the fast and the slow pathway approaches for management of AVNRT in 50 patients.[105] The primary success rates of both techniques were similar. All patients who failed the initial approach were successfully treated by the alternative approach without developing high-grade AV block. Only one of the 50 patients developed complete AV block, and this was the result of RF energy delivered posteriorly to modify the slow pathway.

This study demonstrated that it was safe to cross over from one technique to the other as long as AVNRT persisted. "Slow pathway ablation is preferred because of a lower incidence of producing AV block, a greater likelihood of maintaining a normal PR interval during sinus rhythm, and its efficacy in the atypical forms of AVNRT."[15] Rarely, fast pathway modification may be used when the slow pathway approach has failed.

Conclusions

Radiofrequency catheter modification has proven to be a safe, efficacious, and cost-effective form of therapy for AVNRT. The preferred technique for modifying the AV node to cure both typical and atypical AVNRT is modification of the slow pathway. The most effective method for slow pathway modification appears to be the use of an integrated anatomic and electrogram-guided approach. Radiofrequency application at an effective site usually results in the development of accelerated junctional rhythm. Noninducibility of AVNRT is an acceptable endpoint for AV nodal modification. Using the integrated approach, the success rate is usually greater than 95% and the incidence of inadvertent complete AV block is less than 2%. The recurrence rate is usually less than 5%. The outcome of repeat modification for recurrent tachycardia has also been excellent. Rarely, fast pathway modification may be attempted when the slow pathway approach has failed.

References

1. Josephson ME. Paroxysmal supraventricular tachycardia: an electrophysiologic approach. Am J Cardiol 1978;41:1123–1126.
2. Wu D, Denes P, Amat-y-Leon F, et al. Clinical, electrocardiographic and electrophysiologic observations in patients with paroxysmal supraventricular tachycardia. Am J Cardiol 1978;41:1045–1051.
3. Bar FW, Brugada P, Dassen WR, et al. Differential diagnosis of tachycardia with narrow QRS complex (shorter than 0.12 second). Am J Cardiol 1984;54:555–560.
4. Holman WL, Ikeshita M, Lease JG, et al. Alteration of antegrade atrioventricular conduction by cryoablation of peri-atrioventricular nodal tissue. J Thorax Cardiovasc Surg 1984;88:67–75.
5. Ross DL, Johnson DC, Denniss AR, et al. Curative surgery for atrioventricular junctional (AV nodal) reentrant tachycardia. J Am Coll Cardiol 1985;6:1383–1392.
6. Cox JL, Holman WL, Cain ME. Cryosurgical treatment of atrioventricular node reentrant tachycardia. Circulation 1987;76:1329–1336.
7. Fujimura O, Guiraudon GM, Yee R, et al. Operative therapy of atrioventricular node reentry and results of an anatomically guided procedure. Am J Cardiol 1989;64:1327–1332.
8. Goy JJ, Fromer M, Schlaepfer J, et al. Clinical efficacy of radiofrequency current in the treatment of patients with atrioventricular node reentrant tachycardia. J Am Coll Cardiol 1990;16:418–423.
9. Lee MA, Morady F, Kadish A, et al. Catheter modification of the atrioventricular junction with radiofrequency energy for control of atrioventricular nodal reentry tachycardia. Circulation 1991;83:827–835.
10. Calkins H, Sousa J, El-Atassi R, et al. Diagnosis and cure of the Wolff-Parkinson-White syndrome or paroxysmal supraventricular tachycardias during a single electrophysiologic test. N Engl J Med 1991;324:1612–1618.
11. Jazayeri M, Hempe S, Sra J, et al. Selective transcatheter ablation of the slow pathway for the treatment of atrioventricular nodal reentrant tachycardia. Circulation 1992;85:1318–1328.
12. Langberg J, Harvey M, Calkins H, et al. Titration of power during radiofrequency catheter ablation of atrioventricular nodal reentrant tachycardia. PACE 1993;16:465–470.
13. Mitrani RD, Klein LS, Hackett FK, et al. Radiofrequency ablation for atrioventricular node reentrant tachycardia: comparison between fast (anterior) and slow (posterior) pathway ablation. J Am Coll Cardiol 1993;21:432–441.
14. Chen S, Chiang C, Tsang W, et al. Selective radiofrequency catheter ablation of fast and slow pathways in 100 patients with atrioventricular nodal reentrant tachycardia. Am Heart J 1993;125:1–10.

15. Kottkamp H, Hindricks G, Willems S, et al. An anatomically and electrogram-guided stepwise approach for effective and safe catheter ablation of the fast pathway for elimination of atrioventricular node reentrant tachycardia. J Am Coll Cardiol 1995; 22:974–981.

16. Haissaguerre M, Gaita F, Fischer B, et al. Elimination of atrioventricular nodal reentrant tachycardia using discrete slow potentials to guide application of radiofrequency energy. Circulation 1992;85:2162–2175.

17. Jackman W, Beckman K, McClelland J, et al. Treatment of supraventricular tachycardia due to atrioventricular nodal reentry by radiofrequency catheter ablation of slow-pathway conduction. N Engl J Med 1992; 327:313–318.

18. Wathen M, Natale A, Wolfe K, et al. An anatomically guided approach to atrioventricular node slow pathway ablation. Am J Cardiol 1992;70:886–889.

19. Moulton K, Miller B, Scott J, et al. Radiofrequency catheter ablation for AV nodal reentry: a technique for rapid transection of the slow AV nodal pathway. PACE 1993;16: 760–768.

20. Wu D, Yeh S, Wang C, et al. A simple technique for selective radiofrequency ablation of the slow pathway in atrioventricular node reentrant tachycardia. J Am Coll Cardiol 1993;21:1612–1621.

21. Kay G, Epstein A, Dailey S, et al. Role of radiofrequency ablation in the management of supraventricular arrhythmias: experience in 760 consecutive patients. J Cardiovasc Electrophysiol 1993;4:371–389.

22. Akhtar M, Jazayeri MR, Sra J, et al. Atrioventricular nodal reentry: clinical, electrophysiological, and therapeutic considerations. Circulation 1993;88:282–295.

23. Trohman RG, Pinski SL, Sterba R, et al. Evolving concepts in radiofrequency catheter ablation of atrioventricular nodal reentry tachycardia. Am Heart J 1994;128: 586–595.

24. Epstein LM, Lesh MD, Griffin JC, et al. A direct midseptal approach to slow atrioventricular nodal pathway ablation. PACE 1995;18:57–64.

25. Kay G, Epstein A, Dailey S, et al. Selective radiofrequency ablation of the slow pathway for the treatment of atrioventricular nodal reentrant tachycardia. Circulation 1992;85:1675–1688.

26. Strickberger S, Kalbfleisch S, Williamson B, et al. Radiofrequency catheter ablation of atypical atrioventricular nodal reentrant tachycardia. J Cardiovasc Electrophysiol 1993;4:526–532.

27. Kalbfleisch SJ, Calkins H, Langberg JJ, et al. Comparison of the cost of radiofrequency catheter modification of the atrioventricular nodal and medical therapy for drug-refractory atrioventricular node reentrant tachycardia. J Am Coll Cardiol 1992;19: 1583–1587.

28. Man KC, Kalbfleisch SJ, Hummel JD, et al. The safety and cost of outpatient radiofrequency ablation of the slow pathway in patients with atrioventricular nodal reentrant tachycardia. Am J Cardiol 1993;72: 1323–1324.

29. Tawara K. Die topographie und histologie der bruckenfasern: ein beitrag zur lehre von der bedeutung der purkinjeschen faden. Zentralbl Physiol 1906;19:70–76.

30. Koch WL. Weitere mitteilunger ueber den sinus-knoten des herzens. Verh Dtsch Ges Pathol 1909;13:85–92.

31. Zipes DP. Genesis of cardiac arrhythmias: electrophysiological considerations. In Braunwald E, ed. Heart Disease: A Textbook of Cardiovascular Medicine. W.B. Saunders, Philadelphia, 1992, pp 588–621.

32. Truex R, Smythe M. Reconstruction of the human atrioventricular node. Anat Rec 1967;158:11–20.

33. James T. Morphology of the human atrioventricular node, with remarks pertinent to its electrophysiology. Am Heart J 1961;62: 756–771.

34. Becker A, Anderson R. Morphology of the human atrioventricular junctional area. In Wellens H, Lie K, Janse M, eds. The Conduction System of the Heart: Structure, Function and Clinical Implications. Lea & Febiger, Philadelphia, 1976, pp 263–286.

35. Racker DK. Atrioventricular node and input pathways: a correlated gross anatomical and histological pathways study of the canine atrioventricular junctional region. Anat Rec 1989;224:336–354.

36. Racker DK. Sinoventricular transmission in 10 M K+ by canine atrioventricular nodal inputs. Superior atrionodal bundle and proximal atrioventricular bundle. Circulation 1991;83:1738–1753.

37. Josephson ME, Kastor JA. Paroxysmal supraventricular tachycardias: Is the atrium a necessary link? Circulation 1976;54: 430–435.

38. Josephson ME, Miller JM. Atrioventricular nodal reentry: Evidence supporting an intranodal location. PACE 1993;16:599–614.

39. Jackman WM, Nakagawa H, Heidbuchel H, et al. Three forms of atrioventricular nodal (junctional) reentrant tachycardia: differential diagnosis, electrophysiological characteristics, and implications for anatomy of

the reentrant circuit. In Zipes DP, Jalife J, eds. Cardiac Electrophysiology: From Cell to Bedside. WB Saunders, Philadelphia, 1995, pp 620–637.

40. Olgin JE, Ursell P, Kao AK, et al. Pathological findings following slow pathway ablation for AV nodal reentrant tachycardia. J Cardiovasc Electrophysiol 1996;7:625–631.

41. Ho SW, McComb JM, Scott CD, et al. Morphology of the cardiac conduction system in patients with electrophysiologically proven dual atrioventricular nodal pathways. J Cardiovasc Electrophysiol 1993;4:504–512.

42. Zhu DWX, Maloney JD. Radiofrequency catheter ablative therapy for atrioventricular nodal reentrant tachycardia. In I Singer, ed. Interventional Electrophysiology. Baltimore, Williams & Wilkins, 1997, pp 275–316.

43. Doig JC, Saito J, Harris L, et al. Coronary sinus morphology in patients with atrioventricular junctional reentry tachycardia and other supraventricular tachyarrhythmias. Circulation 1995;92:436–441.

44. Widran J, Lev M. The dissection of the atrioventricular node, bundle branches in the human heart. Circulation 1951;4:863–867.

45. McGuire MA, Johnson DC, Robotin M, et al. Dimensions of the triangle of Koch in humans. Am J Cardiol 1992;70:829–830.

46. Bharati S, Lev M. The morphology of the AV junction and its significance in catheter ablation. PACE 1989;12:879–882.

47. Ueng KC, Chen SA, Chiang CE, et al. Dimension and related anatomical distance of Koch's triangle in patients with atrioventricular nodal reentrant tachycardia. J Cardiovasc Electrophysiol 1996;7:1017–1023.

48. Zhu DWX, Sun H. Radiofrequency catheter ablation of atrioventricular nodal reentrant tachycardia in a patient with heart transplantation. J Interven Cardiac Electrophysiol 1998;2:87–89.

49. Leitch JW, Klein GJ, Yee R, et al. Syncope associated with supraventricular tachycardia: An expression of tachycardia rate or vasomotor response? Circulation 1992;85:1064–1071.

50. Fisch C, Mandrola JM, Rardon DP. Electrocardiographic manifestations of dual atrioventricular node conduction during sinus rhythm. JACC 1997;29:1015–1022.

51. Moe GK, Preston JB, Burlington H. Physiologic evidence for a dual AV transmission system. Circulation Res 1956;4:357–375.

52. Schuilenburg RM, Durrer D. Atrial echo beats in the human heart elicited by induced atrial premature beats. Circulation 1968;37:680–693.

53. Denes P, Wu D, Dhingra R, et al. Dual atrioventricular nodal pathways. A common electrophysiologic response. Br Heart J 1975;37:1069–1076.

54. Rosen KM, Mehta A, Miller RA. Demonstration of dual atrioventricular nodal pathways in man. Am J Cardiol 1974;33:291–294.

55. Denes P, Deleon W, Dhingra RC, et al. Demonstration of dual A-V nodal pathways in patients with paroxysmal supraventricular tachycardia. Circulation 1973;48:549–555.

56. McGuire MA, Robotin M, Yip ASB, et al. Electrophysiologic and histologic effects of dissection of the connections between the atrium and posterior part of the atrioventricular node. J Am Coll Cardiol 1994;23:693–701.

57. Josephson ME, Miller JM. Atrioventricular node reentry tachycardias: Is the atrium a necessary link? In Touboul P, Waldo A, eds. Atrial Arrhythmias: Current Concepts and Management. St. Louis, Mosby Year Book, 1990, pp 311–329.

58. Schuger CD, Steinman RT, Lehman MH. The excitable gap in atrioventricular nodal reentrant tachycardia: characterization with ventricular extrastimuli and pharmacologic intervention. Circulation 1989;80:324–334.

59. Gamache M, Bharati S, Lev M, et al. Histopathological study following radiofrequency current ablation of the slow pathway in a patient with atrioventricular nodal reentrant tachycardia. PACE 1994;17:247–251.

60. Zhu DWX, Sun H, Arnold DJ, et al. The implication of multiple slow pathways on catheter ablation of atrioventricular nodal reentrant tachycardia [Abstract]. Eur Heart J 1997;18:465.

61. Wu D, Denes P, Leon F, et al. An unusual variety of atrioventricular nodal re-entry due to retrograde dual atrioventricular nodal pathways. Circulation 1977;56:50–59.

62. Sung R, Waxman H, Saksena S, et al. Sequence of retrograde atrial activation in patients with dual atrioventricular nodal pathways. Circulation 1981;64:1059–1067.

63. Keim S, Werner P, Jazayeri M, et al. Localization of the fast and slow pathways in atrioventricular nodal reentrant tachycardia by intraoperative ice mapping. Circulation 1992;86:919–925.

64. McGuire MA, Bourke JP, Robotin MC, et al. High resolution mapping of Koch's triangle using sixty electrodes in humans with atrioventricular junctional (AV nodal) reentrant tachycardia. Circulation 1993;88:2315–2328.

65. Benditt DG, Pritchett ELC, Smith WM, et

al. Ventriculoatrial intervals: Diagnostic use in paroxysmal supraventricular tachycardia. Ann Intern Med 1979;91:161–166.

66. Man KC, Brinkman K, Bogun F, et al. 2:1 atrioventricular block during atrioventricular node reentrant tachycardia. J Am Coll Cardiol 1996;28:1770–1774.

67. Sung RJ, Styperek JL, Myerburg RJ, et al. Initiation of two distinct forms of atrioventricular nodal reentrant tachycardia during programmed ventricular stimulation in man. Am J Cardiol 1978;42:404–415.

68. Man KC, Niebauer M, Daoud E, et al. Comparison of atrial-His intervals during tachycardia and atrial pacing in patients with long RP tachycardia. J Cardiovasc Electrophysiol 1995;6:700–710.

69. McGuire MA, Alex SB, Yip SB, et al. Posterior (atypical) atrioventricular junctional reentrant tachycardia. Am J Cardiol 1994; 73:469–477.

70. McGuire MA, Lau KC, Johnson DC, et al. Patients with two types of atrioventricular junctional (AV nodal) reentrant tachycardia: evidence that a common pathway of nodal tissue is not present above the reentrant circuit. Circulation 1991;83:1232–1246.

71. Sra JS, Jazayeri MR, Blanck Z, et al. Slow pathway ablation in patients with atrioventricular node reentrant tachycardia and a prolonged PR interval. J Am Coll Cardiol 1994;24:1064–1068.

72. Deshpande S, Jazayeri M, Dhala A, et al. Selective transcatheter modification of the atrioventricular node. In Zipes DE, ed. Catheter Ablation of Arrhythmias. Armonk, NY, Futura Publishing Co. Inc, 1994, pp 151–186.

73. Sheahan RG, Klein GJ, Yee R, et al. Atrioventricular node reentry with smooth AV node function curves: a different arrhythmia substrate? Circulation 1996;93:969–972.

74. Hirao K, Otomo K, Wang X, et al. Para-Hisian pacing: a new method for differentiating retrograde conduction over an accessory AV pathway from conduction over the AV node. Circulation 1996;94:1027–1035.

75. Bogun F, Knight B, Weiss R, et al. Slow pathway ablation in patients with documented but noninducible paroxysmal supraventricular tachycardia. J Am Coll Cardiol 1996;28:1000–1004.

76. Guidelines for clinical intracardiac electrophysiological and catheter ablation procedures: a report of the American College of Cardiology/American Heart Association Task Force on Practice Guidelines (Committee on Clinical Intracardiac Electrophysiologic and Catheter Ablation Procedures). Circulation 1995;92:673–691.

77. Haissaguerre M, Warin JF, Lemetayer P, et al. Closed chest ablation of retrograde conduction in patients with atrioventricular nodal reentrant tachycardia. N Engl J Med 1989;320:426–433.

78. Epstein LM, Scheinman MM, Langberg JJ, et al. Percutaneous catheter modification of the atrioventricular node: a potential cure for atrioventricular nodal reentrant tachycardia. Circulation 1989;80:757–768.

79. Langberg JJ. Radiofrequency catheter ablation of AVN nodal reentry: the anterior approach. PACE 1993;16:615–622.

80. Weber HP, Kaltenbrunner W, Heinze A, et al. Laser catheter coagulation of atrial myocardium of ablation of atrioventricular nodal reentrant tachycardia: first clinical experience. Eur Heart J 1997;18:487–495.

81. Zhu DWX. Radiofrequency catheter ablative therapy for anteroseptal and midseptal accessory atrioventricular pathways. In Singer I, ed. Interventional Electrophysiology. Baltimore, Williams & Wilkins, 1997, pp 253–273.

82. Fenelon G, d'Avila A, Malacky T, et al. Prognostic significance of transient complete atrioventricular block during radiofrequency ablation of atrioventricular node reentrant tachycardia. Am J Cardiol 1995; 75:698–702.

83. Jentzer JH, Goyal R, Williamson BD, et al. Analysis of junctional ectopy during radiofrequency ablation for atrioventricular node reentrant tachycardia. J Am Coll Cardiol 1993;22:1706–1710.

84. Langberg JJ, Kim YN, Goyal R, et al. Conversion of typical to "atypical" atrioventricular nodal reentrant tachycardia after radiofrequency catheter modification of the atrioventricular junction. Am J Cardiol 1992;69:503–508.

85. Strickberger SA, Zivin A, Daoud EG, et al. Temperature and impedance monitoring during slow pathway ablation in patients with AV nodal reentrant tachycardia. J Cardiovasc Electrophysiol 1996;7:295–300.

86. Willems S, Shenasa H, Kottkamp H, et al. Temperature-controlled slow pathway ablation for treatment of atrioventricular nodal reentrant tachycardia using a combined anatomical and electrogram guided strategy. Eur Heart J 1996;17:1092–1102.

87. Thakur R, Klein G, Yee R, et al. Junctional tachycardia: a useful marker during radiofrequency ablation for atrioventricular node reentrant tachycardia. J Am Coll Cardiol 1993;22:1706–1710.

88. Hintringer F, Hartikainen J, Davies W, et al. Prediction of atrioventricular block during radiofrequency ablation of the slow path-

way of the atrioventricular node. Circulation 1995;92:3491–3496.

89. Niebauer MJ, Daoud E, Williamson B, et al. Atrial electrogram characteristics in patients with and without atrioventricular nodal reentrant tachycardia. Circulation 1995;92:77–81.

90. Willems S, Weiss C, Hofmann T, et al. Subthreshold stimulation in the region of the slow pathway during atrioventricular node reentrant tachycardia: correlation with effect of radiofrequency catheter ablation. J Am Coll Cardiol 1997;29:408–415.

91. Sra J, Jazayeri M, Natale A, et al. Termination of atrioventricular nodal reentrant tachycardia by premature stimulation from ablating catheter. Circulation 1995;91:1095–1100.

92. Tai CT, Chen SA, Chiang CE, et al. Complex electrophysiological characteristics in atrioventricular nodal reentrant tachycardia with continuous atrioventricular node function curves. Circulation 1997;95:2541–2547.

93. Zhu WX, Nitta J, Maloney JD. Impact of slow pathway modification on ventricular rate control during atrial fibrillation [Abstract] PACE 1995;18:1162.

94. Natale A, Klein G, Yee R, et al. Shortening of fast pathway refractoriness after slow pathway ablation: effects of autonomic blockade. Circulation 1994;89:1103–1108.

95. Li H, Klein G, Stites H, et al. Elimination of slow pathway conduction: an accurate indicator of clinical success after radiofrequency atrioventricular node modification. J Am Coll Cardiol 1993;22:1849–1853.

96. Baker J, Plumb V, Epstein A, et al. Predictors of recurrent atrioventricular nodal reentry after selective slow pathway ablation. Am J Cardiol 1994;73:765–769.

97. Tebbenjohanns J, Pfeiffer D, Schumacher B, et al. Impact of the local atrial electrogram in AV nodal reentrant tachycardia: ablation versus modification of the slow pathway. J Cardiovasc Electrophysiol 1995;6:245–251.

98. Lindsay B, Chung M, Gamache M, et al. Therapeutic end points for the treatment of atrioventricular node reentrant tachycardia by catheter guided radiofrequency current. J Am Coll Cardiol 1993;22:733–740.

99. Chen SA, Wu TJ, Chiang CE, et al. Recurrent tachycardia after selective ablation of slow pathway in patients with atrioventricular nodal reentrant tachycardia. Am J Cardiol 1995;76:131–137.

100. Manolis AS, Wang PJ, Estes M, III. Radiofrequency ablation of slow pathway in patients with atrioventricular nodal reentrant tachycardia: Do arrhythmia recurrences correlate with persistent slow pathway conduction or site of successful ablation? Circulation 1994;90:2815–2819.

101. Tondo C, Bella PD, Carbuchicchio C, et al. Persistence of single echo beat inducibility after selective ablation of the slow pathway in patients with atrioventricular nodal reentrant tachycardia: relationship to the functional properties of the atrioventricular node and clinical implications. J Cardiovasc Electrophysiol 1996;7:689–696.

102. Chen SA, Wu TJ, Chiang CE, et al. Recurrent tachycardia after selective ablation of slow pathway in patients with atrioventricular nodal reentrant tachycardia. Am J Cardiol 1995;76:131–137.

103. Hummel JD, Strickberger SA, Williamson BD, et al. The course of recurrences of atrioventricular nodal reentrant tachycardia after radiofrequency ablation of the slow pathway. Am J Cardiol 1995;75:628–630.

104. Englestein ED, Stein KM, Markowitz SM, et al. Posterior fast atrioventricular node pathways: implications for radiofrequency catheter ablation of atrioventricular node reentrant tachycardia. J Am Coll Cardiol 1996;27:1098–1105.

105. Langberg JJ, Leon A, Borganelli M, et al. A randomized comparison of anterior and posterior approaches to radiofrequency catheter ablation of atrioventricular nodal reentry tachycardia. Circulation 1993;87:1551–1556.

106. Kalbfleisch S, Strickberger S, Williamson B. Randomized comparison of anatomic and electrogram mapping approaches to ablation of the slow pathway of atrioventricular node reentrant tachycardia. J Am Coll Cardiol 1994;23:716–723.

107. Kalbfleisch SJ, Morady F. Catheter ablation of atrioventricular nodal reentrant tachycardia. In Zipes DP, Jalife J, ed. Cardiac Electrophysiology: From Cell to Bedside. Philadelphia, W.B. Saunders Company, 1995, pp 1477–1487.

108. Scheinman MM. Patterns of catheter ablation practice in the United States: results of the 1992 NASPE survey. PACE 1994;17:873–875.

109. Hindricks G, on behalf of the Multicenter European Radiofrequency Survey (MERFS) Investigators. Incidence of complete atrioventricular block following attempted radiofrequency catheter modification of the atrioventricular node in 880 patients: results of the Multicenter European Radiofrequency Survey (MERFS). Eur Heart J 1996;17:82–88.

Chapter 9

Ablation of Atrial Tachycardias

Jeffrey E. Olgin, William Miles

Introduction

Over the last 5 years ablative techniques to cure a variety of atrial arrhythmias have been developed and refined. Just a short time ago, patients with atrial tachycardias resistant to medical therapy underwent complete atrioventricular (AV) junction ablation and pacemaker insertion. The invasive electrophysiology era has led to a better understanding of the mechanism, substrate, and varieties of atrial tachycardias that in turn have led to specific curative catheter ablation approaches. Thus, many of these tachycardias can now be successfully eliminated with radiofrequency (RF) ablation.

Atrial tachycardias have been clasified by a variety of schemes based variously on mechanism, substrate, surface ECG pattern, or clinical presentation. The specific mechanism of an atrial tachycardia (reentrant, automatic, or triggered) can often be very difficult to define in a given individual, and ambiguous results are common during the search for a mechanism. The use of the surface ECG or clinical presentation alone is inadequate in classifying atrial tachycardias. For example, a macroreentrant atrial tachycardia resulting from a surgical scar in the atrium may have an ECG appearance similar to typical atrial flutter. Likewise, patients with repaired congenital heart disease may develop typical atrial flutter. In addition, the division of atrial flutter into subtypes based on a variety of criteria is not uniform in the literature.

For the purpose of this review, we will adopt a general classification of atrial tachycardia based on a combination of the above features. The general techniques for mapping and ablation are common to each group of tachycardias. As we learn more about specific mechanism and anatomic substrate, this scheme will likely become more sophisticated and refined.

Macroreentrant atrial tachycardias utilize large circuits in the atria; examples are atrial flutter and atrial tachycardias due to surgical scars. Entrainment can be easily demonstrated by pacing during these tachycardias and is useful in localizing the tachycardia circuit. Mapping involves identifying conduction barriers and isthmuses, and ablation is accomplished by transecting the isthmus. *Focal atrial tachycardias* arise from a localized area of abnormal atrium and may be due to microreentrant, automatic, or triggered mechanisms. Mapping is largely based on identifying the earliest site of activation and these tachycardias can be eliminated by a focal ablation lesion. Examples include sinus node reentry, ectopic atrial

From Singer I, Barold SS, Camm AJ (eds): Nonpharmacological Therapy of Arrhythmias for the 21st Century: The State of the Art. Futura Publishing Co, Inc., Armonk, NY, © 1998.

tachycardias, and automatic atrial tachycardias. *Atrial fibrillation* remains largely an ECG diagnosis. However, knowledge of the mechanism underlying atrial fibrillation is likely to expand rapidly over the next few years as specific ablative techniques for atrial fibrillation are developed. Atrial fibrillation is a heterogeneous entity and will likely be further categorized into different types as we learn more about underlying mechanisms.

Macroreentrant Atrial Tachycardias

The common feature of these tachycardias is that they utilize a macroreentrant circuit somewhere in the atria, and generally (though not always) involve structural barriers that define the reentrant path. What varies is the specific nature and location of those barriers. In addition, given a *potential* reentrant circuit, *actual* reentrant excitation can revolve in one of two possible directions. Atrial flutter is the prototypic macroreentrant atrial tachycardia.

Definitions

Prior to the current era of catheter ablation, the nomenclature used to define the term atrial flutter was somewhat confusing. However, since the only therapy was drugs, the distinction between various types of atrial flutter had little clinical applicability. Thus, the term atrial flutter had been used to describe a variety of different atrial tachycardias. What is sometimes referred to as atrial flutter after reparative surgery for congenital heart disease (Mustard, Senning, or Fontan operations, atrial septal defect repair, etc.) has a different reentrant circuit than the typical, classic, common, usual, type I, type A, or orthodromic atrial flutter involving counterclockwise reentry (in the frontal plane) through an isthmus in the low right atrium.[1–3] Such typical atrial flutter does not require prior surgical incisions in

the atrium. Though typical atrial flutter had been defined by electrocardiographers as a regular atrial tachycardia with an atrial rate between 250 and 350 beats per min and a sawtooth pattern on ECG, flutter can be considerably slower in some patients, particularly those on antiarrhythmic drugs or with abnormal atria. Even more confusing, perhaps, is the division of atrial flutter into subtypes[3,4] based variously on rate; surface ECG morphology; ability to terminate with overdrive pacing from the high right atrium; and/or endocardial activation sequence. Thus, we have atypical, uncommon, rare, antidromic, clockwise, type II, type B, unusual, fast, slow, left atrial, and reverse atrial flutter. In this chapter, the definitions in Table 1, which classifies macroreentrant atrial tachycardias largely based on known substrates, will be used. The prototypic macroreentrant atrial tachycardia is typical atrial flutter. The principles of mechanism, mapping, and ablation of all these arrhythmias are exemplified by typical atrial flutter.

Typical Atrial Flutter

Animal Models

Much of our current understanding of the role of barriers in macroreentrant atrial tachycardias has originated from animal models. Rosenblueth and Garcia-Ramos developed a canine model of atrial flutter by creating a crush lesion between the orifices of the venae cavae.[5] This lesion produced an atrial tachycardia that was identical to atrial flutter in both rate and morphology.[5] Frame et al. used a similar model of atrial flutter as that of the Rosenblueth and Garcia-Ramos lesion with a Y-shaped lesion in the right atrium between the venae cavae and a connecting lesion extending toward the right atrial appendage.[6,7] Mapping revealed that reentry occurred around the tricuspid annulus and not around the lesion itself.[6,7] The Y-shaped lesion served as a barrier to conduction, protecting the tissue

Table 1
Classification of Atrial Flutter

Type	ECG	Characteristics	Circuit	Mapping Techniques	Ablation Site
Typical Atrial Flutter					
Counterclockwise	Negative Fl waves II, III, aVF; Predominantly negative V6	Macroreentrant in right atrium with regular rate (usually 250–350 bpm)	Around tricuspid annulus anterior to CT and ER	Anatomic, activation, and entrainment to confirm critical isthmus	TA to IVC (ER)
Clockwise	Positive/notched Fl waves in II, III, aVF; Predominantly positive in V_6	Rate, regularity, and circuit same as counterclockwise but opposite rotation around TA	Around tricuspid annulus anterior to CT and ER	Anatomic, activation, and entrainment to confirm critical isthmus	TA to IVC (ER)
Atypical Flutter	Variable	Rate usually faster than typical, often more irregular	Unknown (?pulmonary veins, portion of CT, functional barriers)	Activation sequence inconsistent with typical flutter; often difficult to entrain	???
Incisional Reentry (atrial tachycardia in repaired congenital heart disease)	Variable	After surgical repair of congenital heart disease. Rates variable depending on barriers, atrial disease and length of circuit	Repair of congenital defects. Circuit often involves surgical scars or prosthetic material. May also involve subeustachian isthmus.	Identify lines of block with split potentials; activation mapping to identify early sites; entrainment mapping to identify critical isthmus	Variable, but must sever an isthmus from one barrier (surgical or anatomic) to another.

CT = crista terminalis; ER = eustachian ridge; TA = tricuspid annulus; IVC = inferior vena cava.

between the lesion and the tricuspid annulus from being excited from an inferiorly spreading wavefront, thus remaining excitable when the reentrant wavefront arrived. These studies have demonstrated the importance of not one, but two barriers between which reentry can occur, with a second barrier to "protect" the circuit from excitation by wavefronts other than the reentrant wavefront (i.e., short circuiting). Other animal models have emphasized the importance of barriers in atrial flutter.[8–12]

Substrate for Typical Atrial Flutter

Typical atrial flutter has a characteristic pattern on 12-lead ECG, with superiorly directed flutter waves and rates in a range of 200–350 beats per minute (Figure 1). The uniformity of these characteristics among patients with varied cardiac pathology suggests a common substrate for the arrhythmia. As had been hypothesized since early in this century,[13] it is now well established that atrial flutter is a reentrant arrhythmia confined to the right atrium.[1,3,14] The unique endocardial anatomy of the right atrium, with its many orifices and distinct structures around which reentry could occur, likely explains the consistency of atrial flutter from patient to patient.

Two recent reviews discuss in detail the role of barriers in macroreentrant atrial tachycardias.[15,16] It appears that, as was shown in the animal models of flutter, anatomic barriers are essential for establishing a circuit large enough that the circulating

COUNTERCLOCKWISE FLUTTER   **CLOCKWISE FLUTTER**

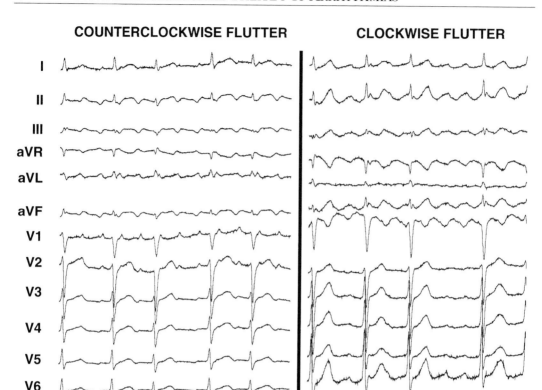

Figure 1. Twelve-lead ECG of a patient with both counterclockwise (left) and clockwise (right) atrial flutter. Counterclockwise flutter has the characteristic negative flutter waves in leads II, III, aVF, and V_1. In clockwise flutter, the upright and notched flutter waves in II, III, and aVF are seen as well as the positive flutter wave in V_6.

wavefront does not impinge on its own tail of refractoriness. Several studies have now demonstrated that the crista terminalis and eustachian ridge form the posterior barriers of the typical flutter circuit and the tricuspid annulus forms the anterior barrier.[17–19] A critical isthmus has been identified in the low right atrium bordered by the tricuspid annulus and the eustachian ridge between the inferior vena cava and the coronary sinus os.[3,17–21] The reentry may occur in a counterclockwise or in a clockwise rotation in the frontal plane around the tricuspid annulus.[19,22–24] While these anatomic structures are present in everyone, it appears that what separates those with the substrate for clinical typical atrial flutter from those without this arrhythmia is either very poor or absent transverse coupling along all or most of the length of the crista terminalis.[25]

Mapping

The electrophysiological evaluation of the patient with atrial flutter begins with identifying the type of atrial flutter, which then helps establish the appropriate site for ablation. This is accomplished by examining the morphology of the flutter wave on the surface ECG, activation mapping and entrainment mapping to identify a critical isthmus.

The surface ECG provides strong clues as to the type of flutter that is present. Typical counterclockwise atrial flutter produces the classic atrial flutter described by early electrocardiographers, with predominantly negative flutter waves in leads II, III, and aVF and predominantly positive flutter waves in lead V_1 (Figure 1). When the flutter waves are recorded during sufficient AV block such that they are not distorted by the QRS or T waves, there is often a positive portion (probably resulting from both craniocaudal activation on the right atrial free wall as well as the left atrium) following the predominant negative component that results from caudocranial activation up the septum and posterior atrial wall. Clockwise atrial flutter also produces characteristic flutter waves that are positive in leads II, III, and aVF, usually notched, and predominantly negative in lead V_1 (Figure 1).[23,26] Because the circuit is identical, atrial rates for clockwise and counterclockwise flutter are nearly the same in a given patient.[22,23]

Atypical flutter has variable characteristics on 12-lead ECG, and the flutter morphology may mimic that of typical flutter.[23,27] By careful use of activation and entrainment mapping (see below), one can demonstrate that these arrhythmias are distinct from typical atrial flutter.[23] The rates of atypical flutters are often faster than those of typical flutter, though there is a large overlap and rate alone cannot be used as a distinguishing feature.[23] Because the barriers and circuit responsible for atypical flutter are not known (and may vary from patient to patient), they are currently not amenable to ablative therapy. It is important to distinguish atypical from typical atrial flutter, since ablation in the subeustachian isthmus will have no effect on atypical flutter.

Activation Mapping

Multipolar mapping catheters such as a 20-pole halo catheter (Cordis-Webster, Miami, FL) are very useful not only for identifying the type of atrial flutter but also in aiding in the evaluation of the ablation (below). The halo catheter is placed around the tricuspid annulus such that the distal pole is located near the coronary sinus os; thus, the activation sequence around the majority of the tricuspid annulus can be

recorded (Figure 2). Care should be taken that the catheter is positioned along the tricuspid annulus anterior to the crista terminalis, since the atrium posterior to this structure is not part of the reentrant circuit in typical atrial flutter.[17] Using these catheters, typical atrial flutter is identified by its counterclockwise or clockwise sequence as shown in Figure 3. Atypical flutter and incisional reentry are often inconsistent with either of these sequences.

A multipolar catheter placed in the coronary sinus such that the proximal pole is at the os is also useful both in the mapping of atrial flutter and in the evaluation of the success of ablation (see below). In counterclockwise typical flutter, this site is near the exit from the isthmus and usually corresponds to the onset of the flutter wave.[17,19–21] Atrial activation recorded from the coronary sinus during typical atrial flutter travels from the os toward the distal pole near the lateral left atrium. Many atypical atrial flutters do not exhibit this sequence, with a left-sided electrode being activated prior to the coronary sinus os. Therefore, a coronary sinus catheter can be useful to distinguish typical from atypical flutter.

Although halo catheters are used at the authors' institutions for most patients with atrial flutter because they are relatively easy to place, any multipolar catheter or series of catheters placed within the typical atrial flutter circuit to map as much of the complete circuit as possible can be used.

Split Potentials

During activation mapping of atrial flutter, split potentials, defined as discrete electrograms separated by an isoelectric phase, have been frequently recorded.[3,17,19,28–30] While controversy exists as to whether isolated split potentials may indicate disparate endocardial and epicardial activation or merely slowed conduction, in many cases they undoubtedly indicate activation on either side of a line of

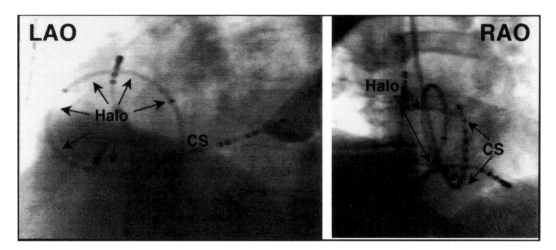

Figure 2. Fluoroscopy of halo catheter positioned along the tricuspid annulus. Catheters are shown in the left anterior oblique (LAO) and right anterior oblique (RAO) view. CS = coronary sinus. Used with permission from Olgin J, et al.[22]

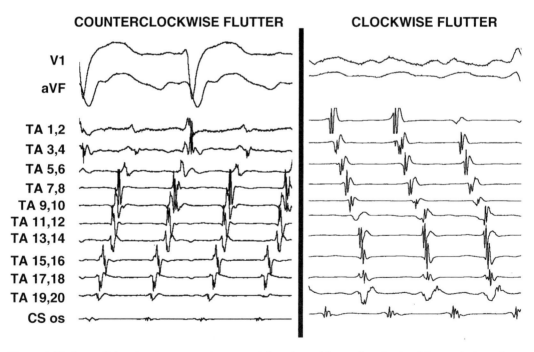

Figure 3. Endocardial activation sequence around the tricuspid annulus obtained from a halo catheter in a patient with counterclockwise and clockwise atrial flutter. Halo distal poles tricuspid annulus 1, 2 are positioned in the low lateral right atrium while the proximal poles tricuspid annulus 19, 20 are positioned on the septum near the His position. In counterclockwise flutter the activation is seen to proceed from the coronary sinus os up the septum to tricuspid annulus 19, 20 in a counterclockwise fashion to tricuspid annulus 1, 2. For clockwise flutter, the activation sequence is the opposite, with activation from the coronary sinus os proceeding first to tricuspid annulus 1, 2 on the low lateral right atrium then in a clockwise fashion toward the tricuspid annulus 19, 20. Notice that in both cases the tricuspid annulus is activated in a sequential manner.

CLOCKWISE　　　　**COUNTERCLOCKWISE**

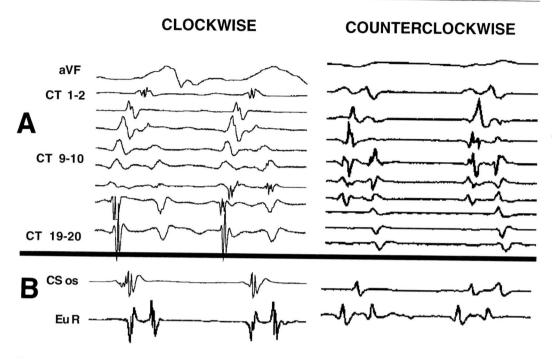

Figure 4. Split potentials recorded along the crista terminalis (**A**) and eustachian ridge (**B**) in counterclockwise and clockwise (typical) flutter. These structures were mapped under intracardiac echo guidance to ensure catheter location. Each component of the split potentials along the crista is activated in opposite sequence. Used with permission from Olgin J, et al.[17]

block.[11,17,19,29,30] Therefore, the finding of split potentials may be a useful adjunct in defining boundaries of the reentrant circuit.

These split potentials have been recorded over the length of the crista terminalis and the eustachian ridge during typical flutter, the known barriers in typical flutter (Figure 4).[16,17,19,23] Because the circuit for typical flutter is constant and well defined, a lengthy search for these barriers is not necessary in each individual case. However, in incisional reentry where the circuit is variable, the identification of split potentials to aid in defining the barriers of the reentrant circuit is very useful in guiding the ablation.[31]

Entrainment Mapping

Transient entrainment was first described in 1977 to demonstrate that atrial flutter was a reentrant arrhythmia.[32] Subsequently, concealed entrainment was described, dem-

onstrating the importance of pacing site on the characteristics of entrainment.[33] With multi-electrode endocardial recordings of entrainment from the subeustachian isthmus during atrial flutter, we now understand there to be endocardial fusion which is not present on the surface ECG because it occurs in a protected isthmus. The work by Stevenson et al. in ventricular tachycardia has further contributed to our understanding of entrainment and has provided techniques for mapping atrial reentrant circuits to identify critical components suitable for ablation.[17,18,31,34,35]

A detailed discussion of entrainment is beyond the scope of this chapter, but several reviews on this topic have recently been published.[16,17,34] Entrainment is the acceleration of a reentrant tachycardia by pacing into the circuit. Entrainment does not affect the reentrant circuit and when pacing ceases, the tachycardia continues unchanged. This allows one to identify critical

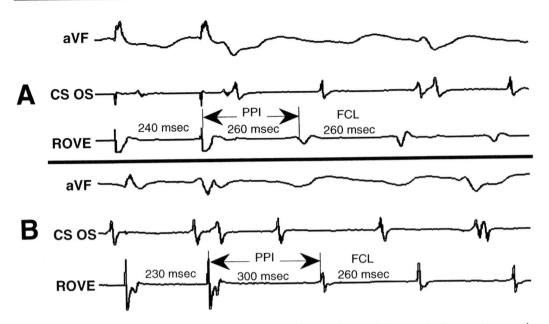

Figure 5. Entrainment of atrial flutter from two different sites. (**A**) Pacing is from a site on the inferior aspect of the tricuspid annulus in the subeustachian isthmus. The post pacing interval (PPI) is equal to the flutter cycle length (FCL). Therefore, this site is within the reentrant circuit. (**B**) Pacing is from the right atrial appendage. The post-pacing interval is longer than the flutter cycle length. Therefore, this site is not within the reentrant circuit. Used with permission from Olgin J, et al.[17]

components of the reentrant circuit. Entrainment is accomplished by pacing slightly faster (i.e., 10–30 ms) than the tachycardia cycle length, to minimize possible decrements within the circuit.[36] Comparing the post-pacing interval, defined as the interval from the last entrained beat to the first spontaneous beat measured at the pacing site, to the spontaneous tachycardia cycle length indicates whether a site is inside or outside the reentrant circuit (Figure 5).[17,31,34,35] Sites within the reentrant circuit will have post-pacing intervals equal to the tachycardia cycle length, while those outside the circuit will have post-pacing intervals longer than the tachycardia cycle length. The presence of concealed fusion entrainment without fusion on the surface ECG indicates that the pacing site is within a protected isthmus.[16,17,34,35] With atrial flutter, p wave fusion on the surface ECG can often be difficult to determine, especially if AV conduction is good. Therefore,

the use of multi-electrode catheters, such as the halo catheter, can be useful to identify parts of the circuit that are antidromically and orthodromically captured. Entrainment mapping can also be useful to identify the extent of a protected isthmus by examining the activation time from pacing stimulus to the flutter wave on the last entrained beat.[17,20,31,34] Entrainment from the entrance would produce a long stimulus to flutter wave interval while entrainment from the exit would produce a short interval.

In a patient with atrial flutter, entrainment mapping is useful to confirm that the flutter is typical (i.e., involves the subeustachian isthmus) and to define the extent of the isthmus.[17] Therefore, limited and targeted entrainment mapping is usually sufficient in typical flutter. For other macroreentrant arrhythmias where the location of a critical isthmus is more variable, entrainment techniques are invaluable in targeting sites for ablation.[31,34,35]

Induction of Flutter

Patients who are referred for atrial flutter often present to the laboratory in sinus rhythm. Although ablation can be performed in sinus rhythm (see below), it is useful to confirm the diagnosis of typical atrial flutter and perform limited endocardial mapping to guide ablation. Several studies have shown that the induction of atrial flutter with programmed stimulation is highly specific.[37,38] In large groups of patients undergoing programmed stimulation, only in those with a clinical history of or risk factors for flutter could atrial flutter be induced.[37,38] However, in a given patient, atrial flutter is very difficult to induce, with only 6.2% of 838 induction attempts in 10 patients with clinical atrial flutter producing atrial flutter.[22]

Because the circuit for both counterclockwise and clockwise flutter are the same, the site from which flutter is induced with programmed stimulation determines which direction the flutter rotates.[22] Pacing from the smooth right atrium posterior to the crista terminalis and eustachian ridge induces counterclockwise flutter while pacing from the trabeculated right atrium anterior to these structures produces clockwise flutter.[22] This site dependence exists because the initiating unidirectional block occurs in the subeustachian isthmus.[22]

In our laboratory, flutter is induced prior to attempted ablation to confirm the presence of typical flutter and electrophysiologically guide the ablation by confirming what sites lie within the critical isthmus. However, once this is done, the ablation and confirmation of success can be performed in sinus rhythm as detailed below.

Ablation

The early studies of catheter ablation for typical flutter utilized a combination of mapping techniques described above. Saoudi et al., utilizing direct current abla-

tion in 14 patients, targeted sites from which they recorded fragmented electrograms that were shown to be critical to the circuit by demonstrating concealed entrainment.[2] These sites were predominantly in the low posterior septal region of the right atrium. The acute success rate of this technique was only 50%. A higher success rate of 83% in 12 patients was obtained by targeting sites in the low posterior right atrium that demonstrated concealed fusion during entrainment.[20] Cosio et al. took an anatomic approach, by ablating in a line from the tricuspid annulus to the inferior vena cava (IVC), yielding a success rate of 78%.[39]

From these early studies, debate spawned as to whether electrophysiological targeting of ablation sites was necessary for typical flutter, since the critical isthmus is consistently located between the tricuspid annulus and the IVC/eustachian ridge. This anatomic approach seems reasonable since all of the human mapping studies of typical flutter identified an isthmus of conduction in the low right atrium between the tricuspid annulus and IVC/eustachian ridge, from the IVC laterally to the coronary sinus os medially.[3,17–21,40] Although no randomized trial has been performed directly comparing the two approaches, recent studies at experienced centers demonstrate that acute success rates for both techniques appear to be the same (80%–100%).[41–45] In our laboratory, limited electrophysiological mapping is performed to confirm that typical flutter is present (i.e., the subeustachian isthmus is critical to the reentrant circuit and roughly determine the extent of the isthmus), and then an anatomic approach is used.

The ablation line can be drawn anywhere in the isthmus from the lateral border of the IVC and tricuspid annulus to the septal border between tricuspid annulus and coronary sinus os. However, in some instances the eustachian ridge does not form a complete line of block from the IVC to the coronary sinus os. This has been shown both electrophysiologically and with pathologic examination of human hearts.[17,46] Olgin et al., using intracardiac echo to identify the eustachian ridge, demonstrated that in some patients the exit to the isthmus is posterior to the coronary sinus os.[17] Adachi et al. performed autopsy examinations of the flutter isthmus and found that the eustachian ridge was "incomplete" in some individuals.[46]

Nakagawa et al. demonstrated that an ablation lesion from the tricuspid annulus to the coronary sinus os was insufficient to eliminate typical flutter in 13 of 27 patients.[19] An additional line of ablation from the coronary sinus os to the eustachian ridge was successful in 12 of the patients.[19] Several other factors are important in determining where in the isthmus (i.e., lateral, mid, medial) to create the ablation line in typical flutter. The subeustachian isthmus can be very wide, particularly in patients with dilated atria, and is usually narrowest at the septal aspect. In addition, the subeustachian isthmus is not a smooth endocardial surface but has many peaks and valleys, making the creation of long ablation lines difficult. Most importantly, the line must be complete from the tricuspid annulus to the IVC/eustachian ridge. Therefore, the ablation lesion should be made wherever in the isthmus optimal catheter tissue contact is best over the entire distance from tricuspid annulus to IVC.

Endpoint Testing

Although high acute success rates at terminating typical atrial flutter with ablation can be achieved, there appears to be a high recurrence rate (up to 25%) of the flutter in earlier studies.[41-45] In these studies, acute success was defined as the termination of flutter with the ablation and the inability to re-induce the flutter after ablation. However, as described above, atrial flutter is not easily or repeatedly inducible in a given patient, even prior to ablation.[22] Therefore, re-inducibility is an inadequate endpoint for ablation and may explain the high recurrence rate in these early studies.

PACING FROM THE CS OS DURING RADIOFREQUENCY ABLATION

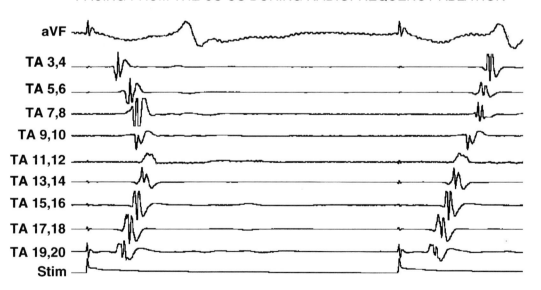

Figure 6. Demonstration of isthmus block during RF ablation of a patient with atrial flutter. After flutter was terminated, pacing from the coronary sinus os was performed during RF ablation. Two paced beats are shown during RF energy application. On the left, activation of the halo catheter proceeds in both the clockwise and counterclockwise direction with fusion of the wavefronts near tricuspid annulus 11, 12. On the next beat, conduction block in the isthmus had been completed as evidenced by activation of the halo catheter in a counterclockwise direction only.

PACING FROM THE LOW LATERAL RIGHT ATRIUM

A   **B**

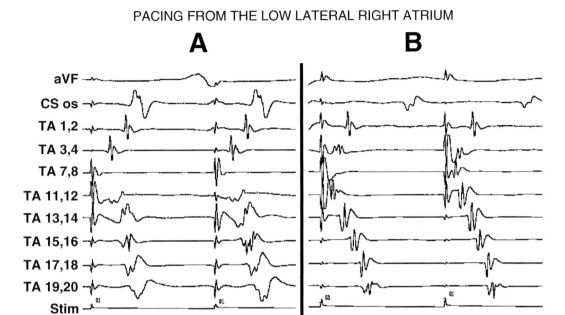

Figure 7. Demonstration of bidirectional block in the patient shown in Figure 5. Pacing from the low lateral right atrium in the region of TA5–6 prior to ablation (**A**) demonstrates activation of the coronary sinus os through the flutter isthmus (TA 3, 4 activated before tricuspid annulus 1, 2 which is activated before coronary sinus os). (**B**) Following ablation, pacing from the low lateral right atrium demonstrates that the coronary sinus os is activated after tricuspid annulus 19, 20 confirming block in the flutter isthmus.

Several investigators have recently described a new technique to demonstrate whether the ablation lesion has severed the subeustachian isthmus with pacing techniques. This is accomplished by initiating pacing during sinus rhythm on one side of the ablation lesion and demonstrating that activation does not proceed across the isthmus lesion (Figures 6 and 7). For example, during pacing from the coronary sinus os pre-ablation, activation will proceed through the subeustachian isthmus to activate the low lateral right atrium (Figure 6). However, after successful ablation, activation cannot proceed through the isthmus and the low lateral right atrium is activated late, after the high lateral right atrium. A halo catheter is very useful to demonstrate this change in activation after successful ablation. Several studies have now confirmed that the demonstration of complete, bidirectional block in the subeustachian isthmus is a more reliable indicator of long-term success with recurrence rates near 0%.[19,24,47–49] Because those patients in whom only unidirectional or rate-dependent block was achieved had a significantly higher recurrence rate, it is important to pace at slower rates and on both sides (i.e., low lateral right atrium and coronary sinus os) of the lesion to establish the presence of bidirectional, rate-independent conduction block.[47,48]

This technique of confirming conduction block not only provides a better endpoint for ablation, but also allows one to ablate the flutter in sinus rhythm.[47] In fact, in our laboratory this is preferred because one can more readily identify the development of conduction block.

Atypical Flutter

Atypical atrial flutters do not appear to use the same circuit as typical atrial flutter.

The rates and endocardial activation are inconsistent with either clockwise or counterclockwise flutter. Although the barriers are unknown for this type of atypical flutter, there are preliminary data to suggest that at least some of these arrhythmias are due to reentry around a portion of the crista terminalis.[23] Other forms of atypical flutter may be due to macroreentry in the left atrium, where the role of anatomic barriers such as the pulmonary veins or mitral annulus is still to be explored. Because the circuit for these flutters are unknown, there is no specific ablation for atypical flutter.

Incisional Reentry

Animal Models and Substrate

Recently, animal models of incisional reentry have been developed in canines, simulating the Mustard and the Fontan procedures.[50,51] In the canine model of the Mustard procedure, suture lines were placed mimicking those placed during placement of the baffle, including an atriotomy, septectomy, and in the usual baffle location.[50] Most of the tachycardias revolved around the tricuspid annulus or around the atriotomy incision.[50] Rarely the tachycardias involved both atria or revolved around the mitral annulus.[50] In the canine model of the Fontan operation, a suture line simulating a cavopulmonary connection suture line is placed through an atriotomy.[51] In this model, induced atrial tachycardias all involved an isthmus created by the lateral margin of the cavopulmonary suture line.[51]

These arrhythmias can occur in any patient who has undergone an atriotomy, usually as part of a surgical repair of congenital heart disease. The atriotomy scar and any other suture lines may be a potential substrate for macroreentry. Reentrant arrhythmias have been reported in patients following atrial septal defect repair, Mustard procedure, Fontan repair, Senning procedure, and the Rastelli procedure.[31,52] The substrate for this group of arrhythmias is

variable and is determined by the surgical scars as well as artificial and natural obstacles in the atrium. The reentrant circuit can involve one or more of these artificial obstacles as well as anatomic obstacles such as those involved in typical flutter (i.e., crista terminalis, subeustachian isthmus); in these patients reentrant arrhythmias involving the typical flutter isthmus may have different activation sequences and surface p waves due to the distorted atrial anatomy. Since the subrate for reentry is so variable and isthmuses can be wide at points, extensive mapping is necessary in each case to identify appropriate ablation targets. The principles of mapping atrial flutter as described above (split potentials and entrainment mapping) are applicable to this patient population. Mapping and ablation are further complicated by the potential for multiple tachycardias in an individual patient.

Mapping and Ablation

Several series have now demonstrated the effectiveness of ablation of reentrant atrial tachycardias following repair of congenital heart disease.[31,52–54] Mapping techniques are similar to those described above for atrial flutter. Because the barriers are variable among patients and isthmuses can be wide, entrainment mapping and recording of split potentials are particularly useful to define barriers in individual patients.[31,52–54] Ablation is targeted to isthmuses that are demonstrated to be critical to the reentrant circuit using entrainment techniques.[31,52,54] These patients may have multiple atrial reentrant circuits[55] and that in general, studies to date have involved ablation of clinical arrhythmias only.[31,52–54] Using this approach, RF ablation has an 80%–93% acute success rate. However, the long-term success rate appears to be less, with a recurrence rate around 40%.[31,52–54] Since these patients may have multiple circuits for atrial reentry, it is unclear whether these recurrences are new tachycardias or true recurrences.[55] In addition, unlike atrial flutter, the endpoint for ablation of these tachycardias may be inadequate, since it is difficult to confirm conduction block produced by the ablation lesion. Therefore, successful ablation is defined as termination of the tachycardia and inability to re-induce the same tachycardia. Other tachycardias, however, may often remain inducible. Newer technologies such as basket catheters or electrospatial mapping may provide improved techniques for mapping, ablation, and endpoint testing in this population.

Focal Atrial Tachycardias

Substrate

The mechanism of ectopic or focal atrial tachycardia is heterogeneous and may include enhanced automaticity, triggered activity, or microreentry.[56–58] However, these arrhythmias have in common that they originate from a single discrete focus and includes atrial tachycardias as well as sinus node reentry. It is this focal nature (rather than the electrophysiological mechanism) that directs the mapping and ablation technique.

A number of studies have shown that focal atrial tachycardias have a highly characteristic anatomic distribution.[59–62] In the left atrium, common sites include the ostia of the pulmonary veins and the left atrial appendage. For right atrial tachycardias the atrial tachycardia foci cluster along the crista terminalis, within the right atrial appendage and near the region of the coronary sinus ostium.[53,59–62] This distribution in the right atrium has been confirmed with electrophysiological-anatomic mapping using intracardiac echocardiography.[63] In addition, Mallavarapu et al. have reported left atrial tachycardias arising from near the mitral annulus.[64] In other rare instances, atrial tachycardias may arise from abnormal atrial structures such as tumors or abnormal trabeculations.[65]

Mapping and Ablation

The 12-lead ECG can in many instances provide information about the anatomic location of the atrial tachycardia focus.[66] The p wave vector in leads aVL and V_1 are useful in differentiating right from left atrial foci and leads II, III, and aVF are useful in differentiating superior from inferior foci.[66] There are, however, some problems with and exceptions to this approach. In many focal atrial tachycardias, AV conduction is usually 1:1 and therefore identification of a "pure" p wave isolated from the t wave is usually difficult. The use of adenosine is not only useful in differentiating atrial tachycardias from AV reentrant tachycardias, but is often useful to reveal "pure" p waves. In addition, left atrial tachycardias arising from the right pulmonary veins often have p wave vectors suggestive of right atrial foci (or are ambiguous). This occurs because the right pulmonary veins lie directly behind the right atrium and are anatomically rightward structures (see below).[65]

Several methods for mapping atrial tachycardias have been reported.[53,59,60,67,68] Activation mapping is the most useful means of mapping atrial tachycardias. Sites with local activation prior to the onset of the surface p wave (15–60 ms) have been demonstrated to be good targets for ablation.[53,59,60] In addition, fragmented electrograms have been recorded from areas near successful ablation sites in some patients.[53] As atrial tachycardias may not be sustained during the electrophysiology study, mapping of monomorphic PACs or nonsustained atrial tachycardia is occasionally necessary. When high-degree AV block is not present and the p wave morphology and onset not apparent, the use of intracardiac surrogate markers for p wave onset is often useful.

Unlike mapping of accessory pathways where mapping is limited to the two-dimensional structure of the AV valves, mapping of focal atrial tachycardias involves mapping in the complex three-dimensional structure of the atria. Mapping techniques for atrial tachycardias have included leapfrogging two mapping catheters in attempt to localize sites of earliest activation.[53,59] Other investigators have proposed using pacemapping to match either p wave morphology or endocardial activation sequence.[67] Pacemapping using p wave morphology is frequently difficult in the absence of high-degree AV block. Pacemapping using endocardial activation sequence is limited by the number of intracardiac recording sites.

Knowledge of the characteristic distribution (along the crista terminalis and pulmonary veins) of atrial tachycardias can expedite mapping. Kalman et al. have described a mapping technique whereby a multipolar catheter is placed along the crista terminalis under intracardiac echo to guide initial mapping.[63] Intracardiac echo is used to identify the crista and guide placement of this 20-pole catheter along its entire extent (Figure 8). Intracardiac echo is necessary as the course of the crista terminalis can be quite variable.[69] This provides an initial road map for guiding the mapping.[63] For those tachycardias arising from the crista terminalis, the earliest site of activation along the multipolar CT cath-

eter facilitates mapping with the ablation catheter (Figure 9). For tachycardias arising away from the crista terminalis, activation of this multipolar CT catheter lacks dispersion of activation times and is relatively late in relation to the surface p wave. This technique is useful for mapping both sustained tachycardias as well as single PACs.

Intracardiac echo is useful in demonstrating the complex anatomy of the atria and is especially helpful in guiding mapping to distinguish right pulmonary vein tachycardias from right atrial tachycardias arising from the high crista terminalis.[63] As mentioned before, the right upper pulmonary vein lies directly posterior to the crista terminalis and is a rightward structure. Using intracardiac echo to guide fine mapping between the crista terminalis and the posterior right atrium opposite the pulmonary vein, one can distinguish between tachycardias originating from these sites (Figure 10).[63] This region is often small and requires mapping in relation to anatomy over 1 cm or less. Therefore, intracardiac echo is useful for providing an anatomic-based electrophysiological mapping of focal atrial tachycardias.

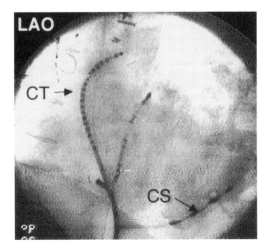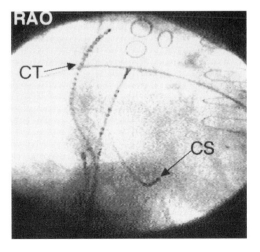

Figure 8. Fluoroscopy of 20-pole catheter positioned along the crista terminalis using intracardiac echo. Catheters are shown in the left anterior oblique (LAO) and right anterior oblique (RAO) view. CS = coronary sinus. Used with permission from Olgin J, et al.[17]

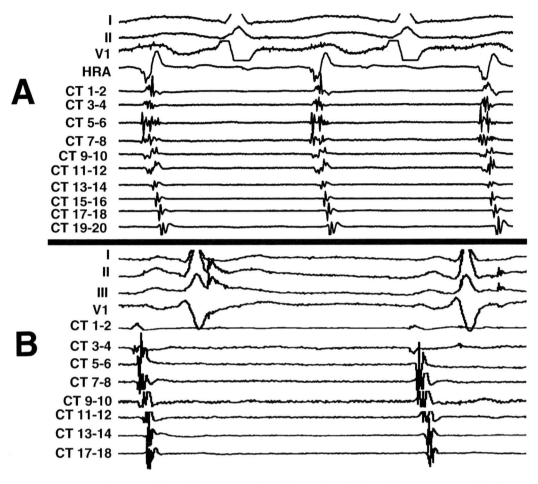

Figure 9. Intracardiac recordings from a 20-pole catheter placed along the crista terminalis during atrial tachycardia (**A**) and during sinus rhythm (**B**). During atrial tachycardia, earliest activation is in the mid-crista terminalis near poles 7–8. This serves to guide initial mapping in the region of these bipoles along the crista. CT = crista terminalis; HRA = high right atrium; CT 1–2 = distal poles positioned superiorly on the crista terminalis; CT 19–20 = proximal poles positioned inferiorly on the crista terminalis.

Another technique, using electrospatial mapping with a computer-based system to localize a mapping catheter in three-dimensional space has been described.[70] This technique is currently limited to mapping regular, sustained tachycardias and is not widely available.[70] Multipolar basket catheters have also been used for mapping atrial tachycardias.[55] However, the electrogram quality can be poor in many electrodes because the baskets do not easily conform to the complex shape of the atrium and localization of individual electrodes can be challenging.

Inappropriate Sinus Tachycardia

The syndrome of inappropriate sinus tachycardia is characterized by an increased resting sinus rate and/or and exaggerated increase in sinus rate with minor exertion.[71–73] The precise mechanism for this is not well understood, but is distinct from focal atrial tachycardias originating from the crista terminalis, such as sinus node reentry.[71,72,74] The anatomic substrate for this tachycardia appears to be based on the electrophysiology of the sinus mechanism, which lies within the crista terminalis. Several studies have demonstrated that the entire crista terminalis is responsible for the sinus mechanism, with faster rates arising from the superior portion and slower rates arising from the lower portions.[25,73,75–77] The relationship between heart rate and site of impulse origin within the crista terminalis in response to autonomic inputs has been well documented.[25,75,76,78] Vagal stimulation produces a sinus slowing associated with an inferior shift in the dominant pacemaker (Figure 11). Sympathetic activation produces a faster sinus rate associated with

a cranial and anterior shift in the dominant pacemaker (Figure 11).[25,75–78]

For patients who are symptomatic and unresponsive to medical therapy, RF modification of the sinus pacemaker can be performed. The feasibility of modifying the rapid sinus rates arising from the superior portions of the crista terminalis has been described in both animals and humans.[73,77] A combined anatomic and electrophysiological approach was used. Mapping is performed much as described for focal atrial tachycardias with a multipolar catheter placed along the crista terminalis under intracardiac echo guidance. Ablation is targeted at the superior sites along the crista terminalis under maximal autonomic stimulation (isoproterenol and atropine) with ablation gradually progressing inferiorly until a 25%–30% reduction in rate is

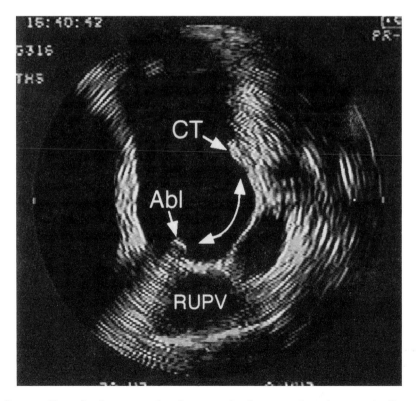

Figure 10. Intracardiac echo demonstrating fine mapping between the crista terminalis and the right atrial wall opposite the right upper pulmonary vein. This technique is useful in distinguishing tachycardias arising near the crista terminalis from those arising from the right pulmonary vein. CT = crista terminalis; Abl = ablation catheter; RUPV = right upper pulmonary vein.

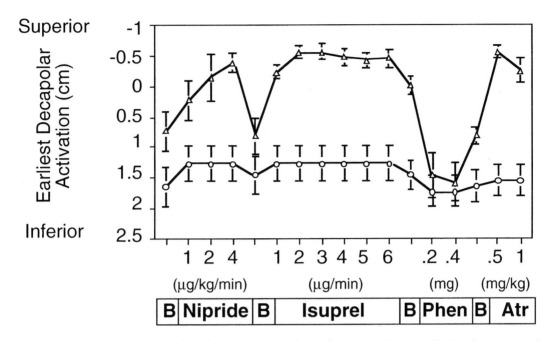

Figure 11. Shift in sinus focus along the crista terminalis with autonomic manipulation demonstrated with a 20-pole catheter placed along the crista terminalis under intracardiac echo guidance. Earliest activation at the second bipole was taken as the 0 cm reference point and distances from this location were calculated according to the bipole distance along the catheter. Before sinus node modification (upper curve △) the sinus focus shifted over a distance of up to 2 cm, moving superiorly with sympathetic stimulation (nipride and isoproterenol) and inferiorly with parasympathetic stimulation (atropine). After sinus node modification (lower curve ○), the earliest activation site was shifted inferiorly and no significant movement occurred in response to sympathetic stimulation. B = baseline; Phen = phenylephrine; At = atropine. Used with permission from Kalman JM, et al.[77]

achieved.[73,77] Care must be taken not to damage the right phrenic nerve; ablation pulses should not be delivered if pacing from the ablation catheter stimulates the diaphragm.

While this approach has been shown to have good results acutely with a low incidence of permanent pacemaker requirement, long-term results appear to be poor with a 68% recurrence rate of symptoms.[79] It is unclear whether sinus tachycardia is present in all patients with symptomatic recurrences. In some patients a more extensive sinus node ablation may be needed.

Atrial Fibrillation

There has recently been intensive research to develop a catheter-based proce-

dure to cure atrial fibrillation. The principles of catheter ablation to cure atrial fibrillation have been demonstrated in the surgical Maze procedure[80]—the creation of lines of conduction block in the atria to prevent atrial fibrillation. Two recent reports in humans suggests that indeed this is feasible.[81,82] In these studies, standard ablation catheters were used to create linear ablation lesions by dragging the catheter over the endocardial surface during RF energy application.[81,82] These procedures were moderately effective (60%–80%) at reducing symptomatic atrial fibrillation but were complicated by macroreentrant atrial tachycardias and required very long procedures.[81,82] Technology must evolve to enable the ablationist to create continuous linear lesions more effectively and efficiently. Newer catheters with multiple ablation coils have

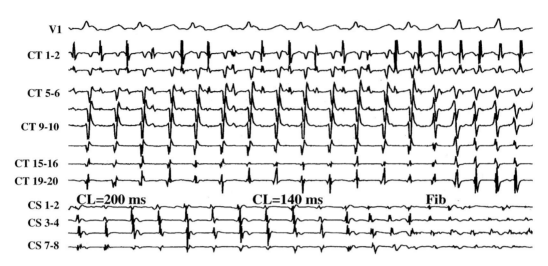

Figure 12. Intracardiac recordings from a patient with focal atrial fibrillation. On the left part of the tracing a regular, rapid atrial tachycardia at a cycle length of 200 ms is seen. This was a stable rhythm for 20 minutes prior to this tracing. The tachycardia suddenly speeds to a cycle length of 140 ms and then results in atrial fibrillation.

been developed that enable creation of linear transmural lesions that produce conduction block.[83] In addition, specially designed long vascular sheaths have been developed to improve catheter stability during drag lesions.[81] Since the linear lesions will likely in part be anatomically determined, intracardiac echo and/or electrospatial mapping may be useful to guide lesion placement and confirm lesion contiguity.[83]

There also appears to be a population of patients with atrial fibrillation who have a focal mechanism that is amenable to standard ablation.[84] Jais et al. have described nine patients with atrial fibrillation who were found to have rapid focal atrial tachycardias that were successfully ablated with RF energy.[84] We have found similar patients at our institution. The foci appear to be in the usual distribution described above and are mapped similarly. However, mapping may be challenging if the atrial tachycardia degenerates into atrial fibrillation rapidly (Figure 12).

References

1. Klein G, Guiraudon G, Sharma A, et al. Demonstration of macroreentry and feasibility of operative therapy in the common type of atrial flutter. Am J Cardiol 1986;57:587–591.
2. Saoudi N, Atallah G, Kirkorian G, et al. Catheter ablation of the atrial myocardium in human type I atrial flutter. Circulation 1990; 81:762–771.
3. Cosio FG, Lopez GM, Goicolea A, et al. Electrophysiologic studies in atrial flutter. Clin Cardiol 1992;15:667–673.
4. Waldo AL, Wells JL Jr, Plumb VJ, et al. Studies of atrial flutter following open heart surgery. Ann Rev Med 1979;30:259–268.
5. Rosenblueth A, Garcia-Ramos J. The influence of artificial obstacles on experimental auricular flutter. Am Heart J 1947;33: 677–684.
6. Frame L, Page R, Hoffman B. Atrial reentry around an anatomic barrier with a partially refractory excitable gap: a canine model of atrial flutter. Circ Res 1986;58:495–511.
7. Frame LH, Page RL, Boyden PA, et al. Circus movement in the canine atrium around the tricuspid ring during experimental atrial flutter and during reentry in vitro. Circulation 1987;76:1155–1175.
8. Boineau JP, Schuessler RB, Mooney CR, et al. Natural and evoked atrial flutter due to circus movement in dogs: role of abnormal atrial pathways, slow conduction, nonuniform refractory period distribution and

premature beats. Am J Cardiol 1980;45: 1167–1181.

9. Inoue H, Toda I, Saihara S, et al. Further observations on entrainment of atrial flutter in the dog. Am Heart J 1989;118:467–474.

10. Yamashita T, Inoue H, Nozaki A, et al. Role of anatomic architecture in sustained atrial reentry and double potentials. Am Heart J 1992;124:938–946.

11. Feld GK, Shahandeh RF. Mechanism of double potentials recorded during sustained atrial flutter in the canine right atrial crush-injury model. Circulation 1992;86:628–641.

12. Feld GK, Shahandeh RF. Activation patterns in experimental canine atrial flutter produced by right atrial crush injury. J Am Coll Cardiol 1992;20:441–451.

13. Lewis T. Observations upon flutter and fibrillation as it occurs in patients. Heart 1921; 8:193.

14. Olshansky B, Wilber DJ, Hariman RJ. Atrial flutter—update on the mechanism and treatment. PACE 1992;15:2308–2335.

15. Boyden R. Models of atrial reentry. J Cardiol Electrophysiol 1995;6:313–324.

16. Olgin J, Kalman J, Lesh M. Conduction barriers in atrial flutter—correlation of electrophysiology and anatomy. J Cardiovasc Electrophysiol 1996;7:1112–1126.

17. Olgin J, Kalman J, Fitzpatrick A, et al. The role of right atrial endocardial structures as barriers to conduction during human type I atrial flutter: activation and entrainment mapping guided by intracardiac echocardiography. Circulation 1995;92:1833–1848.

18. Kalman J, Olgin J, Saxon L, et al. Activation and entrainment mapping defines the tricuspid annulus as the anterior barrier in typical atrial flutter. Circulation 1996;94:398–406.

19. Nakagawa H, Lazzara R, Khastgir T, et al. Role of the tricuspid annulus and the eustachian valve/ridge on atrial flutter: relevance to catheter ablation of the septal isthmus and a new technique for rapid identification of ablation success. Circulation 1996;94: 407–424.

20. Feld GK, Fleck RP, Chen PS, et al. Radiofrequency catheter ablation for the treatment of human type 1 atrial flutter: identification of a critical zone in the reentrant circuit by endocardial mapping techniques. Circulation 1992;86:1233–1240.

21. Olshansky B, Okumura K, Hess PG, et al. Demonstration of an area of slow conduction in human atrial flutter. J Am Coll Cardiol 1990;16:1639–1648.

22. Olgin J, Kalman J, Saxon L, et al. Induction of atrial flutter in man: site dependence and site of unidirectional block. J Am Coll Cardiol 1997;29:376–384.

23. Kalman J, Olgin J, Saxon L, et al. Electrocardiographic and electrophysiologic characterization of atypical atrial flutter in man: use of activation and entrainment mapping and implications for catheter ablation. J Cardiovasc Electrophysiol 1997;8:121–144.

24. Poty H, Saoudi N, Abdel Aziz A, et al. Radiofrequency catheter ablation of type 1 atrial flutter: prediction of late success by electrophysiological criteria. Circulation 1995;92: 1389–1392.

25. Kalman J, Olgin J, Saxon L, et al. Electrophysiologic of the crista terminalis in normal human atria. PACE 1996;19:578.

26. Kall J, Glascock D, Kopp D, et al. Characterization and catheter ablation of the antidromic form of typical atrial flutter [Abstract]. Circulation 1995;92:I-84.

27. Lesh M, Kalman J. To fumble flutter or tackle tach? Toward updated classifiers for atrial tachyarrhythmias. J Cardiovasc Electrophysiol 1996;7:460–466.

28. Puech P, Latour H, Grolleau R. Le Flutter et ses limites. Arch Mal Coeur 1970;63:116–144.

29. Olshansky B, Okumura K, Henthorn R, et al. Characterization of double potentials in human atrial flutter: studies during transient entrainment. J Am Coll Cardiol 1990;15: 833–841.

30. Cosio F, Arribas F, Barbero J, et al. Validation of double spike electrograms as markers of conduction delay or block in atrial flutter. Am J Cardiol 1988;61:775–780.

31. Kalman JM, VanHare GF, Olgin JE, et al. Ablation of 'incisional' reentrant atrial tachycardia complicating surgery for congenital heart disease: use of entrainment to define a critical isthmus of conduction. Circulation 1996;93:502–512.

32. Waldo AL, McLean WAH, Karp RB, et al. Entrainment and interruption of atrial flutter with atrial pacing: studies in man following open heart surgery. Circulation 1977;56: 737–745.

33. Okumura K, Henthorn RW, Epstein AE, et al. Further observations on transient entrainment: importance of pacing site and properties of the components of the reentry circuit. Circulation 1985;72:1293–1307.

34. Stevenson W, Sager P, Friedman P. Entrainment techniques for mapping atrial and ventricular tachycardias. J Cardiovasc Electrophysiol 1995;6:201–216.

35. Stevenson W, Khan H, Sager P, et al. Identification of reentry circuit sites during catheter mapping and radiofrequency ablation of ventricular tachycardia late after myocardial infarction. Ciculation 1993;88:1647–1670.

36. Waldo A, Carlson M, Biblo L, et al. The role of transient entrainment in atrial flutter. In

Waldo A, ed. Atrial Arrhythmias. Mount Kisco, NY, Futura Publishing Co, Inc, 1993, pp 210–228.

37. Watson RM, Josephson ME. Atrial flutter. I. Electrophysiologic substrates and modes of initiation and termination. Am J Cardiol 1980;45:732–741.

38. Brignole M, Menozzi C, Sartore B, et al. The use of atrial pacing to induce atrial fibrillation and flutter. Int J Cardiol 1986;12:45–54.

39. Cosio FG, Lopez GM, Goicolea A, et al. Radiofrequency ablation of the inferior vena cava-tricuspid valve isthmus in common atrial flutter. Am J Cardiol 1993;71:705–709.

40. Cosio FG, Lopez GM, Arribas F, et al. Mechanisms of entrainment of human common flutter studied with multiple endocardial recordings. Circulation 1994;89:2117–2125.

41. Lesh M, Van Hare G, Epstein L, et al. Radiofrequency catheter ablation of atrial arrhythmias: Results and mechanisms. Circulation 1994;89:1074–1089.

42. Calkins H, Leon AR, Deam AG, et al. Catheter ablation of atrial flutter using radiofrequency energy. Am J Cardiol 1994;73:353–356.

43. Kirkorian G, Moncada E, Chevalier P, et al. Radiofrequency ablation of atrial flutter: efficacy of an anatomically guided approach. Circulation 1994;90:2804–2814.

44. Fischer B, Haissaguerre M, Garrigues S, et al. Radiofrequency catheter ablation of common atrial flutter in 80 patients. J Am Coll Cardiol 1995;25:1365–1372.

45. Saxon LA, Kalman JM, Olgin JE, et al. Results of radiofrequency catheter ablation for atrial flutter. Am J Cardiol 1996;77:1014–1016.

46. Adachi M, Igawa O, Tomokuni A, et al. Anatomic characteristics of the eustachian ridge, a barrier to conduction during common type atrial flutter. Circulation 1996;94:I-380.

47. Poty H, Sauodi N, Nair M, et al. Radiofrequency catheter ablation of atrial flutter—further insights into the various types of isthmus block: application to ablation during sinus rhythm. Circulation 1996;94:3204–3213.

48. Cauchemez B, Haissaguerre M, Fischer B, et al. Electrophysiological effects of catheter ablation of inferior vena cava-tricuspid annulus isthmus in common atrial flutter. Circulation 1996;93:284–294.

49. Fischer B, Jais P, Shah D, et al. Radiofrequency catheter ablation of common atrial flutter in 200 patients. J Cardiovasc Electrophysiol 1996;7:1225–1233.

50. Cronin CS, Nitta T, Mitsuno M, et al. Characterization and surgical ablation of acute atrial flutter following the Mustard procedure: a canine model. Circulation 1993;88:461–471.

51. Rodefeld M, Bromberg B, Schuessler R, et al. Atrial flutter after lateral tunnel construction in the modified fontan operation: a canine model. J Thorac Cardiovasc Surg 1996;111:514–526.

52. Triedman J, Saul J, Weindling S, et al. Radiofrequency ablation of intra-atrial reentrant tachycardia after surgical palliation of congenital heart disease. Circulation 1995;91:707–714.

53. Lesh MD, Van Hare GF, Epstein LM, et al. Radiofrequency catheter ablation of atrial arrhythmias: results and mechanisms. Circulation 1994;89:1074–1089.

54. Baker B, Lindsay B, Bromberg B, et al. Catheter ablation of clinical intraatrial reentrant tachycardias resulting from previous atrial surgery: localizing and transecting the critical isthmus. J Am Coll Cardiol 1996;28:411–417.

55. Triedman J, Jenkins K, Colan S, et al. Intra-atrial reentrant tachycardia after palliation of congenital heart disease: characterization of multiple macroreentrant circuits using fluoroscopically based three-dimensional endocardial mapping. J Cardiovasc Electrophysiol 1997;8:259–270.

56. Chen S, Chiang C, Yang C, et al. Sustained atrial tachycardia in adult patients. Electrophysiological characteristics, pharmacological response, possible mechanisms and effects of radiofrequency ablation. Circulation 1994;90:1262–1278.

57. Engelstein E, Lippman N, Stein K, et al. Mechanism-specific effects of adenosine on atrial tachycardia. Circulation 1994;89:2645–2654.

58. Haines D, DiMarco J. Sustained intraatrial reentrant tachycardia: clinical, electrocardiographic and electrophysiologic characteristics and long-term follow-up. J Am Coll Cardiol 1990;15:1345–1354.

59. Kay G, Chong F, Epstein A, et al. Radiofrequency ablation for treatment of primary atrial tachycardias. J Am Coll Cardiol 1993;21:901–909.

60. Walsh E, Saul J, Hulse J, et al. Transcatheter ablation of ectopic atrial tachycardia in young patients using radiofrequency current. Circulation 1992;86:1138–1146.

61. Sanders W, Sorrentino R, Greenfield R, et al. Catheter ablation of sinoatrial node reentrant tachycardia. J Am Coll Cardiol 1994;23:926–934.

62. Shenasa H, Merrill J, Hamer M, et al. Distribution of ectopic atrial tachycardias along the crista terminalis: an atrial ring of fire [Abstract]? Circulation 1993;88:I-29.

63. Kalman J, Olgin J, Karch M, et al. "Cristal tachycardia": origin of right atrial tachycardias from the crista terminalis identified by intracardiac echocardiography. JACC 1998; 31:451–459.

64. Mallavarapu C, Schwartzman D, Callans DJ, et al. Radiofrequency catheter ablation of atrial tachycardia with unusual left atrial sites of origin: report of two cases. PACE 1996;19:988–992.

65. Kalman J, Olgin J, Karch M, et al. Use of intracardiac echocardiography in interventional electrophysiology. PACE 1997;20: 2248–2262.

66. Tang CW, Scheinman MM, Van Hare GF, et al. Use of P wave configuration during atrial tachycardia to predict site of origin. J Am Coll Cardiol 1995;26:1315–1324.

67. Tracy C, Swartz J, Fletcher R, et al. Radiofrequency catheter ablation of ectopic atrial tachycardia using paced activation sequence mapping. J Am Coll Cardiol 1993;21:910–917.

68. Poty H, Saoudi N, Haissaguerre M, et al. Radiofrequency catheter ablation of atrial tachycardias. Am Heart J 1996;131:481–489.

69. Weiss C, Hatala R, Carpinteiro L, et al. Topographic anatomy and in vitro fluoroscopic imaging of the crista terminalis: an attempt to more precisely localize the origin of ectopic atrial tachycardia [Abstract]. Circulation 1994;89:I-595.

70. Gepstein L, Hayam G, Ben-Haim SA. A novel method for nonfluoroscopic catheter-based electroanatomical mapping of the heart: in vitro and in vivo accuracy results. Circulation 1997;95:1611–1622.

71. Morillo CA, Klein GJ, Thakur RK, et al. Mechanism of 'inappropriate' sinus tachycardia. Role of sympathovagal balance. Circulation 1994;90:873–877.

72. Krahn A, Yee R, Klein G, et al. Inappropriate sinus tachycardia: evaluation and therapy. J Cardiovasc Electrophysiol 1995;6: 1124–1128.

73. Lee RJ, Kalman JM, Fitzpatrick AP, et al. Radiofrequency catheter modification of the sinus node for "inappropriate" sinus tachycardia. Circulation 1995;92:2919–2928.

74. Bauernfeind R, Amat Leon F, Dhingra R, et al. Chronic nonparoxysmal sinus tachycardia in otherwise healthy persons. Ann Intern Med 1979;91:702–710.

75. Boineau J, Schuessler R, Hackel D, et al. Widespread distribution and rate differentiation of the atrial pacemaker complex. Am J Physiol 1980;239:H406-H415.

76. Boineau J, Schuessler R, Roeske W, et al. Quantitative relation between sites of atrial impulse origin and cycle length. Am J Physiol 1983;245:H781-H789.

77. Kalman JM, Lee RJ, Fisher WG, et al. Radiofrequency catheter modification of sinus pacemaker function guided by intracardiac echocardiography. Circulation 1995;92: 3070–3081.

78. Jones S, Euler D, Hardie E, et al. Comparison of SA nodal and subsidiary atrial pacemaker function and location in the dog. Am J Physiol 1978;234:H471-H476.

79. Shinbane J, Lesh M, Scheinman M, et al. Long-term follow-up after radiofrequency sinus node modification for inappropriate sinus tachycardia [Abstract]. J Am Coll Cardiol 1997;29:199A.

80. Cox J, Schuessler R, D'Agostino J, et al. The surgical treatment of atrial fibrillation: development of a definitive surgical procedure. J Thorac Cardiovasc Surg 1991;101:569–583.

81. Swartz J, Pellersels G, Silvers J, et al. A catheter-based curative approach to atrial fibrillation in humans [Abstract]. Circulation 1994; 90:I335.

82. Haissaguerre M, Jais P, Shah D, et al. Right and left atrial radiofrequency catheter therapy of paroxysmal atrial fibrillation. J Cardiovasc Electrophysiol 1996;7:1132–1144.

83. Olgin J, Kalman J, Chin M, et al. Electrophysiologic effects of long linear atrial lesions placed under intracardiac ultrasound guidance. Circulation, in press.

84. Jais P, Haissaguerre M, Shah DC, et al. A focal source of atrial fibrillation treated by discrete radiofrequency ablation. Circulation 1997;95:572–576.

Chapter 10

Atrial Fibrillation:
Future Perspectives

Pierre Jaïs, Michel Haïssaguerre, Dipen C. Shah, T. Lavergne,
Stéphane Garrigue, Mélèze Hocini, Atsushi Takahashi,
Jacques Clémenty

Introduction

Atrial fibrillation, the most common sustained cardiac rhythm disturbance, affects more than 2,000,000 Americans with an overall prevalence of 0.89% in the United States.[1] The prevalence increases rapidly with age to 5.9% over the age of 65[1] and is associated with manifestations ranging from palpitations to cardiac failure. The most dreaded complication is stroke; in 30% of patients over the age of 65,[2] it is due to atrial fibrillation. Catheter techniques for ventricular rate control (atrioventricular junction ablation, atrioventricular nodal modification)[3–7] have been shown to be effective but the persistence of atrial fibrillation and the frequent requirement for a permanent pacemaker are significant disadvantages. Curative therapies have therefore been developed both by surgeons[8–13] and cardiologists based on studies demonstrating the co-existence of several reentrant wavelets in a critical mass of atrial tissue responsible for perpetuating atrial fibrillation.[14–18] Linear ablative lesions created by applications of radiofrequency (RF) energy or by the surgeon's knife have been shown to be effective in patients with atrial flutter and paroxysmal or chronic atrial fibrillation.[19–29] This chapter will focus on catheter-based atrial fibrillation ablation.

Biatrial Dimensions Relevant to Catheter Ablation

Atrial contours and dimensions are critical for designing appropriate catheters for successful, precise, and directed ablation lesions in order to treat atrial fibrillation.[30] Therefore a biatrial foam cast model obtained from 10 cadaver hearts was used for different measurements of potential lines in both atria as shown in Figure 1. The lines are connected at least to one anatomic area of block because we think it is important in vivo to avoid a macroreentrant circuit around the line of block. Interestingly, line number 3 in the right atrium, which is common flutter's ablation line, exhibited a wide range from 15 mm to 65 mm. The variability (expressed by the wide SD) of biatrial morphology and shape is impressive and represents a challenge for true linear catheter ablation in the atria.

From Singer I, Barold SS, Camm AJ (eds): Nonpharmacological Therapy of Arrhythmias for the 21st Century: The State of the Art. Futura Publishing Co, Inc., Armonk, NY, © 1998.

Anteroposterior view of right atrium (RA) and left atrium (LA)

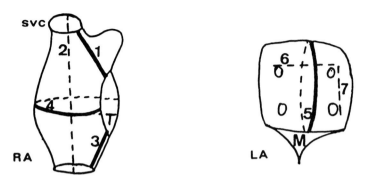

	Right atrium				Left atrium		
line	1	2	3	4	5	6	7
mean	44	54	32	147	139	43	38
SD	10	7	16	27	11	8	7
range	26-64	38-70	15-65	88-177	120-155	31-55	25-46

All values are in millimeters

Figure 1. Biatrial dimensions derived from 10 cadaver hearts. The extreme variability of biatrial morphology and shape (especially in the right atrium) is a challenge for true linear multi-electrode catheter ablation in the atria.

Mapping of Human Atrial Fibrillation

The mechanism of atrial fibrillation is thought to be multiple reentrant wavelets as initially hypothesized by Moe et al.[14] and confirmed later by Allessie et al.[15] Nevertheless, experimental data suggest that wavelets occurring during atrial fibrillation are homogeneously distributed in the atria. In order to address this hypothesis, we investigated the spatial and temporal distribution of complex electrical activity, defined as continuous electrical activity or electrograms with FF intervals less than 100 ms.[31] The duration of complex activity was assessed for 60 sec (expressed as a percentage of time) using a 14-pole catheter sequentially positioned in different regions. Twenty-five males and two females (mean age: 49 ± 11 years) suffering from paroxysmal atrial fibrillation for 5 ± 6.2 years, despite the use of a mean of 3.6 ± 1.7 antiarrhythmic drugs, were studied. With the exception of amiodarone, all antiarrhythmic

drugs were discontinued for five half-lives before the mapping study. The results illustrated in Figure 2 indicate that trabeculated regions (lateral and anterior) in the right atrium had less frequent complex electrograms than the smooth regions extending to the crista terminalis region (septum and intercaval segments) (Figure 3). In contrast, electrograms recorded from the majority of the left atrium were complex except near the appendage, also a trabeculated region. The band of atrial tissue bordering the mitral annulus (and the coronary sinus) was sometimes organized in contrast with the remainder of the left atrium. Whereas the proximal (septal coronary sinus) was usually fibrillating, its posterior and lateral distal parts could be organized despite fibrillating activity in the neighboring endocardial region, showing that regular coronary sinus activity is not a reliable indicator of left atrium activity. It is tempting to consider the most disorganized areas (the smooth parts of the atria) as preferential targets for catheter-based atrial fibrillation ab-

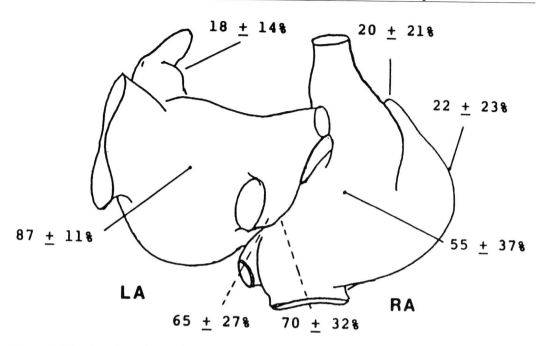

Figure 2. The duration of complex electrical activity (CEA) (either continuous electrograms or FF intervals <100 ms) assessed over 60 sec is expressed as a percentage (±SD). NB = CEA time of the septum has been assessed from the right and left sides.

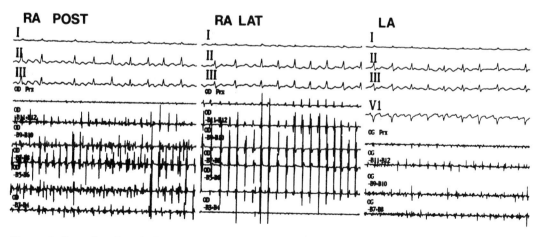

Figure 3. Complex electrical activity recorded from a multipolar catheter placed horizontally across the septum and posterior regions of the right atrium (RA post) and left atrium (lateral RA, and LA). While the electrograms in the lateral right atrium are clearly organized, the vast majority of the left atrium exhibits complex electrical activity with short FF intervals and intermittent continuous electrical activity. RA post = posterior right atrium; RA lat = lateral right atrium; LA = left atrium. Paper speed = 25 mm/sec.

lation. Such very short FF intervals were believed to be strongly associated with very short effective refractory periods (ERPs) or marked uncoupling.

In a recent study, Li et al. demonsrated that the most disorganized electrical activity with the shortest FF intervals exhibited in fact the longest refractory periods.[32] Whatever the respective contribution of the functional and anatomic determinants, we believe it is likely that the regions exhibiting the most temporally prevalent complex electrical activity are most arrhythmogenic and/or associated with the most pathologically affected tissues.[33] Some experimental studies support this concept.[32,34]

Experimental Studies

Different animal models of atrial fibrillation have been recently developed including creation of tricuspid or mitral regurgitation, sterile pericarditis, or chronic rapid atrial pacing mainly in the canine heart. In various dog models of atrial fibrillation, linear transmural atrial lesions produced mainly by endocardial RF current application have been shown to reduce the inducibility and duration of atrial fibrillation. The majority of these have been in the right

atrium and have been based on an anatomic approach. Thus, with few exceptions, none of these studies have used mapping data obtained during atrial fibrillation to guide placement of atrial lesions. The results of right atrial ablation in these models have been quite good with success rates varying from 57% to 100% (Table 1).[32,34–39] High success rates with relatively localized and directed ablation in the right atrium have also been reported. Tondo et al. described the efficiency of a single midseptal line[37] in normal dogs. In the sterile pericarditis model, Nakagawa et al.[38] from the same group performed successful ablation in the region of Bachmann's bundle after mapping data from Waldo's group suggested that about half of reentrant wavelets traversed this area.[38] Nevertheless, one can argue that if Bachmann's bundle ablation can be effective, the consequences for interatrial conduction can also be deleterious. As alluded to earlier Li et al.[32] used two different canine models of atrial fibrillation and described definite spatial patterns of atrial electrogram heterogeneity, a finding also reported in humans.[31] They showed that linear right atrial ablation in the posterior intercaval right atrium (which was shown to have mainly disorganized electrograms

Table 1
Summary of Experimental Results Using Energy Applications to Prevent Induction
of Sustained Atrial Fibrillation

Study	Model of AF	Target Site(s)	Success
Avitall et al.[35]	Sterile pericarditis	RA:SVC to IVC	6/6 (100%)
		SVC-to tricuspid valve	
Elvan et al.[36]	Vagal stimulation	RA + LA + coronary sinus	23/23 (100%)*
Li et al.[32]	Sterile pericarditis	RA:SVC to IVC	4/7 (57%)
	Chronic rapid pacing	RA:SVC to IVC	1/6 (17%)
Tondo et al.[37]	Normal dogs	Right atrial septum	8/9 (89%)
Nakagawa et al.[38]	Sterile pericarditis	Bachman's bundle	8/9 (89%)
Morillo et al.[34]	Chronic rapid pacing	Left atrial posterior wall	9/11 (82%)
Haines et al.[39]	Mitral regurgitation	RA	0/7 (0%)
		LA	4/7 (57%)

N.B. = definition of noninducibility and success varies in the different studies.

* At low-level vagal stimulation.

AF = atrial fibrillation; IVC = inferior vena cava; LA = left atrium; RA = right atrium; SVC = superior vena cava.

but the longest ERP) abolished or greatly attenuated the duration of induced atrial fibrillation. Right atrial ablation rendered atrial fibrillation noninducible in 4 of 7 dogs (57%) with sterile pericarditis versus 1 of 6 dogs (17%) of the rapid pacing model. Also, Morillo et al. terminated atrial fibrillation in the rapid pacing model by cryosurgical applications confined to the left posterior atrium[34] where the shortest atrial fibrillation cycle length was recorded. In the mitral regurgitation model, Haines et al.[39] observed that successful ablation was only achieved by left atrial lines.

Some of the previous results support the concept of using electrophysiological data to guide atrial ablation in contrast to the surgical strategy used for the maze procedure. Other studies indicate the possible role of the atrial fibrillation model in determining the efficacy of ablation depending on the targeted atrium. Ablation in the right atrium seems sufficient in either normal dogs or those with sterile pericarditis. Ablation in the left atrium seems to be required in the rapid pacing and mitral regurgitation models.

One relatively consistently described feature has been the "proarrhythmic" effects of certain locations and kinds of lesions resulting in the induction of "new" atrial flutters. Avitall et al. found that discontinuous lesions were as frequently associated with this phenomenon as full linear lesions[40]; also linear intercaval lesions have been found to stabilize and prolong macroreentrant right atrial flutter.[32] One significant limitation of animal models is the small size of the atria, rendering induction of fibrillation more difficult and more importantly making termination easier (i.e., with smaller lesions), and therefore hampering extrapolation to the clinical context. Also, there is no currently available in vivo model with a reproducible and spontaneous initiation of atrial fibrillation to allow study of triggering events. Nevertheless, Fenelon et al.[41] recently reported a dog model of heart failure (produced by rapid ventricular pacing) with atrial arrhythmias due to a focal source

from the right atrium as well as the pulmonary veins. This very preliminary work needs further confirmation.

Various technical means of achieving linear transmural continuous lesions have been explored in different laboratories. Two main approaches to endocardial catheter ablation of atrial fibrillation are being pursued: either the catheter drag technique with or without a guiding sheath, or the use of multi-electrode catheters. Different configurations of multiple closely spaced ring electrodes, coils, ribbons, and balloons are under investigation for this purpose, some with additional features such as saline irrigation, or simultaneous multi-electrode energy delivery.[36,38,39,42] Whatever the technique, the following steps are required to create and ensure complete linear lesions: (1) positioning the catheter at desired locations; (2) ensuring adequate tissue contact all along the electrode surfaces; (3) delivering enough energy (with temperature control) to create lesion continuity and transmurality without formation of thrombi/char; and (4) verifying linear conduction block. Some authors have suggested the possibility of assessing placement, tissue contact, and lesion size using intracardiac echo guidance.[43] Also the in vivo assessment of the achieved lesions in terms of continuity and transmurality has involved correlation with electrogram changes (amplitude and dv/dt), pacing thresholds and altered activation sequences as well as altered echo characteristics. We found that the simple recording of electrograms along the line after ablation (with orthogonal spontaneous/paced atrial activation) is reliable in predicting linear block in the presence of double potentials separated by isoelectric interval. A gap on the line is indicated by a local single or a continuous electrogram straddling the isoelectric interval of adjacent double potentials.[21,44,45]

A number of techniques include an irrigation system that cools the distal tip to minimize the risk of coagulum both on the electrode and on the endocardium, thus allowing higher power delivery. We assessed the efficacy and safety of a dragging technique with high power delivered through an irrigated tip catheter in 10 anesthetized animals (4 dogs, 6 sheep). RF current was applied during sinus rhythm to create a continuous line using a 4-mm tip (Sprinklr, Medtronic Inc.) ablation catheter. A *single passage* was performed point by point along a predetermined course (50 W at each point with four incremental steps of RF durations). The catheter was withdrawn a small distance under fluoroscopy after each application in order to ensure lesion continuity. Ten lines were performed in the right atrium and six in the left atrium after transseptal catheterization. A mean of 10 ± 3 RF applications lasting 20 sec (4 lines), 40 sec (6), 60 sec (3), and 90 sec (3) were delivered. Most lesions were transmural in the free wall with little endocardial alteration. One septal lesion extended nontransmurally into the ascending aorta. No line was fully continuous and the lesions varied from multiple discrete punctate ones to large and discontinuous linear segments up to 3 cm in length. Four pops (3%) were recorded (the catheter was noted to be entrapped), all after 40 sec or more of RF application. No coagulum was found except in three trabeculated sites (2%). Three endocardial craters were noted only at sites where pops occurred. Acute macroscopic examination of the heart showed there was no hemopericardium attributable to RF.

Therefore, high RF energies delivered through an irrigated 4-mm tip catheter are relatively safe on acute evaluation with a low incidence of coagulum formation. However, a single drag line is unable to create a linear lesion and several passages (and/or an additional sheath) seem to be required to create a continuous transmural line.

right atrial flutter resistant to conventional ablation in the inferior vena cava-tricuspid annulus isthmus. For this study, we define resistant flutter as the inability to achieve complete bidirectional isthmus block after more than 21 (i.e., our mean + 2 SD RF applications) conventional 4-mm tip temperature-controlled, sequential applications of 90 sec (target temperature = 70°, maximal achievable power = 70 W). Four patients (age: 51 ± 9 years) with symptomatic and drug-resistant atrial flutter (at least four antiarrhythmic drugs unsuccessfully tried) have been studied so far. The ablations were performed in flutter (n = 3) or during low lateral right atrial pacing using an irrigated tip catheter (Sprinklr) with a flow rate of 17 cc/min. RF current was applied using a Stockert (Cordis) generator in the temperature mode with a maximal temperature setting of 50° and a maximal power limit of 50 W for 40 sec at each point. This protocol was demonstrated to be safe in previous animal experiments. The inferior vena cava-tricuspid annulus isthmus was targeted and the mean achieved temperature at this flow rate was actually 40°C whereas the temperature of 50°C was occasionally reached. The procedure was successful in all patients. In two of these cases, a single application of RF (40–50 W achieved power) was successful at the identical sites where conventional temperature-guided RF applications with a 4-mm tip electrode catheter (target 70°C) had failed.

Complete bidirectional isthmus block was achieved in all patients without any complication. To date there has been no recurrence. Moderately high RF energies delivered with an irrigated tip catheter using this protocol seem to be safe and may be particularly useful in ablation of resistant flutter.

Use of Irrigated Tip in Resistant Flutter

We are investigating the use of an irrigated tip catheter in patients with common

Role of Arrhythmogenic Foci

Typically atrial fibrillation is believed to result from the simultaneous existence of multiple migratory reentrant wavefronts of activation in both atria. A focal mechanism is thus considered to be very unlikely on the basis of experimental studies and surgical human mapping data.[14–18] However, we observed that a focal mechanism was critical for some patients with paroxysmal atrial fibrillation.

Focal Atrial Fibrillation

We have described a small and uncommon group of patients who have the surface ECG features of atrial fibrillation, not due to random reentry but to a single rapidly discharging focus.[46] Our series now includes 15 patients for whom atrial fibrillation has been cured by discrete RF ablation of the focus. All patients (39 ± 8) were suffering from daily resistant atrial fibrillation (multiple daily bouts of varying duration in some patients) (Figure 4) since a mean of 9 ± 7 years.

The ablation site was determined on the basis of earliest bipolar activity relative to a stable atrial electrogram reference during atrial fibrillation. If the rate was slow enough to allow P wave identification on the surface ECG, the earliest bipolar activity was relative to the P wave onset. Mapping during different types of atrial arrhythmias showed that they were due to the same focus firing irregularly (Figure 5). Most of the patients also had isolated extrasystoles that exhibited the same activation pattern as tachycardias. Long cycle lengths were responsible for the organized monomorphic tachycardia or focal flutter (Figure 6) whereas at short cycle lengths (between 160 and 130 ms), an ECG pattern of atrial fibrillation was observed. In order to facilitate mapping and ablation of the arrhythmia, flecainide infusion (0.5–1 mg/kg) was used in three patients. In most patients, the atrial activity during atrial fibrillation was organized (suggesting type I atrial fibrillation). Four foci were found to be located in the right atrium: two near the sinus node, one at the ostium of the coronary sinus, and one in the right appendage. Others were located in the left atrium, at the ostium of the right superior pulmonary vein (6) or right infe-

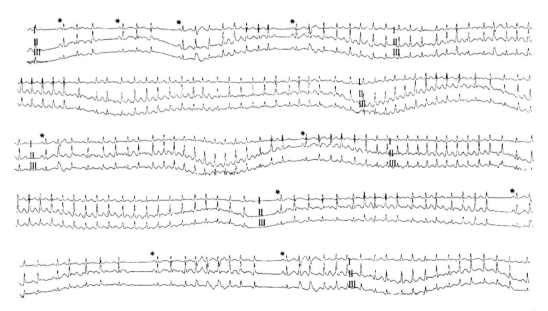

Figure 4. Continuous recording of three surface ECG leads (I, II, III) with multiple initiations of various atrial arrhythmias with isolated intervening sinus beats (asterisk). The atrial arrhythmias range from salves of extrasystoles to flutter and fibrillation. Such behavior is characteristic and must suggest a focal source. Paper speed = 25 mm/sec.

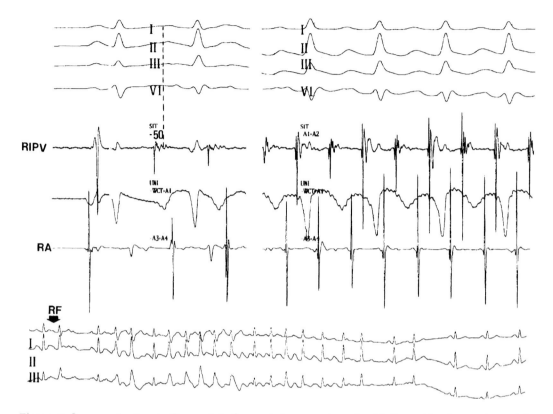

Figure 5. Same patient as in Figure 4. Left panel shows a sinus beat followed by two extrasystoles originating from the right inferior pulmonary vein (RIPV) local bipolar activity precedes the extrasystolic P wave by 50 ms. Note the characteristic P on T ECG pattern. The activation sequence during a focal tachycardia (right panel) is similar to that observed on the left panel. Bottom: RF delivery during arrhythmia which is promptly interrupted with restoration of sinus rhythm. Paper speed = 100 mm/sec.

rior pulmonary vein (3) and at the ostium of the left superior pulmonary vein (3). One patient had two foci (right superior pulmonary vein and right inferior pulmonary vein). All patients were treated with a mean of 4 ± 4 RF pulses, three patients had a clinically documented recurrence 7 days (two patients) and 20 days (one patient) after an initially successful procedure. Two of them underwent a definitively successful second ablation procedure. The third patient had in fact only one episode of arrhythmia which never recurred with a follow-up of 6 months without any antiarrhythmic drug.

All of these patients have a distinctive clinical profile: they are young of either sex, and without structural heart disease. They usually have very frequent episodes of intermittent atrial fibrillation along with epi-

sodes of an irregular atrial tachycardia and monomorphic atrial extrasystoles with contours similar to the P wave during tachycardia. This observation must lead to an early electrophysiological study at the time of spontaneous episodes of tachycardia, thereby allowing mapping and successful ablation of the focus.

Arrhythmogenic Foci Identified after Linear Radiofrequency Ablation of Common Atrial Fibrillation

In patients undergoing linear ablation for common paroxysmal atrial fibrillation, the organization of atrial activity shortened or prevented episodes of atrial fibrillation, allowing the unmasking of foci of extrasystolic activity which were triggers of episodes of atrial fibrillation before ablation. These foci manifest as isolated runs of extrasystoles or trigger bouts of atrial fibrillation. They are identified in at least 40% of patients. This was not evident before the procedure because of continuing and long-lasting paroxysmal atrial fibrillation. This figure may be an overestimate because of the selection of patients with repetitive episodes of atrial fibrillation, but on the other hand, additional patients may have had similar foci manifesting only infrequently. These foci acted as a prominent trigger of paroxysmal atrial fibrillation but such discharges occurring during atrial fibrillation may also contribute to the maintenance of fibrillation. They required organization of the atrial activity by ablation lines to be recognized and mapped. In most cases, they originate from the pulmonary veins (but a few cases have been identified in the right atrium). In the pulmonary veins, the focus could be tracked from its source inside the veins to its atrial exit and shown to have a long conduction time. These foci probably originate from atrial muscular bundles extending up to 5 cm inside the pulmonary veins. In most cases, those bundles are identified during sinus rhythm by a spike potential following the nearfield atrial activity. During extrasystoles, or in some cases, focal flutter, the sequence is inverted and the spike potential originating from the venous bundle precedes the nearfield atrial activity by up to 180 ms. Successful ablation of the focus is usually associated with disappearance of the spike potential in sinus rhythm (Figure 7). Ablation of these foci is predictive of a successful clinical outcome. The present results contrast with surgical mapping studies performed both in experimental animals and in humans. This is probably due to the fact that mapping studies are mostly epicardial and usually limited to the anterolateral free wall of right and left atrium whereas most of the foci are located

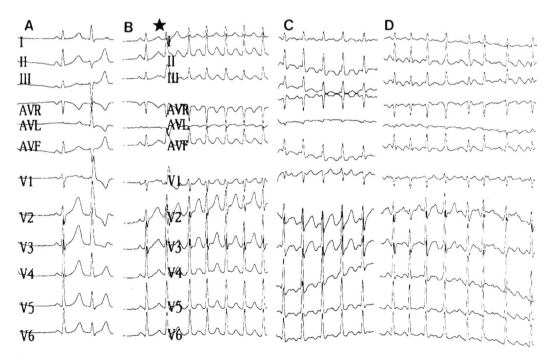

Figure 6. Twelve-lead surface ECG recordings of the same patient as in Figures 4 and 5. **A:** Isolated extrasystole (P on T pattern) with contours similar as the tachycardia initiating beat in panel B. **B** and **C:** Two recordings of flutter like ECGs due in fact to the same focal source. **D:** A tachycardia with a faster, irregular, and pleomorphic surface ECG pattern, close to atrial fibrillation.

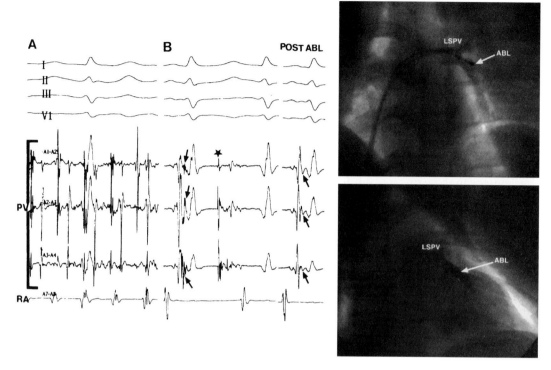

Figure 7. A: Tracings recorded from a quadripolar ablation catheter placed deep inside the left superior pulmonary vein (LSPV) as shown in the angiogram (top = AP view; bottom = LAO 60°). During a bout of arrhythmia, the local activity is rapid and irregular (recordings of bipoles 1–2, 2–3, 3–4 in the pulmonary veins of the ablation catheter, PV). **B**: In sinus rhythm, a spike (arrows) follows the nearfield atrial electrogram. This sequence is inverted during a focal extrasystole originating from the LSPV (asterisk). Post-abl = disappearance of the spike potential after successful ablation (arrows) resulting in complete abolition of atrial arrhythmias. Paper speed = 100 mm/sec.

posteriorly, septally, and near the ostia of great vessels. Moreover, the maps are usually performed during ongoing atrial fibrillation and not at initiation; the time windows used for mapping being probably too short to record this very intermittent phenomenon. Finally, animal models of atrial fibrillation may not be relevant to human pathology. Nevertheless, a recent dog atrial fibrillation model due to high-rate ventricular pacing has been reported. Foci originating from pulmonary veins were demonstrated and successfully ablated.[41]

Atrial Fibrillation Ablation Using Linear Lesions

Two case reports in 1994 demonstrated the feasibility of catheter ablation of atrial

fibrillation in humans. Lesions restricted to the right atrium were successful for a patient with paroxysmal atrial fibrillation[19] using a multi-electrode catheter, whereas in the other report, the catheter-based biatrial maze procedure was performed in a patient with chronic atrial fibrillation.[20] We therefore began a study to assess the efficacy of ablation limited to the right atrium in 45 patients with daily paroxysmal atrial fibrillation.[21] Three groups of 15 patients each underwent increasingly complex lesion patterns in the right atrium. Ablation led to stable sinus rhythm during the procedure in 18 patients (40%) but atrial fibrillation noninducibility using burst pacing was achieved in only five patients (11%). Final success rates with all three types of lesion patterns were similar: 13% without drug increasing to 40% in combination with antiarrhythmic drug therapy. A new typical atrial flutter was observed in 70% of cases after linear ablation in the right atrium requiring subsequent ablation sessions targeting the inferior vena cava tricuspid annulus. No factor predictive of success using right atrial lines was recognized. In view of this unimpressive success rate, the combination of two right atrial lines (one septal and one cavo-tricuspidian) and three to four left atrial lines performed through a transseptal access were performed, initially in 10 patients, with significantly improved results (Figure 8). All lines were connected to anatomic structure except in the roof to avoid isolation of the posterior left atrium. In a total series of 38 patients to date, stable sinus rhythm was obtained in 35 and sustained atrial fibrillation was rendered noninducible in 75% at the end of the session. For the last resistant cases, we

have used an irrigated tip ablation catheter (Sprinklr) to perform the procedure using the protocol (i.e., target temperature = 50°, power limit = 50 W, static ablation duration = 40 sec). This preliminary experience suggests this protocol was found to be as effective as the regular procedure and decreases by 40% the procedure and fluoroscopic duration without any adverse changes in the side effect profile. The use of electrode irrigation during RF delivery may spare the endocardium and avoid char, thus reducing the potential for embolic events.

At least two ablation sessions were required in most cases (75%) to treat arrhythmogenic foci or new left atrial flutters.[45] Left atrial flutters were defined by activation sequence mapping of both atria and the coronary sinus and the response to resetting. A site with a post-pacing interval within 10 ms of the tachycardia cycle

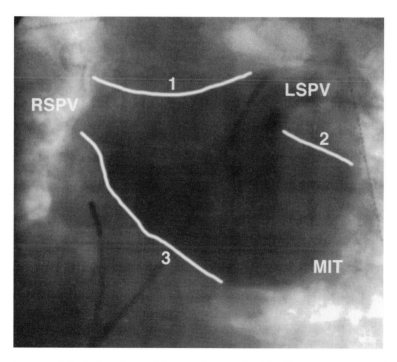

Figure 8. Angiogram of the left atrium with superimposed white lines representing the three linear RF lesions. Line 1 is connecting the right superior pulmonary vein (RSPV) to the left superior pulmonary vein (LSPV). Lines 2 and 3 are joining the superior pulmonary veins to the mitral annulus (Mit). Note that line 3 is clearly longer than line 2. In some cases, the RSPV is connected to the left aspect of the fossa ovalis. This left atrial ablation schema is performed together with a right septal line joining superior vena cava to inferior vena cava and a cavotricuspid line.

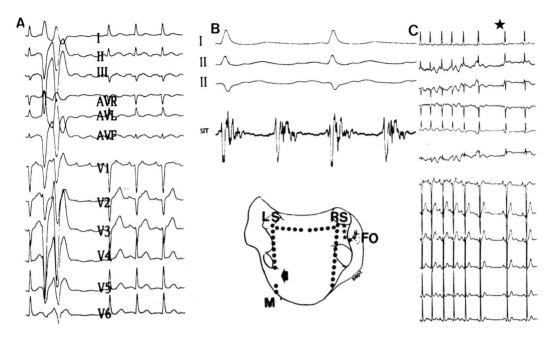

Figure 9. Twelve-lead surface ECG of atypical left flutter (**A**) occurring after biatrial linear RF ablation for atrial fibrillation. This flutter was found to propagate through a gap (arrow) in the left superior pulmonary vein (LS) to mitral (M) line. **B:** The ablation site (sit) exhibits a fractionated and long duration electrograms straddling the interval of double potentials recorded above and below the gap. RF ablation (**C**) delivered at this site interrupted the flutter (star). RS = right superior pulmonary vein; FO = fossa ovalis.

length was considered a part of the circuit. In all sites in the right atrial free wall, the post-pacing interval was more than 40 ms outside the tachycardia cycle length. During sustained left atrial flutter, the linear lesion produced by previous ablation was located by the presence of relatively widely separated double potentials and the line was traced from one end to the other. We looked for a single atrial electrogram or long duration fractionated potentials, bridging the double potentials recorded a few millimeters away on the line. Such activity was attributed to a gap in the line. This suggests the presence of incompletely ablated or recovered functional myocardium. Flutters were usually found to revolve around the pulmonary veins and/or in the septum. In all cases, they were found to propagate through the previous ablation lines. Gaps were encountered in each of the four left atrial lines but more frequently in the right superior pulmonary vein-mi-

tral line, which is the longest. All flutters were interrupted by filling in these gaps using RF (Figure 9). The high incidence of left atrial flutters indicates that significant improvements in catheter design are required to optimize lesion characteristics to prevent these flutters.

Conclusion

Curative catheter ablation of atrial fibrillation is feasible and successful, particularly when a focal mechanism for atrial fibrillation is identified or when linear ablations are performed in the left atrium. However, the procedures are prolonged and it is difficult with current technology to consistently achieve a linear conduction block. The challenge remains to perfect, optimize, and facilitate this still investigational technique and transform it into a routine procedure.

References

1. Feinberg WM, Blackshear JL, Laupacis A, et al. Prevalence, age distribution, and gender of patients with atrial fibrillation: analysis and implications. Arch Intern Med 1995;155: 469–473.

2. Wolf PA, Abbott RD, Kannel WB. Atrial fibrillation: a major contributor to stroke in the elderly: the Framingham Study. Arch Intern Med 1987;147:1561–1564.

3. Scheinman MM, Morady F, Hess DS, et al. Catheter-induced ablation of atrioventricular junction to control refractory supraventricular arrhythmias. JAMA 1982;248: 855–861.

4. Gallagher JJ, Svenson RH, Kasell JH, et al. Catheter technique for closed chest ablation of the atrioventricular conduction system: a therapeutic alternative for the treatment of refractory supraventricular tachycardia. N Engl J Med 1982;306:194–200.

5. Langberg JJ, Chin M, Schamp DJ, et al. Ablation of the atrioventricular junction with radiofrequency current energy using a new electrode catheter. Am J Cardiol 1991;67: 142–147.

6. Huang SK, Bharati S, Graham AR, et al. Closed chest catheter dessication of the atrioventricular junction using radiofrequency energy: a new method of catheter ablation. J Am Coll Cardiol 1987;9:349–358.

7. Williamson BD, Man KC, Daoud E, et al. Radiofrequency catheter modification of atrioventricular conduction to control the ventricular rate during atrial fibrillation. N Engl J Med 1994;331:910–917.

8. Williams JM, Ungerleider RM, Lofland GK, et al. Left atrial isolation: a new technique for the treatment of supraventricular arrhythmias. J Thorac Cardiovasc Surg 1980; 80:373–380.

9. Cox JL, Canavan TE, Schuessler RB, et al. The surgical treatment of atrial fibrillation II: Intraoperative electrophysiologic mapping and description of the electrophysiologic basis of atrial flutter and fibrillation. J Thorac Cardiovasc Surg 1991;101:406–426.

10. Cox JL, Boineau JP, Schuessler RB, et al. Five year experience with the Maze procedure for atrial fibrillation. Ann Thorac Surg 1993;56: 814–824.

11. Defauw JJ, Guiraudon GM, Van Hemel NM, et al. Surgical therapy of paroxysmal atrial fibrillation with the corridor operation. Ann Thorac Surg 1992;53:564–571.

12. Shyu KG, Cheng JJ, Chen JJ, et al. Recovery of atrial function after atrial compartment operation for chronic atrial fibrillation in mitral valve disease. J Am Coll Cardiol 1994; 24:392–398.

13. Kosakai Y, Kawaguchi AT, Isobe F, et al. Modified Maze procedure for patients with atrial fibrillation undergoing simultaneous open heart surgery. Circulation 1995;92:II-359–364.

14. Moe GK, Rheinboldt WC, Abildskov JA. A computer model of atrial fibrillation. Am Heart J 1964;14:200–220.

15. Allessie MA, Lammers WJEP, Bonke FIM, et al. Experimental evaluation of Moes' multiple wavelet hypothesis of atrial fibrillation. In Zipes DP, Jalife J, eds. Cardiac Electrophysiology and Arrhythmias. Orlando, FL, Grune & Stratton, 1985, pp 265–276.

16. Cox JL, Canavan TE, Scheussler RB, et al. The surgical treatment of atrial fibrillation: intraoperative mapping and description of the electrophysiologic basis of atrial flutter and atrial fibrillation. J Thorac Cardiovasc Surg 1991;101:402–426.

17. Konings KTS, Kirchhof CJHJ, Smeets JRLM, et al. High density mapping of electrically induced atrial fibrillation in humans. Circulation 1994;89:1665–1680.

18. Misier ARR, Opthof T, Van Hemel NM, et al. Increased dispersion of refractoriness in patients with idiopathic paroxysmal atrial fibrillation. J Am Coll Cardiol 1992;19: 1531–1535.

19. Haïssaguerre M, Gencel L, Fischer B, et al. Successful catheter ablation of atrial fibrillation. J Cardiovasc Electrophysiol 1994;5: 1045–1052.

20. Swartz JF, Pellersels G, Silvers J, et al. A catheter-based curative approach to atrial fibrillation in humans. Circulation 1994;90:I-335.

21. Haïssaguerre M, Jaïs P, Shah DC, et al. Right and left atrial radiofrequency catheter therapy of paroxysmal atrial fibrillation. J Cardiovasc Electrophysiol 1996;12:1132–1144.

22. Ching Man K, Daoud E, Knight B, et al. Right atrial-radiofrequency catheter ablation of paroxysmal atrial fibrillation. J Am Coll Cardiol 1996;26:188A.

23. Natale A, Tomassoni G, Kearney MM, et al. Catheter ablation approach on the right side only for paroxysmal atrial fibrillation therapy. Circulation 1996;92:I-266.

24. Cosio FG, Lopez-Gil M, Goicolea A, et al. Radiofrequency ablation of the inferior vena cava-tricuspid valve isthmus in common atrial flutter. Am J Cardiol 1993;71:705–709.

25. Lesh MD, Van Hare GF, Epstein LM, et al. Radiofrequency catheter ablation of atrial ar-

rhythmias: results and mechanisms. Circulation 1994;89:1074–1089.

26. Scheinman MM, Olgin J. Catheter ablation of cardiac arrhythmias of atrial origin. In Zipes DP, ed. Catheter Ablation of Arrhythmias. Armonk, NY, Futura Publishing Company Inc., 1994, pp 129–149.

27. Fischer B, Haïssaguerre M, Garrigues S, et al. Radiofrequency catheter ablation of common atrial flutter in 80 patients. J Am Coll Cardiol 1995;25:1365–1372.

28. Fischer B, Jaïs P, Cauchemez B, et al. Double potentials recorded in the cavo-tricuspid isthmus with radiofrequency applications in human atrial flutter. NASPE 1996;19:648 [Abstract].

29. Cauchemez B, Haïssaguerre M, Fischer B, et al. Electrophysiological effects of catheter ablation of inferior vena cava-tricuspid annulus isthmus in common atrial flutter. Circulation 1996;93:284–294.

30. Jaïs P, Coste P, Shah DC, et al. Biatrial dimensions relevant to catheter ablation [Abstract]. Eur JCPE 1996;6(1):87.

31. Jaïs P, Haïssaguerre M, Shah DC, et al. Regional disparities of endocardial atrial activation in paroxysmal atrial fibrillation. PACE 1996;19(pt II):1998–2003.

32. Li H, Hare J, Mughal K, et al. Distribution of atrial electrogram types during atrial fibrillation: effect of rapid atrial pacing and intercaval junction ablation. JACC 1996;27:1713–1721.

33. Avitall B, Hartz R, Bharati S, et al. The correlation of local histology with fractionated local electrical activity during atrial fibrillation in patients undergoing the Maze procedure and mitral valve replacement [Abstract]. PACE 1996;19(Pt II):725.

34. Morillo CA, Klein GJ, Jones DL, et al. Chronic rapid atrial pacing: structural, functional and electrophysiologic characteristics of a new model of sustained atrial fibrillation. Circulation 1995;91:1588–1595.

35. Avitall B, Hare J, Mughal K, et al. Ablation of atrial fibrillation in a dog model. J Am Coll Cardiol 1994;484:276A.

36. Elvan A, Pride HP, Eble JN, et al. Radiofrequency catheter ablation of the atria reduces inducibility and duration of atrial fibrillation in dogs. Circulation 1995;91:2235–2244.

37. Tondo C, Otomo K, Antz M, et al. Successful radiofrequency catheter ablation of atrial fibrillation by a single lesion to the inter-atrial septum. Circulation 1995;92(8):I-265.

38. Nakagawa H, Kumagai K, Imai S, et al. Catheter ablation of Bachmann's bundle from the right atrium eliminates atrial fibrillation in a canine sterile pericarditis model. PACE 1996;19:581A.

39. Haines DE, McRury IA. Primary atrial fibrillation ablation (PAFA) in a chronic atrial fibrillation model. Circulation 1995;92:I-265.

40. Avitall B, Helms RW, Chiang W, et al. Nonlinear atrial radiofrequency lesions are arrhythmogenic: a study of skipped lesions in the normal atria. Circulation 1995;92:I-265.

41. Fenelon G, Shepard RK, Turner A, et al. Evidence of a focal origin as the mechanism of atrial tachycardia in dogs with ventricular pacing-induced congestive heart failure. PACE 1997;20(Pt II):1095.

42. Mackey S, Thornton L, He DS, et al. Simultaneous multipolar radiofrequency ablation in the monopolar mode increases lesion size. PACE 1996;19:1042–1048.

43. Olgin J, Kalman JM, Maguire M, et al. Electrophysiologic effects of long linear atrial lesions placed under intracardiac echo guidance. PACE 1996;19:581–583.

44. Shah DC, Haïssaguerre M, Jaïs P, et al. Directed catheter ablation of recurrent common atrial flutter. Circulation 1997;96:2505–2508.

45. Jaïs P, Haïssaguerre M, Shah DC, et al. Catheter therapy of multiple left atrial flutters following atrial fibrillation ablation. PACE 1997;20(Pt II):1181.

46. Jaïs P, Haïssagerre M, Shah DC, et al. A focal source of atrial fibrillation treated by discrete radiofrequency ablation. Circulation 1997;95:572–576.

Chapter 11

Ablation of Idiopathic Left Ventricular Tachycardia and Right Ventricular Outflow Tract Tachycardia

William M. Miles, Jeffrey E. Olgin

Introduction

Ventricular tachycardia (VT) is most commonly associated with coronary artery disease. The efficacy of radiofrequency (RF) ablation for VT associated with coronary artery disease has been limited by several factors: (1) difficulty in the RF energy penetrating scarred endocardium or clot; (2) intramyocardial or epicardial origin of VT; (3) difficulty identifying an appropriate ablation site to eliminate the complex VT circuit; (4) the existence of multiple VT morphologies and/or sites in a single patient; (5) the hemodynamic instability of VT in many patients precluding adequate mapping; and (6) the progressive nature of the underlying disease leading to the emergence of new VTs over time. Therefore, although ablation techniques continue to improve, ablation is usually not considered a first-line therapy in patients with VT due to coronary artery disease[1-4]; antiarrhythmic drug therapy or implantable cardioverter-defibrillator (ICD) therapy is more commonly used. In contrast, VT in patients with no apparent structural heart disease (idiopathic VT),[5-8] although not as frequently encountered as VT in patients with coronary artery disease,

can be eliminated by RF ablation in a high percentage of patients[9,10] (Table 1). In idiopathic VT, the limitations listed above are absent; these tachycardias are usually uniform, hemodynamically stable, focal in origin, and there is no underlying cardiac pathology to interfere with delivery of ablation energy to the site of VT origin. Thus, ablation may be considered a potential first-line therapy for patients with symptomatic idiopathic VT. The only other VT for which ablation is considered a first-line therapy is bundle branch reentrant VT.[11,12] This VT usually occurs in the setting of significant myocardial disease but is characterized by a well-defined macroreentrant circuit involving the bundle branches and intervening myocardium. Once the diagnosis is established and the macroreentrant circuit defined, it is relatively easy to ablate a bundle branch to eliminate the arrhythmia, although patient survival is limited by the underlying myocardial pathology.

Characteristics of Idiopathic Ventricular Tachycardia

Idiopathic VT[5-8] accounts for up to 10% of patients referred to specialized electro-

From Singer I, Barold SS, Camm AJ (eds): Nonpharmacological Therapy of Arrhythmias for the 21st Century: The State of the Art. Futura Publishing Co, Inc., Armonk, NY, © 1998.

Table 1
Catheter Ablation for Ventricular
Tachyarrhythmias (VT)

Arrhythmia	Ablation Efficacy
Idiopathic VT	+ + +
Bundle branch reentry	+ + +
Sustained VT (incessant)	+ +
Sustained VT (inducible/stable)	+
Sustained VT (unstable)	−
Polymorphic VT	−
Ventricular fibrillation	−

+ + + = consider as first-line therapy.
+ + = reasonable success if drugs fail.
+ = acceptable therapy for particularly refractory or recurrent cases.
− = catheter ablation not indicated.

physiology centers. Related, but not synonymous, terms include right ventricular tachycardia, repetitive monomorphic VT, catecholamine-sensitive VT, exercise-induced VT, adenosine-sensitive VT, and verapamil-sensitive VT. Buxton et al.[13] reported that 27% of their patients with idiopathic VT were asymptomatic, 40% presented with palpitations, 43% dizziness, and 23% syncope. Cardiac arrest has been reported but is rare. Because of incomplete understanding of tachycardia mechanisms, a universally accepted classification of these tachycardias has not yet been developed. The VT may be classified by the clinical pattern such as repetitive monomorphic VT (multiple episodes of mostly nonsustained and self-terminating VT interrupted by occasional sinus beats) or paroxysmal sustained VT (episodes of sustained VT separated by periods of sinus rhythm). The site of VT origin can be used for classification; 70% of cases arise from the right ventricle (mostly the right ventricular outflow tract) and have a QRS morphology resembling a left bundle branch block. Idiopathic VT arising from the left ventricle has a right bundle branch block QRS morphology. In addition, idiopathic VT may be classified by its response to pharmacological or physiological manipulations including exercise, cate-

cholamines, verapamil, and adenosine. Potential mechanisms include reentry, abnormal automaticity, and triggered activity due to afterdepolarizations. Abnormalities of autonomic innervation have been reported[14]: in nine patients with a structurally normal heart and VT, five patients (55%) had regional left ventricular sympathetic denervation demonstrated with ^{123}I-MIBG scintigraphy, compared with zero of nine control patients with a structurally normal heart ($P = 0.029$). Five patients underwent right ventricular RF ablation of VT, and sympathetic denervation was adjacent to the ablation site in one of these patients. The role of regional cardiac sympathetic denervation in arrhythmogenesis remains to be determined, but could be related to the frequent provocation of idiopathic VT by exercise or catecholamines. Of interest, regional abnormalities of left ventricular sympathetic innervation have been reported in 83% of patients with arrhythmogenic right ventricular dysplasia.[15]

Patient evaluation including physical examination, ECG, and echocardiogram are normal. In selected patients, left and right ventriculography, coronary angiography, magnetic resonance imaging, and endomyocardial biopsy may be performed to exclude structural heart disease. Carlson et al.[16] have reported right ventricular abnormalities in 21 of 22 patients with right ventricular outflow VT using cine magnetic resonance imaging. These abnormalities included fixed focal wall thinning, excavation, and decreased systolic thickening localized to the right ventricular outflow tract. Echocardiography showed abnormalities in only two of 21 patients.

Repetitive monomorphic VT[17,18] generally occurs in young or middle-aged patients. These patients may present with dizziness or (rarely) syncope but are frequently asymptomatic. The arrhythmias are often associated with physical or emotional stress, but exercise may suppress the arrhythmia in some patients. ECG features include repetitive runs of nonsustained VT interspersed with sinus rhythm (Figure 1).

There are usually frequent premature ventricular contractions (PVCs) and couplets. Ventricular tachycardia usually has the morphology of a left bundle branch block with a normal or right axis (right ventricular outflow tract VT). These patients usually do not have inducible VT with programmed ventricular stimulation.

Patients with paroxysmal sustained monomorphic VT[19] present with symptoms similar to repetitive monomorphic VT, but in the former group VT tends to be episodic and sustained and therefore more symptomatic. This type of VT is more often inducible with programmed stimulation, often during isoproterenol infusion. Lerman et al.[19] demonstrated that these patients frequently have VT initiated and terminated by programmed stimulation; VT induction is often facilitated by isoproterenol (Figure 2); VT can be terminated with adenosine (Figure 3), verapamil, the Valsalva maneuver, or carotid massage; beta blockade either terminates VT or prevents VT induction in these patients. The mechanism is therefore felt to be cyclic AMP-mediated

triggered activity. The prognosis is generally good for these patients, but they may occasionally have syncope, and rare deaths have been reported.

Patients with idiopathic left ventricular tachycardia[20-26] are generally young and usually symptomatic with sustained VT. Ventricular tachycardia has the morphology of a right bundle branch block with a leftward axis (Figure 4) and is usually inducible with programmed ventricular stimulation. The origin of the VT is usually at the inferior left ventricular midseptum or apex in the region of the posterior fascicle, although occasionally it may originate from the anterior septum and have a rightward axis.[27,28] Ventricular tachycardia is unresponsive to beta blockers or adenosine but frequently responds to verapamil. The prognosis is generally good, but these patients may be highly symptomatic. Syncope may occur and, again, rare sudden deaths have been reported. Although the mechanism of this tachycardia may not always be uniform, investigators have found that idiopathic left ventricular tachycardia can be

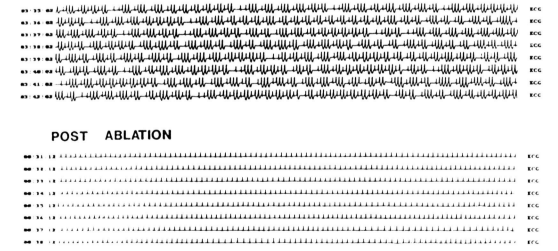

Figure 1. Tracings from a patient with no structural heart disease who presented with repetitive monomorphic VT. The spontaneous arrhythmia (top tracing) is illustrated prior to ablation. After ablation (bottom tracing) all spontaneous ventricular arrhythmia was eliminated. Reproduced with permission from Klein LS, et al.[10]

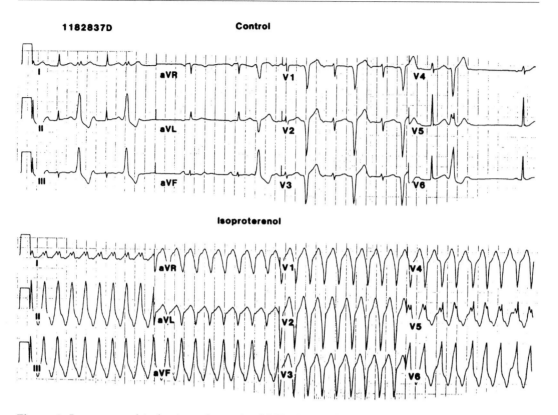

Figure 2. Isoproterenol induction of sustained VT. Two scalar 12-lead ECGs from a patient with exercise-induced VT are illustrated. The top tracing is taken at rest when the patient is having only ventricular extrasystoles. The bottom tracing shows sustained VT that occurred spontaneously during isoproterenol infusion. The QRS morphology of the VT is typical for right ventricular outflow tract VT. Note that the PVCs that occurred at rest are identical in morphology to the VT. Often, PVCs are all that can be induced at electrophysiology study, and they can be used successfully as a target to ablate VT. Reproduced with permission from Klein LS, et al.[54]

entrained, suggesting reentry as a mechanism.[29] The reentrant circuit may involve the distal left specialized conduction system, since ablation experience has shown that distinct fascicular potentials are often recorded prior to ventricular activation at successful sites. However, the detailed anat-omy of the reentrant circuit in this arrhythmia has not been defined.

Pharmacological management for idiopathic VT usually involves beta blockers or calcium blockers, depending on which has been demonstrated to be effective in any particular patient. Membrane-active antiar-

Figure 4. Scalar ECG from a patient with verapamil-sensitive left ventricular tachycardia. The QRS morphology is that of a right bundle branch block with extreme left axis deviation. This patient did not have structural heart disease. The spontaneous episode of VT is shown in the top half of the figure. The bottom half of the figure is a pacemap at the time of electrophysiology study; it shows a QRS morphology during pacing from the successful ablation site similar to that of VT. Used with permission from Klein LS, et al.[56]

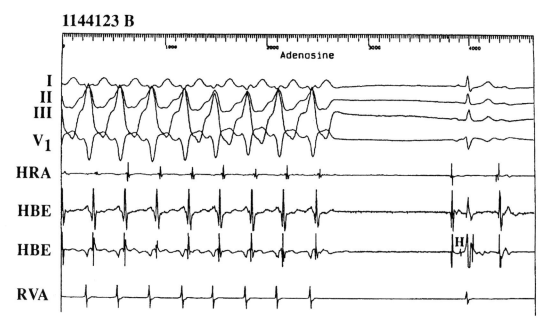

Figure 3. Termination of VT with intravenous adenosine. Sustained VT arising from the right ventricular outflow tract is present on the left of the figure. Fourteen seconds after the administration of intravenous adenosine, VT stops and sinus rhythm is restored, consistent with adenosine-sensitive VT. HRA = high right atrium; HBE = His = bundle electrogram; RVA = right ventricular apex. Reproduced with permission from Miles WM, et al.[55]

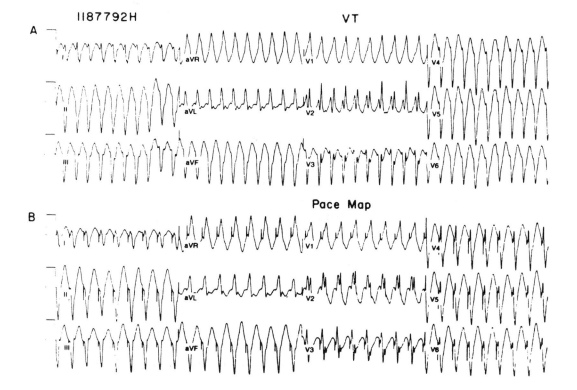

rhythmic drugs from class I or class III are often effective, but the risk:benefit ratio may not warrant use of these medications because these varieties of VT are rarely life-threatening and because of the availability of effective ablation techniques. Catheter ablation is indicated for patients in whom antiarrhythmic drugs have been ineffective or are not tolerated. In addition, catheter ablation may be the therapy of first choice in patients who wish to avoid long-term drug therapy. Ablation has been reported to be effective in patients to eliminate frequent, severely symptomatic, monomorphic, drug-refractory ventricular ectopy,[30,31] but should not be considered for most patients with benign ventricular ectopy.[32] The safety and efficacy of VT ablation in the right ventricular outflow tract of children over age 6 is probably comparable to that in adults.[33] However, studies of RF lesions in the ventricles of infant lambs have suggested that these lesions enlarge over time.[34] Therefore, the safety of VT ablation in very young children is unknown.

Patients with idiopathic VT provide the potentially simplest substrate for VT ablation; that is, they have a stable monomorphic VT that is usually tolerated long enough for mapping, and there is no scar, fibrosis, hypertrophy, or other abnormality of the cardiac muscle to interfere with adequate delivery of the ablation energy to the VT focus. In addition, most of these patients do not have progressive myocardial disease that would be associated with subsequent appearance of new VT foci in the future. However, an occasional patient thought to have idiopathic VT arising from the right ventricle, especially if VT is not arising from the right ventricular outflow tract, may instead have an early form of arrhythmogenic right ventricular dysplasia[35] (Table 2). In these patients, electrophysiological study may reveal more than one VT morphology. Ablative therapy, although still possibly effective, will have a lower success rate because of the multiple VT foci and because progressive myocardial disease may allow appearance of new VT foci in the future. In

Table 2
Arrhythmogenic Right Ventricular Dysplasia (ARVD) vs. Idiopathic Ventricular Tachycardia

The following features favor ARVD:
1. Family history of VT
2. History of resuscitation
3. ECG:
   a. Terminal rightward conduction delay in V1 (epsilon wave)
   b. Anterior T wave inversions
4. Late potentials on signal-averaged ECG
5. Multiple VT morphologies
6. Right ventricular dilatation or wall motion abnormalities

VT = ventricular tachycardia.

addition, thinning of the right ventricular wall in arrhythmogenic right ventricular dysplasia may pose an increased risk of perforation during the ablation procedure. Therefore, although ablation has been clinically successful in patients with arrhythmogenic right ventricular dysplasia, it is not considered a primary therapy if this diagnosis is entertained, and ablation is often more a palliative rather than a curative procedure.[36]

Techniques for Ablation of Idiopathic Ventricular Tachycardia Arising from the Right Ventricle

In patients with no apparent structural heart disease who present with VT having a left bundle branch block morphology, the site of origin of the VT and subsequent ablation site is usually the right ventricle.[10,37,38] This is in contrast to patients who have coronary artery disease and previous infarction (particularly inferior infarction), in whom VTs arising from the left ventricle may have a left bundle branch block morphology because of a septal origin of the tachycardia with initial exit of the circuit toward the right side of the septum.

Ventricular tachycardia arising from the right ventricular outflow tract usually has a relatively narrow QRS duration (approximately 140 ms). There is a typical left bundle branch block configuration in lead V_1 with the precordial transition in the mid to lateral precordial leads (usually V_4 to V_5). The frontal plane QRS axis is close to 90° (or occasionally rightward) with very tall upright QRS complexes in leads II, III, and aVF and low amplitude (or negative) QRS complexes in lead I (Figure 5). In the second most common site of right ventricular tachycardia,

the right ventricular inflow region close to the bundle of His, the precordial QRS complexes are similar to those described above, and the QRS complexes in the inferior leads are also positive but not as tall as those in right ventricular outflow VT.

A newly recognized entity is VT having an inferior axis (tall R waves in leads II, III, and aVF) and a left bundle branch block pattern (rS) in V_1, but with an early precordial R wave transition (usually prominent R

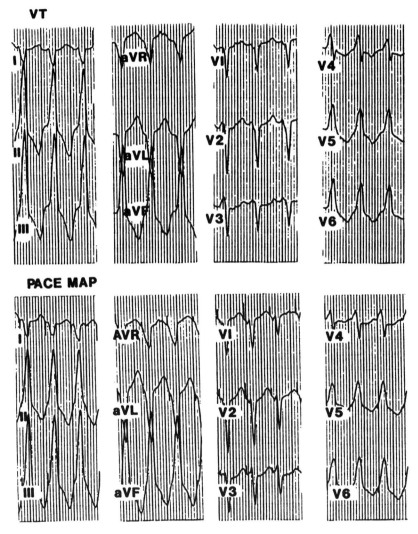

Figure 5. ECGs of VT (top) and a pacemap from the successful ablation site (bottom) are shown in a patient whose VT arose from the right ventricular outflow tract. The site of the best pacemap was the successful ablation site. This was the same site at which earliest endocardial activation was recorded during VT. Used with permission from Klein LS, et al.[10]

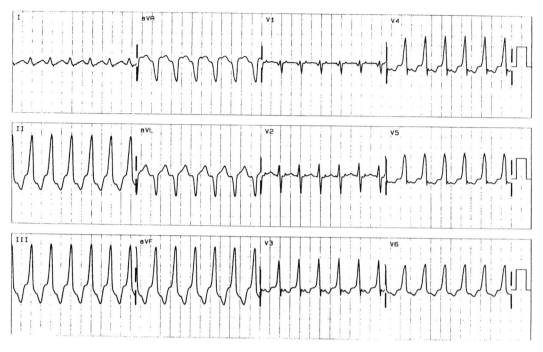

Figure 6. Twelve-lead ECG of a VT that superficially resembles a right ventricular outflow origin (left bundle branch block pattern in lead V_1 and an inferior axis). However, note the early precordial transition to a large R wave in V_2 and predominantly positive QRS complex in V_3. This VT was septal in origin and was eliminated by ablation from the anterobasal left ventricle. Reproduced with permission from Miles WM et al.[55]

wave lead V_2)[39–41](Figure 6). In our experience, ablation from the right ventricular outflow tract may occasionally alter the QRS morphology but not eliminate these VTs, and they appear to arise from the anterobasal left ventricle. Only two of six of these VTs for which RF ablation was attempted from the left ventricle were ablated successfully (both from the left ventricular outflow tract).[39] Thus, an early precordial QRS transition zone distinguishes VT arising distant from the typical right ventricular outflow location despite similar ECGs. These VTs may be arising from the subepicardial region or deep within the interventricular septum, explaining the lower success rate using current RF ablation techniques. Care must be taken in this area because of the proximity of the left main and proximal left anterior descending coronary arteries as well as the His bundle.[40,42] Friedman et al.[42] reported abrupt occlusion

of the left main coronary artery following RF energy delivery to ablate idiopathic VT arising from the high anteroseptal left ventricular outflow tract just beneath the aortic valve; patency of the artery was restored with a stent without evidence of myocardial infarction. Radiofrequency ablation of these VTs from the coronary venous system has been reported.[40]

Induction of Ventricular Tachycardia

Idiopathic right ventricular tachycardias may be difficult to induce consistently in the electrophysiology laboratory. An occasional patient may have very frequent episodes of VT just prior to or following the procedure, but VT is unable to be induced in the laboratory. In some patients, atrial or ventricular drive trains or burst pacing may induce VT whereas premature ventricular extrastimuli do not (Figure 7), suggesting the possibility of a triggered mechanism.[21] As mentioned above, many of these VTs (both those that are inducible by programmed ventricular stimulation and those that are not) are sensitive to adrenergic stimulation. Isoproterenol in doses of 1–6 μg/min is commonly used to facilitate the occurrence of spontaneous VT or its induction by programmed ventricular stimulation. In patients in whom VT is infrequent or nonsustained, infusion of isoproterenol may produce sustained VT, frequent runs of nonsustained VT, or PVCs that can be used for mapping and as target arrhythmias for ablation. In an occasional patient, adrenergic stimulation may increase the sinus rate and decrease the frequency of VT. If

isoproterenol does not increase the VT frequency or duration, infusion of epinephrine (0.01–0.03 μg/kg/min) may increase the VT, implying that alpha-adrenergic stimulation may be important in some patients. Many patients will have more spontaneous VT when they are in the awake and alert (and probably anxious) state rather than after sedation. In these patients, it may be useful to reverse sedation with narcotic or benzodiazepine antagonists if VT is difficult to induce after sedation. Once a dose of isoproterenol or epinephrine has been demonstrated to facilitate spontaneous or inducible VT, the infusion is usually maintained throughout the procedure to provide as much arrhythmia as possible so that activation mapping can be performed effi-

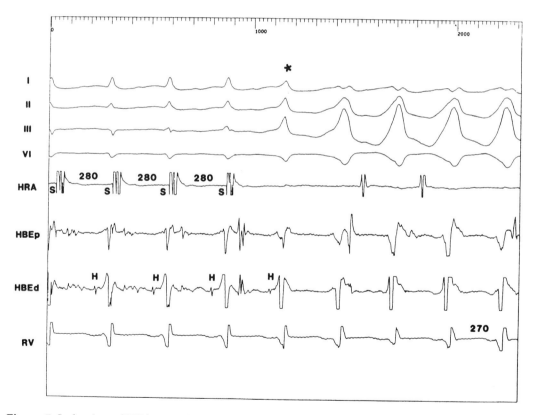

Figure 7. Induction of VT by atrial pacing. Surface leads I, II, III, and V_1 are displayed along with intracardiac leads from the high right atrium (HRA), proximal His = bundle region (HBE$_p$), distal His = bundle region (HBE$_d$), and right ventricle. Rapid atrial pacing at a cycle length of 280 ms results in induction of VT after a fusion beat (*). Reproduced with permission from Klein LS, et al.[54]

ciently and the efficacy of ablation can be quickly assessed. In some patients, only uniform PVCs with a morphology identical to that of their VT are present at the time of study; if frequent, these can be used effectively for mapping and assessment of ablation efficacy for VT.

Activation Mapping

The two techniques commonly used for localization of an appropriate site for ablation are activation mapping and pacemapping. Unlike the electrograms in patients with VT associated with coronary artery disease, the local electrograms at successful sites in patients with idiopathic VT are usually not fractionated. Therefore, fractionated potentials or mid-diastolic potentials are not useful for mapping. However, because these tachycardias appear to be focal (rather than macroreentrant) in origin, searching for the site of earliest ventricular activation during sustained VT, nonsustained VT, or frequent isolated PVCs (having the same morphology as VT) is effective (activation mapping, Figure 8). Local ventricular activation during VT occurs 20–50 ms prior to the onset of the QRS complex at the successful ablation site. In most patients, the final successful ablation site is the site recording earliest endocardial activation. It is difficult in many patients to define precisely the onset of the QRS in the surface leads. It is important to display many surface leads simultaneously in order to ascertain the onset of ventricular activation relative to the surface QRS. A subtle deviation from the isoelectric baseline may occur 20–30 ms prior to the onset of the first sharp QRS deflection. This may be because when VT originates in the right ventricular outflow tract where there are no specialized conduction fibers, initial conduction of the impulse from the VT focus is from ventricular cell to ventricular cell, giving rise to a slow initial QRS deviation prior to the more rapid QRS deflection after the Purkinje system is activated. Therefore, in any individual patient the eventual successful ablation site is that with the earliest activation, although how early this needs to be varies from patient to patient and is dependent on operator selection of the QRS onset during VT.

Pacemapping

Pacemapping is more useful for guiding ablation of idiopathic VT than it is in patients with VT associated with coronary artery disease.[1–4] Because the right ventricular wall is thin and these tachycardias are focal in origin, pacing from the endocardium at the site of tachycardia origin results in QRS complexes on a 12-lead ECG that almost exactly mimic those of the VT (Figures 5 and 9). Pacemapping may be per-

Figure 8. Examples of activation mapping in two different patients with right ventricular tachycardia. (**A**) The site of successful ablation corresponds to the site of earliest ventricular activation that occurs in the ablation catheter electrogram and precedes the QRS complex by 35 ms. Surface leads: I, II, III, and V$_1$. Electrogram leads: ABLATION = ablation catheter; HRA = high right atrium; HBEP = proximal His bundle; HBED = distal His bundle; RV = right ventricle. This VT is arising from the right ventricular outflow region. Reproduced with permission from Miles WM et al.[55] (**B**) Early endocardial activation is displayed in a patient with VT arising from a right posterolateral free wall location under the tricuspid valve. Local ventricular activation at the successful site precedes the onset of the QRS in the surface electrogram by 80 ms. Note the difference in the QRS morphology between panels A and B. Surface leads: I, II, III, and V$_1$. Electrogram leads: ABLATION = ablation catheter; HRA = high right atrium; HBEP = proximal His bundle; HBED = distal His bundle; RV = right ventricle. Used with permission from Miles WM, et al.[55]

formed as an adjunct to activation mapping or may be used as the primary mapping technique in patients whose arrhythmia frequency is low at the beginning of the procedure or diminishes as the procedure progresses. In an occasional patient, if only a single run of VT or a PVC having the tachycardia morphology occurs, the procedure can be guided wholly by pacemapping. However, pacemapping using only reference ECGs of VT recorded at a previous setting (for example, in the emergency room)

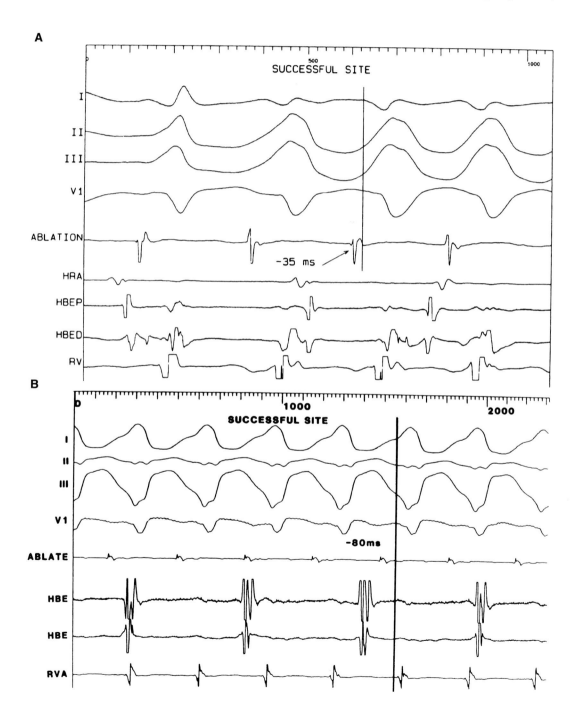

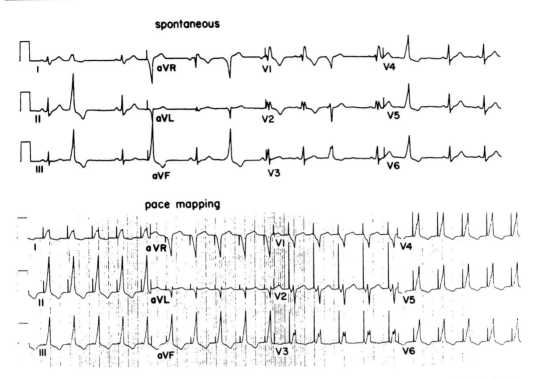

Figure 9. A 12-lead ECG of PVCs (top tracing) and a pacemap from the successful VT ablation site (bottom tracing) are shown. The paced QRS complexes and the PVCs have nearly identical morphology. VT gradually subsided during the study but PVCs having the same morphology as the VT occurred repeatedly and were used for mapping. Reproduced with permission from Klein LS, et al.[10]

are not adequate for ablation mapping because of the differences in lead placement. Pacemapping is relatively tedious, but newer versions of computerized electrophysiological recording systems may decrease the time required for pacemapping by allowing stored VT reference ECGs to be compared quickly with paced QRS complexes.

In patients with right ventricular tachycardia, the pacemap at the successful site is an almost exact match with that during VT, including the frontal plane axis, the precordial transition, and subtle notches on the QRS complexes. Any pacemap that fails to resemble the VT to this extent probably reflects an inadequate ablation location. Pacemapping should be performed at a cycle length near that of the VT so that rate-related changes in the QRS morphology are minimized between VT and the pacemap.

Care must be taken during pacemapping that the pacing does not induce a run of the VT that is then mistaken for an excellent pacemap. An advantage of pacemapping is that the existence of ventricular capture during pacing from the ablation catheter confirms adequate catheter-tissue contact for ablation and also confirms that the catheter is located below the pulmonic valve.

We have performed pacemapping using a pacing amplitude of 10 mA and a pulse width of 2 ms delivered in a bipolar fashion between the 4-mm distal ablating electrode and a ring electrode located 2 mm more proximally on the ablating catheter.[10] In theory, it may be advantageous to use unipolar rather than bipolar pacing and to use lower pacing outputs in order to minimize the volume of tissue depolarized directly by the pacing current and therefore obtain a more precise pacemap[2]; however, possibly because the distal ablation electrode is so large, we have found that bipolar pacing is adequate.

Catheter Positioning

The appropriate catheter position to ablate right ventricular outflow tachycardia can usually be established using the posteroanterior fluoroscopic view, although the right and left anterior oblique views may also be useful (Figure 10). A deflectable catheter is introduced into the femoral vein and advanced across the tricuspid valve. Using catheter deflection and torque, the catheter can be advanced to the right ventricular outflow tract just under the pulmonic valve. If the catheter crosses the pulmonic valve, the ventricular electrogram will suddenly diminish in amplitude. The catheter usually points toward the patient's left, just below the pulmonic valve, although the exact position of the catheter within the outflow tract may vary from patient to patient. This region of the right ventricle is very smooth, and it is often difficult to stabilize the catheter just under the pulmonic valve, although this can usually be accomplished from the femoral approach. Occasionally the superior vena caval approach or stabilization with a long sheath may help. Temperature monitoring during RF ablation is advantageous to confirm adequate catheter-tissue contact and prevent an impedance rise. Excessive heating in this thin-walled region can result rarely in cardiac perforation.

The second most common site of idiopathic right ventricular tachycardia is the right ventricular inflow, near where His bundle activation is recorded (Figure 11).[10] Care must be exercised while performing VT ablation at this site so that heart block does not occur. The catheter may be positioned across the tricuspid annulus to record a His bundle potential and then advanced slightly and deflected superiorly to identify an early site of activation during VT having no His bundle or right bundle branch potential. Occasionally, right bundle

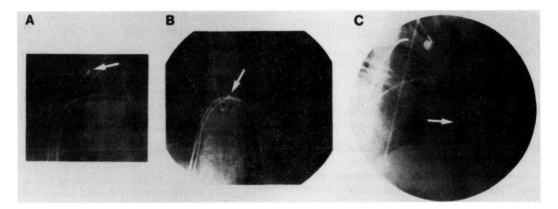

Figure 10. Radiographs of typical catheter positions. (**A**) Left anterior oblique radiograph of catheter position in a patient whose VT arose from the right ventricular outflow tract. Arrows point to the electrode used for successful ablation. (**B**) Right anterior oblique radiograph of catheter position at the successful ablation site in a patient whose VT arose from an anteroseptal region just across the tricuspid valve and adjacent to the His bundle. Tip of the ablation catheter is shown (arrow) with a distal loop adjacent to the His bundle catheter. The tip of this catheter was across the tricuspid valve and in the right ventricle. (**C**) Right anterior oblique radiograph of an ablation catheter in the left ventricle to ablate a posterior fascicular tachycardia. The ablating tip (arrow) is in the posteroseptal region at the mid left ventricular level; this was the successful ablation site. Used with permission from Klein LS, et al.[10]

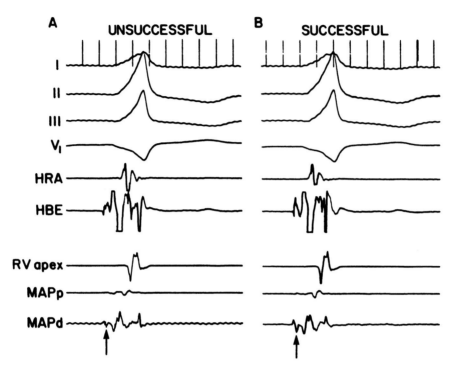

Figure 11. Intracardiac recordings from a patient with a right ventricular inflow origin of VT. Shown are surface leads I, II, III, and V_1 and intracardiac recordings from the high right atrium (HRA), His bundle region (HBE), right ventricular apex (RVA), and bipolar recordings from the proximal poles (MAP_p) and from the distal poles (MAP_d), and from the distal poles (MAP_d) of the quadripolar ablation catheter. This figure illustrates the importance of catheter contact with endocardium. On the left, an early electrogram (arrow) is recorded from the site of a good pacemap, but delivery of RF energy in this region failed to eliminate spontaneous VT. On the right, an equally early electrogram is recorded from this same region. Catheter contact may be better here as evidenced by the larger amplitude of the early portion of the electrogram from this region. Delivery of RF energy here eliminated VT. Note how early the ventricular electrogram is in the His bundle region, consistent with the right ventricular inflow location of the VT. Used with permission from Klein LS, et al.[10]

branch block may occur with the successful energy delivery.

Techniques for Ablation of Idiopathic Left Septal Ventricular Tachycardia

Idiopathic left septal VT is usually sensitive to verapamil and arises in the region of the left posterior fascicle (left posterior fascicular VT, verapamil-sensitive VT).[20–29,] [43,44] Idiopathic left septal VT usually has the QRS morphology of a right bundle branch block and left axis deviation. Rodriguez et

al. have described two distinct groups of idiopathic left septal VT.[45] Ventricular tachycardia in one group had a left axis and more narrow QRS, originated from the inferoposterior left ventricle, and mapping revealed activation of a Purkinje potential prior to ventricular activation in most cases. Ventricular tachycardica in the other group had a left superior axis and a wider QRS, originated from the inferoapical left ventricle, and no Purkinje activity was recorded at the successful ablation site. Our experience is that the former variety is more common. Because these VTs are often able to be entrained by ventricular pacing,[29] they are probably due to reentry utilizing His-Purkinje fibers for at least part of the circuit. The exact circuit is unknown but may involve several centimeters of the left ventricular septum,[46] and ablation guided by an early Purkinje potential may be successful with or without a perfect pacemap.[27,47]

Suwa et al. described a false tendon in the left ventricle of a patient with idiopathic left ventricular tachycardia in whom VT was eliminated by surgical resection of the tendon.[48] Using transthoracic and transesophageal echocardiography, Thakur et al. found false tendons extending from the posteroinferior left ventricle to the left ventricular septum in 15 of 15 patients with idiopathic left ventricular tachycardia but only 5% of control patients.[49] They speculated that the false tendon may be involved with tachycardia either by providing a conduction pathway or producing stretch in the Purkinje fiber network on the septum. Lin et al.[50] also found that 17 of 18 patients with idiopathic left ventricular tachycardia had this fibromuscular band, but also found it in 35 of 40 control patients. They concluded that the band was a common echocardiographic finding and was not a specific anatomic substrate for idiopathic left ventricular tachycardia, although they could not exclude the possibility that the band was a potential substrate for VT.

Ablation is performed by introducing a catheter via the retrograde transaortic approach across the aortic valve into the left ventricle. Left ventricular endocardial mapping during tachycardia is performed in the posteroapical left ventricular septal region.[27,43] The left anterior oblique fluoroscopic view is used to guide the catheter toward the septum, and the right anterior oblique view to guide the catheter posteriorly and toward the apical third of the septum. While mapping the distal left ventricular septum, earliest ventricular activation during VT is usually preceded by a distinct fascicular potential, preceding the QRS by 15–40 ms (Figure 12). A fascicular potential can be recorded during sinus rhythm not only at this site, but also at sites near fascicles that are not associated with the VT focus. The successful ablation site is usually that having the earliest fascicular potential during VT, not necessarily that with earliest ventricular activation. This is because the site of VT origin within the fascicle may be different from where the impulse "exits" or activates ventricular tissue (QRS onset). Pacemapping at this site may result in QRS complexes that closely resemble those of VT but an exact match is not always obtained, probably because pacing in the region of the early fascicular potential may also activate local ventricular myocardium. In addition, a pacemap having a QRS complex identical to that of VT may not necessarily represent a successful ablation site because of the possibility of capture of the Purkinje fiber network at a site remote from the origin of the tachycardia.

Figure 12. Left posterior fascicular tachycardia. Surface leads I, II, III, and V_1 are displayed along with ablation (ABLATION), high right atrium (HRA), proximal His bundle (HBEP), distal His bundle (HBED), and right ventricular (RV) electrograms. An arterial pressure recording is also illustrated. (A) The ablation catheter is positioned in the left posteroseptal region two-thirds of the way toward the apex. A fascicular potential (P) is recorded before the ventricular (V) electrogram. The ventricular electrogram precedes the QRS complex by 10 ms, and the fascicular potential precedes it by 50 ms. Reproduced with permission from Klein LS, et al.[57] (B) This illustrates elimination of the fascicular tachycardia. RF current is turned on in the middle of the figure, and the left posterior fascicular tachycardia terminates abruptly. The tachycardia was no longer inducible in this patient after delivery of this RF pulse. Surface leads I, II, III, and V_1 are displayed along with ablation (ABLATION), high right atrium (HRA), proximal His bundle (HBEP), distal His bundle (HBED), and right ventricular (RV) electrograms. Reproduced with permission from Klein LS, et al.[57]

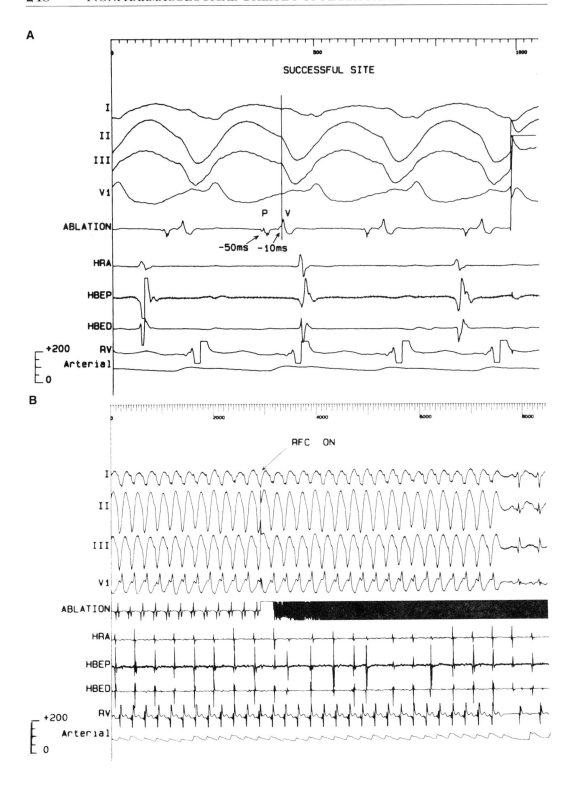

Results of Ablation for Idiopathic Ventricular Tachycardia

We performed RF ablation in 73 patients with idiopathic VT referred to Indiana University Hospital between March 1990 and May 1995.[51] There were 40 men and 33 women with a mean age of 41 years, ranging from 6 to 70 years. The presenting symptoms included palpitations in 31 patients, presyncope in 34, and syncope in eight. Thirty-eight patients had sustained VT as the presenting arrhythmia, 33 patients had nonsustained VT, and two had only symptomatic PVCs. The techniques of ablation were those described above. Ventricular tachycardias was mapped to the right ventricle in 55 (75%) and to the left ventricle in 18 (25%) of the 73 patients. Of the right ventricular tachycardias, 46 originated from the right ventricular outflow tract, seven from the right ventricular inflow region, and two from the right ventricular free wall. Of the left ventricular tachycardias, 13 mapped to the left ventricular posterior septum in the region of the posterior fascicle, and five mapped to other left ventricular sites, including three anterolateral basal, one anteroseptal, and one apical. No patient had more than one VT focus targeted for ablation.

Adrenergic Stimulation

Nine patients did not require adrenergic stimulation for induction of sustained VT. Isoproterenol was administered to 64 (88%) of patients for enhancement of spontaneous VT or facilitation of VT induction. Isoproterenol enhanced or facilitated VT induction in 46 of these 64 patients (71%), had no effect in 14 (22%) patients, and suppressed VT in four patients (7%). Nine patients received epinephrine after isoproterenol either suppressed or failed to enhance VT; epinephrine enhanced VT or facilitated its induction in five out of the nine patients.

Ablation Efficacy

Overall, idiopathic VT was successfully eliminated in 61 of the 73 (84%) patients. There was a higher ablation success rate with VT arising from the right ventricular outflow tract than any other site: 45 of 46 (98%) patients. Ventricular tachycardia was successfully ablated in only three of nine (33%) patients in whom VT arose from right ventricular sites other than the outflow tract (right ventricular inflow tract in two, right ventricular free wall in one). This difference in success rate depending on right ventricular site of origin has been reflected by other authors[52] and may either represent site specific technical differences or may reflect patients with an early form of arrhythmogenic right ventricular dysplasia.

Ventricular tachycardia rising from the left ventricle was eliminated in 13 of 18 (72%) patients. Ten of 13 (77%) patients with left ventricular septal tachycardia had VT successfully ablated, whereas three of five patients with VT arising from other left ventricular sites were successfully ablated (one of three from the anterolateral base, one of one from the anteroseptal region, and one of one from the apex). Therefore, ablation in patients with idiopathic VT is most successful in patients in whom the VT arises either from the right ventricular outflow tract or to a lesser extent from the left ventricular septum.

Nine of 61 (14%) patients who had initially successful VT ablations had recurrent arrhythmia and required two ablation sessions for elimination of VT. Five of these had right ventricular outflow VT, two had right ventricular inflow VT, and two had left posterior fascicular VT. All but one of these patients presented with recurrent VT within 4 weeks after ablation; however, one patient who underwent a left posterior fascicular VT ablation had recurrent arrhythmia 1½ years after a presumed successful ablation.

Complications

Four of the 73 (5%) patients had a procedure-related complication. Three patients developed pericardial effusions due to cardiac perforation; two of the three patients required emergent pericardiocentesis. Two of these patients had manipulation of a monophasic action potential catheter during the procedure that was probably responsible for the perforation. The third patient had perforation of the right ventricular outflow tract during RF energy delivery. Approximately 25 sec into energy delivery, an audible "pop" occurred, and the patient had hemodynamic collapse several minutes later. Echocardiography revealed a pericardial effusion with hemodynamic compromise, and successful pericardiocentesis was performed. The patient recovered, but VT persisted. The audible pop probably represented escape of intramyocardial gasses due to excessive deep tissue heating that occurs when the catheter tip is well cooled by the blood pool.[53] A death from pericardial tamponade during attempted ablation of a right ventricular outflow tract tachycardia has been reported.[38]

One patient who underwet successful ablation of a left posterior fascicular VT had an asymptomatic inferior wall motion abnormality noted on two-dimensional echocardiogram 24 hours after the procedure.

There was no evidence of myocardial infarction on serial ECGs. There was a moderate elevation of CPK MB fraction. Six weeks post ablation, the patient had normal regional wall motion and no evidence of ischemia on stress echocardiography. The transient wall motion abnormality may have been due to myocardial "stunning" from the ablation pulses.

Conclusion

Idiopathic VT can be ablated safely using RF energy and in many cases ablation may be used as a primary therapy. Adrenergic stimulation is often required to provide adequate frequency of arrhythmia for an ablation target. The site of origin of the VT correlates with the success of ablation, with right ventricular outflow tract VT having the highest success rates. Both endocardial activation mapping and pacemapping are useful for right ventricular tachycardias, and recording of an early Purkinje potential is useful in the left posteroseptal VTs. If ablation is acutely successful and clinical follow-up at 4–6 weeks is negative, a long-term success is likely.[51]

References

1. Morady F, Harvey M, Kalbfleisch SJ, et al. Radiofrequency catheter ablation of ventricular tachycardia in patients with coronary artery disease. Circulation 1993;87:363–372.
2. Stevenson WG, Khan H, Sager P, et al. Identification of reentry circuit sites during catheter mapping and radiofrequency ablation of ventricular tachycardia late after myocardial infarction. Circulation 1993;88:1647–1670.
3. Kim YH, Sosa-Suarez G, Tranton TG, et al. Treatment of ventricular tachycardia by transcatheter radiofrequency ablation in patients with ischemic heart disease. Circulation 1994;89:1094–1102.
4. Wilber DJ, Kopp DE, Glascock DN, et al. Catheter ablation of the mitral isthmus for ventricular tachycardia associated with inferior infarction. Circulation 1995;92:348–349.
5. Wellens HJJ, Rodriguez LM, Smeets JL. Ventricular tachycardia in structurally normal hearts. In Zipes DP, Jalife J, eds. Cardiac Electrophysiology: From Cell to Bedside. 2nd ed. Philadelphia, W.B. Saunders, 1995, pp 780–788.
6. Brooks R, Burgess JH. Idiopathic ventricular tachycardia: a review. Medicine 1988;67: 271–272.
7. Belhassen B, Viskin S. Idiopathic ventricular tachycardia and fibrillation. J Cardiovasc Electrophysiol 1993;354:356.
8. Mont L, Seixas T, Brugada P, et al. The electrocardiographic, clinical, and electrophysiologic spectrum of idiopathic monomorphic ventricular tachycardia. Am Heart J 1992;124:746.
9. Morady F, Kadish AH, DiCarlo L, et al. Long-term results of catheter ablation of idiopathic right ventricular tachycardia. Circulation 1990;82:2093–2098.
10. Klein LS, Shih H-T, Hackett FK, et al. Radiofrequency catheter ablation of ventricular tachycardia in patients without structural

heart disease. Circulation 1992;85:1666–1671.

11. Caceras J, Jazayeri M, McKinnie J, et al. Sustained bundle branch reentry as a mechanism of clinical tachycardia. Circulation 1989;79:256.

12. Blanck Z, Dhala A, Deshpande S, et al. Bundle branch reentrant ventricular tachycardia: cumulative experience in 48 patients. J Cardiovasc Electrophysiol 1993;4:253.

13. Buxton AE, Waxman HL, Marchlinski FE, et al. Right ventricular tachycardia: clinical and electrophysiologic characteristics. Circulation 1983;68:917–927.

14. Mitrani R, Klein LS, Miles WM, et al. Regional cardiac sympathetic denervation in patients with ventricular tachycardia in the absence of coronary artery disease. J Am Coll Cardiol 1993;22:1344–1353.

15. Wichler T, Hindricks G, Lerch H, et al. Regional myocardial sympathetic dysinnervation in arrhythmogenic right ventricular cardiomyopathy: an analysis using ^{123}I-meta-iodobenzyguanidine scintigraphy. Circulation 1994;89:667–683.

16. Carlson MD, White RD, Trohman RG, et al. Right ventricular outflow tract ventricular tachycardia: detection of previously unrecognized anatomic abnormalities using cine magnetic resonance imaging. J Am Coll Cardiol 1994;24:720–727.

17. Rahilly GT, Prystowsky EN, Zipes DP, et al. Clinical and electrophysiology findings in patients with repetitive monomorphic ventricular tachycardia and otherwise normal electrocardiogram. Am J Cardiol 1982;50:459–468.

18. Lerman BB, Stein K, Engelstein ED, et al. Mechanism of repetitive monomorphic ventricular tachycardia. Circulation 1995;92:421–429.

19. Lerman BB, Belardinelli L, West GA, et al. Adenosine-sensitive ventricular tachycardia: evidence suggesting cyclic AMP-mediated triggered activity. Circulation 1986;74:270–280.

20. Belhassen B, Rotmensch HH, Laniado S. Response of recurrent sustained ventricular tachycardia to verapamil. Br Heart J 1981;46:679–682.

21. Zipes DP, Foster PR, Troup PJ, et al. Atrial induction of ventricular tachycardia: reentry versus triggered automaticity. Am J Cardiol 1979;44:1–8.

22. Lin FC, Finely CD, Rahimtoola SH, et al. Idiopathic paroxysmal ventricular tachycardia with a QRS pattern of right bundle branch block and left axis deviation: a unique clinical entity with specific properties. Am J Cardiol 1983;52:95–100.

23. German LD, Packer DL, Bardy GH, et al. Ventricular tachycardia induced by atrial stimulation in patients without symptomatic cardiac disease. Am J Cardiol 1983;52:1202–1207.

24. Ward DE, Nathan AW, Camm AJ. Fascicular tachycardia sensitive to calcium antagonists. Eur Heart J 1984;5:896–905.

25. Sung RJ, Keung EC, Nguyen NX, et al. Effects of β-adrenergic blockade on verapamil-responsive and verapamil-irresponsive sustained ventricular tachycardias. J Clin Invest 1988;81:688–699.

26. Ohe T, Shimomura K, Aihara N, et al. Idiopathic sustained left ventricular tachycardia: clinical and electrophysiological characteristics. Circulation 1988;77:560–568.

27. Wen MS, Yeh SJ, Wang CC, et al. Radiofrequency ablation therapy in idiopathic left ventricular tachycardia with no obvious structural heart disease. Circulation 1994;89:1690–1696.

28. Bogun F, El-Atassi R, Daoud E, et al. Radiofrequency ablation of idiopathic left anterior fasicular tachycardia. J Cardiovasc Electrophysiol 1995;6:1113–1116.

29. Okumura K, Matsuyama K, Miyagi H, et al. Entrainment of idiopathic ventricular tachycardia of left ventricular origin with evidence for reentry with an area of slow conduction and effect of verapamil. Am J Cardiol 1988;62:727–732.

30. Gursoy S, Brugada J, Souza O, et al. Radiofrequency ablation of symptomatic but benign ventricular arrhythmias. PACE 1992;15:738–741.

31. Zhu DW, Maloney JD, Simmons TW, et al. Radiofrequency catheter ablation for management of symptomatic ventricular ectopic activity. J Am Coll Cardiol 1995;26:843–849.

32. Wellens HJJ. Radiofrequency catheter ablation of benign ventricular ectopic beats: a therapy in search of a disease? J Am Coll Cardiol 1995;26:850–851.

33. O'Conner BK, Case CL, Sokoloski MC, et al. Radiofrequency catheter ablation of right ventricular outflow tachycardia in children and adolescents. J Am Coll Cardiol 1996;27:869–874.

34. Saul JP, Hulse JE, Papagiannis J, et al. Late enlargement of radiofrequency lesions in infant lambs. Implications for ablation procedures in small children. Circulation 1994;90:492–499.

35. Fontaine G, Fontaliran G, Lascault G, et al. Arrhythmogenic right ventricular dysplasia. In Zipes DP, Jalife J, eds. Cardiac Electrophysiology: From Cell to Bedside. W.B. Saunders, Philadelphia, 1995, pp 754–769.

36. Leclercq JF, Chouty F, Cauchemez B, et al.

Results of electrical fulguration in arrhythmogenic right ventricular disease. Am J Cardiol 1988;62:220–224.

37. Wilber DJ, Baerman J, Okshansky B, et al. Adenosine-sensitive ventricular tachycardia: clinical characteristics and response to catheter ablation. Circulation 1993;87:126–129.

38. Coggins DL, Lee RJ, Sweeney J, et al. Radiofrequency catheter ablation as a cure for idiopathic tachycardia of both left and right ventricular origin. J Am Coll Cardiol 1994;23:1333–1341.

39. Krebs ME, Krause PC, Engelstein ED, et al. Differentiation of right ventricular outflow tract and left basal ventricular tachycardia: electrocardiographic criteria [Abstract]. J Am Coll Cardiol 1997;29:293A.

40. Callans DJ, Menz V, Schartzman D, et al. Repetitive monomorphic tachycardia from the left ventricular outflow tract: electrocardiographic patterns consistent with a left ventricular site of origin. J Am Coll Cardiol 1997;29:1023–1027.

41. Arruda M, Chandrasekaran K, Reynolds D, et al. Idiopathic epicardial outflow tract ventricular tachycardia: implications for RF catheter ablation [Abstract]. PACE 1996;19:611A.

42. Friedman PL, Stevenson WG, Bittl JA, et al. Left main coronary artery occlusion during radiofrequency catheter ablation of idiopathic outflow tract ventricular tachycardia [Abstract]. PACE 1997;20:1184A.

43. Nakagawa H, Beckman KJ, McClelland JH, et al. Radiofrequency catheter ablation of idiopathic left ventricular tachycardia guided by a Purkinje potential. Circulation 1993;88:2607–2617.

44. Wellens HJJ, Smeets JLRM. Idiopathic left ventricular tachycardia: cure by radiofrequency ablation. Circulation 1993;88:2978–2979.

45. Rodriguez L-M, Smeets JLRM, Timmermans C, et al. Predictors for successful ablation of right- and left-sided idiopathic ventricular tachycardia. Am J Cardiol 1997;79:309–314.

46. Aizawa Y, Chinushi M, Kitazawa H, et al. Spatial orientation of the reentrant circuit of idiopathic left ventricular tachycardia. Am J Cardiol 1995;76:316–319.

47. Page RL, Shenasa H, Evans JJ, et al. Radiofrequency catheter ablation of idiopathic recurrent ventricular tachycardia with right bundle branch block, left axis morphology. PACE 1993;16:327–336.

48. Suwa M, Youeda Y, Nagao H, et al. Surgical correction of idiopathic paroxysmal ventricular tachycardia possibly related to left ventricular false tendon. Am J Cardiol 1989;64:1217–1220.

49. Thakur RK, Klein GJ, Sivaram CA, et al. Anatomic substrate for idiopathic left ventricular tachycardia. Circulation 1996;93:497–501.

50. Lin F-C, Wen M-S, Wang C-C, et al. Left ventricular fibromuscular band is not a specific substrate for idiopathic left ventricular tachycardia. Circulation 1996;93:525–528.

51. Mandrola JM, Klein LS, Miles WM, et al. Radiofrequency catheter ablation of idiopathic ventricular tachycardia in 57 patients: acute success and long term follow-up [Abstract]. J Am Coll Cardiol 1995;25:19A.

52. Calkins H, Kalbfleisch SJ, El-Atassi R, et al. Relation between efficacy of radiofrequency catheter ablation and site of origin of idiopathic ventricular tachycardia. Am J Cardiol 1993;71:827–833.

53. Nakagawa H, Yamanashi WS, Pitha JV, et al. Comparison of in vivo tissue temperature profile and lesion geometry for radiofrequency ablation with a saline-irrigated electrode versus temperature control in a canine thigh muscle preparation. Circulation 1995;91:2264–2273.

54. Klein LS, Miles WM. Ventricular tachycardia in patients with normal hearts. Cardiol Rev 1993;1:336–339.

55. Miles WM, Klein LS. Radiofrequency ablation of idiopathic ventricular tachycardia and bundle branch reentrant tachycardia. In Singer I, ed. Interventional Cardiology. Williams and Wilkins, Baltimore, 1996.

56. Klein LS, Miles WM, Zipes DP. Ablation of idiopathic ventricular tachycardia and bundle branch reentry. In Zipes DP, ed. Catheter Ablation of Arrhythmias. Futura Publishing Co, Inc, Armonk, NY, 1994, p 263.

57. Klein LS, Miles WM. Ablative therapy for ventricular arrhythmias. Progr Cardiovasc Dis 1995;37:236.

Chapter 12

Radiofrequency Catheter Ablation of Ventricular Tachycardia in Patients with Coronary Artery Disease

Ross D. Fletcher, Pamela Karasik

Introduction

One of the earliest tachyarrhythmias to be addressed by catheter ablation was ventricular tachycardia (VT) often in patients with coronary artery disease. The first intracardiac target structure to be ablated using percutaneous catheters was the atrioventricular node,[1,2] to improve rate control during atrial fibrillation. Soon thereafter, catheter ablation was shown to be effective in ablating VT. Even though the initial series was only three cases, the authors[3,4] informally postulated that the success in these cases would dramatically change the way we treated VT. This prediction has not yet been realized in part because of the effectiveness of newer antiarrhythmic drugs and antitachycardia/defibrillation devices. In retrospect, it seems that one of the cases may well have been bundle branch reentry, which has proven an easy target for ablation. At the same time surgical and electrophysiology teams in Paris[5] and Philadelphia[6] were demonstrating success against VT using surgical procedures. The success of the endocardial "Philadelphia Peel" resection further encouraged those in the field

determined to use catheters for mapping and ablation. Several investigators amassed a sizable experience in catheter ablation with direct current (DC) shocks, called "fulguration" by Guy Fontaine et al.[7,8] The success rates for DC shock may well be due in part to the large lesion size. The use of catheters in the catheterization laboratory eliminated the risks of anesthesia and cross-clamp times present in the operating room. This allowed both increased time for careful mapping of sustained arrhythmia and the ability to readily return to the catheterization laboratory to ablate a recurrence. However, the use of DC shock, while effective, was always intrinsically dangerous and was proven to have more hemodynamic and arrhythmia complications than other energy sources for creating endocardial lesions.[9] In the early days balloon pumps were on standby in the laboratory in case a DC shock produced cardiogenic shock. Our lab used echocardiograms during the shocks to rapidly detect wall motion abnormalities or perforation. Despite these risks, this technique was life-saving for patients in incessant VT unresponsive to pharmacological agents. Indeed, in our institution, catheter

From Singer I, Barold SS, Camm AJ (eds): Nonpharmacological Therapy of Arrhythmias for the 21st Century: The State of the Art. Futura Publishing Co, Inc., Armonk, NY, © 1998.

ablation has always been used to reverse incessant VT before declaring failure. Incessant tachycardia was the indication that encouraged catheter ablation of VT before many other arrhythmias were attempted.

Indications

In patients with coronary disease, incessant VT, unresponsive to all other forms of therapy, remains one of the primary indications for ablation therapies. Indeed, in one study a multivariate analysis showed incessant tachycardia as the only consistent predictor for success. Frequent recurrent VT is a common additional indication, but the advent of advanced antiarrhythmic pharmacological agents such as intravenous and oral amiodarone and advanced antitachycardia/defibrillation devices have made ablation therapy for VT less necessary. On the other hand, the use of implantable devices has provided new indications. Recurrent VT unresponsive to pacing therapy and requiring frequent cardioversions often is a target for ablation therapy. Slow sustained VT, occurring at rates which overlap the sinus rates, cannot be specifically detected by an implanted device. The device cannot be set to detect and treat only the slow VT without also detecting and treating sinus tachycardia. Pacing therapies may be uncomfortable and inappropriate antitachycardia therapy for sinus tachycardia can induce ventricular fibrillation or VT. These slow VT rhythms are therefore best managed as targets for ablation therapy. In some patients, the sinus rhythm post-shock can rise above the tachycardia rate; in this case inappropriate therapy will be delivered on sinus tachycardia. The explanations for post-shock sinus tachycardia, include response to pain, fear of further shocks, compensation for a period of hypotension, and possibly inhibition of endocardial vagal innervation.

The success rate of many investigators[10–13] for ablation of individual "target" VT morphologies is high. Although these patients may have VT recurrence, it is often greatly modified or is a previously unrecognized arrhythmia. Thus, a new definition for success has been established: if recurrent VT is less frequent and easily reverted by the device, or the target VT does not recur, the ablation procedure is considered successful.

A familiarity with the pathophysiology of VT in coronary disease is important for achieving successful ablations. Most of the cases of VT in coronary artery disease consist of reentrant circuits within or around scarred myocardium or aneurysms that will be discussed in detail under the section on arrhythmia localization.[14,15] Neural hormonal modulation and increased stretch enhance the circuits in the fixed substrate in coronary disease. These factors can facilitate the circuits and produce clinical events that would not be possible without increased sympathetic influence or dilated ventricles secondary to heart failure.

Preparation

The success of ablating VT is dependent on a careful analysis of all data prior to the procedure, a well-defined coordinated plan for executing mapping, and a clear knowledge of the ablating device. Most investigators arrive at the laboratory with a clear idea of the probable location of the target VT. Standard ventriculography and coronary arteriography reveal discrete aneurysms or scars. The most important data are the 12-lead ECG during spontaneous VT. The morphology allows recognition of the target VT when it occurs in the electrophysiological laboratory. All monomorphic sustained VTs induced during the procedure need to be considered possible future clinical problems and may have caused episodes in the past, which were not clinically documented. Differing morphologies may also represent alternative exit sites from the same reentrant circuit.

Common rules that predict location have been defined in the surgical ablation experi-

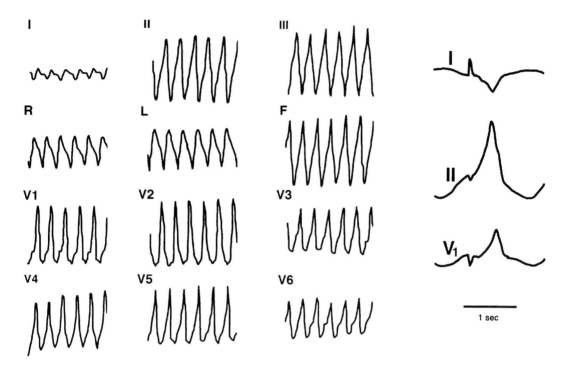

Figure 1. Ventricular tachycardia in a patient after repair of tetralogy of Fallot. The VT has an inferior axis and RBBB morphology in V_1. While this usually represents LV origin, in this patient the pacemap from the outflow of the RV right reproduced the I, II, and V_1 morphology of the VT. This RBBB morphology VT emanates from the repaired outflow of the RV. Used with permission from Singer I, ed.[58]

ence. In general, if V_4, V_5, and V_6 are negative, the tachycardia arises from the apical half of the ventricles. If V_4, V_5, and V_6 are positive, the tachycardia arises from the basal half of the ventricles. If V_1 is positive, the tachycardia is from the left ventricle (LV).[16,17] We have had exceptions to these rules. A patient with a large right ventricle (RV) due to repaired tetralogy of Fallot and persistent pulmonary insufficiency is an example of a VT with right bundle branch block (RBBB) configuration in V_1 (Figure 1). The V_1 during tachycardia and pacemapping from the RV outflow showed a similar upright QRS in V_1. A negative QRS in V_1 that appears like left bundle branch block (LBBB) usually indicates origin in the septum, but RV origin occurred in 36%. A wide (>0.04) small R in V_1 before the deep S may indicate RV free wall origin. While uncommon, the origin of the VT from the RV does occur in coronary artery disease and should be considered if all areas in the LV map are inappropriately late. Negative QRS in II, III, and aVF usually indicate a site on the inferior surface of the heart. As the QRS in these leads becomes more positive, the origin is higher in the ventricle.

Electrophysiology Laboratory: Overview

After the preliminary data have been fully analyzed and suspected sites of altered anatomy are well in mind, the electrophysiological laboratory is prepared for the case. Despite the wide range of equipment available in a modern electrophysiology laboratory, a careful plan for recording and pacing must be established so that mapping proceeds quickly and methodically. While patience and tenacity are the best qualities for success, systematic rapid recording and analyzing of sites are essential. Knowledge of the coronary anatomy, the ventricular anatomy, and the ejection fraction are critical for a safe, successful procedure. The VT ideally should be hemodynamically tolerated with the patient free from angina, and a systolic blood pressure greater than 90 mm Hg. Patients are prepared for the ablation in much the same way as for a diagnostic electrophysiology procedure, with some important exceptions. While antiarrhythmic medications are typically withheld for a diagnostic study, if an otherwise unstable VT is rendered slower and more suitable for mapping, the drug should be continued. Ideally, the target VT must be hemodynamically stable. However, if the tachycardia is more difficult to induce, then the drug should be discontinued for five half-lives. Patients are brought to the laboratory in the fasting nonsedated state. In our laboratory all patients have an indwelling Foley catheter both for patient comfort during what is often an extended procedure, and to better monitor volume status. Conscious sedation is provided using a combination of midazolam, fentanyl, and propofol. In a large series of ablation patients reported by O'Brien et al.,[18] doses of midazolam were 0.5–7 mg total, 25–100 μg of fentanyl, and propofol given as a continuous infusion of 20–130 μg/kg/min. This can be performed by nurses trained in administration of conscious sedation or by anesthesiology personnel. The incidence of requiring mechanical ventilation is approximately 1%.

Venous access is obtained via the right and left femoral veins and arterial access is obtained via the right femoral artery. Continuous arterial monitoring is performed in every patient either via the femoral sheath side arm or through a radial arterial line.

Intracardiac recordings are made from the His position and the RV apex. Often a catheter is placed in the high right atrium as well. The RV catheter is critical for both recording and providing a site for VT induction. Although standard quadripolar cathe-

ters are suitable for this purpose, in our laboratory we use a monophasic action potential catheter with orthogonal pacing. A separate quadripolar catheter is placed in the inferior vena cava for unipolar recording or pacing when combined with the ablation catheter. If a catheter has been placed initially in the high right atrium, it can be withdrawn or advanced to either vena cava and used as the indifferent electrode. In the past, unipolar electrodes were placed proximally on pacing catheters to achieve convenient unipolar pacing. New catheter designs promise to include proximal electrodes for unipolar pacing or recording. Unipolar pacing most accurately reflects events at the tip of the catheter. Pacing near threshold with the ablation tip negative (cathodal polarity), is rarely inaccurate and produces fewer artifacts on the recording channels.[19]

For mapping and ablating, a steerable quadripolar catheter with a 4-mm electrode tip is most commonly used. Early on in ablation therapy, 1- and 2-mm tip catheters produced inadequate lesions and quickly developed coagulum associated with high impedance rises.[20] Larger electrodes such as 8 mm have been used. These create larger and more effective lesions but should be used with caution because they can create larger and deeper lesions and generally require more power than is commonly available on standard RF generators. Ablation catheters come in a variety of curves. A short radius is required for sites in the outflow tract and a long radius curve may be more valuable in seeking sites on the free wall or under the mitral valve.

The retrograde aortic approach is most commonly used to access the LV, but the transseptal approach may be more convenient for some locations. Arterial access is obtained via the right femoral artery. This allows for a retrograde approach to the LV. Care should always be given to crossing the aortic valve, as the structure can be damaged by aggressive manipulation. This is the most common method of mapping the LV; however, in certain patients a transseptal approach may be necessary. A variety of transseptal sheaths are available. In our laboratory we use a standard Mulllins or selected Swartz directional sheath.

Once the LV has been accessed, all patients are anticoagulated with 5,000 uits of heparin. We administer 1,000–2,000 units/heparin per hour for the duration of the procedure to maintain an activated clotting time of 300.

After the catheters are properly positioned, attempts are made to induce the clinical VT. We use standard programmed electrical stimulation protocols, beginning with the least aggressive. The ability to induce the relevant tachycardia may present the biggest impediment to a successful procedure. If the standard protocol is unsuccessful at inducing the tachycardia, several maneuvers can be attempted. First, if the patient is overly sedated, allow them to wake up. Isuprel and special pacing techniques described later may be necessary for induction.

At times tachycardias are induced that do not appear to be the clinical tachycardia. These are frequently induced in patients with coronary artery disease. On rare occasions the "dominant" VT does not allow a second, often slower VT to be expressed. Usually we do not try to ablate VT unless it has been documented to have clinical significance. On some occasions a "new" morphology is easily induced after an initial apparently successful ablation. These may merely represent a new exit for the original tachycardia. We will proceed to ablate these new sites, particularly if they are closely related to the original ablation site. We have encountered patients in whom a nonclinical VT becomes incessant after the primary VT has been ablated. Those patients require ablation of the second focus.

Radiofrequency (RF) generators for ablation may be manually controlled or have thermistor feedback with automatic temperature or wattage control. These devices are helpful in that they will automatically power off in case the impedance rises, thereby minimizing the risk of coagulum

formation on the catheter tip. The temperature data are useful in assessing the degree of myocardial contact. If adequate temperature cannot be reached, there is usually poor contact between the myocardium and the ablation catheter. If the output drops to very low wattage, this suggests that the tip of the catheter is too deeply imbedded in the myocardium and is not being adequately cooled by the blood pool. In some patients the impedance remains high despite absence of coagulum formation. A second indifferent electrode placed on the thorax may lower the impedance and allow for adequate heating.

There is other information available to assess catheter contact. As previously mentioned, the unipolar electrogram recorded between the mapping catheter and a catheter placed in the inferior vena cava with low-frequency settings of 0.05–1 Hz will record the ST segment at the point of contact. As pressure on the myocardium increases, the ST segment will initially elevate. Elevations greater than 1–2 mV herald perforation of the ventricular wall. If a perforation occurs, the ST segment will depress and the usually negative QRS will become positive (Figure 2).[21] There are areas in the RV cavity near the base that produce S-T depression with initial contact and not elevation. These areas should not be interpreted as perforation. During RF energy delivery some patients experience discomfort. Those patients may require deeper anesthesia to prevent movement leading to displacement of the catheter.

We prefer to deliver RF during the VT. If no effect is seen within 20 sec, energy delivery is terminated and mapping continues. If the VT terminates, RF delivery is continued for 60–120 sec. Attempts at re-induction are done after termination of the tachycardia. If no further VT is induced, we wait 30–60 min and repeat the induction protocol. At the conclusion of the procedure, an activated clotting time is measured. When less than 150, the sheaths are removed, and the patient is transferred to the medical intensive care unit. We no longer measure

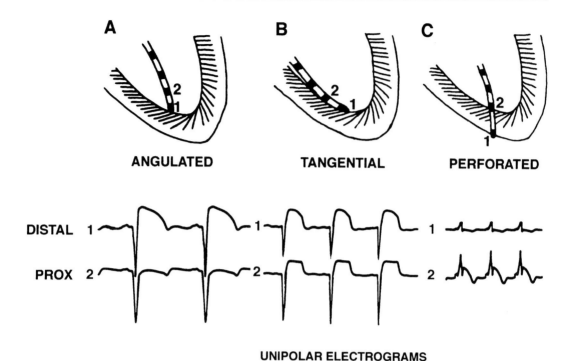

Figure 2. ST segment deviation is higher on the tip than the proximal electrode when the tip is against the ventricular wall. (**A**) The ST may be elevated in both leads when they are equally against the ventricular wall. (**B**) If the catheter perforates the ST will invert and the QRS becomes upright as in **C**. Used with permission from Singer I, ed.[58]

CPK after ablation, as our experience has been that few patients will leak enzyme after delivery of RF energy. Some centers will perform an electrophysiology study the next day, while others will wait for a clinical event.

Recording, Pacing, and Fluoroscopic Technique

The ability to safely manipulate the exploring catheter throughout the left ventricle and achieve consistent contact on left ventricular sites is usually the most difficult part of the procedure and requires persistence. At times a fresh operator will "find" the spot when more experienced operators have fallen into a routine that prevents access to the correct location.

Recognizing when the catheter is in a good location is much easier than getting it

there. The use of electrogram recordings and the classic responses to pacing identify fruitful ablation sites. The commonly used criteria are based both on reliable models of reentrant VT and systematic studies of success rates. The common pathway of a reentrant VT circuit is identified by these techniques. If it exists on a narrow isthmus, the tachycardia can be eliminated with RF energy administered to an electrode as small as 4 mm. Before RF, DC shocks were effective in part because they created a larger lesion.[22] Mapping techniques could be less precise. The earliest successful ablation using open heart surgery excised a 1 cm^2 patch of endocardium and also allowed less precise mapping.[23] The techniques used in these early methods for ablation have been adapted and refined for the more precise mapping required for RF ablation.[24,25] In good hands, the success rates with RF are as good as with DC ablation.

A systematic exploration requires the ability to place each catheter site on a general map of the LV and RV endocardium. Several maps have been developed for endocardial mapping. These include two apical, five mid, and five basal locations. These are located on three septal, five inferior and posterolateral walls, and four anterior positions (Figure 3).[26,27] Frame-grabbing fluoroscopic images in two planes, left anterior oblique (LAO) and right anterior oblique (RAO) or frontal and lateral, are the most helpful when determining the location of the catheter. Ideally, biplane fluoroscopy can be used. Analyzing the catheter locations is especially helpful when dealing with failure or a recurrence. The exact degree of LAO or RAO should be used for each new catheter position so that catheter positions can be superimposed on

each other to create a real image map. For example, 30° RAO and 60° LAO provide convenient orthogonal views. The exact degree of RAO and LAO used is not as important as consistently using the same angle in a given case. Each view needs to be numbered and related to recording sites. Modern electrophysiology computerized recorders allow frame-grabbing of a digital fluoroscopic image to be automatically placed in the record at the time the electrophysiology tracings are recorded. When this feature is not available, placing incremental radiopaque numbers in the fluoroscopic or cine path for each site can number sequential cine film recordings. Usually a small area of interest contains many mapped sites. Relatively minor changes can obtain a more ideal pacemap during either sinus rhythm or earlier,

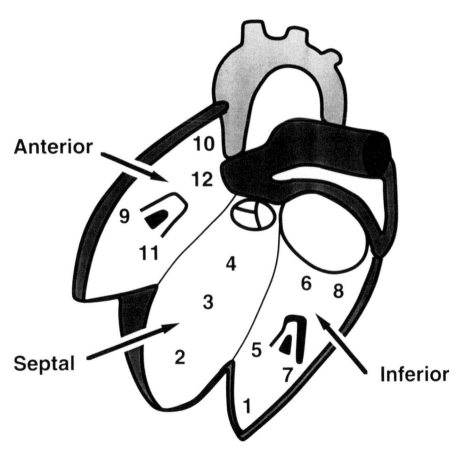

Figure 3. An example of LV positions for endocardial mapping after Josephson.

more discrete electrograms during VT, or better pacemapping during VT. Identifying regions in the heart that are not close to good ablation sites allows the team to focus on more fruitful areas. Systematic mapping allows one to determine when no LV site is present, and directs attention to the right ventricle. Right ventricular VT accounts for small but distinct percentage of successful ablation sites in coronary artery disease.

With modern recorders there is virtually no limitation of leads. The VT should be recorded with the 12 leads as they have been placed in the electrophysiology laboratory. Note that arm leads on the shoulders and leg leads on the hips do not reproduce exactly the 12-lead ECG that was recorded in the emergency room or critical care unit (CCU) during the clinical VT. As often as possible, the electrophysiology lab should place its leads in the standard 12-lead positions. When anterior defibrillating pads are placed low, the V_1 and V_2 are displaced laterally. If special leads were used in the CCU, these can be included as a bipolar lead at standard ECG recording frequencies such as a 0.05-Hz low-frequency setting. The MCL_1 lead is a bipolar monitoring lead whose positive electrode is on the V_1 position and whose negative electrode is on the left shoulder. This lead is commonly used in the CCU to simulate V_1 but will often be different from a standard recording of V_1. Note the critical difference in the standard V_1 and MCL_1 in Figure 4. A major clinical error was made in this case as the clinicians assumed the rsR' in MCL_1 indicated a supraventricular origin of the tachycardia. The early rise to peak in the true V_1, on the other hand, would favor VT with 1:1 retrograde conduction to the atrium.

Before pacing, always test threshold using a pulse width of 2 ms. Set the output to twice threshold. Make certain the ventricle is sensed before pacing to avoid pacing in the vulnerable period. Many programmed stimulators sense in sinus rhythm but pace S_1s at a fixed rate. Custom stimulators made for our lab and some commercial units could sense a premature ventricular beat during the S_1 drive and reset the S_1 count to 1 or continue at the next expected number. At the very least, all stimulators should sense the last QRS before pacing and pace at an interval likely to miss the vulnerable period. In VT patients, recurrent inadvertent inductions with paced R on T can cause the patient to rapidly deteriorate.

Ventricular tachycardia induction for purposes of ablation, especially in coronary artery disease, should be done as mildly as possible with longer S_1 drive cycles (600 ms) and as few extrastimuli as possible. The least aggressive protocol induces the slowest VT, and is unlikely to induce nonclinical arrhythmias. One needs the target VT, and whatever technique is required should be used. At times this means not just S_2, S_3, and S_4, but occasionally an S_5 and commonly the use of isuprel. When isuprel is required to induce the target VT, it is given initially as 0.5 mcg/min and increased gradually to a maximum of 3 mcg/min or a change in sinus rate of greater than 20 beats per minute. Caffeine (125 mg IV) may be helpful. On occasion, a long setup cycle in the drive train aids tachycardia induction. This is achieved by setting the S_1 intervals to seven cycles at 600 ms. The S_1S_2 is set to a long interval, which is limited by the atrial rate. Ventricular pacing must be pure on the eighth beat. The S_2S_3 on the stimulator is the first premature beat and therefore is the true S_1S_2. The S_3S_4 is likewise the S_2S_3. This long setup cycle before the premature beats extends refractory periods to allow unidirectional block and reentrant VT.[28]

When the target VT occurs, it is recorded in the lab with 12 leads and used as the reference morphology for all future pacing studies. Copies should be easily seen, both by those manipulating catheters and those monitoring and recording events. The ablation catheter should be moved to a suspected area. The onset of the earliest QRS on any of the 12 leads is determined. The lead, which shows the clearest and earliest break from baseline, is chosen to measure the onset of QRS in all subsequent interventions. It is important that this QRS

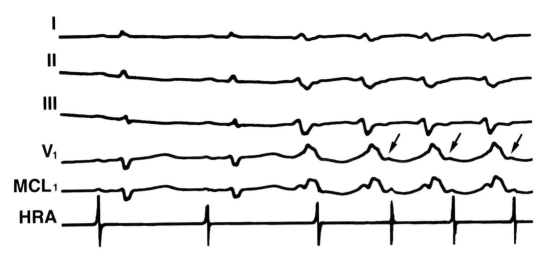

Figure 4. While the MCL$_1$ showed rSR' the V$_1$ recorded simultaneously in an EP lab showed early rise to peak revealing the true nature of its ventricular origin as confirmed by intracavitary recordings. Used with permission from Singer I, ed.[58]

onset be easily seen and reproduced. Always record the 12 lead at a high-frequency filter setting of 100 Hz. The ECG technician's temptation to provide "smooth" tracings with 50- or even 25-Hz high-frequency filters should be discouraged. The onset of the electrogram record on the ablation catheter and the time relationship with the earliest QRS onset is measured. If the VT is hemodynamically tolerated, the catheter is slowly manipulated to obtain an earlier electrogram site. When the VT is no longer tolerated or the mapping is complete, the VT is reverted with the pacing technique least likely to produce VF or polymorphic VT.

Once VT can be reliably induced and reverted by pacing, diagnostic pacing during the VT is started. Typically, pacing at twice threshold requires <1 milliampere (mA). Pacing from the standard 4-mm tip of an ablation catheter usually requires 3–5 mA to capture, but in areas of scar it may require current as high as 12–15 mA. Some investigators recommend high outputs, such as 35–45 mA, when pacemapping scars. This level is rarely necessary, and it may cause pacing of sites remote to the electrode position.

The S$_1$ of the stimulator is set 20–50 ms shorter than the measured VT cycle length (VTCL). Pacing is attempted during VT, always sensing the first QRS to avoid unduly premature pacing intervals. Short pacing intervals not only run the risk of R on T starting rapid polymorphous tachycardia, but more likely, and as important, short pacing intervals may revert the tachycardia or cause misleading delays between stimulus and QRS. At pacing intervals close to the VTCL, it frequently requires eight S$_1$s to assure full capture. Late partial capture with a large component of the VT morphology can give the erroneous impression that the paced QRS is identical to the VT. If the QRS morphology changes during pacing, the pacing site is not in the final common pathway.

Mapping and Pacing Response

The expected electrograms and response to pacing depend on current models for VT in coronary artery disease.[29] Most frequently, ablatable reentrant circuits require a substrate of scar caused by a myocardial infarction. This scar may or may not be an anatomic aneurysm, but the substrate

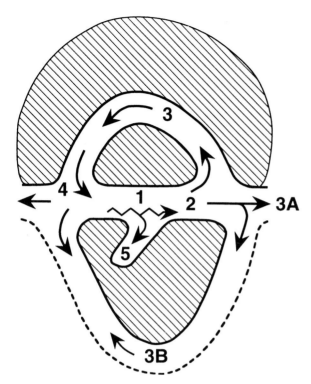

Figure 5. Ventricular tachycardia reentrant circuit (modified from Stevenson) shows the common pathway (1) exiting (2) to an inner loop (3), which reenters at the entrance (4) of the common pathway. The impulse passes from the exit (2) to exit pathway (3A) and simultaneously travels around an outer loop (3B) back to the entrance of the common pathway.

should contain both the barriers and the areas of slow conduction necessary for monomorphic reentrant VT.[30,31] The models recently presented by Stevenson et al. are legitimate simplifications of what is often a more complex electrophysiological source of clinical VT.[32–34] They make the most theoretical sense of the findings during VT mapping and help localize targets for ablating VT. The target of ablation therapy is the common pathway, which has an exit and an entrance connected by an inner loop (Figure 5). Other loops with longer paths or slower conduction can also connect the exit of the common pathway with the entrance but the pathway that leaves the common pathway first and returns to the entrance earliest will be the dominant inner loop. If this loop is ablated, the tachycardia could be sustained through a slower outer loop at a longer cycle length. The exit from the common pathway often branches into several exit pathways before the QRS on the external ECG is inscribed. Ablating after the exit from the common pathway but before

the QRS does not stop the tachycardia but may change the QRS morphology. On the other hand, when the common pathway is ablated, the tachycardia cannot be sustained.

As stated earlier, the common pathway is most amenable to ablation therapy when it narrows to a small isthmus and can be bridged by the 4-mm tip of an ablation catheter. Thus, the earliest sites may not be in as narrow a region as electrograms in mid-diastole. Some[35] have recommended an electrogram-to-QRS (EGM-QRS) no earlier than 70% of the VTCL (Figure 6[1]). On the other hand, electrograms that are quite early with an EGM-QRS of <30% of the VTCL are often recorded from areas emanating from the exit from the common pathway (Figure 6[2]) and includes exit pathways and the early portions of the inner and outer loops. Only rarely does ablating a site with these shorter EGM-QRS times revert to the VT and prevent its induction. The exact onset of the electrogram in the common pathway can be misinterpreted if the gain on the amplifier is relatively low. High gain is important to record the onset of consistent, small electrograms often seen in the common pathway. Appropriate gain is more important on modern digital recorders than it was in analog recorders. Many feel the onset of the electrogram is more important than whether the electrogram is discrete or continuous but isolated diastolic potentials may imply a narrow discrete isthmus amenable to ablation by 4-mm electrode ablating surfaces.[36,37]

Pacing during the tachycardia provides better lcalization. If the paced QRS is identical to the target VT in all 12 leads, the catheter is in the reentrant circuit or in a bystander circuit. Capture of the common pathway is determined by noting that the stimulus-to-QRS (S-QRS) equals the EGM-QRS and that these intervals are longer than 30 ms.

Bystander circuits can have intermediate EGM-QRS simulating common pathway recordings (Figure 6[5]), but stimulation from the exploring catheter during VT will indicate the origin of the electrogram to be outside the reentrant circuit. In such instances there will be a mismatch between recorded EGM-QRS and S-QRS. Conduction into a bystander pathway will make the recorded electrogram of the bystander pathway appear closer to onset of the QRS. It will be closer to the QRS by the amount of time it takes to conduct from the bystander pathway's origin in the common pathway to the recording site in the bystander pathway. When paced, the S-QRS will include the time it takes to conduct from the site on the bystander pathway to the common pathway. It also includes the time it takes to conduct from this point through the common pathway, to its exit. Finally, the S-QRS includes the relatively short time it takes to transmit from the exit of the common path-

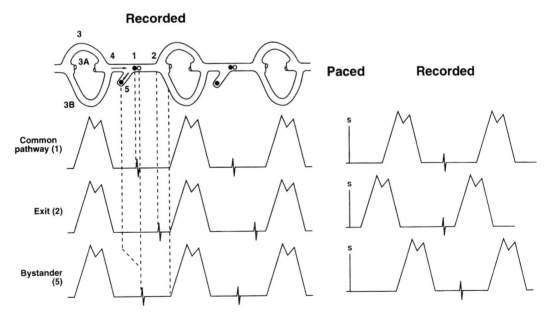

Figure 6. The loop diagram made continuous horizontal to depict several beats of VT. Classic recordings from the common pathway (1), exit pathway (2), and a bystander pathway (5) correspond to their respective positions in the continuous loop. Note the EGM-QRS of the bystander pathway appears earlier than the common pathway but is due to the conduction time from the common pathway to the recording spot on the bystander circuit. While the paced vs. recorded right panel shows that the S-QRS is equal to the EGM-QRS in the common pathway (1) and the exit site (2), the S-QRS is longer than the EGM-QRS in the bystander pathway (5). Used with permission from Singer I, ed.[58]

way to the subsequently inscribed QRS. Recording in the common pathway, on the other hand, always has an S-QRS equal to the EGM-QRS. When the S-QRS and the E-QRS are equal (<20 ms), the catheter is in the reentrant circuit.

Pacing from the recording site during VT not only allows a comparison S-QRS with EGM-QRS, but it also allows one to assess entrainment.[38,39] The VT was entrained when the VT continues after the pacing is stopped and the last paced QRS is the same morphology as the VT. Entrainment can often occur when the paced area is either in the VT circuit or if the excitable gap of the VT circuit is entered from a site outside the reentrant circuit.[40,41] More rapid pacing during VT, as much as 100 ms less than the VTCL, is often done to confirm no change of QRS and therefore no progressive fusion. Entrainment with fusion indicates catheter sites at either the entrance or the exit of the

slow zone, or that the pacing has engaged the excitable gap from outside the tachycardia circuit.[42] Concealed[43] entrainment is present if when pacing at 20–50 ms less than the VTCL, the VT morphology is unchanged, and the return beat is advanced (Figure 7A). If the paced QRS is not identical to the VT, fusion may be occurring. Fusion is more likely to be seen with pacing at faster intervals such as 100 ms shorter than the VT cycle. If the QRS is altered more with a more rapid pacing rate, progressive fusion is present.[44] When progressive fusion is present in classic entrainment, it specifically indicates a site in the outer loop or entrance to the common pathway. Even when progressive fusion occurs with entrainment the last paced QRS is always similar to the tachycardia (Figure 7B). This is because the fusion occurs between the previous orthodromically conducted beat in the VT circuit and depolarization of ventricular myocar-

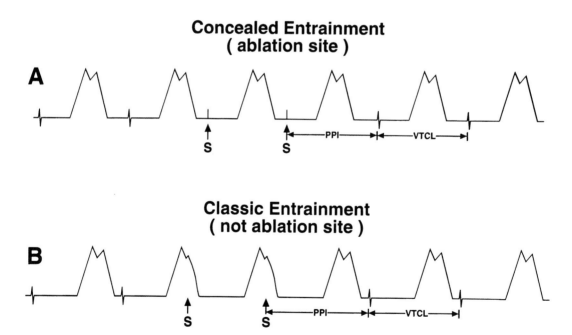

Figure 7. The top panel shows: (A) Pacing during concealed entrainment advances the QRS with no change in QRS morphology and indicates a position of the catheter in the common pathway. The post-pacing interval (PPI) is equal to the VT cycle length (VTCL); (B) stimulation with entrainment and fusion. The first paced beat fuses with the prior VT reentrant beat and advances the next QRS. The last paced beat fuses with the previous QRS but causes normal VT complex on the last paced beat. A faster pace rate would cause more fusion (progressive fusion). The PPI is >VTCL. This does not represent a good ablation site. Used with permission from Singer I, ed.[58]

dium conducted antidromically from the stimulation site. The stimulation itself also enters the tachycardia circuit and conducts orthodromically the next QRS. If pacing is continued, this orthodromically conducted QRS will fuse with antidromic conduction from the next stimulus. The last stimulus in the train will fuse with the previous QRS and conduct orthodromically a QRS, which contains no antidromic component and therefore is identical to the QRS of the native VT. Thus, for all types of entrainment the last paced QRS is the same as the QRS of the VT. Since progressive fusion with entrainment usually does not indicate a position in the common pathway. It is important to view the next to the last paced QRS to determine if an exact morphology match has been achieved. If pacing produces a QRS morphology identical to the VT but at the faster pacing rate and there is no change in QRS even at faster paced rates, entrainment is concealed and the pacing is occurring in the common pathway.

Once concealed entrainment without fuson is established, the interval between the last stimulus and the local electrogram of the first VT QRS is measured as the post-pacing interval (PPI) and compared to the VTCL. If the catheter is in the circuit, the first PPI will be equal to the VTCL. The circuit includes the common pathway, its exit, the inner loop, and its entrance. If the pacing site is not in the VT circuit, the PPI will usually be more than the VTCL. This includes bystander sites, exit pathway, and sites distant from the reentry loop. While the common pathway, the exit, inner loop, and the entrance sites all have a PPI equal to the VTCL, they are distinguished from each other by the EGM-QRS duration.

While there are many possible recordings and pacing responses to specific areas in and around the VT circuit, the only response that must be remembered during mapping is the response when in the common pathway. All other responses are not in the common pathway. Recognizing a good position is usually easy if the VT can be initiated and is hemodynamically stable.

Table 1 suggests an orderly assessment of recording and pacing (1). The first step is to search for exact 12-lead pacemap while pacing in sinus rhythm (2). When exact or close, induce the VT and search for the earliest electrogram during VT (3). Then pace during VT at 20–50 ms less than the VTCL. When consistent capture is achieved, match the paced 12-lead QRS morphology with the target VT. When the paced QRS is an exact match in all 12 leads of the external ECG, compare the EGM-QRS to the S-QRS to see if they are within 20 ms. If VT is sustained when pacing is stopped, entrainment has probably occurred. Measure the PPI and compare with the next VT cycle. If they are equal (<30 ms) the catheter is in the reentrant circuit and therapeutic ablation should proceed (4). Pacing at a more rapid rate, 100 ms shorter than the VTCL, excludes progressive fusion. The catheter often requires adjustment by small amounts to closely match the VT in all 12 leads of the external ECG. The first pacing intervention, a pacemap in sinus rhythm, can be quite valuable for general localization. Pacing in sinus rhythm may not match the VT morphology in all 12 leads. In sinus rhythm, the paced rhythm may propagate both retrogradely or antidromically, and antegradely or orthodromically from the area of slow conduction, and thus may not produce a fusion of the QRS produced at the exit and the entrance of the slow zone. In one series the site of concealed entrainment rarely produced an exact pacemap during sinus rhythm.[11] On the other hand, when pacing well into the common pathway of slow conduction during VT, the returning waveform of the VT prevents antidromic conduction. Orthodromic conduction proceeds slowly, but when it exits the common pathway, the QRS is early and exactly matches the clinical tachycardia in all 12 leads. This event is concealed entrainment. No amount of prematurity is likely to create any of the progressive fusion seen in classic entrainment. When entrainment is concealed, a position well within the common pathway is likely and the site is a good site for ablation.

Table 1

Summary of Different Responses to Pacing during NSR and Ventricular Tachycardia According to Catheter Placement within the Circuit

Site	Distant (6)	Common Pathway (1) Ablate	Exit (2)	Inner Loop (3)	Exit Path (3A)	Outer Loop (3B)	Entrance (4)	Bystander Pathway (5)
Sinus Rhythm								
(1) Pacemap								
QRS in 12-lead match	no	yes/no	yes/rarely no	yes/no	no close match	no	yes/rarely yes	yes/rarely no
Ventricular Tachycardia								
(2) Record								
Earliest EGM <70% VTCL	after QRS	before QRS −30 to −70% VTCL	before QRS −30 to 0% VTCL	before QRS	before QRS	after QRS	before QRS	before QRS shorter than S-QRS
(3) Pace - 50 ms shorter than VTCL *Ablation Criteria*								
QRS in 12-lead match	no	yes	yes	yes	no (minor)	no	yes	yes
S-QRS equals EGM QRS	>>	=	=	= or <	=	>	= or <	>
PPI equals VTCL		=	= or >	=	= or >	=	=	>
(4) Pace - 100 ms shorter than VTCL								
QRS in 12-lead match	no	yes	yes	yes	no	yes/no	no (fusion)	yes
PPI equals VTCL	>	=	=	> or =	>	=	=	>

PPI = post-pacing interval; VTCL = ventricular tachycardia cycle length.

The negative findings that mandate repositioning include an electrogram that is in or after the QRS onset or is exceedingly short such as 20–30 ms. The catheter is not on the common pathway. If the paced QRS during VT does not match exactly, concealed entrainment has not occurred and the catheter needs to be repositioned. If the S-QRS is greater or less than the EGM-QRS, or the PPI is greater than the VTCL, the catheter is not in the reentrant circuit. When one of these negative findings are present, the catheter should be repositioned to a better location.

All the measurements can be made using a simple four-beat analysis at the termination of pacng during VT (Figure 8). Once the catheter is guided to a probable VT site by pacemap, the VT should be induced. Then pace at 20–50 ms less than the VTCL.

Be certain that pacing captures the QRS. When the QRS stops walking through the stimulation artifact, capture is likely. After termination of pacing, freeze the last two intervals paced and the first two intervals not paced. Measure the first two QRS intervals to confirm the R-R is less than the VTCL and equal to the S-S interval. Compare the last two paced beats with the first two post-pacing beats of the VT. Compare the paced QRS in all 12 leads with the adjacent VT morphology. Note whether the electrogram is isolated or continuous. Compare the S-QRS and the EGM-QRS. If the paced and VT QRS match and these intervals do not differ more than 20 ms, the circuit was paced. If the first PPI equals the next interval, which is the VTCL, the circuit was paced. The PPI will not equal the VTCL if a bystander pathway was paced. Once as many positive attributes as possible have been identified, an attempt to ablate the site is made. In the best of hands, the perfect site may not be recorded and paced. The lack of a perfect site, with all criteria met, does not mean the rhythm will not be ablated. Carefully sample the area where the majority of the criteria are met. Ablation with RF can be successful in these suites and should be attempted. At times more than one lesion is required at closely related sites. Creating a continuous lesion toward fixed nonconductive structures such as the mitral valve may prove successful where exact criteria cannot be recorded.

Stevenson et al.,[33] Fitzgerald et al.,[45] and Bogun et al.,[46] have reported systematic studies. The most reliable positive findings as documented with percentage of times the VT was terminated by ablation are shown in in Table 2.

The higher percentage of patients with concealed entrainment and with sucess after ablation reported by Bogun et al.[46] is probably because their patients had a high percentage with slow VT (mean VTCL = 500 ms), and incessant tachycardia (50%). Most were treated with antitachycardia devices (72%) and were on antiarrhythmic medications. Their success rates were higher and the rate of success with each criteria was likewise higher but the relative value of the several criteria was similar. The only criteria that was not proportionately

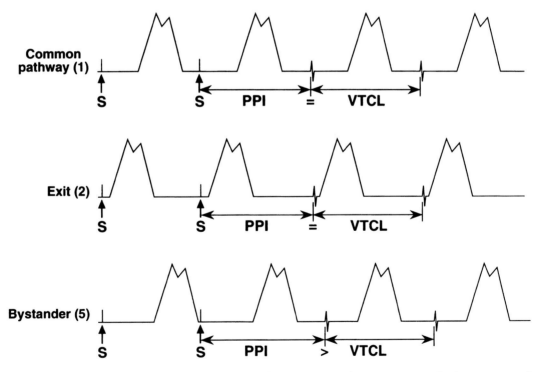

Figure 8. A simple analysis when pacemapping during VT is to freeze on screen the last two paced beats and the first two beats of the VT. This allows comparison of the morphology of paced and VT beats, a comparison of the S-QRS and EGM-QRS and a comparison of the PPI and the VTCL. Since the last paced beat in entrainment is always the VT morphology, the next to last paced beat or first beat in the four-beat analysis should be compared with the VT morphology to detect fusion forms. The common pathway has identical QRS morphology with intermediate EGM-QRS, S-QRS = EGM-QRS, and PPI >VTCL. The exit pathway is the same beat with short EGM-QRS and S-QRS. The bystander has good pacemapping but S-QRS is >EGM-QRS and PPI >VTCL. Used with permission from Singer I, ed.[58]

Table 2
Termination of Ventricular Tachycardia

	Stevenson	Bogun
Pacing during VT at long cycle lengths which has:		
Reproduces VT morphology in 12 leads and shows CE	17%	54%
S-QRS >60 msec, <70% VTCL and CE	36%	71%
EGM-QRS equal to the S-QRS (<20 ms) and CE	24%	82%
Has PPI = VTCL (<30 ms) and CE	25%	45%
Mid-diastolic isolated potential and CE	45%	67%
Not dissociated from VT	NA	89%

CE = concealed entrainment; VTCL = ventricular tachycardia cycle length.

similar was the PPI = VTCL. As discussed by the authors, this may be due to a variation in technique. Stevenson et al.[33] took care to pace and record unipolar signals while Bogun et al.[46] used a separate bipolar pair to pace and record. Nonetheless, the two studies are largely in agreement as to the relative value of the criteria for successful ablation.

An alternative method for pacing during VT is the use of single premature paced beats. A single premature paced beat can fuse with the previous beat of the tachycardia and advance the next beat of the tachycardia when entrainment has occurred. When concealed entrainment has occurred, only the advanced beat of the tachycardia is seen. When the premature paced beat has an S-QRS equal to EGM-QRS and has a PPI equal to the VTCL, the catheter is on the common pathway. A particularly close localization is indicated when further prematurity does not capture the ventricle but extinguishes the tachycardia. This is thought always to be due to concealed conduction in the common pathway and is confirmed by several labs to be a sign of a successful ablation site.[46–51]

Single paced premature beats from the RV apex have been used during VT to reset the tachycardia and their associated isolated diastolic potential.[53] If a premature beat from the RV captures the ventricle and then advances a QRS identical to the VT, entrainment has occurred. If the ablation catheter records the isolated diastolic potential with an EGM-QRS of the entrained VT beat, identical to the EGM-QRS of the spontaneous VT, the isolated diastolic potential is associated with the VT circuit. Ablation of these sites produces excellent results (72% successful). When the EGM-QRS of the paced QRS is not the same, the electrogram is dissociated and ablation produced no success. Because the recording catheter is not the pacing catheter, this technique has the advantage of easily seeing the electrogram during pacing. While this is a newly reported technique and isolated diastolic potentials are not found in all patients, it adds to our armamentarium for identifying ablation sites by pacing during tachycardia.

Ablation with Radiofrequency

Once a site is mapped, RF current is the therapy of choice at this time. All machines at 500–750 kHz designed for electrocautery have worked well in the unipolar mode in human arrhythmia ablation. Modern equipment designed for human ablation should allow rapid switching from recording and pacing to ablation. This is important because the catheter position identified may not be stable. An unchanging electrogram often indicates good contact. ST elevation from a unipolar low-frequency electrogram also indicates good contact. Unchanging steady rise in thermistor temperature also indicates good contact. The thermistor temperature of 60° assures cell death. Avoiding temperatures above 90° prevents coagulation and inordinate rises in impedance. An effective standard dose for VT is 30 watt-seconds for 1 minute. Whenever possible, ablation should begin with the patient in VT. When VT reverts during RF, the application is commonly successful. Reversion of VT usually occurs in <20 sec. If VT has not reverted in 30 sec, further energy rarely causes reversion. A 60-sec application should be used when the ablation energy reverts the VT.

A common practice is to create a second lesion in the same area. If the site was well chosen and the VT reverted early (<10 sec), a second application is not necessary. Attempts to re-induce the tachycardia in the next few minutes should be made before the catheter is moved. Since the catheter pressure on a well chosen site can itself prevent VT, a second attempt to re-induce should be made after the catheter has been moved.

If the impedance rises greater than 100 ohms, the catheter should be removed and the coagulum at the tip cleaned before it is re-inserted. Electrical stunning from energy in a site near the common pathway may recover in 60 min and allow the VT to be induced. Edema and transient inability of cells to be excited from the ablation may clear at a later date and allow the VT, which had been noninducible to be inducible. Recurrence is seen and is itself available for further mapping and ablation most of the time. If the VT target is no longer inducible, the ablation procedure is stopped.

On occasions other monomorphic tachycardia become inducible, or, on rare occasions, slower, incessant VT appears. If the tachycardia is incessant, an attempt to locate its origin and ablate it should be made. If a monomorphic VT is seen that was not recorded clinically, there is a good chance it may become clinically significant. All clinical targets should be ablated. A new VT, which is not incessant and is difficult to induce, could be ignored until it becomes clinically significant. After the ablation, the pa-

tient can be returned to the monitored bed. Monitoring post-procedure will assess success and allow rapid response to any new VT or old VT if it recurs.

The evaluation of the patient post-ablation is difficult. Partial successes are very important for individual patients. Absence of the clinical VT is an obvious success. No recurrence of the target VT is important if the target was relatively slow and prevented adequate recognition by antitachycardia pacing/defibrillating devices. If VT with a similar morphology and rate does not recur, the ablation procedure is considered a success. If VT recurs but can be suppressed with drugs that were not previously effective, a partial success has occurred.

Case Studies

Patient W

An interesting example of the application of principle of ablation of patients with coronary disease, is patient W who had recurrent VT for 6 months. The patient had no response to standard antiarrhythmic drugs and only a partial response to amiodarone. The VT could be induced after amiodarone but at a slower rate. Due to side effects, the dose was reduced to 100 mg every other day. The amiodarone was discontinued 2 weeks before coronary artery bypass surgery. The same monomorphic VT recurred in the postoperative period. Amiodarone was restarted. An electrophysiology study 10 days later failed to induce VT. Amiodarone again was not tolerated and discontinued. One month after discharge, the patient had an episode of clinical VT. Two distinct morphology types had been seen clinically, both at relatively slow rates. An antitachycardia device could be used, but the rate of the tachycardia would overlap with the patient's sinus rate, making detection and treatment difficult. An electrophysiology study for ablation initially reproduced two morphologically distinct VT events, VT-1

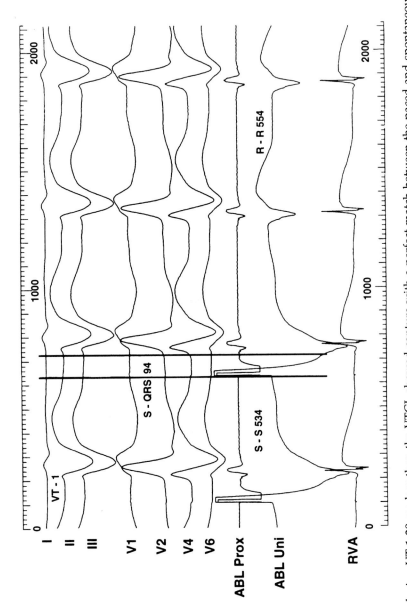

Figure 9. Pacing during VT-1 20 ms less than the VTCL showed capture with a perfect match between the paced and spontaneous VT QRS. The S-QRS was an intermediate 94 ms equal to the electrogram recorded shortly thereafter. Used with permission from Singer I, ed.[58]

and VT-2, both seen clinically. Pacemapping during sinus rhythm rapidly demonstrated a good morphological match in all 12 leads for VT-1. The fluoroscopic image of the ablation catheter position in RAO and LAO placed the site on the inferior septum (Figure 10A). VT induction showed a relatively early EGM-QRS. During concealed entrainment the S-QRS was 94 ms (Figure 9) which was equal to the EGM-QRS. Pacing from this site reverted to VT-2 without capturing the ventricle (Figure 11). Radiofrequency delivery for 30 W for 60 sec also reverted to VT-2 (Figure 12). VT-1 was no longer inducible. VT-2 was an LBBB morphology with a more horizontal axis.

Pacemapping high under the tricuspid valve from the right ventricle produced an exact morphology map but with short EGM-QRS (36 ms) and S-QRS (40 ms) (Fig-

ure 13). Ablation at this probable exit site did not prevent induction of VT. On the LV septal wall opposite the RV exit site a long S-QRS was seen with a perfect 12-lead match of VT-1 morphology (Figure 14). Pacing from this site extinguished VT-2 without capturing the ventricle and then captured with a VT-1 morphology (Figure 15). The catheter positions for the previous attempt at extinguishing VT-2 from the RV and the new position in the LV are quite close (Figure 10B). The decision to ablate this site despite the inability to induce VT-1 at this time was based on the fact that VT-2 could be reverted by pacing from this site without capturing the myocardium and intermediate diastolic potentials at the previous ECG-QRS interval were recorded during pacing. In addition, VT-1 became noninducible before RF in VT-1 position in-

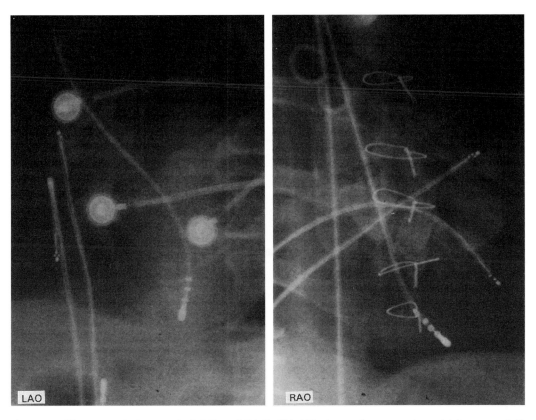

Figure 10. Fluoroscopic images in LAO and RAO: (**A**) Ablation catheter on site, which successfully ablated VT-1.

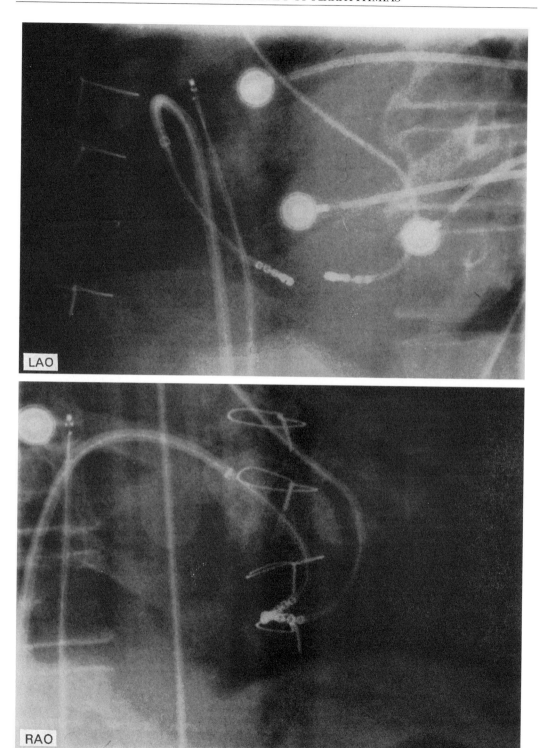

Figure 10. *(Continued)* **(B)** RV catheter at unsuccessful site near exit of VT-2 with LV catheter on site where VT-2 was ablated from the LV.

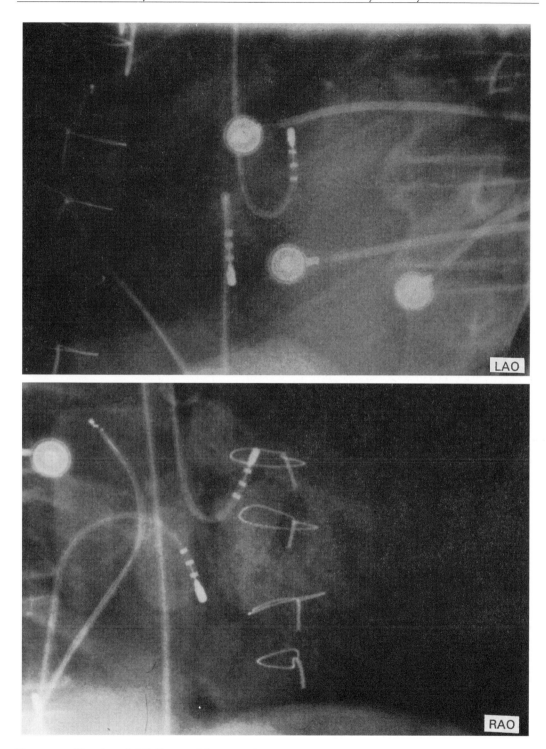

Figure 10. *(Continued)* **(C)** Shows ablation catheter in LV outflow with close but not exact pacemap for VT-3.

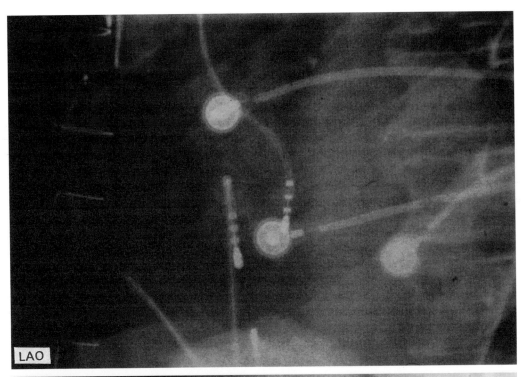

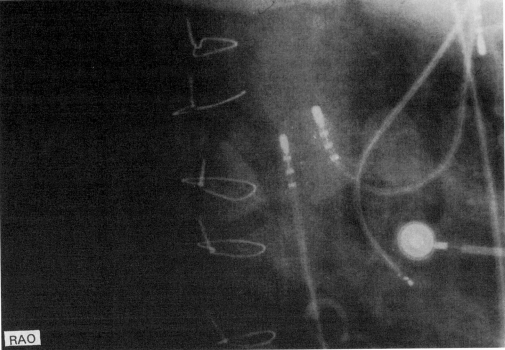

Figure 10. *(Continued)* **(D)** Shows ablation catheter in medial LV outflow where VT-3 had an exact pacemap during VT and concealed entrainment and was ablated. Used with permission from Singer I, ed.[58]

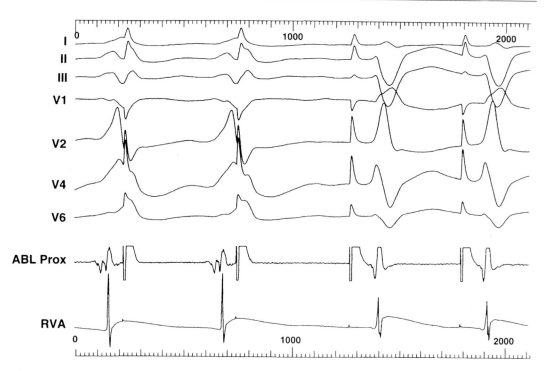

Figure 11. VT-2 stops after the second stimulus, which failed to capture the ventricle. The third and fourth reproduce exactly the morphology of VT-1 with an S-QRS of 100 ms. Used with permission from Singer I, ed.[58]

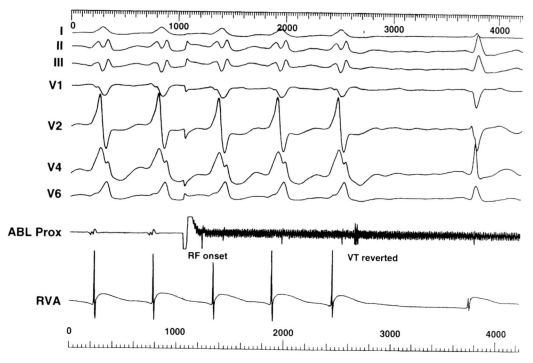

Figure 12. VT-2 stops after 1.8 sec of RF at VT-1 site. VT-1 could not be induced after catheter placement. (Catheter position, Figure 10A.) Used with permission from Singer I, ed.[58]

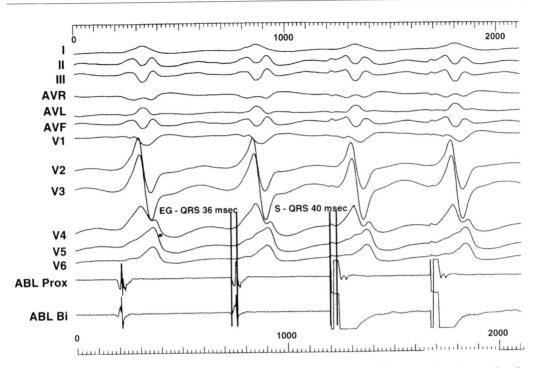

Figure 13. VT-2 morphology was closely matched by pacing in the RV under the tricuspid valve with a short S-QRS (40 ms) approximately equal to the EG-QRS (36 ms) . (RV catheter position, Figure 10B.) Used with permission from Singer I, ed.[58]

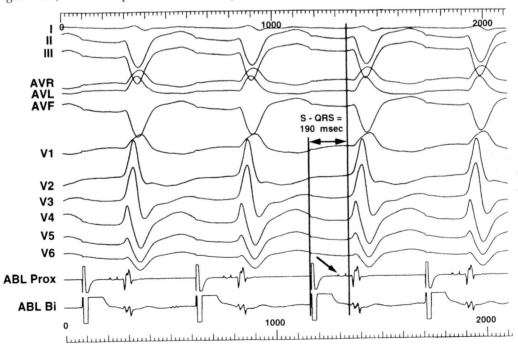

Figure 14. From the opposite side of the septum pacemap produced exact match of VT-1 with S-QRS of 190 ms and clear diastolic potentials (see arrow). (LV catheter position, Figure 10B.) Used with permission from Singer I, ed.[58]

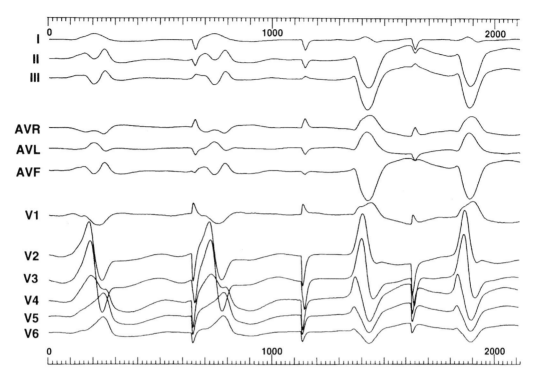

Figure 15. Pacing stopped VT-2 without capture and then produces an exact match of VT-1 with long (200 ms) S-QRS. (LV catheter position, Figure 10B.) Used with permission from Singer I, ed.[58]

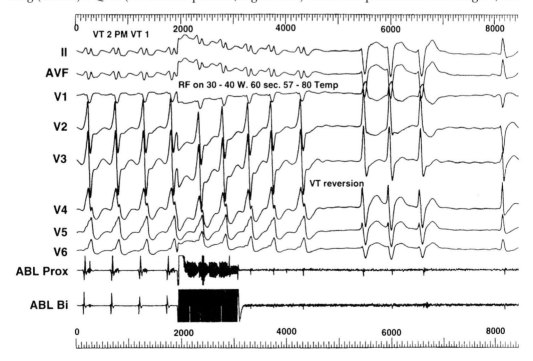

Figure 16. An RF 30 W for 60 sec with temperature 68° reverts VT-2 after which it could not be induced. (LV catheter position, Figure 10B.) Used with permission from Singer I, ed.[58]

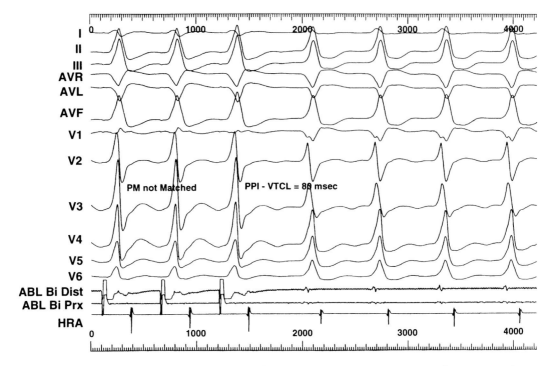

Figure 17. Pacemap during VT was not matched in V_1, I and the PPI-VTCL of 80 ms. (Catheter position, Figure 10C.) Used with permission from Singer I, ed.[58]

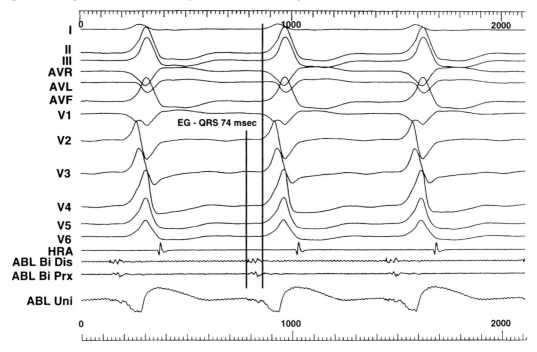

Figure 18. An earlier electrogram was present at a medial lower site. The EG-QRS was 74 ms. Used with permission from Singer I, ed.[58]

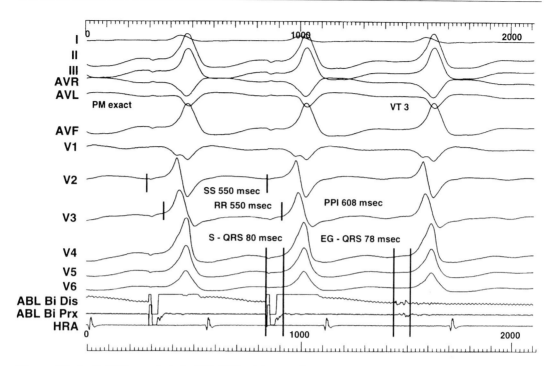

Figure 19. An S-QRS equaled the EG-QRS with a perfect pacemap for VT-3. Used with permission from Singer I, ed.[58]

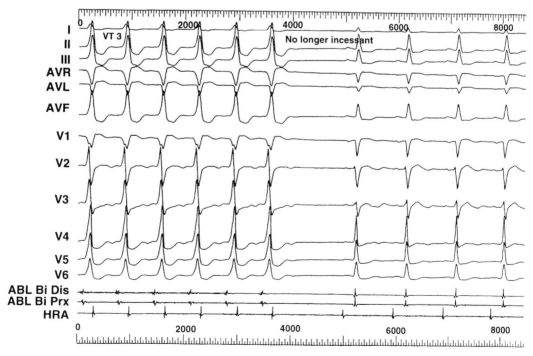

Figure 20. The incessant VT-3 stopped during RF ablation, after which no VT could be induced. (Catheter position, Figure 10D.) Used with permission from Singer I, ed.[58]

dicating possible temporary mechanical injury of the reentrant circuit. After RF energy at the LV site, VT-2 was reverted (Figure 16) and neither VT-1 nor VT-2 could be induced. However, a new slow, incessant VT (VT-3) was evident at 95 bpm. An attempt to map VT-3 to the lateral outflow that did not produce a successful map (Figure 17) (and the catheter position is depicted in Figure 10C). After a change of catheters to one with a shorter radius, VT-3 was mapped to the medial LV outflow tract (Figure 10D). A perfect pacemap was achieved with electrogram. QRS was equal to the S-QRS (Figures 18 and 19). The incessant VT-3 stopped during ablation (Figure 20). After all three VT sites were ablated, no VT could be induced with or without isuprel. Thus, a good clinical result was achieved despite three separate VT morphologies. All three probably originated from different levels of the same scar. VT-1 and VT-2 were quite closely

linked with one exiting the left septum and the other exiting the right. The slower VT-3 may have been facilitated through an outer loop after the inner loop was ablated. It is important to recognize and discard catheter-induced tachycardia, which occurred in this case (Figure 21). The rates are often irregular with large early electrograms and associated ST deviation on the ablation catheter. While the case was not "classic," many of the standard principles were used to achieve a good clinical outcome.

Patient M

Mr. M is a patient who had recurrent VT reverted by 0.6-joule biphasic shocks. Pace-out of his VT was successful only at rapid rates. The farfield electrogram from his device displayed first VT, and then post-shock sinus tachycardia (Figure 22). The sinus tachycardia was also shocked needlessly.

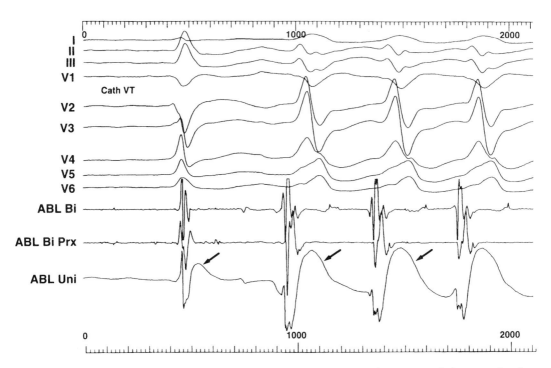

Figure 21. One of many examples of catheter-induced VT during this case with large early electrogram and associated ST elevation on the unipolar recording from the tip of the catheter. These VTs are frequently irregular and can be more difficult to distinguish when the catheter is close to a VT site. Used with permission from Singer I, ed.[58]

Before VT

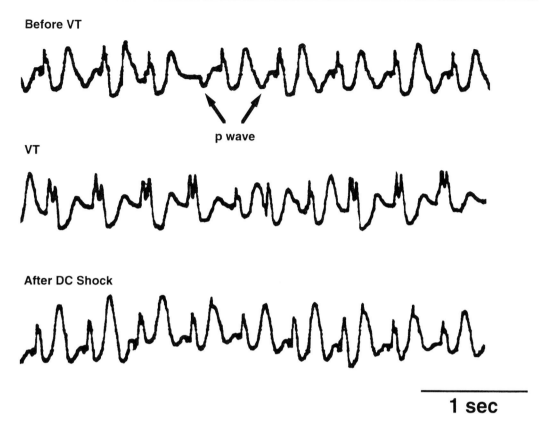

p wave

VT

After DC Shock

1 sec

Figure 22. The patient's implantable defibrillator was capable of recording and storing a farfield ECG in which P waves could be seen and the conducted QRS morphology defined (top panel), with the onset of VT close to the sinus tachycardia rate the defibrillator recognized the event and shocked (middle panel). Immediately post-shock, the patient's sinus tachycardia accelerated (lower panel), causing the defibrillator to shock the patient inappropriately two more times. Used with permission from Singer I, ed.[58]

Later this VT became incessant. Thus, this patient had two indications for ablation of this target VT: the first was the inability to distinguish sinus tachycardia from VT; and the second was that the tachycardia became incessant. Catheters were manipulated until an early EGM-QRS was found (Figure 23). Radiofrequency at 30 W for 60 sec reverted the VT (Figure 24). The patient has never had a recurrence of his VT after the successful ablation in 3 years of follow-up.

Patient AG

Mr. AG is a 63-year-old man with coronary artery disease who presented with sustained VT 3 months after a large anterior myocardial infarction. The ejection fraction was 35%. He was initially treated with amiodarone, with a subsequent negative EPS. However, he developed mild pulmonary toxicity and after discontinuing amiodarone he received a nonthoracotomy defibrillator. Over the next year he experienced an increasing number of defibrillating shocks. Amiodarone was restarted. He then experienced recurrences of a slow sustained tachycardia with rates that overlapped with his sinus mechanism. It was then decided to take the patient for ablative therapy to eliminate the dominant clinical tachycardia. The clinical tachycardia, which could only be induced when the patient was awake, had a superior axis and deep negative forces out to lead V_6 (Figure 25). As expected the tachy-

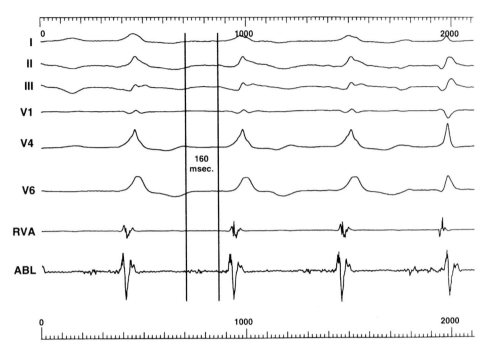

Figure 23. An early electrogram was recorded during incessant VT. Used with permission from Singer I, ed.[58]

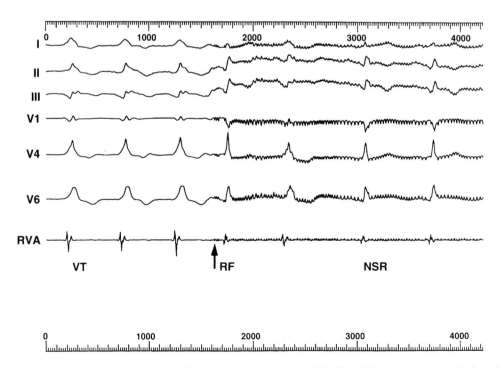

Figure 24. The incessant VT reverted shortly after onset of RF. The VT never recurred after this successful ablation. Used with permission from Singer I, ed.[58]

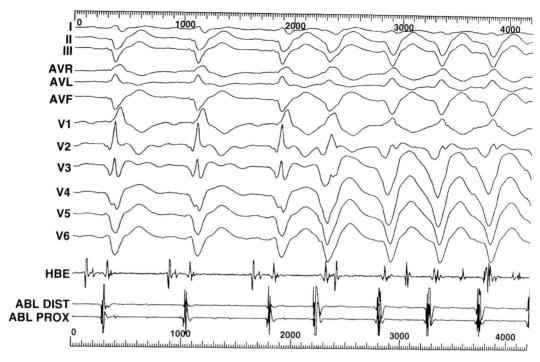

Figure 25. The clinical VT occurred spontaneously when the patient was awake. The morphology of the VT was consistent with an apical position.

cardia was mapped to the left ventricular apex along the septum (Figure 26). Complicating the ablation was the appearance of what seemed to be a second wide complex tachycardia at the same rate as the clinical arrhythmia (Figure 27). Closer scrutiny revealed that the QRS morphology was identical to the normal QRS and that a His bundle recording and then a P wave preceded each beat. This was a supraventricular tachycardia, which overlapped with the VT. In this case it was difficult to find an ideal pacemap and the best site still had a PPI<VTCL (Figure 28). Despite that, the VT terminated with RF energy (Figure 29). The patient has not had a recurrence of sustained VT in 10 months.

Patient JB

Mr. JB was a 45-year-old man with coronary artery disease and an old inferior wall myocardial infarction. He presented with VT to another institution and underwent an ablation. He did well until 9 months later when he presented to our hospital with a recurrence of his clinical arrhythmia. At that time coronary angiography demonstrated patent arteries and a fixed inferior wall defect. Several sites were mapped to the LV. Initially a good 12-lead morphological match was found, but note that the activation sequence during pacing was not identical to that during the clinical tachycardia (Figure 30). During pacemapping, QRS onset to proximal coronary sinus time was 37 ms, compared to 15 ms during the tachycardia. Further mapping then identified a site where the activation map was identical during pacing as well as during the spontaneous arrhythmia (Figure 31). Radiofrequency delivery at this site terminated the arrhythmia within 7 sec (Figure 32). There has not been a recurrence in several years.

Limitations

As with any procedure there may be limitations, which affect success. Investigators

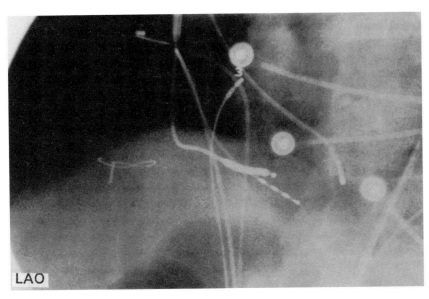

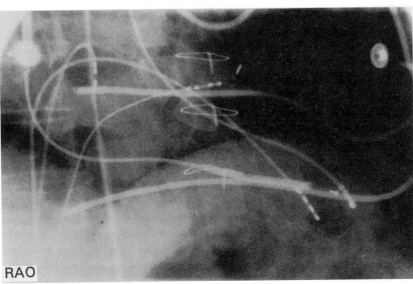

Figure 26. Radiographs in the LAO and RAO projection showing the apical and inferior position of the ablation catheter.

have reported success rates as low as 50% and as high as 80% and recurrences can be as frequent.[52] A key to success is often careful choice of the appropriate patient. The hemodynamically compromised patient who has difficulty tolerating VT may not be the ideal candidate. Recognizing that the nature of the disease is one of multiple VT morphologies with a high recurrence rate is crucial. The intracardiac anatomy is such that identifying the exact position with a small 4-mm tip catheter may be difficult, and although the procedure is considerably safer than DC current ablation there are reports in the literature of complications due to RF ablation.[53] Procedural complications have been reported both with DC and with RF ablation. Pericardial tamponade second-

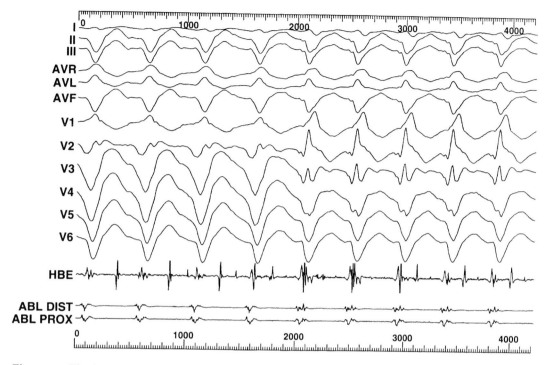

Figure 27. The left side of the tracing shows the clinical VT. There is a morphology change at beat 5. Careful scrutiny of the HBE channel shows an atrial and His bundle deflection proceeding each subsequent beat consistent with a supraventricular tachycardia.

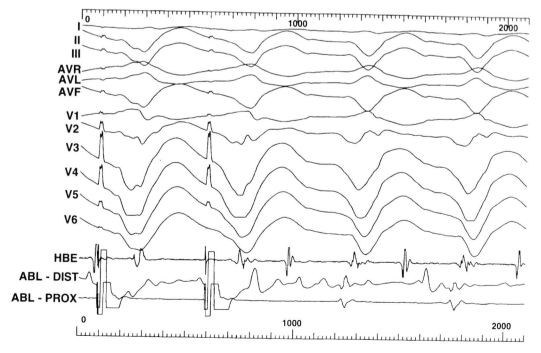

Figure 28. Pacemapping during VT. Note subtle differences in lead II.

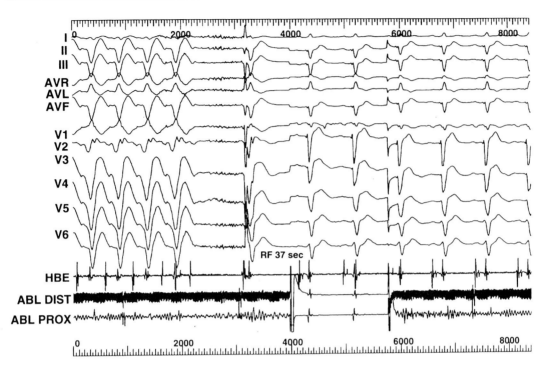

Figure 29. Termination of VT with RF energy.

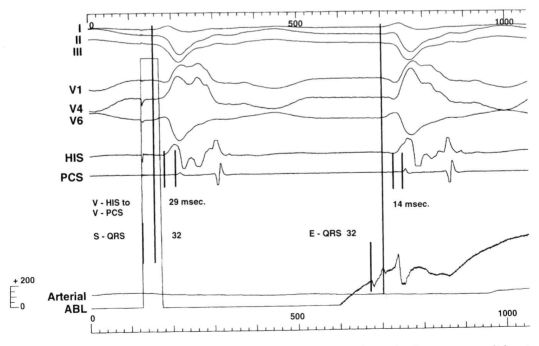

Figure 30. Pacemapping during VT showed a good match, but the activation sequence did not. Note the QRS onset to PCS was 29 ms during pacing, and QRS to PCS was 14 ms during tachycardia.

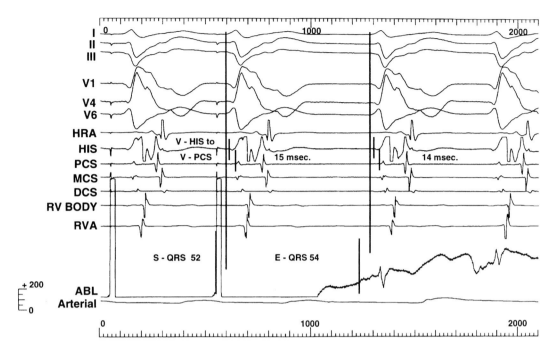

Figure 31. This site shows identical pacemap as well as activation sequence. Note the time V-HIS to V-PCS is 15 ms during pacing and 14 ms during tachycardia. The stimulus to S-QRS = 52 ms; the EGM-QRS = 54 ms.

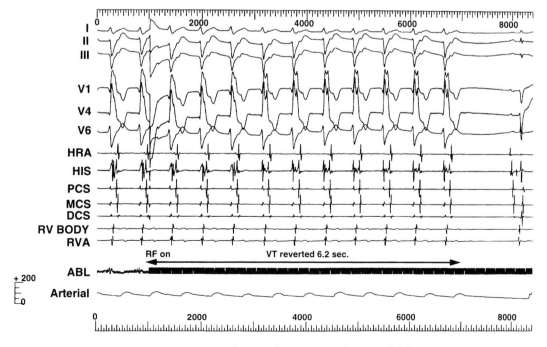

Figure 32. Termination of VT within 6.2 sec of onset of RF energy.

ary to perforation leading to patient death has been reported.[54-56] Perforation when it occurs is as commonly due to catheter manipulation in an anticoagulated patient as due to the actual ablation energy. Transient heart block has been seen in patients who receive RF to the basal septum. There have been reports of sudden death in patients who have had RF ablation.

Conclusion

Ablation of VT in patients with coronary artery disease has been life-saving, especially when the VT is incessant and unresponsive to antiarrhythmic therapy. As a primary therapy, ablation has not been used because of its intermediate success rate (50%–70%). As specific locations are identified, the procedure may be used earlier. For example, VTs that use a narrow isthmus of conducting tissue between scars from myocardial infarction and the mitral valve fibrous ring are ablated when a line of RF block can be placed on this isthmus.[57] Patients with one or two monomorphic VTs can be ablated and should be attempted earlier when one of the VTs prevents adequate antitachycardia pacing. New catheter developments may allow fine adjustment and "roll" to difficult locations or have a longer ablation surface or use energies designed to create larger lesions. New mapping systems are becoming commercially available which use a "locating catheter" and computer programs to identify sites of earliest activation, hoping to limit the need for fluoroscopy. In addition, the ablation site can be determined from short runs of VT. Catheters able to map the venous system of the ventricles may improve our ability to localize tachyarrhythmias. These developments may allow ablation to be the therapy of choice for monomorphic VT. As with all procedures, the more frequently those VTs are addressed, the more likely these necessary advances will occur.

References

1. Scheinman MM, Morady F, Hess DS, et al. Catheter-induced ablation of the atrioventricular junction to control refractory supraventricular arrhythmias. JAMA 1982;248: 851–855.
2. Gallagher JJ, Svenson RH, Kasell JH, et al. Catheter technique for closed-chest ablation of the atrioventricular conduction system. N Engl J Med 1982;306:194–200.
3. Hartzler GO. Electrode catheter ablation of refractory focal ventricular tachycardia. J Am Coll Cardiol 1983;2:1107–1113.
4. Hartzler GO, Giorgi LV. Electrode catheter ablation of refractory focal ventricular tachycardia: continued experience [Abstract]. J Am Coll Cardiol 1984;3:512.
5. Guiradon G, Fontaine G, Frank R, et al. Encircling endocardial ventriculotomy: a new surgical treatment for life-threatening ventricular tachycardias resistant to medical treatment following myocardial infarction. Ann Thorac Surg 1978;26:438.
6. Josephson ME, Harken AH, Horowitz LN. Long-term results of endocardial resection for sustained ventricular tachycardia in coronary disease patients. Am Heart J 1982;104: 51–57.
7. Fontaine G, Frank R, Tonet JL, et al. Catheter ablation of ventricular tachycardia [Abstract]. Eur Heart J 1984;5(Suppl):I-127.
8. Fontaine G, Frank R, Tonet J, et al. Identification of a zone of slow conduction appropriate for ventricular tachycardia ablation: theoretical considerations. PACE 1989;12: 262–267.
9. Lee B, Gottdiener JS, Fletcher RD, et al. Transcatheter ablation: comparison between laser photoablation and electrode shock ablation. Circulation 1985;71(3):579–584.
10. Morady F, Scheinman MM, DiCarlo LA, et al. Catheter ablation of ventricular tachycardia with intracardiac shocks: results in 33 patients. Circulation 1987;75:1037–1049.
11. Morady F, Frank R, Kou WH, et al. Identification and catheter ablation of a zone of slow conduction in the reentrant circuit of ventricular tachycardia in humans. J Am Coll Cardiol 1988;11:775–782.
12. Morady F, Kadish A, Rosenheck S, et al. Concealed entrainment as a guide for catheter ablation of ventricular tachycardia in patients with prior myocardial infarction. J Am Coll Cardiol 1991;17:678–689.
13. Morady F, Harvey M, Kalbfleisch SJ, et al.

Radiofrequency catheter ablation of ventricular tachycardia in patients with coronary artery disease. Circulation 1993;87:363–372.

14. DeBakker JM, VanCapelle FJ, Janse MJ, et al. Reentry as a cause of ventricular tachycardia in patients with chronic ischemic heart disease: electrophysiologic and anatomic correlation. Circulation 1988;77:589–606.

15. Kay GN, Epstein AE, Plumb VJ. Region of slow conduction in sustained ventricular tachycardia: direct endocardial recordings and functional characterization in humans. J Am Coll Cardiol 1988;11:109–116.

16. Josephson ME, Horowitz LN, Farshidi A, et al Recurrent sustained ventricular tachycardia. Circulation 1978;57:431–438.

17. Kienzle MG, Miller J, Falcone RA, et al. Intraoperative endocardial mapping during sinus rhythm: relationship to site of origin of ventricular tachycardia. Circulation 1984;70:957–965.

18. O'Brien JJ, Fallon SL, Tracy CM. Anesthetic methodology during radiofrequency catheter ablation [Abstract]. PACE 1996;1996(Pt II):219a.

19. Kadish AH, Childs K, Schmaltz S, et al. Differences in QRS configuration during unipolar pacing from adjacent sites: implications for the spatial resolution of pacemapping. J Am Coll Cardiol 1991;17:143–151.

20. Langberg JJ, Calkins H, El-Atassi R, et al. Temperature monitoring during radiofrequency catheter ablation of accessory pathways. Circulation 1992;86:1469–1474.

21. Fletcher RD, Swartz JF, Lee B, et al. Advances in catheter ablation: use of unipolar electrograms. PACE 1989;12(Pt II):225.

22. Garan H, Kuchar D, Freeman C, et al. Early assessment of the effect of map-guided transcatheter intracardiac electric shock on sustained ventricular tachycardia secondary to coronary artery disease. Am J Cardiol 1988;1018–1023.

23. El-Sherif N, Mehra R, Gough WB, et al. Reentrant ventricular arrhythmias in the late myocardial infarction period: interruption of reentrant circuits by cryothermal techniques. Circulation 1983;68:644–656.

24. Gallagher JD, Del Rossi AJ, Fernandez J, et al. Cryothermal mapping of recurrent ventricular tachycardia in man. Circulation 1985;71:733–739.

25. Downar E, Harris L, Mickleborough LL, et al. Endocardial mapping of ventricular tachycardia in the intact human ventricle: evidence of reentrant mechanisms. J Am Coll Cardiol 1988;11:783–791.

26. Josephson ME, Horowitz LN, Spielman SR, et al. Role of catheter mapping in the preoperative evaluation of ventricular tachycardia. Am J Cardiol 1982;49:207–220.

27. Josephson ME. Clinical Cardiac Electrophysiology. Lea & Febiger, Philadelphia, 1993, p 789.

28. Littmann L, Svenson RH, Gallagher JJ, et al. High grade entrance and exit block in an area of healed myocardial infarction associated with ventricular tachycardia with successful laser photoablation of the anatomic substrate. Am J Cardiol 1989;64:122–124.

29. El-Sherif N, Scherlag B, Lazzara R, et al. Reentrant ventricular arrhythmias in the late myocardial infarction period. 1. Conduction characteristics in the infarction zone. Circulation 1977;55:686–702.

30. Debakker JM, VanCapelle FJ, Jansen MJ, et al. Reentry as a cause of ventricular tachycardia in patients with chronic ischemic heart disease: electrophysiologic and anatomic correlation. Circulation 1988;77:589–606.

31. Downar E, Kimber S, Harris L, et al. Endocardial mapping of ventricular tachycardia in the intact human heart. II. Evidence for multiuse reentry in a functioning sheet of surviving myocardium. J Am Coll Cardiol 1992;20:869–878.

32. Stevenson WG, Weiss JN, Wiener I, et al. Slow conduction in the infarct scar: relevance to the occurrence, detection, and ablation of ventricular reentry circuits resulting from myocardial infarction. Am Heart J 1989;117:452–464.

33. Stevenson WG, Nademanee K, Weiss JN, et al. Programmed electrical stimulation at potential ventricular reentry circuit sites. A comparison of observations in humans with predictions from computer simulations. Circulation 1989;80:793–806.

34. Frazier DW, Stanton MS. Resetting and transient entrainment of ventricular tachycardia. PACE 1995;18:1919–1946.

35. Stevenson WG, Khan H, Sager P, et al. Identification of reentry circuit sites during catheter mapping and radiofrequency ablation of ventricular tachycardia late after myocardial infarction. Circulation 1993;88:1647–1670.

36. Stevenson W, Weiss J, Wiener I, et al. Resetting of ventricular tachycardia: implications for localizing the area of slow conduction. J Am Coll Cardiol 1988;11:522–529.

37. Brugada P, Abdollah H, Wellens HJJ. Continuous electrical activity during sustained monomorphic ventricular tachycardia. Am J Cardiol 1985;55:402–411.

38. Waldo AL, Henthorn RW. Use of transient entrainment during ventricular tachycardia to localize a critical area in the reentry circuit for ablation. PACE 1989;12:231–244.

39. MacLean WA, Plumb VJ, Waldo AL. Tran-

sient entrainment and interruption of ventricular tachycardia. PACE 1981;4:358–366.

40. Mann D, Lawrie G, Luck J, et al. Importance of pacing site in entrainment of ventricular tachycardia. J Am Coll Cardiol 1985;5:781–787.

41. Anderson KP, Swerdlow CD, Mason JW. Entrainment of ventricular tachycardia. Am J Cardiol 1984;53:335–340.

42. El-Sherif A, Gough W, Restivo M. Reentrant ventricular arrhythmias in the late myocardial infarction period: mechanisms of resetting, entrainment, acceleration, or termination of reentrant tachycardia by programmed electrical stimulation. PACE 1987;10:341–371.

43. Rosenthal ME, Stamato NJ, Almendral JM, et al. Resetting of ventricular tachycardia with electrocardiographic fusion: Incidence and significance. Circulation 1988;77(3):581–588.

44. Henthorn RW, Okumura K, Olshansky B, et al. A fourth criterion for transient entrainment: the electrogram equivalent of progressive fusion. Circulation 1988;77:1003–1012.

45. Fitzgerald DM, Friday KJ, Yeung Lai Wah JA, et al. Electrogram patterns predicting successful catheter ablation of ventricular tachycardia. Circulation 1988;77:806–814.

46. Bogun F, Bahu M, Knight BP, et al. Comparison of effective and ineffective target sites that demonstrate concealed entrainment in patients with coronary artery disease undergoing radiofrequency ablation of ventricular tachycardia. Circulation 1997;94:183–190.

47. Ruffy F, Friday KJ, Southworth WF. Termination of ventricular tachycardia by single extrastimulation during the ventricular effective refractory period. Circulation 1983;67:457–459.

48. Shoda M, Kasanuki H, Ohnishi O, et al. Electrophysiologic properties of substrate critical to perpetuation of reentrant ventricular tachycardia: Observations based on termination of tachycardia by a non-propagated extrastimulus. Circulation 1992;86(4):I-132.

49. Garan H, Ruskin JN. Reproducible termination of ventricular tachycardia by a single extrastimulus within the reentry circuit during the ventricular effective refractory period. Am Heart J 1988;116:546–550.

50. Podczeck A, Borggrefe M, Martinez-Rubio A, et al. Termination of re-entrant ventricular tachycardia by subthreshold stimulus applied to the zone of slow conduction. Eur Heart J 1988;9:1146–1150.

51. Duffy R. Termination of ventricular tachycardia by nonpropagated local depolarization: further observations on entrainment of ventricular tachycardia from an area of slow conduction. PACE 1990;13:852–858.

52. O'Callaghan PA, Ruskin J, McGovern BA, et al. Resetting of mid-diastolic potentials localizes successful sites for radiofrequency ablation in patients with ventricular tachycardia due to coronary artery disease. JACC 1996;27:76A.

53. Morady F, Harvey M, Kalbfleisch SJ, et al. Radiofrequency catheter ablation of ventricular tachycardia in patients with coronary artery disease. Circulation 1993;87(2):363–372.

54. Kim YH, Sosa-Suarez G, Trouton TG, et al. Treatment of ventricular tachycardia by transcatheter radiofrequency ablation in patients with ischemic heart disease. Circulation 1994;89:1094–1102.

55. Borggrefe M, Breithardt G, Podczeck A, et al. Catheter ablation of ventricular tachycardia using defibrillator pulses: eletrophysiological findings and long-term results. Eur Heart J 1989;10:591–601.

56. Belhassen B, Miller HI, Geller E, et al. Transcatheter electrical shock ablation of ventricular tachycardia. J Am Coll Cardiol 1986;6:1347–1355.

57. Wilber DJ, Kopp DE, Glascock DN, et al. Catheter ablation of the mitral isthmus for ventricular tachycardia associated with inferior infarction. Circulation 1995;92:12.

58. Singer I, ed. Interventional Electrophysiology. Baltimore, Williams & Wilkins, 1997, pp 416–441.

Chapter 13

Catheter Designs for Interventional Electrophysiology

Boaz Avitall, Gopal Gupta, Scott Millard, Ray Helms

Introduction

Transcatheter approach for cardiac ablation has become a common procedure and is the primary mode of treating many cardiac arrhythmias. The rapid clinical acceptance of this procedure has resulted in heightened interest from industry as well as clinicians in improving the current technology. Although the success rate for atrioventricular nodal reentry tachycardias and accessory pathway ablation is approaching 100% in many centers, the rate is significantly lower for most other forms of cardiac arrhythmias. Furthermore, the lengthy procedure associated with the ablation of atrial flutter, atrial fibrillation (AF), and ventricular tachycardias is in part directly related to the current catheter technology used. Both ablation and mapping technology are undergoing evolutionary changes that will allow the operator to rapidly predict the ablation site, to maneuver to it quickly using computerized systems, and to use highly mobile catheters to perform multi- site ablation.

This chapter summarizes the determinants for effective cardiac tissue ablation and new catheter designs for both mapping and ablation that may decrease procedure time, improve safety, and increase success rates.

Lesion Generation

Evaluating Electrode-Tissue Contact

Both temperature and impedance can provide useful insight into the status of electrode-tissue contact[1] and lesion formation.[2–4] Though they cannot be directly measured in the clinical setting, electrode-tissue contact and lesion width and depth maturation can be indirectly estimated by tracking changes in temperature and impedance.

Initial Impedance Level

Both in vitro and in vivo studies have shown that increased electrode-tissue contact results in increased initial impedance levels. In a study of isolated pig myocardium using a specially designed catheter with 4-mm tip and ring electrodes, Remp et al. found that impedance could be used to distinguish between contact with blood versus myocardium.[5] In addition, they con-

From Singer I, Barold SS, Camm AJ (eds): Nonpharmacological Therapy of Arrhythmias for the 21st Century: The State of the Art. Futura Publishing Co, Inc., Armonk, NY, © 1998.

cluded that increasing contact pressures were associated with increasing impedances and lesion volumes. Strickberger et al. used 2-W pulses during ablations in humans with standard 4-mm tip ablating electrodes catheters to determine whether the impedance might differ for poor versus firm contact.[6] With firm contact the average impedance level was 22% ± 13% higher versus poor contact (139 ± 24 Ω vs. 113 ± 16 Ω).

Impedance Trend

Impedance trends for four different contact levels while applying 20 W of radiofrequency (RF) power are shown in Figure 1.[1] With increasing electrode-tissue contact, the rate and level of impedance decrease is magnified. With poor electrode-tissue contact, the maximum impedance decreases with 20 W and 30 W were 6 ± 6 Ω and 9 ± 5 Ω, respectively, and the impedance pla-

teaued after a few seconds of power application. With the electrode in good contact, the maximum impedance decreases with 20 W and 30 W were 25 ± 2 Ω and 20 ± 6 Ω, respectively, and the rate of the impedance decrease required 40 sec of power application to reach a plateau.

Several in vitro studies have investigated the relationship between impedance and electrode-tissue contact. Grogan et al. studied impedance in an in vitro, saline perfused model.[7] Power levels of 3–20 W were applied to saline-perfused left ventricular tissue or to saline alone. A 10% decrease in impedance was recorded during application to the tissue, whereas no decrease was noted during the applications to saline alone. In perfused pig heart preparation, Dorwarth et al. compared impedance trends for constant power (8, 12, and 17 W for 10–80 sec) versus temperature-controlled (70°, 80°, and 90°C for 30–90 sec) RF energy delivery.[8] During the constant

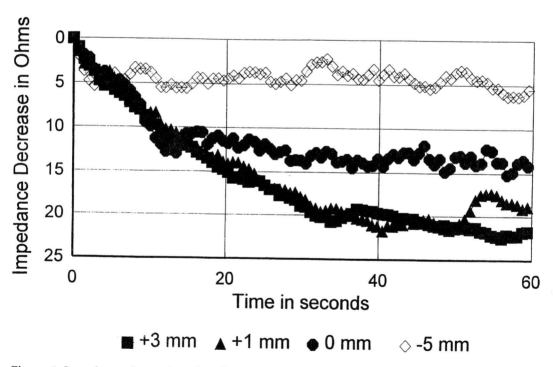

Figure 1. Impedance change from baseline vs. time during the first 60 sec using 20 W of power with the electrode floating in blood (−5), lightly touching the epicardium (0), in good contact (+1), and in very good contact (+3). Used with permission from Avitall B, et al.[1]

power applications, an initial drop in impedance (82 ± 8 Ω to 71 ± 6 Ω) was found to correlate with the induced lesion size. During the temperature- controlled ablations, there was no significant increase or decrease in the impedance.

In a clinical study of 24 patients, Harvey et al. measured impedance during ablations to determine the usefulness of continuous impedance monitoring.[2] An initial drop in impedance of 10 Ω was found to be 78% sensitive and 88% specific for predicting evidence of tissue heating, as gauged by interruption of conduction or a rapid impedance rise due to coagulum formation. This same study concluded that initial values of voltage, current, or impedance were not predictive of effective versus ineffective applications. In a 24-patient investigation, Strickberger et al. found impedance monitoring to be an effective substitute for temperature monitoring during the ablation of accessory pathways.[6] The ablation procedure was successful in all 12 of the temperature monitoring procedures and unsuccessful in one of 12 patients in the impedance monitoring protocol. Otherwise, there was no significant difference in procedure duration, fluoroscopic time, or the number of applications that resulted in coagulum formation.

Temperature

In an in vitro investigation, Chan et al. studied the power requirements needed to create lesions using temperature control set at a target temperature of 80°C for various contact pressures (0, 1, 20, 50, and 100 g).[9] The power required to ablate the tissue at 80°C increased as the contact pressure decreased at each of five superfusate flow rates (0, 1, 2, 4, and 8 L/min). This corroborates with the in vivo epicardial findings of Avitall and associates in their study which found that as the electrode-tissue contact increases, the amount of temperature rise also

increases as shown in Figure 2.[1] With the electrode floating in blood, the average maximum temperature increase with 20 W and 30 W was only $7° \pm 1$°C and $11° \pm 2$°C, respectively, and the temperature plateaued shortly after the initiation of power application. With good electrode-tissue contact, the temperature increase within the first 10 sec was significantly greater than the temperature increase with poor contact and reached a maximum of $60° \pm 1$°C after 60 sec of power application.

Correlation of Width and Depth with Temperature and Impedance

In addition to providing insight into electrode-tissue contact, the impedance decrease and temperature increase also correlate well with both lesion width and depth according to Avitall and associates Figure 3.[1] They found the best correlation between the lesion width and the maximum average temperature increase ($R2 = 0.9$). Lesion depth, however, correlated better with maximum average impedance decrease ($R2 = 0.68$ for impedance vs. $R2 = 0.44$ for temperature).

Biobattery as an Indirect Measure of Temperature and Contact

In in vitro and in vivo studies, He et al. evaluated the use of a biobattery galvanic current model to predict the temperature at the electrode- temperature interface.[10,11] In both investigations, catheters with 4-mm tip electrodes with thermocouples were used to ablate tissues with a generator capable of measuring galvanic current. In the in vitro study the correlation between the measured temperature and the galvanic current was 0.98 for temperatures between 36°C and 75°C. In the in vivo study, the correlation between temperature and galvanic current was 0.98 and 0.97 for two standard catheters from different manufacturers. Since temperature provides insight into electrode-tissue contact and lesion formation, this bio-

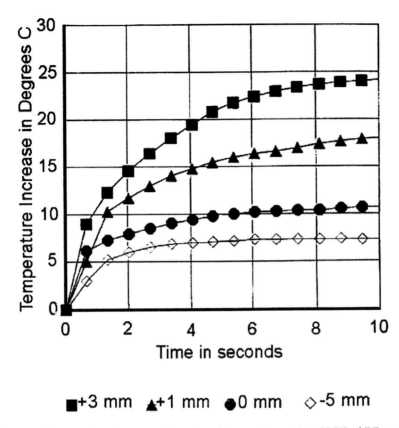

Figure 2. Average temperature increase above baseline vs. time using 20 W of RF power with the electrode floating in blood (-5), lightly touching the epicardium (0), in good contact ($+1$), and in very good contact ($+3$). Used with permission from Avitall B, et al.[1]

battery technique might be helpful in generating lesions using nontemperature- controlled catheters.

Intracardiac Ultrasound Use in Evaluating Electrode-Tissue Contact and Orientation

Recent studies have described the use of intracardiac ultrasound (ICE) to enhance maintenance of adequate electrode-tissue orientation and contact. Kalman et al. reported that ICE can detect changes in tip location and stability and, therefore, can be used to help establish good electrode-tissue contact.[12] In another study, Kalman et al. compared the use of ICE, fluoroscopy and electrocardiograms (ECGs) to the use of only fluoroscopy and ECGs in evaluating contact prior to lesion generation.[13] They

defined three levels of contact: poor, average, and good. In 27% of the RF applications with good contact as determined by fluoroscopy and ECG, ICE found that the contact conditions were actually poor. The size of the lesions generated with good contact were considerably larger than those generated with average or poor contact. The authors suggest that ICE can aid in obtaining good contact, and, therefore, lesion size can be maximized.

The orientation of the ablating electrode in reference to the tissue may have a significant effect on lesion size. Chan et al. evaluated the difference in lesion maturation for perpendicular versus parallel orientations in canines.[14] They evaluated lesions created with 4-, 6-, 8-, 10-, and 12-mm electrodes and found that larger lesions were created

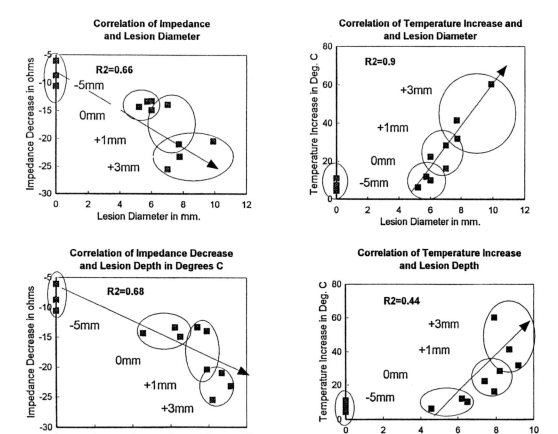

Figure 3. Impedance and temperature vs. lesion width and depth using 20 W of power with the electrode floating in blood (-5), lightly touching the epicardium (0), in good contact ($+1$), and in very good contact ($+3$). The correlation value (R2) is shown on each panel. Used with permission from Avitall B, et al.[1]

with the electrodes oriented parallel to the tissue. This study concluded that ICE could be used to determine orientation and ensure proper contact to maximize lesion size.

Power and Energy

Numerous investigations have analyzed the relationship between lesion dimensions and the amplitude and duration of power delivery with both 2-mm and 4-mm electrodes. With 2-mm electrodes there is a higher probability that the electrode will be fully embedded within the tissue, with little or no exposure to the blood. If this is the case, all the power will be dissipated within the tissue. With larger electrodes much of the electrode may be bathed in fluid. Therefore, some of the power will be shunted through the blood rather than into the tissue and the flowing blood will cool the electrode. This contact scenario is probably common with 4-mm electrodes, especially when the catheter is not imbedded within ventricular trabeculations.

In Vitro Studies

2-mm Electrodes

Hoyt et al.[15] and Hoffman et al.[16] both performed in vitro studies with short power duration using 2-mm electrodes. Using excised bovine left ventricles, Hoyt et al. concluded that pulse power and duration were the most significant variables influencing myocardial damage.[15] They created lesions with 1–50 W of power applied for 2–20 sec and found that diameter and depth both increased as power amplitude and duration increased (Figure 4). Hoffman et al. studied the effects of power amplitude (17, 29, 32, 41, and 57 W for 10 sec) and duration (3, 6, and 9, sec at 57 W) on lesion generation in excised pig myocardium in a circulating blood bath.[16] For these relatively short application times, they concluded that the lesion depth was influenced more by the amplitude of the power, whereas the lesion area was affected more by the duration of power delivery. The short duration of power application in these two studies did not allow for full depth maturation, thus making the depth a function of power. Haines applied RF power for much longer and found that at least 35–45 sec of power delivery were required to obtain maximal lesion size in an in vitro preparation using a 1.6-mm electrode.[17]

In Vivo Studies

In the intact heart, the ability to control lesion dimensions by adjusting power delivery is limited due to the variable nature of the convective cooling effects of circulating blood. Furthermore, in contrast to in vitro studies in which contact or contact pressure may be carefully controlled, the electrode- tissue contact may vary significantly in in vivo studies.

2-mm Electrodes

In an in vivo epicardial study, Bardy et al. evaluated lesion volume while varying the duration (5, 10, 15, and 20 sec) and amount of RF voltage delivered (20, 40, and 60 V).[18] They concluded that lesion volume rises as a function of time and power (Figure 5). At each voltage level, the lesion depth, diameter, and volume increased as the du-

ration increased from 5 to 15 sec. Increasing the duration to 20 sec at 40 V did not result in increased lesion diameter. Furthermore, at 60 V neither lesion depth nor diameter increased significantly when the duration was increased from 15 to 20 sec. A study by Wittkampf et al.[19] used power levels of up to 9 W and created lesions for 5, 10, 20, 30, and 60 sec in canine ventricles using an endocardial approach. They concluded that lesion size (measured as a composite of length, width, and depth) matured within 20 sec and increased in size with higher power for all exposure duration.[19]

Lesion Maturation with 4-mm Electrodes

Simmers et al.[20] evaluated the effects of pulse duration (5, 10, 20, 30, and 60 sec) on lesion dimensions with 4-mm electrodes at a fixed level of 25 W. They concluded that 90% of maximum dimensions were reached within 20 sec of the initiation of power delivery. Lesion depth was found to have matured within the first 10 sec, while lesion diameter required more time, approximately 30 sec.

These results are in contrast to those described by Avitall et al.,[1] who noted that the lesion depth matures much slower than the width and required 30- 40 sec and 90 sec for the lesion depth to mature. It would be prudent for the user of this technology to apply RF power for 60–90 sec if full lesion maturation is desired.

Atrial Tissue

Recently, great energy has been focused on the development of technology for the ablation of atrial arrhythmias. Because the atrial walls are much thinner than the ventricles, the power requirements are different. The power required to create transmural lesions in the atria are much less than for ventricular tissues. Avitall and associates used fixed power levels of 1, 5, 10, 15, 20, and 30 W for 30 sec to create epicardial lesions with a standard 4-mm tip electrode.[21] The lesion diameter increased with increasing power. For power levels of 20 W

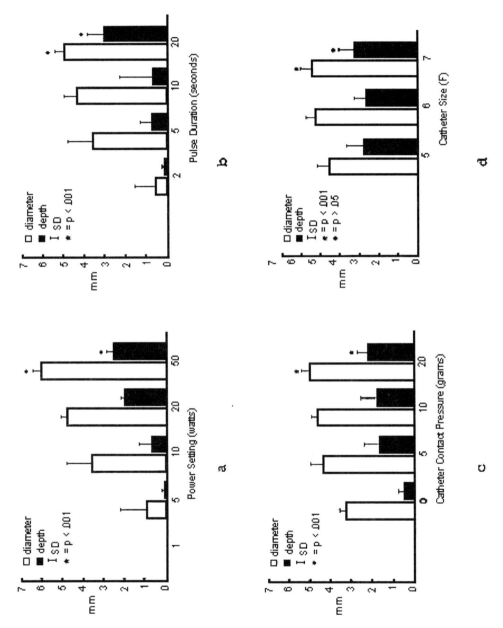

Figure 4. Lesion depth and diameter vs. power, pulse duration, contact pressure, and catheter size. Lesions were created with 1–50 W of power applied for 2–20 sec in an in vitro preparation using 2-mm electrodes. Used with permission from Avitall B, et al.[1]

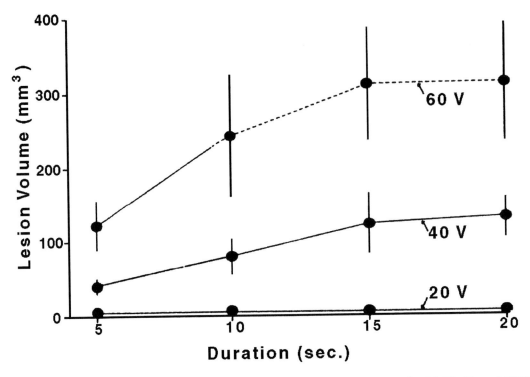

Figure 5. Lesion volume vs. power and pulse duration. Lesions were created with 20, 40, and 60 V applied for 5, 10, 15, and 20 sec in an in vivo preparation using 2-mm electrodes. Used with permission from Avitall B, et al.[1]

and 30 W, all lesions were completely transmural.

Unipolar Versus Bipolar Energy Delivery

Most RF lesions are created by applying energy in a unipolar fashion between an ablating electrode touching the myocardium and a grounded reference patch electrode placed externally on the skin. The goal of cardiac tissue ablation is to eliminate arrhythmogenic foci with the least amount of tissue damage. The unipolar configuration is best suited to this goal because it creates a highly localized lesion, with the least amount of surface injury. Energy can also be applied in a bipolar mode between two endocardial electrodes. This method may prove to be useful in increasing the efficiency of creating long linear lesions for the ablation of AF. Haines et al. compared the delivery of RF energy in unipolar and bipo-

lar modes in the generation of lesions at the tricuspid-inferior vena cava isthmus using two 3-mm electrodes spaced 3 mm apart.[22] Unipolar energy was found to generate lesions that were longer (14.9 ± 1.6 mm vs. 9.2 ± 1.5 mm) and wider (8.1 ± 1.8 vs. 5.6 ± 1.5) than bipolar energy. Anfinsen et al. used a different electrode configuration to test the lesion dimensions created with unipolar versus bipolar RF energy delivery to the right atrial free wall in pigs.[23] Energy was applied via the distal 4-mm tip electrodes of two standard 7F catheters placed 6–8 mm apart on the endocardial surface. In contrast to the Haines study, the lesions generated via bipolar power delivery were longer and wider than those created via unipolar delivery, though the depth of the lesions did not differ between the two methods. In a similar but in vitro investigation by Anfinsen et al. bipolar energy delivery was found to provide a greater lesion length than unipolar delivery, but width and depth were not found to be significantly different between the two methods.[24]

Reference Patch Electrode Location and Size

The standard method of ablating cardiac tissues involves applying RF power in a unipolar fashion from an electrode on a catheter to a reference patch placed on the patient's back. Tomassoni et al. investigated lesion dimensions for standard and nonstandard locations of the reference electrode.[25] The reference electrode was either placed directly opposite the catheter tip on the thorax or placed in a simple anterior or posterior position. Placing the electrode patch opposite the catheter resulted in increased lesion surface area, depth, and volume. Otomo et al. studied lesion dimensions for two different reference patch electrode sizes in a canine thigh muscle preparation.[26] They compared a 252-cm^2 patch (two standard patches) to a 63-cm^2 patch (1/2 standard patch). Lesions were created with a 4-mm electrode with 20 W of power for 60 sec. In the preparation with the larger patch, the lesion depth and volume were significantly increased versus with the smaller patch (depth = 7.4 ± 0.8 mm vs. 5.1 ± 1.1 mm, volume = 368 ± 131 mm^3 vs. 152 ± 50 mm^3). These results suggest that the RF current path and skin reference electrode interface present significant impedance for the ablation current flow, therefore dissipating part of the power. Increasing the patch size and placing the reference patch at the path of least resistance for the ablation current provides for increased heating at the electrode-endocardial interface and thus increased ablation efficiency.

Closed-Loop Automatic Temperature Control

Maintaining the temperature at the electrode-tissue interface below 100°C results in significantly less coagulum formation on the ablation electrode and a decreased incidence of impedance rises and tissue tearing

Figure 6.[27–29] Monitoring the temperature at the electrode-tissue interface to prevent overheating can allow for longer power application and increased lesion dimensions.[28] Therefore, the application of RF power using closed-loop automatic temperature control has become a useful ablation technique. Haines et al. applied RF power to maintain electrode tip temperature at 80°C for 120 sec in an isolated RV free wall preparation.[30] As shown in Figure 7, tip temperature was found to correlate closely with lesion depth (r = 0.92) and width (r = 0.88). In addition, tip temperature was a better predictor of lesion size than measurements of power, current, or energy. The temperature measured at the electrode-tissue interface does not necessarily reflect the temperature within the tissue itself. With increasing distance lateral to the electrode-tissue interface, the maximum temperature decreases rapidly (Figure 8).[30] Because circulating blood cools the tissue near the interface, the temperature measured by a thermistor or thermocouple at the electrode-tissue interface tends to be cooler than within the tissue directly below the electrode.[31–33] The tissue underneath the electrode may be 15°–20°C hotter than the measured temperature within the electrode. The orientation of the temperature- measuring element affects the degree of this difference.[32] Fleischman et al. showed that the temperature measured from a sensor placed at the electrode tip provides a closer estimate of the actual tissue temperature than a centrally located sensor (Figure 9).[33] The measured temperature is affected by the sensor's position, the electrode-tissue contact, and the degree of cooling by intracavitary blood flow. Thus, when using an automatic closed-loop temperature control system the target temperature should be set at 70°–80°C and maintained for 1–2 min to maximize lesion maturation while avoiding impedance rises and popping due to overheating at the electrode-tissue interface.

Cooled-Tip Technology

With the development of cooled-tip technology, it is possible to deliver higher en-

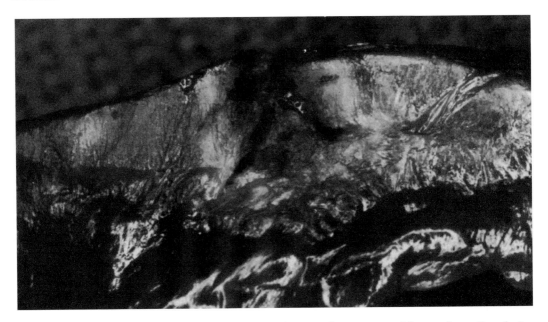

Figure 6. Intramural shredding of tissues resulting from explosions caused by gas formation during boiling with 30 W applied via a 4-mm electrode pressed 3 mm into the epicardium. Used with permission from Avitall B, et al.[1]

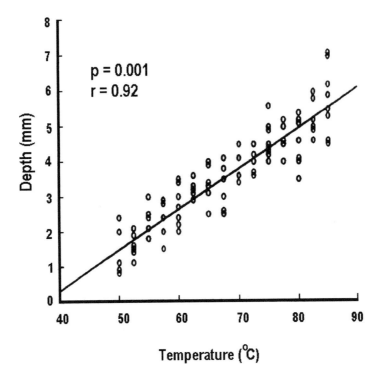

Figure 7. Lesion depth vs. temperature. At a target electrode-tip temperature of 80°C, RF power was applied for 120 sec to create 104 lesions. There is a strong linear relationship between lesion depth and temperature. Used with permission from Avitall B, et al.[1]

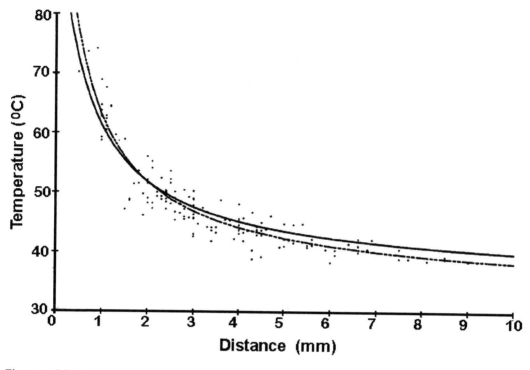

Figure 8. Maximum temperature vs. distance from the ablating electrode. At a target electrode-tip temperature of 80°C, RF power was applied for 120 sec to create 104 lesions. The temperature measured 2 mm below the epicardium decreased rapidly as a function of distance from the ablating electrode. Used with permission from Avitall B, et al.[1]

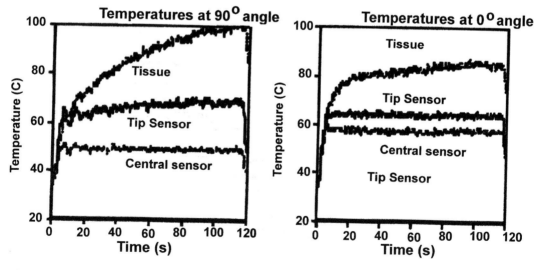

Figure 9. Temperature vs. time for a perpendicular electrode-tissue orientation. In this in vitro preparation, power was adjusted to maintain a target temperature of 50°C at the central sensor. The temperature measured from a sensor placed at the electrode tip provides a closer estimate of the tissue temperature than a centrally located sensor, though neither closely estimates the actual tissue temperature. The tissue temperature was measured 1 mm below the electrode-tissue interface. Used with permission from Avitall B, et al.[1]

ergy levels for longer periods of time while avoiding overheating leading to a rapid impedance rise and subsequent coagulum formation. This allows for the creation of much larger lesions than can be generated with standard technology.

Generator Frequency

Most standard RF generators produce signals in the range of 500–750 kHz. Some recent studies have investigated the lesion dimensions that can be produced using higher frequencies. Kovoor et al. compared lesion dimensions for frequencies of 100, 600, 1,200, and 2,000 kHz.[52] Lesions were generated with a 1-mm long electrode (diameter = 0.8 mm) using temperature control at a setting of 90°C. They found that lesion width was not statistically different for the various frequencies, but the depth increased with increasing frequency. Bru et al. generated lesions to create AV block in sheep with a generator frequency of 27 MHz and an electrode of unknown size.[53] The power levels required for successful ablation were between 30 W and 100 W, and the generated lesions ranged from 3–45 mm in diameter and 1–15 mm in depth. The utility of RF generators with frequencies other than 500–750 kHz with standard catheter technology (4-mm electrodes) remains to be explored.

Pulsed Power Application

By applying power in a pulsatile manner, the convective cooling blood currents may aid in avoiding overheating at the electrode-tissue interface and subsequent rapid impedance rises, therefore allowing the creation of larger lesions. An in vitro study by Nakagawa et al. investigated the creation of lesions using pulsed power delivery with a saline-irrigated electrode.[54] A fixed level of 70 V was applied via three techniques for 180 sec or until a popping sound was heard. Power was applied in one of three ways: continuously, on for 5 sec then off for 5 sec, or on for 4 sec then off for 5 sec. The largest lesion diameter (16.5 ± 1.7 mm) and depth

(10.3 ± 1.1 mm) were generated with the 5-on/5-off method of power delivery; the comparable dimensions with continuous power delivery were 13.1 ± 1.8 and 6.5 ± 1.0, respectively. With continuous power delivery 24/24 applications resulted in a popping sound while the popping frequency decreased to 5/36 and 0/13 for the 5-on/5-off and 4-on/5-off methods, respectively. The use of pulsed power delivery may allow for the creation of larger lesions because the power may be applied over a longer period of time allowing the lesion to mature more completely.

Electrode Morphology

Size and Shape

If the RF power level were adjusted to maintain a constant current density, lesion width would increase proportionally to the electrode-tissue contact area. However, this assumes that the electrode-tissue contact, tissue heat dissipation, and blood flow are uniform throughout the electrode-tissue interface. As the electrode size increases, the likelihood that these assumptions are true diminishes due to variability in cardiac chamber trabeculations and curvature, tissue perfusion, and intracardiac blood flow, which will affect the heat dissipation and contact. These factors will result in unpredictable lesion size and uniformity for electrodes greater than 8 mm long. The character of lesions created with temperature control depends on the placement of the temperature sensor or sensors relative to the portion of the electrode that is in contact with the tissue. Thus, the orientation of the ablating electrode and its temperature sensors will determine the appropriate target temperature required to create maximal lesions while avoiding coagulum formation due to overheating at any location within the electrode-tissue interface.

In vitro studies have shown that lesion formation can be influenced by the size of the electrode-tissue interface.[15,34] Hoyt et al.

reported that increasing the electrode diameter (5F, 6F, 7F) results in a significant increase in lesion diameter but not depth in an in vitro study.[15] This study only used power applications of 20 sec, so the lesions were not allowed to fully mature. Haines and associates evaluated the correlation between electrode radius and lesion transmural (depth) and transverse radii.[34] Lesions were created in a perfused RV free wall using temperature control at a setting of 60°C for 90 sec. As shown in Figure 10, a strong correlation was noted between electrode radius and lesion transmural ($r = 0.89$) and transverse radii ($r = 0.85$).

Theoretically, longer electrodes would be expected to create larger lesions if the power level was increased accordingly to maintain a constant current density. Lang-

berg et al. investigated the effects of distal electrode length (2, 3, 4, 6, 8, and 10 mm) on ventricular lesion volume in vivo.[35] Instead of attempting to maintain a constant current density, a constant power of approximately 13 W was applied until a maximum of 500 J of energy had been delivered or a rapid impedance rise occurred. For this power level, the optimum electrode length was 3–4 mm. Increasing the electrode length from 2 mm to 3 or 4 mm more than doubled the lesion volume (from 143 mm^3 to 303 mm^3 and 326 mm^3, respectively), but increasing the length beyond 4 mm resulted in smaller lesions, presumably because of decreasing current density.

Studies utilizing temperature control have shown that 8-mm electrodes optimize lesion dimensions in ventricular myocar-

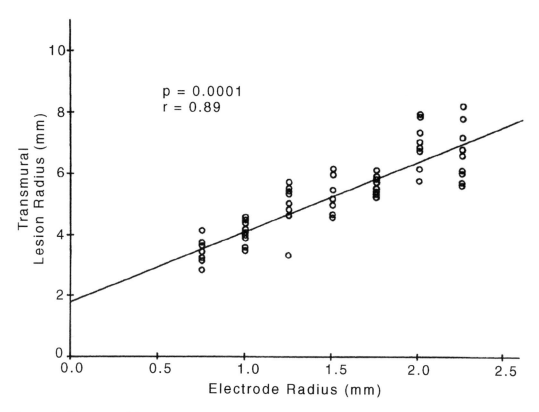

Figure 10. Transmural lesion radius (depth) vs. electrode radius. Power was adjusted to maintain a target temperature of 60°C in this in vitro preparation. Electrodes with larger surface areas require higher powers to maintain the target temperature, and can create deeper lesions at a fixed target temperature. Used with permission from Avitall B, et al.[1]

dium. Langberg et al. compared the use of 8-mm and 12-mm electrodes versus standard 4-mm electrodes at a target temperature of 80°C for 60 sec.[36] Lesions created with 8-mm electrodes were nearly twice as deep and four times as large as lesions made with 4-mm electrodes. The 12-mm electrodes produced lesions with depths and volumes that were smaller than with 8-mm electrodes and slightly larger than with 4-mm electrodes. In addition, the 12-mm electrodes were associated with charring and crater formation. McRury and associates evaluated 4-, 8-, and 10-mm electrodes delivering up to 150 W with temperature controlled at 65°, 80°, and 90°C.[37] The lesion volume more than doubled when increasing the size from 4 mm to 8 mm for each of the target temperatures. The volume increase from 8 mm^3 to 10 mm^3 at each target temperature was minimal.

In a canine thigh muscle preparation, Otomo and associates compared lesions created with 4-mm versus 8-mm tip electrodes with power delivered for 60 sec under temperature control.[26] The target temperature was set at 60°C for a perpendicular electrode-tissue orientation and 90°C for a parallel orientation. The larger (8-mm) electrode produced significantly deeper lesions than the 4-mm electrode in both preparations (7.8 ± 0.8 mm vs. 6.6 ± 0.5 mm at 60°C target; 8.3 ± 0.7 mm vs. 7.2 ± 0.5 mm at 90°C target).

Chan et al. investigated the creation of atrial lesions with electrodes of various sizes (4, 6, 10, and 12 mm) with parallel versus perpendicular orientations.[14] The temperature at the electrode-tissue interface was maintained at 75°C for 60 sec with up to 65 W of power. Lesion area increased with increasing electrode length and was maximized at 10 mm for parallel orientation (55 ± 78 mm vs. 31 ± 12 mm with a 4-mm electrode) and 12 mm for perpendicular orientation (70 ± 40 mm vs. 59 ± 38 mm with a 4- mm electrode).

In attempting to create long lesions in the atria, several investigators have evaluated the use of coiled wire electrodes.[38–42] Long coiled electrodes are advantageous because they do not inhibit catheter flexibility versus the long ring electrodes. Experiments using multiple coils in the range of 4–12.5 mm at various interelectrode distances have concluded that these electrodes can create long atrial lesions, but they are limited in their ability to consistently create completely contiguous and transmural lesions.

Hoey and associates reported using a catheter with a tip that can be actively screwed into ventricular tissue from the endocardium.[43,44] After the tip is screwed into the tissue, saline is infused during RF energy application creating a "virtual electrode" that can be visualized via fluoroscopy. Lesions measuring 10 × 10 × 9 mm were created using 50 W of RF power for 2 min. With power applied for 4 min, the lesion size increased to 17 × 15 × 14 mm. There was no evidence of thrombus formation, desiccation, or wall perforation.

Multi-Electrode Arrays and Segmented Electrodes

Since ventricular tachycardia ablations may require large, deep lesions, several investigations have studied the application of RF energy to multiple electrodes to increase lesion dimensions.

In two investigations, Oeff and associates applied bipolar RF power (7–35 W) between the proximal, middle, and distal pairs of electrodes on a catheter with four 2-mm electrodes.[45,46] The catheter was removed so that it could be cleaned and then the process was repeated 9–11 times at each target site. The surface area and volume of these lesions were much greater than for lesions created with single applications. The average lesion volume was 0.84 ± 0.38 versus 0.12 ± 0.06 cm^3, and the average lesion surface area was 3.7 ± 1.2 versus 0.29 ± 0.15 cm^2.

Chang et al. placed two separate catheters with 4-mm tip electrodes horizontally next to one another to create lesions in isolated bovine myocardium.[47] They compared lesion generation at a fixed level of 30 V in bipolar versus unipolar mode and with one versus both electrodes. Lesion volumes were calculated for interelectrode distances ranging from 2 mm to 7 mm. Lesions produced by simultaneous delivery to both electrodes were twice the size of lesions created with one electrode. Lesion volume and depth decreased with increasing interelectrode distance. In addition, for a given power level, bipolar delivery produced larger lesions than unipolar power application.

Two studies using unipolar RF power via multiple electrodes have been reported. Avitall and associates used a catheter with a distal 2-mm electrode and three additional 2-mm electrodes spaced 0.5 mm apart on its shaft to create lesions in the LV of five dogs.[48] Lesions were made by applying 10 W then 20 W then 30 W of power for 60 sec or until an impedance rise occurred. Lesion dimensions were compared for the use of electrodes 1 and 2 versus 1, 2, 3, and 4. While the depth was not significantly different, the length and width were greater for the 1–2–3–4 method versus the 1–2 method (length = 13 ± 3.7 mm vs. 9.3 ± 2 mm, width = 8.7 ± 2 mm vs. 6.7 ± 0.8 mm).

In a study using a quadripolar catheter, Mackey et al. compared lesions created in vitro and in vivo with a distal 4-mm electrode versus simultaneous application via the distal 4-mm electrode and three 2-mm electrodes placed 2 mm apart on the shaft.[49] The power was set at 12 W for the distal tip ablations and 35 W for the quadripolar applications. These power settings were defined based on preliminary studies documenting the highest power levels with impedance rise rates less than 20%. In both the in vivo and in vitro studies, the lesions were twice as long with the four electrodes than with just the distal electrode. There was a trend toward increasing lesion depth with the quadripolar applications in both sets of experiments with a more substantial increase in the in vivo experiment.

Baal and associates compared the use of a 4-mm distal tip electrode alone versus si-

multaneously ablating with the distal electrode and a 3.5-mm electrode on the catheter shaft using temperature control.[50] The target temperature was set at 80°C and maintained for 60 sec. Using electrodes 1–2 versus 1 alone significantly increased the lesion depth (4.9 ± 0.7 mm vs. 4.5 ± 0.5 mm) and volume (210 ± 61 mm^3 vs. 123 ± 43 mm^3).

Material

Platinum electrodes have been the standard for most RF ablation catheters, but the use of gold electrodes allows for greater power delivery without an impedance rise to create deeper lesions. Because gold has nearly four times the thermal conductivity of platinum, Simmons et al. investigated the use of gold versus platinum electrodes. This in vitro study used both 6F 2-mm and 7F 4-mm electrodes.[51] The power was initiated at 4 W for the 2-mm studies and 12 W for the 4-mm applications and increased in 2-W increments until an impedance rise occurred. In both the 2-mm and 4-mm ablations, the maximum power that could be applied was higher for the electrodes made of gold versus platinum (2 mm: 8 W vs. 6 W; 4 mm: 20 W vs. 14 W). For the 2-mm electrodes, only the lesion depth was significantly increased for the gold versus platinum electrodes. In the 4-mm experiments, lesion depth, length, and volume were significantly increased for the gold electrodes (depth = 7.2 ± 1.4 mm vs. 5.8 ± 0.7 mm, length = 8.0 ± 0.9 mm vs. 6.5 ± 0.8 mm, volume = 195 ± 0.69 mm^3 vs. 115 ± 39 mm^3).

Catheter Design

One of the most important factors that has led to the widespread use of RF ablation has been the development of deflectable catheters that can be guided by localized electrical activity, fluoroscopy, or echocardiographic imaging. However, difficulty in maneuvering catheters to desired anatomic locations is still common, and, therefore, some procedures may last several hours. New catheter technology is needed to allow the operator to adapt the catheter to the cardiac structure. These catheters should allow the operator to map local electrical activity and to apply ablative energy to the appropriate electrode without the need to maneuver the catheter.[55] In this section, we explore catheter design characteristics and special catheters that adapt to specific cardiac anatomic structures.

Left-Sided Accessory Pathway

Left-sided accessory pathways can be approached by inserting the ablation catheter retrogradely through the aortic valve and positioning the tip under the mitral valve leaflets or over the AV ring on the atrial side (Figure 11–1,2). Another approach is to insert the ablation catheter from the right atrium through the atrial septum where the catheter tip is then placed above the AV ring (Figure 11–3). The deflectable tip must allow the operator to map the AV ring and localize the position of the accessory pathway with minimal error. Currently, most electrophysiologists are using a single deflectable catheter for the mapping and ablation of left-sided accessory pathways. Because of the diversity of anatomic positions of accessory pathways, there may be an optimal catheter design that allows the operator to position the ablation electrode with the least amount of difficulty. Since the majority of left-sided accessory pathways are located at the posterior half of the AV ring, this area of the ring should be subdivided into four sections for analysis: posterior septal (PS), posterior (P), posterior lateral (PL), and lateral (L).

Several parameters can be defined to characterize the deflectable catheter shape and size for the different locations of accessory pathways on the left atrioventricular ring (Figure 12). These parameters include:

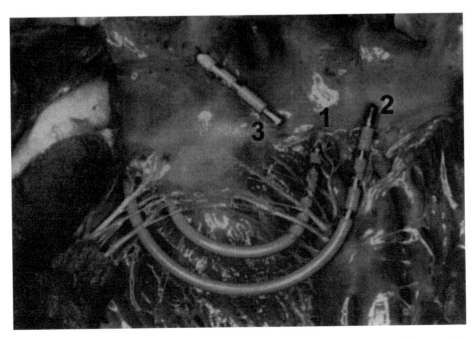

Figure 11. Ablation of bypass tracts can be approached retrogradely with the ablation catheter tip placed either under the mitral valve in the ventricle (1), or just above the valve in the atrium (2). Ablation via a transseptal approach with the catheter introduced through the atrial septum (3). Used with permission from Avitall B, et al.[77]

length of the deflected portion of the wire (TL), tip to shaft distance (T-SH), vertical curvature (R)—the curvature of the wire end along the shaft, and lateral curvature (L-DEF)—the deflection of the end of the wire to either side of the wire shaft.

Examples of wire positioning at the posterior septal, posterior lateral, and lateral sites for the retrograde subvalvular approach are shown in Figure 13. The retrograde supravalvular position approach is shown in Figure 14, and the transseptal supravalvular position is shown in Figure 15.

The data presented in Table 1 demonstrate that the shape of an ablation catheter is similar for posterior septal and posterior pathways for both transseptal and retro-

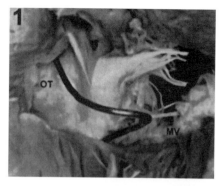

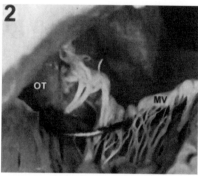

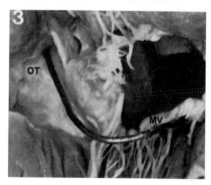

Figure 13. Retrograde approach with the wire tip positioned under the mitral leaflets. OT = left ventricular outflow tract; MV = mitral valve posterior leaflet. Used with permission from Avitall B, et al.[77]

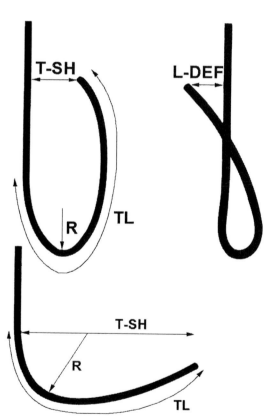

Figure 12. The wire shape was measured in the following manner: 1. Length of the deflected portion of the wire (TL), 2. Tip to shaft distance (T-SH), 3. Vertical curvature (R), and 4. Lateral curvature (L-DEF). Used with permission from Avitall B, et al.[77]

grade approaches. These pathways require a significantly shorter deflectable tip length (TL) (except for posterior lateral from the transseptal approach) and smaller vertical curvature (R) than a catheter used for posterior lateral and lateral pathways. The posterior septal and posterior accessory pathways require a catheter that has a lateral curvature (L-DEF) capability of at least 15

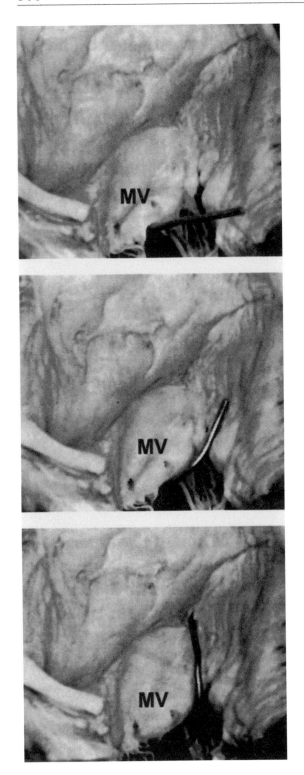

Figure 14. Retrograde supravalvular approach. MV = mitral valve posterior leaflet. Used with permission from Avitall B, et al.[77]

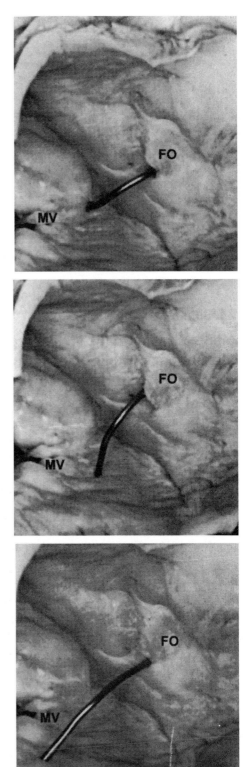

Figure 15. Transeptal approach. FO = foramen ovale; MV = mitral valve posterior leaflet. Used with permission from Avitall B, et al.[77]

Table 1

Measurements (mm) of Different Parameters of Deflectable Catheters for Different Approaches to the Left Atrium

	TL	T-SH	R	L-DEF
PS Retro	45 ± 7	12 ± 3	8 ± 1	10 ± 4
PS Trans	38 ± 6	#18 ± 5	8 ± 1	8 ± 4
P Retro	48 ± 6	19 ± 6	10 ± 1	15 ± 6
P Trans	#36 ± 8	26 ± 7	10 ± 3	#4 ± 3
PL Retro	*52 ± 9	*36 ± 5	*18 ± 4	7 ± 10
PL Trans	#39 ± 11	#29 ± 7	*19 ± 6	*1 ± 2
L Retro	*59 ± 8	*42 ± 5	*24 ± 7	*0.5 ± 2
L Trans	*52 ± 13	*40 ± 9	*27 ± 6	*3 ± 8

* P <0.01 vs Retro, Trans PS and P.

# P <0.01 Trans vs. Retro.

TL = tip length; T-SH = tip to shaft distance; R = vertical curvature; L-DEF = lateral curvature.

Retro = retrograde; Trans = transseptal.

Used with permission from Avitall B, et al.[33]

mm. Catheters used in a transseptal approach require a shorter deflection tip length (TL) than catheters used for a retrograde approach.

As shown in Figure 16, the posterior septal position of the AV ring can be reached only with the short tip (5 cm) catheter when approached retrogradely (top picture) or transseptally (bottom picture), whereas the longer tip (7 cm) catheter is better for the lateral position.

Variable Deflection Length, Lateral, and Bidirectional Deflection

The optimal catheter deflection length cannot always be established prior to catheter insertion. Therefore, a variable deflection length catheter and lateral movement control has been developed (Medtronic Inc.). These catheters may decrease procedure time and increase ablation success rates. The current technology has yet to establish itself in the marketplace and the utility and efficacy of such catheters need to be defined.

Pigtail-Type Mapping and Ablating Electrode

Figure 17 shows a 7F deflectable catheter placed just above the mitral valve in a pa-tient with a lateral accessory pathway. Although the catheter tip is stable above the mitral ring during ventricular systole, during diastole, the anterior leaflet of the mitral valve exerts a downward force on the catheter causing the catheter tip to dislodge from its position above the mitral ring. The anatomic junction of the mitral ring, the atrium, and the ventricle create a depression in the atrium just above the mitral ring. A catheter with a pigtail-type end equipped with six 4-mm long electrodes (used for both recording and ablation) has constructed to fit the left atrium just above the mitral ring.[56] To assess mobility around the mitral ring and stability of recording and ablation, this catheter was inserted into the left ventricle of an intact dog heart under fluoroscopic guidance with the pigtail end positioned retrogradely across the mitral valve on the atrial side of the AV ring Figure 18. The pigtail and a secondary curve allow the catheter to cross the mitral valve apparatus and adapt to the curvature of the atrial mitral ring structure. The secondary curve stabilizes the deflectable tip across the valve so that the opening and closing of the leaflets only minimally affect the catheter's position. The catheter is secured in the mitral ring and is less prone to drop back into the ventricle.

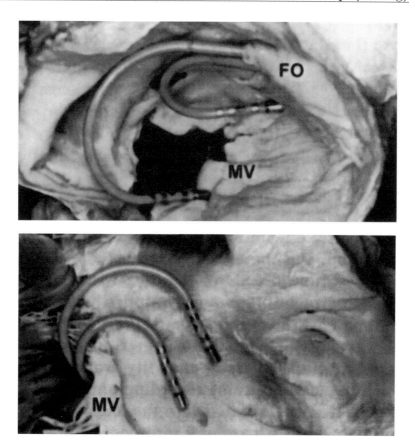

Figure 16. Posterior septal position of the mitral valve AV ring approached retrogradely (top picture) or transseptally (bottom picture). MV = mitral valve; FO = foramen ovale. Used with permission from Avitall B, et al.[77]

As shown in Figure 19, the electrograms from the electrodes on the pigtail portion of the catheter show the transition from the atrium to the ventricle across the mitral ring. Torquing the catheter shaft results in the rotation of the pigtail and the ability to map and apply lesions around the mitral ring. This catheter can be used with a standard 8F introducer.

Deflectable Loop

Ablation of right-sided accessory pathways, modification of AV nodal reentry tachycardia, and His bundle ablation all require mapping and ablation along the perivalvular atrial tissues of the tricuspid ring. Since the tricuspid valve ring is directly ac-

cessible to catheters introduced from the major veins, it provides the setting for a loop-type structure that adapts to the valve ring. The most effective approach for ablation around the tricuspid ring would be to map and then apply RF power through the recording electrode that identified the desired area for ablation. A deflectable loop catheter equipped with 16 electrodes (4 mm long, spaced 4 mm apart) can be used for both recording and ablation (Figure 20 A,B). The distal portion of the catheter is equipped with a small secondary loop. The catheter, introduced into the right atrium from the femoral vein, is capable of adapting to the shape of the tricuspid ring when opened and is also capable of rotation across the valve plane by a separate deflec-

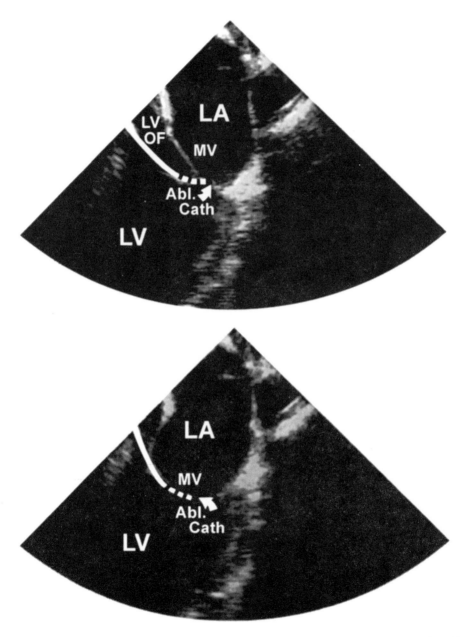

Figure 17. Transesophageal echo with the ablation catheter positioned at the lateral wall of the LA/AV junction during ventricular systole (top) and diastole (bottom) showing the anterior leaflet forcing the catheter tip off the AV junction. LVOF = left ventricular outflow tract; LA = left atrium; MV = mitral valve; ABL. cath = ablation catheter. Used with permission from Avitall B, et al.[77]

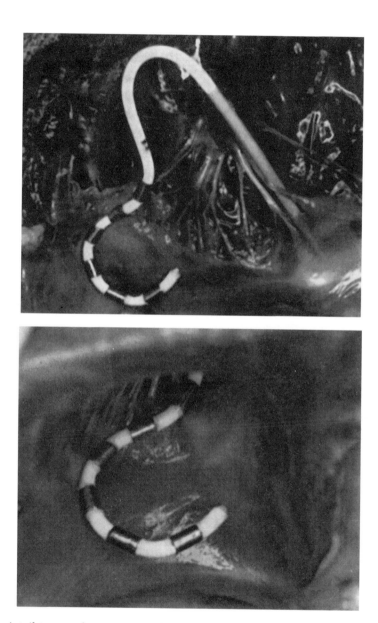

Figure 18. A pigtail-type catheter equipped with 4-mm ablation ring electrodes. Top: the pigtail positioned in the left atria on the AV ring of a dog heart. Bottom: the same heart was opened to expose the mitral apparatus. Used with permission from Avitall B, et al.[77]

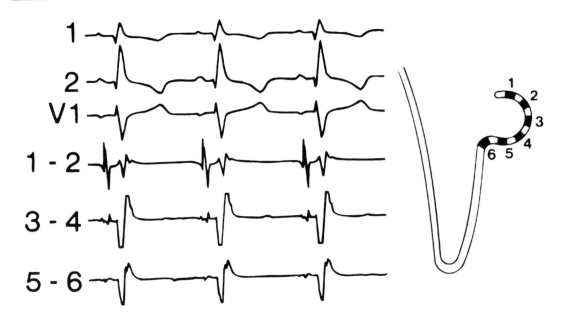

Figure 19. The electrograms recorded from the pigtail portion of the catheter show the transition of the atrial and ventricular electrograms across the mitral ring. The upper three tracings show the scalar leads I, II, and V_1 and the bottom four tracings show the bipolar recordings from the 4-mm ring electrodes shown on the right. Used with permission from Avitall B, et al.[77]

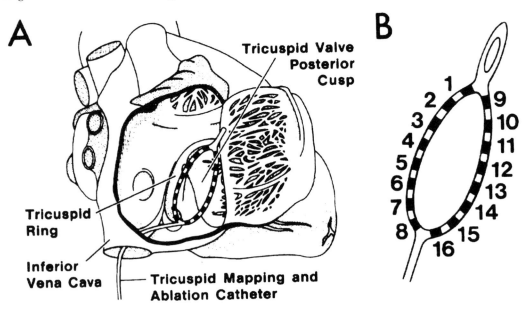

Figure 20. The loop catheter is introduced from the femoral vein into the inferior vena cava and across the tricuspid valve (**A**). The loop is equipped with 16, 4-mm long electrodes spaced 4 mm apart. The most distal portion of the catheter is equipped with a small secondary loop (**B**). Used with permission from Avitall B, et al.[77]

tion control.[57] The smaller secondary loop is anchored in the RV outflow, and the proximal end is anchored by the inferior vena cava as shown in Figure 21. Simultaneous recordings from the electrodes can show both atrial and ventricular electrograms (Figure 22). Adjustments can be made by moving the catheter vertically, by rotating it, and/or by changing the deflection angle of the loop. As shown in Figure 23 (left panel), the mapping/ablation electrodes on the loop catheter adapt well to the tricuspid ring orifice. Discrete, sequential, perivalvular, atrial lesions were produced around the tricuspid valve without the need to readjust the catheter Figure 23 (right panel) (Table 2).

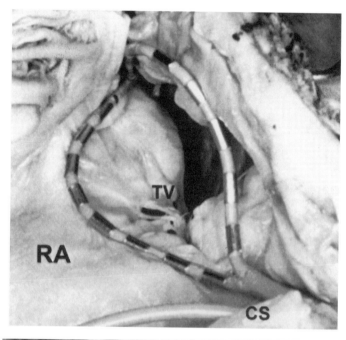

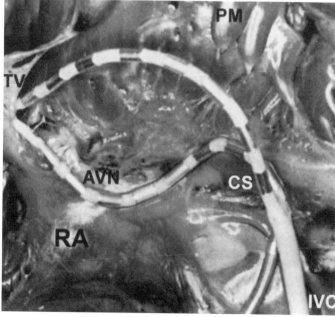

Figure 21. Top: The loop catheter is positioned in a human cadaver heart with an intact tricuspid orifice. Bottom: A dog heart with the orifice open showing the septal leaflet of the tricuspid ring. RA = right atrium; TV = tricuspid valve; CS = coronary sinus; AVN = atrial ventricular node; IVC = inferior vena cava; PM = papillary muscle. Used with permission from Avitall B, et al.[77]

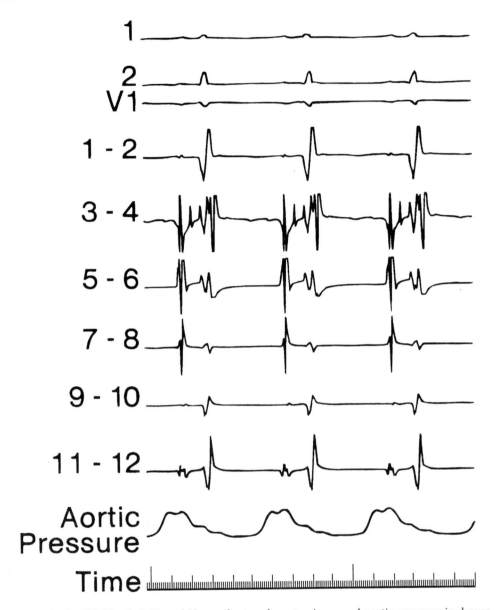

Figure 22. Scalar ECG leads I, II, and V$_1$ are the top three tracings, and aortic pressure is shown on the bottom tracing. Simultaneous recordings from the ring electrode: 1–2, 3–4, 5–6, and 7–8 are from the posterior septum, and 9–10 and 11–12 are from the anterior wall. Used with permission from Avitall B, et al.[77]

Cooled-Tip Mapping and Ablation and Thoracoscopic Cryoablation

Cryoablation would be a desirable means of tissue destruction. Temporary tissue cooling prior to tissue ablation can provide an additional means to ascertain the appropriate application of ablative energy and subsequent freezing of the tissue causes membrane cleavage and cell death with minimal inflammatory response that is seen with tissue heating. During the era of surgical open-chest mapping and cryoablation of accessory pathways and ventricular tachy-

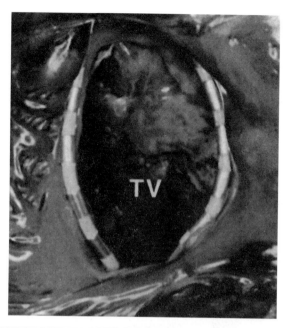

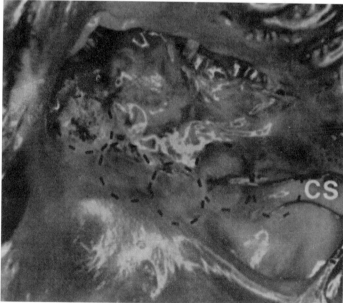

Figure 23. The loop catheter is seen from the open right atrium at the tricuspid valve (TV) orifice of a dog heart (top panel). Discrete perivalvular atrial sequential lesions were produced around the tricuspid valve (bottom panel). Used with permission from Avitall B, et al.[77]

cardia large cryoprobes were used to freeze the tissues to temperatures of −40°C for 3 min. The delivery of a refrigerant cooling to accomplish tissue freezing using an acceptable size catheter is currently not available. However, several patents and catheter prototypes have been published (Peter Freedman patent).[58] An additional concept is the use of the Paltier effect to cool the tip of the

catheter. Novoste Corporation has introduced such a catheter, which was capable of decreasing the temperature of the ablative electrode that causes local electrophysiological alteration of the tissues in contact with the catheter tip. If the local response post cooling indicates appropriate catheter location, RF power is applied to complete the ablation (Novoste patent).[59] Because of the

Table 2
Lesion Measurements (mm) Using Various Electrode Configurations

	2 + 2	2 + 2 + 2	2 + 2 + 2 + 2	4 mm
Length	11.4 ± 1.6	11.9 ± .9*	12.3 ± 0.7*	9.1 ± 0.4
Width	7.8 ± 1.1#	6.5 ± 1.1	5.4 ± 0.2	6.9 ± 1.2
Depth	7.1 ± 1.4*	7.1 ± 1.2*	6.8 ± 1.3	5.3 ± 0.6

* P <0.05 vs. 4 mm.
# P <0.05 vs. 2 + 2 + 2 + 2.
Used with permission from Avitall B, et al.[33]

significant cooling limitation with intracardiac catheter technology, several investigators have proposed the application of such technology using thoracoscopic techniques to introduce cryoprobes into the pericardial space and guiding the probes using standard electrophysiological mapping techniques to the arrhythmogenic area which would initially cooled without freezing. If the probes are proven to be at the proper location (i.e., arrhythmia termination, preexcitation block, etc.), the tissue is frozen by lowering the temperature to −40°C, which is possible with this technique since the probes are not bathed in rapidly flowing blood. In an animal ventricular tachycardia model, this technology has been applied with 100% success in ablation of the VT in this model.[57,58] Furthermore, the cryolesions were transmural as shown in Figure 24.

The Ablation of Atrial Fibrillation

Atrial fibrillation ablation presents the greatest challenge in the development of safe and effective catheter technology. Based on the work of Cox et al.[59,60] we have made an initial assumption that the ablation of AF is likely to require lesions that in some respect mimic the surgical maze procedure. These lesions are linear, contiguous, and transmural. They must end in a fashion preventing the formation of atrial flutter. However, the current acceptable catheter and RF power technology is unlikely to allow the design flexibility capable of creating lesions similar to the surgical maze without inflating production costs, compounding complexity, and compromising safety. In pursuing such an ablation system, we further assume that not every patient with AF requires a full set of maze lesions. In addition, a successful AF ablation system may not totally eliminate the arrhythmia but may provide an increase in susceptibility to drugs, a decrease in the length of time and incidence of paroxysmal AF, or conversion of sustained AF to paroxysmal AF. Since there is much to be learned about the mechanism of AF, a simple safe technology that provides the operator with mapping and ablation capability should be used initially. Such a technology will maximize the information input and increase our understanding of this arrhythmia. In addition, it will allow us to refine the AF ablation tools and ablation techniques. In this section, we have defined the mechanical, electrical, and physiological requirements for AF ablation using RF power, and we have described a system that meets many of the critical design criteria.

Having multiple ablation electrodes on a single shaft allows for minimal catheter manipulation in creating long linear lesions and, therefore, is likely to reduce both thromboembolic risk and radiation exposure. To justify exposing the patient to this procedure, the recovery of atrial mechanical function after the procedure is imperative. Theoretically, AF can be terminated by ablating the majority of the atrial tissues.

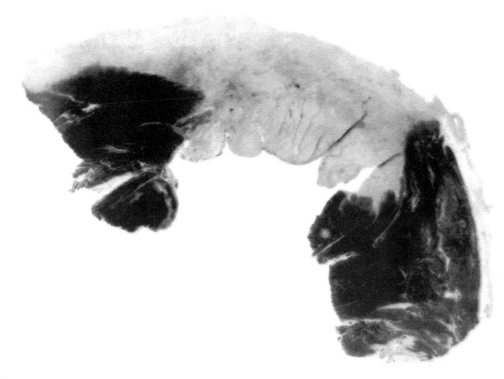

Figure 24. Trichrome stain of a cyrolesion in the left ventricular freewall of a dog with monomorphic ventricular tachycardia. The lesion is transmural and there is a sharp demarcation between the cryoablated region and the myocardium. Used with permission from Avitall B, et al.[77]

However, if mechanical function is not restored, the risk of thromboembolic stroke will remain high, requiring continuous anticoagulation. Furthermore, other than rate control, no mechanical benefit will be provided to the patient. If this is the outcome of a catheter-based AF intervention, AV node modification or AV node or His ablation followed by permanent pacer insertion and continued anticoagulation may be a more appropriate therapy for those highly symptomatic patients whose medical therapy has failed. Such approach presents with minimal acute risk and often is rewarding.[61]

The Design of Multi-Electrode Catheter Ablation

The primary guiding forces for such technology must be safety and to a lesser extent efficacy. The most devastating nonfatal complication of an ablation procedure is the development of thromboembolic stroke, which may totally disable a patient who was functional before the intervention. Such a stroke may result from either excessive catheter dragging which could dislodge an existing fibrin clot or from boiling tissues and blood, causing the formation of char which is loosely adherent to the ablating electrode and/or the endocardium. Once the catheter is moved, this material may be dislodged and could cause a stroke, a myocardial infarct, or a peripheral infarct. There are many other complications that need to be avoided, including:

- Perforation leading to tamponade.
- Injury to the AV valves.
- Injury to ventricular tissues and coronaries.

- Sinus node injury/dysfunction.
- AV node and/or His ablation requiring the insertion of a permanent pacemaker.
- Excessive radiation exposure for both the patient and the operator.
- Development of a new rhythm disturbance, such as incessant atrial flutter, which may be more difficult to treat than the AF for which the patient initially received the intervention.
- The amount of tissue ablated should be the minimum necessary to convert and maintain the atria in sinus rhythm while allowing for effective recovery of atrial transport.

The goal of catheter-based ablation of AF should be safe minimal tissue destruction allowing for the restoration of sinus rhythm under autonomic nervous system control combined with recovery of atrial mechanical transport to prevent the development of a thromboembolic event and provide hemodynamic benefits for the patient.

Technological Assumptions and Goals

When using RF power, the most important factor involved in the creation of an effective linear lesion is the contact between the ablating electrode(s) and the tissue. Based on this primary principle, a safe and effective catheter-based system to ablate AF must meet various design goals including:

- Ability of the catheter to establish and maintain good, continuous contact with the atrial tissues while delivering energy or recording electrical activity.
- Ability of the catheter to adapt to the curvature of the atrium.
- Ability to deliver RF energy to create transmural, continuous linear lesions with minimal tissue destruction.

- Minimization of the need for catheter manipulation to reduce thromboembolic risk and radiation exposure.
- Ease in placement of the catheter in specific anatomic orientations with effective control over the degree and direction of deflection.
- Titration of RF power using closed-loop temperature control and local electrical activity monitoring, to define the formation of an effective lesion and prevent overheating and char formation.
- Ability to retrieve discrete localized recordings from multiple electrodes to assess electrophysiological changes during energy application.
- Simplicity of construction and operation to ensure safety.

Having multiple ablation electrodes on a single shaft can minimize catheter manipulation and may reduce both thromboembolic risk and radiation exposure. A catheter should be atraumatic, having a sufficiently soft tip as to prevent perforations and other injuries to structures. The catheter should not be able to become hooked on atrial tissues or valvular structures. In order to prevent tissue and blood overheating, the ideal power control should be a temperature-sensing unit that limits the power automatically via a closed-loop control system. Finally, during an era of cost-cutting measures where severe limits are placed on medical expenditures, the design of an ablation system must be simple to construct, and the overall cost of the procedure must be minimized.

The Design of the Atrial Fibrillation Ablation Catheter System

Because the atrial chambers, especially the left atrium, are globular structures, we hypothesized that a catheter system that creates adjustable loops is most likely to be able to adapt to the atrial structure. Furthermore, since the atrial tissues are only a few millimeters thick and are elastic, controlled expansion of the loop will force effective continuous contact over the entire length of the ablation portion of the shaft. We developed a catheter system that met each of the design goals noted above. This AF ablation system is capable of safely creating continuous, transmural, linear lesions with minimal tissue destruction.[62-67]

The catheter system consists of:

- **Catheter:** Two versions of a loop-type catheter system were tested. Both consisted of a 7F catheter with 24 4-mm ring electrodes spaced 4 mm apart along the deflectable portion of the catheter. Thus, the total ablation section measures 19 cm. The first catheter is a monorail system with a ring at the distal end of the catheter. A guidewire equipped with a ball-like protrusion (diameter = 2 mm) at its distal end can be inserted through the ring. When the guidewire is retracted, this ball prevents the ablation catheter ring from sliding off the guidewire as the catheter's distal end bends to form a loop. The second version (Figure 25) has a guidewire permanently attached to the catheter's distal tip. In both versions the size of the loop can be adjusted by varying the length of the catheter shaft extending out of a long guiding sheath. We have tested this second system with and without 24 thermocouple temperature sensors placed under the center of each of the ring electrodes along the outer surface of deflection.
- **Guidewire:** A long, soft guidewire is attached to the distal tip of the catheter.
- **Sheaths:** The system utilizes 70-cm long 11F guiding sheaths with a 30° angular bend at the distal end. The sheath is equipped with a central port and a locking hemostatic seal mechanism capable of accommodating the 7F catheter and the guidewire. The sheath also has a sidearm infusion port.

Figure 25 shows the fixed wire catheter system in various degrees of deflection. When placing the catheter for mapping and ablation, it is inserted into a guiding sheath and threaded into the atrial chamber. With the catheter in the atrium, the guidewire can be retracted into the sheath causing the distal tip to bend and create an adjustable loop. Depending on the magnitude of the guidewire retraction and the size of the catheter portion extending from the sheath, the electrode portion of the catheter can bend to create loops of various sizes. The body of the catheter can be forced against the atrial wall with the aid of the sheath. The body of the catheter is flexible enough to adapt to the curvature of the atrial walls, yet stiff enough to force the thin atrial walls to stretch around the catheter and maintain consistent electrode-tissue contact along the entire length of the ablation portion of the catheter. Since the forces that are applied to the atrial walls are distributed along the catheter shaft around the entire loop, no single point is exposed to very high forces. Once the catheter is placed, a locking mechanism attached to the guiding sheath holds the guidewire and catheter firmly in place. Hence, once it has been properly placed, this catheter can be used to generate long linear lesions without the need to move the catheter.

This ablation system was placed in 49 dogs with no mechanical injuries to the atrial or ventricular tissues, no damage to the valvular structures, and no entanglement of the catheter system with tissues. However, as mentioned previously, if an additional catheter is introduced into the cardiac chamber after the deployment of the AF ablation catheter, this second catheter should be retracted prior to the removal of the AF catheter. With this system, there is the potential for mechanical injury to occur across the intra-atrial septum. Once the

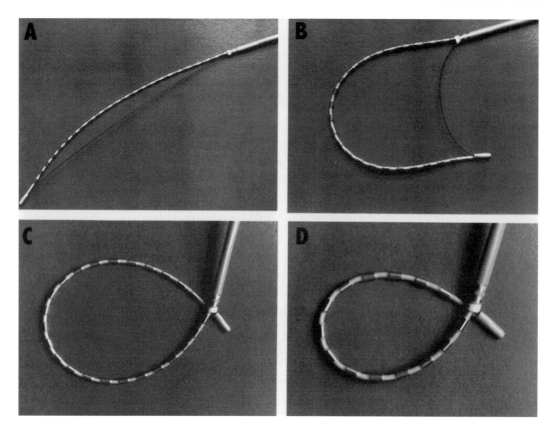

Figure 25. The AF ablation catheter. (**A**) Extended, (**B**) deflected to form a semicircular loop, (**C**) forming a large circular loop, and (**D**) forming a small circular loop. Used with permission from Avitall B, et al.[77]

guiding sheath is placed across the septum, it must be maintained at this position, particularly during catheter manipulation. If the sheath is not kept in the left atrium, the expansion of the catheter loop can result in septal tearing.

Positioning

Placement of this system in specific anatomic locations in this animal model usually required less than a minute. Once the catheter is in place, no further manipulation is needed and a long linear continuous lesion can be generated. Although this system naturally creates loops at the points of maximal diameter, by placing the guiding sheath at different levels within the atria or rotating the sheath, a variety of loops can be placed

in various anatomic locations (Figure 26). For the anatomic locations tested in this investigation, this catheter system is capable of consistently reproducing placements. The operator has the ability to adjust the catheter placement in case of poor contact without significantly changing the location of the lesion.

Lesion Formation

The most important factor involved in the creation of an effective lesion is the contact between the ablating electrode(s) and the tissues. Using the variable loop concept, the globular shaped atrial chambers will adapt around the loop providing continuous contact. These studies have established the feasibility of using ring electrodes placed on

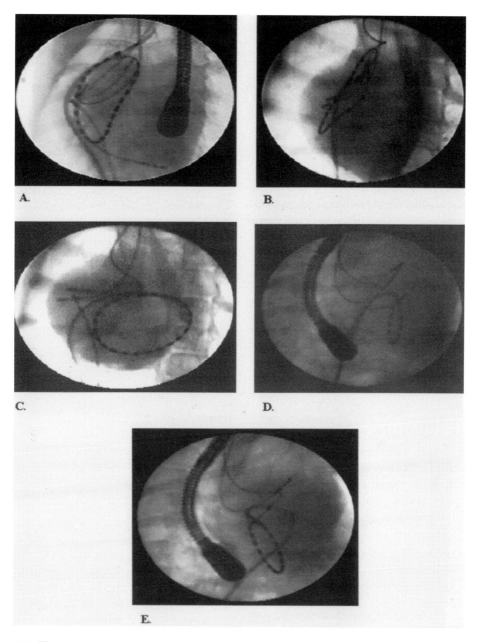

Figure 26. Fluoroscopic images of the catheter positioned in the right and left atria. (**A**) RA loop: A right atrial circular lesion extending from the anterior septal tricuspid valve to the RA appendage to the SVC and circling back to the IVC. (**B**) RAI: An RA isthmus lesion where the catheter is looped into the RV with the ablation electrodes across the tricuspid valve ring and the IVC. (**C**) LAH: A circular horizontal lesion placed under the pulmonary veins in the mid left atrium, parallel to the mitral valve. (**D**) LAV1: A vertical lesion extending from the mitral valve annulus medial of the pulmonary veins. (**E**) LAV2: A vertical linear lesion extending from the mitral valve to the LA appendage, lateral of the pulmonary veins. Panels A, B, D, and E also show a transesophageal echocardiography probe. Standard catheters are shown including a coronary sinus catheter (panel A) and a high right atrium catheter (panels A, C, and D). The two endocardial pacing wires can be seen descending from the superior vena cava into the right atrium in all five panels. Used with permission from Avitall B, et al.[77]

Table 3
Summary of Parameters from Linear Lesion Generation with Power
Titrated to Maintain 70°C for 60 Seconds*

	RA Loop	LAH
Total Individual Lesions	68	42
Maximum Power (W)	21 ± 14	11 ± 6*
Maximum Temperature (°C)	73 ± 8	70 ± 6
% Decrease LEA	65 ± 42	66 ± 19
% Contiguous	98	93
% Transmural	98	92
% Char	8	0
Width (mm)	6 ± 2	6 ± 2
Individual Lesion Length (mm)	6 ± 1	6 ± 1
Impedance (Ω)	131 ± 20	132 ± 12
Total Linear Lesion Length (cm)	12.4 ± 1.3	16 ± 1.1**

** = $P \leq 0.05$
RA Loop = circular lesion in the right atrium; LAH = horizontal lesion in the left atrium.
% Decrease LEA = percent decrease in amplitude of local electrical activity post lesion creation.
* The table only includes data from procedures in which all of the listed parameters were documented.
Used with permission from Avitall B, et al.[33]

the shaft of the catheter to create contiguous lesions. When using this technology equipped with temperature control, good tissue contact between the ablation electrodes along the shaft of the catheter enabled the creation of contiguous and transmural lesions in over 90% of the lesions created in both atria (Table 3). The average total length of these lesions measured 12.4 ± 1.3 cm in the right atrium and 16 ± 1.1 cm in the left atrium, and the lesions measured 6 ± 2 in width. With temperature control, the incidence of impedance rises was minimized, with 3% of total individual power applications in the left atrium and 6% in the right atrium. Although ablating consecutive individual ring electrodes made each linear lesion, one can envision a closed-loop ablation system that is capable of delivering RF power to multiple electrodes simultaneously and maintaining the temperature at a predetermined level.

Such a system will further reduce the procedure time significantly.

Recordings

Using 4-mm ring electrodes separated at 4-mm intervals allows for discrete localized recording of the electrical activity before, during, and after ablation. Such recording provides for online monitoring of the lesion formation. A reduction of greater than 50% in the recorded electrogram is an indication of lesion formation with type 3 lesions generated when the local electrical activity decreased by $67\% \pm 34\%$. It was further noted that if lesions are created during sinus rhythm or flutter, the formation of double potentials and fragmented electrical activity signify transmural lesion creation. The mechanism of this observation is likely related to the formation of a split atrial depolarization wavefront around the catheter as a result of the lesion. Since these recordings are made from two adjacent electrodes, the destruction of the tissue under and between these electrodes results in marked diminution of the recorded electrical activity. Further confirmation of tissue destruction is noted by the significant increase in the pacing threshold. The ability to retrieve discrete localized recordings from multiple electrodes provides additional safety and procedure features with regard to safeguarding the integrity of the His bundle and the additional capability of mapping. Furthermore, as has been shown in the example provided, online changes in AF may predict the efficacy of the ablation procedure.

The MECA System and Its Power Control

Similar to the loop catheter, placing ablation ring or coil electrodes on the catheter shaft expands the utility of such catheters from a single ablation point to a series of electrodes. However, these electrodes must be in firm contact with the tissues to allow for effective ablative lesions. To address the need for the creation of linear contiguous lesions in the atria for the ablation of AF, a catheter system has been proposed that consists of multiple coils (from 3–14 coils) 12.5 mm long and 2 mm apart which are mounted on bidirectional deflection catheters.[68] The catheter shafts are precurved to allow the ablation portion to address specific locations within the left and right atria (Figure 27). Since much of the current den-

sity in this type of electrode has been shown to concentrate at the edges of the electrodes, the thermocouple sensors are placed at the two edges of each electrode. The RF power is adjusted to maintain a preset temperature at the thermocouple that detects the highest temperature. Since the catheter distal end deflection size and curvature are not adjustable, several catheters are needed. This catheter system is likely to require significant catheter manipulation to complete the lesions. Since this system does not allow for the application of uniform pressure over the length of the distal portion of the catheter where the electrodes are mounted, it is likely that the electrode-to-tissue contact is unpredictable, resulting in nonuniform lesions. The large surface area of the electrodes and the likelihood that portions of the electrodes are in flowing blood necessitate the application of high RF power (>50 W) to reach the desired temperature. Noncontiguous lesions are likely to create the proper conditions for flutter formation. Because of the large electrodes, localized electrogram activity reflects a summation of a large tissue mass, which makes His bundle recordings and atrial flutter mapping difficult and less localized. The lower recording resolution of the catheter may result in inadvertent His bundle ablation. Advantages of

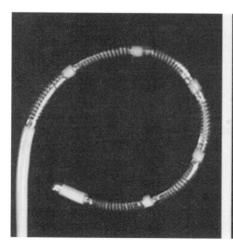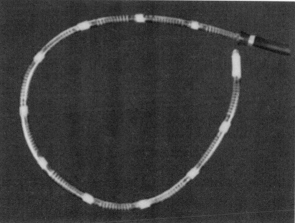

Figure 27. Catheters consisting of multiple coils (from 3 to 14) which are 12.5 mm long and spaced 2 mm apart mounted on (**A**) bi-directional deflection catheter and (**B**) a loop electrode with guidewire. Used with permission from Avitall B, et al.[77]

this system include the use of current deflection technology with which the practicing electrophysiologist is familiar and the ability for complete temperature control to prevent overheating and char formation.

Saline-Perfused Virtual Electrode Catheter

Cardiac Pathways Inc. has been testing a catheter system that consists of several balloon-type membranes that are filled with highly concentrated saline. The membrane has small holes that allow the saline to leak out.[69] RF power is applied to electrodes, which are mounted within the membrane chambers. This technology is delivered into the cardiac chamber over a guidewire that creates a loop within the chamber allowing the saline-filled membrane to contact the chamber walls. The RF power heats both the saline within the chamber and dissipates along the path of least resistance at the membrane-to-tissue interface as well as into the blood. Linear lesions are created by applying RF energy to each of the virtual electrodes and moving the catheter to a new adjacent location. It is yet unclear whether this technology is capable of creating linear lesions by ensuring that the current density is uniform along the saline-perfused membrane. Further concern is the amount of highly concentrated saline that the patient will receive in the course of the ablation procedure with this technology.

Sheath-Guided Catheter Ablation of Atrial Fibrillation

In multiple presentations and in a patent, Swartz et al.[70] have introduced the concept of multicurved sheaths to guide a standard ablation catheter to the desired locations within the right and left atria to aid in the creation of sequential lesions (the drag technique) (Figure 28). Using this technique it has been shown that the ablation of AF is possible. Relying on the findings of the maze procedure, discrete ablation tracks within the left and right atria are created using precurved left and right atria guiding introducers. Precise positioning of catheters within the heart is especially difficult due to the physiology of the heart and the inherent motion of the beating heart. A rigid sheath that is shaped for guiding an ablation or mapping catheter to a specific location in the heart greatly assists the creation of predefined ablation tracks and the mapping of well-known locations. With the precurved guiding introducer holding the ablation catheter in a predetermined location, the ablation catheter ablates on a predetermined ablation track. More than one passage may be necessary to fully ablate the track. After the ablation is complete, the first shaped guiding introducer is withdrawn and a second is inserted in place to create the next ablation track. This is repeated until all the preselected ablation tracks are completed in the heart. In the work of Swartz et al.,[70] nine predetermined ablation tracks are prescribed based on the experimental data from the maze procedure. The creation of each track is facilitated by a precurved guiding introducer. Four tracks are prescribed in the right atria and five tracks in the left atria. However, this technique requires many hours of catheter manipulations and x-ray exposure and most often a second session of this procedure is needed to ablate atrial flutters that are likely the result of incomplete linear lesions (Swartz abstracts and patent). Similarly, Haissaguerre et al.[71,72] have ablated chronic AF in humans by creating sequential lesions in the left atrium and the right atrium by dragging the catheter in a predetermined path similar to the maze procedure. Although no clear pathological evidence has been presented as to the linearity and contiguity of the lesions, the users of this technique have reported success in ablating AF and paroxysmal AF in humans. The data presented thus far indicate that many of the patients required a

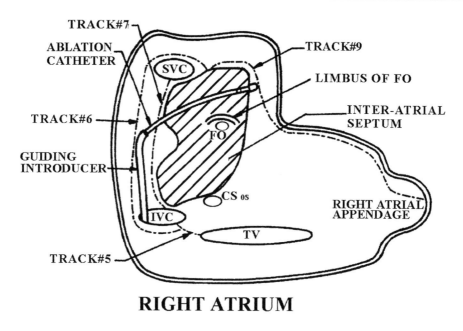

RIGHT ATRIUM

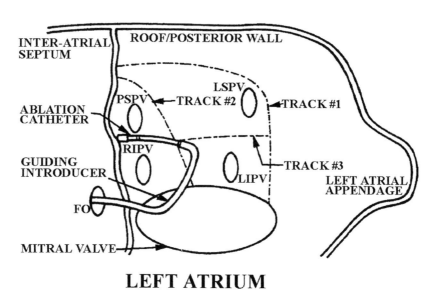

LEFT ATRIUM

Figure 28. The concept of multicurved sheaths to guide standard ablation catheters to the desired locations within the (**A**) right, (**B**) left atria to aid in the creation of sequential lesions to cure AF is shown in these two panels. Used with permission from Swartz JF, US Patent.

second procedure to ablate recurrent AF and atrial flutter.

The major attribute of this approach is its immediate availability. However, such an approach requires long procedure and radiation exposure times, since the catheter is dragged in small increments. Moving the catheter from one point to another over trabeculated tissues is unlikely to result in linear, contiguous lesions. This may lead to the formation of flutter circuits.[64] Furthermore, when dragging the catheter, it is possible that the catheter tip will force free a clot that may result in a stroke. The ideal system should be a catheter system that adapts to the tissues to be ablated and creates the lesion without excessive scraping movements. In order to create the lesions, several different preshaped sheaths have to be used that necessitate several sheath replacements during the procedure.[70] Since the catheter uses temperature control, it is likely that overheating and boiling can be avoided. Furthermore, it is yet unclear whether the elimination of the AF is a result of large atrial tissue debulking and whether atrial mechanical function is restored so as to justify this procedure by benefiting the patient with atrial mechanical contribution to cardiac output.

Saline-Perfused Multi-Electrode Ablation Catheter

Similar to the cooled-tip ablation catheter design, supra-cooling the ablation electrodes along the shaft of the catheter's design to create linear lesions would provide for increasing power application and larger lesion depth and width. In a design presented by Nakagawa et al. (personal communication), a multi-electrode catheter design was equipped with central saline infusion tubing with an opening between each of the ablation electrodes. The saline leaks out of the catheter and cools the ablation area. The investigators were able to show that this catheter design is capable of generating larger and deeper lesions compared to the lesions created without saline infusion.

Thoracoscopic Atrial Fibrillation Ablation Using RF Power

Other approaches to the effective treatment of AF have included delivering RF energy to create linear atrial lesions via a thoracoscopic intrapericardial approach. This is also a feasible way to create transmural and contiguous lesions in the atria without ex-

tensive catheterization. In a study reported by Avitall et al., thoracoscopic ports were placed in the fourth and fifth right intercostal spaces.[73] Under thoracoscopic visual control, RF energy (50 W for 30 sec) was applied via a 10-mm electrode on a handheld probe to create four different types of linear lesions similar to those in the maze procedure in both atria. After generation of all four lesions, sustained AF was no longer inducible. The lesions were also transmural and continuous. However, a purely thoracoscopic approach is limiting in the fact that it is difficult to maneuver and certain lesions cannot be created due to accessibility. However, it may prove to be useful in conjunction with transcatheter ablation technologies and in patients who are at high risk for the open-chest maze procedure.

Mapping and Catheter Localization Technology

Effective rapid and accurate identification of the arrhythmogenic tissues to be ablated represent another important issue in cardiac interventional electrophysiology that is undergoing changes with new emerging technologies. The use of powerful computer graphics technology allows for three-dimensional representation of the cardiac chambers and the electrical activity within them. Several of such technologies have been undergoing testing and others are still in the development stages.

Basket Mapping Catheters

Several variations of a basket catheter have been introduced in recent years, all consisting of several soft spines that are collapsed into an introducer sheath and flares out by using a preshaped curve on each spine or can be expanded by pulling a string that is attached to the dome of the basket

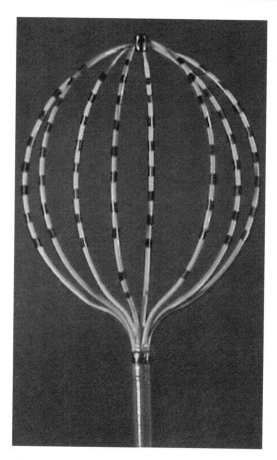

Figure 29. A basket catheter with eight soft collapsible spines that expand in the atria for mapping or pacing with the multiple electrodes on each spine. Used with permission from Avitall B, et al.

(Figure 29).[74] Each spine has multiple electrodes spaced along the shaft either in pairs or are equidistant. The number of electrodes is limited by the ability to insert the conducting wires into each spine and maintaining the total catheter size within 9F–10F. The position of the spines within the cardiac chamber is defined by marker rings. This technology can now guide an ablation catheter to a specific anatomic location by using a high-frequency signal that is emitted by the ablation catheter tip and is received by the electrodes on the spine which in turn identify the location of the ablation tip with respect to the closest electrodes on the spine.

Transcoronary Mapping (CARDIMA)

Although much of the development of cardiac electrophysiology mapping has been intracardiac, significant information can be collected by mapping the coronary tree. Since the coronary tree is often distributed in specific territories, the introduction of miniature recording multi-electrode wires into the coronary veins or arteries is expected to record the electrical activity from these territories. Although most ischemia-related ventricular arrhythmias are originated from the endocardium, such technology can provide important guidance during an ablation procedure. However, most electrophysiologists are reluctant to cannulate the coronary arterial tree.

Noncontact Mapping System

A novel catheter-based technology used to acquire simultaneous data to create unique maps of endocardial activation has been described.[75] Using a noncontact balloon catheter, an endocardial map was created without endocardial contact. A catheter-mounted multi-electrode array consisting of a wire braid on the surface of an 8-mL balloon is introduced into the right atrium. Using the inverse solution mathematics (boundary element method), 3,360 "virtual" electrograms were reconstructed onto a shell model of the endocardium (Figure 30). This technology provides extensive simultaneous data without the need to make adequate contact with the endocardium.

Nonfluoroscopic Electromagnetic Catheter Tip Localization System

A major limitation of the current methods of cardiac mapping is the inability to accurately relate local electrograms to their spatial orientation. Gepstein and associates (Biosense Inc.) have created a system for nonfluoroscopic, catheter-based endocardial mapping that enables the generation of

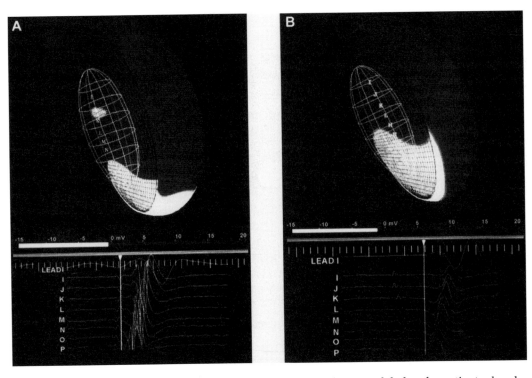

Figure 30. An isopotential map of the left ventricular endocardium modeled to the patients chamber dimensions during (**A**) sinus and (**B**) fasicular tachycardia. The location of the multi-electrode array is represented by the smaller ellipsoid. Used with permission from Gepstein L, et al.[47]

three-dimensional electroanatomic maps of the cardiac chambers.[76] The system is composed of a miniature passive magnetic field sensor just proximal to the tip electrode of an 8F deflectable tip catheter and a locator pad positioned beneath the operating table that generates ultra-low magnetic fields from three coils. Each coil generates a magnetic field that decays as a function of distance from the respective coil. The sensor in the catheter tip measure the strength of the magnetic field, thus giving an accurate indication of where the catheter is in relation to the three coils and in space. By dragging the catheter against the epicardium in different locations of the atria and ventricle while recording local electrograms, a three-dimensional anatomic model of the heart was created with the local electrical activity mapped directly upon it (Figure 31). The accuracy of the system was found to be highly reproducible.

Sonographic Catheter Localization

Mounting a transmitting sonographic crystal at the distal end of an ablation electrode and placing receiving crystals mounted on the chest provides a three-dimensional configuration of the intracardiac movement of the catheter. The distances between the transmitting crystal and each of the external crystals is calculated online and creates a map of the intracardiac anatomic structure and catheter location.

Conclusions

The goal of RF arrhythmia ablation is to minimize the amount of tissue damage while eliminating the arrhythmogenic foci. A variety of technologies are currently used to maximize the ability to create effective lesions, and future technology will likely

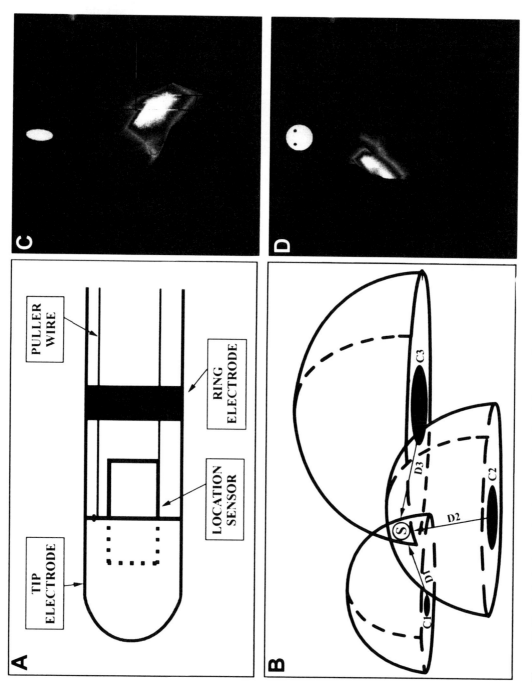

Figure 31. Typical electroanatomic maps of swine left ventricle created by the nonfluoroscopic mapping method. Both were constructed using 60 sampling points. The white areas show the points of earliest activation in the (**A**) right lateral view of left ventricle during right ventricular midseptal pacing and of (**B**) left ventricle during sinus rhythm. Used with permission from Gepstein L, et al.[47]

further increase ablation efficacy while minimizing patient risks.

Lesion Generation

There are numerous factors involved in determining the size of lesions generated using RF power. The most important of these are: electrode size, shape, and material; electrode-tissue contact; electrode-tissue orientation; RF power level and duration; and temperature at the electrode-tissue interface. Adjustments in any of these variables can significantly impact the dimensions of generated RF lesions. Other tools that can be useful in ensuring adequate lesion formation include the monitoring of temperature and impedance changes during power application, the use of intracardiac ultrasound, and possibly galvanic current monitoring.

Catheter Design

In recent years, many unique ablation and mapping catheter systems have been developed. The use of cooled-tip technology allows the formation of larger and deeper lesions. Catheters with segmental and multi-electrodes arrays provide flexibility in lesion size and enable the creation of long linear lesions. Preshaped catheters have been designed to improve catheter mobility and tissue contact for specific tissue targets such as the left atrium and the tricuspid isthmus. New tools that allow for higher density mapping and cooled-tip mapping provide increased precision in identifying the tissue to be ablated. Noncontact mapping systems and systems using electromagnetic and sonographic technology are capable of defining the cardiac chamber anatomy while tracking the ablation catheter tip. Each of these technologies can increase the efficacy and efficiency of cardiac ablation procedures.

Ablation of Atrial Fibrillation

Because of the success that has been achieved in treating chronic AF with surgical procedures, the creation of RF atrial fibrillation ablation technology has been rapidly progressing. This chapter discusses the physiological and technological considerations for the design of catheter technology for the ablation of AF. Several catheter designs have been presented, including a multipolar loop catheter that can create variable sized loops within the right and left atria that force the tissues to create consistent contact enabling the generation of transmural contiguous linear lesions. Other designs include preshaped multi-electrode catheters, a saline-perfused virtual electrode catheter, a sheath-guided system using standard ablation catheters, and thoracoscopic ablation using cryotechnology or RF power.

The Future

Similar to the field of angioplasty 15 years ago, the technology of ablative catheters and energy sources is still in its infancy. As newer generations of catheters are introduced, ablative procedures may become easier, safer, and more successful. Catheters that allow for better mapping and ablation results will reduce radiation exposure time. Electrophysiological testing and therapeutic ablation in a single session are already being done, resulting in decreases in morbidity rates and length of hospital stay. The rapid technological and methodological advancement that has taken place since the introduction of coronary and peripheral angioplasty will likely occur with the treatment of cardiac arrhythmias. Innovative investigators in both industry and medicine will provide practitioners with an assortment of catheters and techniques that will enhance the currently available modalities and provide insight as to the safest and most effective approach for cardiac arrhythmia ablation.

References

1. Avitall B, Mughal K, Hare J, et al. The effects of electrode-tissue contact on radiofrequency lesion generation. PACE 1997:12:2899–2910.
2. Harvey M, Kim Y, Sousa J, et al. Impedance monitoring during radiofrequency catheter ablation in humans. PACE 1992;15:22–27.
3. Hoffman E, Remp T, Gerth A, et al. Does impedance monitoring during radiofrequency catheter ablation reduce the risk of impedance rise? Circulation —Suppl) 1993; 88:I-165.
4. Strickberger S, Hummel J, Vorperian V, et al. A randomized comparison of impedance and temperature monitoring during accessory pathway ablation. Circulation 1993; 88(4):I-295.
5. Remp T, Hoffman E, Dorwarth U, et al. A new catheter design for validation of preablation impedance as a marker for contact. JACC 1997;29(2):1021-68:333A.
6. Strickberger S, Vorperian V, Man K, et al. Relation between impedance and endocardial contact during radiofrequency catheter ablation. Am Heart J 1994:128(2):226–9.
7. Grogan EW, Nellis SH, Subramanian R. Impedance changes during catheter ablation by radiofrequency energy: a potential method for monitoring efficacy of lesion generation. JACC 1987;9:95A.
8. Dorwarth U, Mattke S, Muller D, et al. Impedance monitoring during constant power and temperature-controlled radiofrequency catheter ablation. Circulation 1993; 88(4):#0877;I-165.
9. Chan R, Johnson S, Packer D. The effect of ablation electrode length and catheter tip/endocardial orientation on radiofrequency lesion size in the canine right atrium. PACE 1994;17:225;797.
10. He D, Marcus F, Lampe L, et al. Temperature monitoring during RF energy application without the use of thermistors or thermocouples. PACE 1996;19:2344;626.
11. He D, Sharma P, Marcus F, et al. In vivo experiment of radiofrequency (RF) energy application using bio-battery-induced temperature monitoring. JACC 1997;29(2):913–123; 32A.
12. Kalman J, Fitzpatrick A, Chin M, et al. Efficiency of heating with radiofrequency energy is related to stability of tissue contact: evaluation by intracardiac echocardiography. Circulation 1994;90:1454;I-270.
13. Kalkman J, Fitzpatrick A, Olgin J, et al. Biophysical characteristics of radiofrequency lesion formation in vivo: dynamics of catheter tip-tissue contact evaluated by intracardiac echocardiography. Am Heart J 1997;133(1): 8–18.
14. Chan R, Johnson S, Seward J, et al. Effect of ablation catheter tip/endocardial surface orientation on radiofrequency lesion size in the canine ventricle. JACC 1997;29(2):727-6; 76A.
15. Hoyt R, Huang S, Marcus F, et al. Factors influencing trans-catheter radiofrequency ablation of the myocardium. J App Cardiol 1986;1:469–486.
16. Hoffman E, Haberl R, Pulter R, et al. Biophysical Parameters of radiofrequency catheter ablation. Int J Cardiol 1992;13:213–222.
17. Haines D. Determinants of lesion size during radiofrequency catheter ablation: the role of electrode-tissue contact pressure and duration of energy delivery. J Cardiovascu Electrophysiol 1991;2:509–515.
18. Bardy G, Sawyer P, Johnson G, et al. Radiofrequency ablation: effect of voltage and pulse duration on canine myocardium. Am J Physiol 1990;258:H1899–H1905.
19. Wittkampf F, Hauer R, de Medina R. Control of radiofrequency lesion size by power regulation. Circulation 1989;80(4):962–968.
20. Simmers T, Wittkampf F, Hauer R, et al. In vivo ventricular lesion growth in radiofrequency catheter ablation. PACE 1994;17(II): 523–531.
21. Avitall B, Hare J, Silverstien E, et al. Radiofrequency ablation of atrial tissues: power requirements. JACC (Suppl) 1994:276A.
22. Haines D, McRury I, Whayne J, et al. Radiofrequency ablation at the tricuspid-inferior vena cava isthmus: unipolar versus bipolar delivery. Circulation 1994;90(4):3202;I-594.
23. Anfinsen O, Kongsgaard E, Foerster A, et al. Radiofrequency catheter ablation of pig right atrial free wall: larger lesions but similar incidence of lung injury and diaphragmal paresis with two-catheter bipolar compared to unipolar electrode configuration. Circulation 1995;92(4):3260;I-557.
24. Anfinsen O, Kongsgaard E, Aass H, et al. Radiofrequency current ablation of thin-walled structures: an in vitro study comparing unipolar and bipolar electrode configuration. PACE 1996;19:594;714.
25. Tomassoni G, Jain M, Dixon-Tulloch E, et al. Ground patch location significantly effects radiofrequency ablative lesion dimensions. JACC 1997;29(2):750–6;203A.
26. Otomo K, Arruda M, Tondo C, et al. Why does a large tip electrode make a deeper lesion? Circulation 1995;92(8):3814;I-793.

27. Haines D, Verow A. Observations on electrode-tissue interface temperature and effect on electrical impedance during radiofrequency ablation of ventricular myocardium. Circulation 1990;82:1034–1038.

28. Haines D. The biophysics of radiofrequency catheter ablation in the heart: the importance of temperature monitoring. PACE 1993;16:586–591.

29. Hoffmann E Mattke JS, Dorwarth U, et al. Temperature-controlled radiofrequency catheter ablation of AV conduction: first clinical experience. Eur Heart J 1993;14:57–64.

30. Haines D, Watson D. Tissue heating during radiofrequency catheter ablation: a thermodynamic model and observations in isolated perfused and superperfused canine right ventricular free wall. PACE 1989;12:962–976.

31. McRury I, Whayne J, Mitchell M, et al. Electrode size and temperature effects on lesion volume during temperature-controlled RF ablation in vivo. JACC 1997;29(2):928-28; 123A.

32. Kongsgaard E, Steen T, Amlie J. Temperature guided radiofrequency catheter ablation: cathcter tip temperature underestimates tissue temperature. Circulation 1994; 90(4):1457;I-271.

33. Fleischman S, Panescu D, Whayne J, et al. In vitro study of temperature sensor placement during temperature-controlled radiofrequency ablation. PACE 1995;18:293;869.

34. Haines D, Watson D, Verow A. Electrode radius predicts lesion radius during radiofrequency energy heating. Validation of a proposed hemodynamic model. Circ Res 1990; 67(1):124–129.

35. Langberg J, Lee M, Chin M, et al. Radiofrequency catheter ablation: the effect of electrode size on lesion volume in vivo. PACE 1990;13:1242–1248.

36. Langberg J, Gallagher M, Strickberger S, et al. Temperature-guided radiofrequency catheter ablation with very large distal electrodes. Circulation 1993;88:245–249.

37. McRury I, Whayne J, Haines D. Temperature measurement as a determinant of tissue heating during radiofrequency catheter ablation: an examination of electrode thermistor positioning for measurement accuracy. JCVE 1995;6(4):268–278.

38. Strickberger S, Davis J, Maguire M. Radiofrequency ablation of the atrium using sequential coil electrodes. JACC 1996;27(2):1037-3; 400A.

39. Mitchell M, McRury I, Haines D. Results of linear right atrial radiofrequency ablation with a temperature controlled, multiple coil electrode catheter. JACC 1996;27(2):1037-3; 400A.

40. Fleischman S, Thompson R, Panescu D, et al. Flexible electrodes for long atrial lesions. Circulation 1996;94(8):3952;I-676.

41. Panescu D, Haines D, Fleischman S, et al. Atrial lesions by temperature-controlled radiofrequency ablation. Circulation 1996; 94(8):2891;I-493.

42. Whayne J, Haines D, Panescu D, et al. Ring and coil electrodes for ablation of atrial fibrillation. Circulation 1996;94(8);2891;I-493.

43. Hoey M, Mulier P, Shake J. pre-test mapping with cold Ringer's solution via screw-tip catheter before radiofrequency ablation. Circulation 1995;92(8):3813;I-793.

44. Hoey M, Mulier P, Shake J. Intramural ablations using screw-tip catheter and saline electrode produces predictable lesion sizes. Circulation 1995;92(8):3818;I-794.

45. Oeff M, Langberg J, Chin M, et al. Ablation of ventricular tachycardia using multiple sequential transcatheter application of radiofrequency energy. PACE 1992;15(8): 1167–1176.

46. Oeff M, Langberg J, Franklin J, et al. Effects of multipolar electrode radiofrequency energy delivery on ventricular endocardium. Am Heart J 1990;119:599–607.

47. Chang R, Stevenson W, Saxon L. Increasing catheter ablation lesion size by simultaneous application of radiofrequency current to two adjacent sites. Am Heart J 1993;125: 1276–1284.

48. Avitall B, Hare J, Mughal K, et al. Segmented ablation electrode: a system for flexible lesion size. Circulation 1994;90:671;I-126.

49. Mackey S, Thornton L, He D, et al. Simultaneous multipolar radiofrequency ablation in the monopolar mode increases lesion size. PACE 1996;19:1042–1048.

50. Baal T, Chen X, Kottkamp H, et al. Radiofrequency catheter ablation: improving lesion size achieved with conventional catheters. Circulation 1994;90:1463;I-272.

51. Haines D, Watson D. Tissue heating during radiofrequency catheter ablation: a thermodynamic model and observations in isolated perfused and superperfused canine right ventricualr free wall. PACE 1989;12:962–976.

52. Kovoor P, Eipper V, Dewsnap B, et al. The effect of differing frequencies on lesion size during radiofrequency ablation. Circulation 1996;94:3953;I-677.

53. Bru P, Lauribe P, Rouane A, et al. Catheter ablation using very high frequency energy: a new method without limitation due to impedance rise. Circulation 1994;90:2608;I-485.

54. Nakagawa H, Wittkampf F, Imai, et al. Pulsed current delivery combined with saline irrigation produces deeper radiofre-

quency lesions without steam "pop". JACC 1997;29:786-3;374A.

55. Avitall B, Hare J, Lessila C, et al. New generation of catheters for mapping and ablation: a rotating tip and lateral deflectable catheters. Circulation 1991;84(Suppl II):II-96.

56. Avitall B, Hare J, Krum D, et al. A new pigtail type catheter for retrograde atrial left-sided accessory pathway mapping and ablation. Circulation 1993;88:(Suppl):I-63.

57. Avitall B, Hare J, Khan M, et al. A new catheter for mapping and radiofrequency ablation of the AV node and right-sided accessory pathways. J Am Coll Cardiol 1993;21(Suppl A):418A.

58. Caceres JA, Akhtar M, Werner P, et al. Cryoablation of refractory sustained ventricular tachycardia due to coronary artery disease. Am J Cardiol 1989;63(5):296–300.

59. Cox JL, Boineau JP, Schussler RB, et al. Five-year experience with the Maze procedure for atrial fibrillation. Ann Thorac Surg 1993;56: 814–824.

60. Cox JL, Boineau JP, Schuessler RB, et al. Surgical interruption of atrial reentry as a cure for atrial fibrillation. In Olsson S, Alessie M, Campbell R, eds. Atrial Fibrillation. Futura Publishing Company, Armonk, NY, 1994, pp 373–404.

61. Feld K. Radiofrequency catheter ablation versus modification of the AV node for control of rapid ventricular response in atrial fibrillation. JCE 1995;6(3):217–228.

62. Avitall B, Hare J, Mughal K, et al. A catheter system to ablate atrial fibrillation in a sterile pericarditis dog model. PACE 1994;17(2): 774–778.

63. Avitall B, Hare J, Helms R. Vagally mediated atrial fibrillation in a dog model can be ablated by placing linear radiofrequency lesions at the junction of the right atrial appendage and the superior vena cava. PACE 1995;18:245;857.

64. Avitall B, Helms R, Chiang W, et al. Nonlinear atrial radiofrequency lesions are arrhythmogenic: a study of skipped lesions in the normal atria. Circulation 1995;92:1263;I-265.

65. Avitall B, Helms R, Chiang W, et al. The impact of transcatheter generated atrial linear radiofrequency lesions on atrial function and contractility. PACE 1996;19:530;698.

66. Avitall B, Helms R, Kotov A, et al. The use of temperature versus local depolarization amplitude to monitor atrial lesion maturation during the creation of linear lesions in both atria. Circulation 1996;94:3263;I-904.

67. Avitall B, Kotov A, Helms R. New monitoring criteria for transmural ablation of atrial tissues. Circulation 1996;94:2889;I-904.

68. Whayne JG, Haines DE, Panescu D, et al. Catheter system designs to facilitate RF ablation of atrial fibrillation. PACE 1996;19:650; I-339.

69. Cardiac Pathways

70. Swartz JF, Pellersels G, Silvers J, et al. A catheter-based curative approach to atrial fibrillation in humans. Circulation 1994;90;I-335.

71. Haissaguerre M, Gencel L, Fischer B, et al. Successful catheter ablation of atrial fibrillation. JCE 1994;5(12):1045–1052.

72. Haissaguerre M, Jais P, Shah D, et al. Right and left atrail radiofrequency catheter therapy of paroxysmal atrial fibrillation. JCE 1996;7(12):1132–1144.

73. Avitall B, Hare J, Mughal K, et al. Transcutaneous thoracoscopic intrapericardial cryoablation: an effective approach for mapping and ablation of ventricualr tachycardia. Circulation 1994;90(4):2609;I-485.

74. Panescu D, Greenspon AJ, Hsu SS, et al. Novel device for discrete navigation of conventional endocardial electrodes and simultaneous multisite mapping and pacing. PACE 1997;20:623;1205.

75. Peters NS, Jackman WM, Schilling RJ, et al. Human left ventricualr endocardial activation mapping using a novel noncontact catheter. Circulation 1997;95:1658–1660.

76. Gepstein L, Hayam G, Ben-Haim SA. A novel method for nonfluoroscopic catheter-based electroanatomical mapping of the heart. Circulation 1997;95:1611–1622.

77. Avitall B, et al. PACE 1994;17:908–916.

Section II

Implantable Cardioverter-Defibrillators

Section Editor: Igor Singer

Indications for Implantable Cardioverter-Defibrillator Therapy: Present and Future

Igor Singer

Introduction

The history of the implantable cardioverter-defibrillator (ICD) is perhaps the most remarkable story in modern clinical electrophysiology.[1] This unique innovation is remarkable for its conceptual simplicity and elegance. The ICD embodies many technologically challenging and complex innovations in computer hardware, software, lead technology, microcircuitry, and engineering innovations unforeseen by the ICD inventor, Michel Mirowski, when the concept of a standby ICD was initially proposed.[2] It is worth remembering this fact when one contemplates the evolution of the ICD as a therapeutic strategy. Consensus of experts regarding indications for ICD implantations is evolving in parallel to the advancements in ICD technology. Scientific evidence and accumulated clinical experience with the ICD serves to define present and possible future applications of ICD therapy. Impact of other competing or complementary therapeutic strategies, such as interventional catheter techniques for ventricular tachycardia (VT) ablation, may affect timing and sequencing of ICD therapy in the overall scheme of therapy for patients with lethal ventricular arrhythmias. Discussion of current indications for ICD therapy should be viewed, therefore, as a starting point from which future applications are likely to emerge.

Current Indications for ICD Therapy

Guidelines for the use of ICDs were published in 1991 by two expert panels: one from North American Society for Pacing and Electrophysiology (NASPE)[3] and the other from the American College of Cardiology and American Heart Association Joint Task Force.[4] These guidelines serve as a useful framework on which to base the present discussion. Importantly, however, since the publication of these guidelines, a number of randomized studies have been completed that have either corroborated or modified these recommendations. The NASPE panel recommended the following classification[3]:

1. *Class 1*: ICD therapy is indicated, based up the consensus of experts.

From Singer I, Barold SS, Camm AJ (eds): Nonpharmacological Therapy of Arrhythmias for the 21st Century: The State of the Art. Futura Publishing Co, Inc., Armonk, NY, © 1998.

2. *Class 2*: ICD is a therapeutic option, but the consensus does not exist.
3. *Class 3*: ICD therapy is not indicated.

It should be emphasized at this juncture that *consensus* of experts does not represent anything more or less than what the word suggests: a general agreement among the experts. Departures from the accepted consensus frequently result in scientific progress and evolution of new concepts. In fact, the development of the ICD represented a major departure from the existing "consensus" when first proposed.[5] Thus, the consensus statement should be viewed as only a starting point for discussion.

Class 1 Indications

Class 1 indications are listed in Table 1. It is now accepted beyond all reasonable doubt that ICD therapy is superior to all other available antiarrhythmic therapy for treatment of aborted sudden cardiac death.

Table 1
Class 1 ICD Indications

1. One or more episodes of spontaneous sustained VT or VF in a patient in whom EP testing and/or spontaneous arrhythmia cannot be used accurately to predict efficacy of other therapies.
2. Recurrent episodes of spontaneous sustained VT or VF in a patient despite antiarrhythmic drug therapy (guided by EP testing or Holter).
3. Spontaneous sustained VT or VF in a patient in whom antiarrhythmic drug therapy is limited by intolerance or noncompliance.
4. Persistent inducibility of clinically relevant sustained VT or VF at EP study, on best available drug therapy or despite surgical or catheter abalation, in a patient with spontaneous VT or VF.
5. Asymptomatic nonsustained VT in patients with coronary artery disease and left ventricular dysfunction (LVEF <.36) who have inducible sustained VT at EP study not suppressed with intravenous procainamide.

ICD = implantable cardioverter-defibrillator; VT = ventricular tachycardia; VF = ventricular fibrillation; EP = electrophysiological. Modified from references 3 and 4.

The puerile debate that existed in the literature between those arguing that ICD therapy, though remarkably effective for terminating ventricular fibrillation (VF) and VT, may not necessarily prolong life[6] and those arguing that the overwhelming accumulated clinical evidence supports ICD superiority[7] has been settled recently by the publication of the Antiarrhythmic Versus Implantable Defibrillator (AVID) trial results confirming the superiority of ICD.[8] This NIH-supported randomized prospective clinical trial compared the outcome of patients treated with amiodarone or sotalol with patients treated with ICD after documented aborted sudden cardiac death. It was stopped prematurely following demonstration of 38% improved survival at 1 year in patients randomized to ICD. Therefore, it can now be categorically stated that patients who present with aborted sudden cardiac death documented to be due to hemodynamically destabilizing VT or VF not due to reversible causes, such as acute myocardial infarction or electrolyte imbalance, should be treated with an ICD in preference to antiarrhythmic therapy. Unfortunately, AVID failed to address the role of concurrent antiarrhythmic therapy with an ICD. Answers to this and related questions may emerge from other ongoing clinical trials comparing outcome of patients concurrently treated with class III antiarrhythmic drugs (sotalol, dofetalide, and azimilide) or placebo in patients with implanted ICDs, for drug-refractory sustained VT.[9–11]

Ventricular Tachycardia or Fibrillation Refractory to Antiarrhythmic Therapy

The electropharmacological approach to VT has been the time-honored approach for patients presenting with VT or VF. The rationale for this approach was derived from studies supporting improved outcome in patients who are electrophysiologically inducible in whom sustained VT or VF are induced at electrophysiological (EP) study with programmed ventricular stimulation, and in whom antiarrhythmic drug therapy is demonstrated to suppress EP inducibility.[12] This approach was developed prior to the availability of transvenously implanted ICDs. An alternative approach, implanting an ICD as the initial therapy prior to demonstrating single or multiple drug failures, has not been tested as a viable alternative. The concept of implanting an ICD after antiarrhythmic drugs have failed introduces the bias that ICD therapy is somehow less desirable, and should, therefore, be relegated to a second tier choice. It also presumes that if antiarrhythmic therapy is shown to be effective, that it is preferable to ICD therapy. There are several arguments that question the validity of this approach: (1) An effective drug regimen can often be identified in only a minority of patients who present with VT or VF.[13,14] (2) Effectiveness of some antiarrhythmic drugs in the EP laboratory can be reversed by isoproterenol infusion, suggesting that sympathetic stimulation may overcome demonstrated therapeutic effectiveness of antiarrhythmic drug(s) by EP criteria.[15] (3) Serum concentrations of antiarrhythmic drugs achieved in the EP laboratory during testing can seldom be achieved and consistently maintained in clinical practice due to poor patient compliance, drug intolerance, fluid and electrolyte shifts, alterations in drug clearance and metabolism, drug interactions, or other possible mechanisms. (4) Multiple antiarrhythmic drug trials in an in-hospital setting are economically and logistically no longer viable in the United States, and may well be more expensive than implanting an ICD. (5) Finally, it is likely, though still unproven by randomized trial evidence, that an "ICD first" approach may improve survival beyond that expected from the electropharmacological approach.

Patients in whom VT cannot be suppressed by antiarrhythmic drugs (class I and sotalol) using an EP-directed electropharmacological approach, have been shown to have substantially increased mortality risk.[16–18] It is generally agreed by most experts that ICD therapy is indicated in this patient population. EP inducibility in patients treated with amiodarone is somewhat more controversial.[19] Noninducibility on amiodarone has been shown to confer better prognosis.[20] However, continued inducibility on amiodarone, particularly if significant VT slowing or hemodynamic tolerance can be demonstrated, may not portend a significantly worse outcome.[21] Another related issue is the most appropriate timing for EP testing of patients on amiodarone. Given the extremely long half-life of the drug (30–60 days), the full therapeutic effect may not be apparent for up to 6 months. Clearly, the value of EP study in predicting outcome in hospitalized patients first "loaded" with amiodarone is therefore suspect. This had led some investigators to propose other criteria for assessing amiodarone efficacy (Holter),[22] and others to rely primarily on empirical evidence for efficacy.[23] Based on the best available evidence, it is the author's approach to use amiodarone as an alternative to ICD for patients who refuse ICD as a therapeutic option, or for patients with limited life expectancy due to concurrent disease processes expected to decrease the life expectancy to less than 6 months, and patients with psychiatric or other medical contraindications to ICD. Amiodarone or other antiarrhythmic drug therapy can be used concurrently with ICDs to decrease frequency and duration of nonsustained VT episodes, prevent VT recurrence, and modify VT characteristics. Slowing tachycardia rate results in improved hemodynamic tolerance during VT and improves antitachycardia pacing effectiveness.[24] Since frequent ICD therapies, particularly cardioversion and defibrillation, are unpleasant and sometimes painful, it is the author's philosophy to use antiarrhythmic drugs adjunctively whenever frequent nonsustained VT episodes are documented by Holter or other noninvasive ECG monitoring techniques. Acceptance of ICD therapy, when VT is suppressed effectively with antiarrhythmic drugs, is considerably enhanced in patients in whom this strategy is used. An additional benefit of this approach is extension of ICD pulse generator longevity.

The relative role of surgical and catheter ablative therapy vis a vis ICD therapy is still insufficiently defined. What is clear, however, is that only a subset of patients presenting with sustained VT or VF, can be considered for ablative surgical therapy.[25] Detailed discussion of this issue is considered elsewhere in this book. Briefly, for ablative therapy to be successful, several conditions must exist: (1) VT must be mappable and arise from an anatomic focus accessible to a surgeon or to the ablating catheter, for example, a ventricular aneurysm. (2) Left ventricular function must be relatively well preserved, permitting ablative therapy to be effective without causing critical impairment in the left ventricular function. (3) Operative mortality must be acceptable (operative mortality in the 7%–15% range). (4) Surgical experience and volume must be sufficient in a given clinical center to favor a good surgical outcome. (5) Operative procedure is preferred when other surgical interventions are required, e.g., coronary artery bypass surgery, valvular replacement, etc. Even though surgical ablative therapy offers a potential for cure for VT, the operative risk in the best hands is much higher than the operative mortality of ICD surgery (7%–15% vs. <1% for ICD), suggesting that the ICD therapy is likely to be the preferred option for the majority of patients. Still, since ablative therapy is potentially curative, it represents an attractive therapeutic option in a selected subset of VT patients.

Catheter ablative therapies are still evolving. Therefore, the relative place of VT catheter ablation in the overall therapeutic strategy is still uncertain. It is likely that with improved multipolar basket catheter technologies and other technological enhancements, that catheter abalation may become a viable alternative to ICD in a subset of patients presenting with monomorphic VT.

Recurrent Episodes of Sustained VT or VF Despite Antiarrhythmic Therapy

Recurrent episodes of VT or VF despite EP or Holter-guided antiarrhythmic drug therapy are not uncommon events even when these modalities indicate likelihood of a favorable response. The Electrophysiologic Study Versus Electrocardiographic Monitoring (ESVEM) study reported late arrhythmia recurrences in approximately 40% of patients treated with class I antiarrhythmic drugs and 20% for sotalol in the first year of follow-up. The incidence of sudden cardiac death was somewhat lower: 10% at 1 year and 24% at 4 years. When contrasted with the anticipated sudden cardiac death mortality with ICD of <2% per year and 6% at 5 years,[26–28] it becomes clear that ICDs must be regarded as the preferred therapy over antiarrhythmic drugs even for patients with seemingly suppressible VT by EP or Holter-guided therapy. Thus, although the consensus statement[3,4] regards ICD therapy as indicated for late drug recurrences (with which there is little or no disagreement among the clinicians), the author would argue that in the light of the presently available evidence, the ICD should be regarded as the therapy of choice even when antiarrhythmic drugs show VT suppression in the EP laboratory. As previously stated, the author would regard antiarrhythmic therapy preferable to ICD only when contraindications to ICD therapy exist, or if this represents patient's preference.

Antiarrhythmic Drug Intolerance or Noncompliance

Drug intolerance or noncompliance are not unusual in the VT patient population. Side effects are common with antiarrhythmic medications. Up to 40% of patients taking class I antiarrhythmic drugs discontinue their use due to side effects or proarrhythmia.[29] In the ESVEM trial, up to 32% of patients were unable to tolerate the antiarrhythmic medications. Sotalol was the best-tolerated drug, but despite this, it was discontinued in 13% of patients acutely and 7% chronically.[17,18]

Arguably, the most effective antiarrhythmic drug for therapy of VT, amiodarone, is associated with potentially troublesome and potentially life-threatening side effects, which include pulmonary and hepatic toxicity. Several troublesome side effects have also led to the drug's discontinuation chronically, including thyroid dysfunction, skin pigmentation, optic neuritis, proximal myopathy, and central nervous system side effects. The most serious side effect, pulmonary toxicity, occurred in 10% of patients in the Conventional Versus Amiodarone Drug Evaluation (CASCADE) study[30]. In more recent clinical trials, CAMIAT[31] and EMIAT[32,33] over 40% drop-out rate was seen due to frequent side effects.

Another less discussed but a significant issue is the cost of antiarrhythmic drugs, which is prohibitive for some patients, at least in the United States, and frequently results in patients either overtly or surreptitiously failing to take the prescribed medications. For these and other reasons already discussed, it is the author's opinion that the expert panel's recommendations should be modified with respect to the relative role of ICD in the therapeutic cascade.

Sudden Aborted Cardiac Death Survivors Who Are Noninducible at EP Study

Patients who present with sudden cardiac death and are noninducible nevertheless have high incidence of sudden death if left untreated. Up to 40% recurrence rates have been reported in noninducible patients.[30,34,35] Clearly then, ICD therapy is indicated for these patients whether they are inducible at EP study or not, unless a reversible cause can be identified (e.g., ischemia, acute myocardial infarction, proarrhythmia, electrolyte imbalance, etc.). Still, more impressively, recurrent VT or VF occur in up to 50% of patients, with over one-half not surviving the second recurrence.[34,35]

Since presence or absence of inducibility at EP study is not used as a criterion for ICD implantation in sudden cardiac death survivors, some investigators have questioned the need for an EP study in general

in this subset of patients. It is the author's opinion that although the yield of EP study in this specific situation is rather limited, it is still useful and necessary to exclude possible abnormalities of the conduction system, presence of accessory tracts, and to characterize VT. These data are useful in subsequent decision making process regarding the most optimal ICD therapy. EP-derived data such as VT cycle length, hemodynamic tolerance of VT, value of antitachycardia pacing therapies are used to formulate ICD programming strategy. Another possible use of the EP study is to assess the possible role for ablative therapy.

Nonsustained Ventricular Tachycardia in Patients with Coronary Artery Disease and Impared Left Ventricular Function

The results of Multicenter Automatic Defibrilltor Trial (MADIT) became available recently.[36] The MADIT trial tested the hypothesis that implantation of an ICD in patients with coronary heart disease, left ventricular dysfunction (LVEF <0.36), and unsustained VT will result in a significant reduction in all-cause mortality to conventional therapy. To be eligible for inclusion in this protocol, patients had to have had a Q wave myocardial infarction, be less than 75 years of age, and have asymptomatic, unsustained VT (3–30 beats), and be in NYHA functional class I-III. If these patients were found to be inducible to monomorphic VT with up to three extrastimuli at two cycle length drives (600 and 400 ms) or if they had a very short cycle length VT induced <230 ms, multiform VT or VF induced with one or two extrastimuli, they were given intravenous procainamide (loading dose 15 mg/kg and maintenance dose of 4 mg/min), with programmed stimulation repeated. If inducible on procainamide, these patients were randomized to receive an ICD or were assigned to "conventional therapy." Conventional therapy was left to the discretion of the electrophysiologist and could include no therapy, sequential electropharmacological assesment to find the best antiarrhythmic drug to suppress VT, or were assigned to amiodarone. The patients were then followed, and all-cause mortality was used as the endpoint for study analysis. MADIT was prematurely stopped when 54% better overall survival was demonstrated for the ICD-treated patients compared to the best conventional therapy. It should be pointed out that three-quarters of the patients in the control limb were treated with amiodarone. At 1 year the ICD patients had 87% lower mortality, which remained 60% better over 3 years. Clear superiority was demonstrated for the ICD (hazard ratio-0.46; 95% CI = 0.26–0.82; $P = .009$).

Based on these rather stunning results suggesting overwhelming superiority for the ICD, the FDA has recommended that for the patient population described by the MADIT study variables, ICD therapy now represents the best treatment choice. This is a new indication, not covered by the NASPE or the ACC/AHA panel recommendations but included in the most recent.[3,4] This study has an added significance in that for the first time it has been demonstrated in a randomized prospective trial that ICD is useful for primary sudden cardiac death prophylaxis in a subset of patients at increased arrhythmic risk.

Some questions still remain. MADIT did not have a true control limb (no therapy). Therefore, it is not clear if *no therapy* would have resulted in a better or worse outcome than ICD therapy, a legitimate scientific question. It could, for example, be argued that the better results with ICD therapy are actually due to premature deaths caused by the adverse effects of antiarrhythmic drugs, rather than to the beneficial effect of the ICD. Although this conclusion seems unlikely, legitimate scientific doubt must remain in absence of a control arm in the study. These questions may be resolved by the still ongoing MUSTT clinical trial, where a similar patient population was randomized to no therapy or to the "best" antiarrhythmic therapy based on a similar EP study stratification as in MADIT.[37] The best

antiarrhythmic therapy in MUSTT included either antiarrhythmic drug therapy found to render patient noninducible by electropharmacological testing, or by ICD, if no antiarrhythmic drug or drugs could be found that successfully suppressed EP inducibility. Thus, MUSTT is likely to provide useful complementary information to the MADIT study. Until this study's results are finally published, we will not know whether ICD therapy or no therapy is the superior approach for this patient population. In the absence of these data, some electrophysiologists have adopted the MADIT approach, while others still remain on the sidelines until this issue is clarified.

Patients with Coronary Artery Disease, Left Ventricular Dysfuction and Positive Signal Averaged ECG Undergoing Coronary Artery Bypass Surgery

The results of the CABG PATCH trial were recently published and indicate that prophylactic implantation of an ICD at the time of the coronary artery bypass surgery in patients with LV dysfunction (LVEF <0.36) and positive signal averaged ECG does not improve all-cause mortality.[38] Since these patients did not undergo EP testing prior to or after the surgical intervention, it is not known how EP inducibility or lack of EP inducibility affects outcome. However, based on the study results, prophylactic ICD implantation cannot be recommended for this patient population at increased risk of arrhythmic events based on these criteria exclusively. Further, it suggests that left ventricular dysfunction and signal-averaged ECG by themselves are not sufficently powerful predictors of arrhythmic mortality, particularly when ischemic risk is diminished by surgical revascularization procedures.

Class II Indications

Class II indications are summarized in Table 2. Patients who present with syncope

Table 2
Class 2 ICD Indications

1. Syncope of undetermined cause in a patient with clinically relevant sustained VT or VF induced at EP study in whom antiarrhythmic therapy is limited by inefficacy, intolerance or noncompliance.
2. Hemodynamically significant sustained VT.

ICD = implantable cardioverter-defibrillator; VT = ventricular tachycardia; VF = ventricular fibrillation; EP = electrophysiological. Modified from references 3 and 4.

and have sustained VT induced at EP study, particularly if VT is hemodynamically unstable or requires cardioversion for termination, should be considered for ICD therapy. In this case, an assumption is made that the cause of syncope is most likely due to VT, given the EP inducibility. This assumption may not always be correct. Nevertheless, the relatively high frequency of sudden cardiac events in this population group justifies consideration of ICD therapy. Further data confirming the correctness of this therapeutic rationale is likely to emerge from the ongoing clinical studies.

Contraindications to ICD Therapy

Table 3 lists contraindications to ICD therapy. Reversible causes of VT and VF should be excluded prior to deciding that ICD is the therapy of choice. These include ischemia, acute myocardial infarction, and severe electrolyte and metabolic disturbances. Proarrhythmia due to antiarrhythmic drug toxicity should be suspected in patients who are on antiarrhythmic therapy for another indication (e.g., atrial fibrillation) at the time when the initial episode of VT or VF is first documented. In these patients, antiarrhythmic drug(s) should be discontinued and the patient reevaluated after the antiarrhythmic drug washout (greater than $5\frac{1}{2}$ half-lives of the drug have elapsed). Coronary arteriography is recom-

mended to exclude significant coronary occlusive disease in virtually all patients.

Uncontrolled VT or VF with recurrent, incessant episodes of ventricular arrhythmias represents a clear contraindication to ICD therapy. Stabilization of arrhythmia with antiarrhythmic therapy, revascularization procedures (where indicated), and surgical intervention (in suitable cases) or catheter ablation is required prior to the consideration of ICD therapy.

Patients who present with unwitnessed syncope in whom sustained VT cannot be induced at EP study should not be considered for ICD therapy unless a clear documentation of VT or VF exists. Since causes of syncope are legion, it is more likely that under these circumstances ICD therapy may not be appropriate. Therefore, if doubt exists as to the cause of syncope, particularly in absence of structural cardiac abnormalities, ICD should not be implanted.

There are many possible medical contraindications to ICD, including chronic infection, underlying malignancy, or other concurrent chronic medical conditions that might reasonably be expected to limit patient's life expectancy. Psychiatric illness with past history of psychoses, drug or alcohol dependency, or severe depression contraindicate ICD therapy. Family and social

Table 3
Contraindications to ICD Therapy

1. Sustained VT or VF in the context of acute myocardial ischemia or infarction, or due to metabolic disturbance, severe electrolyte abnormalities, or antiarrhythmic drug toxicity.
2. Incessant VT or VF.
3. Syncope of undetermined etiology in a patient without inducible sustained VT at EP study.
4. VF induced by rapid AV conduction through a bypass tract in a patient with Wolf-Parkinson-White syndrome amenable to surgical or catheter ablation.
5. Medical, surgical, or psychiatric contraindications.

ICD = implantable cardioverter-defibrillator; VT = ventricular tachycardia; VF = ventricular fibrillation; EP = electrophysiological. Modified from references 3 and 4.

support structure are necessary prerequisites for a successful long-term therapy.

New Indications for ICD Therapy

Future applications of ICD therapy are contemplated for patients with paroxysmal recurrent atrial fibrillation (AF), patients with dilated cardiomyopathy and as a bridge to transplantation (Table 4). These new applications will have to await outcomes of the ongoing clinical trials evaluating the ICD for new indications, as well as the evaluation of competing approaches for management of these conditions.

Atrial Defibrillators

Atrial fibrillation is the most common arrhythmia requiring hospitalization.[39] AF can occur as an isolated abnormality or it may be associated with other cardiac diseases. It is most commonly associated with congestive heart failure, regardless of etiology, rheumatic valvular disease, hypertensive cardiac disease, and hypertrophic cardiomyopathy. AF adversely impacts on survival and on patient well-being. The loss of atrial contraction affects ventricular filling and impairs cardiac output, causing irregular heart rate, which at times can be extremely rapid, depending on the AV nodal conduction characteristics, shortening filling time, and further compromising cardiac function.

By far the most devastating complication of AF is embolic stroke. The most recent clinical trials studying incidence of strokes in patients with AF have all shown the beneficial effects of anticoagulation for patients with AF.[40–43] Patients treated with coumadin versus placebo have shown reduction in stroke incidence from 37% to 86%. While warfarin substantially reduced the incidence of strokes, the case for aspirin was less convincing. Though the incidence of strokes is reduced by anticoagulation, a significant number of patients were excluded from taking anticoagulants due to bleeding complications or other contraindications (AFASAK[40] 30%, SPAF[42] 53%). In a significant number of patients, warfarin was discontinued due to complications (BAATAF 10%, AFASAK 38%, SPAF 11%). It therefore appears, based on the results of these studies, that maintenance of sinus rhythm is desirable because it could avoid use of anticoagulants for chronic AF.

Antiarrhythmic Drug Therapy

Antiarrhythmic drugs and external cardioversion are currently the mainstay of therapy for AF. The usual strategy involves an intervention to achieve the following goals: (1) to block AV conduction in order to decrease ventricular rates during AF; (2) to decrease recurrence rates by altering tissue conduction and refractoriness in the atrium; and (3) to prevent strokes by using warfarin and occasionally aspirin.

The first objective may be achieved by beta blocking or calcium channel blocking drugs or the use of digoxin. Class III antiarrhythmic drugs are also effective in this regard. An alternative approach is to ablate AV node and pace with either a VVIR or a DDDR pacemaker, depending on the circumstances. Ablation strategy may be attractive for patients who are either intolerant or noncompliant with antiarrhythmic drugs, although it should be emphasized that this strategy renders the patient pacemaker-dependent.

Antiarrhythmic drugs have well-known limitations: (1) limited effectiveness (range

---

Table 4
Possible Future ICD Indications

1. Paroxysmal recurrent atrial fibrillation
2. ICD as a bridge to transplant
3. Dilated cardiomyopathy (class II and III heart failure)

ICD = implantable cardioverter-defibrillator.

11%–52%), [43-46] (2) proarrhythmia,[47] (3) side effects form antiarrhythmic drugs,[48] and (4) drug-drug interactions.[49]

Ablative Options

Recently, a great deal of interest has been generated by the reports that AF may be cured by operative ablation.[50] Though curative, the surgical maze procedure is associated with significant morbidity and some operative mortality.[51] Despite "maze," some patients may require pacing therapy for chronotropic incompetence, although less frequently with modified maze procedure.[52] A great deal of interest has been generated recently with attempts to apply the principles of the surgical maze procedure to catheter ablative techniques. It is still too early to evaluate the relative role of either operative or catheter-based maze procedures, or the relative role that either procedure is likely to play in the overall therapy of AF.

Atrial Defibrillators

Preliminary data regarding the use of atrial defibrillator suggest that standby defibrillation in the atrium may be a viable therapeutic option.[53] The main limitation in application of this technology is that the energies required to terminate AF are still approximately 1–2 joules, and in some cases up to 5 joules. Although these energy levels are relatively small compared to the energies required for defibrillation in the ventricles, the shocks are unpleasant and painful to most patients. Since AF is not an immediately life-threatening rhythm, the acceptability of this therapy is therefore questionable.

Although the use of implantable atrial defibrillators as stand-alone devices for AF may not be acceptable in their present state of development, it may be acceptable in combination with an ICD to provide atrial and ventricular defibrillation, and dual chamber pacing support. Thus, incorporating atrial defibrillation functionality into the existing ICD and possibly combining it with antitachycardia pacing options in the atrium would potentially extend the therapeutic usefulness of the ICDs considerably. Thus, patients who present with VT, but also have paroxysmal AF or flutter and conduction abnormalities or chronotropic incompetence, would be able to benefit from a combination device providing dual chamber pacing and ATP, with standby defibrillation.

Implantable Cardioverter-Defibrillator as a Bridge to Transplant

Severe left ventricular dysfunction is associated with high mortality, of up to 40% per year. It is estimated that up to one-half of deaths are due to arrhythmic deaths, the majority due to VT or VF, and others due to asystole or advanced AV block. Furthermore, due to the shortage of donor hearts, approximately 20% of patients die awaiting cardiac transplantation. Given the high mortality due to lethal tachy- or bradyarrhythmias in this patient population, and no conclusive evidence that antiarrhythmic drug therapy is effective for this subset of patients, several investigators have proposed that ICD may be used to prevent sudden cardiac death during the time that the patients are awaiting cardiac transplantation. In the Survival Trial of Antiarrhythmic Therapy in Congestive Heart Failure (CHF STAT) study, empirical amiodarone offered no benefit to placebo.[54] The DEFIBRILAT study was therefore proposed to test the hypothesis that prophylactic use of ICD therapy will reduce all-cause mortality in patients heart failure (NYHA class III) due to coronary artery disease who have been accepted for transplantation.[55] DEFIBRILLAT will enroll patients who are <65 years of age, have coronary artery disease, LVEF <0.30, NYHA class III heart failure, and an unsustained VT in a 24-hour ECG monitoring. Patients who qualify would undergo EP study, and if inducible, would be randomized to either ICD or to no antiarrhythmic therapy.

DEFIBRILAT is considering sequential design. The alpha error is set at 0.05 (two-sided) and the power of 0.85. For the sample size calculation, the 1-year cumulative mortality rate was assumed to be about 45% in the control group and 22% in the group assigned to ICD therapy. Using these assumptions, the sample size was calculated to be 300 patients. This study will have significant obstacles, including recruitment, early sensoring due to heart transplantation, and likely significant drop-in and drop-out rates. If ICD benefit is demonstrated, however, it is likely that the loss of patient lives due to attrition while waiting for a donor heart could be diminished by the prophylactic ICD implantation.

Primary Prevention of Sudden Cardiac Death in Patients with Heart Failure with ICD

The rationale for prophylaxis of sudden cardiac death in patients with heart failure is based on the evidence suggesting an increase in the arrhythmic risk in the patient population with class II and III NYHA heart failure. This risk is estimated to be 40%–50% in 2 years, with approximately 40% of the deaths assumed to be due to arrhythmic death (predominantly VT and VF, but also bradyarrhythmias).[56–58] Since modern ICDs incorporate pacing functions as well as anti-tachycardia pacing, cardioversion, and defibrillation, they may be expected to benefit patients regardless of the causes of arrhythmic death. Therefore, selected patients with heart failure might benefit from prophylactic ICD therapy. Two ongoing clinical trials are examining this hypothesis.[59–61]

Dilated Cardiomyopathy Trial

The Dilated Cardiomyopathy Trial is testing the hypothesis that prophylactic implantation of an ICD in patients with dilated cardiomyopathy and severe left ventricular dysfunction will improve the survival due to the prevention of sudden death in this patient population. Inclusion criteria are left ventricular dysfunction with LVEF <0.31 and NYHA class II or III. Patients are excluded if they have significant coronary artery disease, valvular heart disease, are likely to undergo cardiac transplantation in 6 months after enrollment, history of sustained VT or cardiac arrest, and dilated cardiomyopathy longer than 9 months. The patients are randomized to receive an ICD with the control group receiving no additional therapy other than conventional treatment for congestive heart failure. A pilot study of 100 patients has been organized. However, it is likely that a larger sample size may be required to obtain meaningful statistics. The investigators have estimated a 1-year mortality rate of 30%, with 40% of deaths due to arrhythmic deaths. ICDs are expected to reduce the mortality rate to 24%.[62]

Sudden Cardiac Death in Heart Failure Trial (SCDHefT)

The SCDHefT clinical trial is testing the hypothesis that implantation of an ICD in patients with impared left ventricular function (LVEF <0.36) and class II or III heart failure will improve prognosis relative to the best anticongestive heart failure strategy or amiodarone. The amiodarone and ICD therapy patients will also have their therapy optimized relative to the heart failure therapy, including the use of angiotensin-converting enzyme inhibitors, diuretics, and so on. No arrhythmia discriminator is used to qualify patients. The primary endpoint of the study is all-cause mortality. It is hypothesized that ICD will reduce mortality rate by 25% compared to the control arm of the study. It is anticipated, based on these assumptions and a power of 0.90 and the alpha level of 0.05, that 2,500 patients will have to be randomized. Potential problems for SCDHefT are that the event rates in the placebo arm may have been overestimated, and that LVEF alone may not be a sufficient indicator of risk. Also, based on CHF-STAT results, it is not clear that amiodarone has any role in this population subset.

Conclusions

ICD therapy continues to evolve, as well as alternative approaches to tachyarrhyth-mia management. Therefore, it should be anticipated that the indications for ICD will continue to evolve over time. An exciting new era of primary prophylaxis of sudden death is at hand, accelerated by the technological developments in the ICD and new insights based on controlled clinical trials as well as accumulated clinical experience.

References

1. Mower MM. Clinical and Historical perspective. In Singer I, ed. Implantable Cardioverter Defibrillator. Futura Publishing Co., Armonk, NY, 1994, pp 3–12.
2. Mirowski M, Mower MM, Staewen WS, et al. The development of the transvenous automatic defibrillator. Arch Intern Med 1972; 129:773–779.
3. Lehmann MH, Saksena S. Implantable cardioverters defibrillators in cardiovascular practice: report on Policy Conference of the North American Society of Pacing and Electrophysiology. PACE 1991;14:969–979.
4. Dreifus L. Guidelines for implantation of cardiovascular pacemaker and antiarrhythmia devices: report of the American College of Cardiology/American Heart Association Task Force on the assessment of diagnostic and therapeutic cardiovascular procedures (Committee on Pacemaker Implantation). J Am Coll Cardiol 1991;18:1–13.
5. Mirowski M, Mower MM, Gott VL, et al. Feasibility and effectiveness of low energy catheter defibrillation in man. Circulation 1973; 47:79–85.
6. Kim S. Implantable defibrillator therapy: Does it really prolong life? How can we prove it? Am J Cardiol 1993;71:1213–1218.
7. Singer I, Nisam S. There should never be another Antiarrhythmic Versus Implantable Defibrillator (AVID) Trial. Am J Cardiol 1997;80:766–768.
8. Hallstrom A, Zipes D. Preliminary results of AVID (Antiarrhythmics versus Implantable Defibrillator Trial). Oral presentation during Clinical Trials Update. 18th Annual Scientific Sessions of North American Society of Pacing and Electrophysiology (NASPE), New Orleans, LA, May 8, 1997.
9. Placebo-Controlled Evaluation of the Efficacy and Safety of Oral dl-Sotalol in Patients with Life-Threatening Ventricular Arrhythmias and Implanted Cardioverter Defibrillators (Protocol no. 106–104), 1996.
10. A Randomized, Double-Blind Study of Orally Administered Dofetalide and Placebo in Patients with an Implanted Arrhythmia Control Device (Protocol no. 115- 113), 1994.
11. A Multicenter Double-Blind, Placebo-Controlled Study to Evaluate the Efficacy and Safety of 35 mg, 75 mg, and 125 mg/day Doses of Oral Azimilide Hydrochloride in Patients with an Implantable Cardioverter Defibrillator for the Treatment of Ventricular Arrhythmia (Proctor and Gamble), 1996.
12. Wilber DJ, Garan H, Finklestein D, et al. Out of hospital cardiac arrest. Use of electrophysiologic testing in the prediction of long-term outcome. N Engl J Med 1998;318:19–24.
13. Spielman SR, Schwartz JS, McCarthy DM, et al. Predictors of success or failure of medical therapy in patients with chronic recurrent sustained VT: a discriminant analysis. J Am Coll Cardiol 1983;1:401–407.
14. Swerdlow CD, Gong G, Echt DS, et al. Clinical factors predicting successful electrophysiologic-pharmacologic study in patients with ventricular tachycardia. J Am Coll Cardiol 1983;1:409–415.
15. Calkins H, Sousa J, El-Atassi R, et al. Reversal of antiarrhythmic drug effects by epinephrine: quinidine versus amiodarone. J Am Coll Cardiol 1992;19:347–352.
16. Tchou PJ, Kadri N, Anderson J, et al. Automatic implantable cardioverter defibrillator and survival of patients with left ventricular dysfunction and malignant ventricular arrhythmias. Ann Intern Med 1988;109: 529–534.
17. Mason JW for the ESVEM Investigators. A comparison of electrophysiologic testing with Holter monitoring to predict antiarrhythmic drug efficacy for ventricular tachyarrhythmias. N Engl J Med 1993;329: 445–451.
18. Mason JW for the ESVEM Investigators. A comparison of seven antiarrhythmic drugs in patients with ventricular tachyarrhythmias. N Engl J Med 1993;329:452- 458.
19. Hamer AW, Finerman WB Jr, Peter T, et al. Disparity between the clinical and electrophysiologic effects of amiodarone in treatment of recurrent ventricular tachyarrhythmias. Am Heart J 1981;102:992–1000.
20. Horowitz LN, Greenspan AM, Spielman RS,

et al. Usefulness of electrophysiologic testing in evaluation of amiodarone therapy for sustained ventricular tachyarrhythmias associated with coronary artery disease. Am J Cardiol 1985;55:367–371.

21. Nademanee K, Singh BN, Cannom DS, et al. Control of sudden recurrent arrhythmic deaths: role of amiodarone. Am Heart J 1983; 106:895–901.

22. Kim S, Felder SD, Figure I, et al. Value of Holter monitoring in predicting long- term efficacy and inefficacy of amiodarone used alone and in combination with class Ia antiarrhythmic agents in patients with ventricular tachycardia. J Am Coll Cardiol 1987;9: 169–174.

23. Morady F, Scheinmann MM, Hess DA. Amiodarone in management of patients with ventricular tachycardia and ventricular fibrillation. PACE 1983;6:609–615.

24. Yazaki Y, Haffajee C, Gold RL, et al. Electrophysiologic predictors of long-term clinical outcome with amiodarone for refractory ventricular tachycardia secondary to coronary artery disease. Am J Cardiol 1987;60: 293–297.

25. Miller JM, Rothman SA, Addonizzio P. Surgical techniques for ventricular tachycardia ablation. In Singer I, ed. Interventional Electrophysiology. Baltimore, Williams and Wilkins,1987, pp 641–684.

26. Bocker D, Block M, Isbruch F, Weitholt D, et al. Do patients with implantable defibrillator live longer? J Am Coll Cardiol 1993; 1683–1644.

27. Powell A, Finklestein D, Garan H, et al. Influence of implantable cardioverter- defibrillators on long-term prognosis of survivors of out-of-hospital cardiac arrest. Circulation 1993;88:1083–1092.

28. Schlepper M, Neunzner J, Pitschner H. Implantable cardioverter defibrillator: effect on survival. PACE 1996;18:569–578.

29. Velebit V, Podrid P, Lown B, et al. Aggravation and provocation of ventricular arrhythmias by antiarrhythmic drugs. Circulation 1982;65:836–894.

30. The CASCADE Investigators. Cardiac arrest in Seattle: conventional versus amiodarone drug evaluation. Am J Cardiol 1991;67: 578–584.

31. Cairns J, Connolly S. Canadian Amiodarone Myocardial Infarction Arrhythmia Trial (CAMIAT). Oral presentation during 45th annual scientific sessions. American College of Cardiology, Orlando, March 26, 1996.

32. Camm AJ, Julian D, Janse G, et al. The European Myocardial Infarct Amiodarone Trial (EMIAT). Am J Cardiol 1993;72:95F-98F.

33. Swartz P, Camm AJ. European Myocardial Infarction Arrhythmia Trial (EMIAT). Oral presentation during 45th annual scientific sessions, American College of Cardiology, Orlando, March 26, 1996.

34. Swerdlow CD, Winkle RA, Mason JW. Determinants of survival of patients with ventricular tachyarrhythmias. N Engl J Med 1983; 308:1436–1444.

35. Eldar M, Suave MJ, Scheinmann MM. Electrophysiologic testing and follow-up in patients with aborted sudden death. J Am Coll Cardiol 1987;10:291–298.

36. Moss A, Hall J, Cannom D, et al. Improved survival with an implanted defibrillator in patients with coronary artery disease at high risk of ventricular arrhythmias. N Engl J Med 1996;335:1933–1940.

37. Bigger JT. Primary prevention of sudden cardiac death using implantable cardioverter-defibrillators. In Singer I, ed. Implantable Cardioverter Defibrillator. Armonk, NY, Futura Publishing Co, 1994, pp 515–546.

38. Bigger JT Jr. Should defibrillators be implanted in high risk patients without a previous sustained ventricular tachyarrhythmias? In Naccarelli GV, Veltri EP, eds. Implantable Cardioverter-Defibrillators. Boston, Blackwell Scientific Publications, Inc, 1993, p 284–317.

39. Bialy D, Lehmann MH, Schumacher DN, et al. Hospitalization of arrhythmias in the United States: importance of atrial fibrillation. J Am Coll Cardiol 1992;19:41A.

40. Peterson P, Boysen G, Godtfredsen J, et al. Placebo-controlled, randomized trial of warfarin and aspirin for prevention of thromboembolic complications in chronic atrial fibrillation: the Copenhagen study. Lancet 1989; 1:175–179.

41. Boston Area Anticoagulation Trial for Atrial Fibrillation Investigators. The effect of low dose warfarin on the risk of stroke in patients with nonrheumatic atrial fibrillation. N Engl J Med 1990;323:1505–1511.

42. Stroke Prevention in Atrial Fibrillation Investigators. Stroke prevention atrial fibrillation study. Circulation 1991;84:527–539.

43. Lau C, Leung W, Wong CK. A randomized double-blind crossover study comparing efficacy and tolerability of flecainide and quinidine in the control of patients with symptomatic atrial fibrillation. Am Heart J 1992; 124:645–650.

44. Andersen JL, Gilbert E, Alpert BL, et al. Prevention of symptomatic recurrences of paroxysmal atrial fibrillation in patients initially tolerating antiarrhythmic therapy. Circulation 1989;80:1557–1570.

45. Reimold SC, Cantillon CO, Friedman Pl, et al. Propafenone versus sotalol for suppres-

sion of recurrent symptomatic atrial fibrillation. Am J Cardiol 1993;71:558- 563.

46. Juul-Moller S, Edvardsson N, Rehnqvist-Ahlberg N. Sotalol versus quinidine for the maintenance of sinus rhythm after direct current cardioversion of atrial fibrillation. Circulation 1990;82:1932–1939.

47. Flacker GC, Blackshear JL, Mc Bride R, et al. Antiarrhythmic drug therapy and cardiac mortality in atrial fibrillation. J Am Coll Cardiol 1992;20:527–532.

48. Crijns HF, Van Gelder IC, Van Gilst WH, et al. Serial antiarrhythmic drug treatment to maintain sinus rhythm after electrical cardioversion for chronic atrial fibrillation or atrial flutter. Am J Cardiol 1991;68:335–341.

49. Jaillon P, Ferry A. How do kinetics relate to toxicity of antiarrhythmic drugs? Eur Heart J 1988;9(Suppl B):45–50.

50. Cox JL. Surgical treatment of atrial fibrillation IV. Surgical technique. J Thorac Cardiovasc Surg 1991;101:584–592.

51. Ferguson TB Jr. Surgical approach to atrial flutter and fibrillation. In Interventional Electrophysiology. Singer I, ed. Baltimore, Williams and Wilkins, 1997, pp 895–639.

52. Cox JL. The Maze III procedure for treatment of atrial fibrillation. In Sabiston DC, ed. Atlas of Cardiothoracic Surgery. Philladelphia, WB Saunders,1995, pp 460- 475.

53. Keane D, Sulke N, Cooke R, et al. Endocardial cardioversion of atrial flutter and atrial fibrillation. PACE 1993;16:928.

54. Singh SN, Fletcher RD, Fisher SG, et al for the Survival Trial of Antiarrhythmic Therapy in Congestive Heart Failure. Amiodarone in patients with congestive heart failure and asymptomatic ventricular arrhythmia. N Engl J Med 1995;333:77–82.

55. DEFIBRILLAT Study Group. Actuarial risk of sudden death while awaiting cardiac transplantation in patients with atherosclerotic heart disease. Am J Cardiol 1991;68:545–546.

56. Packer M. Sudden unexpected death in patients with congestive heart failure: a second frontier. Circulation 1985;72:681–685.

57. Bigger JT Jr. Why patients with congestive heart failure die: arrhythmias and sudden cardiac death. Circulation 1987;75(Suppl IV): 28–35.

58. Kjekshus J. Arrhythmias and mortality in congestive heart failure. Am J Cardiol 1990; 65:421–481.

59. The German Dilated Cardiomyopathy Study Investigators. Prospective studies assessing prophylactic therapy in high risk patients. The German Dilated Cardiomyopathy Study (GDCMS) - study design. PACE 1992;15: 697–700.

60. The Cardiomyopathy Trial Investigators. Cardiomyopathy trial. PACE 1993;16: 576–581.

61. SCD-Heft Study Manual. 1997.

62. Hauser RG. Atributes of a prophylactic implantable cardioverter defibrillator: how close are we? PACE 1993;16:582–585.

Chapter 15

Implantable Cardioverter-Defibrillator Implantation Techniques

Ramakota K. Reddy, Gregory K. Jones, Gust H. Bardy

Introduction

The evolution of the implantable cardioverter-defibrillator (ICD) has paralleled that of the pacemaker but at an accelerated pace. Initial pacemakers used epicardial leads, were nonprogrammable, and provided only ventricular pacing.[1,2] In addition, they were relatively large, 110 cm^3, 250 g, and required implantation by surgeons in an abdominal position. Current pacing generators are much smaller, 20–25 g and 20 cm^3, are programmable, and are capable of pacing both atrium and ventricle. They are nearly all placed subcutaneously in the pectoral position using endocardial transvenous leads by cardiologists. Similarly, initial ICDs were implanted by surgeons via thoracotomy with epicardial patches and used large, 180 cm^3, abdominally placed shock-only pulse generators. Current ICDs are <60 cm^3 in size and allow pectoral placement by cardiologists in virtually all adult patients. In the majority of cases, only a single transvenous lead is required to provide effective defibrillation. Current ICD pulse generators are equipped with sophisticated programming and recording capabilities, and are capable of single and dual chamber pacing and defibrillation. The purpose of this chapter is to describe the equipment and techniques required for safe and effective ICD implantation.

Facilities and Staffing Requirements

Surgery Location

Implantation of an ICD requires a sterile environment and the same sterile technique that is routinely used in the operating room for any hardware implantation. Because early generation ICD implantations were performed by cardiac surgeons and required general anesthesia, they were performed only in the operating room.

Technological advances have made lengthy and complex surgical procedures unnecessary, and it is now very reasonable for nonsurgeons to implant ICDs in less than an hour. Because of easier accessibility, the electrophysiology (EP) lab or cardiac catheterization laboratory have, for many cardiologists, become locations of choice for ICD implantation. These locations have the advantage of generally superior fluoroscopic equipment, support personnel familiar with potential complications surround-

From Singer I, Barold SS, Camm AJ (eds): Nonpharmacological Therapy of Arrhythmias for the 21st Century: The State of the Art. Futura Publishing Co, Inc., Armonk, NY, © 1998.

ing implantation, and availability of arrhythmia recording equipment necessary for implantation. Delays in access commonly associated with use of operating rooms is also an important consideration in the use of EP and cath labs because they reduce hospital stays and cost.

Before embarking on ICD implantation in a setting outside of the operating room, however, some potential drawbacks must be addressed. Laminar air flow, present in most operating rooms, but absent in the typical EP/cath lab, poses a theoretical increased risk of infection. This has not been observed in large published reports[3–7] and directing air conditioning flow across the surgical field addresses this issue in a cost-effective manner. Education of support personnel in proper sterile technique is critical. Given the limited dissection needed for subcutaneous ICD implantation, one or two portable surgical lights should provide sufficient lighting, and the instruments available in a standard surgical tray are usually adequate.

Equipment

The basic equipment required for ICD implantation are listed in Tables 1 and 2. Elec-

---

Table 1
Minimal Lab Equipment

Patient Monitoring
  Multichannel telemetry monitor
  Arterial blood pressure monitor
  Peripheral O_2 saturation monitor
  End expiratory CO_2 monitor
Procedural Equipment
  Oxygen supply
  Overhead surgical lighting
  Multipositional fluoroscopy unit
  Suction apparatus
  Electrocautery unit
  External device testing system and cables
  Surgical instrument tray
Emergency Equipment
  Two external cardioverter defibrillators
  Pericardiocentesis tray
  Intubation tray
  Portable oxygen canisters

---

trocardiogram and intracardiac electrogram monitoring systems that are capable of multichannel display (with recall) are recommended but not strictly required for implantation. Fluoroscopy systems that are capable of multiple angle views are advisable in that confirmation of endocardial lead placement is often enhanced with the right anterior oblique and left anterior oblique projections, in addition to the standard anteroposterior projection. Adequate ceiling-attached or portable surgical lights are especially important. For cephalic dissection, it is preferable to have at least two portable overhead lights because the dissection can be deep and the cephalic vein difficult to visualize.

For patient monitoring, in addition to ECG monitoring, facilities for peripheral pulse oximetry and CO_2 monitoring are needed to provide safe conscious sedation or general anesthesia. For blood pressure monitoring, direct arterial monitoring is ideal, although noninvasive blood pressure monitoring may be adequate in uncomplicated cases. The capability to monitor and measure right heart pressures is not routinely advisable because of associated risk and cost, but may be necessary in rare cases where cardiac function is tenuous.

Two working external defibrillation systems are recommended for safe implantation of ICDs. The patient is attached to adhesive defibrillation pads in an anteroposterior fashion (right posterior paraspinal and left anterior apical) with an additional backup set of pads or hand-held defibrillation system available. Two orthogonal systems are optimal because there are occasional cases of ventricular fibrillation (VF) that become difficult or refractory to standard external defibrillation. A backup biphasic waveform transthoracic defibrillation system may be especially helpful.[8] Simultaneous or sequential external defibrillation, coupled to internal defibrillation can be life-saving in these cases.[9]

Preparation for other potential emergent situations should be routine. A pericardiocentesis and chest tube tray should be avail-

Table 2
Surgical Instruments

Instrument	Use
Blades	
#10 Scalpel	Incision
#11 Scalpel	Cephalic venotomy
Forceps	
Adson	Subcutaneous skin closure
DeBakey	General use
Deitrich	To hold cephalic vein during venotomy
Retractors	
Weitlander	General retraction
Richardson (large and small)	To retract skin for pocket formation
Army/Navy	To aid in cephalic vein dissection
Rake	Skin and subcutaneous tissue retraction
Vein retractor	To aid in cephalic vein dissection
Scissors	
Tenotomy scissors	Cephalic venotomy incision
Metzenbaum	General use/blunt dissection
Clamps	
Mosquito	General use
Right angle	To place ties across cephalic vein
Towel clips	To approximate skin edges during DFT testing
Needle holders	Suturing
Nonabsorbable suture	Anchor leads
Absorbable suture	Subcutaneous tissue and skin closure
Slowly absorbing suture	Anchor pulse generator

DFT = defibrillation threshold.

able for the rare but inevitable cases of right ventricular perforation and pneumothorax. Consideration should be given to how an emergency echocardiogram might be performed to assess perioperative hypotension. In addition, an intubation tray and bag-valve mask should be immediately available in cases where conscious sedation is used; with general anesthesia, a ventilator is obviously necessary.

Personnel

All individuals who are involved in ICD surgery should be thoroughly familiar with all equipment, in particular the external defibrillators. In addition to the implanting cardiologist/electrophysiologist support staff should include someone facile with the operation of an external programmer/ defibrillator for the ICD. If conscious seda-

tion is to be used, a nurse trained in delivery of analgesia should be available to monitor the patient's airway, oxygenation, and level of sedation. If general anesthesia is used, an anesthesiologist or nurse anesthetist is necessary. A nurse or technician is generally responsible for running the external defibrillator as well as ensuring that the needed supplies and instruments are available. An individual familiar with the operation of the external programmer, often the manufacturer's technical representative, is responsible to test the lead implant parameters, set programming, and initiate ventricular fibrillation under the guidance of the implanting physician. Although not strictly necessary, the availability of a scrub nurse familiar with the surgical procedure is helpful in expediting the surgery.

The physician implanting the ICD can be either a cardiac surgeon, cardiologist, or electrophysiologist; the technical skills involved with current generation devices are simple enough that they could be mastered by reasonable training and experience. Moreover, the complications associated with ICD implantation are now quite few and are medical in nature, such as worsened heart failure or electrical storm, rather than surgical. The practice in a given hospital is primarily based on past history and politics. It is likely that cost considerations will lead to an increased proportion of cardiologists performing the procedure in the EP or cath lab.

Preoperative Patient Evaluation and Anesthesia

Preoperative Patient Preparation

Part of the preoperative assessment is the evaluation of the patient's body habitus to determine the appropriateness of pectoral implantation. In this assessment, concern should be directed at subcutaneous space, any pectoral or chest wall deformities that may present problems for placement, positioning of the device, and an estimation of lead length. A decision can also be made as to whether to perform a submuscular or subcutaneous implantation. The problem of too much lead redundancy should not be overlooked because this could potentially interfere with optimal pocket size and device fit and could lead to unnecessary kinking of the lead, with the potential for subsequent fracture. If there is a reason to suspect a left subclavian vein anomaly or obstruction, a Doppler study or venogram may be warranted to establish patency or plan a different approach. If the left side cannot be used, a right-sided approach is reasonable before proceeding to thoracotomy. Although the right-sided approach is very similar to a left-sided one, defibrillation efficacy may be worse due to less current deliverable to the left ventricle.

To minimize risk of infection, clipping hair over the region of implantation should be done the night before surgery. Using clippers rather than a razor avoids local inflammation and skin abrasions that may serve as a nidus for skin infection. Antibiotics that are appropriate for gram-positive infection, e.g., cefazolin or vancomycin, 1 gram IV, should be administered just prior to incision. A single dose of intravenous antibiotics should be sufficient, although some suggest continuation of intravenous antibiotics for 24 hours following surgery (there is no definitive data to support either approach). In those patients who are anticoagulated, an INR should be less than 1.6 at time of surgery to allow proper hemostasis. Heparin should be stopped for 4 hours prior to incision.

Anesthesia

Individuals familiar with techniques for transvenous pacemaker implantation will find many of the technical aspects of ICD implantation described below familiar. The major departure is the need for efficacy testing of the ICD which requires induction of ventricular fibrillation and shock delivery. For this reason, the choice of anesthetic method and management of sedation is significantly different for ICD implantation in comparison to pacemaker implantation. A patient who would require general anesthesia even for pacemaker implantation, perhaps due to airway management problems, will, of course, also require general anesthesia for ICD implantation. Other reasons to consider general anesthesia include potentially better management of emergencies and intraoperative pain control.

However, for the patient who can reasonably be managed with conscious sedation during the surgical portion of the procedure, brief deeper anesthesia can be administered at times of VF induction and shock. The use of local anesthesia with conscious sedation has the significant advantage of general availability, less cost, shorter procedure times, and rapid postsurgical recovery. For this approach, light conscious sedation with midazolam and fentanyl and local lidocaine, similar to that used for EP studies or pacemaker implantation, should be adequate for most of the cases. At the time of VF induction and shock, an ultrashort-acting anesthetic agent can be used, with proper attention to airway management. Brevital at a dose of 0.6–1.5 mg/kg should provide about 5–7 min of anesthesia. This is ample time for VF induction and treatment. An alternative, which provides even shorter anesthesia time, albeit with some mild negative inotropic effect, is propofol, 0.8-1.0 mg/kg. If the adrenergic outflow from a delivered transvenous or transthoracic shock appears to awaken the patient, a small dose of midazolam post-shock will provide amnesia for the event. The importance of proper attention to airway management and ability to emergently ventilate and/or intubate the patient cannot be overstated with this approach.

Hardware Selection

Choice of Lead System

There are several lead systems available that can provide adequate defibrillation. To deliver a defibrillation shock, at least two locations must be available between which the current can be delivered. If two locations are used, obviously one will act as the cathode and one as the anode. If a system is chosen with more than two electrodes, two or more electrodes must be combined to act as a single, discontinuous, virtual electrode. Optimal defibrillation will occur when the majority of the heart is contained within the voltage field created between the two electrodes or virtual electrodes. Defibrillation has been predicted to be successful, based on animal studies, when more than 95% of the ventricular myocardium is subjected to a field strength of 6 V/cm (with biphasic waveforms).[10]

For example, a simple system consisting of two electrode positions, one at the right ventricular apex and the other in the left pectoral location, provides reasonable field strength to both ventricles, as can be seen in Figure 1. If this system fails to provide effective defibrillation, addition of a third electrode location, for example in the superior vena cava (SVC), may improve field coverage of the heart, as seen in Figure 2. Alternatively, such a change may worsen current delivery to the left ventricle (LV) and make defibrillation more difficult. In this case, one may elect to use a subcutaneous patch or array along the left thorax or consider a change in the waveform characteristics (e.g., a change in biphasic tilt or duration).

There are several issues to keep in mind when selecting locations from which to defibrillate: (1) Keep it simple. Since a lead will need to be placed in the right ventricle (RV) to provide sensing, a defibrillation lead location in the RV is an obvious and essential location, and is nearly always proximal to the sensing electrodes of the lead made by all manufacturers. Also, since a pulse generator needs to be implanted, the pulse generator can itself can act as an electrode, thus providing the two locations from which to defibrillate. Most manufacturers now use this technology. (2) Consider the patient's anatomy. If a patient has a very large and posteriorly displaced LV, failure to defibrillate with an RV to pectoral position may be due to insufficient coverage of the posterior portion of the LV. In this case, addition of a coronary sinus lead, a posterior thoracic subcutaneous patch, or subcutaneous array may improve defibrillation. On the other hand, if the patient has a very large RV, providing better field coverage to the anterior of the heart with an SVC lead might be expected to be beneficial. (3) Do not outsmart yourself. Attempts to predict defibrillation efficacy, based on clinical grounds, are seldom useful.[11] In general, an approach that starts with a simple system and escalates in complexity as the case requires is better than starting with a multi-lead complex system. (4) More is not always better. Additional leads, e.g., an SVC electrode, are often con-

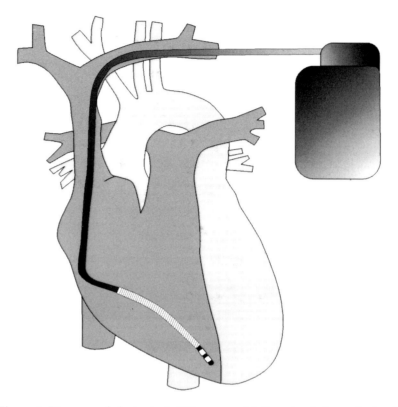

Figure 1. Diagram of electrode in RV apex and left pectoral electrode (can).

sidered beneficial because a larger virtual electrode should create a field that better covers the heart. However, if an additional lead allows shunting of current away from the LV, defibrillation may in fact become worse rather than better. It is the LV, not the SVC that needs current.

It is important to remember that the choice of which RV lead to use has a significant effect on sensing. The lead choices currently available are diagrammed in Figure 3. The use of "integrated bipolar" sensing is a sensing compromise that allows lead design with one less conductor than is required for "true bipolar" sensing. Compared to true bipolar sensing, however, integrated bipolar sensing is more susceptable to noise, farfield artifacts, and post-shock undersensing.[12] If an SVC coil is considered necessary for a given patient, the disadvantage of integrated bipolar sensing would suggest the use of a quadripo-

lar lead. Now one is faced with accepting the increased lead complexity and cost, or use of a separate SVC coil, with its associated need for an additional venapuncture.

In patients who are able to have a subcutaneous left pectoral location for their pulse generator, our general approach is to try the RV-CAN system first, using a tripolar lead with true bipolar sensing. In the rare instances when this fails to defibrillate effectively, the first approach should be to reposition the RV lead. If still ineffective and waveform programming changes or polarity switches are unavailable or ineffective, use of an additional lead could be entertained. Because it involves less surgery, we favor implantation of an SVC lead in this setting. Other options, particularly for patients with difficult venous access, include placement of a subcutaneous patch or array.

The final lead-related decision to be

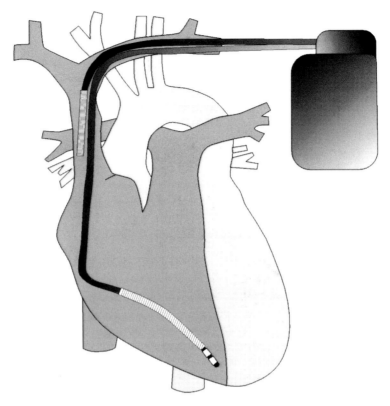

Figure 2. Diagram of electrode in RV apex and SVC + left pectoral. Note that there are higher currents on the right side with use of an SVC electrode, but some areas of the heart have lower current due to shunting.

made is which type of venous access should be used to insert the RV lead. Since defibrillation leads are large and complex, they are certainly susceptable to lead fracture and crush injuries, particularly at the first rib/clavicular junction and at the anchoring sleeve sites. In an effort to avoid first rib/clavicular crush, we favor an attempt at left cephalic cutdown for lead placement if possible, and reversion to subclavian vein cannulation only if the cephalic vein is small or cannot be isolated.

Choice of Pulse Generator Location

The default location for the pulse generator for most people will be the left pectoral region. If the left shoulder region is anatomically inaccessible for ICD placement, the right pectoral location can be used. It should be noted that the right pectoral location is a suboptimal location for an elecrode to defibrillate the heart, thus an active unipolar can in this location may be less effective. That said, RV- CAN usually works from the right side.[13] One, nevertheless, should consider use of an SVC lead or a single lead that incorporates both an SVC and an RV coil under these circumstances. In difficult right-sided cases, one may resort to use of a coronary sinus lead or simply abandon a transvenous approach altogether and proceed to an epicardial lead system.

For patients with a very small body habitus, a subpectoral location for the pulse generator may be considered. There are several concerns with this approach, including increased risk of bleeding, potential for damage to the thoraco-acromial neurovascular

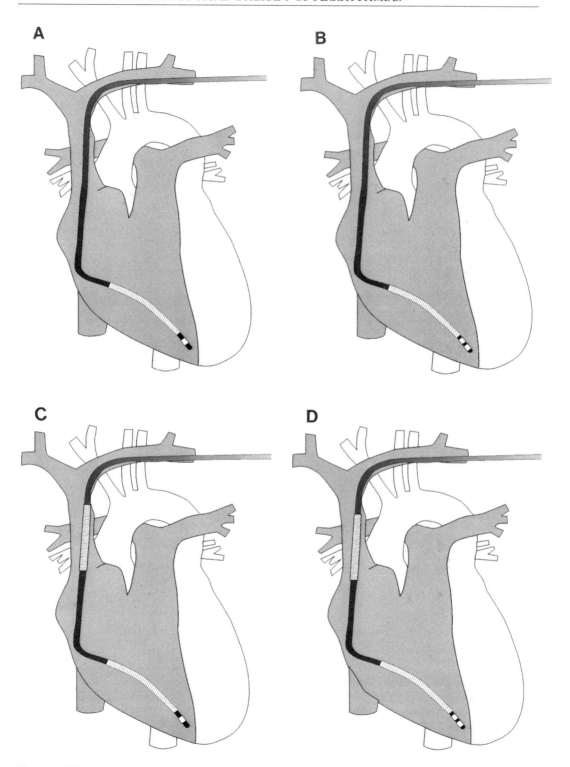

Figure 3. Diagram of four possible RV leads of increasing complexity. **A**: Bipolar with integrated sensing. **B**: Triploar with true bipolar sensing. **C**: Triploar with two coils and integrated sensing. **D**: Quadripolar with two coils and true bipolar sensing.

bundle with subsequent pectoralis major atrophy, and difficulty in subsequent pulse generator replacement. These problems, though, are generally modest and this approach may minimize risk of pocket erosion in the few patients for which today's pulse generators are still too big. Description of this approach is beyond the scope of this chapter and has been described elsewhere.[14]

A final alternative is the use of an abdominal pulse generator. This approach requires two incisions and tunneling of one or two leads from the subclavian region to the abdomen. The abdominal dissection may require a surgeon. The surgery is longer and often is best done with general anesthesia. Long-term disadvantages of this approach, known from earlier defibrillator experience, include higher risk of lead dislodgement and lead fracture due to the longer lead length, infection, and risk of peritoneal erosion of the pulse generator. This approach has become mostly of historic interest, as manufacturers limit production of the long, fracture prone, and difficult to use leads. The surgical technique, as described below, will focus on the subcutaneous implantation of a single lead ICD system in the left pectoral region.

Surgical Technique

Preoperative Preparation

In the operating room, EP lab or cath lab, prior to surgical scrub, appropriate ECG monitoring should be established, and adhesive defibrillation pads for backup defibrillation applied. We recommend the routine placement of a peripheral arterial line, which proves especially valuable in management of complications that unpredictably occur and for assessing the hemodynamic consequence of ventricular tachycardia if it is induced. The surgical site is prepped in the usual manner with sterile towels followed by an ioban cover. General anesthesia or conscious sedation is initiated.

For local anesthesia, the site of incision is infiltrated with lidocaine and bupivicaine.

Initial Incision and Pocket Formation

Defibrillator lead implantation is generally performed through an incision made in the left infraclavicular region. The incision should be sufficiently large, 5–6 cm long, to accommodate the pulse generator and must be made and carried down to the prepectoralis fascia, generally using electrocautery to form a proper pocket. The incision is made approximately 4 cm below the clavicle, extending from the midclavicular region to just above the delto-pectoral groove. The lateral extent of the incision is designed to allow for cephalic vein dissection or lateral puncture of the subclavian vein.

The pocket is fashioned for placement of the pulse generator, typically before lead placement to avoid lead interference with the pocket dissection or inadvertent lead dislodgement. We prefer to make the pocket just above the prepectoralis fascia, using cautery to minimize bleeding. If a unipolar active can system is to be used, the position of the pulse generator becomes relatively important since it serves as a defibrillation electrode. The can should lie approximately in or slightly more lateral to the midline of the clavicle. Care must be given to the lateral margin of the can, which should be at least 2 cm from the delto-pectoral groove to avoid mechanical limitation of shoulder motion, especially during adduction. This position is a compromise between patient comfort and defibrillation efficacy because the ideal can location for defibrillation is probably along the anterior axillary line. The defibrillator pulse generator can be placed in the pocket without an anchoring suture. We prefer an anchoring tie to avoid generator drift, but it is our practice to tie this suture loosely to prevent tenting or levering of the inferior aspect of the can against the skin and to allow the can a modest degree of freedom to find its "home."

Lead Implantation

Use of the cephalic vein for venous access is preferred as a means to avoid first rib/clavicular crush injury. After the initial incision is made and the pocket formed, the cephalic vein is identified by using blunt dissection along the delto-pectoral groove fat pad that overlies the vein (Figure 4). Care must be taken in the dissection because the cephalic vein may lie superficially and is often associated with a small venous plexus. Once the vein is identified and cleaned of adventitial tissue, loose ties are applied proximally, and distally 2–3 cm. The distal tie can be ligated. With light tension applied to the proximal or distal tie of the cephalic vein, a small incision (approximately one-third of the width of the vein) is made in the vein with tenotomy scissors or a #11 scalpel. The RV lead tip is then advanced into the vein and positioned near the RV apex. If the lead cannot be easily passed, a guidewire often helps straighten the vein and facilitates lead passage. Once in the RV, the lead is tested for pacing and sensing characteristics, and repositioned as necessary to achieve a pacing threshold of <1.0 V and an R wave amplitude of >5.0 mV. When the cephalic vein cannot be identified or cannulated, the modified Seldinger technique can be used for lateral subclavian vein access. An attempt should be made to stay in the lateral one-third of the subclavian vein in an effort to minimize the risk of subclavian crush injury of the lead.

If, after defibrillation testing, the system is thought inadequate, repositioning the RV lead further toward the RV apex or closer to the septum often results in improved defibrillation efficacy. If use of a second lead is found necessary, some patients have a ce-

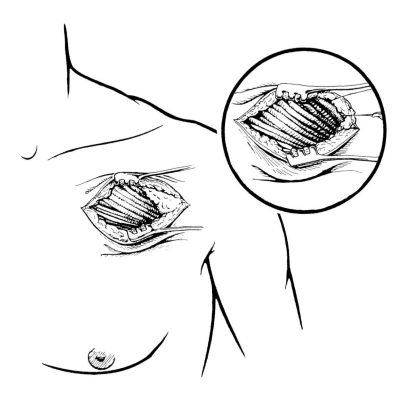

Figure 4. This figure shows the location of the cephalic vein. Used with permission from Singer I, ed.[14]

phalic vein that will accommodate both, otherwise a modified Seldinger approach can be used to puncture the subclavian vein for an SVC lead (presuming a subcutaneous patch or array is not preferred). Care should be taken when the modified Seldinger technique is used to cannulate the subclavian vein after a lead has been implanted via the cephalic vein, since such cannulation carries the risk of lead injury. The SVC lead is then positioned such that the proximal coil lies at the jugular vein/SVC junction for a better field distribution across the left ventricle (Figure 5).

Proper lead anchoring is important for avoidance of lead fracture. Figure 6 shows the leads exiting the cephalic vein and entering the header block. The lead(s) should be anchored to the prepectoralis fascia in such a way that a gentle curve exists at the exit site of the vein to avoid kinking of the lead with the attendant risk of subsequent fracture. The leads should be positioned to gently curve around the ICD pulse generator and enter a medially directed header block. In contrast to pacemaker pulse generators, ICD pulse generators can be implanted with the engraving side up or down without loss of efficacy or concern over pectoralis stimulation during pacing. Two or three interrupted 1–0 sutures moderately firmly applied to the anchoring sleeve are usually sufficient to secure the leads. Excessive compression of the anchoring sleeve with sutures applied too tightly can lead to insulation breeches and conductor fractures years after implantation. Once the lead is secured, the patient is ready to proceed to defibrillation threshold (DFT) testing. Once DFT testing is completed, the pocket can be

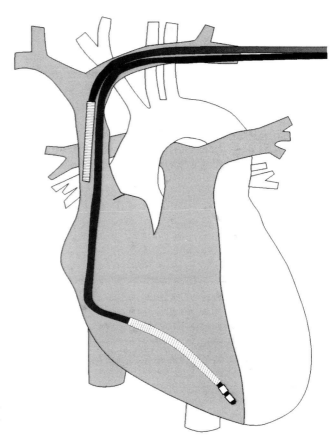

Figure 5. This figure shows the ideal location for the superior vena caval lead.

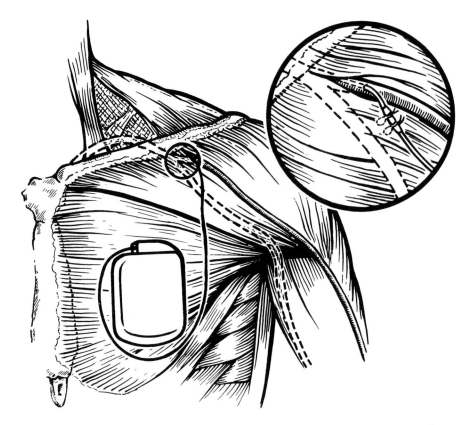

Figure 6. A single lead entering the cephalic vein; the lead is nicely wrapped around pulse generator. Used with permission from Singer I, ed.[15]

closed in two layers using absorbable suture and steri-strips.

Defibrillation Testing

Testing of the ICD system requires induction of ventricular fibrillation and testing of the lead system. Prior to starting, the rescue transthoracic defibrillation system must be verified as working. We deliver a 5-joule synchronized transthoracic test shock to be certain that all connections are intact, observing the patient move with the shock.

Induction and testing of therapy can be performed using either an emulator or the ICD itself. Although an emulator allows one to abandon a case or choose a different pulse generator based on testing results, it is somewhat more difficult to do and may not precisely reflect the ICD response.

Given the very high likelihood of success with current devices (>98%), anticipating a successful implant by testing with the implanted ICD itself is preferable. Moreover, one can almost always reconfigure the lead system for successful defibrillation if the initial test with the ICD fails.

After placing the ICD in the pocket and expelling any air, the pocket can be closed temporarily with towel clips or with a deep skin closure. VF can then be induced. We have found T wave shocks with a three-beat drive train at 400 ms followed by a 0.6 to 1.0 J monophasic shock delivered at 310 ms to be quite effective in creating VF. These intervals may have to be modified for the patient on amiodarone or other antiarrhythmic drugs. Also effective in inducing VF is AC current or high-frequency pacing.

An initial energy is chosen at least 10 J less than the maximal energy deliverable by the device. If the device is successful in terminating VF with this energy, successful implant is virtually assured. Further testing with lower energies can be pursued in an effort to minimize the energy needed for the first shock, the principal benefit of which is to reduce the time to the first shock. The number of VF inductions will be determined by the precision with which the DFT needs to be measured. If the patient is only under local anesthesia or would benefit from a brief surgery, two successful terminations of VF are sufficient. If, however, one would like to treat with the minimal energy in an effort to more rapidly intervene into VT or VF and avoid syncope, multiple inductions may be necessary in order to document a low DFT. In order to allow an adequate safety margin for therapy, the first programmed therapy for VF should be at least 10 J greater than the lowest energy found to successfully terminate VF.

Postsurgical Management

Most patients can be managed as outpatients with 4–6 hours of postoperative observation. Given the stored electrograms and RR intervals available with current devices, even postoperative telemetry monitoring is not strictly necessary. Factors to be considered in deciding the appropriateness of inpatient observation are generally not subtle. Decompensated congestive heart failure, ischemic ECG changes in patients with known coronary disease, adverse reactions to anesthesia, the presence of mechanical valves requiring anticoagulation, or postoperative arrhythmias are the more common issues warranting longer inpatient observation. Management of pain is usually adequate with oral narcotics for 48 hours following surgery. At discharge, patients should be instructed to notify the physician immediately if excessive pain, swelling, or

bleeding occur, or if there is a fever, periincisional redness or warmth suggesting an infection. A chest x-ray with posteroanterior and lateral views to verify proper lead positioning is mandatory prior to releasing the patient.

For current endocardial lead systems, long-term management is approaching the simplicity of long-term pacemaker management. Because patients may have silent events that may warrant programming or medication changes, we encourage clinical visits for follow-up device interrogations every 4 months. This also affords the opportunity to evaluate lead integrity with pacing thresholds and electrogram interrogation. Lead stability and integrity are also evaluated by chest x-ray every 8–12 months. These follow-up schedules may be liberalized in stable patients as transtelephonic monitoring becomes available.

Summary

The once complex and risky procedure of ICD implantation has matured to a nearly routine, often outpatient, procedure. With the technique described above, ICD therapy can be safely applied to nearly any patient. ICD therapy will continue to evolve with smaller pulse generators, longer battery life, lower cost, more programmable features, more memory, improved detection algorithms, improved treatment algorithms (possibly including pre-event interventions based on insight obtained from pre-event RR intervals and electrograms), and incorporation of advanced pacemaker functions. Ongoing improvements in lead technology will improve longevity, optimize current delivery, and provide for easier placement and removal. Perhaps most importantly, ongoing clinical trials will provide better identification of patients who will benefit from this therapy and improve management of patients who have an ICD implanted.

References

1. Parsonnet V, Manhardt M. Permanent pacing of the heart: 1952 to 1976. Am J Cardiol 1977;39:250–256.
2. Parsonnet V. Permanent transvenous pacing in 1962. PACE 1978;1:2562.
3. Bardy GH, Hofer B, Johnson G, et al. Implantable transvenous cardioverter- defibrillators. Circulation 1993;87:1152–1168.
4. Brooks R, Garan H, Torchiana D, et al. Determinants of successful nonthoracotomy cardioverter-defibrillator implantation: experience in 101 patients using two different lead systems. J Am Coll Cardiol 1993;22:1835–1842.
5. Fitzpatrick AP, Lesh MD, Epstein LM, et al. Electrophysiological laboratory, electrophysiologist-implanted, nonthoracotomy-implantable cardioverter/defibrillators. Circulation 1994;89:2503–2508.
6. Strickberger SA, Hummel JD, Daoud E, et al. Implantation by electrophysiologists of 100 consecutive cardioverter defibrillators with nonthoracotomy lead systems. Circulation 1994;90:868–872.
7. Strickberger SA, Niebauer M, Ching MK, et al. Comparison of implantation of nonthoracotomy defibrillators in the operating room versus the electrophysiology laboratory. Am Heart J 1995;75:255–257.
8. Bardy GH, Marchlinski FE, Sharma AD, et al. Multicenter comparison of truncated biphasic shocks and standard damped sine wave monophasic shocks for transthoracic ventricular defibrillation. Circulation 1996;94:2507–2514.
9. Cohen TJ. Innovative emergency defibrillation methods for refractory ventricular fibrillation in a variety of hospital settings. Am Heart J 1993;126:962–968.
10. Ideker RE, Zhou X, Knisley SB. Correlation among fibrillation, defibrillation, and cardiac pacing. PACE 1995;18:512–525.
11. Raitt MH, Johnson G, Dolack GL, et al. Clinical predictors of the defibrillation threshold with the unipolar implantable defibrillation system. J Am Coll Cardiol 1995;25:1576–1583.
12. Natale A, Sra J, Axtell K, et al. Undetected ventricular fibrillation in transvenous implantable cardioverter-defibrillators: prospective comparison of different lead system-device combinations. Circulation 1996;93:91–98.
13. Bardy GH, Yee R, Jung W, for the Active Can Investigators. Multicenter experience with a pectoral unipolar transvenous cardioversion-defibrillation. J Am Coll Cardiol 1996;28:400–410.
14. Jones GK, Bardy GH. Implantation of ICDs in the electrophysiology laboratory. In Singer I, ed. Interventional Electrophysiology. Baltimore, Williams & Wilkins, 1997.
15. Bardy GH, Raitt MH, Jones GK. Unipolar defibrillation systems. In Singer I, ed. Implantable Cardioverter-Defibrillator. Armonk, NY, Futura Publishing Co, Inc., 1994, p 369.

Chapter 16

Defibrillation Waveforms

Jian Huang, Xiaohong Zhou, Randolph A.S. Cooper,
Gregory P. Walcott, Raymond E. Ideker

Waveform Shape and Duration

The shape of the defibrillation waveform has a marked effect on defibrillation efficacy. For example, Schuder et al.[1] have shown that for external defibrillation in the dog, a waveform consisting of an ascending ramp has a much higher success rate for defibrillation than a descending ramp waveform of the same strength (Figure 1). However, since waveforms similar to the descending ramp are much easier to generate with an electronic circuit small enough to fit into an implantable cardioverter-defibrillator than are waveforms similar to an ascending ramp, the descending ramp type of waveform is used clinically even though it is much less efficient for defibrillation.

The waveforms used in internal cardioverters-defibrillators decay exponentially (Figure 2). They are generated by charging a capacitor and allowing it to discharge through the resistance of the leads and the body of the patient. Based on data of the type shown in Figure 1, it is commonly thought that the long, low tail of the exponential waveform shown in Figure 2A refibrillates the heart,[2] and is thus ineffective

for defibrillation. For this reason truncated exponential waveforms of the type shown in Figure 2 B and C are used clinically. However, recent evidence suggests that truncation is not necessary for waveforms with time constants similar to those used clinically. The time constant of an exponentially decaying waveform is defined as the time necessary for the shock voltage to decrease to 37% of its starting value. As shown in Figure 3, defibrillation threshold voltage does not increase even when the waveform is allowed to discharge for three time constants, at which time 95% of the voltage has been delivered to the patient.

Both the time constant and the tilt of the truncated exponential waveform influence the shock strength required for defibrillation.[3,4] Waveform tilt is the percentage of the leading edge voltage of the shock waveform that is still present at the trailing edge of the shock. It is calculated as the difference between the leading and trailing edge voltages divided by the leading edge voltage and multiplied by 100. Waveform tilt can be altered either by changing the duration of waveforms with the same time constant or, as shown in Figure 2 B and C, by changing the time constant without altering the waveform duration. Of course, tilt can also

Supported in part by the National Institutes of Health Research Grant HL-42760.

From Singer I, Barold SS, Camm AJ (eds): Nonpharmacological Therapy of Arrhythmias for the 21st Century: The State of the Art. Futura Publishing Co, Inc., Armonk, NY, © 1998.

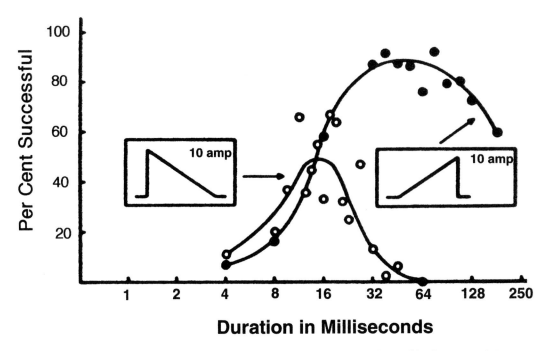

Figure 1. Relation between percent success of transthoracic ventricular defibrillation and duration of 10-amp triangular shocks in dog. The ascending ramp waveform (closed circles) has a higher success rate for defibrillation than a descending ramp waveform (open circles). Used with permission from Schuder JC, et al.[1]

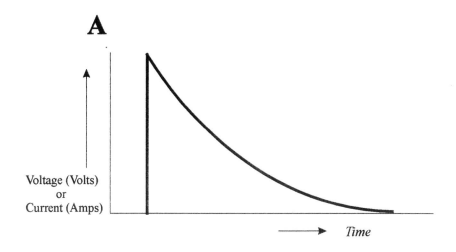

Figure 2. (A) Monophasic capacitive discharge (exponential decay) waveform.

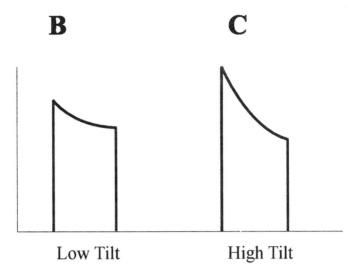

Figure 2. *Continued.* (**B**) Low-tilt monophasic truncated exponential waveform. (**C**) High-tilt monophasic truncated exponential waveform with duration equal to waveform B.

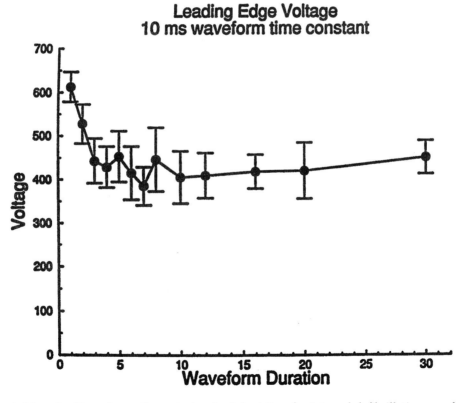

Figure 3. Mean leading edge voltage ± standard deviation for internal defibrillation as a function of waveform duration for a monophasic waveform with a time constant of 10 ms in dogs. The defibrillation threshold decreases to a constant minimum value as waveform duration increases, even for very long waveforms with a low voltage tail.

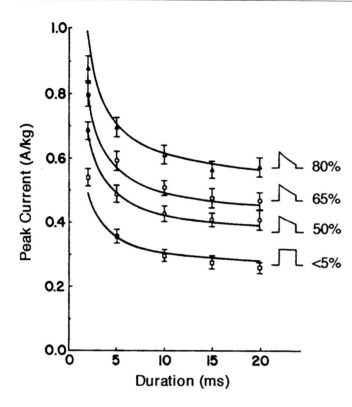

Figure 4. Relationship of waveform tilt and duration to internal defibrillation threshold in dogs. Threshold peak current per unit of body weight in amps/kg versus waveform duration in ms. Percent tilt is given at the right of the figure. The mean ± the standard error (N = 30) is given for each combination of tilt and duration. Used with permission from Wessale JL, et al.[5]

be altered by changing both the time constant and the waveform duration. Similarly, waveform time constant and duration can simultaneously be altered in such a way that the waveform tilt remains constant, generating the data shown in Figure 4.[5] The data in that figure show that: (1) for a constant tilt, the defibrillation threshold decreases as the waveform duration increases; and (2) for a constant duration, the defibrillation threshold decreases as the tilt decreases.

Biphasic Waveforms

A biphasic truncated exponential waveform can be created with a single capacitor by using switches to reverse the polarities that are delivered to the shock electrodes during the shock pulse. Thus, the electrode that was an anode during the first phase is a cathode during the second phase and vice versa. Some biphasic waveforms have a markedly lower defibrillation threshold than do monophasic waveforms,[6] as shown in Figure 5. As shown in this same figure, other biphasic waveforms have significantly higher defibrillation thresholds than monophasic waveforms. An important variable related to the defibrillation efficacy of biphasic waveforms is the relative amount of charge delivered during each phase. Biphasic waveforms with the lowest defibrillation thresholds deliver more charge during the first phase than during the second phase of the waveform. With a few exceptions,[7] this typically means that the biphasic waveforms with the lowest defibrillation thresholds have a second phase that is equal to or shorter than the first phase (Figure 5). As the second phase duration gets considerably longer than the first phase duration, the defibrillation threshold increases until it is higher than for the first phase waveform delivered alone as a monophasic shock (Figure 6).[8] Thus, the strength-duration relationship for the second phase of a biphasic waveform is not the same as that for a monophasic waveform. For either a nontruncated (Figure 3) or a truncated (Figure 4) monophasic exponential waveform, as the duration of the shock is increased, the defibrillation threshold first decreases and then remains nearly constant at its lowest value. In contrast, for the second phase of the biphasic waveform, the defibrillation threshold first decreases as the duration of the second phase increases, but subsequently the defibrillation threshold rises markedly as the second phase duration is further increased (Figure 6).

A simple model has been developed that can be used to predict whether a monophasic or biphasic waveform will have a low defibrillation threshold.[4,9] This model consists of a resistor and a capacitor in parallel (Figure 7). The values of the resistor and capacitor are such that the time constant of the circuit is 2.8 or 3.0 ms.[4,10] These values were obtained by fitting the experimental data obtained from several experiments in dogs for defibrillation with electrodes on or in the heart.[8,11] It is not known how well this resistor-capacitor circuit corresponds to the behavior of the cell membrane and the transmembrane potential during a shock.

To defibrillate, the model assumes that the shock waveform, either the monophasic

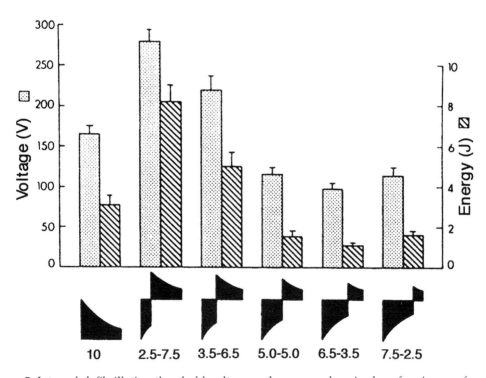

Figure 5. Internal defibrillation threshold voltage and energy values in dogs for six waveforms of the same total duration (10 ms), demonstrating that the defibrillation threshold is lowest for those biphasic waveforms in which the second phase is smaller than the first phase. The mean values and standard deviations are shown. Diagrams of the waveforms are shown below the bar graphs. The biphasic waveform with a second phase duration equal to the first phase (5–5 ms, first phase duration - second phase duration) or shorter than the first phase (6.5–3.5 and 7.5–2.5 ms) had significantly lower leading edge voltage and energy requirements than other waveforms tested. The biphasic waveforms with shorter first phases than second phases (2.5–7.5 and 3.5–6.5 ms) had significantly higher voltage and energy requirements than the other waveforms tested, including the 10 ms monophasic waveform. The 2.5–7.5 biphasic waveform had significantly higher defibrillation voltage and energy requirements than the 3.5–6.5 ms biphasic waveform. Used and modified with permission from Dixon EG, et al.[6]

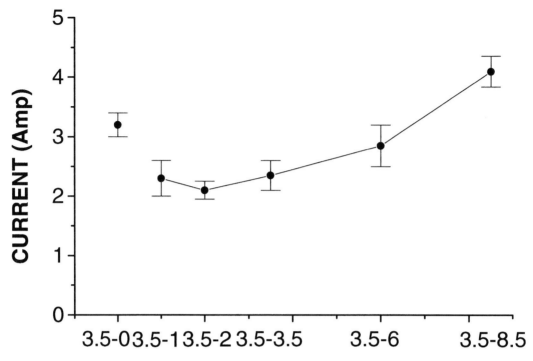

Figure 6. Scatterplots of internal defibrillation threshold current versus phase-two duration in dogs. Mean values ± the standard deviation are shown. As long as the first phase (3.5 ms) was longer than the second phase, the current threshold decreased as the second phase-two duration increased. As the second phase duration got longer than the first phase duration, the defibrillation threshold increased. Used and modified with permission from Feeser SA, et al.[8]

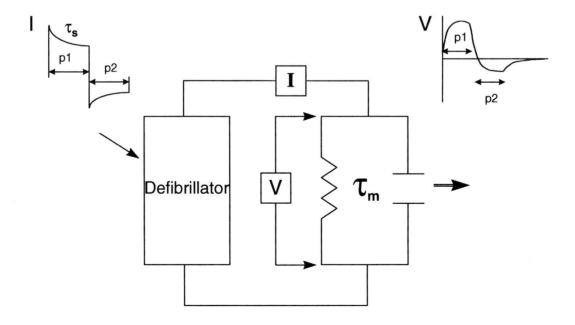

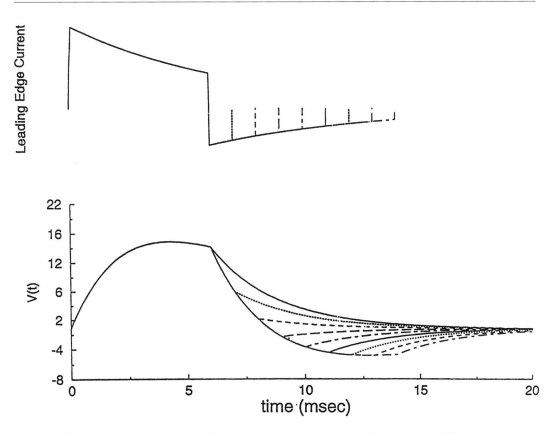

Figure 8. The RC model response to a biphasic truncated exponential waveform with a time constant of 7 ms. Leading edge current of the input waveform was 10 A. Panel **A** shows the shape of the input waveforms. Phase one was truncated at 6 ms. Phase two was truncated after 0, 1, 2, 3, 4, 5, 6, 7, and 8 ms. Panel **B** shows the model response, V(t). The model response does not change polarity until phase two duration is longer than 2 ms. Used with permission from Walcott GP, et al.[4]

waveform or the first phase of the biphasic waveform, must create a certain minimum potential difference across the resistor-capacitor network.[4] The model assumes that the optimum second phase of a biphasic waveform is one that brings the potential difference across the resistor-capacitor circuit quickly back to or slightly past its starting value at the beginning of the first phase.[4,10] Figure 8 indicates the response of the model to a family of biphasic wave-

forms in which the first phase is a constant 6 ms and the second phase varies from 0 ms (i.e., a 6-ms monophasic waveform) to 8 ms. As can be seen in the figure, a second phase of 2 ms brings the potential back to its starting level and a second phase of 3 ms brings the voltage slightly below the starting level. Experimental data show that for biphasic waveforms with this same time constant, the 6–2 ms and 6–3 ms waveforms have lower defibrillation

Figure 7. Diagram shows a parallel resistor-capacitor (RC) circuit. Model to predict defibrillation efficacy of different biphasic waveforms. The RC circuit has a time constant, τ_m, of 2.8 ms. The left panel shows the input biphasic waveform with phase one duration p1 and phase two duration p2. τ_s represents the time constant for the shock waveform. The right panel shows the model response (V) to the input waveform (I).

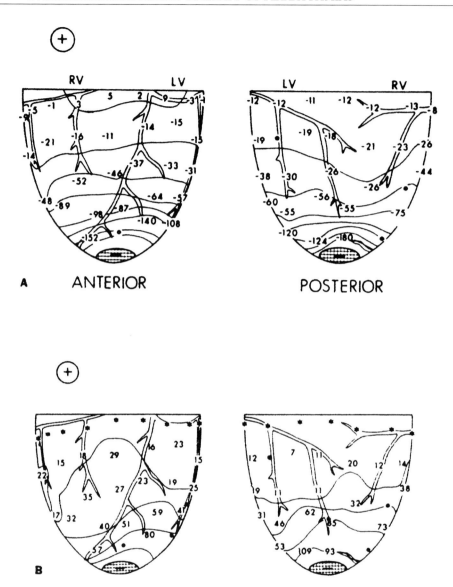

Figure 9. The epicardial potential (panel **A**) and potential gradient (panel **B**) distribution during a very low voltage shock in a dog. The maps are displayed as two complementary projections of the ventricles with the anterior left ventricular (LV) and right ventricular (RV) epicardium shown in the left diagram and the posterior left and right ventricular epicardium in the right diagram. The location of a cathodal defibrillation electrode at the apex is indicated by a minus sign within a cross-hatched circle. The plus sign within a circle indicates that the location of an anodal defibrillation electrode was on the right atrium. Numbers represent the locations of electrodes with satisfactory recordings and give the potential (panel **A**, mV) or potential gradient (panel **B**, mV/cm) for those locations. Closed circles indicate electrode sites where adequate recordings were not obtained. Asterisks indicate electrode sites for which no gradient was calculated because there were neighboring electrodes on only one site. The isopotential lines are 25 mV apart; the isogradient lines are 25 mV/cm apart. Panel **A** shows the isopotential map during a 1 V shock given in electrical diastole during atrial paced rhythm. The voltage drop across the ventricle was 189 mV. The isopotential lines were closer together at the apex than at the base of the heart, indicating a higher gradient at the apex as quantified in panel **B** which shows the isogradient map of the same shock. The higher potential gradient area was near the apex and the lower gradient area was near the base. There was a 102 mV/cm difference between the maximal and minimal gradients on the surface of the heart. Used with permission from Chen PS, et al.[12]

thresholds than the 6–0, 6–1, and 6–4 to 6–8 ms waveforms.[4]

Shock Potential Gradient Field

During a defibrillation shock, a potential gradient field is created through the extracellular space of the heart. This extracellular gradient causes current to enter the myocardial cells, altering the transmembrane potential. It is thought that these changes in the transmembrane potential cause defibrillation.[12–17] For most defibrillation electrode configurations used with implantable cardioverter-defibrillators, the potential gradient field is highly uneven with very high potential gradients adjacent to the defibrillation electrodes and low potential gradients in areas of the heart distant from the electrodes (Figure 9).[12] Both low potential gradients and high potential gradients can cause a defibrillation shock to fail. If the potential gradient is too low, the transmembrane potential may not be sufficiently altered to defibrillate, and activation fronts may appear soon after the shock in the low poten-

tial gradient region that lead to the resumption of fibrillation (Figure 10).[12] If the potential gradient is too large, conduction block occurs for a time period in the tissue exposed to this high potential gradient.[18] At very high potential gradients activation fronts may arise at the border of the blocked region that can refibrillate the heart (Figure 11).[19]

An efficacious biphasic waveform has more beneficial effects than a monophasic waveform of the same total duration at both the low and the high potential gradient regions of the heart (Table 1).[18,20] The minimum potential gradient required for defibrillation is about one-third lower for the biphasic than for the monophasic waveform. If the small change in shock impedance with shock voltage is ignored, the biphasic shock will require approximately two-thirds of the shock voltage required to defibrillate with a monophasic shock. In the regions of high potential gradient around the defibrillation electrode, the biphasic shock potential gradient can be over 10% stronger than the monophasic potential gradient before the detrimental effect of conduction block occurs.

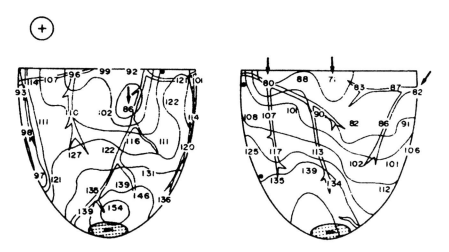

Figure 10. The isochronal map of the first post-shock activation after a 4.9-J unsuccessful defibrillation shock given during electrically induced fibrillation for the electrode configuration shown in Figure 9. The early sites of activation (arrows) appeared 71–86 ms after the shock and were located at the base of the ventricles where the potential gradient was low as shown in Figure 9. Activation spread away from the base so that the apex was the last region to be depolarized. Isochronal lines are spaced 10 ms apart. Used with permission from Chen PS, et al.[12]

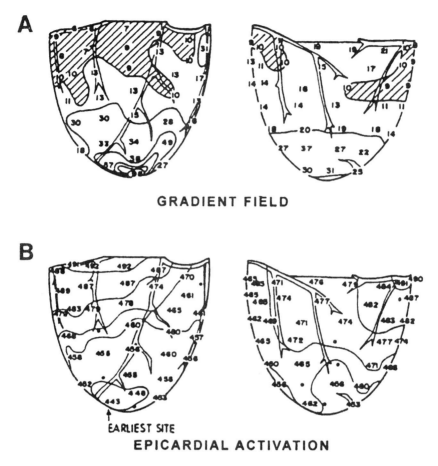

Figure 11. An example of an arrhythmia arising from the tissue adjacent to a defibrillation electrode. Panel **A** shows the potential gradient field for a 284-V shock via a cathode on the left ventricle apex and dual anodes on the right atrium and left ventricle base in a dog. Anterior view to left, posterior to right. Cross-hatched area indicates region where the potential gradient was less than 10 V/cm. Isopotential lines are 10 V/cm apart. Panel **B** shows the isochronal map of the second beat of ventricular tachycardia which arose immediately following the successful defibrillation shock shown in panel A. The origin of the tachycardia was adjacent to the apical shock electrode. The isochronal lines are spaced 10 ms apart. Time zero is the onset of the shock. Used with permission from Wharton JM, et al.[19]

Table 1
Extracellular Potential Gradient Requirements for Stimulation and Defibrillation of Myocardium and Inducing Conduction Block in Myocardium

	Monophasic Waveform	Biphasic Waveform
Stimulation	1 V/cm	?
Defibrillation	6 V/cm	4 V/cm
Conduction Block	64 V/cm	71 V/cm

Used and modified with permission from Frazier DW, et al.,[13] Yabe S, et al.,[18] and Zhou X, et al.[22]

Stimulation and Action Potential Prolongation by Different Waveform

It is intriguing that, even though the biphasic waveform requires a lower potential gradient for defibrillation than does the monophasic waveform, the biphasic waveform is less efficacious in stimulating myocardial tissue. For example, the strength-interval curve for a 2–1 ms biphasic waveform is shifted to the right compared with a 3-ms monophasic waveform, even though the

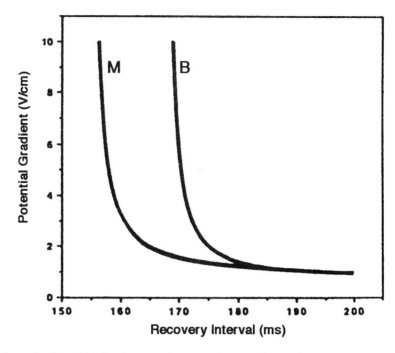

Figure 12. Monophasic and biphasic strength-interval curves for cardiac stimulation in a dog. Biphasic curve (B) is to the right of the monophasic (M) indicating the biphasic waveform is less able to directly excite relatively refractory myocardium. The absolute refractory period is the asymptote of the strength-interval curve parallel to the y axis, and the diastolic threshold is the asymptote parallel to the x axis. The absolute refractory period was 155 ms for the monophasic and 168 ms for the biphasic curve. The monophasic diastolic threshold was 0.7 V/cm, and the biphasic diastolic threshold was 0.6 V/cm. Used with permission from Daubert JP, et al.[21]

biphasic waveform has a significantly lower defibrillation threshold (Figure 12).[21] The shift of the strength-interval curve to the right for the biphasic waveform means that, at a given shock strength, the monophasic waveform can stimulate a new action potential in tissue that is more relatively refractory than can the biphasic waveform. The applicability of this finding, obtained during regular rhythm, to defibrillation is corroborated by the results of a study by Zhou et al. in which the transmembrane potential was measured in open-chest dogs while defibrillation shocks were administered during ventricular fibrillation.[22] This study compared the ability of a 5-ms monophasic shock and a 2.5–2.5 ms biphasic shock, both of which generated potential gradients of 5 V/cm, to stimulate new action potentials when delivered following the same coupling interval from the upstroke

of the last action potential during fibrillation in dogs (Figure 13). This study also demonstrated that the biphasic waveform was less able to stimulate a new action potential than was the monophasic waveform when the shocks were the same strength and were given at the same coupling interval following the previous action potential upstroke.

Many investigators believe that defibrillation efficacy is related to the ability of the shock to cause action potential prolongation and refractory period extension without causing a new action potential.[23–25] An example of such a response is shown in Figure 14. However, Zhou et al.[22] also showed, with floating microelectrode recordings during shocks delivered after 10 seconds of ventricular fibrillation, that at five different coupling intervals following the previous action potential upstroke, the 2.5–2.5 ms bi-

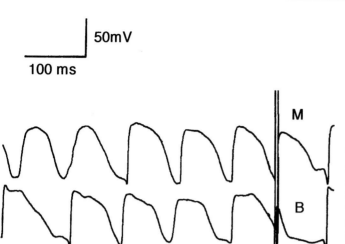

Figure 13. Example of action potentials recorded before and after test shocks during ventricular fibrillation. The voltage and time scales are shown in the top left corner. The response to the monophasic shock is greater than that to the same strength biphasic shock. The monophasic shock induces a new action potential while the biphasic shock merely causes prolongation of the action potential. Used and modified with permission from Zhou X, et al.[22]

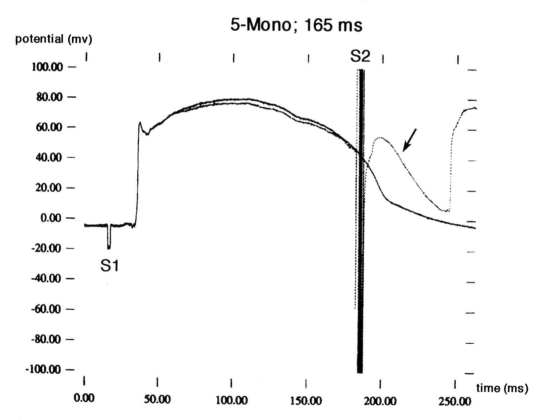

Figure 14. Prolongation of action potential duration following an S_2 shock. At a 165 ms S_1-S_2 interval for a 5-ms monophasic shock, action potential prolongation is observed (arrow). Two S_1-stimulated action potentials are shown. No S_2 was given during the action potential shown by the solid line. An S_2 was given during the action potential indicated by the dotted line. S_1 indicates the S_1 stimulus artifact while S_2 indicates the S_2 shock artifact. Used and modified with permission from Zhou X, et al.[23]

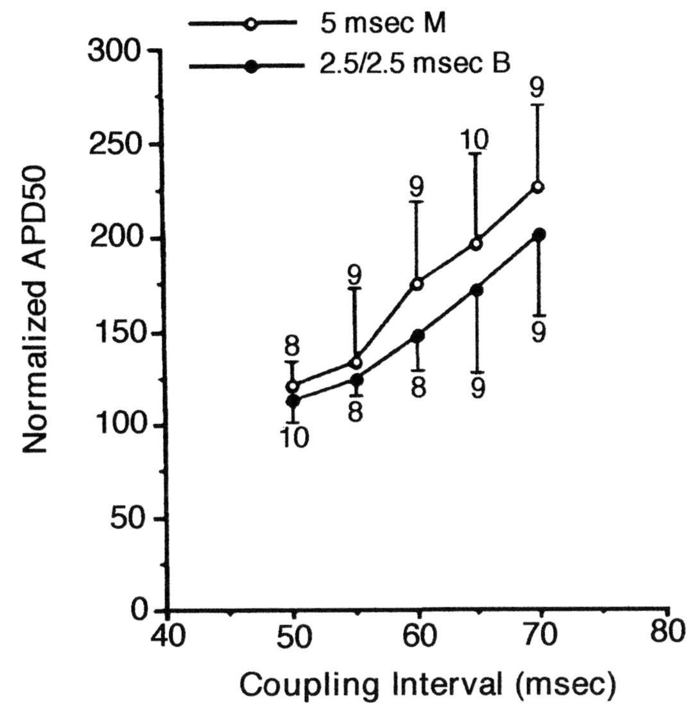

Figure 15. Relation between normalized APD50 (the time from the onset of the S_1-stimulated action potential to the time for the action potential to return to 50% of its maximum value following the S_2 shock) and the S_1-S_2 coupling interval. On the y axis is the APD50 (mean ±SD) expressed as a percent of the APD50 if no S_2 shock is given. The APD50 for the 5-ms monophasic waveform was significantly longer than for the 2.5–2.5-ms biphasic waveform. Used with permission from Zhou X, et al.[22]

phasic waveform caused less action potential prolongation than did the 5 ms monophasic waveform at a shock field strength of 5 V/cm in 10 dogs (Figure 15). Thus, some biphasic waveforms have a markedly lower defibrillation threshold than some monophasic waveforms, yet the biphasic waveforms are less able to stimulate a new action potential or cause action potential prolongation than the monophasic waveforms.

Shock Polarity

While most studies consistently report that the polarity of the shock for internal defibrillation with a monophasic waveform significantly influences the defibrillation waveform,[26–29] there are conflicting reports about whether polarity also significantly influences the defibrillation thresholds of biphasic waveforms.[30–35] The results from one of these studies is illustrated in Figure 16.[34] Defibrillation thresholds were determined for a 6-ms truncated exponential mo-

nophasic waveform and a 6–4 ms truncated exponential biphasic waveform in six pigs. As has been true in almost all studies, the defibrillation threshold for the monophasic waveform was significantly lower when the right ventricular catheter electrode was an anode than when it was a cathode (Figure 16C). However, for the biphasic waveform, polarity did not significantly affect the defibrillation threshold.

Those studies that have reported that polarity influences defibrillation efficacy for biphasic waveforms have found that the defibrillation threshold is lower when the first phase polarity is anodal to the right ventricular electrode.[30,31] No study has yet reported that a cathodal polarity in the right ventricular electrode for a biphasic waveform is uniformly better than an anodal polarity. Therefore, since some of the studies report that polarity makes no difference while the other studies report that an anodal first phase is superior, the prudent choice is to use an anodal first phase polarity to the right ventricular electrode for biphasic

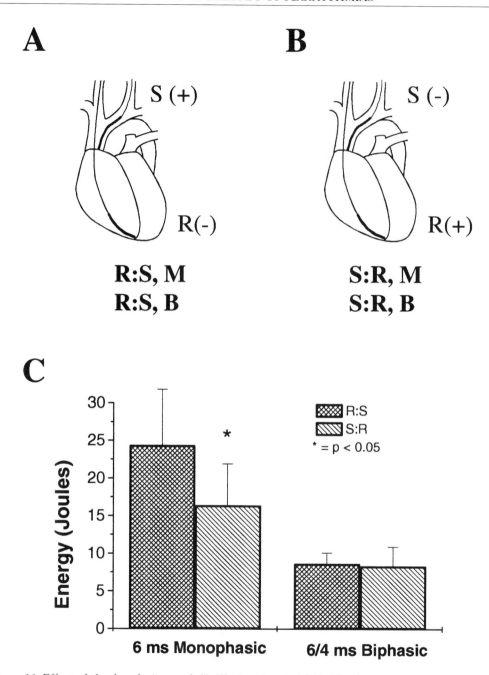

Figure 16. Effect of shock polarity on defibrillation threshold. Defibrillation catheters were placed in the right ventricular apex (R) and at the junction of the superior vena cava and right atrium (S) of six pigs. Four configurations were tested: R cathode (−) to S anode (+), monophasic waveform (R:S, M) (panel **A**); S(−) to R (+), monophasic waveform (R:S, M) (panel **B**); R first phase (−) to S first phase (−), biphasic waveform (R:S, B) (panel **A**); S first phase (+), biphasic waveform (S:R, B) (panel **B**). Mean ± standard deviation of defibrillation threshold energies are shown in panel **C**. For monophasic shocks, the polarity reversal of the RV electrode from cathode to anode caused a significant decrease in voltage. For biphasic shocks, threshold energy was significantly lower than for monophasic shocks. However, polarity reversal of the RV electrode from first phase cathode to first phase anode did not significantly affect defibrillation efficacy. Used and modified with permission from Usui M, et al.[34]

shocks as long as there is no detrimental effect to the patient. Since one of the two polarities must be used at the right ventricular electrode, the polarity used might as well be the one that some studies report as better, even if both polarities actually are equally efficacious.

Atrial and Transthoracic Defibrillation

Biphasic waveforms have been shown to be superior for atrial defibrillation as well as for ventricular defibrillation.[36-38] As shown in Figure 17, in six patients a 3–3 ms

A

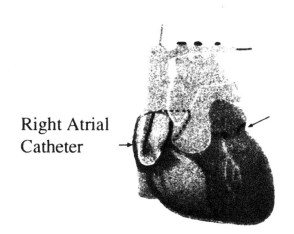

Right Atrial Catheter

Coronary Sinus Catheter Under Left Atrial Appendage

B

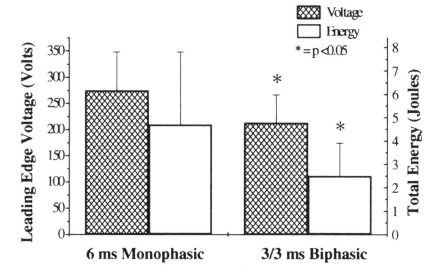

Figure 17. Defibrillation catheters were placed in the right atrium and coronary sinus in six patients (panel **A**). For a 3–3 ms biphasic shock, which was equal in total duration with a 6-ms monophasic shock, atrial defibrillation threshold voltage and energy were both significantly lower than for the monophasic shock (panel **B**). Mean ± standard deviation is shown. Used and modified with permission from Johnson EE, et al.[38]

biphasic waveform had a lower defibrillation threshold, in terms of both energy and voltage, than did a 6-ms monophasic waveform. Recent results also indicate that a truncated exponential biphasic waveform is superior to an Edmark monophasic waveform for external ventricular defibrillation.[39] Thus, the biphasic waveform appears to be more efficacious for defibrillation than the monophasic waveform for internal as well as external defibrillation and for ventricular as well as atrial defibrillation.

Triphasic Waveforms

It remains to be seen if a better waveform than the biphasic waveform can be developed for defibrillation. For example, even though the initial reports about the triphasic waveform reported that it was not as efficacious as a biphasic waveform for defibrillation,[6,40–42] a recent study has reported that one type of triphasic waveform has a slightly lower defibrillation threshold than does a standard biphasic waveform.[43]

References

1. Schuder JC, Rahmoeller GA, Stoeckle H. Transthoracic ventricular defibrillation with triangular and trapezoidal waveforms. Circ Res 1966;19:689–694.
2. Schuder JC, Stoeckle H, Keskar PY, et al. Transthoracic ventricular defibrillation in the dog with unidirectional rectangular double pulses. Cardiovasc Res 1970;4:497–501.
3. Tacker WA Jr, Geddes LA. The automatic implantable defibrillator (AID). In Electrical Defibrillation. Boca Raton, Florida, CRC Press, Inc., 1980, pp 167–178.
4. Walcott GP, Walker RG, Cates AW, et al. Choosing the optimal monophasic and biphasic waveforms for ventricular defibrillation. J Cardiovasc Electrophysiol 1995;6: 737–750.
5. Wessale JL, Boulard JD, Tacker WA Jr, et al. Bipolar catheter defibrillation in dogs using trapezoidal waveforms of various tilts. J Electrocardiol 1980;13:359–366.
6. Dixon EG, Tang ASL, Wolf PD, et al. Improved defibrillation thresholds with large contoured epicardial electrodes and biphasic waveforms. Circulation 1987;76:1176–1184.
7. Swerdlow CD, Fan W, Brewer JE. Charge-burping theory correctly predicts optimal ratios of phase duration for biphasic defibrillation waveforms. Circulation 1996;94: 2278–2284.
8. Feeser SA, Tang ASL, Kavanagh KM, et al. Strength-duration and probability of success curves for defibrillation with biphasic waveforms. Circulation 1990;82:2128–2141.
9. Kroll MW. A minimal model of the monophasic defibrillation pulse. PACE 1993;16: 769–777.
10. Kroll MW. A minimal model of the single capacitor biphasic defibrillation waveform. PACE 1994;17:1782–1792.
11. Tang ASL, Yabe S, Wharton JM, et al. Ventricular defibrillation using biphasic waveforms: the importance of phasic duration. J Am Coll Cardiol 1989;13:207–214.
12. Chen P-S, Wolf PD, Claydon FJ III, et al. The potential gradient field created by epicardial defibrillation electrodes in dogs. Circulation 1986;74:626–636.
13. Frazier DW, Krassowska W, Chen P-S, et al. Extracellular field required for excitation in three-dimensional anisotropic canine myocardium. Circ Res 1988;63:147–164.
14. Krassowska W, Frazier DW, Pilkington TC, et al. Potential distribution in three-dimensional periodic myocardium: Part II. Application to extracellular stimulation. IEEE Trans Biomed Eng 1990;37:267–284.
15. Lepeschkin E, Jones JL, Rush S, et al. Local potential gradients as a unifying measure for thresholds of stimulation, standstill, tachyarrhythmia and fibrillation appearing after strong capacitor discharges. Adv Cardiol 1978;21:268–278.
16. Wharton JM, Rollins DL, Smith WM, et al. Potential gradients generated by defibrillation shocks in humans. Circulation 1989;80: II–44.
17. Witkowski FX, Penkoske PA, Plonsey R. Mechanism of cardiac defibrillation in open-chest dogs with unipolar DC-coupled simultaneous activation and shock potential recordings. Circulation 1990;82:244–260.
18. Yabe S, Smith WM, Daubert JP, et al. Conduction disturbances caused by high current density electric fields. Circ Res 1990;66: 1190–1203.
19. Wharton JM, Wolf PD, Smith WM, et al. Cardiac potential and potential gradient fields generated by single, combined, and sequential shocks during ventricular defibrillation. Circulation 1992;85:1510–1523.

20. Zhou X, Daubert JP, Wolf PD, et al. Epicardial mapping of ventricular defibrillation with monophasic and biphasic shocks in dogs. Circ Res 1993;72:145–160.

21. Daubert JP, Frazier DW, Wolf PD, et al. Response of relatively refractory canine myocardium to monophasic and biphasic shocks. Circulation 1991;84:2522–2538.

22. Zhou X, Wolf PD, Rollins DL, et al. Effects of monophasic and biphasic shocks on action potentials during ventricular fibrillation in dogs. Circ Res 1993;73:325–334.

23. Zhou X, Knisley SB, Wolf PD, et al. Prolongation of repolarization time by electric field stimulation with monophasic and biphasic shocks in open chest dogs. Circ Res 1991;68:1761–1767.

24. Dillon SM. Synchronized repolarization after defibrillation shocks: a possible component of the defibrillation process demonstrated by optical recordings in rabbit heart. Circulation 1992;85:1865–1878.

25. Kwaku KF, Dillon SM. Shock-induced depolarization of refractory myocardium prevents wave-front propagation in defibrillation. Circ Res 1996;79:957–973.

26. Schuder JC, Stoeckle H, McDaniel WC, et al. Is the effectiveness of cardiac ventricular defibrillation dependent upon polarity? Med Instrum 1987;21:262–265.

27. Strickberger SA, Hummel JD, Horwood LE, et al. Effect of shock polarity on ventricular defibrillation threshold using a transveous lead system. J Am Coll Cardiol 1994;24:1069–1072.

28. Bardy GH, Ivey TD, Allen MD, et al. Evaluation of electrode polarity on defibrillation efficacy. Am J Cardiol 1989;63:433–437.

29. O'Neill PG, Boahene KA, Lawrie GM, et al. The automatic implantable cardioverter-defibrillator: effect of patch polarity on defibrillation threshold. J Am Coll Cardiol 1991;17:707–711.

30. Natale A, Sra J, Dhala A, et al. Effects of initial polarity on defibrillation threshold with biphasic pulses. PACE 1995;18:1889–1893.

31. Thakur R, Souza J, Chapman P, et al. Electrode polarity is an important determinant of defibrillation efficacy using a nonthoracotomy system. PACE 1994;17:919–923.

32. Strickberger SA, Man KC, Daoud E, et al. Effect of first-phase polarity of biphasic shocks on defibrillation threshold with a single transvenous lead system. J Am Coll Cardiol 1995;25:1605–1608.

33. Block M, Hammel D, Böcker D, et al. Transvenous-subcutaneous defibrillation leads: effect of transvenous electrode polarity on defibrillation threshold. J Cardiovasc Electrophysiol 1994;5:912–918.

34. Usui M, Walcott GP, Strickberger SA, et al. Effects of polarity for monophasic and biphasic shocks on defibrillation efficacy with an endocardial system. PACE 1996;19:65–71.

35. Huang J, KenKnight BH, Walcott GP, et al. Effect of electrode polarity on internal defibrillation with monophasic and biphasic waveforms using an endocardial lead system. J Cardiovasc Electrophysiol 1997;8:161–171.

36. Cooper RAS, Alferness CA, Smith WM, et al. Internal cardioversion of atrial fibrillation in sheep. Circulation 1993;87:1673–1686.

37. Keane D, Boyd E, Anderson D, et al. Comparison of biphasic and monophasic waveforms in epicardial atrial defibrillation. J Am Coll Cardiol 1994;24:171–176.

38. Johnson EE, Yarger MD, Wharton JM. Monophasic and biphasic waveforms for low energy internal cardioversion of atrial fibrillation in humans. Circulation 1993;88:I-592.

39. Walcott GP, Hagler JA, Walker RG, et al. Comparison of monophasic, biphasic, and the Edmark waveform for external defibrillation. PACE 1992;15:563A.

40. Manz M, Jung W, Wolpert C, et al. Can triphasic shock waveforms improve ICD therapy in man? Circulation 1993;88:I-593.

41. Jung W, Manz M, Moosdorf R, et al. Comparative defibrillation efficacy of biphasic and triphasic waveforms. New Trends Arrhyth 1993;9:765A.

42. Chapman PD, Wetherbee JN, Vetter JW, et al. Comparison of monophasic, biphasic, and triphasic truncated pulses for non-thoracotomy internal defibrillation. J Am Coll Cardiol 1988;11:57A.

43. Huang J, KenKnight BH, Rollins DL, et al. Defibrillation with triphasic waveforms. PACE 1997;20:1056A.

Chapter 17

Dual Chamber Sensing and Detection for Implantable Cardioverter-Defibrillators

Walter H. Olson

Introduction

Dual chamber implantable cardioverter-defibrillators (ICDs) use DDD/R pacing to improve hemodynamics and dual chamber detection algorithms to reduce inappropriate ventricular therapy for supraventricular tachyarrhythmias (SVTs). Inappropriate detection of SVTs by ventricular rate-only algorithms during clinical ICD studies has ranged from 20% to 41%.[1] Inappropriate ATP and shock therapy resulting from these inappropriate detections can be proarrhythmic. Painful inappropriate shocks are frequently repetitive and may result in adverse psychological consequences.[2,3]

Dual chamber ICDs add an atrial lead or at least atrial electrodes on a single pass lead that will undoubtedly increase lead complications. For single chamber ventricular transvenous ICD leads, complications have averaged 6.8% for 13.6 months in 2,152 patients.[4] Implantation of both a single chamber ventricular ICD and a dual chamber pacemaker has been common despite the need to test for device interaction and the number of leads required.[5,6] In part, this has been done to avoid reducing the longevity of the ICD when extensive pacing is needed. The high incidence of heart failure in ICD patients makes the benefits of maintaining atrioventricular (AV) synchrony important.

Sensing of intrinsic atrial and ventricular depolarizations by intracardiac electrodes is the first step in tachyarrhythmia recognition and is also important for inhibition of the pacemaker stimuli.[7] The atrial and ventricular electrogram signals from the leads are processed to determine only the time when the P and R depolarizations occur so they can be compared to the time of other sensed or paced events in both the atrium and the ventricle.

Detection is the process of analyzing the timing of recent atrial and ventricular events to identify sustained tachyarrhythmias that require automatic electrical therapy.[7] This detection of tachyarrhythmias is done by computer algorithms that analyze recent data after every ventricular event. Four ventricular rate-only algorithms were compared using 482 episodes of atrial fibrillation (AF) and 260 episodes of ventricular tachycardia (VT).[8] The algorithm with the best specificity for the VT zone used consecutive counting requiring all R-R intervals to be less than the VT detection interval, even after lengthening this programmable detection interval to maintain sensitivity. To conserve energy, the algorithms may not fully

From Singer I, Barold SS, Camm AJ (eds): Nonpharmacological Therapy of Arrhythmias for the 21st Century: The State of the Art. Futura Publishing Co, Inc., Armonk, NY, © 1998.

analyze the rhythm when the ventricular rate is low.

Dual chamber tachyarrhythmia episodes have the same basic components as single chamber episodes including initial detection, the first therapy preceded by confirmation and synchronization, redetection if therapy is unsuccessful, subsequent therapy, and episode termination after the tachyarrhythmia ends. Stored episode data may include both atrial and ventricular stored electrograms, dual chamber event markers describing all sensed and paced events in both the atrium and the ventricle. Additional messages on the recordings describe progress toward detection or why detection has not occurred. Time intervals, such as P-P, and R-R can be plotted on a vertical cycle length scale for a series of events to illustrate a cardiac rhythm.

When VT detection and therapy were added to basic ventricular defibrillators, concern was expressed that survival from sudden death might be adversely affected by the added complexity. Three large clinical studies with these tiered therapy defibrillators have shown that the complexity did not adversely affect survival.[9] Similarly, concern has been expressed that the added complexity of dual chamber ICDs might somehow have a negative impact on survival. Several more years of dual chamber ICD experience are required to evaluate this concern.

Dual Chamber Sensing Considerations

Reliable sensing of ventricular depolarizations during ventricular fibrillation (VF) is critical to detection of this life-threatening arrhythmia. Bipolar-only ventricular sensing with sensitivities that are about 10 times more sensitive than typical pacemaker sense amplifiers is required and auto-gain control or auto-adjusting sensitivity are needed to avoid T wave oversensing, double counting, and inappropriate detection.[7] A recent direct comparison of single chamber VF sensing by the three major ICDs showed there was significantly less undersensing during VF and less delayed detection by the MicroJewel II™ compared to the Mini II™ and again significantly less undersensing and delayed detection by the Mini II compared to the Cadet™.[10] By personal communication, the authors found these differences to be sustained for a larger series of VF recordings from 47 patients. Time to detection of VF by the dual chamber Ventak AV™ when pacing DDD at 150 bpm was not statistically different when compared to the single chamber Mini™ ICD when pacing VVI at 100 bpm.[11] This comparison showed that the VF detection was not affected by the additional ventricular blanking periods after the ventricular pacing at the higher rate and the additional ventricular blanking after atrial paced events needed to avoid crosstalk in the dual chamber system.

Atrial electrograms have been studied for dual chamber pacing systems. Reliable sensing of AF is not required for bradycardia pacemakers and in fact is undesired to minimize tracking the high atrial rates with high-rate ventricular pacing. The frequency spectra of unipolar and bipolar atrial electrograms have most of the energy in the range from 10–50 Hz.[12,13] Dual chamber defibrillators must sense AF reliably to avoid inappropriate detection of ventricular tachyarrhythmias. Atrial electrograms during AF may be more difficult to sense than VF because atrial electrograms are generally smaller than ventricular electrograms. For bipolar atrial electrograms from the right atrial appendage, Kerr and Mason[14] found in 11 patients that mean peak-to-peak electrogram amplitude in sinus rhythm was 2.6 ± 1.0 mV and not significantly less, 2.3 ± 1.3 mV, during paroxysmal AF. Mean minimum values were 2.0 ± 0.8 mV in sinus rhythm and 1.4 ± 1.1 mV during AF. The smallest value for AF was 0.7 mV. Lower values were found for 25 patients in a more recent study[15] (1.59 ± 1.36 mV sinus vs. 0.77 ± 0.58 mV for AF), however, the proximal pair of quadripolar leads (probably noncontacting) were used and frequencies below 30 Hz were filtered out. Reliable sensing of AF electrograms from 17 patients with acute bipolar electrodes was demonstrated with 0.3-mV sensitivity for 99% of the atrial depolarizations.[16] Only very low-amplitude chronic AF was undersensed, and median atrial cycle lengths were still less than 240 ms. It has been reported that atrial electrogram amplitude decreased by 31% after the onset of induced VF.[17]

Chronic sensing of induced AF in five canines with rate detection required canine specific sensing thresholds set to 10%, 20%, or 30% of the peak amplitude for each recording to achieve 100% sensitivity and at least 95% specificity for detection of AF.[18] No absolute electrogram amplitudes were reported. Sensing and detection of AF in 80 patients during follow-up after implantation of the Jewel AF™ dual chamber ICD was reliable for 109 episodes of induced AF.[19] For 13 patients with programmed sensitivity of 0.4 ± 0.2 mV, 222 of 246 (90%) device detections were appropriate and none of the 222 episodes were prematurely terminated due to atrial undersensing. Device memory recorded 53 episodes greater than 1 hour for a total of 1,290 hours of continuous AF detection.

Oversensing of farfield R waves by the atrial sensing system is avoided in dual chamber pacemakers by postventricular atrial blanking and refractory periods. This must be minimized in a tachyarrhythmia device because the atrial rhythm needs to be sensed reliably during high ventricular rates. Large atrial blanking periods would preclude sensing of most atrial rhythms, especially atrial tachycardias. As bipolar electrode spacing decreases, the size of the farfield R wave relative to the local P waves decreases. Farfield R waves recorded from bipolar atrial leads in 22 patients had peak-to-peak amplitudes that averaged about one-tenth of the P wave amplitude (0.35 ± 0.32 mV vs. 3.28 ± 1.09 mV) and these farfield R waves had slew rates that were one-twentieth of the P waves (0.019 ± 0.017 V/sec vs. 0.53 ± 0.31 V/sec).[20] The unipolar far-

field R waves were four times as large. Two of 17 patients studied had consistent sensing of farfield R waves.[16]

Dual Chamber Pacing in ICDs

Only about 10% of patients indicated for ventricular ICD implantation also have bradycardia that would meet current pacemaker indications. Most ICD patients have the VVI lower rate programmed to 40–50 bpm to avoid unnecessary pacing that may be proarrhythmic in these patients. Combined transvenous implantation of ventricular ICDs and dual chamber pacemakers with separate leads and extensive testing for adverse device-device interactions have been reported. These interactions may give insight into issues for the design of dual chamber ICDs. Fifteen combined implants with integrated bipolar ICD leads (8.2%) were tested and in two patients VF was underdetected due to inappropriate sensing of the pacemaker spikes, three patients had double counting of pacemaker spikes and R waves, and in two patients, pacemaker function was altered after shocks.[5] These problems seen only during implant testing could be eliminated in almost all patients by changing a lead position and programmed device parameters. Another series of 10 combined implants with true bipolar ICD leads (5.3%) and similar testing showed one patient with unipolar ventricular pacing that was sensed by the ICD and required implantation of a bipolar lead, no double counting was observed, and a transient mode change previously described was the only shock effect seen.[6] These combined implants of an ICD and a pacemaker in patients are possible, although the extensive testing for adverse device interactions and the need for at least three leads with special positioning requirements has limited the wide utilization of these combinations in routine clinical practice.

These interactions do indicate some of the requirements for a single device that combines dual chamber pacing with an ICD. Sense amplifier blanking during pacemaker spikes in the opposite chamber is important to avoid oversensing. The ventricular post-pace blanking and the ventricular blanking after atrial pacing spikes should be minimized to allow adequate sensing of ventricular tachyarrhythmias that begin during paced rhythms particularly at the pacemaker upper rate limit. The dual chamber pacing function must not be affected by shocks that may transiently alter the sensing of electrograms in either chamber and shocks may increase pacing thresholds in either chamber. The ICD functions need to operate in all available pacing modes without double counting in either chamber. Automatic mode switching to avoid tracking of atrial tachyarrhythmias should not adversely interact with dual chamber tachyarrhythmia detection.

Timing of Atrial and Ventricular Depolarizations During Ventricular Tachycardia

The ventricular rate during VT is defined as greater than 100 bpm and less than 300 bpm. The beat-to-beat variability for monomorphic sustained VT is usually less than 20–40 ms.[21] The rate of VT or VF may gradually decrease over time particularly with ischemia.[22]

Atrioventricular dissociation, if present is diagnostic for VT. If the ventricular rate is greater than the atrial rate, then VT is present unless a double tachycardia is occurring. During VT, if retrograde conduction to the atrium is present, it may be 1:1, 2:1, or retrograde Wenckebach. Classic studies in supine sedated electrophysiology lab patients showed up to one-third of patients had 1:1 retrograde conduction, but for relatively slow VT. Recently, in 66 ICD patients, 40 had inducible sustained monomorphic VT and occasional ventriculoatrial (VA) conduction was observed in five patients, one patient had 2:1 retrograde conduction,

and no patient had 1:1 retrograde conduction.[23] A larger study with 305 ICD patients had 161 patients with sustained monomorphic VT (cycle length [CL] = 304 ± 61 ms) and 4.4% of these patients with VT had 1:1 retrograde conduction during the VT (median CL = 370, range 280–470 ms).[24] Another study with 105 EP patients had 17 episodes of 1:1 VA conduction during induced VT.[25] Unpublished data from Miller[26] for 388 VTs from 154 patients showed 81% PR dissociation, 5.6% atrial tachyarrhythmia, 3% VA Wenckebach, 5.4% 2:1 Wenckebach, leaving only 4.6% with 1:1 VA conduction.

Dual Chamber Algorithm Concepts

The first algorithm for comparing atrial and ventricular events to discriminate VT versus SVT for most tachyarrhythmias was published in 1979.[27–29] The P-P, P-R, R-P, and R-R intervals were buffered and analyzed by comparing 36 recent atrial and ventricular events. If #R>#P, then VT was diagnosed. If #P>#R, then the atrial rate was used to classify AF (>350 bpm), atrial flutter (>240 and <330 bpm), or atrial tachycardia (<240 bpm). For the 1:1 tachycardias, sudden onset was used for paroxysmal 1:1 tachycardias and if onset was not sudden, then sinus tachycardia was declared. In tests, this algorithm misclassified only one of 22 rhythms as VT because there was retrograde conduction for seven of eight beats.

For another algorithm that used simple VT criterion early after onset of VT and P-R interval tracking, only one of 30 VT episodes tested was underdetected due to concurrent atrial flutter.[30] For differentiating 1:1 tachycardias, a premature atrial extrastimulus delivered 80–120 ms early, failed to alter the R-R intervals by more than 10 ms in 22 VTs, but advanced the ventricular response for SVTs.[31,32] Later, a similar algorithm combined with dual chamber timing[33] was tested on 66 rhythm passages and the only errors described were three slow and regular responses to AFs that were misclassified as atrial flutter. For SVTs, this extrastimulus method may fail if the antegrade premature conduction is too early and blocks at the AV node. It may also fail for slow VT if ventricular capture occurs. Such atrial extrastimuli may be proarrhythmic in either the atrium or the ventricle. Correlation waveform analysis successfully discriminated antegrade from retrograde atrial depolarization waveshapes for 1:1 tachycardias, but required 19 patient-specific thresholds.[34] A special atrial lead with orthogonal electrodes was able to discriminate antegrade from retrograde atrial conduction in all 18 patients studied.[35]

Research studies describe dual chamber detection algorithms that use P and R timing and morphology information in both chambers.[36] A cycle-by-cycle coding system that classified morphology as normal or abnormal and P-P, P-R, and R-R intervals as short, normal, or long was combined with prioritized contextual analysis to detect 34 of 36 rhythm passages correctly. Errors were caused by incorrect associations between atrial and subsequent ventricular events. A similar algorithm was tested on 28 passages of SVT and VT with 99.5% accuracy.[37] A different dual chamber morphology and timing intracardiac classifier (MATIC)[38] used a neural network morphology classifier and a decision tree for timing analysis. This algorithm achieved 99.6% accuracy on a database of 12,483 R waves from 67 patients compared to 75.9% accuracy for the single chamber Guardian ATP 4210® device tested on the same database. A dual chamber detection algorithm was described[39] that used only timing of atrial and ventricular events, a P-R interval ratio and P-R delay creep. A multiway sequential hypothesis testing algorithm calculated a likelihood function from P-R intervals as they were received.[40] For this algorithm, the time to detection can be traded off with the desired accuracy. During testing this algorithm accurately classified 26 of 28 sinus rhythm passages (two called SVT), 31 of 31

passages of SVT, and 41 of 43 passages of VT (two were called sinus).

P-R Logic™ Pattern and Rate Analysis—Gem DR™

The dual chamber detection algorithm in Medtronic dual chamber ICDs utilizes several basic design principles. The high sensitivity of the Jewel™ family of ICDs with ventricular rate-only detection was retained as the underlying basic detection algorithm. Only if dual chamber data can positively identify a particular type of SVT, should this algorithm withhold detection for rhythms with ventricular rates in the VT or VF zones. This design principle is critical to improving specificity of detection without compromising detection sensitivity for life-threatening ventricular tachyarrhythmias. Furthermore, the algorithm must assure prompt detection of VT or VF during ongoing SVT such as AF that may cause the atrial rate to remain above the ventricular rate even after the onset of VT or VF. The algorithm should use at least several beats of the rhythm to make decisions to minimize the effects of undersensing or oversensing in either the atrial or the ventricular channel and to avoid the uncertainty of the onset rhythm which may initially be supraventricular. The physician programmable parameters should be minimal and clinically relevant.

A dual chamber detection algorithm that uses syntactic pattern recognition and contextual timing analysis for rhythm classification was first described in 1995.[41] Atrial and ventricular event pattern and timing for a series of cardiac cycles are used to overrule ventricular rate detection only when specific supraventricular tachyarrhythmias are positively identified.[42]

The pattern analysis, illustrated in Figure 1, analyzes the two previous R-R intervals for each ventricular event. The number of atrial events and their timing relative to the ventricular events are used to assign one of 19 couple codes to the most recent ventricular event (letters A-Q, Y, and Z). Zero, one,

COUPLE CODE SYNTAX ANALYSIS

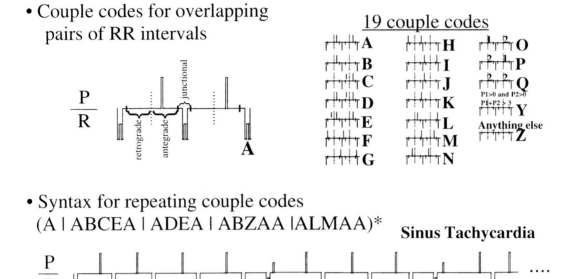

- Couple codes for overlapping pairs of RR intervals

19 couple codes

- Syntax for repeating couple codes
  (A I ABCEA I ADEA I ABZAA IALMAA)*

Sinus Tachycardia

Figure 1. Pattern analysis for P-R logic dual chamber ventricular tachyarrhythmia detection algorithm. For the last two R-R intervals the number and timing of P waves are used to classify the current R wave as one of 19 couple codes represented by the letters of the alphabet shown. P waves may be in the junctional zone from 80 ms before the R wave to 50 ms after the R wave, the antegrade zone from 50% of R-R interval to 80 ms before the R wave, or the retrograde zone from 50 ms after the R wave to 50% of R-R. Pure sinus tachycardia is AAAAA--. Sinus tachycardia is permitted to deviate from pure sinus tachycardia by the syntactic strings of letters such as ABCEA which is one representation for a preventricular contraction as shown on the Marker Channel™ rhythm at the bottom.

two, or more atrial events for each R-R interval are classified within the first half or second half of each R-R interval. If a P wave is within 80 ms before a ventricular event or within 50 ms after a ventricular event, then that P wave should not be related to the ventricular event by either antegrade or retrograde conduction. As the R-R intervals vary, the P-P intervals, P-R intervals, and R-P intervals may or may not change. Note that each R-R interval and its P wave(s) are used twice, first as the most recent R-R interval for one couple code, and then the same R-R interval and its P wave(s) are used again as the second most recent R-R interval for the next couple code. Any cardiac rhythm generates a series of couple code letters as shown for sinus tachycardia at the bottom

of Figure 1. This string of letters is compared to sequences of letters known to occur during sinus tachycardia such as AAA, ABCEA, ADEA, ABZAA, or ALMAA. The pattern ABCEA is typical for a PVC in sinus tachycardia as shown for the rhythm at the bottom of Figure 1. The pattern matching is continuous and analogous to a word processing spelling checker. The sinus tachycardia syntax patterns for sinus tachycardia are like "words" in a spelling checker dictionary. The unknown rhythm being classified is like the stream of new text being evaluated by the spelling checker. Sinus tachycardia is no longer recognized if the string of letters no longer matches the sinus tachycardia patterns and is analogous to the spelling checker stopping for an unknown word. When the pattern is no longer matched, the algorithm does not immediately stop recognizing the SVT for a number of beats to avoid inappropriate detection of VT during the transition between different SVTs. In this way an SVT rhythm must be positively identified almost continuously to withhold VT/VF detection when the ventricular rate is in the VT or VF zones. There are patterns for three groups of SVTs: sinus tachycardia, atrial flutter/fibrillation, and other 1:1 SVTs such as AV nodal tachycardia. The use of these three groups of patterns are independently programmable ON or OFF by the physician. Also, there is a programmable minimum SVT cycle length below which the dual chamber algorithm is not used and ventricular rate-only algorithms apply.

Several new timing measurements are also used by the algorithm to determine the rates in each chamber, a measure of variability, and a measure of P-R dissociation. The median P-P interval and the median R-R interval for the last 12 respective intervals are updated after each ventricular event. The median statistic is not as sensitive to limited undersensing or oversensing as the mean value or other statistics. A new measure of cycle length variability called the modesum is used in several ways. The R-R modesum analyzes the last 18 R-R intervals by putting them into a histogram with 10 ms bins and comparing the sum of the number of intervals in the two largest bins to the total number of intervals. The higher this percentage, the more regular the rhythm. For an irregular rhythm such as the ventricular response to AF or VF, the modesum percentage is low. This measure can tolerate moderate undersensing or oversensing.

A timing measurement of P-R dissociation compares a recent series of P-R intervals. The mean of the most recent eight P-R intervals is computed. An individual P-R interval is judged dissociated if its absolute difference from the average is greater than 40 ms. A rhythm is considered dissociated if at least four of the last eight P-R intervals are dissociated. This algorithm has been tested on a large database of human rhythms and can quickly recognize P-R dissociation.

There are several types of rhythm counters, one for VF, another for VT and a third for AF. The VF rhythm counter nominally requires that 18 of the last 24 R-R intervals be less than the fibrillation detection interval (FDI). This counter is very sensitive to assure rapid detection of VF even if some undersensing occurs. The VT counter nominally requires 16 consecutive R-R intervals be less than the longer tachycardia detection interval (TDI). This counter is much more specific because sensing of VT is rarely a problem and rejection of variable atrial fibrillatory rhythms is important.[8] An up-down atrial evidence counter is used to evaluate atrial tachyarrhythmias. When there are two or more atrial events during an R-R interval, the counter increases by 1. If the previous R-R interval had two or more atrial events, but the most recent R-R interval has 0 or 1 atrial event, then the counter is unchanged. Finally, if both the previous and the current R-R intervals have zero or one atrial events, then the counter counts down by one. This counter cannot be less than zero or greater than 47 and it is used to indicate accumulated evidence for AF because the P and R relationships during AF do not have reliable pattern information.

Possible oversensing of farfield R waves as P waves on the atrial channel is more likely for dual chamber defibrillators than for dual chamber pacemakers because of differences in blanking periods. An algorithm for correctly classifying farfield R waves during sinus tachycardia utilizes consistent alternation of P-P intervals (>30 ms), low R-P interval variability (<50 ms), and consistent R-P intervals (<20 ms from the average R-P). For every R-R interval there must be exactly two atrial events. The consistent alternation of P-P intervals is needed to avoid misclassifying the rhythm as 2:1 atrial flutter. One of the P waves must be close to the R waves (P-R <60 ms or R-P <160 ms). These criteria must be met for 10 of the last 12 R-R intervals to reject P events as farfield R waves.

These building blocks of P and R event pattern analysis and timing analysis are combined to detect and treat ventricular tachyarrhythmias in the Model 7271 Gem DR ICD as shown in Figure 2. All three SVT rejection criteria (ST, AF, other 1:1 SVT) are programmed ON and nominal parameters are used. Then R-R, P-P, R-P, and P-R data are analyzed after each R wave is sensed. If the single chamber Jewel or MicroJewel R-R rate detection criteria for VF/VT/FVT are not met, there is no detection. If R-R rate detection occurs, and the median R-R interval is less than the programmable SVT minimum R-R interval, then VT or VF detection occurs based on fast ventricular rate alone. If not, the possibility of double tachyarrhythmias in both chambers is assessed and if found, then VT or VF is detected. Only then do the atrial fibrillation/atrial flutter, sinus tachycardia, and other 1:1 SVT criteria have the opportunity to withhold detection and therapy if they positively identify an SVT. If none of these SVTs are positively identified, then for safety, VT or VF must be detected.

An example of sinus tachycardia in the VT zone that would have resulted in inappropriate therapy in a single chamber ICD is shown in Figure 3 for the Gem DR. The strip shows atrial and ventricular electrograms, Marker Channel™ (Medtronic Inc.) with numerical values for the P-P and R-R intervals, and a rhythm annotation showing when ventricular rate-only detection is being overruled by the dual chamber detection algorithm. The interval versus time plot shows both the atrial and ventricular cycle lengths versus time for this untreated stored episode. The ventricular events were less than the TDI and are labeled TS (Tachy Sense). On the 16th consecutive TS, VT would have been detected, however, the annotation shows an ST (first arrow) for sinus tachycardia to indicate that the sinus tachycardia rejection criteria is withholding detection. The ST annotations continue until the criteria is no longer withholding detection because one long R-R interval reset the VT counter (second arrow).

Later on the strip the R-R interval increases to values above the TDI as sinus tachycardia slows. The interval plot shows a 1:1 tachycardia in the VT zone that was neither detected nor treated (first and second arrows correspond to the arrows on the strip).

Figure 4 shows a similar strip and interval plot where rejection of atrial fibrillation/flutter prevented inappropriate detection of VT. The atrial tachyarrhythmia at the start of the strip has a 2:1 ventricular response that is in the VT zone and the AF annotations (first arrow) show that the AF rejection criteria is withholding VT detection and therapy. The conduction of AF to the ventricle changes to 3:1 and 2:1 (second arrow) so the ventricular response is no longer consistently in the VT zone and rate detection alone prevented inappropriate detection and the AF annotations stop. The interval plot shows the transition from a 2:1 to a 3:1 ventricular response (arrows again correspond to arrows on the strip). This stored SVT episode demonstrates the rejection of SVTs by the dual chamber detection algorithm.

Detection and treatment of VT with clear P-R dissociation is illustrated in Figure 5. The spontaneous onset of the VT is preceded by a late cycle PVC with the same morphology as the VT. The first TS occurred (first arrow) on the second beat into the VT after the cycle length became less than the TDI. The VT beats 3–8 were classified as VF (TF), but the next 14 beats were in the VT zone. The sum of the VT and VF counters is 21 at detection indicated by the TD (tachycardia detected) marker (second arrow). An antitachycardia pacing burst therapy is shown at the end of the strip. The interval plot shows the detected VT (arrows again correspond to arrows on the strip). The interval plot also shows the 1:1 paced rhythm progressed to VT with a 470-ms initial cycle length that could thwart onset algorithms. Cycle length variability is easily seen on the interval plot. After ATP the rhythm returns to a 1:1 AS-VP rhythm.

The last Gem DR example, shown in Figure 6, is appropriate detection of double

Medtronic GEM DR

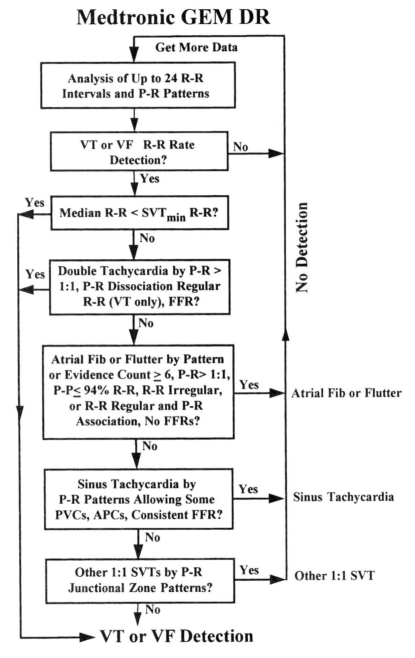

Figure 2. Block diagram for detection of VT or VF by the Gem DR dual chamber ICD. After each new R wave is sensed, at the top, analysis of the R-R, P-P, and P-R patterns and timing occurs, single chamber R-R rate detection is tested and rhythms with median R-R interval less than the programmable SVT minimum cycle length are detected without considering the dual chamber algorithm. If double tachycardia (VF/VT/FVT plus SVT) is not detected, then the three dual chamber criteria for atrial fibrillation/atrial flutter, sinus tachycardia, and other 1:1 SVTs are tested. If any one of these three SVT rhythms is recognized, then inappropriate detection is avoided. However, if none of these SVTs can be positively identified, then detection occurs to maintain high sensitivity for VT and VF detection.

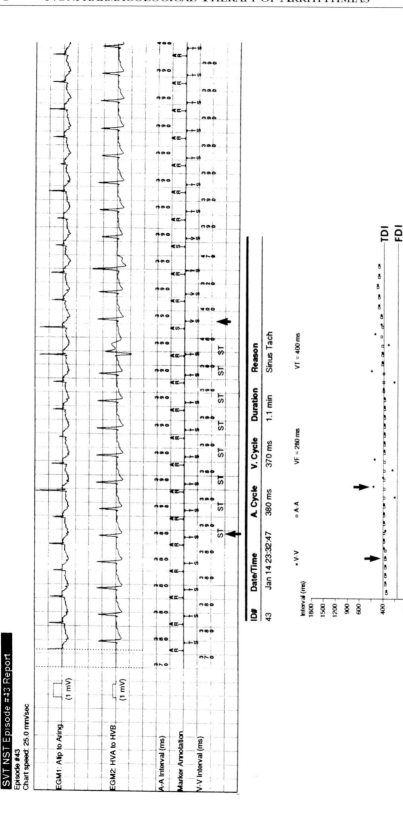

Figure 3. A stored SVT episode from the Gem DR ICD is shown for sinus tachycardia that was not detected as VT because of the sinus tachycardia (ST) dual chamber detection algorithm. The strip shows the bipolar atrial EGM, the RV coil-to-can ventricular EGM and the marker annotations including the rhythm annotations "ST," which begin at the left arrow, show when dual chamber detection is withholding therapy. The "ST" annotations end at the right arrow because the compensatory pause of 480 ms after the PVC resets the VT counter to zero and detection cannot occur again until the VT counter reaches the number of intervals for detection (NID = 16). The interval versus time graph shows the P-P and R-R intervals with a 1:1 rhythm close to the TDI = 400 ms. Arrows on the strip and plot correspond to the beginning and end of this ST episode that was not detected or treated.

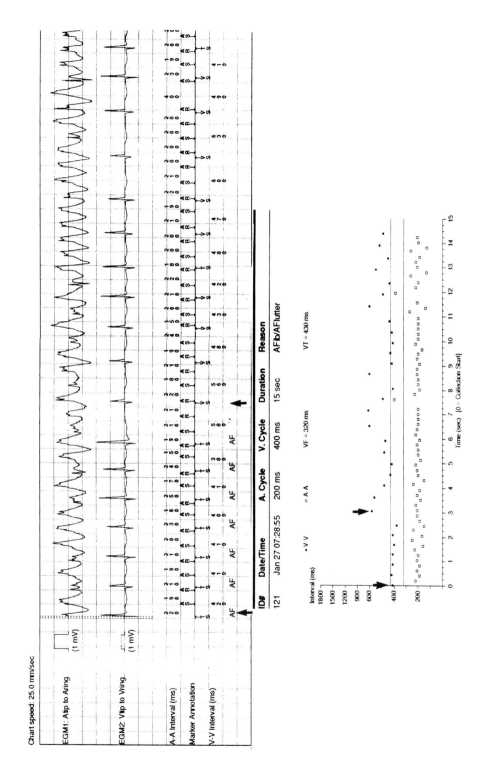

Figure 4. A stored SVT episode from the Gem DR shows dual chamber detection withholding VT therapy because AF was recognized as indicated by the rhythm annotations "AF" (left arrow). The atrial electrogram shows AF and the ventricular electrogram shows the rapid ventricular response in the VT zone less than 430 ms. The ventricular response slows at the right arrow and thereafter the regular consecutive counter for VT avoids inappropriate detection.

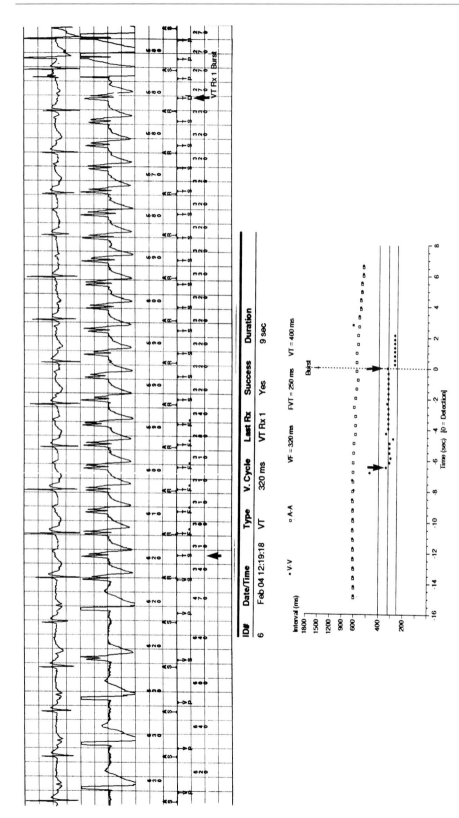

Figure 5. This stored spontaneous episode of VT with undisturbed atrial rhythm used a TDI = 400 ms. The first R-R interval of the VT was not less than the TDI so the onset of this VT was somewhat gradual and might not satisfy onset algorithms (left arrow). Six of the early beats of VT were in the VF zone (TF) and slight variability in VT cycle length seen on the interval plot is associated with morphology changes on the stored electrogram. Detection was met (TD) (right arrow) when the combined VT and VF counter reached 21 beats. Note the wide notched R waves for the VT on the RV coil-to-can ventricular electrogram.

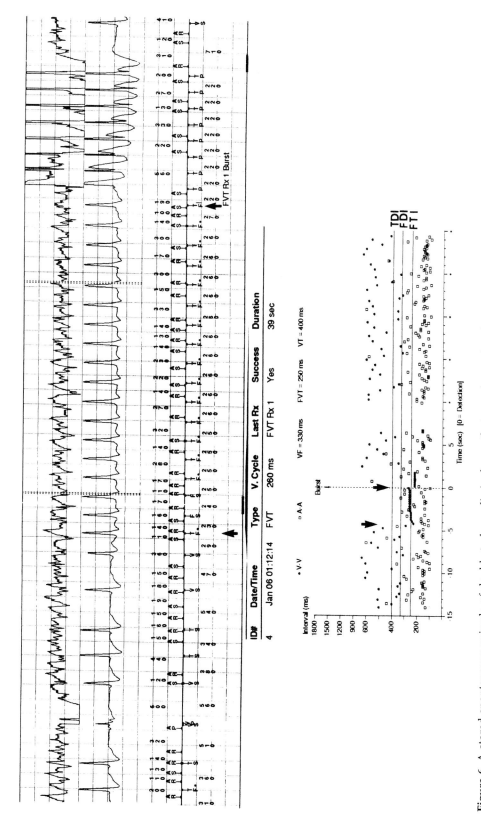

Figure 6. A stored spontaneous episode of double tachycardia is shown that was detected as fast VT (FVT) and terminated by the first sequence of burst antitachycardia pacing. Atrial fibrillation with irregular ventricular response is shown on the left side of the strip. VT begins at the left arrow and was detected after 18 beats at the second arrow. The interval plot shows the detected rhythm between the arrows and successful termination by the burst antitachycardia pacing. The gap in interval data occurred to conserve memory for stored data and was explained on the recorded strip (not shown).

tachycardia consisting of ongoing AF with rapid ventricular responses and spontaneous VT that is promptly detected and terminated with burst antitachycardia pacing. The strip shows AF on the atrial electrogram that is appropriately sensed. Many of the ventricular responses are in the VT zone, but the longer R-R intervals keep resetting the consecutive VT counter to zero. The VT begins at the first arrow and was detected as a fast VT by the dual chamber detection algorithm (second arrow) because the SVT minimum cycle length and the fast tachy interval (FTI) were both programmed to 250 ms. The burst antitachycardia pacing promptly terminated this 260 ms VT and the AF with the same ventricular response continued. The interval plot shows the same events, and the gap in interval data about 7 sec after the time of detection was required to conserve memory for this episode. The episode duration is overestimated at 39 sec because the AF with rapid ventricular response did not promptly satisfy the episode termination criteria. Note that the atrial rate exceeds the ventricular rate throughout this episode of double tachycardia.

Evaluations of the P-R logic algorithm for avoiding inappropriate detection of SVTs as VT were performed using algorithm simulations replicating device operation with prerecorded dual chamber human tachyarrhythmias.[43] Only 20% of 94 AF rhythms were inappropriately detected, 28% of 43 sinus tachycardia rhythms were inappropriately detected, and one of two AV nodal tachycardias were inappropriately detected. Therefore, the overall performance was 25% inappropriate detection compared to 100% inappropriate detection of these rhythms for a comparable ventricular rate-only algorithm.

Clinical evaluation of the P-R logic algorithm for 383 spontaneous detected episodes from 80 patients showed that by stored electrogram and dual chamber interval analysis, only 12% (47 episodes) were inappropriate.[45] This compared favorably to 29% (127 episodes) inappropriate detection for 444 spontaneous detected episodes from a group of 95 patients with comparable single chamber ICDs that use the same kind of rate-only detection (Jewel and Jewel-Plus). Follow-up was less for the dual chamber group, however, history of SVT was much higher (80% vs. 20%) than in the single chamber group. The inappropriate detections despite the dual chamber detection algorithm were caused by sinus tachycardia with first degree AV block (64%), SVT cycle length less than the programmed SVT minimum cycle length (17%), atrial sensing errors detected as P-R dissociation (13%), and AF that conducted rapidly and regularly to the ventricle resulting in inappropriate detection of double tachycardia (6%). No patients had undetected VT or VF so detection sensitivity was 100% for both patient groups.

Atrial Fibrillation Arrhythmia Management Device—Jewel AF™

The Medtronic Jewel AF™ ICD detects and treats tachyarrhythmias in either the atrium or the ventricle with different detection algorithms and different electrical therapies. Figure 7 shows a block diagram of the three major stages of detection for both ventricular and atrial tachyarrhythmias.[46] The dual chamber ventricular detection algorithm (top box, Figure 7), for avoiding inappropriate detection of SVTs as VT or VF, is the same as the ventricular tachyarrhythmia detection algorithm for the Gem DR described in the previous section. For every ventricular event, the VT and VF detection algorithm always has the highest priority. If ventricular detection does not occur, then initial detection of atrial tachyarrhythmias (lower left box) begins. The median P-P interval and the P-R pattern information are used to detect either AF or atrial flutter/tachycardia (AT). The AF and AT detection cycle length zones shown at the bottom of Figure 7 may be programmed to overlap. Atrial cycle length variability is used to discriminate between AT and AF in the overlap autodiscrimination zone. If no atrial

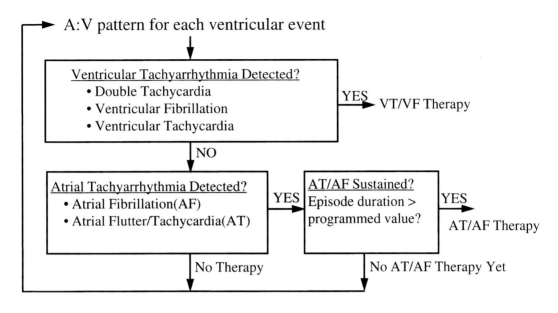

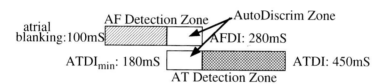

Figure 7. This diagram that explains the Jewel AF™ dual chamber detection algorithm has three major blocks. After each ventricular event, ventricular tachyarrhythmia detection (VT/VF) may result in ventricular antitachycardia pacing or shock therapy. If not, then preliminary atrial tachyarrhythmia (AT or AF), if detected, leads to sustained detection of AT or AF for the programmed duration until atrial antitachycardia pacing or shock therapy. If neither ventricular nor atrial therapy begins, then the algorithm waits for the next ventricular event and the process repeats. The lower panel shows the AF and AT detection zones that may overlap. For atrial rhythms with median P-P intervals in this overlap zone, the irregularity of the P-P intervals determines whether detection is for AT or for AF.

tachyarrhythmia is detected, then no therapy is given and the algorithm waits for more data. If either AF or AT is detected, then a slightly different algorithm is used to determine if AF or AT is sustained (lower right box) until the prescribed time duration to either AT or AF therapy has elapsed.

AF is initially detected if the median atrial cycle length is in the AF zone (100–280 ms nominal) and the AT/AF evidence counter for the P-R patterns reaches 32. The AT/AF evidence counter is an up-down counter that increases when there are two or more Ps in the R-R interval and decreases after the second R-R interval

that has only zero or one P wave. This counter is able to tolerate some undersensing of AF and is specific for greater than 1:1 tachycardias. AT is initially detected if the median atrial cycle length is in the AT zone (180–450 ms nominal) and the AT/AF evidence counter for the P-R pattern reaches 32. If the median atrial cycle length occurs in an overlap between the AF and the AT zones, then an autodiscrimination algorithm decides whether it is AF or AT based on the irregularity of recent P-P intervals. The atrial rhythm is irregular if the difference between the shortest and longest of the last 12 atrial cycle lengths is more than 25% (nominal) of the median atrial cycle length. If the atrial rhythm is irregular for at least six of the last eight ventricular events, then the rhythm is called AF, otherwise it is labeled as AT by the device. Figure 8 shows part of a sustained episode of atrial tachyarrhythmia with ECG, atrial electrogram, and Marker Channel™. On the left side of the strip the atrial electrogram is quite regular and the algorithm classified the rhythm as AT indicated by the tall triple atrial markers and the TD marker label. Just before the middle of the strip the atrial electrogram became irregular and on the right side of the strip became highly irregular with AF characteristics. At the middle of the strip the autodiscrimination algorithm changed its classification from AT to AF as indicated by the shorter triple AF markers and the FD marker label.

The preliminary detection and sustained detection stages for an AT/AF episode are shown in Figure 9. The upper panel plots the median atrial cycle length versus ventricular beat number (time) and has differ-

ent cross-hatching to show the AT and AF zones which do not overlap in this example. The middle panel shows the AT/AF evidence counter and the different thresholds for preliminary versus sustained AT/AF detection. The lower panel shows two horizontal bands depicting the true rhythm classification and the rhythm detected by the Jewel AF™. The rhythm in the first column of panels is 1:1 sinus tachycardia with no progress toward detection. During the second column of panels, preliminary detection of AF occurred as the AT/AF evidence counter rose from 0 to 32 during 58 ventricular beats, 75–133, because of some atrial undersensing. The third, fourth and fifth column of panels show sustained AT/AF detection because the AT/AF evidence counter remains between the maximum value (47), and the minimum threshold 2 (27). The median atrial cycle length remains in the AF detection zone from ventricular beats 133–201, then it crosses into the AT detection zone from ventricular beats 201–231, and returns to the AF detection zone for ventricular beats

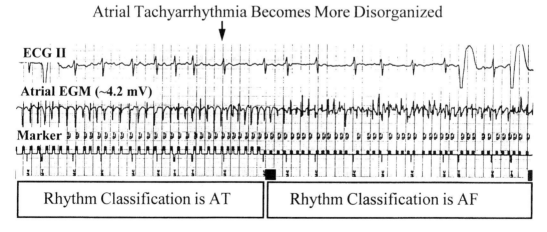

Atrial Tachyarrhythmia Becomes More Disorganized

ECG II

Atrial EGM (~4.2 mV)

Marker

Rhythm Classification is AT | Rhythm Classification is AF

Figure 8. Discrimination of AT and AF. The atrial autodiscrimination algorithm for the overlap between the AT and AF zones shown at the bottom of Figure 7 uses P-P interval irregularity to detect either AT or AF to deliver the appropriate therapy. During sustained detection time-out, the atrial rhythm classification may change as shown in the middle of the strip. Note that the atrial electrogram changes from a regular series of discrete depolarizations with an isoelectric segment on the left to a fractionated disorganized electrogram on the right. The atrial Marker Channel™ shows the rhythm classification changes from AT (large triple marker) to AF (smaller triple marker) in the middle of the strip. The irregular R-R intervals throughout the strip indicate that the flutter-like electrogram on the left may be only local to the sensing electrodes.

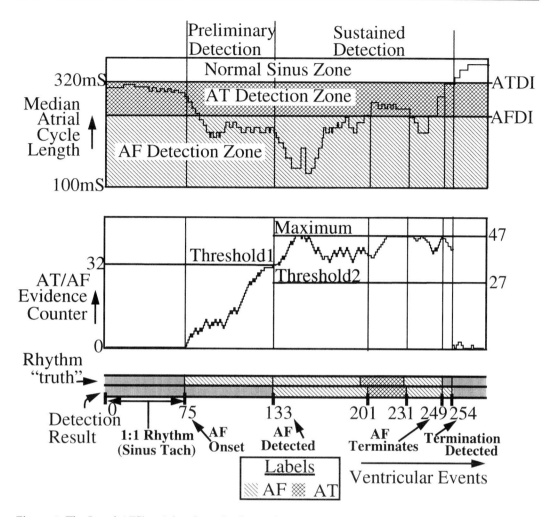

Figure 9. The Jewel AF™ atrial tachyarrhythmia detection algorithm is described in the three panels as a function of over 250 ventricular beats on the common horizontal axis. In the upper panel, the median atrial P-P interval is plotted and the nonoverlapping AT and AF detection zones are shown with different cross-hatching. The median atrial cycle length fluctuates between these two zones. Pattern information is used by the AT/AF evidence counter plotted in the middle panel with different thresholds for preliminary and sustained detection. The bottom panel shows the rhythm truth labeling on the upper band and the device detected rhythm on the lower band. The ventricular beat numbers and the AT or AF rhythm labels are shown. See text for a detailed description of the rhythm changes shown in this example.

231–249. Atrial pacing therapy could have been programmed to begin when the algorithm first detected AT (beat 201) either by atrial rate in the AT zone or by regularity in the overlap zone. In this way the Jewel AF™ may be able to opportunistically pace terminate atrial tachyarrhythmias when they are slower and/or more regular. The transition from detection of AT to AF in Figure 9 at ventricular beat 231 is the type of transition shown on the strip in Figure 8. At ventricular beat 249 the atrial tachyarrhythmia spontaneously terminated. Termination of an atrial tachyarrhythmia is detected when five consecutive ventricular intervals with one P event in the antegrade zone occur or the atrial rhythm is unclassified for 3 min. This strict criterion for detecting atrial episode termination is needed to avoid premature detection of termination during atrial undersensing of AF during sustained duration times up to 24 hours. In Figure 9 the five ventricular beats from 249 to 254 were sufficient to detect spontaneous termination of this episode of atrial tachyarrhythmia.

Figure 10 illustrates a Jewel AF™ stored episode for induced VT with an R-R median of 460 ms. Inspection of the atrial and ventricular markers shows P-R dissociation although the atrial rate is only slightly less than the ventricular rate. The stored electrogram was recorded between the atrial ring and the ventricular ring electrode and clearly shows both the P waves and the R waves in this dissociated rhythm. Some of the atrial sensed P waves are labeled as refractory senses (AR), but this pertains only to the DDD pacing mode. All the atrial and ventricular events are used by the dual chamber detection algorithm. After induction of the VT (not shown on the left), detection was resumed, with a programmer command, and VT markers (TS) begin for R-R intervals less than the tachyarrhythmia detection interval (TDI = 500 ms). VT stability was ON at 40 ms and the 480 ms ventricular beat labeled VS reset the VT counter to zero. The VT was detected 12 beats later at the last beat on the strip (TD) and a ramp ATP terminated the VT (not shown on the right).

An example of atrial tachyarrhythmia detected as atrial flutter by the Jewel AF™ is shown in Figure 11. For atrial tachyarrhythmias the stored electrogram and markers are saved just prior to atrial therapy during sustained detection which for pacing therapy in this example was programmed to 1 min after preliminary detection. The median P-P interval was 190 ms which was in the AT/AF zone overlap so the autodiscriminator determined the atrial rhythm to be very regular. The stored electrogram from atrial tip to ventricular ring shows discrete atrial depolarizations and isoelectric regions. The last two ventricular tachy sense markers (TS) on the figure are followed immediately by atrial tachycardia

markers (TD) that appear to be irregular. These markers are probably delayed by up to 40 ms by temporal competition on the telemetry channel. The actual P-P intervals used inside the device probably were more regular than they appear. The R-R intervals are irregular which may indicate that this locally sensed atrial rhythm is regular, but the global atrial rhythm may be AF.

Detection of AF by the Jewel AF™ is illustrated in Figure 12. Throughout sustained detection of AF the triple atrial markers (FD) are displayed for all atrial sensed events regardless of the P-P interval for a particular P wave. The two long P-P intervals on this strip may be due to atrial undersensing during AF. The stored electrogram was recorded from the atrial tip to ventricular ring electrode. The electrogram deflections that are associated with atrial sense markers have low amplitude and slew rate that may lead to undersensing. The R-R intervals are irregular and some are less than the TDI so they are marked as tachy senses (TS). Four attempts to terminate this atrial tachyarrhythmia with pacing (Ramp, Burst +, 50 Hz Burst, 50 Hz Burst) were all unsuccessful.

Another example of detected AF on a stored strip (Figure 13) shows that if the sustained duration is programmed to zero, then the pre-therapy strip will show preliminary atrial detection. The AF was detected with a median cycle length of 200 ms. The AF and AT detection zones overlap from 170–250 ms. In the autodiscrimination zone, prior to preliminary detection, a short-long marker symbol is used. The short double markers are in the AF only portion of the AF zone (100–170 ms.). The autodiscrimination algorithm found this atrial rhythm to be irregular so AF was detected and 50-Hz burst pacing was attempted. The stored electrogram was recorded from the atrial tip to ventricular ring electrodes and the P waves exhibit large variations in morphology suggestive of AF.

Figure 14 shows a stored strip of a rhythm

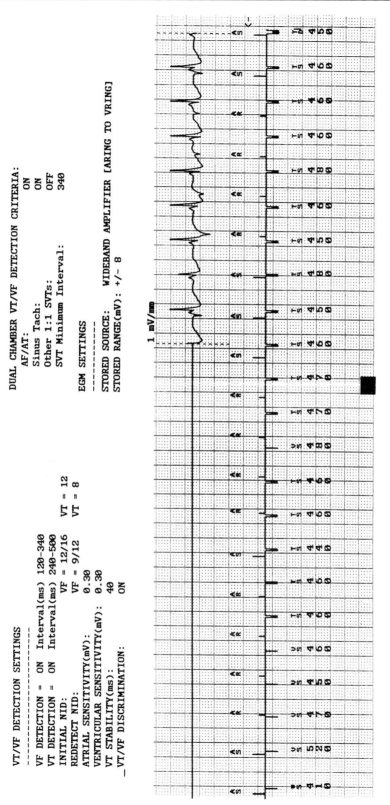

VT/VF DETECTION SETTINGS

VF DETECTION = ON   Interval(ms) 120-340
VT DETECTION = ON   Interval(ms) 240-500
INITIAL NID: VF = 12/16   VT = 12
REDETECT NID: VF = 9/12   VT = 8
ATRIAL SENSITIVITY(mV):   0.30
VENTRICULAR SENSITIVITY(mV):   0.30
VT STABILITY(ms):   40
_VT/VF DISCRIMINATION: ON

DUAL CHAMBER VT/VF DETECTION CRITERIA:

AF/AT: ON
Sinus Tach: ON
Other 1:1 SVTs: OFF
SVT Minimum Interval: 340

EGM SETTINGS

STORED SOURCE: WIDEBAND AMPLIFIER [ARING TO VRING]
STORED RANGE(mV): +/- 8

1 mV/mm

Figure 10. Jewel AF™ detection of induced VT showing resumption of detection, reset of the VT counter by stability, P-R dissociation, and VT detection. The Aring to Vring stored electrogram clearly shows atrial and ventricular depolarizations and P-R dissociation. The SVT minimum interval was 340 ms and neither AF/AT nor sinus tachycardia were recognized so VT detection occurred and ramp antitachycardia pacing terminated the VT on the first attempt (not shown).

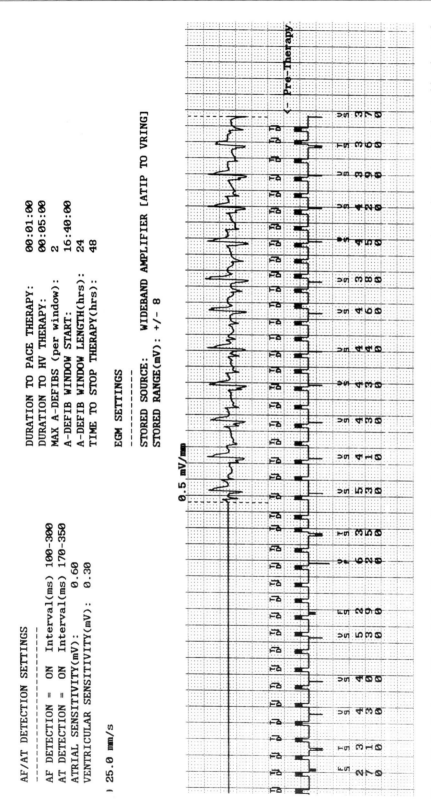

AF/AT DETECTION SETTINGS

AF DETECTION = ON   Interval(ms) 100-300
AT DETECTION = ON   Interval(ms) 170-350
ATRIAL SENSITIVITY(mV):   0.60
VENTRICULAR SENSITIVITY(mV):   0.30

) 25.0 mm/s

DURATION TO PACE THERAPY: 00:01:00
DURATION TO HV THERAPY: 00:05:00
MAX A-DEFIBS (per window):   2
A-DEFIB WINDOW START: 16:40:00
A-DEFIB WINDOW LENGTH(hrs):   24
TIME TO STOP THERAPY(hrs):   48

EGM SETTINGS

STORED SOURCE: WIDEBAND AMPLIFIER [ATIP TO VRING]
STORED RANGE(mV): +/- 8

0.5 mV/mm

Figure 11. Preliminary AT was detected 1 minute earlier and sustained AT detection prior to atrial antitachycardia pacing is indicated by the triple "TD" atrial markers on the strip. The ventricular rate clearly did not satisfy the VT detection algorithm. The stored electrogram recorded from Atip to Vring clearly shows both atrial and ventricular depolarizations. The P-P median cycle length was 190 ms which was in the AT/AF overlap zone from 170–300 ms. in this example, so the atrial autodiscriminator found the rhythm was regular so AT was detected and atrial ATP occurred.

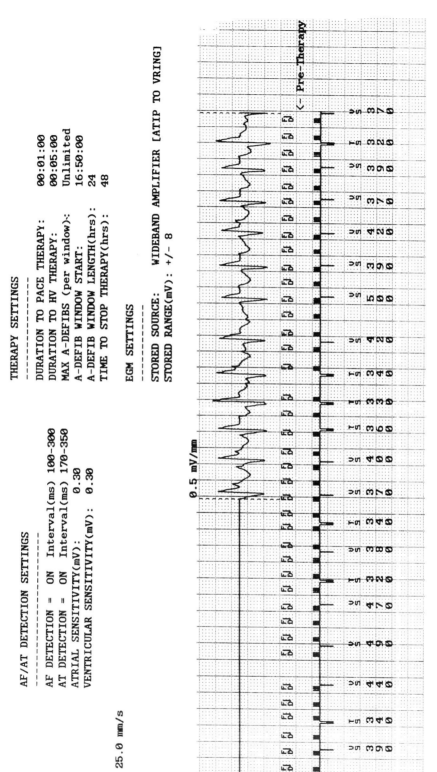

AF/AT DETECTION SETTINGS

AF DETECTION = ON   Interval(ms) 100-300
AT DETECTION = ON   Interval(ms) 170-350
ATRIAL SENSITIVITY(mV):   0.30
VENTRICULAR SENSITIVITY(mV):   0.30

25.0 mm/s

THERAPY SETTINGS

DURATION TO PACE THERAPY: 00:01:00
DURATION TO HV THERAPY: 00:05:00
MAX A-DEFIBS (per window)-:   Unlimited
A-DEFIB WINDOW START: 16:50:00
A-DEFIB WINDOW LENGTH(hrs):   24
TIME TO STOP THERAPY(hrs):   48

EGM SETTINGS

STORED SOURCE: WIDEBAND AMPLIFIER [ATIP TO VRING]
STORED RANGE(mV): +/- 8

0.5 mV/mm

<-- Pre-Therapy

Figure 12. Preliminary AT was detected 11 min before this strip and three prior ATP therapies failed to terminate this atrial tachyarrhythmia. This fourth detection was AF for a median P-P of 200 ms in the overlap between the AT and AF zones. Irregularity in the P-P intervals, undersensing perhaps twice, and the irregular ventricular response support the diagnosis of true AF. The stored electrogram recorded from Atip to Vring has some deflections associated with the P wave sensing, but minimal slew rate. The 50-Hz pacing therapy delivered immediately after this strip was not successful.

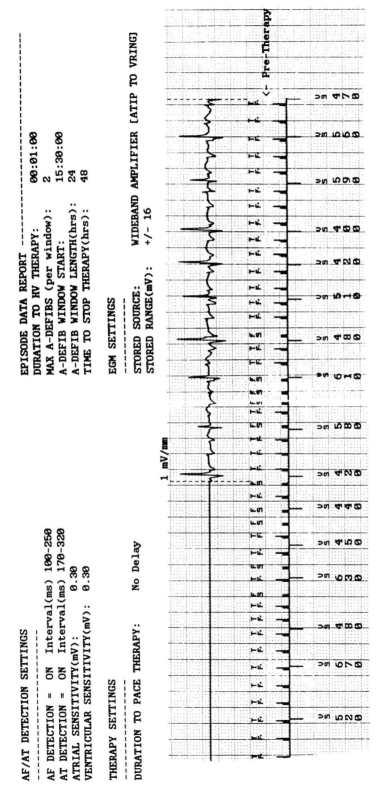

Figure 13. In this example from the Jewel AF™, the sustained detection to first ATP therapy was programmed to zero min so the atrial detection markers show some intervals as AF (short double marker) for P-P<170 ms and some intervals in the overlap zone (short-long marker) 170<P-P<250 ms. No P-P intervals were in the AT zone (long double marker) 250<P-P<320 ms. AF was detected by the device using the last 12 P-P intervals which were sufficiently variable for the autodiscrimination algorithm to detect it as AF rather than AT. The stored electrogram recorded from Atip to Vring has variable P wave morphology and variable R-R intervals that suggest AF as the true rhythm.

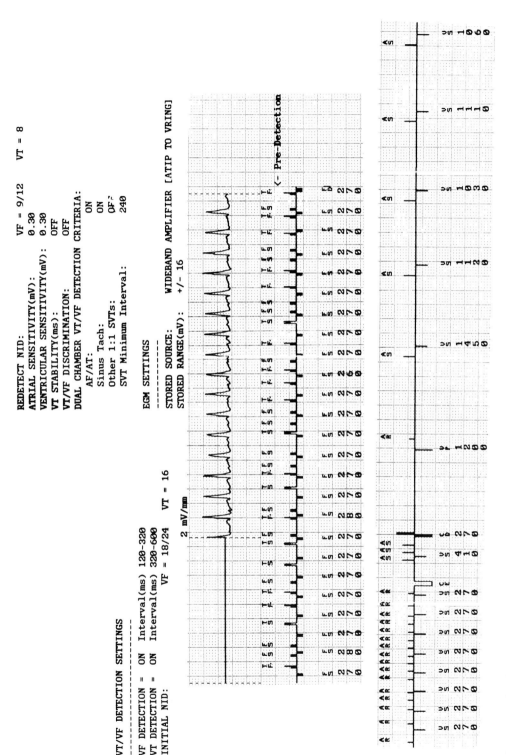

Figure 14. This last example from the Jewel AF™ ICD shows detection of double tachycardia in the VF zone that resulted in the ventricular shock on the Marker Channel™. The ventricular shock marker initially goes down whereas an atrial shock marker initially goes up. The median R-R interval was only 270 ms and the R-R intervals are very regular. The P-P intervals are quite irregular and farfield R wave oversensing if present is not consistent. Atrial deflections on this Atip to Vring stored electrogram are consistent with atrial sensing and certainly verifies the very fast ventricular rate.

that was detected as double tachycardia, so the ventricular detection of VF with median R-R interval of 270 ms prevailed and a 12-J ventricular shock terminated both tachyarrhythmias. The electrogram was recorded per-detection because a ventricular tachyarrhythmia was detected. The SVTmin CL was programmed to 240 ms and the fibrillation detection interval (FDI) for the ventricle was programmed to 320 ms. The atrial rhythm appears to be AF with irregular P-P intervals and some evidence of atrial deflections on the atrial tip to ventricular ring electrogram. The very rapid and very regular ventricular rhythm could be caused by the AF, however, a concurrent rapid ventricular tachycardia cannot be ruled out so detection of double tachycardia occurred. The episode duration was 13 sec.

Evaluation of AF and AT detection for prerecorded atrial tachyarrhythmias showed high sensitivity 98% (89/91) and only one false positive in 62 nonarrhythmic episodes. Some true AFs were inappropriately detected as AT. Prototype testing of the Jewel AF™ in the cardiac electrophysiology laboratory[47] showed detection of AF in 12/12 episodes in nine patients, 19/20 episodes of atrial flutter in 15 patients, and 6/9 episodes of atrial tachycardia in five patients. For non 1:1 atrial tachyarrhythmias, AT/AF was detected in 97% (37/38) of the episodes from 23 patients.

Preliminary clinical evaluation of atrial tachyarrhythmia sensing and detection for 80 patients implanted with the Jewel AF™ dual chamber ICD was performed using stored data and 24-hour Holter telemetry in 30 of these patients.[19] During postoperative testing, 109 episodes of induced AF were all detected in 18 ± 11 sec. For spontaneous AT/AF in 14 patients, 223 of 247 (90%) detected atrial episodes were appropriate. Undersensing of AT/AF caused premature termination of the episode in only one of the 223 episodes initially detected (0.9 mV sensitivity in that case). Continuous detection of AT/AF for a total of 1,290 hours occurred during 53 episodes that each lasted for at least 1 hour. This continuous detection of

AT/AF was validated with Holter telemetry monitoring in three patients for 45 hours. Two patients had 24 inappropriate detections of AT/AF for 2.6 ± 2.0 min due to intermittent farfield R wave oversensing during sinus tachycardia. No patient had symptomatic undetected atrial tachyarrhythmia. The Jewel AF™ detected AT/AF promptly and continuously so that shocks for AF can be programmed for many hours after the onset of AF.

Atrial View™ Enhanced Onset and Stability—Ventak AV™

The Ventak AV dual chamber detection algorithm adds two enhancements, AFib rate threshold and VRate>ARate, to the preexisting single chamber algorithms. The AFib rate threshold enhancement is used in conjunction with the ventricular rate stability and onset algorithms as therapy inhibitors. The VRate>ARate enhancement is an inhibitor override that uses the average atrial rate to overrule all therapy inhibitors including the ventricular rate onset or stability algorithms [48] The physician can program these two enhancements "ON" or "OFF." The diagram in Figure 15 shows the logic used in the Ventak AV for the two new dual chamber enhancements. This algorithm is more sensitive than previously available onset and stability algorithms based solely on ventricular rate.

After initial detection by 8 of 10 fast R-R intervals, at least 6 of 10 R-R intervals must remain fast during the duration time to avoid resetting detection. At the end of the duration time, the last interval must be in the detection zone to complete ventricular rate detection. Once duration is met, each therapy enhancement that is programmed "ON" will provide diagnostic information. The onset algorithm searches backward in time to a pivotal interval defining the onset of the episode. A comparison of the inter-

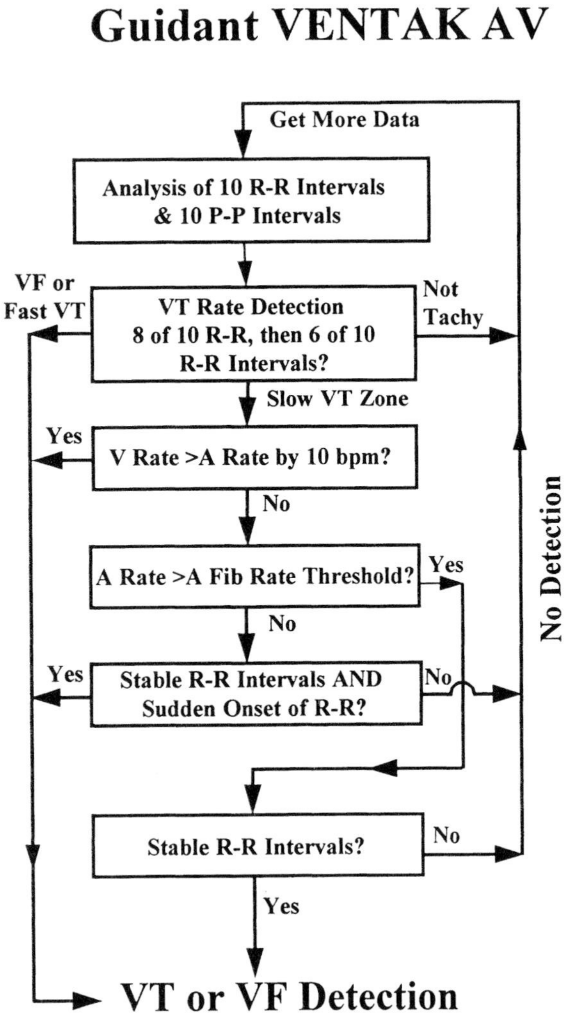

Guidant VENTAK AV

Figure 15. The Ventak AV dual chamber detection algorithm modifies R-R interval stability and onset algorithms using atrial rate information. Figure 15 shows that if all detection enhancements are programmed ON, then for each ventricular event, the 10 most recent P-P and R-R intervals may be analyzed if ventricular rate detection initially finds 8 of 10 R-R intervals in the slow VT zone and then at least 6 of 10 R-R intervals remain in the slow VT zone. If the dual chamber analysis in the slow VT zone finds the ventricular rate is greater than the atrial rate by at least 10 bpm, then detection occurs. Otherwise, if the atrial rate is greater than the atrial fibrillation rate threshold and the R-R intervals are not stable, then detection is withheld. If the atrial rate is not greater than the atrial fibrillation rate threshold, then detection still can be withheld if the R-R intervals are stable and there was sudden onset of the short R-R intervals.

vals on both sides of this pivotal interval is made to assess whether the onset was sudden or gradual. The stability algorithm averages the R-R interval differences. A comparison is made between this average and the programmed stability threshold (6–120 ms) to assess whether the rhythm is stable or unstable. The AFib rate threshold algorithm compares the 10 most recent P-P intervals to a threshold. The AFib rate threshold criterion is met if 6 of 10 (and 4 of 10 thereafter) intervals are greater than the programmed AFib rate threshold.

Once duration is met, the VRate>ARate detection enhancement uses the average of the 10 most recent P-P and R-R intervals to assess which chamber has a faster rate. If the Vrate exceeds the Arate by 10 bpm, the VRate>ARate criterion is met. If the previously described inhibitors collectively recommend to inhibit therapy, they will be overruled if the VRate>ARate criterion is met. The VRate>ARate algorithm analyzes the average atrial and ventricular rates and does not compare the beat-to-beat timing of individual atrial and ventricular events. Sustained rate duration (SRD) will override inhibitors if therapy has been withheld for a time equal to the SRD threshold. It is important to note that all enhancements are calculated and assessed concurrently and not sequentially. All diagnostic information from active therapy inhibitors and inhibitor overrides are used collectively to generate a final therapy decision (inhibit or do not inhibit).

Figure 16 shows a Ventak AV example of atrial flutter and spontaneous VF that was detected promptly, charging occurred, and a shock was delivered that terminated both the VF and the atrial flutter. The strip shows the ECG, atrial electrogram, ventricular electrogram, event markers with intervals, and episode annotations at the bottom. The atrial rhythm was sensed and AF markers show P-P intervals of about 210 ms. There is some atrial undersensing (AS) and atrial sensing within the noise window (AN) during VF. Ventricular sensing as VF with some sensing within the noise window (VN) resulted in initial 8 of 10 detection (Epsd), sudden onset (Suddn) and mode switch (ATR) during VF detection (Detct). The rhythm was judged unstable (Unstb) and charging began (Chrg), was completed (Chrg) and the shock (Shock) was delivered appropriately. The first post-shock beat was paced in both chambers and sensing soon returned.

A second example for VT during atrial flutter in the top panel of Figure 17 shows atrial undersensing and noise sensing again particularly when the atrial and ventricular events are nearly coincident due to the 86 ms cross-chamber atrial refractory period after each ventricular sense. The VT was reliably sensed, initially detected (Epsd), sudden onset and mode switching occurred, and when the duration (Dur) expired, the unstable (Unstab) R-R intervals inhibited detection due to AF (AFib). This continued onto the second panel where the VT became stable, was detected (Detct), charging begins, ends and the shock was appropriately delivered with success.

Atrial fibrillation conducts rapidly enough to the ventricle in Figure 18 to initiate an inappropriate episode (Epsd) (8 of 10 VT beats) and a mode switch from (ATR) (the beginning of ATR precedes this strip)

due to a ventricular episode declaration. Despite two long R-R intervals (742, 842 ms), the 6 of 10 detection criterion remained satisfied and the duration (Dur) expired. The ventricular rhythm was unstable (Unstb) and identified as AF (AFib) for five ventricular beats after which the detection window was closed due to the series of long R-R intervals that did not satisfy the 6 of 10 detection criterion. Near the end of the strip, six more beats were sensed as VT. This process of nearly detecting double tachycardia may occur repeatedly to avoid inappropriate detection.

Two to one atrial flutter rhythms such as the one shown in Figure 19 can result in relatively regular ventricular responses that may be inappropriately detected as VT using stability. On this strip, however, eight VT beats initiated detection (Epsd) and at the end of duration, VT was detected because the rhythm was unstable (Unstb). VT was inappropriately detected because every other P wave was not sensed or sensed as noise (AN), so the AFib rate threshold was not met. Charging occurred and an inappropriate shock was delivered.

Preliminary clinical evaluation of dual chamber sensing and detection by the Ventak AV implanted in 69 patients with ventricular tachyarrhythmias was performed.[51,52] Some of these patients had secondary indications of bradycardia (64%) and intermittent AF (13%). Induced monomorphic VT was detected in all episodes. Induced AF was inhibited in 26 of 29 episodes (89.7%). One patient had insufficient atrial sensing to receive the device. After testing and reprogramming, 56 of 58 patients (97%) had appropriate DDD sensing and pacing.

PARAD™ Atrioventricular Sequence Analysis—Defender™

The dual chamber detection algorithm, called PARAD, used in the ELA Defender™

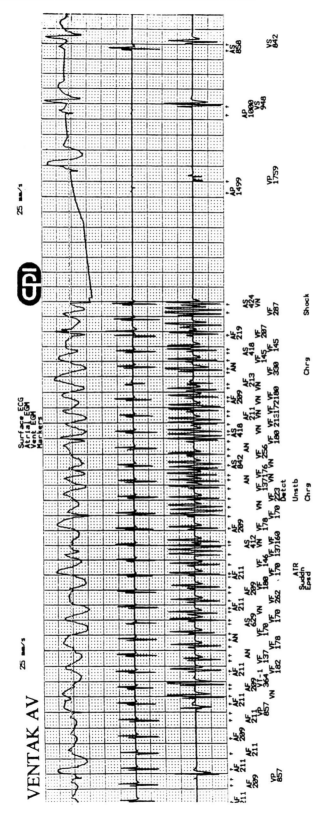

Figure 16. This real-time strip from the Ventak AV shows ongoing atrial flutter, initiation of spontaneous VF that was detected and socked. The channels are: surface ECG, atrial electrogram, ventricular electrogram, sense/pace arrows, atrial markers with P-P intervals, ventricular markers with R-R intervals, and episode annotations. Atrial markers are atrial pace (AP), atrial sense (AS), atrial fibrillation (AF), and atrial noise (AN). Ventricular markers are ventricular pace (VP), ventricular sense (VS), VT-1 zone sense (VT-1), VT zone sense (VT), VF zone sense (VF), ventricular noise (VN), and noise-telemetry (TN). Episode annotation markers are: start/end of episode (Epsd), onset-sudden (Suddn), onset-gradual (Gradl), atrial tachy response mode switch (ATR), duration expired (Dur), stable (Stb), unstable (Unstb), atrial fibrillation met (AFib), V rate faster than A rate (V>A), detection met (Detct), sustained rate duration expired (SRD), start/end of charge (Chrg), shock delivered (Shock), and therapy diverted (Dvrt).

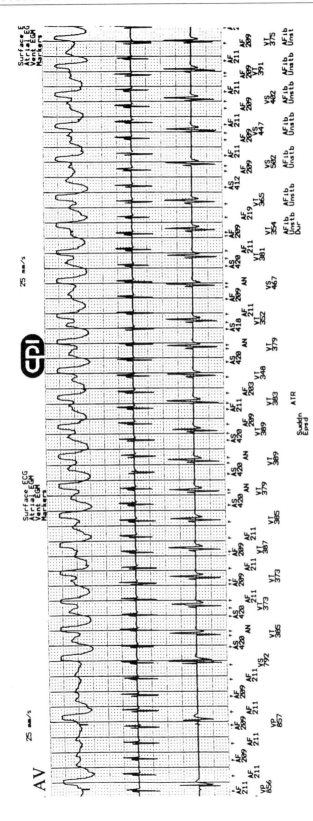

Figure 17. A: Real-time strip showing atrial flutter and spontaneous VT with sudden onset, mode switch, and duration is met for the unstable ventricular rhythm that was initially diagnosed as AF because both the atrial rate is faster than the AFib rate threshold and the ventricular rate is unstable. This strip is continued on the next page. that the ventricular R-R intervals become more regular at 375 ms which causes VT detection, charging, and a shock that terminated both the atrial and the ventricular tachyarrhythmias. Some atrial undersensing is indicated by the AS markers with 420-ms P-P intervals, but at least 4 of 10 atrial markers are AF to maintain the AFib episode annotation markers.

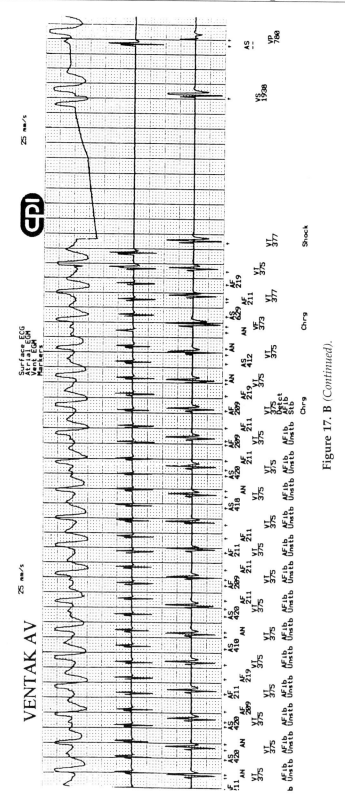

Figure 17. B *(Continued).*

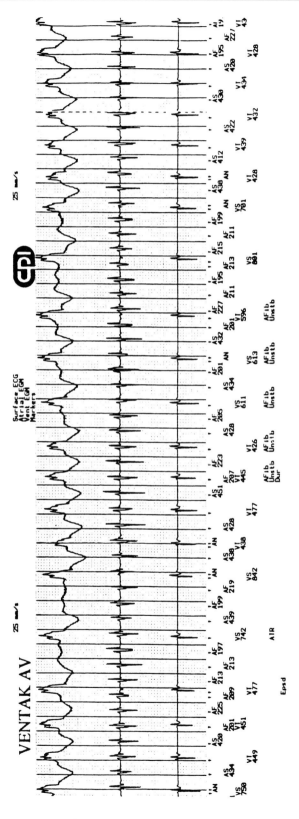

Figure 18. Double tachycardia is almost inappropriately detected for AF that transiently conducts rapidly to the ventricle. Enough beats of VT (8 of 10) are sensed to initiate an episode (Epsd) of VT that despite two long R-R intervals satisfied duration (Dur). The AF is recognized by the unstable ventricular intervals and enough atrial intervals are less than the AFib rate interval threshold. After five beats of AFib detection, the episode ends because there are less than six of the last 10 ventricular events in the VT zone.

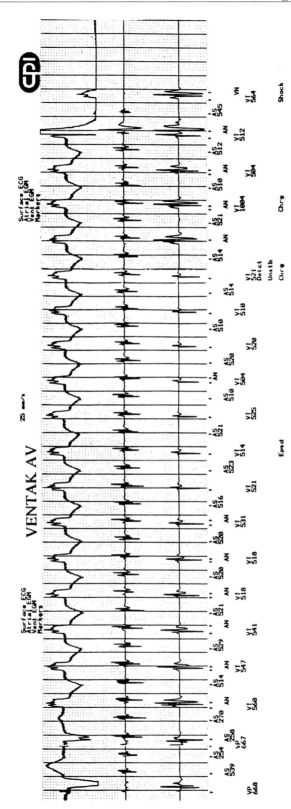

Figure 19. This Ventak AV strip illustrates inappropriate detection of VT and shock for atrial flutter that conducts 2:1 to the ventricle in the VT zone. Eight VT beats met initial detection (Epsd) and after five more VT beats, VT was detected (Detct) despite the R-R intervals being unstable (Unstb). VT detection would not have occurred if simple stability had been used. Inappropriate VT detection occurs due to the additional criterion of ARate >AFib rate threshold which is not satisfied because every other P wave is undersensed. The undersensed P waves appear to be just after the ventricular depolarizations in the fixed 86 ms cross chamber atrial refractory period after each ventricular sense.

ICD uses cycle length zones like other devices, identifies a majority rhythm, which if fast, gets classified as VT, SVT or ST based on R-R stability, then by AV association, and finally if 1:1, then by the chamber of onset.[53-59] A diagram describing this algorithm, shown in Figure 20, analyzes the last 8 R-R intervals (programmable 8–16) and initially classifies the rhythm as sinus rhythm (SR), ventricular tachycardia (VT), or ventricular fibrillation (VF).

For each new R-R interval, one of these three rhythms is identified when 75% (programmable 63%–100%) of the last eight R-R intervals are in the SR, VT, or VF zone, respectively. This rhythm classification can exclude the early intervals of the tachyarrhythmia (programmable 0–8) to allow the rhythm to stabilize, but nominally (0) it does not. Rhythms in the VF zone are shocked and no therapy is given for the SR zone. Analysis continues for rhythms in the VT zone by analyzing R-R stability with a histogram of the R-R intervals using 15.6 ms wide bins for the VT and VF intervals among the last eight intervals. A correlation window that is four bins wide (nominally 63 ms wide) is positioned to maximize the number of R-R intervals in the window. The rhythm is judged unstable and classified as AF with no therapy if less than 75% (nominal) of the R-R intervals are in the window.

If the rhythm is stable, analysis continues for AV association by constructing a similar P-R interval histogram using up to five P-R intervals from each R-R interval. A similar correlation window (nominally four bins wide) is positioned to maximize the number of P-R intervals in the window. The rhythm is associated if this number of stable P-R intervals is at least 75% (nominally) of the number of stable R-R intervals found previously in the R-R histogram. If the rhythm is not associated, then VT is diagnosed and therapy for VT is given (For dissociated rhythms, the PARAD+, Defender™ 9201, algorithm,(not shown, will not detect VT if the last R-R interval is at least 63 ms longer than the average of the last four R-R intervals that are less than the tachycardia detection interval[57]). If the rhythm is associated, then it is classified as 1:1 when the percentage of the number of stable P-R intervals compared to the total number of P-R intervals is at least 75% (nominal). If the association is not 1:1, then it is N:1 and classified as atrial flutter with no therapy. For 1:1 rhythms, the onset of the tachycardia is analyzed to find if there is no acceleration, atrial acceleration, or ventricular acceleration. Acceleration is defined when a VT or VF type R-R interval is shorter than a reference cycle by at least 25% (nominal). The reference R-R interval is defined as the previous R-R interval unless it is a pause or accelerated itself, in which case the average of the last four nonaccelerated R-R intervals are used as the reference R-R interval. An atrial acceleration is defined if both ventricular R-R intervals are preceded by a P-R interval that is between min and max values. Otherwise, the acceleration is ventricular if one or both of the R waves are not conducted, VT is diagnosed and therapy is given. If there is no acceleration or it is atrial in origin, then SVT is diagnosed and no therapy is given. In summary, VT is diagnosed for stable ventricular rhythms that are dissociated or <1:1 and for 1:1 rhythms with ventricular acceleration.

Figure 21 on the left side shows an example of tachycardia with an AV marker recording (EM) that was stable, had 1:1 association with acceleration by the atrium and therefore diagnosed as SVT. Therefore, it was not treated despite a cycle length of 328 ms.[54] This SVT self-terminated after 8 sec. The AV electrogram recording shows a similar R wave morphology for both rhythms and P waves can be seen. The right side of the same figure shows another tachycardia from the same patient with an atrioventricular marker recording that was stable, dissociated, and acceleration was ventricular in origin. The stored electrograms before and after successful ATP show a distinctly different R wave morphology. The stored atrioventricular electrogram of the VT does not have visible P waves to confirm P-R dissociation because of quantization noise on these electrograms.

ELA DEFENDER

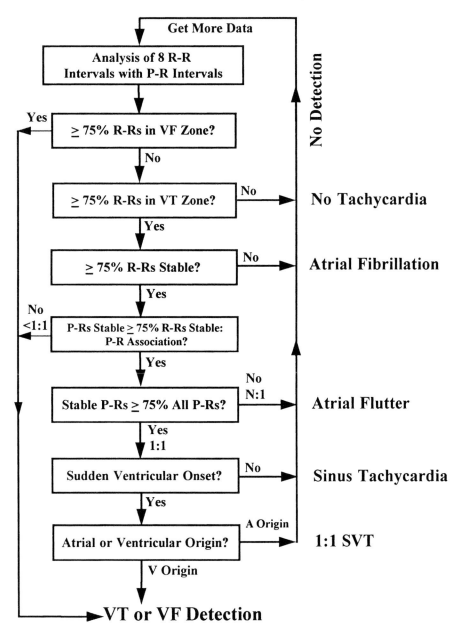

Figure 20. A block diagram for the PARAD dual chamber detection algorithm in the ELA Defender™ ICD with a detection enhancements programmed ON is shown for the processing of each ventricular event. Eight previous R-R intervals are analyzed including up to five P-R intervals for each R-R interval. If at least 75% of R-R intervals are in the VF zone, detection occurs. Analysis proceeds if at least 75% of the R-R intervals are in the VT zone. If the R-R intervals are unstable, then atrial fibrillation is diagnosed and detection is withheld. If a stable rhythm is dissociated, then VT is detected. If at least 75% of all the P-R intervals are stable, then the rhythm is 1:1. If the P-R intervals are unstable, then the rhythm is N:1, such as atrial flutter, and detection is withheld. For 1:1 rhythms, onset acceleration is then measured and if ventricular in origin, then VT is detected.

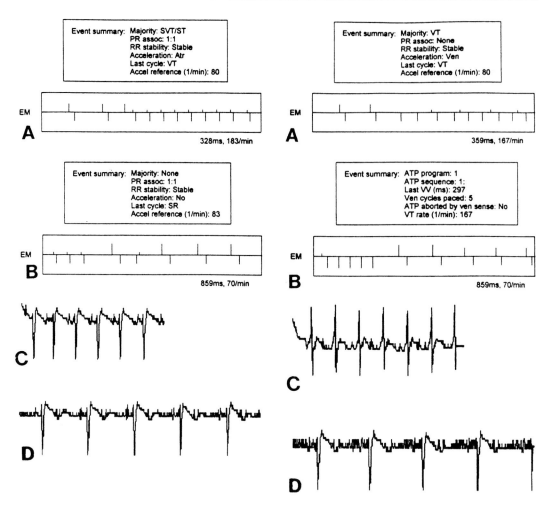

Figure 21. Two example episodes from the Defender™ dual chamber ICD are shown in each column of panels. On the left a stable ventricular rhythm with 1:1 P-R association had onset acceleration with atrial origin so it was diagnosed as SVT. The upper AV marker recording (EM) shows P and R events. The ventricular electrogram during tachycardia has the same morphology as the slower rhythm recorded after spontaneous termination. On the right side of the figure the tachycardia was stable, but had P-R dissociation so it was detected as VT. The upper AV marker recording (EM) shows the P-R dissociation and the stored electrogram morphology was very different for the tachycardia. P waves are difficult to see due to quantization noise particularly for the dissociated VT.

Testing of the PARAD dual chamber detection algorithm prototype for the ELA Defender™ ICD[59] was performed with 156 episodes prerecorded from 50 patients during EP studies. VF sensitivity and specificity were both 100% for 22 episodes with detection times of 2.1±0.4 sec (1.5–2.9 sec). VT sensitivity was 96% for 85 episodes with detection times of 2.6±8 sec (1.8–4.4 sec). The three VTs missed were due to unstable R-R intervals, a low VT rate limit, and oversensing artifacts. Double tachycardia sensitivity was 92% with 1 of 12 episodes underdetected because a N:1 association was found during AF. Inappropriate VT detection occurred for 3 of 12 episodes of AF in three patients with WPW and a very stable fast ventricular response. For atrial flutter, 5 of 12 cases had every other P wave blanked by the postventricular atrial refractory period and were classified as stable with 1:1 association; however, onset testing was not possible. Ten episodes of ST and AT were stable with 1:1 association, but onsets were not available for testing. Clinical results from the ELA Defender™ dual chamber ICD are also described in Chapter 18.

Conclusions and Future Developments

The dual chamber ICD detection algorithms described in this chapter clearly use different methods for analyzing the parallel series of atrial and ventricular events that occur in the wide variety of tachyarrhythmias in patients with various underlying cardiac disease and electrophysiological phenomena. Publications describing the clinical performance of these dual chamber algorithms are limited particularly in the duration of follow-up and the number of patients studied. The number of patients indicated for dual chamber ICDs appears to be greater than the 10% of patients with single chamber ICDs that really needed VVI pacing to treat symptomatic bradycardia.

Some rhythm uncertainties will undoubtedly remain because interpretation disagreements for 12-lead ECGs and even EP studies that lack His recordings are well known. The value of stored electrograms with consistently visible P waves will substantially reduce the number of uncertain diagnoses for spontaneous tachyarrhythmias in patients with ICDs. Atrial sensing problems and rapid regular ventricular responses to atrial tachyarrhythmias are likely to become the major sources of the reduced but remaining inappropriate detections in dual chamber ICDs. Loss of atrial capture, loss of atrial sensing during chronic AF and dislodged atrial leads will undoubtedly cause trouble in selected patients compared to single chamber ICDs. Oversensing of farfield R waves as seen on the atrial lead for some patients is likely to confound some diagnoses as will other types of crosstalk between the two sensing systems. Increased implant time and complications associated with atrial leads may also detract from the benefits of the dual chamber ICDs.

Future developments for dual chamber ICD detection algorithms may include addition of ventricular and even atrial depolarization morphology analysis to compliment the P and R wave timing analysis. Practical chronic recordings from the His bundle or methods to determine the direction of activation in the atrium and/or the ventricle may provide a "third channel" for future algorithms. The use of premature atrial test stimuli proposed 12 years ago.[32] may be utilized to aid the diagnosis of the 1:1 tachyrrhythmias. Finally, advances in signal processing,[60] computational capabilities, and adaptive systems made possible by advances in microelectronics are likely to allow more comprehensive systems to be developed.

Acknowledgments: I am grateful to Jean Hayman for literature research and figure preparation. I appreciate helpful reviews and corrections by Charles D. Swerdlow, MD, Milton Morris from Guidant, Inc., and Remi Nitzsche from ELA Medical, Inc.

References

1. Jenkins JM, Caswell SA. Detection algorithms in implantable cardioverter defibrillators. Proc IEEE 1996;84(3):428–445.
2. Johnson NJ, Marchlinski FE. Arrhythmias induced by device tachycardia therapy due to diagnostic nonspecificity. J Am Coll Cardiol 1991;18(5):1418–1425.
3. Dougherty CM. Psychological reactions and family adjustment in shock versus no shock groups after implantation of internal cardioverter defibrillator. Heart Lung 1995;24(4): 281–291.
4. Lawton JS, Wood MA, Gilligan DM, et al. Implantable transvenous cardioverter defibrillator leads: the dark side. PACE 1996; 19(9):1273–1295.
5. Noguera HH, Peralta AO, John RM, et al. Combined use of non-thoracotomy cardioverter defibrillators and endocardial pacemakers. Heart 1997;78:50–55.

6. Mattke S, Markewitz A, Muller D, et al. The combined transvenous implantation of cardioverter defibrillators and permanent pacemakers. PACE 1997;20(11):2775–2782.

7. Olson WH. Tachyarrhythmia sensing and detection. In Singer I, ed. Implantable Cardioverter-Defibrillator. Futura Publishing Co, Inc., Armonk, NY, 1994, pp 71–107.

8. Anderson MH, Murgatroyd FD, Hnatkova K, et al. Performance of basic ventricular tachycardia detection algorithms in implantable cardioverter defibrillators. PACE 1997; 20(Pt I): 2975–2983.

9. Ellenbogen K, Epstein AE, Wood MA, et al. Are more complex implantable cardioverter defibrillators associated with an increased mortality? Lessons learned from clinical trials. Am J Cardiol 1997;80(7):958–960.

10. Panotopoulos PT, Krum D, Axtell K, et al. Comparison of ventricular fibrillation sensing by implantable defibrillator systems: Is one better than the others? Circulation 1997; 96(Suppl 1):I-696.

11. Khulkamp V, Mortensen PT, Dinberger V, et al. A randomized controlled clinical trial comparing VF detection time between the VENTAK AV acute study device and the VENTAK MINI. PACE 1997;20(4):1094.

12. Kleinert M, Elmquist H, Strandberg H. Spectral properties of atrial and ventricular endocardial signals. PACE 1079;2(1):11–18.

13. Goldreyer BN, Almquist CK, Beck RC, et al. Waveform and frequency analysis of unipolar, bipolar, and orthogonal atrial electrograms. PACE 1986;9(2):283.

14. Kerr CR, Mason MA. Amplitude of atrial electrical activity during sinus rhythm and during atrial flutter-fibrillation. PACE 1985; 8(Pt I):348–355.

15. Wood MA, Moskovljevic P, Stambler BS, et al. Comparison of bipolar atrial electrogram amplitude in sinus rhythm, atrial fibrillation, and atrial flutter. PACE 1996;19(2):150–156.

16. Ruetz L, Yee R, Bardy G, et al. Reliable sensing of human atrial fibrillation. PACE 1993; 16(Pt II):902.

17. Kopp DE, Gilkerson J, Kall JG, et al. Effect of ventricular fibrillation on atrial electrograms. Circulation 1994;90(Pt 2):I-177.

18. Jenkins J, Noh KH, Guezennec A, et al. Diagnosis of atrial fibrillation using electrograms from chronic leads: evaluation of computer algorithms. PACE 1988;11(5):622–631.

19. Swerdlow CD, Sheth NV, Gunderson BD, et al. Rapid continuous detection of atrial fibrillation by a dual-chamber implantable cardioverter-defibrillator. PACE 1998;21(Pt II): 853.

20. Brouwer J, Nagelkerke D, den Heijer P, et al. Analysis of atrial sensed farfield ventricular signals: a reassessment. PACE 1997;20(Pt I): 916–922.

21. Volosin KJ, Beauregard L-AM, Fabiszewski R, et al. Spontaneous changes in ventricular tachycardia cycle length. J Am Coll Cardiol 1991;17(2):409–414.

22. Chen PS. Personal communication, February 1998.

23. Li HG, Thakur RK, Yee R, et al. Ventriculoatrial conduction in patients with implantable cardioverter defibrillators: implications for tachycardia discrimination by dual chamber sensing. PACE 1994;17(Pt I):2304–2306.

24. Militianu A, Salacata A, Meissner MD, et al. Ventriculoatrial conduction capability and prevalence of 1:1 retrograde conduction during inducible sustained monomorphic ventricular tachycardia in 305 implantable cardioverter defibrillator recipients. PACE 1997; 20(Pt I):2378–2384.

25. Brown ML, Gillberg JM, Stanton MS, et al. Retrograde conduction during ventricular tachycardia: implications for dual chamber implantable defibrillators. Circulation 1996; 94(Suppl):I-321.

26. Miller J. Personal communication. July 1997.

27. Jenkins JM, Wu D, Arzbaecher RC. Computer diagnosis of supraventricular and ventricular arrhythmias. Circulation 1979;60(5): 977–987.

28. Jenkins J, Bump T, Glick K, et al. Automated recognition of tachycardias from electrograms: decision rules for diagnosis. Computers Cardiol 1983.

29. Arzbaecher R, Bump T, Jenkins J, et al. Automatic tachycardia recognition. PACE 1984; 7(Pt II):541–547.

30. Schuger CD, Jackson K, Steinman RT, et al. Atrial sensing to augment ventricular tachycardia detection by the automatic implantable cardioverter defibrillator: a utility study. PACE 1988;11(10):1456–1463.

31. Munkenbeck FC, Bump TE, Arzbaecher RC. Differentiation of sinus tachycardia from paroxysmal 1:1 tachycardias using single late diastolic atrial extrastimuli. PACE 1986; 9(Pt I):53–64.

32. Jenkins J, Noh KH, Bump T, et al. A single atrial extrastimulus can distinguish sinus tachycardia from 1:1 paroxysmal tachycardia. PACE 1986;9(Pt II):1063–1068.

33. Arzbaecher R, Polikaitis A. Dual chamber tachycardia identification. PACE 1993;16(Pt II):1110.

34. Throne RD, Jenkins JM, Winston SA, et al. Discrimination of retrograde from antegrade atrial activation using intracardiac electrogram waveform analysis. PACE 1989; 12(10):1622.

35. Gerstenfeld EP, Sahakian AV, Baerman JM,

et al. Detection changes in atrial endocardial activation with use of an orthogonal catheter. J Am Coll Cardiol 1991;18(4):1034.

36. Chiang C-M, Jenkins JM, DiCarlo LA, et al. Real-time arrhythmia identification from automated analysis of intraatrial and intraventricular electrograms. PACE 1993;16(Pt II): 223–227.

37. DiCarlo LA, Lin D, Jenkins JM. Automated interpretation of cardiac arrhythmias. J Electrocardiol 1993;26:53–63.

38. Leong PHW, Jabri MA. Matic: an intracardiac tachycardia classification system. PACE 1992;15:1317–1331.

39. Murphy AJ, Mason D, Bassin D. Dual-chamber rhythm classifier for implantable cardioverter defibrillators. PACE 1993;16(Pt II):928.

40. Thakor NV, Natarajan A, Tomaselli GF. Multiway sequential hypothesis testing for tachyarrhythmia discrimination. IEEE Trans Biomed Eng 1994;41(5):480–487.

41. Kaemmerer WF, Olson WH. Dual chamber tachyarrhythmia detection using syntactic pattern recognition and contextual timing rules for rhythm classification. PACE 1995; 18(Pt II):872.

42. System Reference Guide. Model 7271 GEM$_{DR}$—Dual Chamber Implantable Cardioverter Defibrillator, Medtronic, Inc. Minneapolis, MN.

43. Gillberg JM, Gunderson BD, Brown ML, et al. Dual chamber versus single chamber ventricular tachyarrhythmia detection: a retrograde comparison. PACE 1998;21(Pt II):909.

44. Brown ML, Gillberg JM, Hammill SC, et al. Acute human testing of a dual chamber ventricular tachyarrhythmia detection algorithm at Mayo Clinic. Computers Cardiol 1996;61–64.

45. Swerdlow CD, Sheth NV, Olson WH. Clinical performance of a pattern-based, dual-chamber algorithm for discrimination of ventricular from supraventricular arrhythmias. PACE 1998 in press.

46. System Reference Guide. Model 7250 Jewel AF™—Arrhythmia Management Device, Medtronic, Inc. Minneapolis, MN.

47. Gillberg JM, Brown ML, Stanton MS, et al. Clinical testing of a dual chamber atrial tachyarrhythmia detection algorithm. Computers Cardiol 1996;57–60.

48. Technical Manuals. Models 1810, 1815, Ventak AV Dual Chamber ICD, Guidant Inc. St. Paul, MN.

49. Mehmanesh H, Lange R, Brachmann J, et al. First report on surgical experience with a new implantable cardioverter defibrillator

providing dual-chamber pacing and sensing. PACE 1997;20(Pt II):1079.

50. Butter Ch, Auriccio A, Schwarz T, et al. Clinical evaluation of a dual chamber passive fixation single pass lead for cardioversion/defibrillation. Eur Heart J 1997;18(Suppl):27A.

51. Ruppel R, Langes K, Kalkowski H, et al. Initial experience with implantable cardioverter defibrillator providing dual chamber pacing and sensing. PACE 1997;20(Pt II):1078.

52. Block M, and the Ventak AV Investigators. Dual-chamber implantable cardioverter-defibrillator Ventak AV: first results from the multicenter premarket release study. PACE 1997;20(Pt II):1473.

53. Technical Manual. Model 9001 Defender™—Dual Chamber Cardioverter Defibrillator, Ela Medical, Inc. Montrouge, France.

54. Korte T, Jung W, Wolpert C, et al. A new classification algorithm for discrimination of ventricular from supraventricular tachycardia in a dual chamber implantable cardioverter defibrillator. J Cardiovasc Electrophysiol 1998;9(1):70–73.

55. LaVergne T, Daubert J-C, Chauvin M, et al. Preliminary clinical experience with the first dual chamber pacemaker defibrillator. PACE 1997;20(Pt II):182–188.

56. Saoudi N, Nitzsche R, Kroiss D, et al. Accuracy of rapid automatic identification of supraventricular and ventricular tachyarrhythmias using atrioventricular sequence analysis. In Santini M, ed. Proceedings of the International Symposium, Progress in Clinical Pacing. Futura Media Services, Inc, Armonk, NY, 1997, pp 445–450.

57. Montenero AS, Nitzsche R, De Chillou C, et al. Preliminary assessment of a new algorithm for automatic detection of fast atrial fibrillation in a dual-chamber implantable cardioverter-defibrillator. Europace Proc: 8th Euro Sympos Cardiac Pacing, Athens, Greece, June 1997.

58. Leenhardt A, Thomas O, Coumel P. A new algorithm for arrhythmia detection. In Santini M, ed. Proceedings of the International Symposium, Progress in Clinical Pacing. Futura Media Services, Inc, Armonk, NY, 1997, pp 131–138.

59. Nair M, Saoudi N, Kroiss D, et al. Automatic arrhythmia identification using analysis of the atrioventricular association. Circulation 1997;95:967–973.

60. Shkurovich S, Sahakian AV, Swiryn S. Detection of atrial activity from high-voltage leads of implantable ventricular defibrillators using a cancellation technique. IEEE Trans Biomed Eng 1998;45(2):229–234.

Dual Chamber Implantable Cardioverter-Defibrillator:
A Preliminary Experience

Etienne M. Aliot, M. Limousin, R. Nitzsche, N. Saoudi, T. Lavergne, C. de Chillou, N. Sadoul, and the Defender 9001 Investigator Group

Introduction

Development of the implantable cardio-verter-defibrillator (ICD) represents an outstanding technological achievement. More than 15 years of research and development have produced devices which combine complex diagnostic and therapeutic capabilities with a simple implantation technique. However, although the efficacy of these devices is consistently proven in clinical use, there is no question that two of their principal functions still require improvement: first, better detection to ensure the most acurate identification of an arrhythmia (supraventricular or ventricular) and, second, an improvement in the quality of cardiac pacing, which is often required in patients with malignant ventricular arrhythmias.

Benefits of Dual Chamber Implantable Cardioverter-Defibrillator Devices

These devices may offer some potential advances of substantial clinical relevance.

These major electrical and hemodynamic benefits have been previously highlighted and reviewed.[1] Dual chamber ICDs allow atrioventricular pacing. It is estimated that more than 15% of ICD patients could require concomitant pacing. Dual chamber pacing renders separately implanted pacemaker/ICD systems unnecessary[2] (Figure 1).

Four primary interactions between pacemakers and ICDs have been listed.[3] Failure to sense or capture has been observed immediately following shock. Oversensing of pacemaker stimulus may result in double counting, or, ventricular fibrillation (VF) undersensing may be due to sensing of pacemaker stimulus. Pacemakers can be reset by ICD discharge. All of these interactions could have potential proarrhythmic effects which are reduced with a dual chamber ICD. Finally, a dual chamber ICD may decrease atrial fibrillation (AF) incidence by atrial pacing.

It is acknowledged that inappropriate shock therapy delivered in a patient in whom arrhythmia has been poorly identified by an ICD constitutes an ever-present

From Singer I, Barold SS, Camm AJ (eds): Nonpharmacological Therapy of Arrhythmias for the 21st Century: The State of the Art. Futura Publishing Co, Inc., Armonk, NY, © 1998.

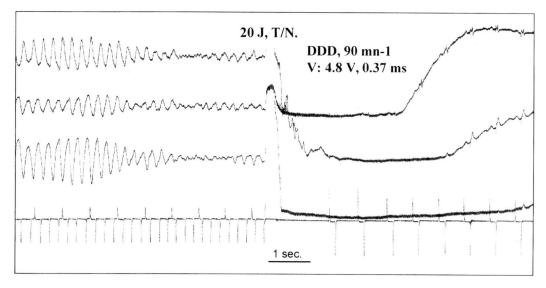

Figure 1. Ventricular fibrillation leading to a 20-J shock. Dual chamber pacing post shock.

problem. Data from the literature suggest that such inappropriate shocks are delivered in more than 30% of implanted patients, and that about one-third of shocks are delivered for sinus tachycardia. It is therefore essential to clearly differentiate ventricular from supraventricular arrhythmias. Currently applied criteria that take into account only ventricular activity have long been criticized for their limits. Atrial activity must henceforth be considered to improve the reliability of ICDs.

Atrial or dual chamber defibrillation may also be considered in the near future. Finally, atrial pacing may improve hemodynamics in patients with poor left ventricular function and reduce the incidence of AF episodes.

Specific Technical Problems Related to Dual Chamber Defibrillators

Whichever cardiac chamber is addressed, the analysis of rhythm disturbances by an implantable device remains complex. This is due to two combined factors: it is currently possible to analyze only changes in rhythm and chronology of events, but this analysis is limited by several artifacts. The device includes protective features (refractory periods) causing blanking periods that may be asynchronous with the event being monitored, resulting in an unacceptable decrease in its sensing capability. Dual chamber sensing, which allows a more accurate determination of the arrhythmic origin, may also be the source of undesirable behavior. Recognition and correction of these iatrogenic behaviors must be incorporated in the device algorithms. Recently developed pacemakers or defibrillators offer diagnostic tools to facilitate the follow-up and allow a better understanding of the rhythm abnormalities. These features are both a complement and a prerequisite for the successful automatic treatment of arrhythmias.

Arrhythmia Recognition

Sensing System

The use of differential amplifiers[4] (the circuit adds up positive input and negative output, thereby eliminating farfield signals with a similar amplitude on each entry but with opposite polarity) provides a significantly better signal to noise ratio. Indeed, the least sensitive the amplifier is to interferences, the greater is the capability of sensing or ampliflying the biological signals of interest. Reliable sensing of fibrillatory signals dictates a programming of the highest available sensitivity in most patients. Bipolar sensing is thus essential,[5] although its systematic use is limited by both the size and the reliability of current electrodes. On the other hand, while bipolar systems may improve sensing, it is not sufficient to eliminate undesirable interferences.[5,7]

Atrial Sensing

Atrial depolarization is known to be associated with large variations in signal amplitude between sinus rhythm, exercise, and arrhythmias[8–10] prompting the systematic programming of the highest sensitivity.[10] Sensing within the atrial chamber is thus susceptible to typical interferences[6] and to sensing the ventricular depolarization.[9,11] It is therefore critical to confirm the atrial origin of all sensed signals. The various elements of atrial sensing by an implantable device will be reviewed.

Refractory Period
A period of absolute blanking is mandatory after each sensed and paced event to prevent repetitive sensing of a single signal. Its duration must be at least 50 ms and 100 ms after sensed and paced events, respectively.

Arrhythmia Detection
Various factors may disturb the detection of arrhythmias, including electrical and electromagnetic interferences, as well as crosstalk from other cardiac chambers. A defibrillator must, therefore, use specific methods to analyze the source of the sensed signal.

Discrimination of interferences may be achieved by the use of recyclable relative refractory periods. By virtue of its higher frequency, a foreign signal has a behavior unlike the sinus node (e.g., 60 Hz occurring 60 times per sec). A minimum protection will, therefore, avoid sensing of all events occurring at a frequency beyond 10 Hz. This protection begins at the end of the absolute refractory period and is recycled with each sensed event, causing thereby an "asynchronous" behavior lasting as long as artifact continues. The sum of both refractory periods (absolute and relative) results in a blanking period of 150 ms after each sensed atrial or ventricular event. One other source of unwanted events consists of spontaneous or paced electrical activity from another cardiac chamber. Ventricular depolarization is quite often sensed by the atrial electrode[9,12] and shares comparable electrical characteristics.[11] This results in double counting,[9] which prevents a correct discrimination of rhythm disturbances. An extension of the atrial refractory period encompassing the PR and QRS intervals is thus necessary. This creates a short atrial refractory period (200–250 ms). This will be of little help in the case of ventricular extrasystoles that may be sensed and interpreted as being of atrial origin since they are not usually preceded by sinus activity. The use of a double chamber system may partially circumvent this problem but may be the source of new problems.[13] Depending on its origin, a spontaneous ventricular depolarization may, indeed, be sensed sequentially in the atrium and in the ventricle.

Crosstalk
Ventricular stimulation offers a different challenge. Atrial refractory periods, triggered by a ventricular pacing stimulus are of long duration, ranging from 200 to 300 ms. No anomalous behavior has been reported with such protection in current pacemakers. However, if the aim is to design a device capable of analyzing rapid atrial rhythms, it becomes essential in a pacemaker-dependent patient to shorten the postventricular atrial refractory period. In

new generation defibrillators, the refractory period that follows ventricular pacing can be kept as short as 100–125 ms. However, in programming the highest atrial sensitivity necessary to reliably sense all episodes of paroxysmal supraventricular tachyarrhythmias, one may also sense in the atrium, near the end of that refractory period, a paced ventricular depolarization that renders an accurate diagnosis impossible. This phenomenon, referred to here as crosstalk, can only be eliminated by refractory periods >140 ms. Special attention must be paid in programming refractory periods since it remains, in all cases, the safest protection against interferences, but excessively long nominal programming becomes a factor limiting the sensing of rhythm disturbances.

Given these preliminary considerations, the special case of tachycardias with a 1:1 atrioventricular relationship is particularly noteworthy. The use of dual chamber defibrillator, as long as atrial and ventricular sensing both remain reliable, will undoubtedly improve the discrimination of atrial and ventricular tachyarrhythmias.[45] The recognition of 1:1 tachycardias remain nevertheless complex. The sudden acceleration of the atrial rate at the onset of the tachycardia has been proposed[14] to separate sinus tachycardia from abnormal rhythms. This criterion is, unfortunately, insufficient by itself since acceleration of sinus rhythm at the onset of exercise may mimic a tachyarrhythmia.[14] Other algorithms have been proposed, for instance, premature atrial stimulation during suspected ongoing tachycardias, allowing the differentiation of atrial tachycardia versus ventricular tachycardia with 1:1 retrograde conduction[16] by examining the stability of the ventricular cycle. These algorithms require extreme precision in the measure of time intervals, and their application is limited to highly stable tachycardias. Finally, in the discussion of 1:1 tachyarrhythmias, mention must be made of pacemaker tachycardia, a classic complication of dual chamber pacing.

Detection of Ventricular Arrhythmias

These considerations pertaining to atrial sensing can be easily applied to ventricular sensed events, except for spontaneous atrial activity that is never detected in the ventricle. Limiting factors consist mostly of sensing of interferences, requiring a specific refractory period, and sensing of atrial pacing stimuli. The latter can be completely eliminated by the systematic use of blanking periods and of safety windows after all atrial pacing stimuli. Signal filtering by specific amplifiers eliminates T wave sensing while preserving electrical characteristics distinct from the QRS of sinus rhythm. This should, therefore, no longer limit the recognition of ventricular arrhythmias.

Template Analysis and Energy Consumption

This discussion has been limited, thus far, to the contraints and limits imposed by rhythm analysis. However, several methods, such as fast Fourier transform, have been proposed to sharpen the recognition of rhythm disorders by morphology analysis.[17,18] Although these various methods are often effective in a laboratory setting, they have never been tested in an implantable device. All require extensive data processing and, therefore, consume much energy. These techniques are inconceivable without the inclusion of a microprocessor in the device. Such components consume as high as 300 to 500 μA per cardiac cycle, which is 20–50 times more than acceptable to guarantee a reasonable device longevity of at least 4–5 years. Some existing devices, however, are based on a variation of this tehnology which consists of powering the microprocessor for only a few milliseconds, just long enough to complete all the calculations needed to handle the cardiac events and the algorithms included in their program.[19] This results in a low usage ratio, which reduces current consumption. Energy drain is reduced to a few μA, consistent with the requirements of technology using traditional components. The implementation of algorithms for morphology analysis will have to be studied, not only from the standpoint of their efficacy, but also from the standpoint of the complexity and repetitiveness of data processing and resulting energy consumption.

Treatment of Rhythm Disturbances

Passive Functions

As discussed earlier, the use of a dual chamber defibrillator in the detection and treatment of arrhythmias may be the source of undesirable behaviors. The device has to recruit a series of functions to protect the ventricles. Indeed, the detection of rapid atrial activity inducing an atrioventricular delay will predictably result in rapid ventricular pacing. The two most common situations consist of pacemaker-mediated reciprocating tachycardia, which requires dedicated methods of diagnosis and treatment, several of which are convincingly efficacious[20,21] versus the development of primary atrial tachyarrhythmias which, in contrast, is more complex because it is not spontaneously suppressible and imposes a ventricular pacing mode switch for the duration of the arrhythmia. Various options have been described ranging from Wenckebach behavior to fallback algorithms or mode switching converting the system to VVI as long as the tachyarrhythmia persists.[22]

Active Functions

Active functions intend to treat arrhythmias rather than to prevent them. Methods can be described as preventive or curative. Preventive methods consist mostly of overdrive VVI pacing,[23] which may suppress the development of ventricular arrhythmias. Likewise, it has been clearly shown that dual chamber pacing, compared to single chamber ventricular pacing, may prevent the emergence of atrial arrhythmias.[24] As for methods of treatment of ongoing arrhythmias, detailed descriptions of various

algorithms are available.[25,26] However, the number of stimulation modes including salvos, long held as the standard autodecremental pacing, subthreshold stimulation,[27] burst scanning,[28] etc., only underlines the persistent complexity of treating arrhythmias by cardiac stimulation. They first imply the capability of consistent capture with a sufficient margin of safety within the range of pacing rates of the antitachycardia program. Furthemore, there is a distinct risk of tachycardia acceleration.[29] Besides this risk which, at the ventricular level, mandates a capability of defibrillation, the issue of long-term efficacy of the antitachycardia algorithm is a recurrent concern because it may vary with known factors, such as drug therapy, or less well understood spontaneous variations in the refractory periods of the areas from which the tachycardia emerges.[30,31]

Follow-Up and Surveillance of Efficacy of Implantable Defibrillator

Regular testing of the chosen antitachycardia pacing protocol is essential. The protocol must be accessible by noninvasive programming of the implanted device which should allow not only to induce the tachycardia in a first step, but also to verify its proper detection and, finally, its automatic interruption by the progam selected. These tests do not, however, guarantee that the tachycardia induced is the same as the one occurring sontaneously and therefore do not guarantee the efficacy of antitachycardia pacing.[30] The automatic treatment of rapid rhythms is particularly relevant in ICDs that offer a large choice of pacing protocols. The device is capable of delivering therapies in sequences and to memorize the successful mode of termination that will be activated first with the next episode of tachycardia. The complexity, not just of the device, but also of its programming, becomes a problem from the standpoint of fully using its capabilities. The device should thus combine this programmability with enough Holter memory to verify the efficacy of the protocol selected, and memorize the information needed to understand the nature of the arrhythmias that have been treated.[32]

Accuracy of Rapid Automatic Identification of Tachyarrhythmias Using Atrioventricular Sequence Analysis

The third generation of ICDs used ventricular intervals or signal morphology to classify tachycardias: rate, PR interval stability, R wave morphology, sudden onset, etc. The criteria allowed a very high sensitivity on monomorphic VT, but many supraventricular arrhythmias were treated, mainly AF and sinus tachycardia.[34–44] Defender 9001 (Ela Médical, France) was the first to use atrial-based criteria to reject supraventricular tachycardia (SVT) from therapy. The activity of dual chamber sensing has been used to differentiate ventricular from supraventricular arrhythmias.[45]

The Algorithm

The algorithm (PARAD, ELA Medical) has been tested and previously published by one of us.[33] It uses atrial and ventricular signals and performs a tiered analysis of the arrhythmia in a three-step fashion: (1) cycle length sorting; (2) majority rhythm identification; and (3) VT/SVT/sinus tachycardia sorting. The algorithm uses four criteria to detect and classify tachyarrhythmias: (a) ventricular rate; (b) stability of the ventricular (V-V) intervals; (c) type of atrioventricular association; and (d) acceleration magnitude and origin.

1. **Cycle length sorting.** This step aims to identify the occurrence of an arrhythmia and to analyze its type. Each ventricular cycle is classified according to its coupling time into one of the following categories: SR (slow rhythm cycle), VT (VT cycle), or VF (VF cycle). The algorithm measures the V-V interval and compares it to two programmable boundaries: the VT cycle length and the VF cycle length. Each cycle is identified as follows: (a) SR cycle, if the corresponding VV interval is longer than both the VT and the VF cycle lengths; (b) VT cycle, if the VV interval is longer than the VF cycle length and shorter than or equal to the VT cycle length; or (c) VF cycle, if the corresponding VV interval is shorter than or equal to the VF cycle length.

2. **Majority rhythm identification.** This uses two programmable parameters: (1) Y number of recent cycles taken into account; and (2) percentage of those cycles. The algorithm identifies three categories of majority rhythm: (a) SR majority is detected when X% of the last Y cycles are classified as SR; (b) VT majority is detected when X% of the last Y cycles are classified as VT or VF; and (c) VF majority is detected when X% of the last Y cycles are classified as VF. This rhythm classification is established after each new cycle and always takes into account the last Y cycles. The values for X and Y are most often programmed to 75% and eight cycles, respectively.

3. **Ventricular tachycardia/supraventricular tachycardia/sinus tachycardia sorting.** Once a VT majority rhythm is identified, this diagnosis is either confirmed or changed to SVT based on stability of the VV intervals and on AV association. Supraventricular tachycardia as defined here includes sinus tachycardia, atrial tachycardia, reentrant SVT, AF, and atrial flutter. The VV intervals are classified as stable if the majority of recent VT or VF intervals

do not vary by more than a programmed maximum limit within. For assessing the AV association, the algorithm measures all the AV intervals within those recent VT or VF cycles. It then identifies whether the AV intervals are stable or unstable. If the intervals are unstable, AV dissociation is diagnosed. In case of stable AV intervals, the next step involves finding the type of AV association i.e., 1:1 or N:1. If there is only one set of stable intervals within the population of analyzed AV intervals, then the AV association is characterized as 1:1. If more than one set of stable AV intervals is found for a given number of VV cycles, the AV association is classified as N:1. The procedure is as follows:

a. VV stablity: to assess this criterion, the algorithm constructs the histogram of VV intervals of cycles classified as VT or VF, out of the last Y ventricular cycles. The algorithm scans the VV interval histogram with a window set to a programmed width (63 ms), looking for the position of the window which encompasses a maximum number of intervals in the histogram. When it finds that position, it counts the number of VV intervals in the window. if this number is greater than or equal to X% of Y (in this case programmed to 75% of 8); the rhythm is classified as stable. In this case, further analysis is done to discriminate VT from SVT. All tachycardias with an unstable ventricular rhythm are classified as AF and no additionnal criterion is required.

b. AV association: this criterion is evaluated only if the assessment of VV stablity leads to the conclusion that VV intervals are stable. To evaluate the atrioventricular association criterion, the algorithm uses the VV interval histogram already constructed for assessing stability and constructs an AV interval histogram corresponding to the cycles stored within the VV histogram. Up to five AV intervals can be stored for each VV cycle. This in fact corresponds to the memorizing capabilities of the device. For example if the ratio is 5:1, 5 AV intervals will be stored for one VV interval. Like the VV histogram, the AV interval histogram is scanned with a 63 ms window. AV association is defined as established when the ratio of the number of stable AV intervals to the number of stable VV intervals is greater or equal to X% (here 75%). When AV association is established, it is further classified as 1:1 when the ratio of the number of stable AV intervals to the total number of AV intervals in the histogram is greater or equal to 75%; otherwise, it is classified as N:1 (Figures 2 and 3).

Analysis of Clinically Induced Tachycardias

This algorithm was prospectively evaluated in 156 episodes of induced sustained (duration of greater than or equal to 6 sec) tachycardias.[33] Among these, 89 episodes from 43 patients were taken from the Ann Arbor electrogram libraries (Ann Arbor, MI). The other 67 arrhythmias were recorded in 50 patients during electrophysiological studies performed for the diagnosis of clinical arrhythmias.

Nominal settings for this study have been chosen as 63 ms for definition of stability and 75% for the value of stable RR because in our previous (unpublished) experience, these were the values for which the sensitivity for VT detection was 100%.

In this study, out of the 85 episodes of VT, a correct diagnosis was made in 82 cases, giving a sensitivity of 96%. The device failed to diagnose VT in three cases. In one case,

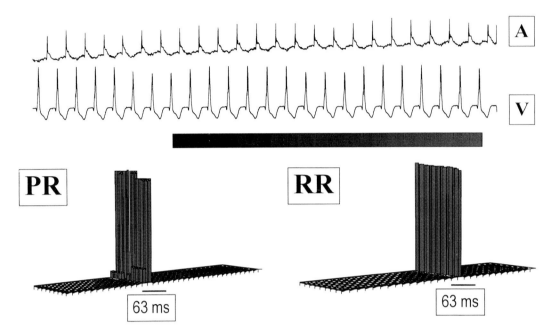

Figure 2. Example of 1:1 AV association. Use of the VV stability criterion (right) resulted in the conclusion that there were stable VV intervals. The number of stable AV intervals in these VV cycles is identified by scanning the AV histogram with a 63-ms window (left) AV association is identified. The ratio of the number of stable AV intervals to the number of VV interval is >75%. the ratio of number of stable AV intervals to the total number of AV intervals is however >75% (8 out of 8) and the association is classified as 1:1.

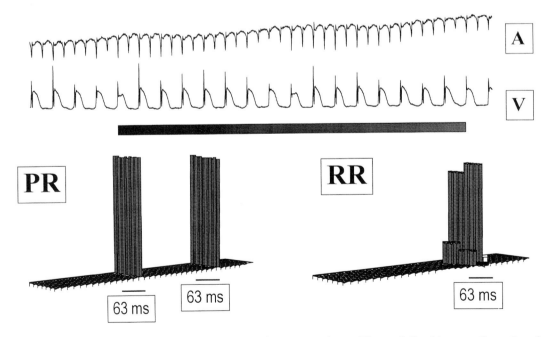

Figure 3. Example of N:1 AV association. Analysis is similar to Figure 2. In this case, the ratio of the number of stable AV to the number of VV intervals is again >75%. The ratio of number of stable AV intervals to the total number of AV intervals in any 63 ms is, however, <75% (8/16) and the association is classified as N:1.

the error was due to a slow VT with a cycle length of 560 ms, whereas the programmed lower limit for VT detection was 500 ms. In another case, VT with a cycle length of 420 ms was erroneously classified because of unstable VV cycles. In the third case, oversensing in the ventricle occurred due to tape artifacts. Three episodes of AF occurring in three patients with WPW syndrome were detected as stable, dissociated, and therefore diagnosed as VT because the rapidity of the ventricular response led to VV interval variations that were less than that required for classification as unstable VV cycles. One case of atrial flutter was wrongly labelled as stable with no AV association, because of noise in the atrial channel. The specificity of the algorithm for diagnosing VT was thus 94%. In none of the episodes, the detection time was more than 5 sec.

All 22 episodes of ventricular flutter or fibrillation were correctly identified, and there was no instance of SVT being misdiagnosed as VF. Thus, the sensitivity and specificity for VF diagnosis were 100%. The mean VF detection time was 2.1 ± 0.4 sec (range 1.5–2.9 sec).

In this study, there were 12 episodes of bi-tachycardia (7 VTs and 2 VFs with AF episodes, and 3 VTs with associated atrial flutter episodes). Out of these 12, 11 were correctly identified as VT. In one case, fast VT (VV cycles = 360 ms) was associated by AF and an N:1 association was detected, leading to erroneous diagnosis of SVT.

Out of the 15 episodes of AF, 12 were correctly identified. As mentioned previously, three episodes in three patients with the WPW syndrome were diagnosed as VT. Their VV cycle length were, repectively, 270, 310, and 330 ms and because the irregularity criterions best applies to relatively lower rhythms, they were detected as stable and dissociated. The mean detection time for AF was 3.1 ± 1.9 sec (range 2.4–6.8 sec).

Out of the 12 cases of atrial flutter, six were correctly identified. In five episodes in four patients, because every second atrial electrogram fell in the postventricular atrial absolute refractory period, the episodes were classified as stable tachycardia having a 1:1 AV association and were not further classified. In another patient, an episode of atrial flutter was detected as stable without AV association because of noise in the atrial channel. The mean detection time for atrial flutter was 2.9 ± 3.1 sec (range 2.2–12.2 sec).

All 10 cases of these arrhythmias were not identified as such but classified as being stable with 1: 1 AV association. The mean detection time in this case was 2.4 ± 0.7 sec (1.7–3.5 sec). Further sorting of these rhythms would require analysis of acceleration magnitude and chamber of origin, which could not be used in this study, as mentioned earlier.

Using an algorithm that incorporated analysis of AV association in addition to the rate and stability criteria, it has been possible to achieve a sensitivity of 97% and a specificity of 98% for the diagnosis of ventricular arrhythmias with nominal programming parameters. This algorithm was also able to identify AF with a positive predictive value of 92% and atrial flutter episodes with a positive predictive value of 86%. Apart from one instance of erroneous diagnosis due to an episode of VT failing to meet the rate criterion and another one due to technically defective signals, the only case of VT in which the diagnosis was erroneous occurred in a patient with fast VT and AF. In this case, N:1 association was detected and the tachycardia was classified as supraventricular. More importantly, except for AF occurring in three patients with WPW syndrome and one case of atrial flutter with noise in the atrial channel, no case of SVT was classified as a ventricular arrhythmia. This should lead to a substantial reduction in the number of inappropriate shocks. In addition, the arrhythmias encountered in the WPW syndrome could have been eliminated from this study since arrhythmias associated with this syndrome represent contraindications to ICD implant.

An added advantage of this algorithm over the previously tested dual chamber analysis has been the ability to accurately classify bi-tachycardias in the VT zone.

Eleven out of 12 episodes of tachycardia were correctly classified in this study. One of the concerns when using complex algorithms has been the possibility of having longer detection times. The mean VT and VF detection times were, however, quite short. In none of the episodes of VT or VF the detection time was more than 5 sec.

Preliminary Clinical Experience with the First Dual Chamber Pacemaker Defibrillator

The initial clinical experience with the first dual chamber pacemaker defibrillator (Defender 9001, ELA Medical, France) has been recently reported.[45a] This device has two leads, one ventricular and one atrial, enabling the identification of arrhythmias on a dual chamber basis before delivering appropriate shock therapy, and also providing dual chamber pacing in the DDD or DDI modes. The combined detection of atrial and ventricular activities makes it possible to classify tachycardias according to the PARAD algorithm described above.[45a,46]

In the context of a French multicenter study,[45a] the new ICD was implanted in 18 patients (15 men, 3 women, mean age of 55 ± 15 years). The indications for implantation were sudden cardiac death secondary to VT, or spontaneous symptomatic ventricular arrhythmias refractory to drug therapy. All patients had a life expectancy longer than 1 year, and their arrhythmias did not stem from any acute, short-lived etiology and were not related to AF. Ten patients suffered from coronary disease (nine with past myocardial infarction), six patients had dilated cardiomyopathy, and another patient had hypertrophic cardiomyopathy. One patient was diagnosed as suffering from arrhythmogenic right ventricular dysplasia. The mean left ventricular ejection fraction was $35\% \pm 11\%$.

All of the devices were implanted abdominally. In most cases, two endocardial leads were sufficient to ensure the success of shock therapies (two successful shocks on VF at 20 J). Three patients required a subcutaneous patch and one an epicardial patch. Furthermore, an old pulse generator connected to epicardial leads and patches was replaced in one patient. The lead system was retained, but supplemented with additional endocardial leads for bipolar atrial detection.

Sixteen of the 18 ICD patients were available to follow-up. One patient died during the implantation procedure, and another, who had received the ICD in spite of high defibrillation thresholds, had to be excluded from the protocol due to an inadequate safety margin.

Post-implantation evaluation using the noninvasive induction of ventricular arrhythmias enhanced the induction of 27 VFs, 8 ventricular flutters, and 38 VTs: all of these arrhythmias were correctly identified by the devices and treated accordingly. Interestingly, during the treadmill test systematically performed after implantation, 13 patients accelerated their heart rate above the rate programmed for VT detection. In all cases, the devices appropriately identified the sinus tachycardia and thus did not deliver VT therapy.

During mean follow-up of 7.1 ± 4.5 months, 176 arrhythmia episodes were stored in the Holter function of the device. All arrhythmias were reviewed by the investigators who diagnosed 7 SVT, 44 sinus tachycardias, and 122 VTs/VFs, with one episode probably related to atrial fibrillation that could not be positively identified. These diagnoses showed that the algorithm had correctly identified 173 of the 175 arrhythmic episodes (Figures 4 and 5). The two poorly identified episodes consisted in AF and flutter with very rapid atrioventricular conduction, which were confused with a VT (stable RR intervals).

Fourteen VFs were efficiently treated by the first shock delivered. Out of the 63 episodes, 51 were interrupted by ATP, whereas 12 required shock therapy after ATP failure. All the symptomatic ventricular arrhyth-

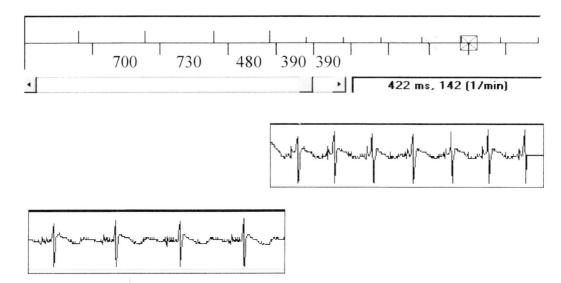

Figure 4. Programmer display demonstrating onset of SVT diagnosed as 1:1. **Top**: atrial markers, (above line) and ventricular markers (below line) events, with calipers. **Middle**: Stored AV electrograms during confirmation. **Bottom**: Electrogram after sinus rhythm resumption.

mias requiring shock therapy were identified as such and treated accordingly.

Complications included two atrial lead displacements and one ventricular oversensing. The latter was due to old defective epicardial detection leads, reused with adapters. These leads were therefore abandoned and a new endocardial lead was used for ventricular detection and pacing. Concerning the lead displacements, only one case required repositioning while the other was treated by reprogramming the device in the VVI mode. At the end of follow-up, 10 devices were programmed in the DDD

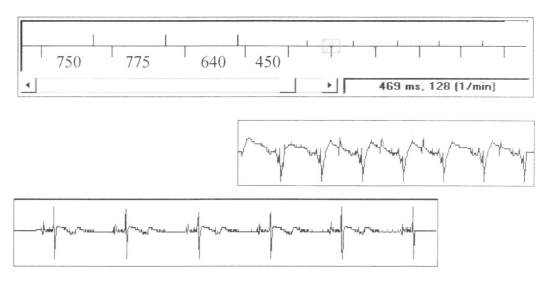

Figure 5. Programmer display demonstrating onset of tachycardia diagnosed as ventricular with 1:1 AV association. Layout as in Figure 4.

mode, five in the DDI mode, and one in the VVI mode.

This study aimed to verify whether a new identification algorithm based on dual chamber atrioventricular detection analysis decreased the number of inappropriately delivered shock therapies. All the ventricular arrhythmias were correctly diagnosed. Only three cases of SVT were mistaken for VTs, with shock therapy being delivered as a result. The percentage of inappropriate therapies was thus 3.8% (vs. 12%–15% in the literature for single chamber ICDs.[46–52] The percentage of patients concerned by this problem was 18% (vs. 34% in the literature[46–52]). In spite of the small number of patients in this series, the results of which can only be considered as preliminary, its seems that the atrioventricular detection of arrhythmias offered by this new algorithm considerably improves the reliability of such devices. The presence of two detection leads obviously increases the risk of lead displacement, as was demonstrated in this series. Furthermore, the algorithm requires some additional improvements, particularly to preclude a diagnosis of VT, when, in fact, the patient is suffering from undersensed AV. Nevertheless, dual chamber pacing represents a notable advance for many patients with a precarious hemodynamic state who required pacing.[53] Hopefully, in the future, this dual chamber pacing will also incorporate rate response.

In March 1997, 70 patients have been implanted with an ICD Defender 9001. Analyzed data are in the process of being published. In summary, 308 tachycardia events were documented by the implanted devices during follow-up; 160 episodes with rapid and highly regular ventricular rates were treated by the device, 13 of which were diagnosed by the physician as AF and atrial flutter. All of those episodes were classified as stable and dissociated tachycardias. Algorithm PARAD has been improved to a new algorithm PARAD+ which will be tested and incorporated in the next Defender generation.

Conclusion

The dual chamber sensing of VTs in the development of implantable defibrillators is an effective improvement. The challenges offered by this technology pertain not only to the proper detection and identification of arrhythmias but also to the choice of antitachycardia algorithms which cannot be guaranteed to remain efficacious. The concept of mutiple programs delivered in sequence until successful treatment seems often necessary. The need for diagnostic functions to study the mechanisms and incidence of arrhythmic episodes, as well as the behavior and response of antitachycardia pacing, is necessary to optimize the follow-up and programming of the device. One should not forget, however, that the very interpretation of the diagnostics depends on the detection (refractory periods) and pacing characteristics. Furthermore, an automatic device can only be conceived under the close surveillance of a physician whose expertise and interpretation of the data cannot be replaced by the existing technology.

References

1. Saksena S, Munsif AN, Prakash A, et al. Future directions for implantable defibrillation devices. In Saksena S, Luderitz B, eds. Interventional Electrophysiology (2nd edition). Futura Publishing Co, Armonk, NY, 1996, p 617.
2. Brooks R, Garan A, McGovern BA, et al. Implantation of transvenous non thoracotomy cardioverter defibrillator systems in patients with permanent endocardial pacemakers. Am Heart J 1995;129:1165–1170.
3. Calkins H, Brinker J, Veltri E, et al. Clinical interactions between pacemakers and AICDs. J Am Coll Cardiol 1990;16:666–673.
4. De Boer H, Kofflard M, Scholtes T, et al. Differential bipolar sensing of a dual chamber pacemaker. PACE 1988;11:158.
5. Mond HG. Unipolar versus bipolar pacing—poles apart. PACE 1991;14:1411.
6. Gross JN, Ritacco R, Andrews C, et al. The clinical relevance of electromyopotential

oversensing in current unipolar devices. PACE 1992;15:2023.

7. Sweesy MW, Batey RL, Forney RC. Crosstalk during bipolar pacing. PACE 1988;11:1512.

8. Waldo AL, Henthorn RW, Plumb VJ. Relevance of electrograms and transient entrainment for antitachycardia devices. PACE 1984;7:588.

9. Barold SS, Falkoff MD, Ong LS, et al. Double sensing by atrial automatic tachycardia-terminating pulse generator. PACE 1987;10:58.

10. Cazeau S, Ritter P, Kojoukharow Y, et al. Is it possible to optimally program a dual chamber pacemaker without performing an exercise test? PACE 1993;16:919.

11. Kleinert M, Elmqvist H, Strandberg H. Spectral properties of atrial and ventricular endocardial signals. PACE 1979;2:11.

12. Shandling HA, Florio S, Castellanet MJ, et al. Physical determinant of the endocardial P-wave. PACE 1990;13:1585.

13. Arzbaecher R, Bump T, Jenkins J, et al. Automatic tachycardia recognition. PACE 1984;7:541.

14. Camm AJ, Davies DW, Ward DE. Tachycardia recognition by implantable electronics devices. PACE 1987;10:1175.

15. Fisher JD, Goldstein M, Ostrow E, et al. Maximum rate of tachycardia development: sinus tachycardia with sudden exercise vs spontaneous ventricular tachycardia. PACE 1986;6:221.

16. Munkenbeck FC, Bump TE, Arzbaecher RC. Differentiation of sinus tachycardia from paroxysmal 1:1 tachycardias using a single late diastolic extrastimulus. PACE 1996;9:53.

17. Throne RD, DiCarlo LA, Jenkins JM, et al. Paroxysmal bundle branch block of supraventricular origin: a possible source of misdiagnosis in detecting ventricular tachycardia using time domain analyses of intraventricular electrograms. PACE 1990;13:453.

18. DiCarlo L, Jenkins JM, Chiang CMJ, et al. Ventricular tachycardia detection using electrogram analysis in specific sites. PACE 1992;15:2154.

19. Jacobson P, Dalmolin R. Procédé et dispositif de commande d'un appareil ou instrument notamment un stimulateur cardiaque implantable (brevet d'invention). In Institut National de la Propriété Industrielle. Imprimerie nationale. Paris, France. #2492262.

20. Limousin M, Bonnet JL, and the Investigators of the Multi-center Study. A new algorithm to solve endless loop tachycardia: a multi-center study of 91 patients. PACE 1990;13:867.

21. Cazeau S, Bonnet JL, Ritter P, et al. Impact of programming short PVARPs on the epidemiology of endless-loop tachycardia in DDD mode. Eur JCPE 1993;3:123.

22. Ritter P, Cazeau S, Kojoukharov Y, et al. Critical analysis of the different algorithms designed to protect the paced patient against atrial tachyarrhythmias. In Aubert AE, Ector H, et al. eds. Cardiac Pacing and Electrophysiology. Kluwer Academic Publishers, Dordrecht, Germany, 1994, p 355.

23. Fischer JD, Teichman S, Ferrick A, et al. Antiarrhythmic effect of VVI pacing at physiologic rates: a crossover controlled evaluation. PACE 1987;10:822.

24. Attuel P, Pellegrin D, Mugica J, et al. DDD pacing: an effective treatment modality for recurrent atrial arrhythmias. PACE 1988;11:1647.

25. Fischer JD, Furman S, Kim SG, et al. Tachycardia management by devices. In Barold S, Mugica J, eds. New Perspectives in Cardiac Pacing. Futura Publishing Co, Armonk, NY, 1991, p 359.

26. Holt P, Cride JCP, Sowton E. Antitachycardia pacing. A comparison of burst overdrive, self-searching and adaptative table scanning overdrive. PACE 1986;9:490.

27. Shenasa M, Cardinal R, Kus T, et al. Termination of sustained ventricular tachycardia by ultrarapid subthreshold stimulation in humans. Circulation 1988;78:1135.

28. Palakurthy P, Slater D. Automatic implantable scanning burst pacemakers for recurrent tachyarrhythmias. PACE 1988;11:185.

29. Fisher JD, Mehra R, Furman S. Termination of ventricular tachycardia with bursts of ventricular pacing. Am J Cardiol 1994;41:97.

30. Vertongen P, Van Wassenhove E, Jordaens L. Antitachycardia pacing for supraventricular tachycardia: limited long-term efficacy due to atrial fibrillation. Eur JCPE 1992;2:90.

31. Ehrlich S, Shandling A, Crump R, et al. Efficacy of pacemaker tachycardia termination algorithm: is electrophysiological testing alone adequate? PACE 1993;16:978.

32. Jung W, Mletzko R, Manz M, et al. Long-term therapy of antitachycardia pacing for supraventricular tachycardia. PACE 1992;15:179.

33. Nair M, Saoudi N, Kroiss D, et al. Automatic arrhythmia identification using analysis of the atrioventricular association: application to a new generation of implantable defibrillators. Circulation 1997;95:967.

34. Kelly PA, Cannom DS, Garan H, et al. The automatic implantable cardioverter-defibrillator: efficacy, complications and survival in patients with malignant ventricular arrhythmias. J Am Coll Cardiol 1988;11:1278–1286.

35. Nunain SO, Roelke M, Trouton T, et al. Limitations and late complications of third generation cardioverter-defibrillators. Circulation 1995;91:2204–2213.

36. CEDARS Investigators. Comprehensive

evaluation of defibrillators and resuscitative shocks (Cedars) study: Does atrial fibrillation increase the incidence of inappropriate shock by implanted defibrillators? J Am Coll Cardiol 1993;21:278A.

37. Swerdlow CD, Chen PS, Kass RM, et al. Discrimination of ventricular tachycardia from sinus tachycardia in a tiered therapy cardioverter-defibrillator. J Am Coll Cardiol 1994;23:1342–1355.

38. Swerdlow CD, Ahren T, Chen PS, et al. Underdetection of ventricular tachycardia by algorithms to enhance specificity in a tiered-therapy cardioverter-defibrillator. J Am Coll Cardiol 1994;24:416–424.

39. Cohen TJ, Liem LB. A hemodynamically responsive antitachycardia system: development and basis for design in humans. Circulation 1990;82:394–406.

40. Schuger CD, Jackson K, Russel TS, et al. Atrial sensing to augment ventricular tachycardia detection by the automatic implantable cardioverter defibrillator: a utility study. PACE 1988;11:1456–1464.

41. Leong PHW, Jabri MA. Arrhythmia classification using two intracardiac leads. IEEE 1992;29:751.

42. Polikaitis A, Arzbaecher R. Sensitivity and specificity of a dual-chamber arrhythmia recognition algorithm for implantable devices. J Electrocardiol 1995;27:78–83.

43. Arzbaecher R, Bump T, Jenkins J, et al. Automatic tachycardia recognition. PACE 1984;7:541–547.

44. Chiang CMJ, Jenkings JM, DiCarlo LA. The value of rate stability and multiplicity measures to detect ventricular tachycardia in the presence of atrial fibrillation or flutter. PACE 1994;17:1503–1508..

45. Saoudi N, Henri C, Brugada P, et al. Automatic ventricular tachycardia recognition during sustained rapid rhythms: superiority of dual chamber over single chamber ventricular monitoring. PACE 1994;17:112A.

45a.Lavergne T, Daubert JC, Chauvin M, et al. Prelimary clinical experience with the first dual chamber pacemaker defibrillator. PACE 1997;20:182–188.

46. Bardy GH, Hofer B, Johnson G, et al. Implantable transvenous cardioverter-defibrillators. Circulation 1993;87:1152–1168.

47. Grimm W, Flores BF, Marchlinski FE, et al. Electrocardiographically documented unnecessary, spontaneous shocks in 241 patients with implantable cardioverter defibrillators. PACE 1992;15:1667–1673.

48. Hook BG, Callans DJ, Kleiman RB, et al. Implantable cardioverter-defibrillator therapy in the absence of significant symptoms: rhythm diagnosis and management aided by stored electrogram analysis. Circulation 1993;87:1897–1906.

49. Fromer M, Brachmann J, Block M, et al. Efficacy of automatic multimodal device therapy for ventricular tachyarrhythmias as delivered by a new implantable pacing cardioverter-defibrillator. Results of a European multicenter study of 102 implants. Circulation 1992;86:363–374.

50. O'Nunain S, Roelke M, Trouton T, et al. Limitations and late complications of third-generation automatic cardioverter-defibrillators. Circultation 1995;91:2204–2213.

51. Bocker D, Block M, Isbruch F, et al. Comparison of frequency of aggravation of ventricular tachyarrhythmias after implantation of automatic defibrillators using epicardial versus nonthoracotomy lead systems. Am J Cardiol 1993;71:1064.

52. Reiter MJ, Mann DE: Sensing and tachyarrhythmia detection problems in implantable cardioverter defibrillators. J Cardiovasc Electrophysiol 1996;7:542–548.

53. Geelen P, Chauvin M, Roul G, et al. The value of DDD pacing in implantable defibrillators [Abstract]. Eur JCPE 1996;6:275A.

Chapter 19

Future Implantable Defibrillator Technologies

Edwin G. Duffin

Introduction

The implantable cardioverter-defibrillator has evolved from a 160-cc, nonprogrammable, shock-only device requiring placement by thoracotomy to a multiprogrammable, antitachy/antibrady pacemaker-like device with extensive data memories and a volume of less than 55 cm³. Figure 1 contrasts defibrillator volume and weight reductions with pacemaker evolution. Longevity has been extended from less than 30 months[1] to projections of 9 years,[2] and electrode systems have progressed from epicardial shock delivery patches with separate unipolar rate-sensing leads to single multifunction catheters. This impressive transformation occurred in a period of about 11 years, and many opportunities for improvement remain. New technology for high-voltage output capacitors will significantly increase energy storage density yielding meaningful reduction in capacitor and generator size. Electronic circuitry will be more densely packed and made to operate on less power to enhance defibrillator longevity and facilitate further size reduction. Lead systems, the weakest link in defibrillator system reliability, are bulky, relatively inefficient, subject to rising thresholds, fractures, and dislodgement[3]; they present considerable opportunity for improvement. Programmers are physically cumbersome, slow, and complex, making manipulation of the devices and processing of the increasing amounts of stored data inconvenient and time consuming. Additional implantable system features are needed to assist with management of the ventricular tachycardia (VT)/ventricular fibrillation (VF) patients' co-morbidities of bradycardia, atrial fibrillation, and heart failure. Up-front therapeutic costs are high. As technology improves, therapy costs decline, and studies beyond MADIT[4] and AVID[5] are completed, it is probable that indications for defibrillator implantation will continue to expand.

Implantable Cardioverter-Defibrillators

Arrhythmia Detection

False positive arrhythmia detections occur in 16%–53% of implantable defibrillator patients,[11,12] and can have serious proarrhythmic consequences with a reported incidence ranging up to 8%.[9] Many of these

From Singer I, Barold SS, Camm AJ (eds): Nonpharmacological Therapy of Arrhythmias for the 21st Century: The State of the Art. Futura Publishing Co, Inc., Armonk, NY, © 1998.

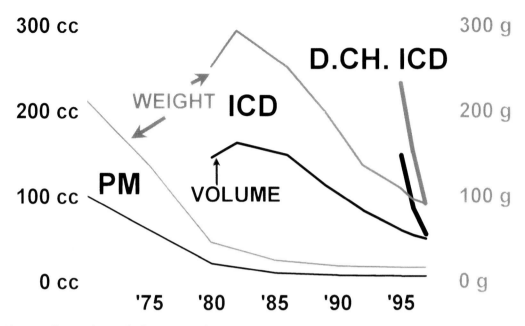

Figure 1. Pacemaker and ICD size trends. Progressive reductions in implantable defibrillator volume and weight are contrasted with the corresponding progress made earlier with implantable pacemakers. The two curves at the lower left of the figure represent pacemaker weights and volumes, the middle pair of curves represent single chamber defibrillator weights and volumes, and the two curves at the upper right represent dual chamber defibrillator weights and volumes.

detection errors can be eliminated by suitable programming.[10] Stability and onset algorithms have been developed to deal with atrial fibrillation and sinus tachycardia, and they help,[11,12] but many physicians are unwilling to apply these algorithms either because of the effort required to determine appropriate settings for the algorithms or for fear that they might reduce sensitivity to VT and VF. An obvious candidate for improving discrimination is morphology analysis. The initial foray into such an approach, the probability density function, has been abandoned. A more recently introduced morphology analysis evaluates the width of sensed ventricular electrograms, and withholds therapy if a percentage of the measured complexes are narrow.[13–15] In the clinical trial this algorithm provided an 88% increase in specificity while reducing VT sensitivity by 2%.[16] More complex morphology analyses present a challenge given the relatively limited processing power of the energy-efficient microprocessors used in implantable devices. However, care in selection of filters and sampling rates[17] and selection of computationally efficient algorithms[18] should permit use of more advanced waveform analyses in future designs.

The detection approach that is most natural and appealing to clinicians is to add atrial electrogram analysis to the detection algorithm, and the introduction of dual chamber implantable defibrillators makes this practicable.[19] Approaches will vary among devices, but one example of a dual chamber arrhythmia detection algorithm demonstrated excellent results in lab tests.[20] Yet despite use of timing and morphology analyses, even this sophisticated approach was imperfect, encountering problems distinguishing sinus tachycardia from paroxysmal supraventricular tachycardia (SVT) or VT and SVT with aberrancy from VT with retrograde atrial activation. And, of course, lab simulations are usually spared the complications of lead dislodgements, and algorithm evaluation in isolation does not reveal limitations imposed by the addition of pacemaker function. Acute testing of a prototype dual chamber implantable defibrillator was accomplished using a large series of recorded human arrhythmias,[21] a method that accounts for some of the pacing system refractory periods and timing restrictions. The algorithm had positive predictive values for diagnosis of atrial fibrillation and flutter of 92% and 86%, respectively. The values for VT and VF were 95% and 100%. Acute human testing in real-time allows evaluation of the entire defibrillator system, including leads, pacing functions, refractory periods, and patient interactions with the device. Such tests of a prototype dual chamber implantable defibrillator[22,23] showed no adverse interactions between pacing and arrhythmia detection processes. Detection was appropriate in 34 out of 35 atrial tachyarrhythmia episodes in 23 patients, and there were no false positive detections of episode termination. VT/VF detection was appropriate in 26 of 26 episodes in 13 patients, and inappropriate detection of VT/VF was prevented in 28 of 37 episodes of SVT. Availability of dual chamber implantable defibrillators will improve arrhythmia detection, but clinicians must remember that these analyses are accomplished by computer algorithms which, however sophisticated, will never replicate the performance of an expert electrophysiologist.

As improved algorithms reduce the incidence of inappropriate shocks for AF, SVT, and sinus tachycardia, increased effort will need to be focused on reducing inappropriate shocks associated with nonsustained arrhythmias,[24-26] since these will become, by process of elimination, a more significant cause of unwarranted therapy.

Fibrillation Therapy

The introduction of various biphasic waveforms was a major contributor to reduced defibrillation thresholds,[27] yet the reasons for their success remain unclear,[28] making the task of optimization difficult. Clearly, manipulation of the energy storage capacitor value,[29] the output voltage, pulse duration, and tilt[30] can vary defibrillation thresholds, but it is not clear that there is one ideal waveform for all lead system configurations and resistances.[31,32] Programmable options might easily be offered, but physicians will be loath to perform the requisite VF inductions to evaluate the combinations and permutations needed to determine the optimum waveform for each patient. Moreover, as lead system impedance changes,[33] the ideal settings may vary, suggesting that the optimization might best be accomplished automatically in real-time by the implanted device using an algorithm that considers capacitor size and lead impedance.[34,35] Research continues, and there is reason to believe that waveform modifications will further reduce threshold.[36-39]

Other therapy modifications to reduce defibrillation thresholds have been proposed or are being investigated. Examples include: timing of shock delivery based on VF electrogram characteristics,[40,41] delivery during a specific respiratory phase,[42] and preconditioning the tissue with a second high-energy shock,[43] or a brief train of 50 Hz pacing pulses.[44] The latter has been reported to reduce canine defibrillation energy thresholds by 20%. It is also conceivable that autonomic manipulation may eventually be used to lower defibrillation thresholds[45] using drug administration systems or electrical stimulation.

Effort will be needed to prevent increases in defibrillator charge times, a natural tendency in the quest for smaller devices. If single-cell power sources with reduced surface area electrodes are used, extra care must be taken to prevent excessive charge times. The drive to the use of lower output devices creates additional pressure on the need to retain short charge times. Charge time typically increases significantly as the implantable defibrillator battery depletes. If the device must cycle more than once to treat an arrhythmia the defibrillation threshold may be significantly higher than the value that was measured at implant, simply because of the longer duration of VF,[46] a factor that has been reported to be pronounced at lower energy levels.[47] Moreover, from a patient's perspective, automobile driving limitations can be a major negative side effect of tachyarrhythmias and implantable defibrillator therapy. Many patients are likely to ignore driving restrictions,[48,49] and a device that allows loss of consciousness can be particularly problematic for them.

It was inevitable that defibrillation therapy would be extended beyond the treatment of sudden death survivors, and major steps have been taken with the initiation of clinical studies of three defibrillators designed to treat atrial fibrillation. One, intended to treat AF only,[50] provides atrial defibrillation capability with shocks of up to 3 J in the original units, and up to 6 J in more recent versions. The other two, one of which is shown in Figure 2, incorporate atrial defibrillation capability of more than 28 J, and also provide DDD antibradycardia pacing, pacing algorithms for prevention

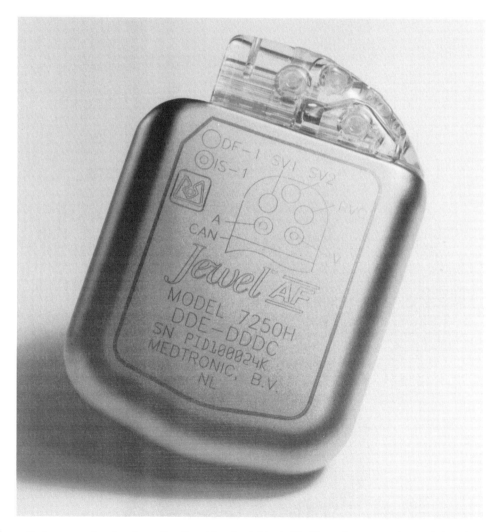

Figure 2. An example of an investigational implantable defibrillator incorporating atrial and ventricular defibrillation capabilities. This 55-cc device also provides antitachycardia pacing algorithms for atrial arrhythmia management and DDD pacing.

and termination of atrial arrhythmias, anti-tachy pacing for VT, and ventricular defi-brillation.[51,52] It is too early to predict the role of implantable atrial defibrillation, but the biggest hurdle will probably be the issue of patient acceptance of painful shocks.[53–55] An alternative painless approach, such as a drug infusion system, might provide significant competition, and a practicable transvenous ablative cure would surely limit the role of both pharmacological and electrical atrial defibrillators.

Arrhythmia Prevention

The ideal therapy would prevent arrhyth-mias yet, despite great interest in this goal, there has been little progress toward a prac-tical approach. Emerging defibrillators with dual chamber pacing capability, either DDD or DDDR, may confer some degree of ar-rhythmia prevention and some investiga-tional devices offer rate stabilization algo-rithms for the atria or ventricles. These stabilization modes accelerate brady pacing rate following early ectopic events and then provide a gradual rate decline to the basal programmed value. Clinical availability of devices embodying such algorithms will fa-cilitate evaluation of these concepts.

Multi-site atrial pacing is currently under investigation as a means for preventing atrial fibrillation,[56–58] though results remain tentative, and much work needs to be done to evaluate the various electrode locations and pacing algorithms that might be used.

Perhaps a combination device[59] offering drug delivery for prevention, but having backup ventricular defibrillation capability will be a viable alternative. As examples, pericardial instillation of amiodarone has been reported to suppress AF,[60] L-arginine has been reported to reduce the severity of ventricular arrhythmias during sympa-thetic stimulation in dogs with acute coro-nary occlusions,[61] and pharmacological blockade of the left stellate ganglion via a drug pump was reported to be successful in the treatment of long QT syndrome.[62]

Bradycardia Therapies

Defibrillators with dual chamber anti-bradycardia pacing are now available com-mercially outside the United States and sev-eral manufacturers are conducting studies of such units in the US. The first DDD im-plantable defibrillator[63] was implanted in early 1995 and had a volume of 148 cc. This was followed in September 1996 by an 85-cc unit.[64] In October 1996 a 69-cc unit was introduced,[52] followed in January 1997 by a 55-cc unit,[65] both adding atrial defibrillation capability. These units will soon be sup-planted with devices offering DDDR pacing (Figure 3), and there will be companion sin-gle chamber rate responsive devices. Inte-grated dual chamber capability facilitates improvement in arrhythmia detection algo-rithms and also eases the transition to atrial tachyarrhythmia therapeutic capabilities.

Defibrillator antibrady functions will be-come as sophisticated as those in standard pacemakers, embracing all of the auto-mated parameter manipulations that have become the norm for pacemakers. Auto-matic adjustment of rate responsiveness, AV intervals, output energy, mode switch-ing, and the like will simplify programming and increase patient safety and comfort.

Monitoring

Implantable defibrillator memories are growing rapidly. Some devices now have random access memories of a quarter of a megabyte, providing substantial documen-tation of patient and device status. Eventu-ally these devices will include complete am-bulatory rhythm recorder/analyzers. Dual chamber electrograms, patient clinical data, programming histories, and expanded troubleshooting data will all be stored in the device memory. But perhaps the most inter-esting new use of memory capability will be in managing patients' co-morbidities.

The majority of defibrillator patients have some degree of pump dysfunction. Indeed, if the implantable defibrillator successfully

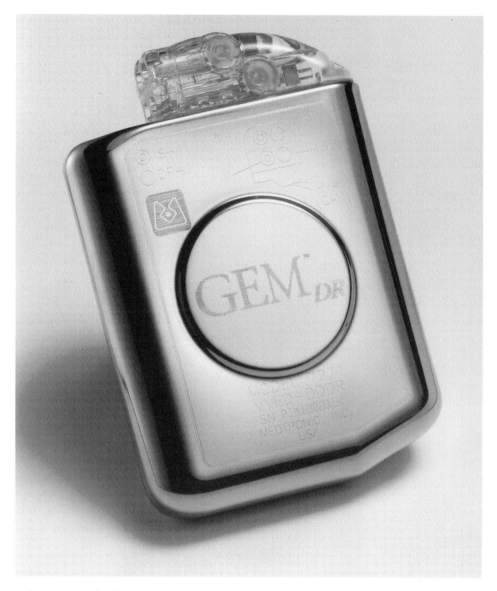

Figure 3. An example of an investigational implantable defibrillator providing DDDR pacing and dual chamber electrogram analysis for arrhythmia detection. This 62-cc device also provides automatic daily painless evaluation of pacing and high-voltage electrodes by means of a subthreshold pulse delivered during the tissue refractory period associated with sensed and paced events.

defers arrhythmic death, the likelihood of progressive heart failure is increased. It would therefore seem appropriate to include mechanisms in the implantable defibrillator to help manage this co-morbidity. Progress is being made in the development of implantable catheters capable of chronic measurement of oxygen saturation and pressure in the right ventricle.[66] Once sensor reliability is assured, consideration of clinical value must be addressed.[67] Early experience with a device intended solely for monitoring heart failure has been encouraging[68,69] and, inclusion of equivalent monitoring capability in future implantable defibrillators is likely. Extension of the parameters beyond oxygen and pressure is also highly probable. One possibility might be a right ventricular catheter-based accelerometer which has been reported to provide data reflecting left ventricular contractility[70] or global ventricular contractility.[71] Respiratory rate and daily activity levels, currently obtained and used for rate-responsive pacing, might also prove useful in evaluating patient status and heart failure therapy efficacy. When fully developed, these advanced implantable systems might spare their bearers the need for invasive monitoring instrumentation when the inevitable hospitalizations occur. A somewhat larger leap of faith would have these systems automatically effecting one or more therapeutic modalities such as instituting a change in pacemaker function and/or controlling an implanted drug administration device.

Telemetry

While implantable defibrillator memory sizes have increased dramatically, the telemetry link between them and the user has changed little. Consequently, interrogation time has grown significantly, and the users' patience is sorely tested. It is inevitable that much faster, more convenient, and more robust telemetry systems will be needed if device memories and functions continue to expand. Moreover, multiple implanted systems may need to be linked electronically to coordinate functions; an implantable defibrillator might trigger a remote drug infusion pump, for example. This concept is not new,[72,73] but the enabling technology has yet to be implemented. With suitable range, newer systems could eventually link into the cellular phone systems and the internet, opening powerful new concepts in patient management.

Troubleshooting/Follow-Up Tools

Patient follow-up will be enhanced as expanded monitoring capabilities add atrial electrograms, documentation of nonsustained events, passive mode documentation of subsidiary detection algorithm performance, and the ability to replay stored episodes to test programming alternatives.

Some systems now perform rudimentary evaluation of stored data, calling the physician's attention to suspect events and making programming change recommendations. These systems may well evolve to the point of automatically adjusting detection algorithms and therapies. Some commercially available devices automatically disable antitachy pacing therapies if they are unsuccessful in four consecutive arrhythmia episodes.

One investigational implantable defibrillator now provides automatic daily evaluations of the pacing and high-voltage lead systems, using very low-voltage pulses that are well below the stimulation threshold. A record of these daily measurements is maintained in the device memory, allowing monitoring of impedance trends that may provide early detection of lead failure.

Many physicians would like to be able to follow defibrillator patients remotely by telephone. Such capability has been demonstrated by several manufacturers,[74,75] but availability has been limited given the problematic economics of providing transmitting equipment to each patient. Ultimately, advanced telemetry systems may make it possible to link implanted devices directly to the phone systems, obviating the need for ancillary patient transmitters. In the interim, a far less expensive alternative, incorporated in an investigational defibrillator,[76] allows the physician to program the device to automatically monitor select parameters (e.g., battery voltage, high voltage and pacing lead impedance, charge time), and to sound a modest duration tone at a specific time of day should one of the monitored conditions occur. The patient is instructed to call the clinic if the device beeps, and to wave a magnet across the device while the technician listens over the phone. With magnet placement, the device emits one of three clearly differentiable tones indicating:

"immediate attention is needed," "attention is needed when convenient," or, "everything is working properly, the patient imagined hearing tones." This system is inexpensive, requiring only a magnet, works anywhere there is a phone, and triggers needed care more promptly than would be the case if the patient had to wait for a scheduled telephone follow-up session.

Electronics

In the quest for smaller defibrillator size, all design aspects are candidates for improvement.[77] As shown in Figure 4, circuitry represents a rather small portion of total implantable defibrillator volume, but further functional integration can reduce the number of discrete components and inte-

grated circuits. As illustrated in Figure 5, integrated circuits will be formed with finer lines, moving from the 3- and 1.5-micron technologies used in early and current units, to a 0.6-micron technology in many of the future digital circuit functions. To a first approximation, halving line size roughly halves current drain and cuts circuit volume by about a factor of four. These smaller integrated circuits combined with thinner circuit substrates will reduce total circuit volume considerably. In addition, these circuits will be designed to operate at lower voltages to further reduce power consumption, thereby reducing battery size needed for a given implantable defibrillator longevity.

Until recently, all implantable defibrillators used cylindrical aluminum electrolytic capacitors to store charge prior to shock delivery. These capacitors are sold widely for many consumer products, but the tradi-

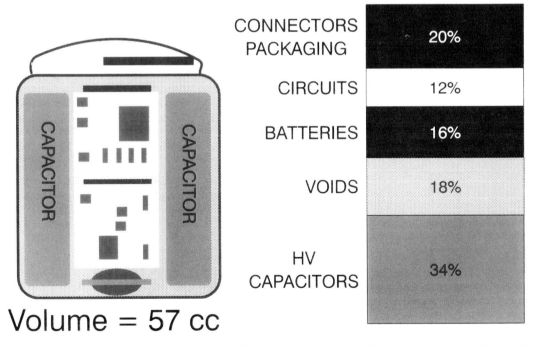

Figure 4. Traditional ICD construction. This figure presents the relative volumes required by each of the major elements of an implantable defibrillator built with traditional tubular aluminum electrolytic capacitors. These capacitors have been the dominant factor in determining defibrillator volume and package morphology.

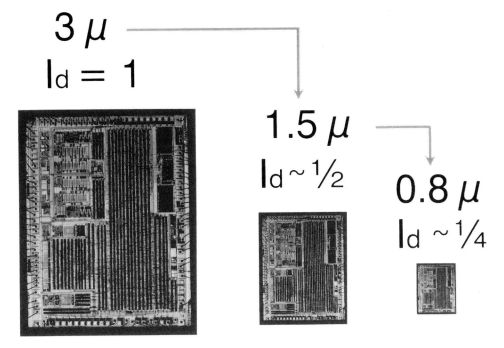

Figure 5. This schematic illustrates the benefits of using fine line widths when manufacturing digital integrated circuits. Halving line width roughly halves current drain and reduces circuit area by a factor of 4. These gains can be used to provide defibrillator size reduction, longevity enhancement, and/or increased functionality.

tional suppliers have little incentive to produce unique devices for implantable defibrillators since the number of capacitors sold for this application is negligible in comparison with other uses. Consequently, these capacitors have not been optimized for implantable use. Off-the-shelf aluminum electrolytic capacitors store approximately 0.2–1.7 J/cm^3,[78] must be used in pairs to meet operating voltage requirements, generally require periodic charging to ensure acceptable charge times, and are available only in a cylindrical shape that is inefficient for packaging purposes.

New capacitor designs, including improved flat aluminum electrolytic, tantalum, ceramic, and metallized polymer films, are being developed specifically for use in implantable defibrillators. These are diagrammed in Figure 6. The ceramic and polymer technologies appear to be the most likely candidates to yield substantial gains in stored energy density, while the aluminum and tantalum technologies seem closest to being practicable.

Recently, a proprietary flat electrolytic capacitor with an energy density of 2.8 J/cc was introduced in a commercially available defibrillator, allowing a stored shock energy of 42 J in a 57-cc device,[79] and flat aluminum electrolytic capacitors with storage densities of 3 J/cc have been reported though not yet realized in implantable form.[80]

A prototype wet tantalum capacitor has been constructed using proprietary cathode preparation, anode formation at working voltages as high as 250 V, and efficient packaging that yields an energy density approaching 4 J/cc. The anode is tantalum with a layer of tantalum oxide (Ta_2O_5) and the cathode is a thin film of ruthenium oxide deposited onto a metallic current collector. The aqueous-based electrolyte contains positive ions that are generally, but not necessarily, hydrogen and negative ions from

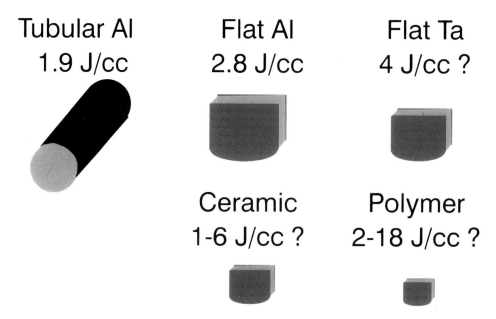

Tubular Al
1.9 J/cc

Flat Al
2.8 J/cc

Flat Ta
4 J/cc ?

Ceramic
1-6 J/cc ?

Polymer
2-18 J/cc ?

Figure 6. This diagram compares the sizes and energy densities of various capacitor technologies that might be incorporated in evolving implantable defibrillator designs. The widely used tubular aluminum capacitors are gradually being replaced by devices capable of storing significantly larger amounts of energy per unit volume. Flat aluminum devices are currently in limited use, flat tantalum capacitors should be available in the very near future, and, farther out, ceramic and polymer technologies may provide extremely high stored energy densities.

an acid. Hermetically sealed in a metal case, this capacitor exhibits very low leakage currents and does not require regular reforming of the anode. A package of three series-connected capacitors capable of storing 32 J and working at 750 V is projected to weigh approximately 50 g and occupy a volume of 8 cc, and further size and weight reductions are possible. The developer, Wilson Greatbatch Limited, is currently preparing to supply these custom capacitors for implantable applications.[81]

It is probable there will be a phased transition from one capacitor technology to another with raw stored volumetric energy densities possibly increasing by 30% to 100% with each new technology. As an added benefit, these designs will yield secondary reductions in implantable device sizes as a consequence of better capacitor shapes and elimination of the need to provide battery capacity for capacitor formation.

Commercially approved implantable de-

fibrillators have more than tripled the packaging density from the early ICDs of 0.23 J/cc to a current value of 0.74 J/cc. Anticipated capacitor, circuit, battery, and packaging technology, illustrated in Figure 7, will eventually push this to 1 J/cc.

Software

A few implantable defibrillator features, such as specific antitachy pacing algorithms, have been implemented in some current implantable defibrillators by means of programmer-delivered instructions that are placed in appropriate locations in the implantable defibrillator's random access memory, and many designs are amenable to the addition of limited amounts of operational code telemetered to the device after implantation. A recently introduced design extends this capability to allow the user to purchase a basic device for initial implantation and then buy and install additional ca-

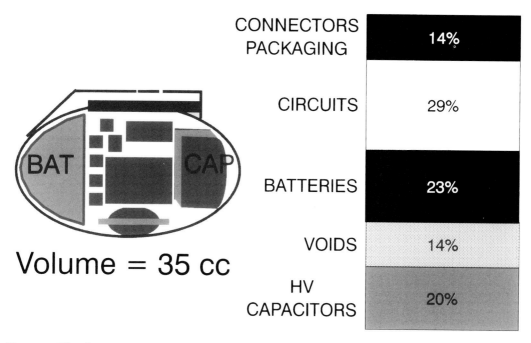

Figure 7. This hypothetical component layout for future defibrillators illustrates the use of high-energy density capacitors, very fine line integrated circuit technology, and smaller lead connectors to provide 35-J stored energy shocks in a 35-cc package.

pabilities noninvasively if the patient needs them. This approach could become especially helpful given the increasing longevity of defibrillator systems and could also provide economic benefits to the healthcare system. However, reimbursement issues need resolution before this can become commonplace.

Leads

Size

Ventricular defibrillation systems have progressed from use of multiple epicardial leads (patches and rate sensing electrodes), to complex transvenous systems (coronary sinus leads, SVC, and right ventricular leads), to the current solitary transvenous right ventricular catheters. Now, as dual chamber defibrillators emerge, there is increased need to emphasize further reduction in lead diameters while enhancing reliability.[82–84] Early transvenous leads required use of a 14F introducer, current systems pass through a 10.5F introducer, and further size reductions are imminent. New conductor designs, new insulation materials, and modified placement technologies will provide significant size reductions and improve ease of use. Smaller lead diameters will complement other design concepts, such as compressible lumens, to increase reliability by reducing the likelihood of crush fractures.

Pacing Efficiency

Defibrillator pacing electrodes will increasingly adopt the beneficial technologies of bradycardia pacing leads, some of which offer extremely low thresholds of 0.5 V with 0.5-ms pulse widths and pacing impedances of more than 1,000 ohms (Ω).[85] Steroid-eluting defibrillator lead systems are now available, and small-geometry high-efficiency electrode tips are being added. These new leads will contribute substantially to increased implantable defibrillator longevity in pacing-dependent patients. Consider that continuous single chamber pacing at 70 pulses per minute with a 5-V output and 0.5-ms pulse width using a 500-Ω lead draws approximately 5.8 μA from the defibrillator. A slightly more efficient lead that allows operation at 4 V and 0.4 ms with a pacing impedance of 800 Ω will reduce the current demand to 2.3 μA. Further modest improvement allowing operation at 3 V and 0.3 ms with an impedance of 1,000 Ω would yield a current of 1 μA. Given that the underlying monitoring current of a typical implantable defibrillator is in the 7- to 10-μA range, the significance of these pacing efficiency improvements is obvious. Figure 8 demonstrates the importance of lead efficiency improvements for implantable defibrillators incorporating dual chamber pacing. If these defibrillators are to be cost-effective, lead improvements will be essential.

Defibrillation Efficiency

Designers will continue to reduce lead conductor resistance and to improve field distribution patterns in order to allow defibrillation with less energy. A 50-Ω defibrillation lead system operating at 750 V delivers a current of nearly 15 amps during shock delivery. Each ohm of resistance in the lead's conducting wire decreases the peak delivered voltage by 15 V. For a typical 34-J system, 1 Ω of wire resistance reduces the energy delivered to the patient by slightly more than 1 J, so it is clearly advantageous to minimize losses within the lead.

New electrode materials are being considered for increased defibrillation efficiency. In animal studies, an electrode formed from electrically conductive carbon fibers demonstrated defibrillation energy thresholds that were roughly 30% lower than that achieved by commercially available metal electrodes.[86]

Smaller, more easily manipulated leads will allow placement in locations that were

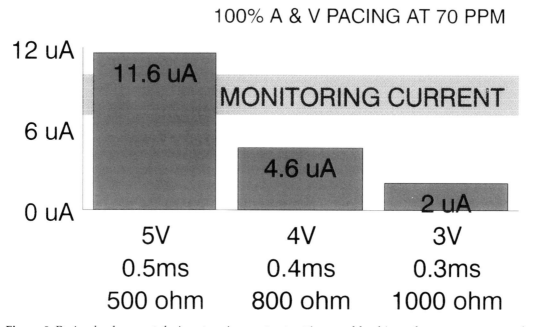

Figure 8. Pacing lead current drains at various output settings and lead impedances are contrasted with the monitoring current of a typical implantable defibrillator. The current drains assume DOO pacing at a rate of 70 pulses per minute. Advances in lead technology can significantly reduce the burden of pacing to dramatically extend device longevity in pacing-dependent patients.

previously inaccessible transvenously, providing enhanced field distribution patterns and further improvements in defibrillation efficacy.

Other Functions

Treatment of implantable defibrillator patients' co-morbidities will be assisted with additional implantable defibrillator capabilities requiring unique leads. Single-pass leads that permit dual chamber pacing and dual chamber defibrillation will be helpful for bradyarrhythmia and tachyarrhythmia management and will also facilitate use of more complex pacing techniques designed to improve hemodynamics. Defibrillator leads with implantable sensor technology will be developed to assist with management of heart failure. Preliminary work is already in progress using implantable hemodynamic monitoring devices that can record pressures and oxygen saturation levels, and additional parameters are being investigated. Other research is in progress on multi-site pacing concepts[87–89] for improving ventricular performance in heart failure.

Connectors

The IS-1/DF-1 connector system used in current implantable defibrillators is not optimized for size or for ease of use and, as generators and leads continue to shrink, the connector module looms as an obvious target for improvement. Various small, in-line, tool-less connector concepts have been proposed for defibrillators yet their adoption by individual manufacturers is hampered by the fear of interbrand compatibility problems. It is highly desirable that a new industry standard be developed. A well thought out flexible system will be crucial when catheter-based sensors are required.

Programmers

Programmers will continue to evolve, growing smaller and lighter yet more powerful. Abetted by defibrillators with greater automaticity, larger memories, and sensors that provide data indicating the status of patients' co-morbidities, programmers will become substantial data management tools. No longer will the user be burdened with interpretation of the raw data collected by the implantable devices. Instead, the programmer will analyze device performance and patient status to present concise reports, making recommendations for changes where appropriate. The supporting raw data will be available on request should there be questions regarding the automated suggestions.

Programmers are currently used primarily to provide information and means to appropriately alter operating parameters in an implantable device, but they are evolving to become powerful information management centers. The omnipresent Internet browser and its extension to the Intranet present natural pathways for linking all facets of patient care. Programmers will be able to use these networks to retrieve patient records, place new data in the charts, obtain data on specific device characteristics, consult technical support functions for troubleshooting, provide remote programming and follow-up, send clinical study data to sponsors' databases, and initiate billing records.

Indications

The FDA has approved the use of implantable defibrillators in patients who are at high risk of sudden death due to VF and/or VT and who have experienced one of the following situations: survival of at least one episode of cardiac arrest (manifested by a loss of consciousness) due to a ventricular tachyarrhythmia; recurrent, poorly tolerated sustained VT that remains inducible despite the most efficacious antiarrhythmic drug therapy that can be tolerated by the patient; and prior myocardial infarction, left ventricular ejection fraction of ≤35%, and a documented episode of nonsustained VT, with an inducible ventricular tachyarrhythmia (patients suppressible with IV procainamide or an equivalent antiarrhythmic have not been studied).[90] Usage is contraindicated in patients with ventricular tachyarrhythmias due to transient conditions such as ischemia, acute infarction, drug toxicity, arrhythmogenic drug response, electrolyte imbalance, hypoxia, or electrocution. These indications have been validated by the AVID and MADIT studies.

As implantable defibrillator systems advance technologically the range of indications will likely broaden. Proposed, though controversial, indications include: patients awaiting cardiac transplant[91–93]; patients with sustained tolerated VT amenable to pace termination[94]; patients who are asymptomatic and have never had an aborted sudden cardiac death yet fall into a range of debatable prophylactic applications,[95,96] such as genetically screened cardiomyopathy patients, congenital long QT syndrome, extensive infarct with ejection fraction <0.40, and recurrent syncope of unknown cause; patients with unexplained syncope; patients with cardiac sarcoidosis[97]; and, of course, patients with atrial fibrillation.[98–101] Costly outcome studies will be needed to substantiate any of these indications. Currently, progress is being made in launching the Sudden Cardiac Death in Heart Failure Trial,[102] a massive study designed to test the hypothesis that amiodarone or an ICD will increase survival over placebo therapy in NYHA class II and class III patients who have left ventricular ejection fractions ≤35%. Ultimately, successful expansion to prophylactic indications will hinge on the development of appropriate risk stratification tools[103] (e.g., ejection fraction, signal-averaged ECG, exercise tests, baroreflex sensitivity, T-wave alternans, heart rate variability) along with requisite cost reductions for implantable systems to create cost-effective solutions.[104]

Cost

Advanced technology is usually a double-edged sword, exacting a price for the advantages conveyed, particularly when low volumes of high-reliability miniaturized devices are involved. Compounding the cost issue is the fact that many suppliers of raw materials will no longer sell to implantable device manufacturers at any price. There has been a 40% drop in the number of suppliers since 1994, a change attributed to the perceived liability risk balanced against the small market which is between 0.002% and 3% of the total market for these materials.[105] Device manufacturers will have to indemnify suppliers or become more vertically integrated. Capacitors developed specifically for implantable defibrillators will be built in small quantities, making them expensive in comparison with off-the-shelf parts. Highly integrated circuit functions are expensive since the manufacturing yield of viable components falls as complexity rises. Rapid evolution of device designs limits the marketing window and manufacturing volumes of each implantable defibrillator model, yielding a smaller base for amortization of development costs. On the other hand, small devices are easier and less expensive to implant,[106,107] and the increasing longevity of newer devices can dramatically reduce the annualized cost of therapy.

Encouraging data were reported in a study[108,109] comparing conventional therapy to early defibrillator implantation in the period from 1989 to 1993. This prospective study demonstrated a cost-effectiveness ratio (dollars per patient day alive) of $87/day for conventional therapy versus $64/day for the implantable defibrillator despite use of a device that required a thoracotomy, patch electrodes, and relatively frequent replacement. The authors also analyzed a hypothetical scenario that assumed a device longevity of 5 years and transvenous pectoral implantation. They predicted a future cost effectiveness ratio of $51/day, a figure that is likely to be improved upon with current technology which is expected to provide implantable defibrillator longevity that is substantially better than the 5-year estimate used in this model.

In another study, total charges were evaluated for 99 consecutive ICD patients, 18 with epicardial systems implanted via thoracotomy, 62 with abdominal transvenous implants, and 19 with pectoral transvenous systems.[110] Costs for the three approaches expressed in 1994 dollars were $99,081, $59,961, and $44,128, respectively. Assuming that modern ICDs will last at least 6 years, the annual cost of therapy, excluding follow-up, is now roughly $7,300.

Conclusion

Smaller, easier to use, more potent and cost-effective implantable defibrillators are a certainty. Given the impressive technological possibilities, we await the future avidly.

References

1. Song S. The Bilitch Report: Part B. Performance of implantable cardiac rhythm management devices. PACE 1994;17:131.
2. System Reference Guide, Micro Jewel^{Tm} II Arrhythmia Management Device. Ref No. UC960158laEN, Medtronic, Inc., Minneapolis, MN, July, 1996.
3. Schwartzman D, Nallamothu N, Callans D, et al. Postoperative lead-related complications in patients with nonthoracotomy defibrillation lead systems. J Am Coll Cardiol 1995;26:776.
4. Moss A, Hall J, Cannom D, et al. Improved survival with an implanted defibrillator in patients with coronary disease at high risk for ventricular arrhythmia. N Engl J Med 1996;335:1933.
5. The AVID Investigators. Antiarrhythmics versus implantable defibrillators (AVID) rationale, design, and methods. Am J Cardiol 1995;75:470.
6. Schmitt C, Montero M, Melichercik J. Significance of supraventricular tachyarrhythmias in patients with implanted pacing cardioverter defibrillators. PACE 1994;17:295.
7. Grimm W, Flores B, Marchlinski F. Electrocardiographically documented unnecessary, spontaneous shocks in 241 patients with implantable cardioverter defibrillators. PACE 1992;15:1667.
8. Stambler B, Wood M, Ellenbogen K. Limitations of tachycardia confirmation and rate classification algorithms in a third-generation implantable cardioverter defibrillator. PACE 1996;19:1618.
9. Pinski S, Fahy G. The proarrhythmic potential of implantable cardioverter-defibrillators. Circulation 1995;92:1651.
10. Callans D, Hook B, Kleiman R, et al. Unique sensing errors in third-generation implantable cardioverter-defibrillators. J Am Coll Cardiol 1993;22:1135.
11. Schaumann A, Muhlen F, Gonska B. et al. Enhanced detection criteria in implantable cardioverter-defibrillators to avoid inappropriate therapy. Am J Cardiol 1996;78:42.
12. Swerdlow C, Chen P, Kass R, et al. Discrimination of ventricular tachycardia from sinus tachycardia and atrial fibrillation in a tiered-therapy cardioverter-defibrillator. J Am Coll Cardiol 1994;23:1342.
13. MicroJewel^{Tm} II System Reference Guide. Publication number UC960158laEN 196803–002, Medtronic Inc., Minneapolis, MN, July, 1996.
14. Ruetz L, Bardy G, Mitchell L, et al. Clinical evaluation of electrogram width measurements for automatic detection of ventricular tachycardia. PACE 1996;19:582A.
15. Barold H, Newby K, Tomassoni G, et al. Prospective evaluation of new and old criteria to discriminate between supraventricular and ventricular tachycardia in the Medtronic 7218C implantable defibrillator. Circulation 1996;94:I-568.
16. Brachmann J, Swerdlow C, Mitchell B, et al., for the Worldwide 7218 ICD Investigators. Worldwide experience with the electrogram width feature for improved detection in an implantable pacer-cardioverter-defibrillator. JACC 1997;29:115A.
17. Morris M, Jenkins J, DiCarlo L. Band-limited morphometric analysis of the intracardiac signal: implications for antitachycardia devices. PACE 1997;20:34.
18. DiCarlo L, Jenkins J, Caswell S, et al. Tachycardia detection by antitachycardia devices, present limitations and future strategies. J Interven Cardiol 1994;5:459.
19. Lavergne T, Daubert C, Chauvin M, et al. Preliminary clinical experience with the first dual chamber pacemaker defibrillator. PACE 1997;20:182.
20. Chiang C, Jenkins J, Caswell S, et al. Augmented two-channel arrhythmia detection: an efficient diagnostic method for implantable devices. PACE 1996;19:1493.
21. Nair M, Saoudi N, Kroiss D, et al. Auto-

matic arrhythmia identification using analysis of the atrioventricular association: application to a new generation of implantable defibrillators. Circulation 1997; 95:967.

22. Gillberg J, Brown M, Olson W, et al. Acute testing of a prototype dual chamber defibrillator at Mayo Clinic. Circulation 1996; 94:I-562.

23. Stanton M, Hammill S, Gillberg J, et al. Clinical testing of a dual chamber combined atrial and ventricular defibrillator. JACC 1997;29:473A.

24. Stambler B, Wood M, Ellenbogen K. Limitations of tachycardia confirmation and rate classification algorithms in a third-generation implantable cardioverter defibrillator. PACE 1996;19:1618.

25. Candinas R, Kramm B, Buckingham T. Inappropriate implantable cardioverter defibrillator shocks due to ventricular extrasystoles despite use of a reconfirmation algorithm. Eur JCPE 1996;6:47.

26. Blanck Z, Biehl M, Sra J, et al. Delivery of noncommitted shocks for nonsustained ventricular arrhythmias by a new implantable cardioverter defibrillator with abortive shock capability. J Cardiovasc Electrophysiol 1997;8:317.

27. Thakur R, Souza J, Chapman P, et al. Direct comparison of monophasic, biphasic, and sequential pulse defibrillation over a single current pathway. Can J Cardiol 1996;12:407.

28. Jones J, Tovar O. Threshold reduction with biphasic defibrillator waveforms. J Electrocardiol 1995;28:25.

29. Swerdlow C, Kass R, Chen P, et al. Effect of capacitor size and pathway resistance on defibrillation threshold for implantable defibrillators. Circulation 1994;90:1840.

30. Lin J, Stotts L, Rosborough J, et al. Comparison of defibrillation efficacy using biphasic waveforms delivered from various capacitances/pulse widths. PACE 1997;20:158.

31. Swerdlow C, Kass R, Davie S, et al. Short biphasic pulses from 90 microfarad capacitors lower defibrillation threshold. PACE 1996;19:1053.

32. Cleland B. A conceptual basis for defibrillation waveforms. PACE 1996;19:1186.

33. Schwartzman D, Hull M, Callans D, et al. Serial defibrillation lead impedance in patients with epicardial and nonthoracotomy lead systems. J Cardiovasc Electrophysiol 1996;7:697.

34. Walcott G, Walker R, Cates A, et al. Choosing the optimal monophasic and biphasic waveforms for ventricular defibrillation. J Cardiovasc Electrophysiol 1995;6:737.

35. Swerdlow C, Fan W, Brewer J. Charge-burping theory correctly predicts optimal ratios of phase duration for biphasic defibrillation waveforms. Circulation 1996;94: 2278.

36. Irnich W. Optimal truncation of defibrillation pulses. PACE 1995;18:673.

37. Walcott G, Rollins D, Smith W, et al. Effect of changing capacitors between phases of a biphasic defibrillation shock. PACE 1996; 19:945.

38. Natale A, Sra J, Krum D, et al. Relative efficacy of different tilts with biphasic defibrillation in humans. PACE 1996;19:197.

39. Block M, Hammel D, Bocker D, et al. Biphasic defibrillation using a single capacitor with large capacitance: reduction of peak voltages and implantable defibrillator device size. PACE 1996;19:207.

40. Hsu W, Lin Y, Heil J, et al. Effect of shock timing on defibrillation success. PACE 1997;20:153.

41. Hsia P, Suresh G, Allen C, et al. Improved nonthoracotomy defibrillation based on ventricular fibrillation waveform characteristics. PACE 1996;19:1537.

42. Yamanouchi Y, Mowrey K, Nadzam G, et al. Effects of respiration phase on defibrillation threshold in nonthoracotomy active can electrode configuration. PACE 1996;19: 736.

43. Sweeney R, Gill R, Reid P. Double-pulse defibrillation using pulse separation based on the fibrillation cycle length. J Cardiovasc Electrophysiol 1994;5:761.

44. Min X, Mongeon L, Warman E, et al. A prospective canine study of high frequency pacing pulses prior to defibrillation shocks for lowering defibrillation thresholds. Circulation 1996;94:I-439.

45. Morillo C, Jones D, Klein G. Effects of autonomic manipulation on ventricular fibrillation and internal cardiac defibrillation thresholds in pigs. PACE 1996;19:1355.

46. Lerman B, Engelstein E. Increased defibrillation threshold due to ventricular fibrillation duration. J Electrocardiol 1995;28:21.

47. Winkle R, Mead H, Ruder M, et al. Effect of duration of ventricular fibrillation on defibrillation efficacy in humans. Circulation 1990;81:1477.

48. Curtis A, Conti J, Tucker K, et al. Motor vehicle accidents in patients with an implantable cardioverter-defibrillator. J Am Coll Cardiol 1995;26:180.

49. Epstein A, Miles W, Benditt D, et al. Personal and public safety issues related to arrhythmias that may affect consciousness: implications for regulation and physician recommendations. A medical/scientific statement from the American Heart Associ-

ation and the North American Society of Pacing and Electrophysiology. Circulation 1996;94:1147.

50. Lau C, Tse H, Lok N, et al. Initial clinical experience with an implantable human atrial defibrillator. PACE 1997;20:220.

51. Model 7250 System Reference Guide, Publication number UC9601584 En. Medtronic Inc., Minneapolis, MN, November, 1996.

52. Schalidach M, Thong T, Revishvili A, et al. Technologie und algorithmen fur implantierbare zweikammer-defibrillatoren. (Technology and algorithms for implantable dual-chamber defibrillators.) Biomedizinische Technik 1996;41:351.

53. Ammer R, Alt E, Ayers G, et al. Pain threshold for low energy intracardiac cardioversion of atrial fibrillation with low or no sedation. PACE 1997;20:230A.

54. Steinhaus D, Cardinal D, Mongeon L, et al. Atrial defibrillation: are low energy shocks acceptable to patients? PACE 1996;19:625A.

55. Tomassoni G, Newby K, Kearney M, et al. Testing different biphasic waveforms and capacitances: effect on atrial defibrillation threshold and pain perception. J Am Coll Cardiol 1996;28:695.

56. Hill M, Mongeon L, Mehra R. Prevention of atrial fibrillation: dual site atrial pacing reduces the coupling window of induction of atrial fibrillation. PACE 1996;19:630.

57. Prakash A, Hill M, Krol R, et al. Long-term atrial pacing for prevention of atrial fibrillation: selection of patients and drug therapy. PACE 1996;19:618.

58. Prakash A, Hill M, Lewis C, et al. Comparative efficacy of high right atrial, coronary sinus, and dual site right atrial pacing in prevention of atrial fibrillation. PACE 1996;19:634A.

59. KenKnight B, Jones B, Thomas A, et al. Technological advances in implantable cardioverter-defibrillators before the year 2000 and beyond. Am J Cardiol 1996;79:108.

60. Ayers G, Rho T, Ben-David J, et al. Amiodarone instilled into the canine pericardial sac migrates transmurally to produce electrophysiology effects and suppress atrial fibrillation. J Cardiovasc Electrophysiol 1996;7:713.

61. Fei L, Zipes D. L-arginine reduces the increased severity of ventricular arrhythmias during sympathetic stimulation in dogs with acute coronary occlusion: nitric oxide modulates sympathetic effects on ventricular electrophysiologic properties. Circulation in press.

62. Eggeling T, Hoepp H, Koulousakis A, et al. Left stellate ganglion blockade using a drug reservoir pump system. A new therapeutic approach in the long QT syndrome. Z Kardiol 1988;77:185.

63. Santini M, Ansalone G, Auriti A, et al. Indications for dual-chamber (DDD) pacing in implantable cardioverter-defibrillator patients. Am J Cardiol 1996;78:116.

64. Instruction Manual for the Physician, Ventak AV 1810/1815. Code:1682-51326. Guidant Corporation, Saint Paul, MN.

65. Jung W. Implantation of an arrhythmia management system for ventricular and supraventricular tachyarrhythmias. Lancet 1997;349:853.

66. Ohlsson A, Beck R, Bennett T, et al. Monitoring of mixed venous oxygen saturation and pressure from biosensors in the right ventricle: a 24-hour study in patients with heart failure. Eur Heart J 1995;16:1215.

67. Van Veldhuisen D, Remme W. Value of simultaneous monitoring of right ventricular oxygen saturation and pressure using biosensors. Eur Heart J 1995;16:1164.

68. Steinhaus D, Lemery R, Bresnahan D, et al. Initial experience with an implantable hemodynamic monitor. Circulation 1996;93:745.

69. Ohlsson A, Bennett T, Ottenhoff F, et al. Long-term recording of cardiac output via an implantable haemodynamic monitoring device. Eur Heart J 1996;17:1902.

70. Rickards A, Corbucci G, Bombardini T, et al. Peak endocardial acceleration (PEA): a new implantable sensor for cardiac contractility monitoring. PACE 1996;19:631A.

71. Bongiorni A, Soldati E, Arena G, et al. Is local myocardial contractility related to endocardial acceleration signals detected by a transvenous pacing lead? PACE 1996;19:1682.

72. U.S. Patent Number 4,987,897: Body bus medical device communication system. H.D. Funke, inventor; Medtronic Inc. assignee. Issued Sept 18, 1989.

73. U.S. Patent Number 5,113,859: Acoustic body bus medical device communication system. H.D. Funke, inventor; Medtronic Inc. assignee. Issued June 25, 1990.

74. Fetter J, Stanton M, Benditt D, et al. Telephonic monitoring and transmission of stored arrhythmia detection and therapy data from an implantable cardioverter defibrillator. PACE 1995;18:1531.

75. Porterfield J, Porterfield L, Easley A, et al. Transtelephonic ICD follow-up: A new patient management tool. PACE 1997;20,1208.

76. Gem DR System Reference Guide, Publication number UC9604326. Medtronic Inc., Minneapolis, MN, May 1997.

77. Warren J, Dreher R, Jaworski R, et al. Im-

plantable cardioverter defibrillators. Proc IEEE 1996;84:468.

78. Takeuchi S, Clark W. Energy storage and delivery. In Estes N, Manolis A, Wang P, eds. Implantable Cardioverter-Defibrillators. Marcel Dekker Inc., New York, 1994, p 123.

79. The Ventritex Flatcap™ capacitor. Publication number 0144A-1 196. Ventritex, Inc., Sunnyvale, CA, November 1996.

80. Lunsmann P, MacFarlane D. High energy density capacitors for implantable defibrillators. 1996 Proceedings of the 16th Capacitor and Resistor Technology Symposium: 277, 1996. Components Technology Institute Inc., Huntsville, AL, March 1996.

81. Holmes CF (for Wilson Greatbatch, Ltd.). Personal communication, April 8, 1997.

82. Block M, Breithardt G. Long term outcome with transvenous (-subcutaneous) defibrillation leads. In Oto AM, ed. Practice and Progress in Cardiac Pacing and Electrophysiology. Kluwer Academic Publishers, Netherlands 1996, p 337.

83. Lawton J, Ellenbogen K, Wood M, et al. Sensing lead-related complications in patients with transvenous implantable cardioverter-defibrillators, Am J Cardiol 1996;78:647.

84. Lawton J, Wood M, Gilligan A, et al. Implantable transvenous cardioverter defibrillator leads: the dark side. PACE 1996; 19:1273.

85. Fogel R, Pirzada F, Casavant D, et al. Initial experience with 1.5-mm² high impedance, steroid-eluting pacing electrodes. PACE 1996;19:188.

86. Alt E, Fotuhi P, Callihan R, et al. Endocardial carbon-braid electrodes: a new concept for lower defibrillation thresholds. Circulation 1995;92:1627.

87. Cazeau S, Ritter P, Lazarus A, et al. Hemodynamic improvement provided by biventricular pacing in congestive heart failure: an acute study. PACE 1996;19:568.

88. Cazeau S, Ritter P, Lazarus A, et al. Multisite pacing for congestive heart failure. PACE 1996;19:568A.

89. Cazeau S, Ritter P, Lazarus A, et al. Multisite pacing for end-stage heart failure: early experience. PACE 1996;19:1748.

90. MADIT FDA Info Pack. Food and Drug Administration. U.S. Department of Health and Human Services, Rockville, MD, May 16, 1996.

91. Grimm M, Grimm G, Zuckermann A, et al. Implantable defibrillator therapy in survivors of sudden cardiac death awaiting heart transplantation. Ann Thorac Surg 1995;59: 916.

92. Sweeney M, Ruskin J, Garan H, et al. Influence of the implantable cardioverter/defibrillator on sudden death and total mortality in patients evaluated for cardiac transplantation. Circulation 1995;92:3273.

93. Saxon L, Wiener I, DeLurgio D, et al. Implantable defibrillators for high-risk patients with heart failure who are awaiting cardiac transplantation. Am Heart J 1995; 130:501.

94. Bocker D, Block M, Isbruch F, et al. Benefits of treatment with implantable cardioverter-defibrillators in patients with stable ventricular tachycardia without cardiac arrest. Br Heart J 1995;73:158.

95. Brugada P, Wellens F, Andries E. A prophylactic implantable cardioverter-defibrillator? Am J Cardiol 1996;78:128.

96. Trouton T, Powell A, Garan H, et al. Risk identification for sudden cardiac death: implications for implantable cardioverter-defibrillator use. Progr Cardiovasc Dis 1993; 36:195.

97. Paz H, McCormick D, Kutalek S, et al. The automatic implantable cardiac defibrillator: prophylaxis in cardiac sarcoidosis. Chest 1994;106:1603.

98. Griffin J, Ayers G, Adams J, et al. Is the automatic atrial defibrillator a promising approach? J Cardiovasc Electrophysiol 1996;7:1217.

99. Heisel A, Jung J, Fries R, et al. Atrial defibrillation: can modifications in current implantable cardioverter-defibrillators achieve this? Am J Cardiol 1996;78:119.

100. Wellens H. Atrial fibrillation: the last big hurdle in treating supraventricular tachycardia. N Engl J Med 1994;331:944.

101. Toubol P. Atrial defibrillator: is it needed? would society pay for it? PACE 1995;18:616.

102. Bardy G, Lee K, Mark D, et al. Sudden cardiac death in heart failure trial: Pilot study. PACE 1997;20,1148A.

103. Camm J, Fei L. Risk stratification after myocardial infarction. PACE 1994;17:401.

104. Bigger T. Prophylactic use of implantable cardioverter defibrillators: medical, technical, and economic considerations. PACE 1991;14:376.

105. Biomaterials availability: a vital health care industry hangs in the balance. Health Industry Manufacturers Association, Washington, DC, April 8, 1997.

106. Cardinal D, Connelly D, Steinhaus D, et al. Cost savings with nonthoracotomy implantable cardioverter-defibrillators. Am J Cardiol 1996;78:1255.

107. Anvari A, Stix G, Grabenwoger M, et al. Comparison of three cardioverter defibrillator implantation techniques: initial results

with transvenous pectoral implantation. PACE 1996;19:1061.

108. Hauer R, Derksen R, Wever E. Can implantable cardioverter-defibrillator therapy reduce healthcare costs? Am J Cardiol 1996; 78:134.

109. Wever E, Hauer R, Schrijvers G, et al. Cost-effectiveness of implantable defibrillator as first-choice therapy versus electrophysiologically guided, tiered strategy in postinfarct sudden death survivors. A randomized study. Circulation 1996;93;489.

110. Cardinal D, Connelly D, Steinhaus D, et al. Cost savings with nonthoracotomy implantable cardioverter-defibrillators. Am J Cardiol 1996;78:1255.

Chapter 20

Atrial Defibrillation for Implantable Cardioverter-Defibrillators:
Lead Systems, Waveforms, Detection Algorithms, and Results

Bruce H. KenKnight, Douglas J. Lang, Avram Scheiner, Randolph A.S. Cooper

Introduction

Supraventricular tachyarrhythmias (SVTs) appear to be more prevalent today than ever before. Such observations are most likely the result of global population expansion, increasing human life span, increased patient awareness and education, and improved arrhythmia detection techniques. The breadth of medical treatments for the symptoms associated with atrial tachyarrhythmias has increased dramatically in recent decades. Effectiveness of these treatments has come under scientific scrutiny during the last half of this century.

Atrial tachyarrhythmias are most commonly treated using pharmacological approaches to control symptoms or facilitate normal sinus rhythm. In general, drugs alone have proven unsatisfactory.[1] Consequently, nonpharmacological techniques have been developed and are being clinically evaluated.[2] It remains unclear whether so-called stand-alone atrial defibrillation therapy will withstand the test of rigorous clinical evaluation. Some physicians believe that the tolerance of atrial defibrillation shock therapy in unsedated patients and the risk of ventricular proarrhythmia are issues that have not yet been fully resolved.[2]

This chapter describes the role of implanted atrial and ventricular cardiac rhythm management devices for the treatment of short-duration, persistent atrial tachyarrhythmia. We first review the therapeutic options typically considered by physicians treating patients afflicted with atrial tachyarrhythmias. In subsequent sections we describe previously published work that focuses on questions related to the effectiveness of specific shock waveforms and lead systems that may be used in implantable cardioverter-defibrillator (ICD) systems capable of delivering atrial defibrillation therapy. Finally, we describe the important issues related to implementation of atrial defibrillation therapy in a conventional ICD platform.

From Singer I, Barold SS, Camm AJ (eds): Nonpharmacological Therapy of Arrhythmias for the 21st Century: The State of the Art. Futura Publishing Co, Inc., Armonk, NY, © 1998.

SVT Therapy: The Emerging Role of Implanted Devices

Recently reported data suggest that SVTs, such as atrial fibrillation (AF), may be more prevalent than previously thought.[3] As the population ages, the number of patients presenting with AF is expected to increase dramatically.[4] The healthcare costs associated with AF have and will continue to motivate improved treatment strategies.[5]

When a patient presents with SVT, the treatment strategy formulated by the physician is heavily influenced by the frequency and severity of symptoms, as well as factors such as patient age, concomitant heart disease, tolerance of treatment side effects, and success of previous treatment regimens. Most often, the initial treatment is the least invasive with the fewest risks and side effects. As the arrhythmia recurs, which is so often true for SVT, more aggressive treatments may be indicated. At the present time, treatment strategies for SVT can be classified as either *established* or *emerging* (see Table 1). Established treatments for SVT include not only electrical or pharmacological cardioversion followed by oral ad-

ministration of antiarrhythmic medicines, but also temporary (drug-induced) and permanent (AV node ablation) ventricular rate control with anticoagulation therapy to reduce risk of stroke. Radiofrequency (RF) catheter ablation in the right atrium for the abolition of typical and atypical flutter can now be considered an established treatment.[6,7] However, more extensive transvenous ablation for AF remains technically challenging.[8,9] Newer treatment strategies have been under clinical investigation in recent years. These "emerging" AF treatment strategies are being evaluated and will require careful clinical trials to compare their safety and effectiveness to established treatment modalities. Their role in the clinical management of patients with AF is being debated.[2]

When established AF therapies fail as a result of frequent arrhythmia recurrence or drug intolerance, additional options may need to be sought. Both catheter ablation and implanted devices are being considered in cases where established treatments have failed to control symptoms. Transvenous catheter ablation for treatment of AF has been suggested as a means to cure AF.[8,9] However, the feasibility and long-term safety of a procedure which at this point in time requires long anesthesia times as well as fluoroscopy exposures times has limited the universal acceptance of this technique. Yet, it seems unlikely in the near future that patients with symptomatic paroxysmal AF will or should be candidates for such a highly invasive "curative procedure" unless this procedure can be simplified and show a clinical benefit over more established and less invasive therapies for paroxysmal AF. In the future, appropriate catheter delivery techniques and energy delivery systems may help simplify the procedure of ablation for AF and permit interventional electrophysiologists to cure AF in selected patients.

Implanted dual chamber ICDs capable of providing automatic or patient-commanded atrial defibrillation therapy may provide clinical benefits that have not yet been fully studied. Two obvious benefits

---

Table 1

Classification of Supraventricular Tachycardia Treatments

Established
- Electrical external cardioversion
- Pharmacological ventricular rate control with chronic anticoagulation therapy
- Pharmacological cardioversion
- Catheter ablation of atrial flutter, focal atrial tachycardia and AV nodal reentrant tachycardia
- Catheter ablation of the AV node, implantation of a pacemaker system and chronic anticoagulation therapy

Emerging
- Electrical internal cardioversion
- Catheter ablation of atrial fibrillation
- Pacing for prevention of SVT recurrence
- Implantable atrial defibrillator
- Implantable cardiac rhythm manager (atrial and ventricular ICD)

---

might be reduction of stroke risk and a restoration of hemodynamics associated with normal sinus rhythm. An additional potential benefit in the ventricular ICD patient population may be derived by limiting the exposure of patients to the possible deleterious consequences of elevated mean heart rate during AF.[10] The contribution of AF to the exacerbation of the electrical instability of the ventricles and, therefore, to the genesis of ventricular arrhythmias is not fully understood. In addition to studies that will more clearly define the clinical utility of SVT therapies in dual chamber ICDs, clinical studies, similar to the AFFIRM trial,[11] which isolate the impact of AF on quality of life and therapy cost-effectiveness, will also need to be performed.

In the following sections, we review research related to atrial defibrillation lead systems and waveforms as well as describe the unique challenges associated with atrial and ventricular rhythm detection and classification.

Lead Systems

Implantable lead systems not only deliver therapeutic shocks, they also transmit electrical information from the heart muscle to the implanted pulse generator. For ICDs that incorporate atrial defibrillation therapy, leads must be positioned in the heart in a manner consistent with sensing intrinsic heart rhythms, delivery of pacing therapy, and delivery of both atrial and ventricular defibrillation therapy. These requirements place constraints on lead system design.

Defibrillation Electrodes

To defibrillate heart tissue, whether atrial or ventricular, ionic current must flow between electrodes positioned near the heart. When ionic current produced by discharging a capacitor between electrodes crosses myocyte membranes, the transmembrane potentials are altered, thereby causing changes in the electrophysiological status (e.g., refractory period extension) of the tissue.[12] The position of the defibrillation electrodes relative to the tissue requiring treatment affects the spatial intensity distribution of the shock field. Figure 1 shows the position of electrodes that have been investigated for defibrillation of the atria using a stand-alone atrial defibrillation system. Figure 2 shows the position of electrodes most likely to be utilized for atrial defibrillation therapy incorporated in a dual chamber ICD.

Studies of ventricular defibrillation have taught us that the lowest defibrillation thresholds (DFTs) result when the largest portion of ventricular mass is situated between the electrodes.[13,14] More recent investigation of factors influencing atrial DFTs produced similar recommendations.[15] In a study by Cooper et al.,[16] atrial DFTs were determined for multiple electrode configurations in a sheep model of acute AF produced by rapid stimulation. In this study, configurations that directed shock current from the right atrium to the left atrium via an electrode positioned in the great cardiac vein consistently had lower peak voltage and delivered energy DFTs compared to configurations having both electrodes on the right side of the heart. In the sheep model of AF, this right-to-left electrode configuration results in mean DFTs of 1–2 J. In humans, a similar electrode configuration requires slightly higher shock energies for acute AF and significantly higher shock energies for chronic AF. In a study by Heisel et al.,[17] eight patients with acute AF and eight patients with chronic AF were subjected to biphasic shocks applied to electrodes in the right atrium and in the coronary sinus. They found that mean delivered energy DFTs for patients with acute AF (38 ± 9 min) were significantly lower (2.0 ± 1.4 J acute vs. 9.2 ± 5.9 J chronic) than for patients presenting with chronic AF (6.6 ± 5.0 months).

Others studies have shown similar dependence of DFT on the duration of AF prior to attempted conversion.[18–21] Re-

RAA → CS   RA → CS+Can

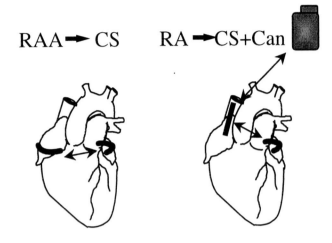

RA/SVC → CS   RA → CS

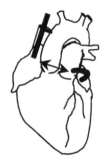
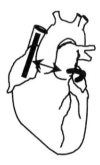

Figure 1. Diagram of electrode positions that have been investigated for use with stand-alone atrial defibrillation systems. The lowest mean atrial DFTs in both animals and humans have been achieved when electrodes are placed in the right atrial appendage (RAA) and in the coronary sinus (CS). RA = right atrium; SVC = superior vena cava; Can = active shell electrode of defibrillation system.

cently, theories concerning calcium overloading of atrial myocytes during AF have been advanced to explain the rise in DFT and early recurrence of AF following successful conversion.[22,23]

Results from both animal and human studies show that the lowest atrial DFTs are obtained when electrodes are placed in the right atrial appendage and in the great cardiac vein adjacent to the left atrial appendage. If this "optimal" lead system had resulted in highly effective therapy that was painless, the clinical benefits of the therapy and the patients' ability to tolerate it would certainly justify the added complexity of ac-

cessing the coronary sinus. However, the studies described in the following sections suggest that atrial defibrillation therapy in the near future, at least, is unlikely to be painless, even for electrode configurations that yield minimum atrial DFTs. Therefore, it would be difficult to justify the addition of the coronary sinus lead if shocks delivered through these optimized atrial defibrillation electrode configurations were just as painful as those delivered through the conventional ICD electrode configurations (e.g., RV → SVC + Can).

To illustrate this point, Min and colleagues[24] performed computational simula-

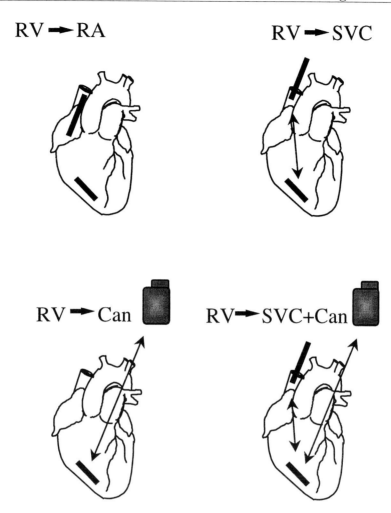

Figure 2. Diagram of electrode positions that have been investigated for use for atrial defibrillation therapy provided by an ICD system. The lowest mean atrial DFTs in humans have been obtained when the active shell electrode (Can) of defibrillation system is incorporated in the defibrillation electrode configuration. See Figure 1 for definition of abbreviations.

tions of atrial defibrillation using finite element methods in a three dimensional model of the human thorax. Realistic tissue conductivities were assigned to isolated tissue volumes obtained from magnetic resonance image slices. Atrial DFTs were computed by determining the peak voltage required to produce an electric field intensity of >5 V/cm throughout 95% of the atrial tissue. Several electrode configurations were evaluated. They concluded that the lowest atrial DFTs were obtained for the configuration having electrodes in the right atrial append-

age and the coronary sinus; similar to the in vivo results from both animal[16,25] experiments and human[26] clinical trials. Further, the model presented by Min et al.[24] predicts that the peak voltage requirement for atrial defibrillation using a conventional ICD shock (RV → SVC + Can) is only about 25% greater than the optimal shock vector (right atrial appendage to coronary sinus). This suggests that the conventional ICD system alone provides an adequate electric field distribution for atrial defibrillation. In fact, clinical data from Heisel et al.[27] reveal that the mean atrial DFT from 27 patients with acutely induced AF was 3.2 ± 1.6 J for biphasic shocks using the TRIAD™ configuration (Guidant Corp., RV → SVC + Can). Indeed, the mean atrial DFT reported by Heisel et al. compares favorably to the optimized atrial DFTs observed for lead systems incorporating electrodes in the great cardiac vein.

Similar results were presented by Saksena et al.[26] in a randomized trial comparing the atrial DFTs of three electrode configurations in 10 patients with a history of drug refractory, chronic AF using a biphasic waveform. Two of the three electrode configurations were similar to contemporary ICD electrode configurations, RV to SVC and RV to right atrium. The third electrode configuration was right atrium to a cutaneous patch located in the left axilla, which was used to emulate an active can electrode. The atrial DFTs for these three configurations were 13.3 ± 5 J for RV to SVC, 16.5 ± 11 J for RV to right atrium, and 20.1 ± 7.4 J for right atrium to left axilla. In a nonrandomized portion of this study in six patients, Saksena and coworkers[26] also tested a right atrium to left pulmonary artery configuration in four patients and right atrium to coronary sinus configuration in two patients. They found that the combined atrial DFT of this small subgroup with chronic AF was 8.9 ± 9 J. Thus, both conventional ICD and more complex electrode configurations yielded atrial DFTs that exceed the pain threshold in unsedated patients with established chronic AF.

A significant variability in atrial DFT exists among electrode configurations in various studies in the literature. In addition to differences in shock distribution, this variability is also a result of variations in the type of AF being defibrillated (i.e., acute vs. chronic) and possibly the degree of electrophysiological derangements[28] present when the defibrillation shock is applied. Most published clinical studies of internal atrial defibrillation recommend the use of a coronary sinus lead to minimize atrial DFTs, but even these shock levels (2–4 J) in

acutely induced AF remain intolerable for most patients. Therefore, it is unclear whether the addition of a coronary sinus lead to an ICD system for atrial defibrillation provides a significant clinical advantage over a standard, less complex ICD lead system. Given that atrial defibrillation shocks will be painful for most unsedated patients, the magnitude of the atrial DFT for dual chamber ICDs may be less important, since the maximum energy stored in the device yields substantial atrial defibrillation safety margins between the output of the device and the DFT.

Waveforms

The term "waveform" in the defibrillation literature is commonly used to refer to a current pulse having a certain shape in the time domain. The shape of a capacitor discharge waveform, commonly used for internal defibrillation, is determined by the rate of voltage decay and the intrapulse switching scheme to control phase duration, polarity and trailing edge truncation point. When a capacitor is discharged between electrodes in the body, the voltage on the capacitor declines at an exponential rate. The time constant (time at which the capacitor voltage declines to a value equal to 1/e [37%] of the initial voltage) is given by the product of the capacitance (units of farads) and the impedance to the shock (units of ohms).

Waveforms affect the peak voltage, peak current, and delivered energy requirements for ventricular[29,30] and atrial[16,31–34] defibrillation. The interactions between waveform shape and effectiveness has been summarized for ventricular defibrillation.[35–37] It is thought that waveforms that are effective for defibrillation of ventricular tissue are also effective for defibrillation of atrial tissue.[38] However, whether the optimal waveform for ventricular defibrillation is identical to the optimal waveform for atrial defibrillation remains unclear.

Empiric Waveform Efficacy Studies

The shock strength required to defibrillate the atria of patients is important because it impacts both the size of implanted devices designed specifically to treat atrial tachyarrhythmias alone and patient acceptance of shock therapy delivered in the absence of sedation.

Much of the empiric atrial defibrillation waveform testing has been motivated by pursuit of "painless" therapy through dramatic reductions in DFT. Atrial defibrillation waveform testing has been substantially influenced by previously published investigations of ventricular defibrillation waveforms associated with ICD development and refinement.[29,30,35] The general rules for optimal ventricular defibrillation waveform definition seem to hold true for atrial defibrillation.[38] Cooper et al.[16] showed that atrial DFTs in sheep were lower for biphasic waveforms compared to monophasic waveforms. It has been demonstrated that atrial DFTs in humans are lower with biphasic compared to monophasic waveforms and that the individual phase durations of these waveforms are important for defibrillation efficacy.[31] More recently, Cooper and colleagues[39] have demonstrated that delivered energy atrial DFTs were reduced 70% when sequential biphasic shocks were applied to dual current pathways. The mean single current pathway (right atrial appendage to distal coronary sinus) DFT was 1.3 ± 0.3 J, whereas the mean sequential shock configuration (right atrial appendage to distal coronary sinus followed by proximal coronary sinus to pulmonary artery) DFT was 0.36 ± 0.13 J. These findings have been verified in clinical studies. Cooper and coworkers,[40] in 12 patients with chronic AF (mean duration 165 ± 187 days), compared the atrial DFT of a single shock/single current pathway configuration (right atrial appendage to distal coronary sinus) to a sequential shock/dual current configuration (right atrial appendage to distal coronary sinus followed by proximal coronary sinus to left subclavian vein).

In this study the atrial DFT for the single shock/single pathway system was significantly higher than the sequential shock/dual pathway configuration (5.1 ± 1.8 J vs. 2.0 ± 0.4 J, $P < 0.05$). While these impressive reductions in atrial DFT move us closer to "painless" atrial defibrillation, demonstration of an incremental clinical benefit with a more complex implanted lead system over that provided by a standard ICD system is needed.

Relationship Between Shock-Induced Pain and Waveform Shape

The meaningful quantification of pain severity is extremely difficult. This difficulty arises from the tremendous subjectivity of pain perception and classification of severity within and among patients. Further, interpretation and comparison of published data concerning pain resulting from noxious stimuli (e.g., defibrillation shocks) is complicated by the lack of standardized methods. However, existing data provide some helpful insights about tolerance to atrial defibrillation shocks. In general, a shock of sufficient strength to reliably defibrillate the atria of humans may range from 200 V to 500 V and may depend on the duration of the AF episode being treated as well as atrial dimensions.[41] Investigators studying therapy tolerance have observed that unsedated patients consistently classified shocks below DFT as "painful."[32] While there are wide variations in the severity of discomfort experienced by individual patients, these data demonstrate that higher voltage (>220 V) shocks cause, on average, more discomfort than low voltage (<220 V) shocks.[41] In addition, for shocks given in pairs, the second shock is likely to be perceived as more painful than the first, independent of the relative strengths of the shocks.[42]

The biophysical mechanisms of pain are complex and multifactorial. For defibrillation shocks, the discomfort experienced immediately after the shock is probably a combination of physical and psychological factors. The biophysics of electrical field interactions with tissues have been well documented.[43] The electrical currents produced by the intracardiac shocks of sufficient magnitude result in pain receptor stimulation and violent skeletal muscle contraction of major muscle groups (e.g., diaphragm, pectoralis major, latissimus dorsi). It remains unclear whether these factors are independent and how they contribute to the perceived level of discomfort. However, one fact is clear from the studies reported thus far; atrial defibrillation shocks applied in the absence of sedation or analgesia are not well tolerated by an overwhelming majority of patients at relatively low shock intensities (below atrial DFT). Further refinements in waveform and delivery method that dramatically reduce DFT are required.[44]

Jung et al.[45] observed that patients typically classified shocks >1 J in strength as "painful" and requested sedation for shocks >2 J. Thus, atrial defibrillation shocks, whether delivered from lead systems that result in the lowest atrial DFT possible (electrodes in right atrium to coronary sinus) or from ICD lead systems using conventional ventricular defibrillation shock vectors, will likely result in intolerable discomfort and apprehension in the majority of patients.

When considering the clinical viability of automatic internal atrial defibrillation, the relationship between pain threshold and atrial DFT must be considered. Murgatroyd et al. showed that the pain threshold is well below the atrial DFT and that the majority of patients requested anesthesia before the DFT was reached in a step-up protocol.[32] Heisel et al. tested the hypothesis that a longer duration high capacitance (500 μF) biphasic waveform would dramatically reduce the voltage DFT compared to a low (60 μF) capacitance waveform.[48] AF was induced with burst pacing in sedated patients. Atrial DFTs were determined for both high-capacitance and low-capacitance waveforms using a step-up protocol. After withdrawal of the anesthesia, two shocks were delivered to the conscious patient, one at the 60-μF waveform DFT and the other at the 500-μF waveform DFT. The order was randomized among patients. Mean peak voltage DFTs for the 60-μF waveform were 191 ± 46 V compared to 73 ± 23 V for the 500-μF waveform, a 62% reduction. Nevertheless, there were no differences in the pain perception scores and the pain thresholds were below the DFT voltage in 11 of 12 patients tested. In one of the patients, testing was stopped after a 55-V (500-μF waveform) shock was declared "intolerable." Heisel et al. also concluded that the second shock was almost always perceived as more painful than the first, independent of the strength.[48] These results are in agreement with the study performed by Steinhaus et al.[42]

Several other groups have also explored the idea that pain perception is predominately related to the peak voltage during the shock. As in Heisel et al.'s study,[48] the hypothesis tested was that longer duration waveforms from higher capacitance devices would cause less pain than shorter duration waveforms using lower capacitance. The data are conflicting. As discussed above, Heisel et al. concluded that both short and long duration shocks were painful, with the second shock almost always more painful than the first, independent of duration. Alt et al.[19] reported that pain scores were lower and patients required lower doses of anesthesia when atrial DFT voltage was reduced about 30% by using longer biphasic (6 ms/6 ms) waveforms compared to the control waveform (3 ms/3 ms biphasic). Tomassoni et al.[46] found that higher capacitance waveforms (120 μF) in humans were associated with a higher atrial DFT energy requirement but a decreased perception of pain in 6 of 10 patients compared to lower capacitance waveforms (50 μF). However, even shocks of less than 0.5 J were considered painful by most patients, despite the low mean atrial DFT in their study (2.0 ± 1.0 J for 120 μF shocks).

Peak voltage can also be reduced by including an inductor in the discharge circuit. The inductor rounds the leading edge of the waveform. Harbinson et al.[47] recently reported that a rounded biphasic waveform had a lower atrial DFT in terms of leading edge voltage, current, and energy compared to a conventional biphasic capacitor discharge waveform. Clinical studies are in progress to determine if rounded biphasic waveforms result in increased tolerance to internal atrial defibrillation shocks.

Atrial Tachyarrhythmia Detection Algorithms

Implanted devices that automatically manage cardiac arrhythmias must be able to discriminate between normal and abnormal rhythms using algorithms that are both highly sensitive and specific. For ventricular tachyarrhythmias, the sensitivity of detection algorithms (percentage of ventricular tachyarrhythmias classified correctly as originating in the ventricle) must be 100%; anything less could prove fatal. In the very earliest ventricular ICD devices, the desired ventricular arrhythmia detection sensitivity was achieved by treating all fast ventricular rhythms. This conservative approach resulted in some "inappropriate" or nonspecific therapy triggered by rapid ventricular response to sinus tachycardia or SVT. In later model ventricular ICD systems, detection enhancement algorithms have been implemented to improve the specificity of therapy delivery, while maintaining the high level of specificity for the patient. As one incorporates atrial tachyarrhythmia therapy into a dual chamber ICD, the relative importance of sensitivity and specificity for atrial treatment is essentially reversed. In these systems, very high sensitivity is required, possibly at the expense of atrial conversion specificity, since these supraventricular rhythms are not likely to be lethal and the high-voltage therapy to treat these rhythms would be classified as "painful" by the patient.

Primary detection for all ICD therapy is based on rate and duration. Detection decisions are based on cardiac cycle length (rate), which is evaluated by the pulse generator on an interval-by-interval (R-R) basis. One of the most fundamental detection concepts underlying the detection architecture of an ICD is the classification of a rhythm as either fast or slow compared to a programmed rate cutoff, or rate threshold. Once a rhythm is diagnosed as rapid, the device verifies that the rhythm continues to be classified as rapid over a programmable time duration before treatment is initiated. This secondary detection criteria of duration assures that an arrhythmia is sustained before it is treated.

Older devices implemented this rate and duration architecture with one rate threshold; current technology uses multiple tiered diagnostic zones to direct ICD therapy based on specific rates. Zone-based detection permits the device to identify specific arrhythmias and quickly initiate appropriate therapy in multiple zones based on the programming of the device, e.g., bradycardia zone, lower ventricular tachycardia (VT) zone, medium VT zone, and high rate VT or ventricular fibrillation zone. Detection enhancements are available within these rate zones to supplement therapy decisions based on rate and duration criteria.[49]

This scheme is rather straightforward for a single chamber ICD in the absence of rate-response pacing. The introduction of dual chamber ICDs[50] required the development of simultaneous, independent sensing and detection of both atrial and ventricular activation rates. Accurate detection of atrial rate permits more specific ventricular therapy and will enable accurate classification and treatment of atrial tachyarrhythmias as well. In the following sections we discuss a few of the technical challenges arising from integration of advanced dual chamber sensing and pacing functionality with ventricular and atrial tachyarrhythmia therapy.

Sensing

Engineers and scientists designing dual chamber ICDs capable of delivering atrial defibrillation shocks face a superset of technical challenges confronted by developers of single chamber ICD systems. Dual chamber systems use bipolar sensing electrodes, bandpass filters and auto-adjusting sense amplifiers (which automatically adjust gain or sensing threshold) to optimize sensing of cardiac depolarizations, minimizing the impact of the natural variations of signal amplitude and extraneous signals, such as myopotentials or farfield depolarizations. Building on pacemaker sensing design, dual chamber systems also incorprate atrial blanking periods to prevent atrial oversensing as a result of farfield signals from intrinsic or paced ventricular depolarizations. To assure the accuracy of atrial sensing, dual chamber ICDs should incorporate automatic gain control on the atrial sensing channel. This strategy assures the most accurate sensing when the P wave amplitudes change from beat to beat. Not only does this improve sensing during atrial arrhythmias, but also allows the device to accurately track atrial depolarizations during nonarrhythmic conditions. Studies have shown that while telemetered P wave amplitudes remain constant over time in controlled clinical settings,[51] they vary with respiration phase,[52] decline markedly during atrial tachyarrhythmias[53] and decline slightly during exercise.[54] Changes in P wave amplitudes and slew rates in response to antiarrhythmic medications also has been reported.[53]

Rhythm Detection and Classification for Dual Chamber ICD Therapy

Single chamber ICD systems previously did not have direct access to information about the atrium and, thus, based their therapy decisions on tiered rate zones with ventricular rate. Besides this basic "ventricle only" mode, dual chamber ICDs can also operate with tiered-rate zones in both the atrium and the ventricle to govern therapy in either chamber. The ability to classify both atrial and ventricular signals allows

the device to identify the rhythm and deliver appropriate therapy.

When this dual atrial and ventricular tiered-rate zone architecture is used to direct ventricular ICD therapy, the atrial rate information is typically used for ventricular rhythms in the lowest VT rate zone. For high specificity, this lowest VT zone requires the greatest flexibility in the number and combination of detection parameters, because it is most likely the zone in which sinus rate crossover or AF can occur. For tachycardias in this lowest VT zone, the dual chamber ICD fine tunes its diagnosis using atrial rate and its comparison to ventricular activity. To provide tiered atrial zones in this lowest VT zone, several programmable atrial rate thresholds have been used (Ventak AV, Guidant Corp., Cardiac Pacemakers, Inc.).[50] One threshold used in the Ventak AV system is the Afib rate threshold (A > Afib), which is useful for diagnosis of AF and its concomitant irregular rapid ventricular rhythm. This "AF zone" can be programmed with Afib rate thresholds ranging from 200 to 300 min⁻¹.

When atrial detection of the Ventak AV is programmed with an AF zone alone, all ventricular rhythms with concomitant atrial rates above this AF threshold would be diagnosed as SVT (or potentially SVT). Under this regimen, slow VTs with atrial rates less than or equal to the Afib rate threshold would be treated, while therapy for VTs with atrial rates faster than Afib would be inhibited. This diagnosis is made more specific in the ventricle by also including the stability criterion in the upper atrial zone to identify irregular ventricular rhythms. With Afib rate threshold *and* ventricular stability, therapy delivery for the treatment of slower VT would be inhibited for A > Afib only during an unstable ventricular rate. Stability would not be invoked for A-rates <Afib.

An alternative atrial rate criterion available in Ventak AV is based on the comparison of average A- and V-rates at the end of a programmable duration, i.e., V > A or A ≥V. This comparison of A- and V-rates can be used alone or in conjunction with the AF zone. When the comparison is used alone, the ICD system operates with a single atrial tachycardia (AT)/AF zone that encompasses all SVTs, ranging from rapid AF, slow-to-moderate-rate ATs, and one-to-one conducted rhythms. When rate comparison is used together with the AF zone, the Ventak AV operates with two atrial tachy zones—a lower-rate AT zone (V ≤ A ≤ Afib) and a higher-rate AF zone (A > Afib).

When this comparison of atrial and ventricular rates is used, slow tachycardias with V-rate > A-rate would be diagnosed as a VT, resulting in the immediate delivery of the programmed therapy sequence. If a tachycardia had concomitant A-rates that were equal to or greater than the V-rate (A ≥ V), which would place the atrial rhythm in the AT/AF zone, a diagnosis of ST or SVT could be made by other detection enhancements, leading to an inhibition of therapy. This SVT/ST diagnosis in the AT/AF zone could also be made more specific by invoking ventricular rate detection enhancements, such as stability and/or onset, to further dictate therapy inhibition. Under this scenario, therapy delivery for the treatment of a slow tachycardia would be inhibited only if the atrial rate fell in the AT/AF zone *and* the programmed detection enhancement(s) in the ventricle were satisfied. Below the AT/AF zone (V > A), detection enhancements would be ignored, since therapy should be administered immediately for fast rhythms occurring solely in the ventricle.

When the Ventak AV is programmed to operate with two atrial tachy zones, the AT and AF zones, rhythm discrimination is based not only on the atrial and ventricular rates, but also on their comparison. In this case, all slow VTs in the lowest VT zone are immediately treated if V rate > A rate, ignoring any detection enhancements that might have been programmed on in this lower VT zone. Slow VTs with concomitant atrial tachycardia rates in the AF zone are diagnosed as SVT, leading to therapy inhibition. When the AF zone is combined with the ventricular stability detection enhance-

ment, therapy would be withheld in the lower VT zone only if atrial rates also fall in the AF zone AND the VT rate is unstable. Rhythms in the AT zone (V ≤ A ≤ Afib) are treated or could be further evaluated with additional detection enhancements to detect and inhibit therapy for ST or SVT.

This fundamental ICD detection architecture, which combines both atrial and ventricular tiered rate zones with different detection enhancements applied only in certain zones, has the potential of improving the specificity of dual chamber ICDs under a "don't treat" condition for therapy to a given chamber. While the example above demonstrates this detection architecture applied to ventricular therapy from a dual chamber ICD, this same detection regimen may be adapted to control electrical therapy for the atria as well. As atrial therapies are integrated into dual chamber ICDs, careful consideration must be made to assure accurate sensing, rhythm detection and classification, and automatic bradyarrhythmia and tachyarrhythmia therapy delivery in both chambers simultaneously. Since, in some cases, an atrial tachyarrhythmia may be coincident with a ventricular tachyarrhythmia, arbitration among atrial and ventricular detection algorithms must be unambiguous. To avoid the potential deleterious consequences of misdiagnosis and incorrect therapy in patients with malignant ventricular arrhythmias, developers of dual chamber ICDs have made the atrial detection algorithms subservient to the ventricular detection algorithms so that ventricular tachyarrhythmia detection sensitivity is not degraded.

From a safety perspective, studies have shown that anticoagulation reduces the risk of stroke following electrical cardioversion in patients that have had AF for greater than 48 hours.[55] Therefore, devices that detect and automatically treat AF should permit physicians to select the duration of the treatment window. If the atrial tachyarrhythmia has not converted prior to expiration of the treatment window, therapy is withdrawn. In addition, high-voltage shocks applied during bouts of AF should be synchronized to either paced or intrinsic ventricular depolarization to avoid ventricular tachyarrhythmia resulting from stimulation during the T wave.[56] While ventricular proarrhythmia is much less likely to be fatal for ICDs since highly effective ventricular therapies are also available, appropriate shock synchronization is important because syncope associated with ventricular arrhythmias is certainly undesirable.

One recent example of the use of a dual chamber tiered architecture for detection and treatment of atrial arrhythmias is the Jewel® AF (Model 7250, Medtronic), which is under clinical investigation.[55] This device provides automatic atrial defibrillation shocks and ramp or burst antitachycardia pacing modes for the treatment of SVTs. Since antitachycardia pacing therapy is thought to be largely ineffective for termination of AF, this device provides two programmable atrial detection zones to prescribe appropriate therapies—the AF zone for AF and the AT zone for atrial tachycardia, atrial flutter and slower AF rhythms. Rhythm detection and classification is performed using various combinations of atrial rate, R:R and P:R patterns (also referred to as coupling codes or A:V syntactical codes), and presence or absence of farfield R wave sensing. Initial detection is declared when 32 ventricular cycles that have P:R patterns consistent with atrial tachyarrhythmia are observed. As P:R patterns for subsequent ventricular events continue to provide evidence of ongoing atrial tachyarrhythmia, a sustained episode detection timer starts. When the episode exceeds the programmed duration (up to 24 hours), the device automatically begins to deliver the therapies that have been selected.

For most patients, shock therapy is likely to be painful. To provide the patient with more control over therapy delivery, the Jewel® AF can be configured to allow the patient to manually enable shock therapy using the Model 9464 Activator. Some patients may specify a preference for shock therapy delivery during certain times of the day or night to avoid the consequences of

therapy delivery in public places or the consequences of shock-induced distraction during activities that require mental concentration (e.g., driving cars, climbing ladders, operating heavy machinery, etc.). To accommodate this, this device allows shock therapy to be enabled continuously or only during certain programmable times.

The first implantation of the Jewel® AF was recently reported[58] and the initial clinical experience has been described.[55] Jung et al.[55] reported that this system was implanted in 28 patients in six European centers. Of these patients, 21 had a history of AF or atrial flutter. The step-up, atrial DFT was determined in 10 patients during predischarge testing. The median atrial DFT was 2 J and ranged from 0.6 J to 16 J. While the clinical follow-up periods are relatively short, Jung et al.[55] reported that three patients experienced 14 spontaneous, sustained episodes of AF or atrial flutter that were successfully treated with automatic therapies.

Summary and Future Issues

Clinical studies are under way to address important questions about atrial defibrillation therapy delivered by ICDs. At this stage, it is too early to conclude that patients will derive significant benefits from automatic atrial defibrillation therapy delivered from an ICD platform. From a theoretical viewpoint, patients in normal sinus rhythm should be expected to do better than patients with paroxysmal or chronic AF since complications associated with anticoagulation and exacerbation of heart failure might be avoided.

As ICDs continue to evolve,[59] they will incorporate features designed to safely and effectively manage a wide spectrum of fast and slow cardiac rhythms originating in the atria or ventricles. It is very likely that, in the future, dual chamber ICDs will provide a platform on which advanced pacing systems designed to also provide hemodynamic improvements to patients suffering from severe congestive heart failure can be clinically evaluated.

References

1. Hohnloser S, Li Y. Drug treatment of atrial fibrillation: what have we learned? Curr Opin Cardiol 1997;12:24–32.

2. Luderitz B, Pfeiffer D, Tebbenjohanns J, et al. Nonpharmacological strategies for treating atrial fibrillation. Am J Cardiol 1996;77: 45A–52A.

3. Psaty BM, Manolio TA, Kuller LH, et al. Incidence of and risk factors for atrial fibrillation in older adults. Circulation 1997;96: 2455–2461.

4. Mackstaller LL, Alpert JS. Atrial fibrillation: a review of mechanism, etiology, and therapy. Clin Cardiol 1997;20:640–650.

5. Gorelick PB. Stroke prevention: an opportunity for efficient utilization of health care resources during the coming decade. Stroke 1994;25:220–224.

6. Feld GK, Fleck P, Chen P-S, et al. Radiofrequency catheter ablation for the treatment of human type 1 atrial flutter: identification of a critical zone in the reentrant circuit by endocardial mapping techniques. Circulation 1992;86:1233–1240.

7. Cosio FG, Arribas F, Lopez-Gil M, et al. Radiofrequency ablation of atrial flutter. J Cardiovasc Electrophysiol 1996;7:60–70.

8. Swartz JF, Pellersels G, Silvers J, et al. A catheter-based approach to atrial fibrillation in humans. Circulation 1994;90:I-335.

9. Haissaguerre M, Gencel L, Fischer B, et al. Successful catheter ablation of atrial fibrillation. J Cardiovasc Electrophysiol 1994;5: 1045–1052.

10. Van Den Berg MP, Tuinenburg AE, Crijns HJGM, et al. Heart failure and atrial fibrillation: current concepts and controversies. Heart 1997;77:309–313.

11. AFFIRM Investigators. Atrial fibrillation follow-up investigation of rhythm management-the AFFIRM study design. Am J Cardiol 1997;79:1198–1202.

12. Dillon SM, Mehra R. Prolongation of ventricular refractoriness by defibrillation shocks may be due to additional depolarization of the action potential. J Cardiovasc Electrophysiol 1992;3:442–456.

13. Ideker RE, Wolf PD, Alferness CA, et al. Current concepts for selecting the location, size, and shape of defibrillation electrodes. PACE 1991;14:227–240.

14. Alt EU, Fotuhi PC, Callihan RL, et al. Endocardial carbon-braid electrodes: a new concept for lower defibrillation thresholds. Circulation 1995;92:1627–1633.

15. Cooper RAS, Alferness CA, Wolf PD, et al. Optimal electrode location and waveform for internal cardioversion of atrial fibrillation in sheep. Circulation 1992;86:I-791.

16. Cooper RAS, Alferness CA, Smith WM, et al. Internal cardioversion of atrial fibrillation in sheep. Circulation 1993;87:1673–1686.

17. Heisel A, Jung J, Neuzner J, et al. Low-energy transvenous cardioversion of atrial fibrillation using a single atrial lead system. J Cardiovasc Electrophysiol 1997;8:607–614.

18. Johnson E, Smith W, Yarger M, et al. Clinical predictors of low energy defibrillation thresholds in patients undergoing internal cardioversion of atrial fibrillation. PACE 1994;17:742A.

19. Alt E, Coenen M, Schmitt C, et al. Intracardiac electrical conversion of atrial fibrillation: Which energies should be used? Circulation 1994;90:I–14.

20. Alt E, Schmitt C, Ammer R, et al. Effect of electrode position on outcome of low-energy intracardiac cardioversion of atrial fibrillation. J Am Coll Cardiol 1997;79:621–625.

21. Levy S, Ricard P, Lau CP, et al. Multicenter low energy transvenous atrial defibrillation (XAD) trial results in different subsets of atrial fibrillation. J Am Coll Cardiol 1997;29: 750–755.

22. Van Wagoner DR, Lamorgese M, Kirian, P, et al. Calcium current density is reduced in atrial myocytes isolated from patients in chronic atrial fibrillation. Circulation 1997; 96:I-180.

23. Pu J, Shvilkin A, Hara M, et al. Altered inward currents in myocytes from chronically fibrillating canine atria. Circulation 1997;96: I-180.

24. Min X, Mongeon LR, Mehra R. Low threshold non-CS electrode systems for atrial defibrillation and compared with CS-RA by finite element human thorax model. Circulation 1997;96:I-529.

25. Cooper RAS, Smith WM, Ideker RE. Early activation sites after unsuccessful internal atrial defibrillation shocks: the effects of electrode configuration. PACE 1996;19:706A.

26. Saksena S, Prakash A, Mangeon L, et al. Clinical efficacy and safety of atrial defibrillation using biphasic shocks and current nonthoracotomy endocardial lead configurations. Am J Cardiol 1995;76:913–921.

27. Heisel A, Jung J, Fries R, et al. Influence of active pectoral can on transvenous atrial cardioversion threshold in patients with implantable cardioverter-defibrillator. J Am Coll Cardiol in press.

28. Goette A, Honeycutt C, Langberg JJ. Electrical remodeling in atrial fibrillation: time

course and mechanisms. Circulation 1997;94: 2968–2974.

29. Jones JL. Waveforms for implantable cardioverter defibrillators (ICDs) and transchest defibrillation. In Tacker WA Jr, ed. Defibrillation of the Heart: ICDs, AEDs, and Manual. Mosby-Year Book, Inc, St. Louis, 1994, pp 46–81.

30. Walcott GP, Walker RG, Cates AW, et al. Choosing the optimal monophasic and biphasic waveforms for ventricular defibrillation. J Cardiovasc Electrophysiol 1995;6: 737–750.

31. Cooper RAS, Johnson EE, Wharton JM. Internal atrial defibrillation in humans: the improved efficacy of biphasic waveforms and the importance of phase duration. Circulation 1997;95:1487–1496.

32. Murgatroyd FD, Slade AKB, Sopher SM, et al. Efficacy and tolerability of transvenous low energy cardioversion of paroxysmal atrial fibrillation in humans. J Am Coll Cardiol 1996;25:1347–1353.

33. Keane D. Impact of pulse characteristics on atrial defibrillation energy requirements. PACE 1994;17:1048–1057.

34. Johnson EE, Yarger MD, Wharton JM. Monophasic and biphasic waveforms for low energy internal cardioversion of atrial fibrillation in humans. Circulation 1993;88:I-592.

35. Schuder JC, McDaniel WC, Stoeckle H, et al. Optimal biphasic waveform morphology for canine defibrillation with a transvenous catheter and subcutaneous patch system. Circulation 1988;78:II-219.

36. Chapman PD, Vetter JW, Souza JJ, et al. Comparative efficacy of monophasic and biphasic truncated exponential shocks for nonthoracotomy internal defibrillation in dogs. J Am Coll Cardiol 1988;12:739–745.

37. Fain ES, Sweeney MB, Franz MR. Improved internal defibrillation efficacy with a biphasic waveform. Am Heart J 1989;117:358–364.

38. Ideker RE, Cooper RAS, Walcott KT. Comparison of atrial and ventricular fibrillation and defibrillation. PACE 1994;17:1034–1042.

39. Cooper RAS, Smith WM, Ideker RE. Internal cardioversion of atrial fibrillation: marked reduction in defibrillation threshold with dual current pathways. Circulation 1997;96: 2693–2700.

40. Cooper RAS, Plumb VJ, Epstein AE, et al. Marked reduction in internal atrial defibrillation thresholds with dual current pathways and sequential shocks in humans. Circulation in press.

41. Levy S, Ricard P, Gueunoun M, et al. Low-energy cardioversion of spontaneous atrial fibrillation: immediate and long-term results. Circulation 1997;96:253–259.

42. Steinhaus DM, Cardinal D, Mongeon L, et al. Atrial defibrillation: Are low energy shocks acceptable to patients? PACE 1996;19:625A.

43. Plonsey R, Barr RC. Bioelectricity: A Quantitative Approach. Plenum Press, New York, London, 1988, p 329.

44. Heisel A, Jung J, Fries R, et al. Atrial defibrillation: can modifications in current implantable cardioverter-defibrilators achieve this? Am J Cardiol 1997;78:119–127.

45. Jung W, Tebbenjohanns J, Wopert C, et al. Safety, efficacy, and pain perception of internal atrial defibrillation in humans. Circulation 1995;92:I-472.

46. Tomassoni G, Newby KH, Kearney MM, et al. Testing different biphasic waveforms and capacitances: effect on atrial defibrillation threshold and pain perception. J Am Coll Cardiol 1996;28:695–699.

47. Harbinson MT, Allen JD, Imam Z, et al. Rounded biphasic waveform reduces energy requirements for transvenous catheter cardioversion of atrial fibrillation and flutter. PACE 1997;20:226–229A.

48. Heisel A, Jung J, Schubert BD. Evaluation of two new biphasic waveforms for internal cardioversion of atrial fibrillation. Circulation 1997;96:I-207.

49. Olson WH. Tachyarrhythmia sensing and detection. In Singer I, ed. Implantable Cardioverter Defibrillator. Futura Publishing Company, Inc., Armonk, NY, 1994, pp 71–107.

50. Jung W, Spehl S, Wolpert C, et al. For the European Ventak AV Investigators: Improved arrhythmia classification with a new pectoral dual-chamber implantable cardioverter defibrillator. Circulation 1997;96:I-579.

51. Platia EV, Brinker JA. Time course of transvenous pacemaker stimulation impedance, capture threshold, and electrogram amplitude. PACE 1986;9:620–625.

52. Shandling AH, Florio J, Castellanet MJ, et al. Physical determinants of the endocardial P wave. PACE 1990;13:1585–1589.

53. Ropella KM, Sahakian AV, Baerman JM, et al. Effects of procainamide on intra-atrial electrograms during atrial fibrillation: implications for detection algorithms. Circulation 1988;77:1047–1054.

54. Fröhlig G, Schieffer H, Bette L. Atrial signal variations and pacemaker malsensing during exercise: a study in the time and frequency domain. J Am Coll Cardiol 1988;11: 806–813.

55. Jung W, Brachmann J, den Dulk K, et al. Initial clinical experience with a new arrhythmia management device. Circulation 1997; 96:I-208.
56. Laupacis A, Albers G, Dunn M, et al. Antithrombotic therapy in atrial fibrillation. Chest 1992;102:426S–433S.
57. Ayers GM, Alferness CA, Ilina M, et al. Ventricular proarrhythmic effects of ventricular cycle length and shock strength in a sheep model of transvenous atrial defibrillation. Circulation 1994;89:413–422.
58. Jung W, Luderitz B. Implantation of a new arrhythmia management system in patients with supraventricular and ventricular tachyarrhythmias. Lancet 1997;349:853–854.
59. KenKnight BH, Jones BR, Thomas AC, et al. Technological advances in ICDs before the year 2000 and beyond. Am J Cardiol 1996; 78:108–115.

Chapter 21

Atrial Defibrillators

S. Mark Sopher, A. John Camm

Introduction

Atrial fibrillation (AF) very frequently recurs in patients in whom the arrhythmia has terminated spontaneously (paroxysmal AF) or has required antiarrhythmic drugs or transthoracic countershock to restore sinus rhythm (persistent AF). Aggressive management strategies designed to restore and maintain sinus rhythm are justified by the results of studies demonstrating the magnitude of the subjective and objective benefits of restoring sinus rhythm, even where the ventricular rate in AF has been "controlled." Furthermore, prompt cardioversion is supported by recent data that over time AF changes atrial electrophysiology in a way that promotes continuation of the arrhythmia ("AF begets AF"). While transthoracic countershock can restore sinus rhythm in the majority of patients with a short history of AF, the efficacy of antiarrhythmic drugs intended to maintain sinus rhythm is limited in both paroxysmal and persistent AF. Furthermore, the tolerability and safety of these drugs is of major concern when treating a relatively benign arrhythmia. The use of pacemakers to maintain sinus rhythm in patients with a history of AF who do not have a conventional indication for pacing is in its infancy and does not appear to be widely applicable. Major cardiac surgical operations have been devised to maintain sinus rhythm, but these have significant morbidity, are expensive, and require specialist resources. New approaches, the value of which remains to be established, are catheter ablation for AF and the use of high-frequency burst stimulation to terminate AF.

Recurrent AF is therefore one of the most difficult arrhythmias to treat. Repeated cardioversions by conventional means is expensive in terms of resources, probably requires long-term anticoagulation unless feasible within a few hours of the onset of AF, and may be unacceptable to patients with frequent recurrences. A well-tolerated therapy that could safely and promptly cardiovert AF out of hospital would thus have great potential for improving the management of a large proportion of patients with AF.

AF is also a particular problem in the population of patients implanted with conventional (ventricular) cardioverter-defibrillators (ICDs). It is a common occurrence in this population and is the most frequent cause of inappropriate therapy. The incorporation into an ICD of the capacity to accurately distinguish AF from ventricular arrhythmia and to treat AF specifically would

From Singer I, Barold SS, Camm AJ (eds): Nonpharmacological Therapy of Arrhythmias for the 21st Century: The State of the Art. Futura Publishing Co, Inc., Armonk, NY, © 1998.

therefore represent a significant therapeutic advance.

"Internal" cardioversion of AF by shocks using intraesophageal or intracardiac electrodes was first reported 30 years ago, and the last decade has seen large-scale investigations of such shocks in animals and in man. The efficiency of the shock energy is considerably increased by focusing the electrical field on the atrial myocardium. Indeed shock waveforms and vectors have been identified that can consistently terminate AF in man with <5 J. Since patients may find such low-energy shocks tolerable without general anaesthesia, these studies suggested the potential value of an implantable device that could recognize and promptly terminate AF using such shocks. Two such devices have now been developed and are undergoing clinical investigation. One is a "stand-alone" atrial defibrillator and the other incorporates prevention, detection, and treatment strategies for supraventricular tachyarrhythmias, including AF, into a conventional ICD. This article discusses the background of the development of these devices and focuses on the important concerns regarding their efficacy, safety, tolerability, and appropriate indications for use.

The Benefits of Sinus Rhythm and Limitations of Conventional Therapies

Studies examining the effects of therapies designed to restore and/or maintain sinus rhythm in patients with a history of AF have tended to focus only on their efficacy rather than providing data allowing an overall cost-benefit analysis. While some data exist that provide an indication of the benefits and risks of such therapies in patients with persistent AF, the difficulties of documenting recurrent arrhythmia in patients with paroxysmal AF make even trials designed only to demonstrate efficacy difficult to conduct and analyze. However, it is common experience that patients with paroxysmal AF are often particularly disturbed by symptoms of the arrhythmia and that drugs used to attempt control of the ventricular rate during AF are generally of limited value in controlling symptoms. Furthermore, both calcium-channel antagonists and digoxin may have effects on atrial electrophysiology that promote AF, although the evidence for an increase in the frequency of episodes attributable to therapy with digoxin is equivocal.[1-4] It is therefore usual practice to use antiarrhythmic rather than rate-controlling drugs in this group. The potential value of antiarrhythmic therapy designed to reduce the frequency of episodes of arrhythmia or, ideally, to abolish recurrence, clearly depends on the underlying frequency of episodes and the symptoms during each episode. There is clear evidence of the efficacy of some antiarrhythmic agents to reduce the frequency of episodes of AF.[5-12]

Following cardioversion of persistent AF by transthoracic countershock, improvements can be seen in symptoms, functional capacity, and left ventricular ejection fraction.[13-16] The prompt restoration of sinus rhythm is further justified by the recent experimental evidence that supports the widely held impression that AF itself alters the electrophysiology of the atrium in such a way as to facilitate further AF (AF begets AF).[17] This process appears to be reversible in the short-term, suggesting that early cardioversion of AF episodes may ultimately lessen the tendency for the arrhythmia to recur. However, following cardioversion of persistent AF, most studies indicate continuance of sinus rhythm in only 30%–50% of patients at 3 months and in around 20%–40% at 12 months.[18-21] This proportion can be increased by treatment with antiarrhythmic agents. The most aggressive strategy published using repeated cardioversions and the sequential use of flecainide, quinidine or sotalol, and amiodarone allowed 63% of patients to remain free of persistent AF and required a mean of 1.8 cardioversions each.[22] While amiodarone may be effective where other agents have failed,[23] it carries the risk of severe and irreversible side effects. In addition to their relative inefficacy, inconvenience and associated financial costs, conventional aggressive strategies to the restoration and maintenance of sinus rhythm in patients with AF may be associated with significant morbidity and possible mortality. Intolerance and induced bradyarrhythmias are common problems, and there is major concern over the risks of ventricular proarrhythmia of all antiarrhythmic agents when used to treat a relatively benign arrhythmia.[24-26] The proarrhythmic risks of quinidine were recognized early on[27,28] and were highlighted by Coplen et al.'s meta-analysis of six selected randomized trials of quinidine used to maintain sinus rhythm following cardioversion of AF.[19] The results of the CAST study[29] serve to remind us of the risks of the widespread use of antiarrhythmic therapy and there is clear evidence that, in patients with AF, these risks are not limited to the use of quinidine, although this drug may be an important culprit.[24] However, it must also be remembered that the proarrhythmic risks of antiarrhythmic drugs are importantly influenced by the presence of structural heart disease, ischemia, and heart failure, and that the majority of patients with paroxysmal AF have none of these.

Thus, while it is clear that in patients with recurrent AF (whether paroxysmal or persistent) there are compelling arguments to support an aggressive approach to the restoration and maintenance of sinus rhythm, conventional therapies are frequently limited by their inefficacy, costs, inconvenience, intolerability, and risks. An implantable device that would terminate an episode of AF within minutes or hours of its onset could be a considerable advantage to patients with recurrent persistent AF if the function of such a device were reliably effective, safe, and tolerable. Such an atrial defibrillator could obviate the need for poorly tolerated and potentially dangerous antiarrhythmic drugs in many patients, and reduce this need in others. Finally, the ability to restore sinus rhythm more rapidly than

is conventionally feasible may limit the electrical remodeling[17] and thus reduce the tendency of the rhythm to recur.

Internal Cardioversion of Atrial Fibrillation

Various attempts have been made to increase the efficiency of shocks used to cardiovert AF by delivering energy closer to the atria. In a canine model, defibrillation thresholds <1.5 J have been obtained with an esophageal catheter.[30] Transoesophageal cardioversion in humans, however, requires 100–200 J to achieve an 80% success rate.[31] Similarly, there are discrepancies between animal and human atrial defibrillation using endocavitary shocks. In dogs, cardioversion can be achieved with less than 5 J using right atrial bipolar or unipolar electrode configurations (the latter with a skin patch acting as indifferent electrode).[32,33] The sheep heart may provide a better model of clinical AF, as it is of similar size to that of humans, and stable fibrillation can be produced by burst pacing alone, without the need for measures such as vagal stimulation or talc-induced pericarditis. Powell et al. obtained 80% success with 2.5-J shocks delivered in sheep between a right atrial spring electrode and a skin patch.[34] However, initial attempts at endocavitary cardioversion in humans were less successful. Nathan et al. delivered shocks between an active electrode positioned in the right atrium or ventricular apex, and an indifferent electrode in the right atrium, superior vena cava, or inferior vena cava.[35] At the low energies used (up to 10 J), these shocks were uniformly unsuccessful in terminating AF. However, Lévy et al. demonstrated the increased efficacy of internal shocks by delivering high energies between a conventional pacing electrode catheter positioned in the low right atrium and a backplate. These shocks were able to terminate AF in patients for whom conventional attempts at electrical and pharmacological cardioversion had failed.[36] However, energies of over

200 J were used, and it is possible that the efficacy of the technique owes as much to barotrauma, caused by arcing from the low electrode surface area,[37] as to a direct electrical effect on the arrhythmia.

Biatrial and Other Shock Configurations and Waveforms

The most efficient defibrillation electrode configuration encompasses a sufficient proportion of the target tissue within its electric field while wasting minimal energy elsewhere. As the entirety of the atrial myocardium is involved in the electrical mechanism of AF, it would seem likely that a successful shock field must involve at least a significant proportion of both atria. A systematic comparison of "biatrial" transvenous lead configurations and shock waveforms was therefore conducted by Cooper et al. in a series of experiments using a pacing-induced model of AF in sheep.[38] This examined four right atrial electrode positions (superior vena cava, right atrial appendage, mid and low right atrium) and three "left atrial" positions (coronary sinus, left pulmonary artery, and a left axillary subcutaneous patch). As expected, the lowest defibrillation thresholds were obtained using left-right atrial configurations, those using an electrode pair in the right atrium and the coronary sinus being somewhat lower than others. Using this configuration and a 3 ms + 3 ms biphasic truncated exponential shock, the mean energy requirement for cardioversion of AF in this sheep model was 1.3 ± 0.4 J. Preliminary data in a dog model of AF suggest that defibrillation thresholds can be reduced still further by incorporating an SVC coil and using a shock configuration of [RA + SVC] to CS.[39]

Following the remarkably low atrial defibrillation thresholds achieved in these animal experiments, several centers have investigated the use of biatrial shocks in patients with paroxysmal and persistent AF. Keane et al. delivered shocks between epicardial paddle electrodes on the surface of each atrium[40] in 21 patients undergoing cardiopulmonary bypass. With 8-ms monophasic shocks, 50% success was obtained at a mean energy of 1.44 J, and with 4-ms + 4-ms biphasic shocks, the mean energy was 0.37 J. However, large surface area paddles were used in this study, and the AF was artificially induced and of short duration. We have reported the use of biatrial biphasic (3 ms + 3 ms) shocks delivered between transvenous electrodes in the high right atrium and coronary sinus[41]: 22 patients with acute AF were studied in the context of electrophysiological investigations: the arrhythmia was induced by catheter manipulation or pacing in 18 and occurred spontaneously in four. Most patients had a history of spontaneous paroxysmal AF. The mean energy requirement for cardioversion was 2.16 ± 1.02 J. Our experience was included in a multicenter trial of this technique in four groups of patients that has recently been reported[42]: AF was (1) chronic (>30 days) in 53; (2) intermediate (>7 days) in 18; (3) acute (7 days) in 50; and (4) induced in 20 patients. Using a maximum leading edge voltage of 400 V (approximately 5 J), cardioversion was successful in 70%, 89%, 92%, and 80% with a mean energy of 3.6 J, 2.8 J, 2.0 J, and 1.8 J, respectively.

Several series have examined atrial defibrillation thresholds using different transvenous lead configurations including those used by conventional ICDs designed for ventricular arrhythmias. Desai et al. was able to terminate induced AF (six patients) and chronic AF (three patients) with mean energies of 1.5 J and 9.3 J, respectively, using the right atrium-coronary sinus configuration, of 4.3 J and 10.4 J using electrodes in the superior vena cava and right ventricle, and of 5.4 J and 12.1 J using a right atrial electrode and a pectoral can.[43] Saksena et al. performed atrial defibrillation using a variety of transvenous defibrillator lead configurations in 10 patients.[44] The mean energy requirements were 10.8 J for a superior vena cava–right ventricle configuration, 10.4 J for a right atrium–right ventricle configuration, and 17.5 J for a right ventri-

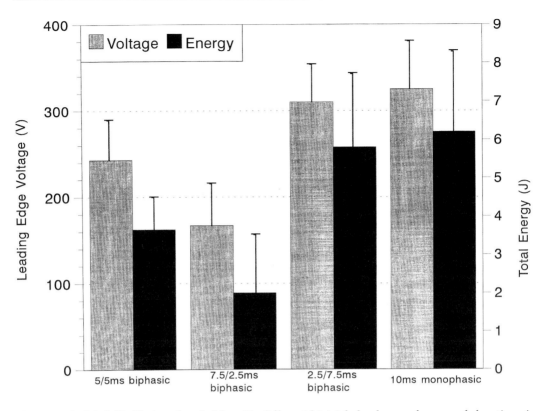

Figure 1. Atrial defibrillation thresholds with different biatrial shock waveforms and durations in man. Mean SD of atrial defibrillation threshold in terms of leading edge voltage and total energy for a monophasic waveform and a symmetrical biphasic waveform compared to two asymetrical biphasic waveforms. Used with permission and modified from Cooper RAS, et al.[45]

cle/patch configuration. These studies indicate that in humans as in animals, the lowest atrial defibrillation thresholds are obtained using lead configurations which encompass the atria. Cooper and colleagues[45] recently extended their earlier work in sheep to human AF in a study examining the effect on defibrillation threshold of altering waveforms and phase duration of biatrial shocks. They demonstrated a dramatic reduction in thresholds with the use of a biphasic compared to a monophasic waveform and that the threshold was also profoundly affected by the duration of each phase (Figure 1). Other investigators have examined the effect of altering the tilt of the biphasic waveform on the atrial defibrillation threshold.[46] No consistent effect was identified, but marked differences in the threshold with a 65% tilt compared to a 50% tilt were seen

in some patients, suggesting that it might be possible to reduce defibrillation thresholds further by optimizing the waveform in each patient.

Applications for Low-Energy Cardioversion and Implantable Atrial Defibrillators

The efficacy of low-energy cardioversion and the lack of requirement for general anesthesia makes the technique potentially valuable in a variety of situations. Several centers already use the technique routinely for AF complicating diagnostic electrophysiological procedures and catheter ablation. The technique may also be extended to acute AF in intensive care settings, such as the management of patients following cardiac surgery and acute myocardial infarction, and to patients in whom general anesthesia may be hazardous, such as the morbidly obese.[47]

Internal shocks can also be used to terminate AF that has been resistant to conventional methods of cardioversion. In a multicenter study following up on the initial experience of Lévy, 112 patients who had failed at least one attempt at electrical or pharmacological cardioversion were loaded with amiodarone and randomized to a further attempt using either high-energy unipolar shocks (200–300 J between the right atrium and a backplate) or repeated external shocks (300–360 J).[48] The success rates were 91% and 67%, respectively (P<0.02). Alt et al. delivered shocks between high-surface area electrodes in the right atrium and the coronary sinus or left pulmonary artery in 14 patients with established AF, six of whom had previously failed external cardioversion.[49] The technique was successful in 10 cases, with shocks of up to 520 V (7.9 J). We achieved success in 8 out of 11 patients with highly resistant AF with the right atrium-coronary sinus configuration with shocks of up to 400 V (6 J).[50] All patients had previously failed to cardiovert with repeated external shocks of up to 360 J delivered using both apex-base and anteroposterior paddle configurations, in many cases while taking adjunctive class III antiarrhythmic medication.

The most exciting potential application of low-energy internal cardioversion is undoubtedly its use in implanted devices. AF occurs in 20%–30% of patients with ICDs,[51–54] and is probably the most common cause of inappropriate therapy.[54,55] Inappropriate shocks cause premature battery depletion,[56] have adverse psychological effects,[57] are proarrhythmic,[58] and can be fatal.[59] The maintenance of sinus rhythm has particular advantages in the ICD population which has a high incidence of ischemic heart disease and impaired ventricular function such that AF may precipitate acute ischemia and is frequently poorly tol-

erated hemodynamically. However, the antiarrhythmic drugs commonly used to maintain sinus rhythm or control the ventricular rate during AF may be particularly unsuitable in this population due to a negative inotropic effect, the increased risk of proarrhythmia associated with structural heart disease and ischemia, and the effect of some antiarrhythmic drugs to increase the ventricular defibrillation threshold as seen most clearly with amiodarone.[60] The ability to reliably discriminate AF from ventricular arrhythmia and to ensure prompt termination of AF in a tolerable fashion would therefore be a major advance in ICD technology. Existing ventricular defibrillation electrode systems can be used for cardioversion, but the energy required is of the order of 5–10 J for paroxysmal AF, and 10–20 J for chronic AF.[43,44] An arrhythmia management device (Figure 2) (Model 7250, Medtronic Inc., Minneapolis, MN) that incorporates atrial sensing and pacing into a conventional ICD and that allows different shock vectors to be delivered for atrial and ventricular defibrillation is undergoing clinical evaluation. In addition to shocks to terminate AF, this device also uses atrial pacing strategies to prevent and terminate atrial tachyarrhythmias. Medtronic Inc. is also planning a generation of such atrial tachyarrhythmia devices for patients who do not have a history of ventricular tachyarrhythmia; however, the devices may incorporate a limited capacity to defibrillate the ventricles to allay fears of a ventricular proarrhythmic risk associated with atrial defibrillation.

A "stand-alone" atrial defibrillator (Metrix®) has already been developed by InControl Inc. (Redmond, WA) (Figure 3) and tested in sheep[61] and man.[62] It uses defibrillation electrodes in the right atrium and coronary sinus, and a conventional ventricular lead for R wave synchronization and backup pacing. Biphasic (3 ms + 3 ms or 6 ms + 6 ms) R wave synchronized shocks of up to around 300 V (equivalent to around 3 J or 6 J) are delivered between the defibrillation electrodes. The testing in sheep has

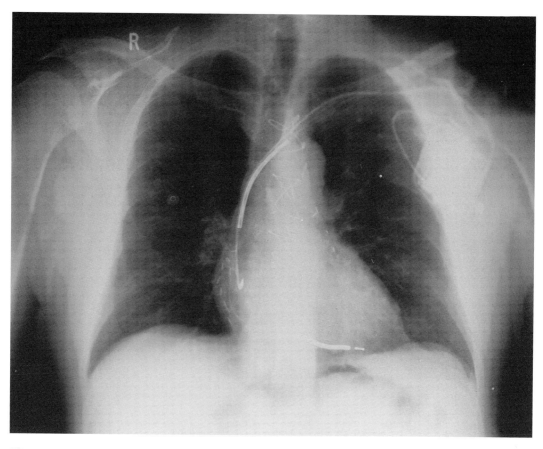

Figure 2. An atrial and ventricular "arrhythmia management device." The generator has been implanted in a left subpectoral pocket with separate pacing/defibrillation electrodes in the right atrium and the right ventricle. The vector of the shocks used for ventricular and atrial defibrillation may be programmed independently and may use any combination of endocardial coils and the "can" (generator casing).

indicated the chronic stability of the lead system and of atrial defibrillation thresholds. The first human implants of this system took place in late 1995, and following presentation to the regulatory authorities of the results of initial clinical investigations, the system has recently been approved for clinical use by the European regulatory authorities.

The technical feasibility of atrial defibrillation is not in doubt, but its clinical utility will depend on the further demonstration of its safety and tolerability, and on a knowledge of the manner in which it alters the natural history of the condition. Although based on similar technology to existing pacemakers and ICDs, the requirements of an atrial defibrillator, especially of the "stand-alone" type, are necessarily very different. In particular, safety is paramount in the treatment of a non-life-threatening arrhythmia, and there is no need for immediate cardioversion. The particular features and operation of these atrial defibrillators are considered below.

Device Size

The size of any implantable defibrillator is principally determined by the dimensions of the battery and capacitor. Several factors

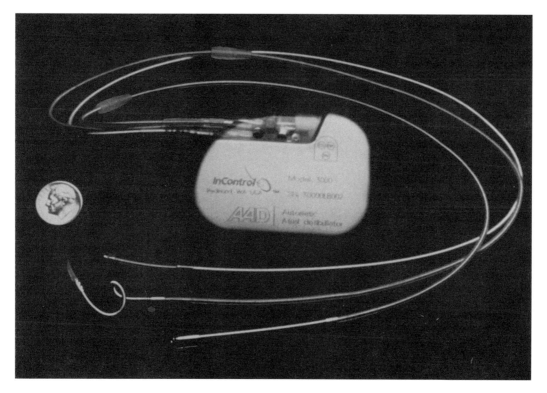

Figure 3A. A stand-alone implantable atrial defibrillator. Defibrillation is achieved by low-energy biphasic shocks delivered between electrodes in the right atrium and the coronary sinus. The coronary sinus lead is designed to adopt a spiral shape on withdrawal of the stylet in order to enhance stability. A lead in the right ventricle is used for sensing and pacing. A 10-cent coin is also shown to indicate the size of the device.

allow the "stand-alone" atrial defibrillator to be smaller than conventional ICDs. The most obvious of these is the energy required for cardioversion, an order of magnitude lower than for ventricular defibrillation. Also important is that AF is not immediately life-threatening and need not be terminated within seconds. A capacitor charge time of the order of a minute can therefore be allowed, which would be out of the question for an ICD. Finally, detection algorithms, which consume considerable current, need not be continuously active. The device can therefore remain inactive for most of the time, waking up for a few seconds at predetermined intervals or at the patient's behest, and only remaining active if AF is detected. The InControl device (Metrix®) has a volume around 50 mls and is thus designed for routine prepectoral im-

plantation. However, the pace of progress in battery and capacitor technology is reflected in the volume of the Medtronic device (Model 7250) which has a volume of only 55 mls despite possessing the capacity for ventricular defibrillation.

Atrial Leads

Minimizing the energy required to defibrillate the atria is a particular priority of the "stand-alone" atrial defibrillator, and the InControl device (Metrix®) therefore uses a right atrial and a coronary sinus lead mounted with a defibrillation coil. Although the coronary sinus has been used for pacing and more recently by conventional ICDs, it is not always simple to achieve a stable position. This difficulty has been ap-

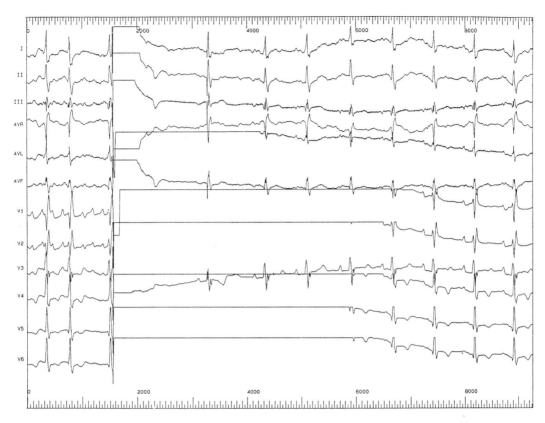

Figure 3B. A 2.2-J shock delivered by this device which cardioverts atrial fibrillation.

proached in a novel way for the InControl device using a lead whose defibrillation coil assumes a helical conformation when its stylet is withdrawn, expanding against the wall of the coronary sinus. Initial experience in sheep[61] and in humans suggests that this lead is highly stable, although it can be foreseen that lead extraction, should it become necessary, may be difficult and dangerous. Recent work has suggested that the device could use a "single-pass" lead with right atrial and coronary sinus coils.[63-65] The Medtronic "arrhythmia management device" may be used with a variety of lead systems: in addition to right ventricular and right atrial leads, a conventional defibrillation lead may also be positioned in the superior vena cava or in the coronary sinus and a subcutaneous patch electrode may also be used. The "can" (generator casing) may be incorporated into any combination of leads

to improve the shock vector and reduce atrial and ventricular defibrillation thresholds.

Detection Algorithms

For conventional ICDs, it is vital that no sustained ventricular arrhythmia is missed by the device. In spite of the many methods used to improve specificity, it is necessary to accept a small risk that therapy will be inappropriately triggered by atrial tachyarrhythmias or oversensing,[51] in order to guarantee a sensitivity around 100%. Conversely, for the "stand-alone" atrial defibrillator, late detection or even nondetection of an episode of AF is not dangerous, while an inappropriate shock given by an atrial defibrillator might carry a risk of proarrhythmia and be unacceptable to the patient. Of paramount importance (see below) is that shock delivery be correctly synchronized with the QRS complex, and avoid short RR intervals. The arrhythmia detection algorithms utilized by the InControl and Medtronic devices are both novel. For QRS detection the InControl device (Metrix®) uses analysis of both the right ventricular bipolar electrogram and the electrogram generated from the right ventricular apical electrode to the coronary sinus electrode (RV-CS). AF detection also depends on two vectors, utilizing both the right ventricular electrogram and the electrogram generated from the right atrial electrode to the coronary sinus electrode (RA-CS). Sophisticated interpretation of these electrograms involving both quiet time and baseline crossing analysis on the RA-CS channel is used with automatic or programmable settings to determine the presence of AF. The Medtronic device utilzes a different strategy to define the presence and nature of any tachyarrhythmia and may classify AF, atrial flutter/tachycardia, sinus and other 1:1 supraventricular tachycardias, ventricular tachycardia, ventricular fibrillation, and "dual" tachycardia/fibrillation (atrial and ventricular co-existing).[66,67] Auto-adjusting atrial and ventricular sensing thresholds and short cross-chamber blanking periods are used to prevent undersensing. The RR interval is divided into four time zones (Figure 4). Atrial event(s) during two successive RR intervals are used to generate interval codes representing the number and timing of P relative to R waves. The succession of interval codes defines the arrhythmia. The detection algorithms are used in a hierarchical fashion to ensure that ventricular tachycardia and ventricular fibrillation detection always take precedence over other possible tachyarrhythmias.

Current Practice and Future Applications for Implantable Atrial Defibrillators

Experience with the InControl "stand-alone" atrial defibrillator has been obtained in highly selected patients with well-described clinical features and patterns of AF. Safety concerns dictated that these patients be of very low risk for proarrhythmia, with little or no structural heart disease. Patients have generally been resistant to, or intolerant of, antiarrhythmic drugs with episodes of AF generally lasting for hours or days, possibly requiring attendance at hospital

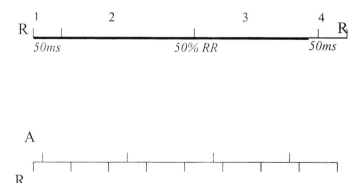

Figure 4. Arrhythmia detection in the dual chamber defibrillator. Each RR interval is divided into four zones: R to R + 50 ms, R + 50 ms to 50%RR interval, 50%RR interval to R-50 ms, R-50 ms to R. During two successive RR intervals, the timing and number of P waves within each of these four intervals is used to define a "couple code." The sequence of couple codes is used to generate a rhythm syntax which defines the detected arrhythmia. In the lower trace, sinus rhythm and ventricular tachycardia co-exist such that there are 0 or 1 detected atrial events in each RR interval and the timing of the atrial event within the RR interval varies.

for cardioversion. Patients have been required to go to the investigational center to have their device activated. With the continued accumulation of data relating to the appropriate functioning of the device and the safety of shocks, the indications will be broadened to include patients with structural cardiac abnormalities, such as left ventricular hypertrophy or heart failure, who may obtain more benefit from the restoration of sinus rhythm because of their increased dependence on atrial transport.

Initial programming of the "stand-alone" atrial defibrillator has also been very conservative in relation to safety. Patients have been admitted to the hospital each time AF occurred to have the device activated, allowing verification of correct functioning and ensuring the absence of adverse consequences of shocks delivered. Again, however, the next phase of investigation will involve the use of the patient-activated mode, allowing patients to activate the defibrillator out of hospital using a magnet, so that it promptly detects and terminates AF episodes. Other modes of function include automatic shocking with the option of a very small preceding "warning" shock. This phase of investigation will allow the very pertinent question of whether prompt termination of AF is antiarrhythmic (i.e., does "sinus rhythm beget sinus rhythm?") to be addressed by comparing arrhythmia-free intervals in patients randomized to prompt defibrillation by the device or to delayed cardioversion.

The Medtronic device also incorporates highly programmable features in the use of atrial defibrillation therapy. A programmable number of high-frequency (50 Hz) bursts lasting 1, 2, or 3 sec may be used in an attempt to terminate AF despite the very limited data that exist to suggest the efficacy of this technique in clinical AF in humans. Shocks to cardiovert AF may be delivered after a programmable duration of AF, during a programmable time window (e.g., only at night), and the tilt as well as the energy of the biphasic shock is programmable. In addition, atrial shock therapy may be automatic or patient activated. At present the device is undergoing clinical investigation in patients who require conventional ICD therapy and may benefit from atrial sensing and/or pacing. Most patients have a history of supraventricular arrhythmia and others are felt to be at particularly high risk of AF (e.g., patients with a cardiomyopathy). The prevention, detection, and treatment capabilities of the device are being closely monitored. This experience will determine the features of the next generation of Medtronic defibrillators designed for atrial or dual chamber defibrillation.

Safety of Transvenous Atrial Defibrillation

The most serious potential drawback to transvenous atrial defibrillation is the possibility that internal shocks delivered to terminate AF may provoke malignant ventricular arrhythmias. This is of particular concern with a "stand-alone" implantable atrial defibrillator, for use out of hospital without the availability of immediate therapy for ventricular tachyarrhythmias. Three factors are likely to determine the risk of ventricular proarrhythmia.

First, as discussed earlier, the electrode configuration determines the energy necessary for atrial defibrillation and therefore both the strength and the distribution of the defibrillation field. The RA-CS configuration appears to be the most efficient, with minimum ventricular involvement in the defibrillation field. Geometric considerations suggest that other electrode configurations, such as those using the left pulmonary artery or a subcutaneous patch, require greater total field strengths and are likely to deliver a higher energy to the ventricles.

Second, the timing of shocks within the cardiac cycle is critical to their safety. External cardioversion shocks falling on the T wave can induce ventricular fibrillation,[68,69] and for this reason shocks are conventionally synchronized to the surface QRS complex or the endocardial R wave. Even with correct synchronization, it is possible that an atrial shock delivered following a short RR interval may fall into the relative refractory period of part of the ventricle and thus initiate ventricular fibrillation. This possibility was systematically investigated by Ayers et al.,[70] using shocks delivered between the right atrium and coronary sinus in sheep, both above and below the atrial defibrillation threshold. Shocks were delivered with a delay of 0–100 ms after the R wave, in paced rhythm, after single and double extrastimuli, and in AF. Four episodes of ventricular fibrillation ensued at the lower energy settings, and seven at the higher. These episodes were all initiated by shocks following RR intervals of 300 ms or less. It was suggested that shocks using this electrode configuration would be safe in humans only if they are reliably synchronous with the QRS complex, and delivered after a minimum RR intervals that exceeded this figure with a safety margin, such as a total of 500 ms.

Finally, the ventricular proarrhythmic risk of atrial shocks is likely to be affected by the susceptibility of the ventricle at a given time in a given patient. The inducibility of ventricular fibrillation, in particular, is determined by functional (ischemia, autonomic tone, electrolyte imbalance, and antiarrhythmic drugs) as well as structural factors.

No individual center has had sufficient experience to demonstrate the absolute safety of such shocks. A co-operative registry has therefore been instituted of researchers known to be investigating biatrial shocks delivered in patients, and reported initially from a 1,000 biatrial shocks.[71] This figure has now exceeded 3,000 shocks. No proarrhythmia has resulted from synchronized shocks delivered following an RR interval that is not short between electrodes in the right atrium and coronary sinus, though unsynchronized shocks and shocks following a short RR interval[72] have triggered ventricular fibrillation. Higher energies delivered between the right atrium and pulmonary artery have occasionally given rise to nonsustained runs of broad complex tachycardia that may represent ventricular ectopy or aberrantly conducted AF. In addition to data in this registry, two cases have been reported of nonsustained ventricular tachycardia caused by synchronous shocks to cardiovert AF delivered between the right atrium and the right ventricle.[73] These were in patients with structural heart disease. The registry has also demonstrated that higher energy (>4 J) biatrial shocks can affect sinoatrial and atrioventricular nodal function, causing slowing of the ventricular rate during AF, and significant pauses after cardioversion.

It is therefore clear that a substantial risk of ventricular fibrillation exists with unsynchronized atrial defibrillation shocks, whatever the electrode configuration. The risk of ventricular proarrhythmia appears to be extremely low with properly synchronized shocks delivered between right atrium and coronary sinus. This risk can be estimated if the assumption is made that the cumulative probability of a proarrhythmic occurrence follows a binomial distribution. The lack of any events following 3,000 synchronized shocks gives an upper 95% confidence interval of the risk per shock of 0.1%. In a device delivering one shock per month on average, this would yield an annual risk comparable to, or lower than, that of antiarrhythmic drugs in a similar group of patients. Other electrode configurations investigated require more energy and deliver a greater proportion of this energy to the ventricles. Such configurations would therefore be expected to have a greater risk but could safely be utilized by a combined atrial and ventricular defibrillator.

Tolerability of Transvenous Atrial Defibrillation

Although the energies used with these techniques are considerably lower than with conventional cardioversion, shocks are far from imperceptible. Unfortunately, there are few data regarding the tolerability of transvenous atrial shocks, largely because few studies have been performed with conscious patients. Nathan et al. did not find any relation between the intensity of intracardiac shocks and symptoms.[35] In the series of Murgatroyd et al., sedation was withheld initially, but allowed at the patients' request as progressively greater energies were delivered. In all patients, discomfort increased with shock intensity, and there was great interindividual variation in the maximum energy tolerated, which was between 0.5 and 1.0 J in most cases.[41] In contrast, in a study of the effect of different right atrial lead positions on defibrillation thresholds, Lok et al. reported that sedation was only required for shocks of over 3–4 J.[74]

Undoubtedly, the perception of discomfort is highly subjective, and data obtained from patients receiving a series of incrementally larger shocks during an electrophysiological study, may not tell us very much about tolerability in a more realistic setting. Patients are likely to tolerate shocks of greater energy if they are familiar with them and associate them with therapeutic benefit. Much remains to be learned regarding the determinants of discomfort from atrial shocks, and how altered lead configuration or shock waveform may improve the relationship between atrial defibrillation threshold and pain threshold. Skeletal muscle contraction is likely to be involved and this may depend on the leading edge voltage of the shock more than shock energy,[75] providing the rationale for the use of rounded biphasic waveforms.[76,77] However, despite much ongoing research, it seems unlikely that atrial defibrillation shocks will become imperceptible in the near future. Therefore, even if safety considerations can be adequately met, few atrial defibrillators are likely to be programmed to an automatic mode for the time being. However, the ability to terminate prolonged symptomatic episodes of AF by activating the device with a magnet would allow patients to control their antiarrhythmic therapy to a degree that is unusual, even if this required attending a hospital or clinic for brief sedation. The confidence that shocks will never be delivered unexpectedly would be a psychological advantage, and would not interfere with activities such as driving.

Summary

The use of high surface area defibrillation electrodes especially in a biatrial configuration, combined with biphasic waveforms, has been shown to dramatically lower the atrial defibrillation threshold. The energy requirement for cardioversion has been reduced by two orders of magnitude, and general anesthesia is no longer required. Although shocks may still remain uncomfortable, modifications to the design and location of electrodes, and possibly to the shock waveform, may improve the tolerability of atrial defibrillation to the extent that it can be routinely performed in unsedated patients. Initial experience suggests that the risk of proarrhythmia is extremely low if shocks are correctly synchronized. Several potential applications for this technique exist in acute situations and for implanted devices. A stand-alone atrial defibrillator has been tested in animals, and the first human implants were performed at the end of 1995. However, this therapeutic modality is still some way from being suitable for widespread use. In the immediate future, experience with the safety of biatrial shocks and the function of the device must be greatly expanded, and improved tolerability of shocks is needed. If these issues are satisfactorily addressed, atrial defibrillators should be certified for more widespread use (Figure 5). Only then can the clinical utility of these devices emerge, as it will be possible to study how they modify the natural history of paroxysmal AF and the quality of life of patients. The parallel development of other nonpharmacological treatments for AF (surgical procedures, catheter ablation, and pacemaker therapy), and the inevitable financial limitations, will determine the fu-

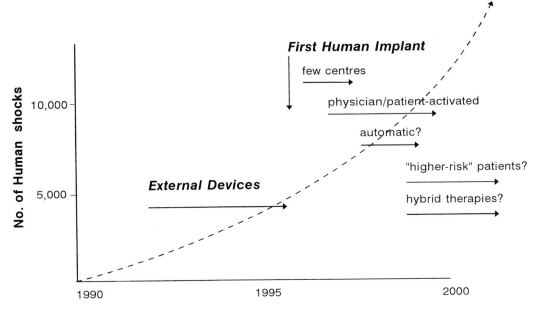

Figure 5. The future of the atrial defibrillator. With increasing experience of the safety of internal cardioversion of AF in man, there is likely to be an expansion in the use of the atrial defibrillator. This experience and that of other new treatments for AF, possibly in combination with the atrial defibrillator as "hybrid" therapy will determine its future.

ture role of implantable defibrillators for the treatment of the most common cardiac arrhythmia. The incorporation of atrial sensing is a major advance in ICD technology as it will substantially reduce the problem of inappropriate detection of ventricular arrhythmia. A significant proportion of ICD patients will also benefit from the incorporation of therapies specifically designed to cardiovert AF.

References

1. Galun E, Flugelman MY, Glickson M, et al. Failure of long-term digitalization to prevent rapid ventricular response in patients with paroxysmal atrial fibrillation. Chest 1991;99:1038–1040.
2. Coumel P. Role of the autonomic nervous system in paroxysmal atrial fibrillation. In Touboul P, Waldo AL, eds. Atrial Arrhythmias: Current Concepts and Management. Mosby-Year Book, St. Louis, 1990, pp 248–261.
3. Rawles JM, Metcalfe MJ, Jennings K. Time of occurrence, duration, and ventricular rate of paroxysmal atrial fibrillation: the effect of digoxin. Br Heart J 1990;63:225–227.
4. Murgatroyd FD, Xie B, Gibson SM, et al. The effects of digoxin in patients with paroxysmal atrial fibrillation: analysis of Holter data from the CRAFT-1 trial. J Am Coll Cardiol 1993;21:203A.
5. Anderson JL, Gilbert EM, Alpert BL, et al. Prevention of symptomatic recurrences of paroxysmal atrial fibrillation in patients initially tolerating antiarrhythmic therapy: a multicenter, double-blind, crossover study of flecainide and placebo with transtelephonic monitoring. Flecainide Supraventricular Tachycardia Study Group. Circulation 1989;80:1557–1570.
6. Connolly SJ, Hoffert DL. Usefulness of propafenone for recurrent paroxysmal atrial fibrillation. Am J Cardiol 1989;63:817–819.
7. Pritchett ELC, McCarthy EA, Wilkinson WE. Propafenone treatment of symptomatic paroxysmal supraventricular arrhythmias: a randomized, placebo-controlled, crossover trial in patients tolerating oral therapy. Ann Intern Med 1991;114:539–544.
8. Cobbe SM. A randomized, placebo-controlled trial of propafenone in the prophy-

laxis of paroxysmal supraventricular tachyarrhythmias. J Am Coll Cardiol 1994;23: 251A.

9. Lau CP, Leung WH, Wong CK. A randomized double-blind crossover study comparing the efficacy and tolerability of flecainide and quinidine in the control of patients with symptomatic paroxysmal atrial fibrillation. Am Heart J 1992;124:645–650.

10. Reimold SC, Cantillon CO, Friedman PL, et al. Propafenone versus sotalol for suppression of recurrent symptomatic atrial fibrillation. Am J Cardiol 1993;71:558–563.

11. Antman EM, Beamer AD, Cantillon C, et al. Therapy of refractory symptomatic atrial fibrillation and atrial flutter: a staged care approach with new antiarrhythmic drugs. J Am Coll Cardiol 1990;15:698–707.

12. Horowitz LN, Spielman SR, Greenspan AM, et al. Use of amiodarone in the treatment of persistent and paroxysmal atrial fibrillation resistant to quinidine therapy. J Am Coll Cardiol 1985;6:1402–1407.

13. Gosselink ATM, Crijns HJ, Van Den Berg MP, et al. Functional capacity before and after cardioversion of atrial fibrillation: a controlled study. Br Heart J 1994;72:161–166.

14. Brand FN, Abbott RD, Kannel WB, et al. Characteristics and prognosis of lone atrial fibrillation: thirty year follow up in the Framingham study. JAMA 1985;254:3449–3453.

15. Kopecky SL, Gersh BJ, McGoon MD, et al. The natural history of lone atrial fibrillation: a population based study over three decades. N Engl J Med 1987;317:669–674.

16. Montoya PT, Brugada P, Smeets J, et al. Ventricular fibrillation in the Wolff-Parkinson-White syndrome. Eur Heart J 1991;I 2: 144–150.

17. Wijffels MC, Kirchhof CJ, Dorland R, et al. Atrial fibrillation begets atrial fibrillation. Circulation. 1995;92(7):1954–1968.

18. Metcalfe MJ, Smith F, Jennings K, et al. Does cardioversion of atrial fibrillation result in myocardial damage? Br Med J 1988;290: 1364A.

19. Coplen SE, Antman EM, Berlin JA, et al. Efficacy and safety of quinidine therapy for maintenance of sinus rhythm after cardioversion: a meta-analysis of randomized control trials. Circulation 1990;82:1106–1116.

20. Falk RH, Podrid PJ. Electrical cardioversion of atrial fibrillation. In Falk RH, Podrid PJ, eds. Atrial Fibrillation: Mechanisms and Management. Raven Press, New York, 1992, pp 181–195.

21. Lundstrom T, Ryden L. Chronic atrial fibrillation: long-term results of direct current conversion. Acta Med Scand 1988;223:53–59.

22. Crijns HJ, Van Gelder IC, Van Gilst WH, et al. Serial antiarrhythmic drug treatment to maintain sinus rhythm after electrical cardioversion for chronic atrial fibrillation or atrial flutter. Am J Cardiol 1991;68:335–341.

23. Gosselink ATM, Crijns HJ, Van Gelder IC, et al. Low-dose amiodarone for maintenance of sinus rhythm after cardioversion of atrial fibrillation or flutter. JAMA 1992;267: 3289–3293.

24. Falk RH. Proarrhythmia in patients treated for atrial fibrillation or flutter. Ann Intern Med 1992;117:141–150.

25. Pritchett ELC, Wilkinson WE. Mortality in patients treated with flecainide and encainide for supraventricular arrhythmias. Am J Cardiol 1991;67:976–980.

26. Cowan JC. Antiarrhythmic drugs in the management of atrial fibrillation. Br Heart J 1993;70:304–306.

27. Selzer A, Wray HW. Quinidine syncope: paroxysmal ventricular fibrillation occurring during treatment of chronic atrial arrhythmias. Circulation 1964;30:17–26.

28. Radford MD, Evans DW. Long-term results of DC reversion of atrial fibrillation. Br Heart J 1968;30:91–96.

29. Ruskin JN. The Cardiac Arrhythmia Suppression Trial (CAST). N Engl J Med 1989; 321:386–388.

30. Yamanouchi Y, Kumagai K, Tashiro N, et al. Transesophageal low-energy synchronous cardioversion of atrial flutter/fibrillation in the dog. Am Heart J 1992;123:417–420.

31. McKeown PP, Croal S, Allen JD, et al. Transesophageal cardioversion. Am Heart J 1993; 125:396–404.

32. Kumagai K, Yamanouchi Y, Tashiro N, et al. Low energy synchronous transcatheter cardioversion of atrial flutter/fibrillation in the dog. J Am Coll Cardiol 1990;16:497–501.

33. Dunbar DN, Tobler HG, Fetter J, et al. Intracavitary electrode catheter cardioversion of atrial tachyarrhythmias in the dog. J Am Coll Cardiol 1986;7:1015–1027.

34. Powell AC, Garan H, McGovern BA, et al. Low energy conversion of atrial fibrillation in the sheep. J Am Coll Cardiol 1992;20: 707–711.

35. Nathan AW, Bexton RS, Spurrell RAJ, et al. Internal transvenous low energy cardioversion for the treatment of cardiac arrhythmias. Br Heart J 1984;52:377–384.

36. Lévy S, Lacombe P, Cointe R, et al. High energy transcatheter cardioversion of chronic atrial fibrillation. J Am Coll Cardiol 1988;12: 514–518.

37. Bardy GH, Coltorti F, Stewart RB, et al. Catheter-mediated electrical ablation: the relation between current and pulse width on voltage

breakdown and shock-wave generation. Circ Res 1988;63:409–414.

38. Cooper RA, Alferness CA, Smith WM, et al. Internal cardioversion of atrial fibrillation in sheep. Circulation 1993;87:1673–1686.

39. Krum D, Hare J, Mughal K, et al. Optimal electrode configuration reduces energy requirements for internal atrial defibrillation. PACE 1997;20:1127.

40. Keane D, Boyd E, Anderson D, et al. Comparison of biphasic and monophasic waveforms in epicardial atrial defibrillation. J Am Coll Cardiol 1994;24:171–176.

41. Murgatroyd FD, Slade AKB, Sopher SM, et al. Efficacy and tolerability of transvenous low energy cardioversion of paroxysmal atrial fibrillation in man. J Am Coll Cardiol 1995;25:1347–1353.

42. Lévy S, Ricard P, Lau CP, et al. Multicenter low energy transvenous atrial defibrillation (XAD) trial results in different subsets of atrial fibrillation. JACC 1997;29:750–755.

43. Desai PK, Mongeon L, Conlon S, et al. Is energy for transvenous defibrillation of atrial fibrillation (AF) with active pectoral can feasible? Circulation 1994;90:I-376.

44. Saksena S, Mongeon L, Krol R, et al. Clinical efficacy and safety of atrial defibrillation using current nonthoracotomy endocardial lead configurations: a prospective randomized study. J Am Coll Cardiol 1994;23:125A.

45. Cooper RAS, Johnson EE, Wharton JM. Internal atrial defibrillation in humans: improved efficacy of biphasic wavforms and the importance of phase duration. Circulation 1997; 95:1487–1496.

46. Sra J, Bremner S, Krum D, et al. The effect of biphasic waveform tilt in transvenous atrial defibrillation. PACE 1997;20:1613–1618.

47. Baker BM, Botteron GW, Smith JM. Low-energy internal cardioversion for atrial fibrillation resistant to external cardioversion. J Cardiovasc Electrophysiol 1995;6:44–47.

48. Lévy S, Lauribe P, Dolla E, et al. A randomized comparison of external and internal cardioversion of chronic atrial fibrillation. Circulation 1992;86:1415–1420.

49. Alt E, Schmitt C, Ammer R, et al. Initial experience with intracardiac atrial defibrillation in patients with chronic atrial fibrillation. PACE 1994;17:1067–1078.

50. Sopher SM, Murgatroyd FD, Slade AKB, et al. Low energy internal cardioversion of atrial fibrillation resistant to transthoracic shocks. Br Heart J 1996;75:635–638.

51. O'Nunain S, Roelke M, Trouton TG, et al. Limitations and late complications of third-generation automatic cardioverter defibrillators. Circulation 1995;91:2204–2213.

52. Neuzner J. Clinical experience with a new cardioverter defibrillator capable of biphasic waveform pulse and enhanced data storage: results of a prospective multicenter study. European Ventak P2 Investigator Group. PACE 1994;17:1243–1255.

53. Wood MA, Stambler BS, Damiano RJ, et al. Lessons learned from data logging in a multicenter clinical trial using a late-generation implantable cardioverter-defibrillator. The Guardian ATP 4210 Multicenter Investigators Group. J Am Coll Cardiol 1994;24: 1692–1699.

54. Brachmann J, Sterns LD, Hilbel T, et al. Acute efficacy and chronic follow-up of patients with non-thoracotomy third generation implantable defibrillators. PACE 1994;17: 499–505.

55. Grimm W, Flores BF, Marchlinski FE. Complications of implantable cardioverter defibrillator therapy: follow-up of 241 patients. PACE 1993;16:218–222.

56. Fogoros RN, Elson JJ, Bonnet CA. Actuarial incidence and pattern of occurrence of shocks following implantation of the automatic implantable cardioverter defibrillator. PACE 1989;12:1465–1473.

57. Lüderitz B, Jung W, Deister A, et al. Patient acceptance of the implantable cardioverter defibrillator in ventricular tachyarrhythmias. PACE 1993;16:1815–1821.

58. Johnson NJ, Marchlinski FE. Arrhythmias induced by device antitachycardia therapy due to diagnostic nonspecificity. J Am Coll Cardiol 1991;18:1418–1425.

59. Birgersdotter-Green U, Rosenqvist M, et al. Holter documented sudden death in a patient with an implanted defibrillator. PACE 1992;15:1008–1014.

60. Guarnieri T, Levine JH, Veltri EP, et al. Success of chronic defibrillation and the role of antiarrhythmic drugs with the automatic implantable cardioverter/defibrillator. Am J Cardiol 1987;60:1061–1064.

61. Ayers GM, Griffin JC, Ilina MB, et al. An implantable atrial defibrillator: initial experience with a novel device. PACE 1994;17: 769A.

62. Lau CP, Tse HF, Lee K, et al. Initial clinical experience with an implantable human atrial defibrillator. PACE 1997;20:220–225.

63. Heisel A, Jung J, Neuzner J, et al. Low-energy transvenous cardioversion of atrial fibrillation using a single atrial lead system. J Cardiovasc Electrophysiol 1997;8:607–614.

64. Sopher SM, Ayers GM, Obel OA, et al. Atrial defibrillation in man by low energy biatrial shocks employing a single-pass transvenous catheter. Circulation 1996;91:I-563A.

65. Tse HF, Lau CP, Ayers GM. Initial clinical experience with a single-pass (solo) dual

electrode lead for an implantable atrial defibrillator. PACE 1997;20:1126.

66. Gillberg JM, Brown ML, Stanton MS, et al. Clinical testing of a dual chamber atrial tachyarrhythmia detection algorithm. Comput Cardiol 1996:57–60.

67. Brown ML, Gillberg JM, Stanton MS, et al. Acute human testing of a dual chamber ventricular tachyarrhythmia detection algorithm at Mayo Clinic. Comput Cardiol 1996: 61–64.

68. King BG. The effect of electric shock on heart action with special reference to varying susceptibility in different parts of the cardiac cycle. Doctoral Thesis. 1934 (Abstract).

69. Wiggers CJ, Wegria R. Ventricular fibrillation due to single, localized induction and condenser shocks applied during the vulnerable phase of ventricular systole. Am J Physiol 1921;128:500–505.

70. Ayers GM, Alferness CA, Ilina M, et al. Ventricular proarrhythmic effects of ventricular cycle length and shock strength in a sheep model of transvenous atrial defibrillation. Circulation 1994;89:413–422.

71. Murgatroyd FD, Johnson EE, Cooper RA, et al. Safety of low energy transvenous atrial defibrillation: world experience. Circulation 1994;90:14A.

72. Barold HS, Wharton JM. Ventricular fibrillation resulting from synchronised internal atrial defibrillation in a patient with ventricular preexcitation. J Cardiovasc Electrophysiol 1997;8:436–440.

73. Saksena S, Krol RB, Varanasi S, et al. Internal atrial defibrillation in symptomatic atrial flutter/fibrillation. Circulation 1994;90:I-377.

74. Lok NS, Lau CP, Lee KLF, et al. Effect of different right atrial lead locations on the efficacy and tolerability of low energy transvenous atrial defibrillation with an implantable lead system. PACE 1996;19:633A.

75. Alt E, Ammer R, Schmitt C, et al. Pain threshold for internal cardioversion with low or no sedation. PACE 1996;19:737A.

76. Gonzalez X, Ayers GM, Wagner DO, et al. Waveforms to reduce peak voltages for internal atrial defibrillation. PACE 1996;19:696A.

77. Harbinson M, Trouton T, Imam Z, et al. Transvenous catheter atrial defibrillation using rounded versus standard biphasic waveforms. PACE 1996;19:696A.

Chapter 22

Quality of Life in Patients with Atrial Fibrillation

Berndt Lüderitz, Werner Jung

Introduction

The efficacy of a therapy has been primarily based on objective criteria such as mortality and morbidity. In addition to these objective criteria, interest has increased in recent years in the measurement of quality of life in relation to health care. Quality of life is now the new "catch phrase" in medicine. Like happiness, it is one of those terms that we all understand but for which adequate definitions do not exist. It is generally agreed that quality of life should be measured as an integral component of most trials, particularly where treatments are given with an intention to palliate or reduce symptoms.[1] The term quality of life suggests an abstract and philosophical approach, but in reality most approaches used in medical contexts do not attempt to include more general notions such as life satisfaction or standard of living, and rather tend to concentrate on aspects of personal experience that might be related to health and health care.[2] The incorporation of quality of life measurements in clinical studies is fortunately receiving a higher priority and often provides information that would be unobtainable by other means. It is important to distinguish the different applications of quality of life measure because instruments that have proven useful when applied in one context may be less appropriate elsewhere. A good research tool may be impractical for clinical uses. Generally, more attention has been given to the use of quality of life instruments in clinical trials than to an examination of their value in routine clinical care, medical audit, or resource allocation.[1–4]

Definition of Quality of Life

Unfortunately, many trials dealing with aspects of quality of life do not assess the construct properly, or they assess only a single or limited aspect of what is really a multidimensional construct (Figure 1). Moreover, multidimensional endpoints such as quality of life present particular problems of design, analysis and interpretation.[2] Although the concept of quality of life is inherently subjective and definitions vary, it can be assessed on the basis of four components[6,7]: physical condition, psychological well-being, social activities, and everyday activity. All four dimensions can be subdivided into various aspects. For instance, physical function includes mobility and self-care, whereas the emotional dimension

From Singer I, Barold SS, Camm AJ (eds): Nonpharmacological Therapy of Arrhythmias for the 21st Century: The State of the Art. Futura Publishing Co, Inc., Armonk, NY, © 1998.

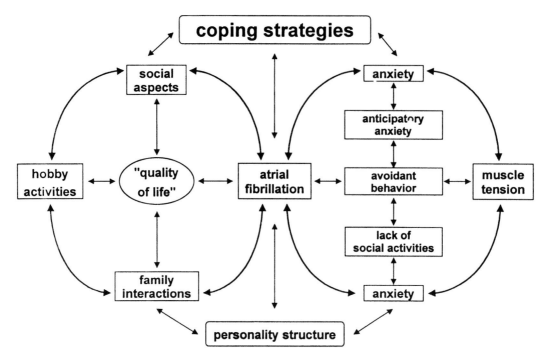

Figure 1. Quality of life in atrial fibrillation as a multidimensional construct. The circle of anxiety shows the interactions between anxiety, muscle tension, and atrial fibrillation (center) influenced by anticipatory anxiety, avoidant behavior, and lack of social activities. Concerning quality of life also family interactions, hobby activities, and social aspects are involved. The symptom atrial fibrillation stands between coping strategies and personality structure.[5]

includes aspects such as anxiety and depression. The social dimension includes aspects such as intimacy, social support, and family contact. Each of these items can be measured in a quantitative way, hence

the selection of appropriate instruments allows an extensive description of quality of life (Table 1). Many instruments consist of a large number of questions in order to consider as many subscales and dimensions as possible. However, the evaluation of each question individually is not useful; it is necessary to assess quality of life scores for specific dimensions. The scores of each scale in a given instrument are summarized and expressed in a total quality of life score.[6–9]

Constructing Scales of Measurement

The measurement of quality of life should address each objective and subjective component that is important to members of the patient population and susceptible to being affected, positively or negatively, by inter-

Table 1
Quality of Life, Medical Outcomes Study
Short-Form Survey (SF-36)

SF-36 Category	US-Norm	Atrial Fibrillation
Mental Health	74,74	58,28
Vitality	60,86	24,29
Physical Functioning	84,15	34,05
Emotional Role Function	80,96	7,15
Physical Role Function	81,26	28,33
Social Role Function	83,28	41,07
Bodily Pain	75,15	44,95
General Health	71,95	48,00

Lower score represents a lower quality of life.
Used with permission from Bubien RS, et al.[9]

ventions. In order to compare quality of life with other patient groups, the use of standardized instruments is strongly recommended. Many new instruments reflect the multidimensionality of quality of life. There are several factors influencing the selection of appropriate instruments to assess quality of life.[3] The first and most important issue when selecting an instrument is how well it will perform in the required situation. This can be assessed from the instrument's psychometric properties. Validity and reliability are necessary for all contexts.

Reliability means that all instruments must produce the same results on repeated use under the same conditions. This can be examined by test-retest reliability, although practically it may be difficult to distinguish measurement error from real changes in quality of life.[2] Reliability is often assessed by examining internal reliability—the degree of agreement of items addressing equivalent concepts. Inter-rater reliability also needs to be established for interview-based assessments.

The *validity* of quality of life measures is more difficult to assess because instruments are measuring an inherently subjective phenomenon. An informal but essential approach is to examine face validity by using instruments that seem to cover the full range of relevant topics. This process may be enhanced by including people with a wide range of backgrounds in the assessment process. In addition, in-depth descriptive surveys of the relevant patient group should be consulted as these provide invaluable evidence of the range of patients' experiences. Once validity has been shown for one purpose, it cannot be assumed for all possible populations or applications. Measures of quality of life that can distinguish between patients at a point in time are not necessarily as sensitive to changes (responsiveness) in patients over time when repeated.

Responsiveness is a measure of the association between the change in the observed score and the change in the true value of the construct. Responsiveness is a crucial requirement for most applications, especially in clinical trials. The absence of a standard against which to assess the measurement properties of a quality of life instrument is a particular problem when examining instruments sensitive to change. Although a measure may be responsive to changes in the true value of the construct, graduations in the metric of the observed score may not be adequate to reflect these changes.

Sensitivity refers to the ability of the measurement to reflect true changes or differences in the true quality of life value. Problems such as an inadequate range or delineation of the response can mask important and therapeutically meaningful changes in quality of life. One of the most important areas for further development is in making quantitative change scores for quality of life more clinically meaningful. To ensure that the quality of life measure used is the most appropriate, the health problem and likely range of impacts of the treatment being investigated need to be carefully considered. Established instruments cannot be assumed to be most appropriate. One approach to improving the appropriateness of quality of life measures is to use instruments that let patients select the dimensions of most concern. Quality of life measures that are to be used routinely should be brief and simple. Brevity may mean, however, that potentially important information about patients' experiences is missed and the validity and responsiveness of shorter instruments need to be studied.[2] In summary, the basic requirement of quality of life assessments are: multidimensional construct, reliability, validity, sensitivity, responsiveness, appropriateness to question or use, and practical utility.

Selecting an Assessment Instrument

Three study designs are most commonly used in quality of life evaluation.[10] The first is the cross-sectional or nonrandomized longitudinal study, which describes predictors of quality of life (for example, speciality vs. primary care). The second common design is the randomized study of a clinical intervention. In these studies, the measures must reflect the nature of the disease, be reponsive to perceptually meaningful changes, and be sensitive to changes within the range of function specific to the disease. The third common design is the study of cost-effectiveness and cost-benefit analysis, which estimates the incremental cost of a program or treatment compared with the program's incremental effects on health, which are usually measured by adjusting a clinical outcome such as survival by the quality of life. The instruments and techniques used to assess quality of life vary according to the identity of the respondent, the setting of the evaluation and the type of the questionnaire used (short form, self-assessment instrument, interview, clinic-based survey, telephone query, or mail-back survey), and the general approach to evaluation.

Generic instruments are used in general populations to assess a wide range of domains applicable to a variety of health states, conditions, and diseases.[10] They are usually not specific to any particular disease state or susceptible population of patients and are therefore most useful in conducting general survey research on health and making comparisons between disease states. Generic instruments have advantages and disadvantages. Many health-related dimensions remove the need to select dimensions for a particular study and allow for the detection of unexpected effects. A further benefit of generic instruments is to facilitate comparisons among different disease groups. A negative aspect is that a broad approach may reduce responsiveness to effects of health care.

Disease-specific instruments focus on the domains most relevant to the disease or condition under study and on the characteristics of patients in whom the condition is most prevalent. Disease-specific instru-

ments are most appropriate for clinical trials in which specific therapeutic interventions are being evaluated. Disease-specific instruments have several theoretical advantages. They reduce patient burden and increase acceptability by including only relevant dimensions. Disadvantages are the lack of comparability of results with those from other disease groups and the possibility of missing effects in dimensions that are not included.[3] Batteries of scales and modular instruments combine the generic and the disease-specific approaches by maintaining a core module of questions applicable to diverse disease states and patient populations to which the questions most relevant to the disease and therapy in question are added as needed. Studies have shown that clinicians' and patients' judgments of quality of life differ substantially and systematic assessment may improve health professionals' judgment.[2] Therefore, self-administered questionnaires or questionnaires administered by interviewers should be used.

Atrial Fibrillation

Atrial fibrillation is a frequent and costly health care problem representing the most common arrhythmia resulting in hospital admission. The high prevalence of atrial fibrillation (2%–4% in people over the age of 65 years) and its clinical complications, the poor efficacy of medical therapy for preventing recurrences, and dissatisfaction with alternative modes of therapy stimulated interest in an implantable atrial defibrillator. Two-thirds of patients with atrial fibrillation report that symptoms such as fatigue, presyncope, palpitations, and dizziness significantly disrupt their lives.[11] Since an implantable atrial defibrillator alleviates symptom burden rather than to cure the underlying rhythm disorder, it is important to assess quality of life in patients with atrial fibrillation who are considered candidates for an implantable atrial defibrillator. Our own experience in patients with malignant

Psychological General Well-Being Scores
(PGWB)

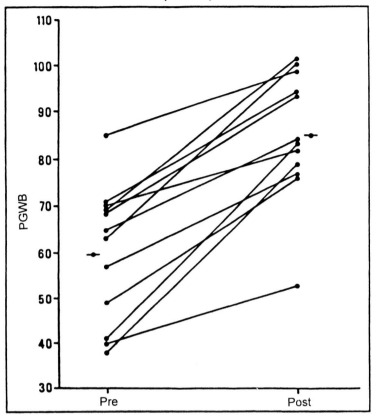

Figure 2. Psychological General Well-Being Index scores in 12 patients before (Pre) and 6 weeks after catheter ablation of the atrioventricular junction and permanent pacemaker implantation (Post). The range of possible scores is 0 to 110, with higher scores representing a greater perception of health and well-being. Used with permission from Kay GN, et al.[17]

ventricular tachyarrhythmias suggests that there is a significant improvement in quality of life 12 months after implantation of a cardioverter-defibrillator in the majority of patients. [12–14] However, the impact of atrial fibrillation on quality of life has not been widely evaluated, and of the relatively few studies in this field,[11,15,16] few have used validated methods (Figure 2, Table 2). Therefore, a worldwide prospective study will address the impact of atrial fibrillation and the atrial defibrillator on patient health-related quality of life using validated generic measures and specific conducted disease scales.

Study Design

Three different patient groups are involved in this prospective multicenter trial. Group 1 will include all patients with atrial fibrillation who meet inclusion criteria and have no exclusion criteria for receipt of the atrial defibrillator. Of group 1, a subset will receive a device, some will be put on a waiting list to receive a device, and the remainder will not receive a device for a variety of reasons unrelated to inclusion or exclusion criteria. Group 2 will include patients with paroxysmal or chronic atrial fibrillation who do not meet criteria for the device, and

Table 2
Percentage Increase in Cardiac Output Acutely after Cardioversion of Atrial Fibrillation

Study	Patients (n)	CO Change at Rest (%)	CO Change with Exercise (%)
Hansen	14	27*	30*
Graettinger	17	10	7
Kahn	10	22*	27*
Morris	11	16*	18*
Rowlands	12	11*	—
Resnekow	15	2	16*
Kaplan	16	15*	—
Shapiro	11	12	15*
Orlando	15	9*	—

* $P < 0.05$; CO = cardiac output.
Used with permission from Crijns HJGM, et al.[18]

group 3 will consist of healthy controls and control patients with heart disease. A total of 158 patients must be recruited in this study in order to answer the primary hypothesis that atrial fibrillation has a negative impact on patient-perceived quality of life compared to controls. The following test instruments are administered at certain time intervals (see Table 3): patient self-reporting instruments including demographic component and predictive scales such as the Life Orientation Test (LOT), the Barsky Somatization Scale, and the Freiburg Questionnaire of Coping with Illness (FQCI). In addition, the following outcome scales will be completed by the patients at baseline, 3-months, 6-months, and 1 year: The Short-Form of the Medical Outcome Study (SF-36), the Specific Activity Scale (SAS), The University of Toronto Defibrillator Scale (UoTDS), the Symptom Checklist (SC), the Illness Intrusiveness Scale (IIS), and the Impact of Event Scale (IES).[19]

Medical Outcome Study Short-Form Health Survey (MOS-SF36)

This instrument assesses patient perceptions related to general health status. The

Table 3
Quality of Life in Atrial Fibrillation: Timing of Questionnaire Administration

Questionnaire	Baseline	Months 3	Months 6	Months 12	Shock	After Atrial Fibrillation
Demographic Data	○					
Clinical Evaluation	○	○	○	○		
Short-Form 36	○	○	○	○		
Specific Activity Scale	○	○	○	○		
Symptom Checklist	○	○	○	○		
Illness Intrusiveness Scale	○	○	○	○		
Life Orientation Test	○					
Barsky Somatization Scale	○					
Atrial Fibrillation Severity Score	○	○	○	○		
Impact of Events Scale					○	○

information helps to evaluate perceptions of physical well-being and the ability of the patient to perform everyday activities. The MOS-SF36 was developed as a brief, simple questionnaire geared to practicality and usefulness. The test is a generic instrument that covers a broad range of quality of life dimensions. It has been translated into German and validated over a large number of different patient populations. The short form of the MOS comprises 36 items, each rated on a 4-point scale measuring physical dimensions of quality of life. It is easy to score and can be divided into different subsets. The MOS-SF36 addresses the following dimensions: physical, social, role functioning, everyday life, patients' perceptions of their general health and well-being, and satisfaction with treatment.

Freiburger Personality Inventory (FPI)

This test was used to examine personality structure before ICD implantation. The inventory comprises 138 questions about personality disorders, attitudes, and behavior. Each question is rated as yes or no.

Implantable Atrial Defibrillator

The acceptance of an implantable cardioverter-defibrillator for the management of ventricular tachyarrhythmias has stimulated the development of an implantable atrial defibrillator. Patients with symptomatic, long-lasting, and drug refractory recurrences of atrial fibrillation are potential candidates for an implantable atrial defibrillator. The number and duration of atrial fibrillation episodes should be taken into account in the indications. Patients with frequent episodes must be excluded as candidates for implantation of an atrial defibrillator because of too frequent discharges, patient discomfort, and rapid battery deple-

tion. Similarly, patients with episodes of short duration and spontaneous termination may not be good candidates. Highly selected patients with infrequent, symptomatic attacks of long-lasting episodes of atrial fibrillation despite antiarrhythmic drug therapy may benefit from an implantable atrial defibrillator.

On April 3, 1996, an implantable atrial defibrillator (Metrix 3000, InControl Inc., Redmond, WA) was successfully implanted at the University of Bonn for the first time in Germany in a 64-year-old female patient with symptomatic, drug refractory atrial fibrillation. The atrial defibrillator has a weight of 79 g and a volume of 53 cc and is combined with three transvenous leads which are positioned in the right atrium, coronary sinus, and the right ventricle. The right ventricular electrode is used for postshock pacing and proper R-wave synchronization. Biphasic shock waveforms are delivered between the two electrodes located in the right atrium and the coronary sinus. A second device was implanted on June 11, 1996 in a 66-year-old male patient suffering from symptomatic drug resistant paroxysmal atrial fibrillation. No complications have occurred thus far in the follow-up. Both patients are in excellent condition and are completely satisfied with this type of treatment.

A recent innovation in the electrical management of cardiac rhythm disorders is the implantable atrioventricular defibrillator (Model 7250, Medtronic Inc.). The first such device to be implanted in the world was implanted successfully also at the University Hospital in Bonn on January 10, 1997, in a 61-year-old female patient. The decisive advancement represented by this new electrical shock system is that it combines two therapeutic principles in one device, in that it automatically detects atrial and ventricular signals and delivers electrical therapy in the appropriate chamber to terminate the arrhythmia.[20,21] Follow-up and quality of life in patients with implantable atrial defibrillators or atrioventricular defibrillators have to be evaluated in the near future.

Summary

The efficacy of antiarrhythmic therapy in patients with atrial fibrillation has been based primarily on objective criteria, such as mortality and morbidity. However, therapies have also come to be evaluated on the basis of quality-of-life issues, because interest in measuring quality of life as it relates to health care has piqued during recent years. Since 1948, when the World Health Organization defined health as being not only the absence of disease and infirmity but also the presence of physical, mental, and social well-being, quality of life parameters have become steadily more important in health care practice and research. Some authors have defined quality of life as an individuals' overall satisfaction with life and the general sense of well-being. Most definitions include several such broad domains as physical function, emotional state, social interaction, and somatic sensation. In some definitions two additional domains are included: personal productivity and intimacy. Personal productivity is the ability to contribute to society (e.g., work or pursuit of a hobby), and intimacy includes sexual functioning as well as the ability to be intimately involved with other individuals. In an ongoing prospective study, we are applying two different types of instruments questionnaires and standardized and validated instruments. The questionnaires were designed specifically to cover the following dimensions: social demographic data including age, education, occupation level, driving behavior, return to work, and sexual activity. In addition, the following standardized instruments are being completed by the patients at preselected times: the Medical Outcome Study Short Form General Health Survey to address generic quality-of-life aspects; the Beck Depression Inventory to assess mood disorders; and a Specific Activity Scale to assess fatigue and exercise tolerability. Realizing that as quality of life is a multidimensional construct, our description of quality of life should take into account many different factors.

References

1. Slevin ML. Quality of life: philosophical question or clinical reality? Br Med J 1992; 305:466–469.
2. Fitzpatrick R, Fletcher A, Gore S, et al. Quality of life measures in health care. I: Applications and issues in assessment: Br Med J 1992;305:1074–1077.
3. Fletcher A, Gore S, Jones D, et al. Quality of life in health care. II: Design, analysis, and interpretation. Br Med J 1992;305:1145–1148.
4. Spiegelhalter DJ, Gore SM, Fitzpatrick R, et al. Quality of life measures in health care. III: Resource allocation. Br Med J 1992;305: 1205–1209.
5. Deister A. Vorhofflimmern - Entscheidungshilfen für die ambulante Therapie. Herz 1995;20(Suppl III):4.
6. Olschewski M, Schumacher M. "Lebensqualität" als Kriterium in der Therapieforschung. Intensivmed 1993;30:522–527.
7. Schumacher M, Olschewski M, Schulgen G. Assessment of quality of life in clinical trials. Stat Med 1991;10:1915–1930.
8. Jung W, Deister A, Lüderitz B. Quality of life, psychological, and social aspects in patients with implantable cardioverter-defibrillators. In Allessie MA, Fromer M, eds. Atrial and Ventricular Fibrillation: Mechanisms and Device Therapy. Futura Publishing Co, Inc., Armonk, NY, 1997, pp 311–320.
9. Bubien RS, Knotts-Dolson SM, Plumb VJ, et al. Effect of radiofrequency catheter ablation on health-related quality of life and activities of daily living in patients with recurrent arrhythmias. Circulation 1996;94:1585–1591.
10. Testa M, Simonson DC. Assessment of quality-of-life outcomes. N Engl J Med 1996;334: 835–840.
11. Hamer ME, Blumenthal JA, McCarthy EA, et al. Quality-of-life assessment in patients with paroxysmal atrial fibrillation or paroxysmal supraventricular tachycardia. Am J Cardiol 1994;74:826–829.
12. Lüderitz B, Jung W, Deister A, et al. Patient acceptance of the implantable cardioverter defibrillator in ventricular tachyarrhythmias. PACE 1993;16:1815–1821.

13. Lüderitz B, Jung W, Deister A, et al. Patient acceptance of implantable cardioverter defibrillator devices: changing attitudes. Am Heart J 1994;127:1179–1184.

14. Lüderitz B, Jung W, Deister A, et al. Quality of life in multiprogrammable implantable cardioverter-defibrillator recipients. In Saksena S, Lüderitz B, eds. Textbook of Interventional Electrophysiology. Futura Publishing Co, Inc., Armonk, NY, 1996, pp 305–314.

15. Brignole M, Gianfranchi L, Menozzi C, et al. Influence of atrioventricular junction radiofrequency ablation in patients with chronic atrial fibrillation and flutter on quality of life and cardiac performance. Am J Cardiol 1994; 74:242–246.

16. Fitzpatrick AP, Kourouyan HD, Siu A, et al. Quality of life and outcomes after radiofrequency His-bundle catheter ablation and permanent pacemaker implantation: impact of treatment in paroxysmal and established atrial fibrillation. Am Heart J 1996;131: 499–507.

17. Kay GN, Bubien RS, Epstein AE, et al. Effect of catheter ablation of the atrioventricular junction on quality of life and exercise tolerance in paroxysmal atrial fibrillation. Am J Cardiol 1988;62:741–744.

18. Crijns HJGM, Van Gelder IC, Tieleman, RG, et al. Why is atrial fibrillation bad for you? In Murgatroyd FD, Camm AJ, eds. Nonpharmacological Management of Atrial Fibrillation. Futura Publishing Co, Inc, Armonk, NY, 1997, pp 3–13.

19. Lüderitz B, Jung W. Quality of life of patients with atrial fibrillation. In Santini M, ed. Progress in Clinical Pacing. Futura Media Services, Inc, Armonk, NY, 1996, pp 253–262.

20. Jung W, Lüderitz B. Intraatrial defibrillation of atrial fibrillation. Z Kardiol 1996;85(Suppl 6):75–78.

21. Jung W, Lüderitz B. Implantation of an arrhythmia management system for patients with ventricular and supraventricular tachyarrhythmias. Lancet 1993;349:853.

Chapter 23

Impact of Implantable Cardioverter-Defibrillators on Survival

Seah Nisam

Introduction

The implantable cardioverter-defibrillator (ICD) is acknowledged to be *the* most effective therapy in terms of protecting patients with malignant ventricular arrhythmias against sudden, arrhythmic death, due to ventricular tachycardia or fibrillation (VT/VF).[1–3] But the majority of patients with a previous history of sustained VT/VF, as well as those highly susceptible to develop them in the future, have serious nonarrhythmic cardiac and noncardiac risk factors. These *competing risks* potentially dilute the ability of the ICD to substantially prolong such patients' lives. Therefore, since the modern pacemaker-like ICD does not itself *contribute* to mortality—the real issue of its impact on survival must focus on whether the patients being selected for ICDs have *competing* risks high enough to essentially undo the sudden death protection. A closely related issue is how the ICD compares to alternative therapies—essentially, antiarrhythmic drugs (AARx)—in terms of protecting patients against all-cause mortality. This chapter will concentrate on these two important aspects of ICD therapy.

ICD Patient Survival in the Modern (Nonthoracotomy) Era

The history and development of the ICD, conceived by Michel Mirowski in 1966, and introduced into clinical practice by Mirowski and colleagues in 1980, is now well known.[4–8] Even the simplest, early devices quickly demonstrated that they were able to do exactly what they were supposed to: rapidly convert sustained episodes of VT/VF to sinus rhythm, achieving therewith a reduction in sudden death to about 1% per year, a standard that has held up through nearly two decades.[9–13] However, patients receiving ICDs in the 1980s had to survive a thoracotomy, required to place the defibrillating "patch" electrodes directly on the heart surface. Meta-analysis indicates that the *perioperative* mortality associated with this procedure was about 3%.[14,15] It has to be said that there were great variances, from 0% to 5% between centers, and the situation was further clouded by the fact that approximately 20%–25% of the thoracotomy procedures were combined with high-risk concurrent cardiac surgery (generally, coronary artery bypass grafting, either alone, or com-

From Singer I, Barold SS, Camm AJ (eds): Nonpharmacological Therapy of Arrhythmias for the 21st Century: The State of the Art. Futura Publishing Co., Armonk, NY, © 1998.

bined with other cardiac surgery); several series have shown substantial differences in perioperative mortality between "ICD alone" versus combined procedures.[13,16–17] For instance, we have observed that patients who underwent bypass graft surgery (but otherwise had similar demographic profiles), had a 3% higher perioperative mortality than those who received the ICD without additional surgery.[13] The end result, in terms of overall survival during this early era (Figure 1), generally showed 85%–90% survival at 1 year and 70%–80% by 5 years.[9–13,15,18]

The perioperative mortality and morbidity was of course substantially reduced with the introduction of transvenous ICD lead systems, at the end of the 1980s.[19,20] It would appear that the elimination of thoracotomy may have enhanced survival even beyond the perioperative period.[13,21] From the CPI clinical data bank, we noted that even if patients with concomitant surgery were excluded, those receiving endocardial systems had a 1.3% lower perioperative mortality compared to the epicardial implants, and this 1.3% improvement at 30 days grew to nearly 5% better survival at 1 year![13] Still, for 3–4 years, until the general availabity of biphasic waveforms, substantial numbers of patients required fairly complex two- and three-lead systems, and large series indicate perioperative mortalities of approximately 1.0%.[13,15,21–23] The "modern" era, using single-lead plus "hot can" (pulse generator housing as an active electrode) systems, implanted pectorally, has resulted in further reductions in perioperative mortality, now ranging from 0% to 0.5%.[24–28] While speculative, the fact that 80%–90% of VT episodes are interrupted by antitachycardia pacing[21,29]—before accelerating to more ominous rapid polymorphic VT or VF—may be a further contributing factor to the overall better survival observed in the "modern era" compared to the earlier series, where antitachycardia pacing was not available. The resulting freedom from all-cause mortality is now 90%–95% at 1 year, and 80%–85% through 4 years.[2,21,23–26] Table 1 lists the 1- and 2-year survival rates from several large, recent ICD series, all im-

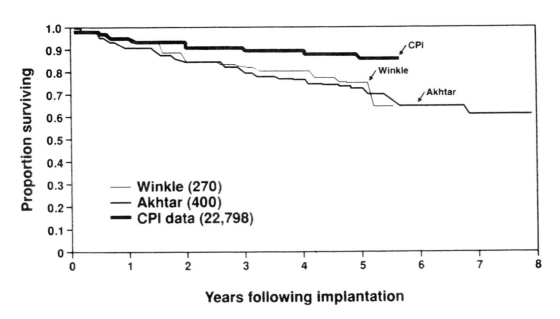

Years following implantation

Figure 1. Kaplan-Meier curves showing freedom from all-cause mortality in two early large independently reported ICD series (Akhtar: N = 400; Winkle: N = 270), and from CPI clinical records data base (N = 22,798). Used with permission from Nisam S, et al.[18]

Table 1
Mortality of ICD Therapy in Patients with Transvenous Defibrillation LeadsΦ

Study*	Block	Bardy	Transvene PCD	ENDOTAK Ventak P	ENDOTAK Ventak P2	All†
Transvenously implanted (%)	95.1	95.2	88.6	NA	97.8	91.0
Subcutaneous patch used (%)	78.1	100	94.8	NA	32.3	85.2
Perioperative mortality (%)	1.1‡	0.0	0.7‡	NA	1.4‡	0.8‡
Actuarial survival						
1 Year (%)	96.0	98.0	93.3	90.8	96.2‡	93.5
2 Years (%)	92.0	NA	NA	NA	NA	92.0
Sudden death rate						
1 year (%)	0.0	0.0	0.5	2.8	1.3§	1.0
2 years (%)	1.6	NA	NA	NA	NA	1.6

* Listed is the first author of a single-center study or lead system and device evaluated in a multicenter study.
† Some patients might be counted in both the single-center and the multicenter studies.
‡ Only patients with successful transvenous implantation
§ 235 days instead of 1 year.
NA. Data not available.
Φ Used with permission from Block M, et al.[15]

planted with transvenous lead systems, showing that outcomes in terms of survival have definitely improved in more recent years, to the extent that, at 2 years, 92% of the patients were still alive.[15] Even more recent series, each with over 200 patients, all implanted subpectorally, quite analogous to pacemakers, shows 2-year freedom from all-cause mortality below 5%.[28,29]

Results with Antiarrhythmic Drugs

In 1980, essentially all patients presenting with VT/VF received AARx therapy; nearly none were prescribed ICDs. In 1996, close to 25,000 patients received ICDs.[30] Figure 2 shows the evolution, both in terms of major technological milestones in ICD therapy, and in numbers of patients. This evolution necessarily complicates any analysis of the impact of drug therapy: with increased physician (and patient) acceptance of ICDs, the patients treated by medical therapy today may differ significantly from those for whom AARx were the primary therapy a few years ago. An example of this difficulty, since we are looking at overall survival, is

that literally thousands of patients were started off on AARx, and then received ICDs following VT/VF recurrences while on those drugs. What would have happened to those patients had they remained on those drugs is only conjecture, but presumably physicians' decisions to stop AARx and implant ICDs must have made some important contribution to their survival.

Accepting the important qualifying comments just above, there are large series of patients treated with AARx, which permit us to examine outcomes. Class I antiarrhythmic agents are now seldom used for patients with ventricular tachyarrhythmias, following evidence that they lead to increased mortality, particularly in patients following myocardial infarctions.[31–34] Figure 3 shows the number of ICD implants (CPI data bank) in the months preceding the CAST results, and in the year thereafter. It appears that CAST had a dramatic impact on physicians' receptiveness to ICD therapy. The ESVEM (Electrophysiologic Study versus Electrocardiographic Monitoring) study demonstrated that, while sotalol was far preferable to class I agents, it was nevertheless associated with very high VT recurrence rates: 20% at 1 year, 50% VT and

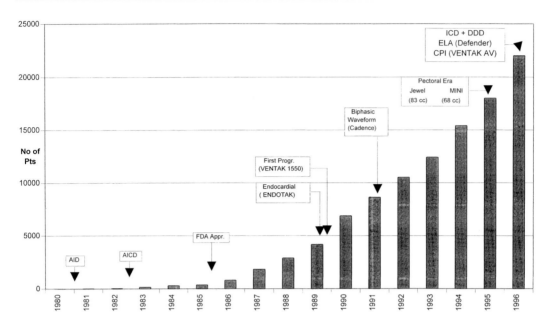

Figure 2. Evolution in ICD technology and accompanying growth in numbers of patients treated with ICD therapy from 1980 through 1996. Adapted and used with permission from Nisam S, et al.[64]

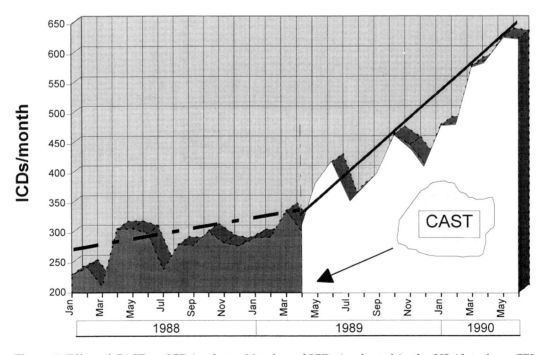

Figure 3. Effect of CAST on ICD implants. Number of ICDs implanted in the US (data from CPI clinical records) in the months preceding and the year following the announcement of the results of the CAST study.[31]

sudden death by 4 years.[34] Böcker et al. performed a matched case control study in 100 patients, comparing electrophysiologically guided d,l-sotalol treatment versus the ICD.[35] They reported an overall mortality rate with sotalol of 26% by 2 years—nearly identical to the ESVEM results—compared to 11% for the ICD ($P = 0.02$). Further evidence in the same direction came from the SWORD (Survival with Oral d-Sotalol) trial, which was stopped after results showing premature harm from sotalol compared to placebo.[36] Lee et al. reported the most recent series of long-term experience with electrophysiologically guided sotalol treatment.[37] Of 133 patients with VT/VF, 66 (50%) were considered "responders" (52 rendered noninducible, 14 with hemodynamically stable inducible VT). Among these 52 responders followed-up for a mean of 36 months, two-thirds were considered to be successfully treated. Among the failures, there were four sudden deaths, two VT recurrences, and six patients withdrawn due to severe side effects.

Amiodarone

For some years, many have considered this drug the most effective AARx for patients with serious VT/VF. The CASCADE (Cardiac Arrest in Seattle: Conventional versus Amiodarone Drug Evaluation) study certainly supports that it is more effective than class I agents, showing lower mortality as well as lower number of syncopes and fewer ICD shocks in patients on amiodarone compared to class I drugs.[32] Nevertheless, the absolute results for patients prescribed amiodarone are not that good, with multiple studies showing approximately 10% sudden death at 1 year, and 20%–25% by 5 years.[9,38–40] For instance, in CASCADE, there was a 22% rate of cardiac mortality at 2 years for patients on amiodarone, leading the investigators to change the study design to recommend ICDs (!) for the last half of the study.[32] Adding to the VT and sudden death recurrences, many patients are forced to discontinue

Table 2
Causes of Cardiac Mortality in Patients with Ventricular Arrhythmias

1. "Primary VF"
2. VT and/or VT $\Rightarrow$ VF
3. Reinfarction
4. VF associated with reinfarction
5. Frank heart failure
6. Heart failure as late sequelae to prolonged or numerous VT episodes
7. Bradyarrhythmias
8. Electromechanical dissociation
9. Perioperative mortality (within 30-days of ICD implant) or during "run-in" period with AARx
10. Proarrhythmia from AARx

VT = ventricular tachycardia; VF = ventricular fibrillation; AARx = antiarrhythmic drugs.

treatment due to serious side effects, with the end result that generally less than half the patients are still alive and on the drug past 4 years.[38–40] But the most powerful confirmation of the limitations of amiodarone come from recent large, prospective, randomized studies indicating mortality *equal to placebo* in coronary patients with poor left ventricular function.[41–43]

Comparing the Impact of Drugs Versus ICDs on Survival

Before examining the critical issue comparing survival benefit of the ICD to that achieved with medical management, it is enlightening to review the different causes of deaths in these high-risk patients (Table 2). Generally about 75% of patients with VT/VF have advanced coronary artery disease, with one or more myocardial infarctions. Most of the remaining patients have some type of nonischemic cardiomyopathy. Certainly less than 5% of such patients—those with "primarily electrical disease," long-QT syndrome, etc.—can be considered void of very significant competing risks. Regarding the third and fourth points listed in the table, revascularization, thrombolytic therapy, and anti-ischemic medical

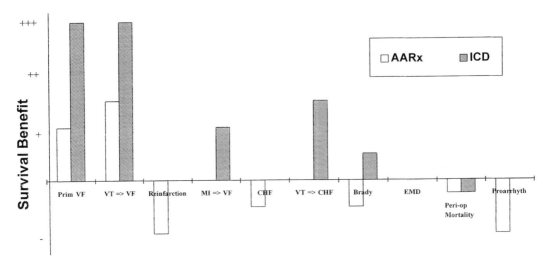

Figure 4. Relative impact on patient survival of ICD compared to AARx. The "survival benefit" is a measure of the protection against each source or risk of death, varying from 0 = no impact to + + + = significant positive impact; values below zero imply harm, i.e., contribute to mortality. The causes of mortality are shown on the horizontal axis: Prim VF = primary VF; VT ⇒ VF = VT degenerating to VF; reinfarction; MI ⇒ VF = VF associated with acute myocardial infarction; CHF = congestive heart failure; VT ⇒ CHF = CHF as a late consequence of prolonged or recurrent VT/VF; Brady = bradyarrhythmias; EMD = electromechanical dissociation; Periop = mortality within 30 days of ICD implant or during run-in period with AARx; Proarrhyth = proarrhythmia; ICD = implantable cardioverter-defibrillator; AARx = antiarrhythmic drug therapy; VT = ventricular tachycardia; VF = ventricular fibrillation; MI = myocardial infarction.

management are of course of primary importance in patients with chronic coronary disease. Nevertheless, despite optimal management of their ischemic problem, such patients remain under the menace of reinfarction and ventricular arrhythmias associated with residual ischemia. Items 5–8 in Table 2 all relate to congestive heart failure (CHF). The great majority of these patients have poor left ventricular function, so many will die from CHF. Their mode of death will be frank heart failure in many and from CHF-associated arrhythmias—VT/VF, bradyarrhythmias, and electromechanical dissociation—in others. The final two items in Table 2 relate to risks directly associated with the drugs themselves. As we will discuss below, this differentiation on the mode of death may be important in understanding the difference in survival impact of ICD therapy versus AARx management.

Upon examining the mechanisms that lead to death in patients with severe cardio-myopathies, ischemic and nonischemic, it becomes quite clear that the effect of the intervention—AARx versus ICDs—is usually quite different (Figure 4). For the first two categories listed, it is evident that one of the primary actions of AARx is of course to prevent VT/VF from occurring; unfortunately, as we have summarized above, multiple series have clearly demonstrated that unacceptably high rates of VT/VF episodes do recur despite AARx.[9,31–43] The ICD's higher rating is simply based on the fact that once such arrhythmias have begun, AARx can do little, while the ICD is extremely effective. The ICD cannot prevent the onset of "primary VF," but it is remarkably potent in terminating it. Furthermore, there is now ample evidence that "primary VF" is almost always really VT degenerating to VF over time[44–45] and here, the ICD's rapid intervention prevents such degeneration in the high majority of episodes.[21,27] Shown next in Table 2 and Figure 4 is reinfarction, which the ICD can, of course, not impact in any direct manner. On the drug side, there is evidence from the European Myocardial Infarction Amiodarone Trial (EMIAT) of *excess* mortality due to reinfarctions in patients randomized to amiodarone compared to placebo.[43] With regard to the fourth cause listed, VF in association with acute myocardial infarction (MI), it has been known for years that defibrillation can effectively terminate VF even during ischemia.[46] so it is highly likely that the ICD, ignorant of the cause of VF, stops it in at least some episodes of acute MI, permitting the patients to arrive in the emergency room for treatment of their infarction.

Deaths from end-stage heart failure are of course a major concern in the population of patients with malignant arrhythmias. With regard to frank heart failure, ICDs obviously have no effect, neither positive nor negative, whereas the negative inotropic effects of AARx may contribute to the final result. This differential effect, shown in Figure 4 to be in favor of the ICD, is unaffected by optimal heart failure management, as this is assumed to be the same irrespective of whether the patients receive AARx or ICDs. Concerning the next cause on the list, late sequelae to CHF, we have postulated that some deaths classified as heart failure deaths, actually originated with long-lasting or multiple bouts of VT, in themselves not immediately fatal, but causing irrevocable, deleterious effects on ventricular function.[47,48] For such scenarios, patients whose VT episodes are interrupted within seconds by the ICD evidently fare better than those treated by AARx, whose arrhythmias may last for hours, sometimes days before cardioversion. Bradyarrhythmias in such patients are surely not helped by antiarrhythmic agents, whose effect is to prolong refractory periods, whereas brady pacing available in ICDs may in some cases reestablish sinus rhythm. On the other hand, deaths due to electromechanical dissociation cannot be prevented with either treatment, so Figure 4 shows neither benefit nor harm for either. Points 9 and 10 in Table 2

and the far right portion of Figure 4 address the risk of the intervention itself: for the intravenous implantation of ICDs, the perioperative risk is < 0.5%; the run-in period for AARx treatment is not without risk, as has been shown by several studies.[12,32,34,37,38] For the purposes of this analysis, we have shown on Figure 4 a small and equal mortality risk for both options. Finally, the risk of proarrhythmia has already sounded the death knoll for class I AARx for the treatment of ventricular arrhythmias, but torsade de point and other iatrogenic rhythms have also been reported with class III agents.[36] ICD proarrhythmia can also occur, for example antitachycardia pacing resulting in acceleration of VT,[49,50] but the device's own defibrillatory mechanism reestablishes sinus rhythm in all but extremely rare cases.[51]

Can the ICD Impact Nonarrhythmic Mortality?

Of course not! Still this is an intriguing question, because there is ample evidence indicating that ICD therapy, compared to AARx, does exactly that (Table 3). The rate of nonarrhythmic deaths in Winkle et al.'s 270-patient ICD series was 21.6% at 5 years.[10] In contrast, the nonarrhythmic rate of death in Herre et al.'s 462 patients treated by amiodarone was nearly double, 41%.[38] The two studies took place over approximately the same time frame, both published in 1989, and the profiles of the patients appear very similar, e.g, left ventricular ejection fraction 34.1% for the ICD patients versus 36% for the amiodarone treated patients. Nevertheless, some researchers have pointed to the disparity in nonarrhythmic deaths as "evidence" that the ICD patients were at lower risk[52] despite the apparent equivalence of the patient profiles. In this respect, Newman et al.'s well-known matched controls study, which followed the above two studies by 3 years, is very important: it matched 60 patients treated with ICDs to 120 patients with equivalent base-

Table 3
Mortality: Total, Arrhythmic, and Nonarrhythmic

Major Series of Patients with VT/VF		Follow-up* (yrs)	Total (%)	Arrhythmic (%)	Nonarrhythmic (%)
Herre[38]	Amiodarone (N = 462)	5	62	21	41
Winkle[10]	ICD (N = 270)	5	26	4.4	21.6
Newman[53]	Amiodarone (N = 120)	3	49	10	39
	ICD (N = 60)	3	22	5	17
Wever[54]	Conv'l AARx (N = 31)	2.25	35.5	12.9	22.6
	ICD (N = 29)	2.25	13.7	3.4	10.3
MADIT[55]	Conv'l AARx (N = 101)	2.25	38.6	12.9	25.7
	ICD (N = 95)	2.25	15.8	3.2	12.6
AVID[56]	AARx (N = 498)	3	35		
	ICD (N = 503)	3	25		

VT/VF = ventricular tachycardia/fibrillation; ICD = implantable cardioverter defibrillator; Conv'l AARx = conventional antiarrhythmic drug therapy; MADIT = Multicenter Automatic Defibrillator Implantation Trial; AVID = antiarrhythmics vs. implantable defibrillator.
* Follow-up times indicated above are *actuarial* in Herre, Winkle, Newman, and AVID series; and *mean* in Wever and MADIT series.
Used with permission from Nisam S.[68]

line variables, who were given amiodarone.[53] The rates of nonarrhythmic deaths were 16.7% for the ICD patients versus 39.2% for those receiving amiodarone, i.e., ratios similar to the Winkle/Herre comparison! There are many other examples where the overall better survival with ICD-treated patients versus those receiving AARx cannot be explained by the far lower sudden death rate alone.

Now there is evidence from recently completed prospective, randomized trials that substantiates the fact that ICD patients also do better in terms of nonarrhythmic mortality, compared to patients treated with AARx. In the Netherlands prospective study of ICDs versus conventional therapy in sudden death survivors, there were seven (22.6%) nonarrhythmic deaths for the AARx group compared to three (10.3%) in the ICD patients.[54] In the Multicenter Automatic Defibrillation Implantation Trial (MADIT), the number of deaths classified as nonarrhythmic or uncertain was much higher in the AARx treated patients, compared to those randomized to ICDs, 26 (25.7%) versus 12 (12.6%), respectively.[55] Table 3 shows this consistently higher rate of nonarrhythmic

deaths cited in the above matched controls studies as well as from randomized, prospective studies. The AVID (Antiarrhythmics vs Implantable Defibrillator) trial was stopped on April 7, 1997 due to evidence of significantly better survival for the ICD patients.[56] With 1,001 patients enrolled at that time, the ICD superiority was 38% at 1 year, $P = 0.02$. Data on the arrhythmic/nonarrhythmic mortality has not yet been published.

How Can the ICD Impact Nonarrhythmic Mortality?

Having noticed this curious disparity some years ago, we speculated on the possible explanations.[47,48] In the meanwhile, there is important data coming out of major randomized trials that provide insights into this question. Looking at two recently completed prospective, randomized trials (EMIAT and MADIT) there is evidence of dramatically different impact of amiodarone therapy compared to ICD therapy. In MADIT, all-cause mortality was 54% higher in the conventional treatment limb patients,

Table 4*
Causes of Deaths in EMIAT and MADIT

	All Causes	Arrhythmic	Nonarrhythmic**
EMIAT placebo (N = 743)	102	50	52
EMIAT amiodarone (N = 743)	103	33	70
MADIT conventional treatment (N = 101)	39	13	26
MADIT ICD (N = 95)	15	3	12

** Includes deaths from *unknown* causes.
* Used with permission from Nisam S.[63]

three-quarters of whom received amiodarone, than in those randomized to ICDs.[55] But only part of this superiority came from the ICD's better prevention of arrhythmic deaths; as stated above, and seen clearly in Table 4 and Figure 5, patients treated with ICDs also suffered far fewer nonarrhythmic (or uncertain) deaths compared to the conventional limb. In EMIAT, also a large (1,500 patients) randomized, prospective trial, the opposite occurred with regard to the impact of amiodarone: it did indeed re-

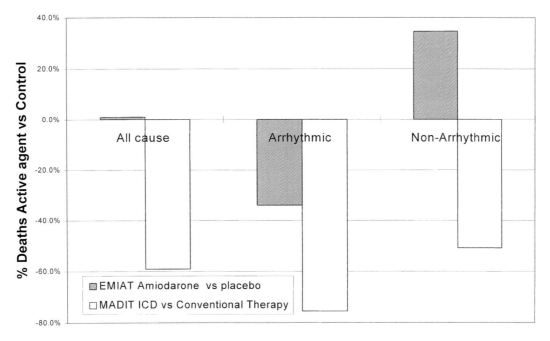

Figure 5. Comparison of amiodarone's impact on mortality in EMIAT versus ICD's impact on mortality in MADIT. "Impact on mortality" was calculated by comparing the percentage increase or decrease in mortality vis-à-vis controls. Impact on mortality of amiodarone in EMIAT compared the percentage of deaths for patients randomized to amiodarone versus placebo, for each category of death (all-cause, arrhythmic, nonarrhythmic). Impact on mortality of ICD in MADIT compared the percentage of deaths for patients randomized to ICD, compared to conventional therapy, for each category of death. Sample calculation: nonarrhythmic mortality in the MADIT study showed 12 of 95 (12.6%) nonarrhythmic deaths for ICD patients vs. 26 of 101 (25.7%) for conventionally treated patients; 12.6% represents a 51.0% reduction for ICD treated patients vis-à-vis those treated conventionally. Used with permission from Nisam S.[63]

Table 5
Potential Causes for Lower *Nonarrhythmic* Mortality in ICD Patients

Possible Cause	*Possible Mechanism*
• negative inotropic effects of AARx	could be contributing to late, nonarrhythmic mortality
• long-lasting VT episodes	in contrast to ICDs terminating them within seconds, can last for hours or days, leading to irreversible CHF
• less regular follow-up	hence, less aggressive attention to CHF or other problems
• drug proarrhythmia	may in itself not be fatal, but could lead to progressive degeneration of cardiac function
• noncompliance	drug withdrawals, for side effects or other reasons, may leave the patient unprotected. This is not possible with ICDs
• lengthy drug trials or "run-in" periods	may render such patients "intrinsically sicker" by the time they are actually discharged on the chosen AARx

AARx = antiarrhythmic drug therapy; ICD = implantable cardioverter defibrillator; VT = ventricular tachycardia; CHF = (congestive) heart failure.

duce arrhythmic deaths compared to placebo, just as it is supposed to; but this beneficial effect was entirely annulled by the fact that patients on amiodarone had *excess* nonarrhythmic mortality.[43] The preliminary data presented on EMIAT indicated excess numbers of deaths due to respiratory problems, reinfarction, and other causes for patients treated with amiodarone, but this can only be a partial explanation for the major divergences observed. We believe that a greater contribution to the differential effects of the ICD vs. AARx comes from the the arrhythmia problems paramount in these patients. When such arrhythmias occur with the ICD present, they are converted within seconds to sinus rhythm without any deterioration of the patient's cardiac function. In the absence of the ICD, the same VT episode lasting many hours, while often not immediately fatal, has to have debilitating effects on that patient's already compromised ventricular function. His or her death during follow-up may appear to be from pump failure, but it is hard to exclude the contribution of long-lasting VT episodes to that final event.

The point that needs to be kept in mind when analyzing this situation is that two treatment strategies are being compared. It then becomes evident that the true explanation of the results showing a benefit due to

the ICD may simply reflect excess nonarrhythmic deaths associated with antiarrhythmic drugs. Table 5 summarizes the reasons that could explain how this observed disparity is real, not some type of artifact: (1) negative inotropic effects of AARx may lead to deaths from nonarrhythmic causes; (2) in the absence of an ICD, VT episodes may last for many hours, eventually leading to death from heart failure; (3) ICD patients may be benefiting from more frequent follow-ups, hence better attention to heart failure compared to those treated by AARx; (4) AARx proarrhythmia, without necessarily producing arrhythmic death, could still lead to worsening cardiac function, with death as the final consequence; (5) high rates of drug discontinuation due to severe side effects, which in turn leaves patients without protection[12,32,34, 37–39,42,43]; and (6) problems associated with lengthy drug trials or "run-in" periods, after which the patients may in fact have become "intrinsically sicker." The latter two points really have to do with what we, as well as Saksena et al., have referred to as the difference in *safety* between managing patients pharmacologically, with reported 3%–5% 30-day mortality rates[2,12,32,34,38,48] compared to near nil mortality with pectoral implantation of ICDs.

In this section where we are focusing on

the difference in both safety and long-term outcome of the two treatment strategies, we are obliged to address the issue termed "not-so-sudden-death."[57] Böcker et al.'s recent article about evidence-based cardiology in the *European Heart Journal*[3] noted that the debate on whether the ICD prolongs life stems largely from "... data from the Montefiore group[58,59] (regarding) ... nonsudden deaths ... causally related to arrhythmias." Böcker et al. conclude that this result "... seems to be a rare finding as it has not been reported in most studies. In our series of 462 patients treated with a third-generation ICD in combination with endocardial leads, we have observed only two cases of arrhythmia-related nonsudden deaths ..."

ICD Versus Antiarrhythmic Drugs: Head-to-Head Comparisons

There are now no less than five head-to-head studies completed, comparing the survival outcome for patients treated with ICDs versus antiarrhythmic drugs (Table 6).

The first three studies shown in the table were randomized, prospective studies, whereas the last two were concurrent, matched case control studies. All but MADIT were studies on patients with previous history of life-threatening sustained VT/VF, while MADIT randomized chronic coronary artery disease patients identified to be at high risk to develop VT/VF, but without previous history of sustained arrhythmias. Amiodarone was the primary or only antiarrhythmic drug used in the MADIT (74%), AVID (93%), and Newman (100%) studies; d-l sotalol was the control drug in the Böcker et al. study. The unequivocal outcome showed statistically significant reductions in all-cause mortality greater than 30% (range, 31%–61%) for patients treated by ICD therapy in all five studies. This improvement in survival remained statistically significant in all five studies through 3 years, although the percentage difference diminished with time. Evidently, given enough time—the survival curves for these highly endangered patients, with high co-morbidity due to

Table 6
Total Mortality, ICD vs. AARx

Study	Patients	Drugs Used	Mortality AARx	Mortality ICD	Reduction due to ICD
Wever et al.[54] (R) (N = 60)	CAD, resuscitated from VT/VF	Class 1 (EP-guided)	35%	13%	61%
MADIT[55]* (R) (N = 196)	CAD, LVEF ≤ 0.35, NSVT, Inducible	amiodarone/sotalol/ Class 1A (74%/7%/10%)	38.6%	15.8%	59%
AVID[56] (R) (N = 1001)	Resuscitated from VT/VF + Sync. VT	amiodarone/sotalol (93%/7%)	22.9%	15.9%	31%
Newman[53] (MC) (N = 180)	Resuscitated from VT/VF	amiodarone	51%**	35%**	31%**
Böcker[35] (MC) (N = 100)	Resuscitated from VT/VF	d-l sotalol	25%**	15%**	40%**

CAD = coronary artery disease; LVEF = left ventricular ejection fraction; VT/VF = ventricular tachycardia/fibrillation; NSVT = nonsustained VT; EP = electrophysiologic; R = randomized, prospective trial; MC = matched case controls; MADIT = multicenter automatic defibrillator implantation trial; AVID = antiarrhythmics vs. implantable defibrillator trial.

* No past history of VT/VF.

** Actuarial survival at 3 years.

their underlying disease—will of course converge.

We have not overlooked the fact that substantial numbers of ICD patients receive adjunctive AARx (often for managing supraventricular arrhythmias). All this means from a treatment strategy point of view is that patients with ICDs, with or without AARx, have far better overall survival than those who are on AARx in the absence of an ICD.

The Role of the ICD in Patients with Heart Failure

Moss et al. emphasized the importance of optimal heart failure therapy, in combination with the ICD, which permitted such a high-risk population as in the MADIT study to achieve such excellent survival rates.[55] Evidently, with the ICD not only preventing arrhythmic deaths, but also minimizing the sequelae from long sustained VT episodes, there was greater opportunity for management with ACE-inhibitors (given to 55% of MADIT patients), diuretics, etc., to keep the patients alive. This is also the explanation of why the "conversion theory," stipulating that all the ICD does is convert arrhythmic death to heart failure death, with little extension of life,[61] *did not happen* in MADIT. In contrast, the equivalent optimal heart failure treatment was not able to prevent a far higher number of pump failure deaths, consequent to such arrhythmias in the drug limb, i.e., in the absence of an ICD.

Much of the above is, admittedly, speculation. What is not speculation is the fact that in MADIT, a randomized, prospective trial with exquisitely balanced baseline variables, over twice as many deaths not directly attributable to arrhythmias occurred in conventionally treated patients as in those randomized to ICDs: *whatever the mechanism*! In fact, these results partially contradict Fogoros' thoughtful review[62] of the competing risks theory. Dr. Fogoros predicted that a population of patients with high co-morbidity would receive little or no

benefit from antiarrhythmic therapy, even a particularly effective one, since they were destined to die of heart failure or another such cause without meaningful prolongation of life.

The MADIT patients certainly fit that description: previous myocardial infarction, with mean LVEF 0.26, and half of them being treated for congestive heart failure at time of enrollment into the study.[55] Yet, in the group randomized to ICDs, three-quarters were still alive after 4 years. What these results show is that, in light of major advances in the treatment of heart failure, combined with an antiarrhythmic modality, the ICD, which not only contributes no risk, but also precludes administration of agents which potentially contribute some risk, the view toward the management of such patients may have to be reexamined.

Addendum

Subsequent to submitting this chapter, the results of two further studies, highly pertinent to the topic, have just been announced: the results of the Cardiac Arrest Study Hamburg (CASH) and the Canadian Implantable Defibrillator Study (CIDS) were both made public by their principle investigators, Karl-Heinz Kuck (Hamburg) and Stuart Connolly (Hamilton, Ontario, Canada), respectively, during the "Update on Clinical Trials" session on March 30, 1998, at the 47th scientific session of the American College of Cardiology meeting.[65–67] CASH had randomized 349 patients resuscitated from cardiac arrest due to VT/VF between amiodarone, metoprolol, propafenone, and ICDs. Whereas the propafenone arm had been discontinued already in 1992 due to 62% higher mortality compared to the ICD arm, the study had continued until December 1997 for the other three limbs. At 2 years of follow-up, the final results showed 37% lower mortality for 99 patients with ICDs compared to 189 patients randomized to amiodarone (n = 92) or metoprolol (n = 97), $P = 0.047$. CIDS had randomized 656 patients following cardiac arrest or syncopal VT to amiodarone versus ICDs, and found 20% lower mortality ($P = 0.072$) for the ICD-treated patients at 4 years of follow-up. Evidently, these results simply reinforce the points made in this chapter, and in particular in the discussion pertaining to Table 6.

Acknowledgment: The author wishes to acknowledge the expert help of Mr. Jack Latucca in setting up several of the figures and tables.

References

1. Lehmann M, et al. The automatic implantable cardioverter defibrillator as antiarrhythmic treatment modality of choice for survivors of cardiac arrest unrelated to acute myocardial infarction. Am J Cardiol 1988;62: 803–805.

2. Saksena S, Madan N, Lewis C. Implantable cardioverter-defibrillators are preferable to drugs a primary therapy in sustained ventricular tachyarrhythmias. Progr Cardiovasc Dis 1996;38:445–454.

3. Böcker D, Block M, Borggrefe M, et al. Defibrillators are superior to antiarrhythmic drugs in the treatment of ventricular tachyarrhythmias. Eur Heart J 1997;18:26–30.

4. Mirowski M, Mower M, Staewen W, et al. Standby automatic defibrillator: an approach to prevention of sudden coronary death. Arch Intern Med 1970;126:158–161.

5. Mirowski M, Mower M. Feasibility and effectiveness of low-energy catheter-defibrillation in man. Circulation 1973;47:79–85.

6. Mirowski M, Reid P, Mower M, et al. Termination of malignant ventricular arrhythmias with an implanted automatic defibrillator in human beings. N Engl J Med 1980;303: 322–324.

7. Kastor J. Historical study. Michel Mirowski and the automatic implantable defibrillator. Am J Cardiol 1989;63:977–982.

8. Mower M, Hauser R. Historical development of the AICD. In Estes M, Manolis A, Wang P, eds. Implantable Cardioverter-Defibrillators. Marcel Decker, Inc., NY, 1994.

9. Fogoros R, Elson J, Bonnet C, et al. The automatic implantable cardioverter defibrillator in drug-refractory ventricular arrhythmias. Ann Intern Med 1987;107:635–641.

10. Winkle R, Mead H, Ruder M, et al. Long-term outcome with the automatic implantable cardioverter defibrillator. J Am Coll Cardiol 1989;13:1353–1361.

11. Akhtar M, Avitall B, Jazayeri M, et al. Role of implantable cardioverter defibrillator therapy in the management of high-risk patients. Circulation 1992;85(I):I-131–139.

12. Powell A, Finkelstein D, Garan H, et al. Influence of implantable cardioverter-defibrilla-tors on the long-term prognosis of survivors of out-of-hospital cardiac arrest. Circulation 1993;88:1083–1892.

13. Nisam S, Kaye S, Mower M, et al. AICD automatic cardioverter defibrillator clinical update: 14 years experience in over 34,000 patients. PACE 1995;18 (pt II):142–147.

14. Mosteller R, Lehmann M, Thomas A, et al. Operative mortality with implantation of the automatic cardioverter-defibrillator. Am J Cardiol 1991;68:1340–1345.

15. Block M, Breithardt M. Long-term follow-up and clinical results of implantable cardioverter-defibrillators. In Zipes D, Jalife J, eds. Cardiac Electrophysiology: From Cell to Bedside. WB Saunders, Philadelphia, 1995, pp 1412–1425.

16. Trappe H, Klein H, Wahlers T, et al. Risk and benefit of additional aortocoronary bypass grafting in patients undergoing cardioverter-defibrillator implantation. Am Heart J 1994;1275–1282.

17. Manolis A, Rastegar H, Estes M. Prophylactic automatic implantable cardioverter defibrillator patches in patients at high risk for postoperative ventricular tachyarrhythmias. J Am Coll Cardiol 1989;13:1367–1373.

18. Nisam S, Mower M, Thomas A, et al. Patient survival comparison in three generations of automatic implantatble cardioverter defibrillators: review of 12 years, 25,000 patients. PACE 1993;16(II):174–178.

19. Saksena S, Parsonnet V. Implantation of a cardioverter/defibrillator without thoracotomy using a triple electrode system. JAMA 1988;259:69–72.

20. Hauser R, Mower M, Mitchell M, et al. Current status of the Ventak PRx Pulse Generator and ENDOTAK Nonthoracotomy Lead System. PACE 1992;15:671–677.

21. Zipes D, Roberts D. Results of the international study of the implantable pacemaker cardioverter defibrillator: a comparison of epicardial and endocardial lead systems. Circulation 1995;92:59–65.

22. Brooks R, Garan H, Torchiana D, et al. Determinants of successful nonthoracotomy cardioverter-defibrillator implantation: experi-

ence in 101 patients using two different lead systems. J Am Coll Cardiol 1993;22: 1835–1842.

23. Böcker D, Block M, Isbruch F, et al. Do patients with an implantable defibrillator live longer? JACC 1993;21:1638–1644.

24. Raviele A, Gasparini G, for the Italian EN-DOTAK Investigator Group. Italian multicenter cliinical experience with endocardial defibrillation: acute and long-term results in 307 patients. PACE 1995;18:559–608.

25. Schlepper M, Neuzner J, Pitschner H. Implantable cardioverter defibrillator: effect on survival. PACE 1995;18:569–578.

26. Klein H, Auricchio A, Huvelle E, et al. Initial clinical experience with a new down-sized implantable cardioverter-defibrillator. Am J Cardiol 1996;78(5A):9–14.

27. Bardy G, Raitt M, Jones G. Unipolar defibrillation systems. In Singer I, ed. Implantable Cardioverter Defibrillator. Futura Publishing Co., Armonk, NY, 1994, pp 365–376.

28. Pacifico A, Wheelan K, Nasir N, et al. Long-term follow-up of cardioverter-defibrillator implanted under conscious sedation in prepectoral subfascial position. Circulation 1997;95:946–950.

29. Rosenqvist M. Antitachycardia pacing: which patients and which methods. Am J Cardiol 1996;78(5A):92–97.

30. Nisam S. Technology update: the modern implantable cardioverter defibrillator. Ann Noninvasive Electrocardiogr 1997;2:69–78.

31. The Cardiac Arrhythmia Suppression Trial (CAST) Investigators. Effect of encainide and flecainide on mortality in a randomized trial of arrhythmia suppression after myocardial infarction. N Engl J Med 1989;321:406–412.

32. The CASCADE Investigators. Cardiac arrest in Seattle: conventional versus amiodarone drug evaluation. Am J Cardiol 1991;7: 578–584.

33. Siebels J, Cappato R, Rüppel R, et al. ICD versus drugs in cardiac arrest survivors: preliminary results of the Cardiac Arrest Study Hamburg (CASH). PACE 1993;16:552–558.

34. Mason J, on behalf of the ESVEM Investigators. A comparison of seven antiarrhythmic drugs in patients with ventricular tachyarrhythmias. N Engl J Med 1993;329:452–458.

35. Böcker E, Haverkamp W, Block M, et al. Comparison of d,l-sotalol and implantable defibrillators for treatment of sustained ventricular tachycardia or fibrillation in patients with coronary artery disease. Circulation in press.

36. Waldo A, Camm J, de Ruyter H, et al. for the SWORD Investigators. Effect of d-sotalol on mortality in patients with left ventricular dysfunction after recent and remote myocardial infarction. Lancet 1996;348:7–12.

37. Lee R, Wong M, Siu A, et al. Long-term results of electrophysiologically guided sotalol therapy for life-threatening ventricular arrhythmias. Am Heart J 1996;132:973–978.

38. Herre J, Sauve M, Scheinman M. Long-term results of amiodarone therapy with recurrent sustained ventricular tachycardia or ventricular fibrillation. J Am Coll Cardiol 1989;13:442–449.

39. Olson P, Woelfel A, Simpson R, et al. Stratification of sudden death risk in patients receiving long-term amiodarone treatment for sustained ventricular tachycardia or ventricular fibrillation. Am J Cardiol 1993;72: 823–826.

40. Weinberg B, Miles W, Klein S, et al. Five-year follow-up of 589 patients treated with amiodarone. Am Heart J 1993;125:109–120.

41. Pfisterer M, Kiowski W, Burckhardt D, et al. Beneficial effect of amiodarone on cardiac mortality in patients with asymptomatic complex ventricular arrhythmias after acute myocardial infarction and preserved but not impaired left ventricular function.

42. Singh S, Fletcher R, Fisher S, et al. for the Survival Trial of Antiarrhythmic Therapy in Congestive Heart Failure (STAT-CHF). Amiodarone in patients with congestive heart failure and asymptomatic ventricular arrhythmia. N Engl J Med 1995;333:77–82.

43. Julian D, Camm J, Frangin G, et al. for the European Myocardial Infarct Amiodarone Trial Investigators. Randomised trial of effect of amiodarone on mortality in patients with left ventricular dysfunction after recent myocardial infarction: EMIAT. Lancet 1997; 349:667–674.

44. Neuzner J, Pitschner H, König S, et al. Stored electrograms in cardioverter/defibrillator therapy: accuracy of rhythm diagnosis in 335 spontaneous arrhythmia episodes. J Ambul Mon 1995;8(1):1–9.

45. Schaumann A, Mühlen V, Herse B, et al. Empiric versus tested antitachycardia pacing in implantable cardioverter defibrillators: a prospective study including 200 patients. Circulation 1998;97:66–74.

46. Pantridge J, Geddes J. A mobile intensive-care unit in the management of myocardial infarction. Lancet 1967;2:271–273.

47. Josephson M, Nisam S. Prospective trials of implantable cardioverter defibrillators versus drugs: are they addressing the right question? Am J Cardiol 1996;77:859–863.

48. Nisam S, Breithardt G. Mortality trials with implantable defibrillators. Am J Cardiol 1997;79:468–471.

49. Cohen T, Chien W, Lurie K, et al. Implanta-

ble cardioverter defibrillator proarrhythmia: case report and review of the literature. PACE 1991;13:1326.

50. Fiksinski E, Martin D, Venditte F. Electrical proarrhythmia with procainamide: a new ICD-drug interaction. J Cardiovasc Electrophysiol 1994;5:144–145.

51. Birgersdotter-Green U, Rosenqvist M, Lindemans F, et al. Holter documented sudden death in a patient with an implanted defibrillator. PACE 1992;15:1008A.

52. Connolly S, Yusuf S. Evaluation of the implantable cardioverter defibrillator in survivors of cardiac arrest: the need for randomized trials. Am J Cardiol 1992;69:959–962.

53. Newman D, Sauve J, Herre J, et al. Survival after implantation of the cardioverter defibrillator. Am J Cardiol 1992;69:889–903.

54. Wever E, Hauer R, Van Capelle F, et al. Randomized study of implantable defibrillator as first-choice therapy versus conventional strategy in postinfarct sudden death survivors. Circulation 1995;91:2195–2203.

55. Moss A, Hall J, Cannom D, et al. for the MADIT Investigators. Improved survival with an implanted defibrillator in patients with coronary disease at high risk of ventricular arrhythmias. N Engl J Med 1996;335:1933–1940.

56. Hallstrom A, Zipes D. Preliminary results of AVID (Antiarrhythmics vs Implantable Defibrillator) Trial. Oral presentation during Clinical Trials Update, May 8, 1997, during 18th annual scientific sessions of North American Society of Pacing and Electrophysiology (NASPE), New Orleans, LA.

57. Guarnieri T, Levine J, Griffith L, et al. When "sudden cardiac death" is not so sudden: lessons learned from the automatic implantable defibrillator. Am Heart J 1988;15:205–207.

58. Kim S, Fisher J, Choue C, et al. Influence on left ventricular function on outcome of patients treated with implantable defibrillators. Circulation 1992;85:1304–1310.

59. Choue C, Kim S, Fisher J, et al. Comparison of defibrillator therapy and other therapeutic modalities for sustained ventricular tachycardia or ventricular fibrillation associated with coronary artery disease. Am J Cardiol 1994;73:1075–1079.

60. National Institute of Health (NIH) Press Release. AVID. April 14, 1997.

61. Sweeney M, Ruskin J. Mortality benefits and the implantable cardioverter defibrillator. Circulation 1994;89:1851–1858.

62. Fogoros R. Impact of the implantable cardioverter defibrillator on mortality: the axiom of overall implantable cardioverter defibrillator survival. Am J Cardiol 1996;78:57–61.

63. Nisam S. Do MADIT results apply only to MADIT patients? Am J Cardiol 1997;79 (6A):27–30.

64. Nisam S, Fogoros R. Troubleshooting of patients with implantable cardioverter-defibrillators. In Singer I, ed. Interventional Electrophysiology. Williams & Wilkins, Inc., Baltimore MD, 1996, pp 793.

65. Siebels J, Cappato R, Ruppel R, et al. Preliminary results of the Cardiac Arrest Study Hamburg (CASH). Am J Cardiol 1993;72:109–113F.

66. Cappato R, Kuck K-H. Study results: implantable heart defibrillator saves lives in patients with previous cardiac arrest. Press release, during Update on Clinical Trials session at the 47th annual scientific sessions of the American College of Cardiology, Atlanta, GA, March 30, 1998.

67. Connolly S. Results of the Canadian Implantable Defibrillator Study (CIDS). Oral presentation during Update on Clinical Trials session at the 47th annual scientific sessions of the American College of Cardiology, Atlanta, GA, March 30, 1998.

68. Nisam S. The ICD cannot impact nonarrhythmic mortality. Or can it? In Raviele A, ed. Proceedings of Cardiac Arrhythmias, Fifth International Workshop, Venice, Oct. 7–10, 1997, Springer-Verlag, Milan.

Chapter 24

Clinical Results with the Fourth Generation and Investigational Implantable Cardioverter-Defibrillators

Werner Jung, Berndt Lüderitz

Introduction

Single chamber ventricular defibrillator implantation has been shown to be an effective and safe treatment for patients with malignant ventricular tachyarrhythmias and to significantly reduce the incidence of sudden cardiac death. However, the high incidence of inappropriate implantable cardioverter defibrillator (ICD) therapy due to supraventricular tachycardias is a major challenge and has been reported to affect up to 25% of patients.[1,2] Enhanced detection criteria such as rate stability, sudden onset, and morphology assessment improve the specificity of ICD therapy, but may place the patient at risk of underdetection of ventricular tachycardia.[3–7] Recently, it has been shown that algorithms using dual chamber sensing may significantly improve differentiation between supraventricular tachycardia and ventricular tachycardia.[8–10] Another beneficial effect of dual chamber ICD may be the opportunity not only to sense in the atrium, but also to pace in this chamber. Special options that are available in modern implantable defibrillators are listed in Table 1. Although the beneficial effects of DDD pacing

are well known, most of the currently available ICDs provide only fixed ventricular antibradycardia pacing. In a recent retrospective study, the need for antibradycardia pacing was analyzed in a consecutive series of 139 ICD patients.[11] The findings of this report indicate that up to 18% of the ICD patients are in need of antibradycardia pacing, with up to 80% of these patients having an indication for DDD pacing. This chapter describes early clinical experience with investigational ICDs capable of dual chamber detection for arrhythmia diagnosis and dual chamber pacing function.

Defender 9001 Dual Chamber Defibrillator

The dual chamber ICD (Defender™ 9001, ELA Medical, Montrouge, France), with a weight of 230 g and a volume of 148 mL, uses a new classification algorithm and performs a tiered analysis of the arrhythmia in three steps: cycle length sorting, majority rhythm identification, and ventricular tachycardia/supraventricular tachycardia/sinus tachycardia sorting. The algorithm

From Singer I, Barold SS, Camm AJ (eds): *Nonpharmacological Therapy of Arrhythmias for the 21st Century: The State of the Art.* Futura Publishing Co., Inc., Armonk, NY, © 1998.

Table 1
Modern Pulse Generators: (Fourth Generation)

- Antitachycardia and antibradycardia (DDD) pacing
- Programmable rate/energy
- Biphasic programmable waveforms
- Tiered therapy
- Noninvasive electrophysiological programmed stimulation
- Sophisticated detection algorithms
- Atrial shock therapy and prevention strategies
- Extended stored electrograms and Marker Channels™
- Low weight (<100 g); small volume (<60 mL)

uses four criteria to detect and classify tachyarrhythmias: (a) ventricular rate; (b) stability of the ventricular (RR) intervals; (c) type of AV association; and (d) acceleration magnitude and origin.[12] Figure 1 depicts the new tachycardia classification algorithm. The Defender device stores statistics including pacing and detection data, the number of delivered and successful tachycardia

therapies, and details of the four most recent tachyarrhythmia episodes that were diagnosed as ventricular and/or sustained. For each of the four episodes the following data are stored: (a) event logs detailing the entire sequence of detection; rhythm diagnosis, therapy delivered, and outcome; (b) atrial and ventricular marker chains documenting the onset of the episode, therapy delivered, and outcome; (c) intracardiac electrograms (recorded between the atrial and ventricular pace/sense electrodes) during diagnosis and after the last therapy delivered during the episode.

Results

The diagnostic accuracy of the new tachycardia classification algorithm was evaluated prospectively in 156 episodes of induced sustained tachycardias on the basis of the stability of the RR cycle lengths and AV association.[13] Eighty-nine tachycardias were taken from the Ann Arbor electrogram

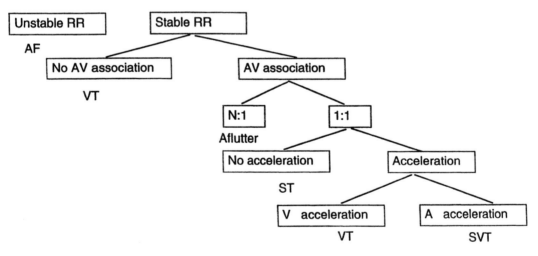

Figure 1. Tachycardia classification algorithm based on three criteria ventricular (RR) stability, atrioventricular (AV) association, and acceleration. An unstable ventricular rhythm is always considered to be atrial fibrillation (AF) and therapy is withheld. A stable ventricular rhythm without AV association is declared as ventricular tachycardia (VT) and is immediately treated. A stable ventricular rhythm with N:1 AV association is interpreted as atrial flutter (Aflutter). A stable ventricular rhythm with 1:1 AV association but without acceleration is considered as sinus tachycardia (ST) and no therapy is delivered. A stable ventricular rhythm with 1:1 AV association and with either acceleration of atrial origin or of ventricular origin is classified as supraventricular tachycardia (SVT) or ventricular tachycardia, respectively.

library; the others were recorded in 50 patients during electrophysiological studies. The atrial and ventricular signals were stored on an external recorder and then injected into an external prototype of a dual chamber ICD (Defender 9001). The algorithm correctly diagnosed 96% of VT episodes, 100% of ventricular fibrillation (VF) episodes, and 92% of double tachycardia episodes. The mean detection time for ventricular tachycardia was 2.6 ± 0.8 sec, and for ventricular fibrillation 2.1 ± 0.4 sec. The positive predictive values for the diagnosis of atrial fibrillation and flutter were 92% and 86%, respectively, and for ventricular tachycardia and ventricular fibrillation 95% and 100%, respectively.

In a recent publication, the sensitivity and specificity of this new tachycardia classification algorithm was evaluated in 18 patients with a mean age of 55 ± 15 years and a mean left ventricular ejection fraction of 35% ± 11% undergoing implantation with the first dual chamber ICD, the Defender 9001.[14] One patient with a defibrillation threshold of 34 J was excluded from the primary follow-up analysis because of protocol violation, and a second patient who developed multiple episodes of ventricular fibrillation at the end of the implantation procedure died in electromechanical dissociation despite many successful internal and external DC shocks and vigorous resuscitation attempts. Over a mean follow-up period of 7.1 ± 4.5 months, 176 spontaneous tachyarrhythmia episodes were recorded in 11 patients in the device memory. The stored data for each episode was reviewed by independent investigators. A diagnosis was reached by consensus in all but one episode. The physician diagnosis was compared with that by the device. All 122 ventricular tachycardia/ventricular fibrillation episodes were correctly diagnosed, as were 51 of 53 supraventricular tachycardias. Two episodes of atrial fibrillation with rapid regular ventricular rates were treated as ventricular tachycardia, and a third episode, treated as ventricular tachycardia, could not be diagnosed with certainty. The time to first therapy delivery was 9.8 ± 3.4 (range, 2.3–14) sec for ventricular fibrillation, and 5.4 ± 1.5 (range, 2.0–9.5) sec for ventricular tachycardia, respectively. All ventricular tachycardia/ventricular fibrillation episodes were successfully treated with the first ICD shock therapy. The mean tachycardia rate for the spontaneous ventricular tachycardia episodes was 153 ± 19 (range, 110–200) beats per minute, for the spontaneous sinus tachycardia episodes was 131 ± 20 (range, 104–180) beats per minute, and for the spontaneous supraventricular tachycardia episodes 136 ± 12 (range, 125–153) beats per minute.

During follow-up two atrial lead displacements occurred. In one patient the lead was replaced and in another patient the device was reprogrammed to ventricular-based pacing and tachycardia detection. One patient developed progressive heart failure and died 8 months after ICD implantation. The patient who was excluded from the primary analysis because of a high defibrillation threshold suffered 19 ventricular tachycardia episodes during follow-up, all of which were detected and treated successfully by antitachycardia pacing or with shock therapy. Three months after ICD implant, the patient died in ventricular fibrillation despite receiving multiple automatically delivered 34-J shocks. At the end of the follow-up period, 10 DDD-ICD devices were programmed in DDD mode, five in DDI mode, and one in VVI mode. By June 1997, 70 patients received the dual chamber ICD, the Defender 9001.[15] The preliminary evaluation of these 70 patients support the promising early experience with this first dual chamber ICD with respect to the accuracy in discriminating supraventricular tachycardia from ventricular tachycardia.

Ventak AV Dual Chamber Defibrillator

The advent of a new small sized dual chamber ICD (Ventak AV, CPI Guidant Inc.,

Table 2
Detection Enhancements in Multizone Configurations

One-zone configuration
  Ventricular fibrillation
  No detection enhancements
Two-zone configuration

Ventricular tachycardia	Ventricular fibrillation	
Onset		
Stability as an inhibitor	No detection enhancements	
Sustained rate duration		
AFib rate/AFib stability		*Stability analysis cannot be
V rate > A rate		programmed as both an
or		inhibitor and an accelerator
Stability as an accelerator*		in the same zone

Three-zone configuration

Ventricular tachycardia-1	Ventricular tachycardia	Ventricular fibrillation
Onset	Stability as an accelerator	No detection enhancements
Stability as an inhibitor		
Sustained rate duration		
AFib rate/AFib stability		
V rate > A rate		

St. Paul, MN), with a weight of 150 g and a volume of 79 mL, offering enhanced detection criteria for arrhythmia classification may allow for an improved discrimination between ventricular tachycardia and supraventricular tachycardia. The new detection enhancements may be programmed as therapy inhibitors, inhibitor overrides, and therapy accelerators. A therapy inhibitor causes a therapy to be delayed or inhibited if certain enhancement criteria are not satisfied at the end of the duration. Onset can be programmed to inhibit therapy if the patient's heart rate increases gradually. The stability parameter can be programmed to inhibit therapy if the ventricular rate is unstable. The AFib rate threshold and corresponding AFib stability criterion can be programmed to inhibit ventricular therapy, if the atrial rhythm is fast and the ventricular rate is unstable. An inhibitor override causes the therapy inhibitors to be bypassed if certain criteria are satisfied. The V Rate > A Rate criterion can be used to override the therapy inhibitors, onset and stability, if the ventricular rate is faster than the atrial rate. The sustained rate duration parameter enables the pulse generator to override the therapy inhibitors, onset and stability, if the

high rate continues over an extended time period. A therapy accelerator accelerates the sequence of a therapy by skipping over or interrupting an antitachycardia schema to initiate charging for the first programmed shock for the rate zone. The stability parameter can be programmed to accelerate delivery of shock therapy if the rhythm is declared to be unstable. The atrial rate may be used to inhibit therapy in the presence of atrial fibrillation and to bypass onset or stability as inhibitors, if the ventricular rate is faster than the atrial rate. Table 2 shows detection enhancements which may be programmed in multizone configurations.

Results

Recently, preliminary results were reported with this dual chamber ICD. A total of 69 patients at 17 centers received the Ventak AV. The AFib rate threshold feature inhibited therapy in 29 episodes (91%) of induced atrial fibrillation in 20 patients. Therapy was delivered appropriately for 64 induced episodes of ventricular tachycardia (100%) in 32 patients. A total of 40 spontaneous episodes occurred in 10 patients.[16] At our institution, 12 patients with a mean age of 57 ± 17 years were implanted with this new dual chamber ICD.[17] The underlying heart disease was coronary artery diease in nine patients and idiopathic dilated cardiomyopathy in three patients. Eight patients had an advanced atrioventricular block and four patients suffered from paroxysmal atrial fibrillation. At implant, the mean ventricular defibrillation threshold was 9.1 ± 3 J (5–15 J). Intraoperatively, the following signals were obtained: atrial pacing threshold 1.58 ± 0.6 V (1.0–2.7 V), P wave 3.9 ± 1.7 mV (2.0–6.9 mV), ventricular pacing threshold 0.6 ± 0.4 V, (0.4–1.7 V), R wave 9.5 ± 3.2 mV (6.7–16.5 mV). In all induced episodes of atrial fibrillation with fast and irregular ventricular response, no inappropriate ICD therapy was delivered. In all episodes in which the ventricular rate was faster than the atrial rate, the therapy inhibitors were overriden and an appropriate ICD therapy was delivered. The new detection enhancement features, AFib rate threshold and V Rate > A Rate in combination with stability and onset, allowed in all induced episodes of atrial fibrillation an accurate discrimination between supraventricular and ventricular tachycardia.

Jewel AF™ Arrhythmia Management Device

Concern has been raised whether or not a stand alone implantable atrial defibrillator is safe enough or should provide ventricular backup defibrillation in the rare case of shock-induced ventricular proarrhythmia. Recently, a new dual chamber defibrillator (Arrhythmia Management Device, AMD, model 7250, Medtronic Inc., Minneapolis, MN) has entered clinical investigation (Figure 2). The 7250 AMD, with a weight of 93 g and a volume of 55 mL, can be programmed to detect four types of arrhythmias: atrial tachycardia, atrial fibrillation, ventricular tachycardia, and ventricular fibrillation. The most important new features of the 7250 AMD system include: dual chamber pacing, a new dual chamber detection criterion for rejection of supraventricular tachycardias, detection and treatment modalities of atrial arrhythmias, prevention strategies for atrial arrhythmias. The dual chamber detection criterion is constantly monitoring the rhythm in the ventricle as well as in the atrium. This new dual chamber detection algorithm is used to improve discrimination of ventricular tachycardia from supraventricular tachycardia by applying pattern recognition methods based on different P-wave positions within RR sequences. The detection algorithm can be used to withhold inappropriate ventricular therapies for atrial tachycardias, atrial fibrillation, sinus tachycardia, 1:1 supraventricular tachycardias, or any combination of these. It should be noted that the device takes a fairly conservative approach: in the case of evidence of a ventricular arrhythmia, particularly ventricular fibrillation, a therapy will be delivered. Two detection zones can be programmed in the atrium. Treatment in these two zones includes antitachycardia pacing (burst and ramp), high frequency (50 Hz) burst pacing and R wave synchronous shock therapies ranging from 0.1 to 27 J. Time to delivery of pacing and shock therapies is independently programmable. Atrial shock therapy can be delivered within a specified time window and the number of shocks can be limited. The 7250 AMD has two prevention strategies for atrial arrhythmias: switchback delay and atrial rate stabilization. The first feature prolongs the time that the device is in DDI pacing mode after mode switching. The latter feature aims to eliminate the short–long PP intervals that often precede atrial arrhythmias. As soon as the device detects such intervals, it starts overdrive pacing in the atrium.

Results

Preliminary results with a prototype dual chamber defibrillator showed that detection of atrial tachyarrhythmias was appropriate

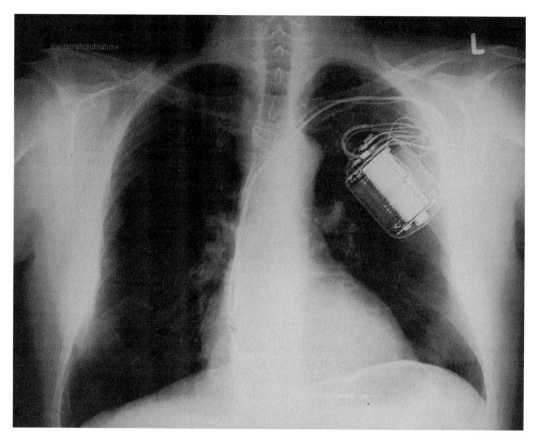

Figure 2. Chest x-ray of a patient with an arrhythmia management device (model 7250). The pectorally implanted active can device is connected with two transvenous electrodes, one located in the right atrial appendage and the other in the apex of the right ventricle.

in 62 of 74 induced and in 43 of 47 simulated episodes. Detection of ventricular fibrillation and tachycardia was appropriate in 50 of 50 induced and in 148 of 164 simulated episodes. Nine of 19 simulated and true dual tachycardias were properly detected as ventricular fibrillation or tachycardia. A revised detection algorithm resulted in 25 of 28 dual tachycardias being properly detected as ventricular fibrillation or tachycardia. High-frequency burst pacing terminated four of five episodes of atrial tachycardia and one of eight episodes of atrial fibrillation. Atrial rate stabilization and automatic mode switching was successfully demonstrated in 16 of 17 patients.[18] On January 10, 1997, a 61-year-old woman suffering from both recurrent, drug refractory supraventricular and ventricular tachycardia was the first patient in the world to receive a multiprogrammable dual chamber implantable defibrillator, the 7250 AMD system, at our institution.[19] The device was implanted in the left pectoral region and connected with transvenous defibrillation leads placed in the apex of the right ventricle (model 6936) and in the appendage of the right atrium (model 6943). The first day after implantation of the new defibrillator, three sustained episodes of atrial fibrillation occurred that were all successfully treated by high-frequency burst pacing, a new option, which allows painless termination of recent onset atrial tachycardias. None of these arrhythmias were inappropriately detected or treated as ventricular episodes.

June 1997

Table 3
Implanted Pulse Generators at the University of Bonn

Patients; Age (years)	321 (m: 264, f: 57); 56 ± 19
Disease:	
• Coronary artery disease	215
• Idiopathic dilated cardiomyopathy	45
• Hypertrophic (non) obstructive cardiomyopathy	8
• Myocarditis	6
• Arrhythmogenic right ventricular dysplasia	8
• Idiopathic ventricular fibrillation	27
• Others	12
Implantable cardioverter defibrillator devices:	459 (138 × replacement)
AICD (60), AICD + Tachylog (6), PRx (17), PRxII (22), PRxIII (6), Ventak P 2 (25), Ventak Mini (21), Ventak AV (11) PCD 7217B (36), 7219B (7), D (24), E (6), C (45), 7220/1 (14), 7218 (65), 7223 (26), Guardian ATP 4211 (4), 4215 (7), Res-Q I (24), Res-Q II (6), Cadence (3), Cadet (3), Sentinel (2), Defender (8), 7250 (5), Metrix (6)	
Transvenous approach:	277
Shocks:	46 ± 29
Antitachycardia pacing	171 ± 81
Months:	23 ± 16

Table 3 provides an overview of the implanted pulse generators at the University of Bonn including fourth generation and investigational devices.

Metrix™ Implantable Atrial Defibrillator

The development of an ICD for the management of ventricular tachyarrhythmias has stimulated investigation of a similar approach to atrial fibrillation. A device for the management of recurring atrial fibrillation should have several characteristics:[20] low thresholds using only transvenous electrodes, small size with several years of implant life, freedom from ventricular proarrhythmia, a minimum of patient discomfort, limited thromboembolic risk, high sensitivity and specificity for atrial fibrillation detection. Furthermore, cost-effectiveness and improvement in quality of life have to be demonstrated when such a device is introduced for clinical management of patients with atrial fibrillation. Patients with symptomatic recurrences of atrial fibrillation despite the use of antiarrhythmic drug therapy represent potential candidates for an implantable atrial defibrillator.[20-23] The number and duration of atrial fibrillation episodes should be taken into account in the indications. Patients with frequent episodes must be excluded as candidates for implantation of an atrial defibrillator because of too frequent discharges, patient discomfort, and rapid battery depletion. Similarly, patients with episodes of short duration and spontaneous termination may not be good candidates. Selected patients with infrequent, symptomatic attacks of long-lasting episodes of atrial fibrillation despite antiarrhythmic drug therapy may benefit from an implantable atrial defibrillator.

Recently, a stand-alone implantable atrial defibrillator (METRIX System, models 3000 and 3020, InControl Inc., Redmond, WA) has entered clinical investigation (Figure 3). The primary objective of this clinical study is to evaluate the device safety in terms of appropriate shock synchronization to avoid shock-induced ventricular proarrhythmia. The secondary endpoint is to assess efficacy in detecting and terminating atrial fibrillation. The METRIX implantable atrial defi-

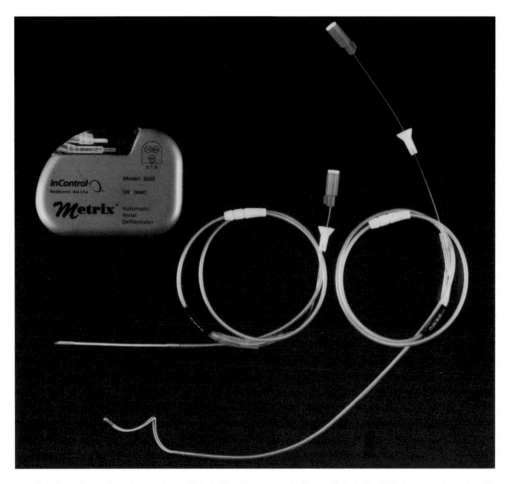

Figure 3. The Metrix implantable atrial defibrillator and the atrial defibrillation leads. The device has a weight of 79 g and a volume of 53 mL, and is implanted in the pectoral region. The defibrillation coils for both the right atrium and the coronary sinus leads are each 6 cm long. The defibrillation lead for the right atrium has a nonretractable screw-in active fixation. The defibrillation lead for the coronary sinus has a preformed spiral shape at the end, designed to stabilize the lead in the coronary sinus.

brillator, models 3000 or 3020, uses a pair of defibrillation leads to detect atrial fibrillation in the coronary sinus and the right atrium.[24] Both are 7F in diameter and the defibrillation coils are each 6 cm in length. The right atrial lead has an active fixation in the right atrium. The coronary sinus lead has a natural spiral configuration for retention in the coronary sinus, and can be straightened with a stylet. A separate bipolar right ventricular lead is used for ventricular pacing and sensing. The device, with a weight of 79 g and a volume of 53 mL, is intended for implantation in the pectoral region like a conventional antibradycardiac pacemaker. Graded shock therapy is available for up to eight shocks (two at each level) for each episode of atrial fibrillation. Biphasic shocks are programmable in 20 V increments up to 300 V (about 3 J in the Model 3000 and 6 J in the Model 3020). The METRIX defibrillator can be used to induce atrial fibrillation by using R wave synchronous shocks and can store intracardiac electrograms (EGMs) for up to 2 min from the most recent six atrial fibrillation episodes.

The device can be programmed into one of four different operating modes: fully automatic, patient-activated mode, monitor mode, or pacing only mode. As atrial fibrillation is not life-threatening, the device is only intermittently active in detecting and treating atrial fibrillation, and this "sleep wake-up" cycle interval is programmable.

A two-staged atrial fibrillation detection algorithm is operative after automatic gain control.[25] The "quiet interval analysis algorithm" is used to discriminate between a sinus and a nonsinus rhythm in the 8-sec EGM segment. The quiet interval is defined as an interval greater than the preselected interval during which no sensed events occur on the right atrium channel and is programmable from 130 to 220 ms. The percent quiet time is calculated by dividing the total time by 8 sec and multiplying by 100%. The percent quiet time is programmable from 10% to 30% in increments of 5%. If the percent quiet time is equal to or rises above the programmed value, the cardiac rhythm is diagnosed as normal sinus rhythm. If the percent quiet time falls below the programmed value, the rhythm is determined to be nonsinus, and the "baseline crossing algorithm" is invoked to detect atrial fibrillation. The "quiet interval algorithm" is highly specific for sinus rhythm. The "baseline crossing analysis" is a configuration analysis method that examines the average number of baseline crossings on the ST-T region. Using a right atrium EGM, a detection window is set beginning 80 ms after the R wave and ending 200 ms later, except in the last R wave. The device then analyzes the filtered right atrium EGM data to count the number of times the signal crosses both the negative and positive baseline crossing thresholds within each detection window. The baseline crossing count is the average number of baseline crossings per R wave. It is programmable from 1.6 to 3.0 in increments of 0.1. If the average baseline crossing count in the 8-sec window exceeds the programmed count, the cardiac rhythm is defined as atrial fibrillation. The "baseline crossing algorithm" is very specific for atrial fibrillation. The METRIX device uses a dual channel synchronization algorithm. This algorithm is designed to ensure that all shocks will be delivered only to correctly synchronized R waves. Before synchronization is attempted, two electrograms are evaluated simultaneously in real time for integrity and data quality. The right ventricular and the right ventricle–coronary sinus channels are used for the synchronization process. The minimal synchronization interval can be programmed from 500 ms to 800 ms. Constraints for shock delivery after long–short cycles are also separately implemented and shocks are avoided for long–short cycles that differ by > 140 ms for cycles < 800 ms.

Results

Initial clinical experience with the METRIX human implantable atrial defibrillator has been recently reported.[24] The device was implanted in three patients with drug refractory paroxysmal atrial fibrillation. The mean implant threshold (ED 50) was 195 V (1.8 J), and minimum voltage at conversion during follow-up assessments at 1, 3, and 6 months were 260 V (2.5 J), 250 V (2.3 J), and 300 V (3.0 J), respectively. Detection of atrial fibrillation was 100% specific and shocks were 100% synchronized, although only a proportion of synchronized R waves were considered suitable for shock delivery primarily because of closely coupled cycle lengths. Three patients had nine spontaneous episodes of atrial fibrillation with eight out of nine (89%) successfully defibrillated by shocks of 260-300 V. Sedation was not used in four out of nine (45%) episodes. Back-up ventricular pacing was initiated by the device in six out of nine (67%) episodes. One patient had more frequent episodes of atrial fibrillation after lead placement, which subsided after a change in medication. There was no ventricular proarrhythmia observed. Initial clinical experience with an implantable atrial defibrillator indicates stable atrial defibrillation thresholds, appropriate R-wave synchronization markers, no shock induced ventricular proarrhythmia, and detection of atrial fibrillation with a specificity of 100%.[24,26,27] Various issues with an implantable atrial defibrillator have to be addressed before such a device will be widely accepted for the clinical management of patients with atrial fibrillation. These issues include: accurate detection of atrial fibrillation, safe and effective termination of atrial fibrillation, patient tolerability, risk of thromboembolism, quality of life, and costs.[28,29]

Summary

Dual chamber ICDs provide equivalent efficacy and safety rates compared to single chamber ICDs. The new detection algorithms significantly improve arrhythmia diagnosis accuracy. In dual chamber ICDs, the new algorithms are highly effective in reducing the number of inappropriate ICD therapies without sacrificing the delivery of appropriate shocks. Major issues which have to be addressed with an implantable atrial defibrillator are pain perception and the potential risk of inducing life-threatening ventricular arrhythmias during delivery of low-energy atrial shocks. At the very beginning, the implantable atrial defibrillator should be restricted to highly selected patients with drug refractory, poorly tolerated, recurrent episodes of atrial fibrillation. The extension of this therapy to wider subsets of patients should be dependent on the initial results with regard to clinical efficacy and safety as well as patient tolerance. Finally, cost-effectiveness as well as quality of life studies are needed to demonstrate the benefit of this specific therapy among other therapeutic strategies available for the management of atrial fibrillation. Early clinical experience with an implantable atrial defibrillator indicates stable atrial defibrillation thresholds, appropriate R-wave synchronization markers, no shock induced ventricular proarrhythmia, and detection of atrial fibrillation with a specificity of 100%. A new arrhythmia management system that combines both detection and treatment in the atrium as well as in the ventricle may represent an important milestone and a significant improvement in the management of patients with both supraventricular and ventricular tachyarrhythmias.

References

1. Hook BG, Marchlinski FE. Value of ventricular electrogram in the diagnosis of arrhythmias precipitating electrical device therapy. J Am Coll Cardiol 1991;19:490–499.

2. Grimm W, Flores BF, Marchlinski FE. Electrocardiographically documented unnecessary, spontaneous shocks in 241 patients with implantable cardioverter-defibrillators. PACE 1992;15:1667–1673.

3. Swerdlow CD, Chen PS, Kass RM, et al. Discrimination of ventricular tachycardia from sinus tachycardia and atrial fibrillation in a tiered-therapy cardioverter-defibrillator. J Am Coll Cardiol 1994;23:1342–1355.

4. Swerdlow CD, Ahern T, Chen PS, et al. Underdetection of ventricular tachycardia by algorithms to enhance specificity in a tiered-therapy cardioverter-defibrillator. J Am Coll Cardiol 1994;24:416–424.

5. Neuzner J, Pitschner HF, Schlepper M. Programmable VT detection enhancements in implantable cardioverter defibrillator therapy. PACE 1995;18:539–547.

6. Schaumann A, von zur Mühlen F, Gonska BD, et al. Enhanced detection criteria in implantable cardioverter-defibrillators to avoid inappropriate therapy. Am J Cardiol 1996; 78:42–50.

7. Higgins SL, Lee RS, Kramer RL. Stability: An ICD detection criterion for discriminating atrial fibrillation from ventricular tachycardia. J Cardiovasc Electrophysiol 1995;6: 1081–1088.

8. Schuger CD, Jackson K, Russel TS, et al. Atrial sensing to augment ventricular tachycardia detection by the automatic implantable cardioverter defibrillator: a utility study. PACE 1988;11:1456–1464.

9. Leong PHW, Jabri MA. Arrhythmia classification using two intracardiac leads. Proceedings of Computers in Cardiology. Los Alamitos, CA IEEE Computer Society Press 1992; 189–192.

10. Polikaitis A, Arzbaecher R. Sensitivity and specificity of a dual-chamber arrhythmia recognition algorithm for implantable devices. J Electrocardiol 1995;27:78–83.

11. Geelen P, Lorga A, Chauvin M, et al. The value of DDD pacing in patients with an implantable cardioverter defibrillator. PACE 1997;20:177–181.

12. Jung W, Wolpert C, Spehl S, et al. Does a dual-chamber detection algorithm really increase the specificity of ICD treatment? Results of Defender clinical trials. In Raviele A, ed. Cardiac Arrhythmias. Springer Verlag, Heidelberg, 1997, pp 41–45.

13. Nair M, Saoudi N, Kroiss D, et al, for the Participating Centers of the Automatic Recognition of Arrhythmia Study Group. Automatic arrhythmia identification using analysis of the atrioventricular association. Circulation 1997;95:973–967.

14. Lavergne T, Daubert JC, Chauvin M, et al. Preliminary clinical experience with the first dual-chamber pacemaker defibrillator. PACE 1997;20:182–188.

15. Jung W, Esmailzadeh B, Wolpert C, et al, for the Defender Clinical Investigational Group 9001. Arrhythmia classification with the first dual-chamber implantable cardioverter-defibrillator. J Am Coll Cardiol 1997;29:48A.

16. Rüppel R, Langes K, Kalkowski H, et al. Initial experience with implantable cardioverter defibrillator providing dual-chamber pacing and sensing. PACE 1997;20:1078A.

17. Jung W, Spehl S, Esmailzadeh B, et al. New detection enhancement for arrhythmia classification with a pectoral dual-chamber implantable cardioverter defibrillator. PACE 1997;20:1168A.

18. Stanton MS, Hammill SC, Gillberg JM, et al. Clinical testing of a dual-chamber combined atrial and ventricular defibrillator. J Am Coll Cardiol 1997;29:473A.

19. Jung W, Lüderitz B. Implantation of a new arrhythmia management system in patients with supraventricular and ventricular tachyarrhythmias. Lancet 1997;349:853–854.

20. Griffin JC, Ayers GM, Adams J, et al. Is the automatic atrial defibrillator a promising approach? J Cardiovasc Electrophysiol 1996;7:1217–1224.

21. Hillsey RE, Wharton JM. Implantable atrial defibrillators. J Cardiovasc Electrophysiol 1995;6:634–648.

22. Jung W, Wolpert C, Spehl S, et al. Implantable atrial and dual-chamber defibrillators. In Schoels W, El-Sherif, eds. Nonpharmacologic Therapy. Futura Publishing Company Inc., Armonk, NY, 1997, pp 327–348.

23. Jung W, Lüderitz B. Implantable atrial defibrillator: Which results and indications In: Raviele A, ed. Cardiac Arrhythmias. Springer Verlag, Heidelberg, 1997, pp 100–105.

24. Lau CP, Tse HF, Lok NS, et al. Initial clinical experience with an implantable human atrial defibrillator. PACE 1977;20:220–225.

25. Sra JS, Maglio C, Dhala A, et al. Feasibility of atrial fibrillation detection and use of a preceding synchronization interval as a criterion for shock delivery in humans with atrial fibrillation. J Am Coll Cardiol 1996;28:1532–1538.

26. Lau CP, Tse HF, Jung W, et al. Safety and efficacy of an human implantable defibrillator for atrial fibrillation. Circulation 1996;94:I-562.

27. Jung W, Kirchhoff PG, Lau CP, et al., for the Metrix System Clinical Investigational Group. Therapy delivery with the METRIX automatic atrial defibrillation system: threshold stability and shock safety. J Am Coll Cardiol 1997;29:78A.

28. Lüderitz B, Jung W. Quality of life of patients with atrial fibrillation. In Santini M, ed. Progress in Clinical Pacing. Futura Media Services Inc., Armonk, NY, 1996, pp 253–262.

29. Jung W, Herwig S, Spehl S, et al. Quality of life in clinical trials and practice. In Vardas PE, ed. Cardiac Arrhythmias: Pacing and Electrophysiology, Kluwer Academic Publishers Dordrecht, Boston, London, 1997, pp 131–140.

Chapter 25

Clinical Trials to Evaluate the Survival Benefit of Implantable Cardiac Defibrillators

J. Thomas Bigger, Jr.

Introduction

Ongoing or recently completed trials address the use of implantable cardioverter-defibrillator (ICD) therapy for secondary or primary prevention of sudden cardiac death in a number of clinically important groups. This chapter will discuss what we have learned from controlled clinical trials of ICDs.

Secondary Prevention of Sudden Cardiac Death

Currently, most ICD therapy is directed at survivors of cardiac arrest or hemodynamically significant ventricular tachycardia (VT). Because electrophysiologically guided antiarrhythmic drug therapy was established as a standard of practice long before ICD therapy became available in 1985, physicians were not willing to randomly allocate patients with malignant ventricular arrhythmias to a nontherapy arm in

a research study. A large-scale, randomized clinical trial that compares ICD treatment with no therapy will never be done in patients who have survived an episode of cardiac arrest. Thus, the magnitude of improvement in overall survival due to ICD therapy will always remain unknown for patients with malignant ventricular arrhythmias. Several ongoing trials are comparing ICD therapy with drug therapy (primarily amiodarone) in patients with malignant ventricular arrhythmias.

Primary Prevention of Sudden Cardiac Death

The Case for Primary Prevention of Sudden Cardiac Death

The poor salvage rate for out-of-hospital cardiac arrest provides a strong rationale for primary prevention of sudden cardiac death. Each year, more than 400,000 cardiac arrests occur in the United States, almost

Supported in part by NIH Grants HL-48159 and HL-48120 from the National Heart, Lung, and Blood Institute, Bethesda, MD and RR-00645 from the Research Resources Administration, NIH; and by funds from Guidant/Cardiac Pacemakers, Inc., and Mrs. Adelaide Segerman, New York, NY.
From Singer I, Barold SS, Camm AJ (eds): Nonpharmacological Therapy of Arrhythmias for the 21st Century: The State of the Art. Futura Publishing Co, Inc., Armonk, NY, © 1998.

one per minute.[1,2] A similar number occur annually in western Europe. Only about 2% of cardiac arrest victims are resuscitated and leave the hospital alive.[3,4] A few well-organized communities, e.g., Seattle, have higher salvage rates, but, even in these communities, more than three-fourths of the cardiac arrest victims die. Survivors of cardiac arrest are treated vigorously, usually with ICDs or with electrophysiologically guided drug therapy. However, the impact of this approach is small because so few patients survive a cardiac arrest to take advantage of modern treatment. The poor salvage rate for patients experiencing cardiac arrest provides strong motivation for prophylaxis. Many sudden cardiac deaths are due to ischemia in previously asymptomatic patients.[5-8] These deaths can be addressed by aggressive treatment of risk factors for coronary heart disease. About three-fourths of sudden cardiac deaths occur in patients with previously recognized heart disease who are available for screening, risk stratification, and prophylaxis.[9,10] If the patients with heart disease who will experience cardiac arrest can be identified, preventive measures could have a substantially larger impact on the sudden cardiac death problem than is currently achieved with the salvage and treat strategy. ICD therapy is an attractive candidate for prophylaxis of high-risk patients. In 1996, MADIT, a randomized, controlled clinical trial, reported that ICD prophylaxis was significantly better than conventional (drug) therapy to prevent death in high-risk subgroup of coronary heart disease patients.[11]

The Case Against Primary Prevention of Sudden Cardiac Death

A strategy of detection and treatment of high-risk patients requires that tests to detect high-risk patients be accurate and that treatments be effective. The tests currently available to identify patients for ICD prophylaxis are not ideal. Tests that predict cardiac mortality and sudden cardiac death include left ventricular ejection fraction (LVEF), spontaneous, unsustained ventricular arrhythmias quantified in 24-hour continuous ECG recordings, RR variability over a 24-hour or shorter interval, baroreflex sensitivity, signal-averaged ECG, T wave alternans, and electrophysiological studies. Individually, these tests have low positive predictive accuracy, about 15% to 30%,[12-28] and at least 70% of the patients in the high-risk group will not have a cardiac arrest during a 2–3 year period of follow-up, i.e., will receive prophylaxis without benefit.

Recent data suggest that signal-averaged ECG, cardiac electrophysiological studies, Holter variables (VPC and RR variability), baroreflex sensitivity, and LVEF can be combined to obtain positive predictive accuracies of about 50%,[27,28] a level of positive predictive accuracy that may warrant prophylaxis, even with a treatment that has significant morbidity and great cost.

How Big an Effect on All-Cause Mortality Could ICD Therapy Have?

Connolly and Yusuf argue that the reduction in all-cause mortality could not be greater than 33%.[29] They point out that less than 50% of deaths are sudden, some of the sudden deaths are not tachyarrhythmic (e.g., cardiac rupture, cerebral hemorrhage, bradyarrhythmias), and some tachyarrhythmic deaths are not prevented by ICD treatment.

Is ICD Therapy Better than Antiarrhythmic Drug Therapy?

We are fortunate that at least three studies are being done to compare ICD therapy with drug therapy in patients with malignant ventricular arrhythmias: the Cardiac Arrest Study of Hamburg (CASH), the Canadian Implantable Defibrillator Study (CIDS), and the Antiarrhythmics Versus Implantable Defibrillators (AVID) trial. A small Dutch study of ICD cost-effectiveness has been completed and suggests, for the sample studied, that first-choice ICD therapy is more cost-effective than electrophysiologically guided antiarrhythmic drug therapy for cardiac arrest survivors. A preliminary report from AVID reported that ICD therapy had more benefit than empiric amiodarone for patients who survive an episode of ventricular fibrillation (VF) or symptomatic sustained VT.

The Cardiac Arrest Study of Hamburg (CASH)

CASH began enrolling in 1987 and completed recruitment in 1996. CASH is testing the hypothesis that ICD therapy is better than drug therapy in patients who had cardiac arrest and have inducible VT or VF. When planning the trial, a 50% 2-year death rate was assumed for untreated patients and a 31% 2-year death rate in the group assigned to ICD therapy. The randomization goal for CASH was 400, 100 each to ICD treatment or to one of three drugs each with a different mechanism of action: propafenone (IC), metoprolol (II), or amiodarone (III).[30]

Details of Treatment

Patients with ischemic ST depression during an exercise test or an abnormal thallium scan were revascularized (angioplasty or CABG). About 20% of the patients in CASH were revascularized. A loading dose of 1,000 mg amiodarone per day was given for 7 days followed by a dose of 400 to 600 mg per day starting on day 8.[31] Metoprolol was started at a low initial dose of 12.5 to 25 mg per day and increased to the maximum tolerated dose or 300 mg per day over 2 weeks. Propafenone was started at 450 mg per day and increased to the maximum tolerated dose or 900 mg per day over 2 weeks. A variety of ICDs manufactured by Cardiac Pacemakers Inc. were implanted in CASH. The rate for VT detection was programmed between 170 and 200 per minute. The primary therapy was a high-energy discharge in all cases. When repeated episodes of documented VT occurred, investigators were permitted to activate antitachycardia pacing, if available. Many patients had recurrences of sustained, but nonfatal ventricular tachyarrhythmias during long-term drug therapy and crossed over to ICD therapy.[31]

Patient Sample

A total of 349 patients were randomized in CASH: 100 to ICD therapy; 95 to amiodarone, 96 to metoprolol, and 58 to propafenone. The average age of CASH patients was 57 years and 80% were male. Seventy-nine percent had coronary heart disease and approximately 15% had no heart disease. The average LVEF, 0.42, was higher than expected for a group of cardiac arrest survivors. The primary endpoint for CASH was all-cause mortality. All-cause mortality or recurrence of nonfatal cardiac arrest was a secondary endpoint. In March 1992, after a total of 229 patients were enrolled, randomization to the propafenone arm was stopped.[31] In 1992, 18% of the propafenone group had experienced sudden cardiac death compared with none in the ICD group.[32] All-cause mortality was 34% in the propafenone group compared with 17% in the ICD group. All-cause mortality or cardiac arrest occurred in 44% of the propafenone group compared with 17% of the ICD group. The results of electrophysiological testing (positive or negative) had no predictive value for death or nonfatal arrhythmic events during follow-up on propafenone therapy. These findings led the CASH investigators to conclude that propafenone treatment should not be recommended in survivors of cardiac arrest even when the drug converts inducible VT to not inducible.[31] Randomization in the other three limbs was completed in 1996. Stopping recruitment early for the propafenone group will complicate the primary analysis which should have been a comparison of the ICD group with the three drug groups combined. The statistical power of CASH was reduced by a series of interim reports of outcome data. Final results are expected to be available late in 1997.

The Canadian Implantable Defibrillator Study (CIDS)

CIDS began enrolling early in 1991 and completed recruitment of 659 patients in 1996. Follow-up ended in December 1997 and the main results should be available soon. CIDS recruited patients who had: VF without myocardial infarction, VT with syncope, or VT with presyncope, a rate >150 bpm, and a LVEF <0.36. Patients also could be enrolled if they had unmonitored syncope and were later documented to have either spontaneous unsustained VT that lasted >10 sec or inducible sustained uniform VT. Patients were randomized in 50:50 proportions to empiric amiodarone therapy or to ICD treatment.[33] Patients who were randomized to amiodarone were given 1,200 or more mg per day for at least a week, 400 or more mg per day for 10 weeks, and then given 300 or more mg per day until the end of the trial. It is recommended that amiodarone not be used in the ICD group to treat patients with AF. Patients who were randomized to ICD therapy could be treated with any available ICD system. When the trial began, the primary endpoint was arrhythmic death as defined by Hinkle and Thaler.[34] CIDS assumed a 15% 3-year mortality rate for the group assigned to amiodarone and was designed to have 80% power to detect a 58% difference in death between the ICD and amiodarone groups. CIDS originally planned to use arrhythmic death as the primary endpoint and to randomize 400 patients and follow them an average of 3 years. After the study was well under way, a consensus developed to use all-cause mortality as the primary endpoint for ICD trials and CIDS changed its primary endpoint to all-cause mortality in 1995. The change in primary endpoint prompted an increase in sample size from 400 patients to 650 patients. Recruitment of 650 patients will give about 80% power to detect a 33% reduction in the 30% mortality rate assumed for the amiodarone group. In the group assigned to ICD treatment, about 20% are taking amiodarone; in the group assigned to amiodarone treatment, about 5% have had ICDs implanted. After AVID reported in May 1997 that patients treated with ICD therapy had significantly better survival than those assigned to amiodarone treatment, the CIDS DSMB met and recommended that the patients randomized in CIDS continue to be followed until the end of 1997. Although CIDS is following about 350 fewer patients than AVID, it should produce about the same amount of outcome information because the average follow-up is so much longer in CIDS than in AVID. Thus, the information available comparing empiric amiodarone with ICD therapy for patients with sustained ventricular arrhythmias will more than double when CIDS and CASH report their results.

Antiarrhythmics Versus Implantable Defibrillators (AVID)

The National Heart, Lung, and Blood Institute (NHLBI) is conducting a trial to determine whether there is a significant difference in efficacy, safety, quality of life, and cost between ICD therapy and drug treatment with either amiodarone or dl-sotalol.[35] The NHLBI trial is called Antiarrhythmics Versus Implantable Defibrillators (AVID). The one-year pilot phase began in June 1993 in 20 clinical centers in the United States; it had a recruitment goal of 200 patients. The purpose of the pilot study was to evaluate feasibility, safety, and procedures for a full-scale trial. The full-scale trial recruited patients in about 50 clinical centers in the United States and Canada. The full-scale trial tested the hypothesis that the policy of implanting an ICD in patients who survive cardiac arrest or an episode of sustained VT will improve survival compared with the

The AVID Trial

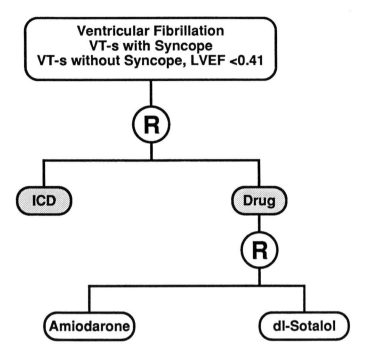

Figure 1. Flow diagram for the Antiarrhythmics Versus Implantable Defibrillators (AVID). The **R** in the circles indicate the points of randomization. The shaded boxes indicate the main comparison for the trial. ICD = implantable cardiac defibrillator; LVEF = left ventricular ejection fraction; VT-s = sustained ventricular tachycardia. Used with permission from Bigger JT Jr.[114]

policy of treatment with amiodarone or dl-sotalol (Figure 1). AVID recruited patients who survived cardiac arrest due to VF or syncope due to documented sustained VT. For these two groups, there was no LVEF criterion to qualify. Patients who had hemo-dynamically compromising sustained VT without syncope were eligible if they had a LVEF <0.41. There were no age restrictions for enrollment. Patients who qualified and lacked exclusions (Table 1) were random-ized with equal probability to ICD treat-ment or drug treatment.

Design Features and Sample Size

AVID was designed as a fixed sample size, randomized clinical trial with group sequential monitoring for safety.[35] Like all of the other ICD trials, AVID was not blinded. Patients who agreed to join the study were randomized with an equal chance of being assigned to ICD or drug therapy. The primary randomization to ICD or drug therapy was stratified on clinical center and primary rhythm disorder (VF versus sustained VT). The primary end-point for the study was all-cause mortality. The primary hypothesis was tested using the intention to treat principle and a Cox regression model. The alpha error was set at 0.05 (2-tailed) and the power between 0.85 and 0.90 to test a 30% difference. The dropin rate (crossover from drug therapy to ICD therapy) was estimated at 20% and the dropout rate at 0%. For the sample size cal-culation, the 2.5-year primary event rate in the group assigned to drug therapy was as-

Table 1
Exclusion Criteria for the AVID Trial Pilot Study

1. Transient or correctable cause of the index arrhythmic event.
2. Index arrhythmic event occurred while on amiodarone.
3. Index event within 7 days of revascularization (CABG or PTCA).
4. CABG surgery performed since index arrhythmic event.
5. Revascularization (CABG or PTCA) is planned and LVEF is >0.40.
6. Inability to undergo thoracotomy or have an ICD implanted.
7. Contraindications to amiodarone.
8. More than 6 weeks of exposure to amiodarone in the last 6 months or maximum plasma level of amiodarone ≥0.2 mcg/mL.
9. Supraventricular arrhythmia requiring antiarrhythmic drug with class I or III action.
10. Less than age of consent.
11. Long QT syndrome.
12. Mechanical device or inotropic drug (excluding digitalis) required for hemodynamic support.
13. NYHA functional class IV (heart failure).
14. On a heart transplant waiting list.
15. Life expectancy <1 year.
16. Chronic serious bacterial infection.
17. Unable to give informed consent.
18. Psychiatric condition likely to limit cooperation.
19. Geographically inaccessible for follow-up.
20. Concurrent use of an investigational antiarrhythmic drug or device.

sumed to be 35% and ICD therapy was assumed to reduce this rate by 30%, i.e., to 24.5%. These parameters yield a sample size of about 1,200 patients, 600 in each group.

Baseline Studies

Clinically indicated baseline tests to define the type and extent of disease and the need for revascularization (CABG surgery or PTCA), e.g., coronary angiography, radionuclide ventriculogram, exercise tests, were done before randomization. Decisions about the use of beta blockers, angiotensin converting enzyme inhibitors, and aspirin therapy also were made before randomiza-

tion. Holter recordings and electrophysiological studies were not required at baseline, but were utilized as needed to establish a diagnosis of the index rhythm or characterize the disease.

Enrollment Cascade

It was anticipated that about half of the patients presenting with malignant ventricular arrhythmias would be eligible for the trial and that about half of the eligible patients would be willing to enroll. A registry was kept of the patients who qualified for randomization to enable a comparison of randomized and nonrandomized patients. A total of 5,915 patients were screened and 4,557 eligible patients were entered into the registry.[36] In April 1997, AVID stopped recruiting patients because survival in the ICD group was found to be significantly better than survival in the drug group. At that time, 1,016 had been randomized, 509 to the drug group and 507 to the ICD group.

Clinical Characteristics of the Randomized Patients at Baseline

The mean age of the 1,016 randomized patients was 65 years; 79% were men, and 87% were Caucasian.[36] Coronary artery disease was the etiologic heart disease in 81% of the patients. Four hundred fifty-five (45%) of the randomized patients qualified with VF and 561 (55%) qualified with symptomatic VT. The qualifying arrhythmia occurred in hospital in 25% of patients and 9% were taking antiarrhythmic drugs at the time of the qualifying arrhythmia. A history of VF was present in 5% and a history of VT was present in 15% of the patients. A history of heart failure was present in 46%, hypertension in 55%, and diabetes in 24% of the patients. CABG surgery or PTCA was performed on 10% of the patients during the hospitalization for the qualifying cardiac arrhythmia. All of these clinical characteristics of the randomized group were similar to those found in the 2,033 patients who were eligible but not enrolled. When AVID started, there was concern that an atypical sample with a low prevalence of VF as the qualifying rhythm would be recruited and result in a low mortality rate and a negative trial.[37-42] This problem did not materialize; the prevalence of VF in the trial was not significantly different from the prevalence overall.

Drug Therapy

Of the 509 patients assigned to drug treatment, 356 went directly to empiric amiodarone and 153 were randomized either to amiodarone or to dl-sotalol (Figure 1).[36] Amiodarone therapy was empiric, but dl-sotalol therapy was guided either by Holter assessment or programmed ventricular stimulation. Patients who were randomized to drug therapy, but could not be assessed by either Holter recordings or electrophysiological studies (<30 ventricular premature complexes per hour and not inducible), were treated empirically with amiodarone. Only 153 patients assigned to the drug arm were randomized: 79 to amiodarone and 74 to dl-sotalol. Only 13 of the 74 patients assigned to dl-sotalol went home on this drug, too few for a comparison of amiodarone and dl-sotalol.

ICD Therapy

AVID used tiered-therapy pulse generators and, whenever possible, transvenous lead systems. When the trial started in June 1993, no ICD systems that included both tiered therapy devices and transvenous leads were marketed. Accordingly, AVID implanted ICD systems under of an Investigational Device Exemption from the Food and Drug Administration. Transvenous leads were used (94%) unless patients were undergoing thoracotomy for revascularization or valvular surgery (4%). The median time from randomization to ICD implantation was 2 days. Before discharge, the final settings were programmed and tested; at least one test of the device against induced

VF was recommended. For patients who qualified with sustained VT, antitachycardia pacing was programmed and tested. The median time from randomization to discharge was 6 days in the ICD group and 7 days in the amiodarone group.

Drug Therapy

Patients assigned to the drug limb were randomized to start dl-sotalol or amiodarone first. Patients assigned to amiodarone were not required to have electrophysiological or Holter assessment. Loading doses of 800–1,600 mg/day of amiodarone were given for 1–3 weeks; it was recommended that a loading dose of 10 gm be achieved before discharge. The median loading dose was 8,800 mg and the median number of days for in-hospital amiodarone loading was 7 days.[36] After loading, doses of 400–800 mg/day were given for 4 weeks. Thereafter, a maintenance dose was given, usually 400 mg/day; the minimum acceptable maintenance dose was 200 mg, 5 days a week. Most patients assigned to amiodarone treatment continued to take the drug long term, 88% at 1 year and 87% at 2 years. The average daily maintenance dose tended to decrease with follow-up time, 390 ± 99 mg at discharge, 330 ± 96 mg at 1 year, and 288 ± 95 mg at 2 years.

dl-Sotalol was started at a dose of 80 mg twice a day. The dose was advanced every 2–3 days to a maximum of 320 mg twice a day. The median number of days for in-hospital loading and testing for dl-sotalol was 6 days; the median dose at discharge was 320 mg per day. dl-Sotalol therapy was guided by Holter recordings or electrophysiological studies, at the investigator's choice. Efficacy by Holter required a ≥75% suppression of ventricular premature complexes and >90% suppression of couplets and unsustained VT. To be evaluated with electrophysiological studies, patients with sustained VT as their qualifying clinical event had to have inducible sustained (uniform) VT. Patients with VF as their clinical event had to have inducible sustained (uniform or multiform) VT, sustained ventricular flutter, or sustained VF. Drug success was defined as inability to induce >15 complexes of unsustained VT. If the first drug tried was not effective or not tolerated, the patient could be crossed over to the other, i.e., dl-sotalol to amiodarone or vice versa. If neither drug was predicted effective and tolerated, investigators were permitted to choose another antiarrhythmic regimen.

Crossovers

AVID recommended that arrhythmias that occurred after ICD implantation be managed by ICD reprogramming alone; addition of antiarrhythmic drug therapy was discouraged. During follow-up, patients who experienced nonfatal cardiac arrest or a recurrence of sustained VT in the drug limb were managed using conventional standards of care. However, investigators were asked to consider whether the patient could be managed by increasing drug doses, changing the drug, or by adding a drug. In fact, by 2 years of follow-up, 20% of the patients assigned to antiarrhythmic drug therapy had had an ICD implanted and 33% of the patients assigned to ICD therapy were taking amiodarone.[36]

Effects of Treatment on Survival

The primary endpoint for AVID was death of any cause. At the time when the main results were reported, the average follow-up was 18 months. Overall survival was 86% at 1 year, 79% at 2 years, and 71% at 3 years.[36] Figure 2 shows that the ICD group had significantly better survival throughout the study. Survival in the ICD group was 89.3% at 1 year, 81.6% at 2 years, and 75.4% at 3 years compared with 82.3%, 75.1%, and 64.7% in the drug (amiodarone) arm. These survival figures represent an unadjusted decrease in mortality rates of 38%, 26%, and 30% and approximately $2\frac{1}{2}$ months prolongation of life. Cause-specific

death will be classified using the CAST definitions,[43,44] but at the time of this report, these data were not yet available. AVID identified a small number of subgroups of interest before the study began: age (<60, 60–69, ≥70), LVEF (≤0.35, >0.35), cardiac diagnosis (coronary heart disease vs other), and qualifying arrhythmia (VF or VT). There was no evidence of interaction between these subgroups and treatment effect, although the power to detect interactions is relatively low because the trial was stopped almost 17 months early. Several variables were significantly different between the treatment groups in a way that gave the ICD group a survival advantage: severity of congestive heart failure, history of atrial fibrillation, LVEF, beta blocker use, and the PR interval. However, multivariate analyses indicated that these differences did not account for the lower mortality rate in the AVID ICD group during follow-up.

What Will We Learn from Trials that Compare ICD and Drug Therapy?

AVID is the first study to show that ICD therapy prolongs life significantly more than empirical amiodarone treatment in patients who have hemodynamically important, symptomatic sustained VT. CIDS, CASH, and AVID can not estimate accurately the magnitude of ICD benefit because each had a positive control group, i.e., ICD treatment was compared to drug therapy. A difference in favor of ICD treatment could indicate a substantial benefit of ICD therapy or a modest ICD benefit combined with a harmful effect of amiodarone. This result is unlikely because in randomized comparisons with placebo, amiodarone shows a trend toward benefit, not harm.[45–54] A difference in favor of amiodarone could occur because of benefits unrelated to an antiarrhythmic action, e.g., an anti-ischemic action or a vasodilator action. The advantage of ICD treatment over propafenone found in the CASH could represent little or no benefit from ICD treatment combined with

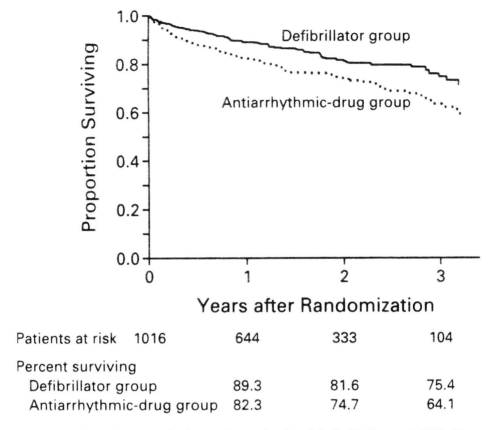

Figure 2. Survival in the Antiarrhythmics Versus Implantable Defibrillators (AVID). The group assigned to ICD therapy showed better overall survival than the group assigned to empirical amiodarone. Used with permission from the Antiarrhythmics Versus Implantable Defibrillators (AVID) Investigators.[36]

substantial harm from propafenone. It would not be surprising if propafenone doubled the all-cause mortality rate in patients with malignant ventricular arrhythmias since this was the magnitude of the adverse effect on mortality seen with encainide and flecainide in the CAST. Alternatively, there could be modest benefit in the ICD group and modest harm in the propafenone group. It should be recognized that antiarrhythmic drug treatment is mostly empiric in all three of these trials so they will not answer how well electrophysiologically guided antiarrhythmic drug therapy would compare with ICD therapy. Nevertheless, AVID indicates, for the first time, that ICD therapy affords significantly greater survival benefit than amiodarone

therapy for patients who have survived cardiac arrest or symptomatic sustained VT and has few adverse effects. Also, a comparison of patients randomized and those eligible but not randomized indicate that the patients recruited for AVID are quite similar to patients treated in clinical practice. AVID is likely to cause a large increment in the use of ICD therapy because physicians who preferred amiodarone therapy to ICD therapy are likely to switch and recommend ICD therapy instead.

Dutch ICD Cost-Effectiveness Study

The Dutch ICD cost-effectiveness study was sponsored by Guidant/CPI and was conducted at the University Hospitals of Utrecht and Groningen.[55,56] Between April 1989 and April 1993, 60 patients <75 years of age with coronary heart disease, previous myocardial infarction, and cardiac arrest were recruited. Patients who were eligible and had no exclusion criteria were randomized to immediate treatment with an ICD or to tiered therapy beginning with electrophysiologically guided antiarrhythmic drug therapy. Follow-up ended for all patients on January 1, 1994. The main finding of this study was that immediate ICD implantation was more cost-effective than electrophysiologically guided arrhythmia control.[57]

Baseline Studies

Baseline studies used to characterize the patients included Holter recording, exercise test, nuclear scintigraphy, coronary angiography, left ventriculography, and electrophysiological study. Programmed stimulation included two basic stimulation rates, two sites for stimulation, and up to three premature stimuli.

Enrollment Cascade

To be eligible for the study, patients had to have a cardiac arrest, be resuscitated and expected to survive, and be less than 75 years of age. Patients had to have a previous myocardial infarction to be eligible for the study and the infarct had to occur at least 4 weeks before recruitment. To participate, patients had to be subject to drug therapy and had to have inducible VT so that drug therapy could be evaluated by programmed ventricular stimulation. Sixty patients were randomized, 54 men and six women, average age 58 years; 51 presented with ventricular fibrillation and nine with rapid VT and syncope.[56,57] Their New York Heart Association classification was: I, 39; II, 20; III, 1; and IV, 0. The average LVEF was 0.30. After the baseline studies, 29 patients were randomized to receive an ICD implant immediately and 31 patients were randomized to

electrophysiologically guided tiered therapy which always started with antiarrhythmic drugs.

Design Features and Sample Size

The hypothesis being tested was: immediate treatment with ICD is more cost-effective than the conventional electrophysiologically guided therapy that was prevalent at the time the study was done. The investigators thought that 60 patients who survived cardiac arrest randomized 50 : 50 to immediate treatment with ICD or electrophysiologically guided tiered therapy would provide adequate power to detect a meaningful difference in cost-effectiveness. To increase the comparability of the groups, randomization was stratified on the number of normal kinetic segments in a quantitative analysis of the left ventricular cineangiogram, <4 versus 4–9 segments.[56] It was recognized that this small number of participants would not provide much power to detect a difference in the two arms of the study with respect to death or arrhythmia recurrence.

ICD Therapy

The 29 patients who were randomized to ICD therapy were scheduled immediately for ICD implantation, but there was an average delay of 12 days between randomization and implantation. All but three patients had epicardial ICD systems implanted by thoracotomy using CPI Ventak P pulse generators. There were two operative deaths and 27 patients were discharged alive with working ICD systems. The median initial hospital stay was 25 days.

Electrophysiologically Guided (Tiered) Therapy

All 31 patients in the tiered therapy group had at least one antiarrhythmic drug trial. The number of drug trials ranged from 1 to 5 per patient and averaged 2.2. Nine patients were judged to have a drug success and two died during drug trials before programmed ventricular stimulation was done to evaluate efficacy. Twenty patients were judged to be drug failures after a series of drug trials. Six of the 20 patients who failed drug therapy had electrophysiologically guided arrhythmia surgery and 14 had an ICD system implanted. There was one operative death after arrhythmia surgery and another patient had an ICD system implanted to treat an arrhythmia recurrence after arrhythmia surgery. Twenty-seven of the 31 patients randomized to tiered therapy were discharged alive: eight on antiarrhythmic drugs only, four who had arrhythmia surgery (two of these were on antiarrhythmic drugs), and 15 who had ICD systems. The median initial hospital stay was 38 days.

Events During Follow-Up

During an average follow-up of 27 months, 62% of the patients randomized to immediate ICD therapy had ICD shocks and eight (28%) were given antiarrhythmic drugs to decrease the frequency of ICD shocks.[56] There were four deaths (14%) in the ICD therapy group (two in hospital and two during follow-up). In the group randomized to tiered therapy, one additional ICD was implanted after cardiac arrest occurred during follow-up; this made a total of 16 (52%) ICDs implanted in the tiered therapy group. In the tiered therapy group, 63% of the patients had an ICD shock and 25% were given antiarrhythmic drugs to decrease the frequency of ICD shocks. There were 11 (35%) deaths in the tiered therapy group (four in hospital and seven during follow-up). The median number of days in hospital during 2 years of follow-up was 34 days for the first-choice ICD group and 49 days for the tiered therapy group.

What Did We Learn from the Dutch ICD Cost-Effectiveness Study?

The Dutch ICD cost-effectiveness study found that ICD therapy was significantly more cost-effective than electrophysiologically guided tiered therapy (drugs-surgery-ICD) even though epicardial ICD systems with ~3.5 year longevity were used.[57] This was the first prospective, randomized cost-effectiveness study, but it generally confirmed the conclusions of previous retrospective studies.[58–60] The results are strictly applicable to cardiac arrest patients and to the therapies that were evaluated. The study was too small to generalize. The difference in favor of immediate ICD therapy is likely to be larger with transvenous lead systems and pulse generators that last almost 7 years. Several ongoing studies have cost-effectiveness substudies and should extend the findings of the Dutch ICD cost-effectiveness study.[35,61,62] Different strategies for screening and for application of ICD and comparative therapies will significantly influence cost-effectiveness. Half of the patients randomized to tiered therapy ultimately had an ICD implant. It is notable that the mortality rate in the group assigned to immediate ICD implant was less than half that of the tiered therapy group. The Dutch ICD cost-effectiveness study was much too small to have an important mortality result, but it is interesting that the mortality advantage for cardiac arrest patients in the Dutch ICD cost-effectiveness study is very similar to the reduction in mortality found in MADIT, which studied ICD prophylaxis in high-risk coronary heart disease patients.

Randomized, Controlled Clinical Trials of ICD Prophylaxis

In the early 1990s, three studies began to evaluate prophylactic use of ICD therapy. The Multicenter UnSustained Tachycardia Trial (MUSTT) aims to determine whether electrophysiologically guided treatment, including drugs and ICD, will improve survival without arrhythmic events.[63] The Multicenter Automatic Defibrillator Implantation Trial (MADIT) compared ICD prophylaxis with conventional treatment for patients who had left ventricular dysfunction and unsustained VT.[11,61] The Coronary Artery Bypass Graft (CABG) Patch Trial compared ICD therapy with no therapy for high-risk patients undergoing CABG surgery.[62] In addition to these, there are three ICD trials being planned for patients with heart failure and ventricular arrhythmias—the CArdiomyopathy Trial (CAT), SCD-HeFT, and MADIT II.

The Rationale for Prophylactic Treatment of Patients with Unsustained VT

Two of the trials we will discuss, MUSTT and MADIT, are evaluating ICD prophylaxis for coronary heart disease patients who have left ventricular dysfunction and unsustained VT. Unsustained VT is an excellent univariate predictor of death in coronary heart disease and, combined with LVEF <0.40, has a positive predictive accuracy of about 40%.[63–66]

Inducible Ventricular Arrhythmias and Arrhythmic Events in Patients with Unsustained VT

A number of studies have been done to determine whether programmed ventricular stimulation can stratify the risk of patients with coronary heart disease and unsustained VT. Kowey et al. reported an overview of 12 studies that published results of programmed ventricular stimulation in patients with coronary heart disease and unsustained VT and also reported arrhythmic events during follow-up.[67] The number of patients in the 12 studies totaled 926; their mean age was 61 years, 80% were male, 88% had coronary heart disease, and 72% had previous myocardial infarction. One-third (n = 302) of the patients had sustained ventricular arrhythmias induced by programmed ventricular stimulation. The studies that limited programmed ventricular stimulation to patients with LVEF <0.40 had higher percentages of positive tests, approximately 45%. During an average follow-up of 19 months, 100 arrhythmic events occurred: 60 sudden cardiac deaths, 39 episodes of spontaneous, sustained VT, and one episode of syncope attributed to VT. The arrhythmic event rate was 17.9% for inducible patients and 7.4% for noninducible patients, a relative risk of 2.4; 251 (83%) of the inducible patients were treated with antiarrhythmic drugs even when no drug was predicted to be effective by electrophysiological studies. The frequent use of antiarrhythmic drugs makes it impossible to determine the natural history of unsustained VT. During follow-up, arrhythmic events were common in the inducible patients despite or because of the high prevalence of antiarrhythmic drug use in this group. The characteristics of programmed ventricular stimulation as a test to predict risk were: sensitivity, 54%; specificity, 70%; positive predictive accuracy, 18%; and negative predictive accuracy, 93%. Taken together, these studies show that programmed ventricular stimulation has considerable merit to identify patients at low risk to arrhythmic events during follow-up and, to a lesser extent, to identify the patients at high risk.

The Predictive Value of Inducible VT for Arrhythmic Events

Overall, uncontrolled data from the pooled studies do not suggest that programmed ventricular stimulation predicts long-term arrhythmic drug efficacy in patients with spontaneous unsustained VT and inducible sustained VT.[67] The study by Wilber et al. is the only one that suggested that programmed ventricular stimulation has merit for evaluating drug therapy.[68,69] In this study, 100 patients with coronary heart disease, LVEF <0.40, and unsustained VT were evaluated with programmed ventricular stimulation. In 57 patients, no sustained ventricular arrhythmia was induced;

these were discharged on no therapy. Forty of the remainder had serial drug evaluation using programmed ventricular stimulation; 20 were suppressed (i.e., not inducible) on a drug and were discharged on the drug predicted to be efficacious. Twenty were not suppressed but were discharged on a drug that increased the cycle length of the induced VT by ≥100 ms and made the tachycardia hemodynamically well tolerated. Sudden death or cardiac arrest, during an average of 16.7 months of follow-up, were the endpoints of the study. The 2-year actuarial rates of sudden death or cardiac arrest for the three groups were: not inducible, 6%; inducible but suppressed, 11%; and inducible but not suppressed, 50%. From this initial experience, Wilber et al. found that only 50% of patients with left ventricular dysfunction and inducible sustained VT responded to drug therapy and that partial responders remained at high risk.[68] In 1991, the authors updated their results after 32.1 months average follow-up.[69] The 2-year actuarial rates of arrhythmic events were: not inducible, 6%; inducible but suppressed, 28%; and inducible but not suppressed, 50%. The authors concluded that electrophysiologically guided antiarrhythmic drug treatment had limited utility in this population whether or not induced arrhythmias are suppressed.[69] This study suggested that electrophysiological testing is excellent for predicting risk, but has limited value for predicting drug efficacy in patients who have unsustained VT.

At this time, there is no clear indication that antiarrhythmic drug therapy guided by results of programmed ventricular stimulation should be used in patients with left ventricular dysfunction and unsustained VT. However, the high risk of this group for arrhythmic events makes it a prime target for studies aimed at preventing lethal or morbid outcomes. The poor prognosis of patients with unsustained VT also provides a rationale for randomized controlled trials to evaluate treatment effects on survival.

The Multicenter Unsustained Tachycardia Trial (MUSTT)

MUSTT will test the hypothesis that electrophysiologically guided antiarrhythmic therapy will reduce the risk of arrhythmic death or cardiac arrest in patients with unsustained VT and left ventricular dysfunction (see Table 2).[63] MUSTT started in October 1991 with 25 clinical centers in North America participating; recruitment ended on October 31, 1996 with 704 patients randomized. Follow-up of patients is expected to end in the fall of 1998. MUSTT enrolled patients with coronary heart disease and age <80 years, LVEF <0.41, and asymptomatic, or minimally symptomatic, unsustained VT. Patients who qualified and lacked exclusions (see Table 3) were offered an electrophysiological study. If sustained ventricular arrhythmias were induced by programmed ventricular stimulation, patients were randomized to no antiarrhythmic treatment or to electrophysiologically guided antiarrhythmic treatment (see Figure 3).

Baseline Studies

When it began, MUSTT excluded patients who had myocardial infarction within 4 weeks of enrollment. This interval was changed to 4 days during the second year of enrollment. Patients who were anticipated to need CABG surgery or angioplasty were excluded. Patients had to have LVEF quantified within 1 year of enrollment by left ventriculogram, radionuclide angiography, or echocardiogram. Unsustained VT (duration, three complexes to 30 sec, rate, ≥100/min) had to be documented electrocardiographically and had to be associated with no symptoms or minimal symptoms. A signal-averaged ECG was obtained to determine its prognostic value. A baseline electrophysiological study was done to identify eligible patients. Patients who had sustained, uniform VT with a cycle length

Table 2

Design Features of ICD Prophylaxis Trials in Patients with Coronary Heart Disease

	MUSTT	MADIT	CABG Patch II
Design	Fixed sample size	Sequential	Fixed sample size
Stratification variable(s)	Center	Center	Center
		Time after MI	LV ejection fraction
Eligibility criteria	Coronary heart disease	Q-wave MI	CABG surgery
	Age <80	Age <75	Age <80
	LVEF <0.41	LVEF <0.36	LVEF <0.36
	Unsustained VT	Unsustained VT	Abnormal SAECG
	Inducible VT	Inducible VT	
Primary Endpoint	Sudden death, cardiac arrest	Death of any cause	Death of any cause
Minimum follow-up (mo)	24	—	24
Average follow-up (mo)	36	26	40
Event Rate			
Control group	15% (24 mo)	30% (26 mo)	>30% (40 mo)
Assumed reduction	33%	46%	26%
Alpha	5%	5%	5%
Power (1-beta)	80%	85%	85%
Drop-in rate	not estimated	<5%	11%
Dropout rate	not estimated	<5%	6%
Sample size (each group)	450	140	400

VT = ventricular tachycardia.

Table 3

Exclusion Criteria for the Multicenter
Unsustained Tachycardia Trial

1. Previous syncope, sustained ventricular tachycardia or fibrillation.
2. Unsustained ventricular tachycardia due to long QT syndrome, acute ischemia, acute metabolic disorder, or drug toxicity.
3. Unsustained ventricular tachycardia symptomatic enough to need treatment.
4. CABG surgery or coronary angioplasty in the previous month.
5. Myocardial infarction in the previous month.
5. Left ventricular ejection fraction >0.40.
6. Patients likely to undergo CABG or valve surgery during the study.
7. History of noncompliance.
8. Patients with uncontrolled congestive heart failure.
9. Patients who have received amiodarone in previous 6 months.
10. Noncardiac disease with likelihood of <2 years survival.
11. Patients who live too far for follow-up visits.

>220 ms induced by ≤3 premature stimuli or sustained, multiform VT or VF induced by ≤2 premature stimuli were eligible to be randomized to antiarrhythmic therapy or no therapy. Patients who had VT with a cycle length ≤220 ms or who have VF induced with triple premature stimuli did not qualify.

Enrollment Cascade

When planning MUSTT, it was assumed that about half of the qualified patients would agree to have an electrophysiological study, about 40% would be inducible, and about 50% of the inducible patients would agree to be randomized. A 70% success rate (VT not inducible or slowed) was expected for those randomized to electrophysiologically guided antiarrhythmic therapy and the 30% with drug failures were expected to be treated with ICDs. Between October 1991 and October 31, 1996, more than 2,203 patients were enrolled into MUSTT and 765 (35%) had inducible ventricular arrhyth-

MUSTT

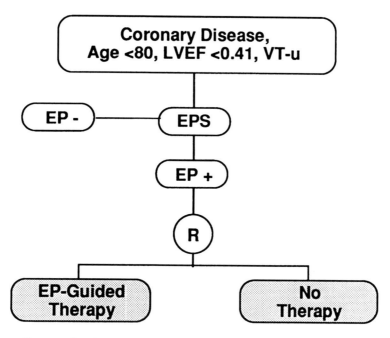

Figure 3. Flow diagram for the Multicenter Unsustained Tachycardia Trial. The **R** in the circle indicates the point of randomization. The shaded boxes indicate the main comparison for the trial. EPS = electrophysiologic study, LVEF = left ventricular ejection fraction, VT-u = unsustained ventricular tachycardia. Used with permission from Bigger JT Jr.[115]

mias that qualified them for randomization[64,65]; half of the qualifying ventricular arrhythmias were induced with three premature stimuli. Of the eligible patients, 704 (about 90%) were randomized. More than 90% of the randomized patients were male and their average LVEF was 0.29. About half of the patients randomized to electrophysiologically guided antiarrhythmic therapy ultimately had ICD implants.

Design Features and Sample Size

MUSTT was designed as a fixed sample size randomized clinical trial with group sequential monitoring for safety. Qualified patients who had inducible, sustained ventricular arrhythmias were randomized 50:50 to be followed 2–5 years without any antiarrhythmic treatment or to be followed on antiarrhythmic treatment guided by the results of electrophysiological studies. Randomization was stratified only by clinical center. The primary endpoint for the study is arrhythmic death and nonfatal cardiac arrest (causing loss of consciousness and requiring cardioversion). The primary hypothesis will be tested using the intention to treat principle. The alpha error (i.e., chance of declaring a significant difference when none exists) is set at 0.05 (two-sided) and the power (the chance of finding a difference when there is one) is about 0.80. No specific estimates were made of the dropin and dropout rates but, given the primary endpoint being used, these rates are likely to be small and accounted for in the conservative estimates of sample size. For the sample size calculation, the 2-year primary event rate was assumed to be 15% and treatment was assumed to reduce this rate by

Table 4
Drugs Used in The Multicenter Unsustained Tachycardia Trial

Drug	Recommended Dose	Target Plasma Concentration
Procainamide	—	8–10 μg/mL
Quinidine	—	3.5–5 μg/mL
Disopyramide	—	3.5 μg/mL
Mexiletine	150–200 mg q 8 h	—
Propafenone	200–300 mg TID	—
Acebutalol	200 mg BID for 2 days, 400 mg BID if tolerated	—
Amiodarone	1,000–2,000 mg/day for 1 week, 400 mg/day maintenance	—

33%, i.e., to 10%. Using these parameters, the sample size was calculated to be 814 patients. If all else were equal, but the 2-year primary event rate were 25%, the total sample size required would be only 460.

Antiarrhythmic Drug Therapy in MUSTT

Seven antiarrhythmic drugs are authorized for use in MUSTT (see Table 4). The sequence of drug therapy is governed by a strategy of rounds. In Round A, any tolerated drug with class IA action can be given or, alternatively, the drug with class IC action, propafenone, can be given. If Round A is unsuccessful, patients continue to Round B. At least two drug trials must be attempted before amiodarone is given. After three or more unsuccessful drug trials, an ICD can be implanted. Drug efficacy is evaluated with programmed ventricular stimulation. To declare a drug successful, the stimulation protocol, including triple premature stimuli, must be completed with <15 consecutive VPC being induced.

What Will We Learn from MUSTT?

MUSTT should tell us whether patients with unsustained VT and reduced LVEF are significantly benefited by prophylactic antiarrhythmic treatment guided by electrophysiological studies. MUSTT will not give a definitive answer about which drugs are more efficacious, better tolerated, or safer, although we may see helpful trends. The chance of finding significant benefit for electrophysiologically guided therapy will be reduced by patients in the treatment group who refused ICD implantation when no effective drug was found. Early experience showed that about half of the patients refused epicardial ICD systems. A much larger percentage accepted transvenous systems. Almost half of the patients randomized to electrophysiologically guided antiarrhythmic therapy ultimately were treated with ICDs, a percentage very similar to that found in the Dutch cost-effectiveness study. We won't be able to estimate definitively the benefit of ICD therapy relative to no treatment or to drug treatment, but trends should suggest relative efficacy and safety for ICD therapy. For example, ICD therapy is likely to be used in the sickest patients, i.e., those not responding to drugs. If patients treated with ICD therapy survive better than drug-treated patients, we can infer that ICD therapy is more effective since the comparison is biased against ICD therapy. From MUSTT, we should learn how good electrophysiological testing is for assessing risk and, for the first time, be able to compare the outcome of noninducible and inducible patients without the confounding effects of antiarrhythmic drug treatment. This comparison will help to interpret the results of The CABG Patch Trial. We should learn how the results of electrophysiological studies correlate with signal-averaged ECG results and determine the relative predictive accuracy of these two tests for arrhythmic events. These data should suggest how the two tests should be used to stratify the risk of patients with left ventricular dysfunction and unsustained VT. Together with MADIT, MUSTT should substantially advance our knowledge of how to evaluate and treat patients with decreased LVEF and unsustained VT.

The Multicenter Automatic Defibrillator Implantation Trial (MADIT)

MADIT tested the hypothesis that implantation of an ICD in high-risk coronary heart disease patients will result in a significant reduction in all-cause mortality when compared to "conventional therapy" using a sequential design (see Table 2).[11,61] MADIT began enrolling in the fall of 1990 in 24 hospitals in the United States and Europe. MADIT-enrolled patients who had a Q wave myocardial infarction, were <75 years of age, had a LVEF <0.36, and had asymptomatic, unsustained VT (3 to 30 consecutive complexes, rate ≥120/min).[61] Patients who qualified and who lacked exclusions (see Table 5) had an electro-

---

Table 5
Exclusion Criteria for The Multicenter Automatic Defibrillator Implantation Trial

1. Previous cardiac arrest or syncopal ventricular tachycardia.
2. New York Heart Association functional class IV.
3. CABG surgery or coronary angioplasty in the previous 6 months.
4. Myocardial infarction in the previous month.
5. Left ventricular ejection fraction >0.35.
6. Patients likely to undergo CABG surgery during the study.
7. Patients with severe cerebral vascular disease.
8. Women with childbearing potential.
9. Noncardiac disease with likelihood of <2 years survival.
10. Patients participating in other clinical trials.
11. Patients who live too far for follow-up visits.
12. Patients unwilling or unable to cooperate with the study.

---

physiological study. Patients who had sustained, inducible ventricular arrhythmias that did not respond to an intravenous procainamide infusion and who consented were randomized to conventional pharmacological therapy or to ICD implantation (see Figure 4).

Baseline Studies

The qualifying Q wave myocardial infarction had to occur ≥4 weeks prior to enrollment. Unsustained VT was documented by 12-lead ECG, telemetry, Holter recording, or an exercise ECG. The VT had to be associated with no or minimal symptoms. LVEF had to be <0.36 and the patient had to be in New York Heart Association functional classes I-III.[61] Patients were not eligible for MADIT if they were candidates for CABG surgery. The electrophysiological study to determine whether patients were inducible used two pacing cycle lengths, 600 and 400 ms, and three premature stimuli. To qualify for MADIT, patients had to be inducible, i.e., uniform VT with a cycle length ≥230 ms, multiform VT, or VF had to be induced. The induced ventricular arrhythmia had to be reproducible, i.e., induced at least twice. Inducible patients were given a loading dose of 15 mg/kg of procainamide intravenously at a rate of 50 mg/min, and then given a maintenance infusion of 4 mg/min. Programmed ventricular stimulation was repeated and patients who remained inducible during procainamide infusion were eligible.[70,71]

Enrollment Cascade

When planning MADIT, it was expected that about half of the patients who qualified would agree to have an electrophysiological study, 40% would be inducible, and 80% of these would not be suppressed by intravenous procainamide infusion.[61] About 50% of the patients who were fully eligible were expected to consent to be randomized.

MADIT

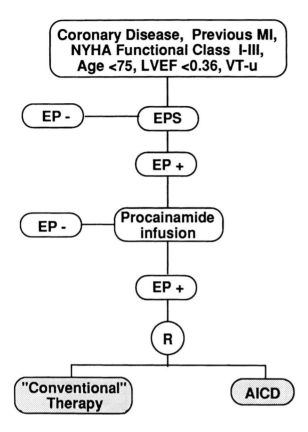

Figure 4. Flow diagram for Multicenter Automatic Defibrillator Implantation Trial (MADIT). The **R** in the circle indicates the point of randomization. The shaded boxes indicate the main comparison for the trial. EPS = electrophysiologic study; LVEF = left ventricular ejection fraction; NYHA = New York Heart Association; MI = myocardial infarction; VT-u = unsustained ventricular tachycardia. Used with permission from Bigger JT Jr.[115]

A total of 253 patients qualified for the study and 196 (78%) of them gave informed consent for enrollment.[11] A few of the MADIT clinical centers followed 85 patients who were eligible except for a negative electrophysiological study and compared them with the 101 patients randomized to the conventional therapy group. The mortality rate for the patients with inducible sustained VT was four times that of a group of patients who were identical except for not being inducible (32% vs. 8%).[72] Of the 196 patients, 95 were randomized to the ICD group and 101 to the conventional therapy group; 48 patients were assigned to transthoracic ICDs implants and 47 were assigned to transvenous implants. Five patients assigned to the ICD group never had an ICD implanted. Only lead systems and pulse generators that were manufactured by Cardiac Pacemakers, Inc. and approved by the U.S. Food and Drug Administration were implanted. Monophasic defibrillating waveforms were provided by 79 pulse generators and biphasic waveforms by 11.

Design Features and Sample Size

Randomization in MADIT was stratified by clinical center and the interval between the most recent myocardial infarction and randomization (<6 months vs. ≥6 months). The primary hypothesis was tested using the intention to treat principle. The primary endpoint for the study was all-cause mortality. To calculate the sample size for MADIT, the 2-year cumulative mortality rate was assumed to be 30% in the control group (20% arrhythmic death and 10% nonarrhythmic death) and ICD treatment was assumed to reduce this rate by 46%, i.e., to 16.3% (4.4% arrhythmic death, 10.4% nonarrhythmic death, and 1.5% operative mortality associated with ICD implantation). The alpha error was set at 0.05 (two-sided) and the power at 0.85. The dropin and dropout rates were estimated to be less than 5%. Using these parameters, it was calculated that about 280 patients would be randomized, 140 in each group. MADIT had a sequential design (rarely used in cardiovascular medicine), and the endpoints were examined monthly. MADIT planned to stop recruiting when the difference in all-cause mortality between the two groups crossed a boundary indicating that the ICD group was significantly better than conventional therapy or a boundary indicating that the trial was unlikely to show benefit for ICD treatment.

Treatment in the Control Group

Patients randomized to the control group were treated with "conventional therapy"; 81% of the patients in the control group were treated with amiodarone (74%) or dl-sotalol (7%) compared with 3% in the ICD group. Beta blocking drugs were given to 15% of the control group compared with 27% in the ICD group.

ICD Therapy Significantly Better than Conventional Therapy

On March 25, 1996, MADIT was stopped because the boundary for ICD benefit had been crossed after an average of 27 months of follow-up. The two groups formed by randomization were remarkably well matched for relevant variables considering the small size for this trial. The crude mortality rates were 39/101 (38.6%) for the conventional therapy group and 15/95 (15.8%) for the ICD group. The Kaplan-Meier survival curves for MADIT are shown in Figure 5. The hazard ratio from the Cox regression analysis was 0.46 with a 95% confidence interval of 0.26 to 0.82. Thus, the point estimate for mortality reduction at 27-months was 54% with a 95% confidence interval of 18% to 74%. Additional Cox regression analyses did not show any evidence that antiarrhythmic therapy (mostly amiodarone or dl-sotalol) had any meaningful influence on the hazard ratio. No difference in benefit was seen between ICDs implanted by thoracotomy or transvenously. Also, no significant difference in benefit was seen among the clinical centers. Because ICD benefit was so striking, patients in the conventional therapy group were offered ICD therapy when the results were announced.

What Did We Learn from MADIT?

In March 1996, with 196 patients randomized, MADIT was stopped because the ICD group had a significantly better survival than the conventional therapy group; a 54% decrease in mortality in the ICD group compared with conventional therapy ($P < 0.01$). MADIT is the first randomized trial to demonstrate that ICD prophylaxis is better than drug therapy for primary prevention of sudden cardiac death. Some of the apparent benefit of ICD therapy may be due to advantages the ICD group had for antiarrhythmic drug or beta-blocker treatment. Also sequential trials can overestimate the magnitude of treatment effect because chance is likely to contribute to a boundary crossing. Even though the ICD benefit may not be as large as the observed 54%, it is likely that the benefit is large, e.g., near the maximum possible benefit of 33% estimated by Yusuf and Connolly. Based on the MADIT results, the FDA quickly gave a new indication for prophylactic ICD implantation.

We now have to judge how to apply the results of MADIT to clinical practice. I recommend that patients like those who were enrolled in MADIT be screened and, if qualified, treated with ICD implantation. Can we simplify the screening process to make

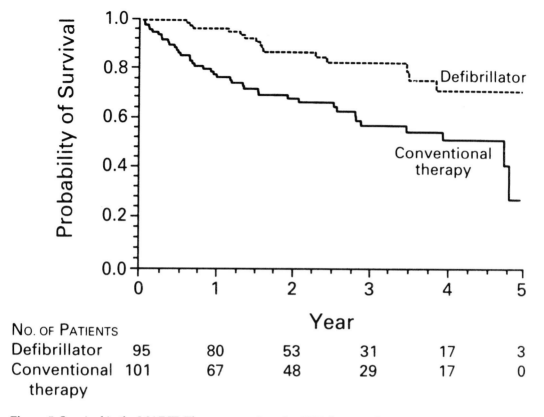

Figure 5. Survival in the MADIT. The group assigned to ICD therapy showed better overall survival than the group assigned to conventional antiarrhythmic drug therapy. Used with permission from Moss AJ, et al.[11]

it less complex and less expensive? The screening procedures to qualify patients for MADIT were complex and expensive. Attempts to simplify screening should be carefully evaluated in controlled studies. Since >90% of patients still had inducible VT during the procainamide infusion, I conclude that this portion of the MADIT electrophysiological protocol is unnecessary. Given the similarities of the patient population in MADIT and The CABG Patch Trial, but the strikingly different reduction in mortality, the results of MADIT should not be extrapolated to other groups.

Cost-effectiveness and quality of life studies are forthcoming from the MADIT data set and will be helpful in making decisions about screening and treating patients with low LVEF and unsustained VT. Because ICD therapy was so effective in

MADIT, it was more cost effective than it was in AVID.

The CABG Patch Trial

The CABG Patch Trial tested the hypothesis that implantation of an ICD in patients with coronary heart disease, left ventricular dysfunction, and an abnormal signal-averaged ECG will reduce the risk of death from all causes.[62] In September 1990, The CABG Patch Trial started a pilot study in five North American clinical centers. In January 1992, enrollment was extended to 13 hospitals in North America and Europe and, in March 1993, The CABG Patch Trial became a cooperative study with the National Heart, Lung, and Blood Institute and enrollment was extended to 37 clinical centers.

Table 6
Exclusion Criteria for The CABG Patch Trial

1. History of sustained VT, VF, or cardiac arrest with inducible VT.
2. Renal dysfunction (creatinine >3 mg/dL).
3. Insulin-dependent diabetes mellitus with significant vascular complications or history of poor control and recurrent infections.
4. Unipolar pacemakers.
5. Previous or concomitant aortic or mitral valve surgery.
6. Concomitant cerebrovascular surgery.
7. Emergency CABG surgery.
8. Thrombolysis in the 2 days prior to CABG surgery.
9. Concomitant arrhythmia surgery or aneurysmectomy.
10. Co-morbidity associated with expected survival <2 years.
11. Lives too far away to return for follow-up visits.
12. Inadequate time to obtain informed consent.
13. Enrolled in another randomized controlled clinical trial.
14. Physician, surgeon, or patient refusal.

The CABG Patch Trial enrolled patients with coronary heart disease who were having elective CABG surgery, were <80 years of age, had a LVEF <0.36, and had an abnormal signal-averaged ECG. Patients with these qualifying characteristics, who lacked exclusions (see Table 6), and signed consent were randomized to ICD therapy or to a control group that received no therapy in addition to their routine CABG surgery (see Figure 6). Randomization of a 900 patient sample ended in February 1996.

The Rationale for Prophylactic ICD Treatment for High Risk CABG Surgery Patients

The planning effort that led to the CABG Patch Trial began in 1988. The planning group realized that there were serious scientific problems with conducting a randomized controlled trial of ICD prophylaxis using a transthoracic approach for implantation of epicardial patch leads. Greater use of diagnostic coronary angiography and revascularization procedures were almost certain to occur in patients randomized to receive ICD therapy and would confound the interpretation of results: benefit due to ICD therapy could not be distinguished from benefit due to revascularization. To avoid confounding, patients at high risk for arrhythmic death who were having CABG surgery were selected for study. Thus, all patients in the experiment were revascularized to avoid confounding by differences in frequency of revascularization in the randomized groups.

Rationale for Policy on Antiarrhythmic Drugs

Aside from beta blockers,[73–76] no antiarrhythmic drug therapy could be recommended. To the contrary, most clinical trials suggested that antiarrhythmic drugs with class I action had a substantial harmful effect and that drugs with class III action have some benefit.[77–86] Therefore, a substantial difference in antiarrhythmic drug use in the two arms of the trial could confound the primary results. The CABG Patch Trial adopted a policy of no treatment of unsustained VT with either class I or class III antiarrhythmic drugs.

High Long-Term Mortality Rates after CABG Surgery in Patients Who Have Left Ventricular Dysfunction

Patients with two- or three-vessel coronary artery disease and reduced LVEF show better long-term survival with surgical treatment than with medical treatment.[87–89] However, after CABG surgery, mortality rates are high for patients with poor left ventricular function. Alderman et al. compared the long-term survival of 231 patients in the CASS registry with LVEF <0.36 who had CABG surgery between 1975 and 1979 with 420 medically treated CASS registry patients who had LVEF <0.36.[90] The average LVEF was 0.30 in both the medical and surgical groups. The 3-year cumulative

The CABG Patch Trial

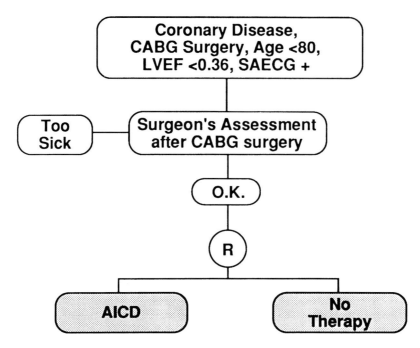

Figure 6. Flow diagram for The CABG Patch Trial. The **R** in the circle indicates the point of randomization. The shaded boxes indicate the main comparison for the trial. CABG = coronary artery bypass graft; LVEF = left ventricular ejection fraction; SAECG = signal-averaged ECG. Used with permission from Bigger JT Jr.[115]

mortality rate was 23% for surgically treated patients and 34% for medically treated patients.

Hochberg et al.[91] reported the surgical mortality and long-term survival of 466 patients with LVEF <0.40 undergoing CABG surgery between 1976 and 1982. All of the patients had previous myocardial infarction and 36% had congestive heart failure. There were 425 patients with LVEF 0.20–0.39 and 41 patients with LVEF 0.10–0.19 in their study. In the group with LVEF of 0.20–0.39, surgical mortality was 11% and the 3-year mortality rate was 40%. In the group with LVEF 0.10–0.19, surgical mortality was 27% and the 3-year mortality rate was 85%. The patients were divided into six groups based on LVEF, each with a 5-point range. The groups with LVEF 0.10–0.14 and 0.15–0.19 had a similar survival experience and the

groups with LVEF 0.20–0.24, 0.25–0.29, and 0.30–0.34 had a similar survival experience that was substantially better than the groups with LVEF 0.10–0.19 and substantially worse than the group with LVEF 0.35–0.39. This study provided the rationale for the use of LVEF in The CABG Patch Trial: requiring a LVEF of 0.36 for eligibility and stratifying randomization at a LVEF of 0.20.

CABG Surgery Does Not Decrease the Prevalence of Ventricular Arrhythmias

In the CASS registry study reported by Alderman et al.,[90] rehospitalization for arrhythmias occurred in 21.2% of the surgical group and in 17.9% of the medical group. This study suggests that CABG surgery does not substantially reduce arrhythmic risk.

Arrhythmic Deaths Are Common after CABG Surgery

There is not much information on the causes of death during long-term follow-up after CABG surgery. Holmes reported the mortality experience during 5 years of follow-up in 11,843 medically treated patients and 8,103 surgically treated patients in the Coronary Artery Surgery Study Registry.[92,93] In the surgically treated patients, death was sudden in 204 patients (25%), not sudden but cardiac in 390 (47%), and not cardiac in 230 (28%).[92] In the CASS database, there were no baseline variables that predicted sudden death better than nonsudden cardiac death after CABG surgery. This study confirmed a previous report by the same authors that CABG surgery reduced sudden cardiac death in the highest risk patients, but that substantial numbers of sudden deaths continue to occur after surgical treatment.[93] Bolooki reported a 35% sudden death mortality after CABG surgery during a follow-up period of 50 months in a relatively small group of patients.[94] Tresch et al. reported the long-term follow-up of 49 patients who had CABG surgery after cardiac arrest.[95] The mean LVEF for the group was 45%. Seven (16%) of the 45 patients discharged alive died during an average follow-up of 55 months. Five of the seven deaths were due to recurrent ventricular fibrillation and two were due to congestive heart failure. This study suggests that CABG surgery alone does not eliminate arrhythmic risk.

Arrhythmic Death after CABG Surgery

The studies summarized above and others indicate that the reported operative mortality for CABG surgery in patients with LVEF <0.36 ranges from 4% to 24%, 3-year all-cause mortality after CABG surgery in patients with LVEF <0.36 ranges from 24%

to 50%, and the percentage of all deaths after CABG surgery that are sudden ranges from 25% to 50%.

The CABG Surgery Survey

Because there was so much variability among the reports in the literature and because most of the relevant studies were 10 to 20 years old, The CABG Patch Trial planning group surveyed seven of their institutions to determine the percentage of patients who had CABG surgery during 1986 who were <80 years of age and had LVEF <0.36 and to determine the survival experience of this high-risk subset. A total of 3,217 CABG operations were done in the participating hospitals in 1986 and 17% were <80 years of age and had LVEF <0.36.[62] The surgical mortality rate for patients with LVEF <0.36 averaged 11.6%. The overall 2-year actuarial mortality rate was 28%. A number of nonfatal cardiac arrests were reported in patients with LVEF <0.36, but the data were too incomplete to permit precise estimates of rates.

The CABG Patch Trial Pilot Study

A 1-year pilot study was undertaken between September 1, 1990 and August 31, 1991 to obtain information needed to plan a full-scale trial.[62] The major objectives of the pilot study were to determine: (1) whether the signal-averaged ECG was a worthwhile arrhythmia qualifier; (2) the percentage of CABG surgery patients who were fully eligible for the trial; (3) the percentage of fully eligible patients who would consent to the study; and (4) the percentage of enrolled patients who could be randomized.

The investigators wanted a marker that would permit them to enroll patients at high risk for arrhythmic events during follow-up. Three tests were considered: (1) signal-averaged ECG, (2) ventricular arrhythmias in 24-hour Holter ECG recordings, and (3) electrophysiological studies. The signal-averaged ECG was chosen based on its feasibility and its high predictive value for arrhythmic events. Most patients were admitted much less than 24 hours before their CABG surgery, making 24-hour ECG recordings or electrophysiological studies less feasible than the signal-averaged ECG, a noninvasive test that can be completed in less than 30 min. Also, the signal-averaged ECG identifies patients at high risk for sudden cardiac death or nonfatal cardiac arrest after myocardial infarction better than ventricular arrhythmias detected by Holter recordings; the average relative risk for an abnormal signal-averaged ECG is 6 to 8.[13,18,20] The planning group thought that an abnormal signal-averaged ECG should have a relative risk of at least 2.0 to be worth using in a full-scale trial.

During the 1-year pilot study, 2,508 patients were screened and 18% of them were less than 80 years of age and had a LVEF <0.36; these percentages are remarkably similar to those found previously in the survey of CABG surgery.[62] Overall, 3.3% of the screened patients were fully eligible and 68% of the eligible patients signed a consent form. Of those who signed a consent form, 80% were randomized. About 65% of the otherwise eligible patients had an abnormal signal-averaged ECG and the relative risk of patients with abnormal signal-averaged ECG for death or cardiac arrest was about 3.0.

The Full-Scale CABG Patch Trial

In March 1993, the full-scale CABG Patch Trial began recruiting in 37 centers, 35 in the United States and two in Germany. All-cause mortality was chosen as the primary endpoint for the full-scale trial.

Baseline Studies

Patients with coronary artery disease scheduled for elective CABG surgery were screened at The CABG Patch Trial clinical centers. All patients had coronary angiography and measurement of LVEF within a year, most within a month of the CABG surgery. Almost 80% of the qualifying LVEF were calculated from RAO views of left ventriculograms. The criterion for a qualifying signal-averaged ECG was any one of the following: (1) a filtered QRS duration of ≥114 ms; (2) a root mean square voltage <20 μV in the terminal 40 ms of the filtered QRS duration; or (3) duration of the terminal filtered QRS complex of >38 ms after the QRS voltage falls below 40 μV.[96] These criteria were selected to exclude low-risk patients while qualifying more high-risk patients than conventional criteria would.

Enrollment Cascade

Five percent of patients scheduled for elective CABG surgery were excluded for age ≥80 and 74% for a LVEF ≥0.36. About half of otherwise eligible patients had a normal signal-averaged ECG. Patients who were fully eligible and who signed consent forms proceeded to CABG surgery. After the bypass grafts were done, the surgeon made the judgment whether the patient was stable enough to implant an ICD and, if so, the patient was randomized and the ICD system implanted and tested in the operating room, usually while patients were on partial cardiopulmonary bypass. More than 90% of patients who signed a consent form and remained eligible were randomized. The CABG Patch Trial completed enrollment in January 1996; >71,000 patients were screened, 1,422 eligible patients were identified, 1,055 were enrolled, and 900 were randomized.[97] Also, about 350 patients were enrolled in the substudy to determine the value of the signal-averaged ECG for predicting death or nonfatal arrhythmic events after CABG surgery.[96]

Design Features and Sample Size

The CABG Patch Trial was designed as a fixed sample size, randomized clinical trial with group sequential monitoring for safety.[62] Qualified patients were randomized 50:50 to ICD therapy or to no therapy. Randomization was stratified by clinical center and LVEF (≤0.20 vs. 0.21–0.35). The average follow-up was expected to be about 40 months. The primary endpoint for the study was all-cause mortality. The primary hypothesis was tested using the intention to treat principle; data were analyzed using the Cox regression model; the significance of differences between groups was tested with the log rank test. The alpha error was set at 0.05 (two-tailed) and the power at about 0.85. The dropin rate was expected to be 11% and the dropout rate was expected to be 6%. For the sample size calculation, ICD treatment was assumed to reduce the 40-month mortality rate by 26%. Using these parameters, the sample size required for the trial was calculated to be about 800 patients, 400 in each group. In October 1994, the Data and Safety Monitoring Board recommended that the sample size be increased to 900 to correct for a lower than expected mortality rate in the control group and a shortening of follow-up time caused by a June 1994 subpoena from the Office of the Inspector General.[98]

Treatment in the Control Group

There was a policy that patients are not to be treated with antiarrhythmic drugs in either group for asymptomatic or minimally symptomatic ventricular arrhythmias. About 15% of the patients in both groups were treated with antiarrhythmic drugs, mostly for atrial fibrillation.[99] Aspirin prophylaxis was recommended for both groups.

Effects of Treatment on Survival

The primary endpoint for the CABG Patch Trial was death of any cause. As of April 30, 1997, when the interim results were summarized, the average follow-up was 32 months. There were 101 deaths in the ICD group and 95 deaths in the control group; the actuarial mortality rate was about 25% in both groups,[99] Figure 7 shows that the ICD group mortality rate was almost identical to that found in the control group. The hazard ratio was 1.07, indicating almost identical mortality rates in the two groups over 4 years of follow-up. Cause-specific death will be classified by an external Events Committee using the modified Hinkle-Thaler definitions, but the results had not been reported at the time of this writing. The CABG Patch Trial specified 10 covariates of interest before the study began: age, gender, heart failure, New York Heart Association (NYHA) functional class, left ventricular ejection fraction, diabetes mellitus, QRS duration >100 ms, angiotensin converting enzyme inhibitors, class I or class III antiarrhythmic drugs, and beta adrenergic blocking drugs. There was no statistically significant interaction between any of these 10 covariates and treatment effect.

What Did We Learn from The CABG Patch Trial?

The CABG Patch Trial showed that ICD prophylaxis did not improve survival of high-risk patients having CABG surgery. These results indicate that not all high-risk groups of coronary heart disease patients will benefit from ICD therapy. Table 7 shows that many characteristics of patients in The CABG Patch Trial and those in MADIT are almost identical: age, gender, etiologic heart disease, prevalence and severity of heart failure, number with multiple previous myocardial infarcts, average LVEF. The two characteristics that differ substantially between these two primary prevention trials are inducible VT and revascularization with CABG surgery.

Why Was There No Benefit from ICD Therapy in The CABG Patch Trial?

Although the patients recruited for The CABG Patch Trial were very similar to those

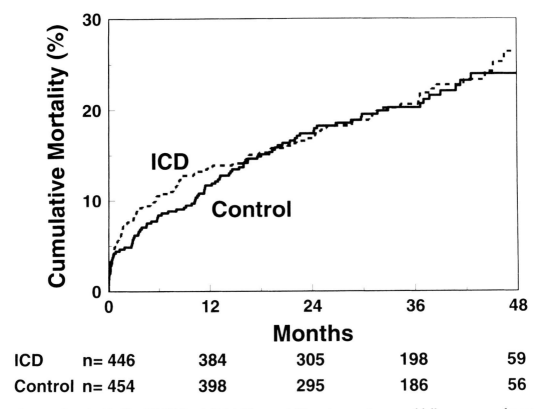

Figure 7. Survival in The CABG Patch Trial. The mortality rate over 4 years of follow-up was almost identical for patients assigned to ICD therapy and those assigned to no antiarrhythmic therapy. Used with permission from Bigger JT Jr for The CABG Patch Trial Investigators.[99]

Table 7
Comparison of Patient Characteristics in MADIT and in The CABG Patch Trial*

	MADIT	CABG Patch Trial
Age in years (mean ± SD)	63 ± 9	64 ± 9
Male	92	84
Coronary heart disease	100	100
LV ejection fraction (mean ± SD)	0.26 ± 0.07	0.27 ± 0.06
History of myocardial infarction	100	85
History of ≥2 myocardial infarctions	31	31
History of heart failure	51	50
CABG surgery	45	100
Coronary angioplasty/atherectomy	22	11
Unsustained ventricular tachycardia	100	30
Abnormal signal averaged ECG (fQRS)	57	100
Abnormal signal averaged ECG (fQRS or LP)	70	100
VT inducible by programmed stimulation	100	—

* Except where indicated, the numbers in the table indicate percentages.
ECG = electrocardiogram; fQRS = filtered QRS; LP = late potential; LV = left ventricular; SD = standard deviation; VT = ventricular tachycardia.

recruited for MADIT (see Table 7), the benefit of ICD therapy was nil in The CABG Patch Trial, but great in MADIT. A likely explanation for the difference in ICD benefit between MADIT and The CABG Patch Trial is that a very small proportion of patients (i.e., ≤0.20) randomized in The CABG Patch Trial had inducible sustained VT contrasted with MADIT in which all patients had inducible sustained VT. Alternatively, if the proportion of patients with inducible VT is large (>0.30) in The CABG Patch Trial, then it can be concluded that CABG surgery uncoupled inducible VT from spontaneous arrhythmic events during follow-up. The former explanation gives electrophysiological studies the dominant role in identifying patients who will benefit from prophylactic ICD therapy. The latter explanation will dictate that CABG surgery play a more important role in the primary prevention of sudden cardiac death. The CABG Patch Trial and upcoming ICD trials in heart failure are the only randomized controlled trials of ICD therapy in which the control group is not given antiarrhythmic treatment. The CABG Patch Trial is the only trial so far that is able to estimate the magnitude of the effect of ICD therapy on survival and on cardiac arrest. The trial has already shown that the signal-averaged ECG predicts early post operative death as well as late death and cardiac arrest in high-risk CABG surgery patients.[62,96] The CABG Patch Trial was not confounded by the effects of thoracotomy or by ischemic events since both the ICD treated group and the control group had thoracotomy and complete surgical revascularization. Since the effect of thoracotomy can be factored out, The CABG Patch Trial should be able to classify the mechanisms of death after CABG surgery better than ever before.

Trials of ICD Therapy in Heart Failure

Three studies are being planned to evaluate ICD therapy in patients with congestive heart failure, the Dilated Cardiomyopathy Trial (CAT), SCD-HeFT, and MADIT II.

The Rationale for ICD Prophylaxis in Patients with Heart Failure

Patients with heart failure classified as New York Heart Association functional class III or IV have a very high mortality rate, e.g., 40% to 50% during 2 years of follow-up and about 40% of this mortality is sudden, presumably arrhythmic, death.[100–103] A higher percentage of the deaths are sudden in class II or III patients than in class IV patients.[103] Selected heart failure patients might benefit from ICD prophylaxis. ICD treatment has been suggested as a bridge to heart transplantation, i.e., as therapy for patients who are accepted for heart transplantation, but who are waiting for a donor heart. About half of the patients accepted for a heart transplant die while on the waiting list.[104,105] Two preliminary studies[106,107] showed that patients on the heart transplant waiting list with LVEF <0.20 tolerated thoracotomy and ICD implantation very well (no operative mortality in 20 patients). Nineteen of 20 patients survived to transplant; 95% used their ICD during the first year after implant. About half of the patients used their ICD >10 times. There was no increase in difficulty of the subsequent transplant operation due to previous ICD implantation. Patients who are evaluated for heart transplantation and not accepted also have a very high mortality rate and ICD treatment could be helpful in this group as well.[108] Because a significant proportion of cardiac arrests in patients with heart failure are due to bradyarrhythmias or electromechanical dissociation, the benefit of ICD therapy is uncertain for this group.[109] Klein et al.[110] studied 81 patients referred for heart transplantation but considered too well for an immediate transplant; 60 had cardiomyopathy and 21 had coronary heart disease. During a mean follow-up of 20 months; 38 patients (47%) died; 45% of the deaths (n = 17) were sudden. In the subgroup of 39 patients selected by presence of spontaneous, complex ventricular arrhythmias, 21 were treated with antiarrhythmic drugs and 18 with ICDs.

There were eight (38%) sudden deaths in the drug treated patients and zero (0%) in ICD treated patients; 94% of the ICD pulse generators discharged during follow-up (an average of four ICD discharges per patient). These authors concluded that drug therapy was unreliable and that ICD treatment was advisable to prevent sudden death in patients with congestive heart failure and complex unsustained ventricular arrhythmias.

The prophylactic use of ICD treatment in heart failure patients should be subjected to randomized controlled clinical trials before this approach is accepted because effectively treating arrhythmic events might not increase survival very much in heart failure patients due to other lethal mechanisms, e.g., pump failure, myocardial ischemia/infarction, and bradyarrhythmias.

Dilated Cardiomyopathy Trial (CAT)

The CAT will test the hypothesis that implantation of an ICD in patients with dilated cardiomyopathy and severe left ventricular dysfunction will reduce the mortality rate.[111,112] The CAT started randomizing patients in a pilot study on July 1, 1991 with nine German centers participating. Patients with dilated cardiomyopathy are eligible if their LVEF is ≤0.30 and they are in New York Heart Association functional class II or III. The following conditions exclude patients from CAT: (1) history of sustained VT or cardiac arrest; (2) coronary atherosclerosis with >70% stenosis of a coronary artery; (3) valvular heart disease; (4) likely to undergo cardiac transplantation in the 6 months after enrollment; and (5) dilated cardiomyopathy present longer than 9 months. Patients who qualify and consent to join the study are randomized to ICD therapy or a control group that receives no formal alternate therapy. A registry is being kept on patients with dilated cardiomyopathy who have LVEF >0.30 or a history of cardiomyopathy for longer than 9 months.

Baseline Studies

A large battery of baseline tests is performed in CAT, bicycle exercise testing, 24-hour continuous ECG recording, signal-averaged ECG, coronary angiography, and programmed ventricular stimulation, but none of them are used to qualify patients or to stratify the randomization.

Enrollment Cascade

Many of the percentages needed to design the CAT are not available. Accordingly, the CAT investigators are conducting a pilot study to enroll 100 patients so they can estimate the critical parameters for the trial. Between May 15, 1991 and June 1996, 90 patients were randomized. The major obstacle to enrollment in the early months of the study was the requirement that the dilated cardiomyopathy be diagnosed within the 6 months prior to enrollment. The interval was changed to 9 months during the course of the pilot study.[112]

Design Features and Sample Size

The design for CAT will not be finalized until after the pilot study, but it is anticipated that CAT will be a fixed sample size, randomized clinical trial. In the pilot study, the only stratifying variable for randomization is clinical center. The alpha error is set at 0.05 and the power at 0.80. The CAT investigators expect a 1-year mortality rate (deaths of all causes) of 30%; 60% of the deaths to be due to heart failure and 40% due to sudden cardiac death. ICD therapy is expected to reduce the 1-year mortality rate to 24% (a reduction of 20%). Originally, the CAT investigators estimated the perioperative mortality to be 5%, but, with the advent of transvenous leads, the mortality rate is much lower. When 100 patients have been recruited, the final design, sample size, and feasibility of CAT will be assessed and the decision made whether a full-scale trial will be conducted.

Therapy in the Control Group

The use of beta adrenergic blocking and calcium channel blocking drugs is not controlled by the protocol. CAT has a policy against using antiarrhythmic drugs in the control group.

What Will We Learn from CAT?

The primary information that will come from the pilot study is whether it is feasible to conduct a full-scale trial. The exclusion for long-standing cardiomyopathy has caused a problem already and may be dropped. Perhaps, the time between documentation of cardiomyopathy and enrollment in CAT will be used to stratify randomization rather than to exclude patients. A positive control group, e.g., amiodarone, may be required to make the trial feasible. If it turns out not to be feasible to do a full-scale trial in this patient group, some controlled information on the safety of implantation of nonthoracotomy ICD systems will be developed. Information on the frequency of ICD firing in patients with NYHA class II and III heart failure will be determined. With 100 patients in the pilot sample, it is unlikely that any useful information will be acquired related to the potential of ICD therapy to reduce mortality. Hopefully, a full-scale trial will be conducted to provide definitive information on the magnitude of the reduction of mortality by ICD treatment in patients with dilated cardiomyopathy and class II and III heart failure.

Sudden Cardiac Death in Heart Failure Trial (SCD-HeFT)

SCD-HeFT is an investigator-initiated trial jointly sponsored by the National Heart, Lung, and Blood Institute and Medtronic Inc. SCD-HeFT will test the hypothesis that implantation of an ICD in patients in New York Heart Association class II or III and with LVEF <0.36 will improve survival. No arrhythmia marker is required to

Table 8
Exclusion Criteria for The SCD-HeFT

1. Age <18 years.
2. Women who are pregnant or have child bearing potential.
3. History of sustained VT or cardiac arrest.
4. Restrictive, infiltrative or hypertrophic cardiomyopathy, valvular or congenital heart disease.
5. LVEF >0.35.
6. NYHA functional class IV (heart failure).
7. Mechanical prosthetic heart valve.
8. Need for antiarrhythmic drugs except digitalis, calcium or beta blocking drugs.
9. Cardiac transplantation expected in <1 year.
10. Expected survival <1 year.
11. Unexplained syncope.
12. Liver function tests 2.5 times normal or serum creatinine >2.5 mg/dL.
13. Implanted pacemaker.
14. Unable to accommodate an ICD pulse generator in the left infraclavicular region.
15. Enrolled in another randomized controlled clinical trial.
16. Unable to provide informed consent.

qualify for the study. SCD-HeFT began recruiting in July 1997 and hopes to randomize 1,000 patients per year in >90 clinical centers. Patients must be ≥18 years of age and must have taken an angiotensin converting enzyme inhibitor for 2 or more weeks before recruited. Also, patients in atrial fibrillation must have warfarin therapy stabilized before recruitment. Exclusion criteria for SCD HeFT are listed in Table 8.

Baseline Studies

Patients must have had coronary angiography done within 2 years of recruitment. A 6-minute walk will be done at baseline to quantify the functional capacity of patients. Baseline measures will be made to permit safety monitoring of amiodarone therapy. Special precautions will be taken for patients with atrial fibrillation, and those taking digoxin or warfarin when medication (amiodarone or placebo) is started.

Design Features and Sample Size

Equal percentages of patients will be randomized to each of three treatment groups: placebo, amiodarone, and ICD therapy. The primary endpoint is all-cause mortality. A 25% mortality rate is expected at an average follow-up of 2.5 years. It is expected that ICD therapy will reduce the mortality rate by 25% (i.e., that sudden cardiac death will be reduced by 50%) when compared to placebo treatment. To calculate the sample size, a power of 0.90 and an alpha level of 0.01 were used. Using these parameters, a sample size of 2,500 was calculated, 833 in each group. The primary comparisons will be each active treatment with placebo using the intention to treat principle.

Treatment Protocol

All patients will be treated with digoxin, diuretics, and converting enzyme inhibitors. Patients randomized to amiodarone will be loaded with 800 mg per day for 1 week and 400 mg per day for 2–4 weeks. Maintenance amiodarone will be adjusted by weight: <150 pounds, 200 mg per day; 150–200 pounds, 300 mg per day; >200 pounds, 400 mg per day. Patients randomized to ICD therapy will have a pectoral implant with a Medtronic "hot can" pulse generator connected to a transvenous lead. A rate of 188 beats per minute (cycle length 320 ms) will be used for detection of ventricular fibrillation. VVI pacing will be set for 50 beats per minute. The stored electrograms collected by the ICDs will be transmitted electronically to a core laboratory.

What Will We Learn from SCD-HeFT?

SCD-HeFT should define the efficacy of ICD prophylaxis in patients with heart failure and severe reductions in LVEF. One group of patients will be randomized to placebo treatment. Comparison of the ICD group with the placebo group will quantify the effect size of ICD therapy. SCD-HeFT plans to capture and analyze electrograms from the ICDs to document the rhythms that are treated in patients with heart failure. SCD-HeFT will compare the cost-effectiveness and quality of life of placebo treatment with amiodarone and ICD therapy.

Conclusions

AVID has shown that ICD therapy is better than empiric amiodarone therapy for secondary prevention of sudden cardiac death. The National Heart, Lung, and Blood Institute estimates that first line use of ICD therapy in survivors of cardiac arrest or hemodynamically significant VT will save an additional 500 lives per year. When CASH and CIDS complete their follow-up, their results should amplify the results recently reported by AVID.

At the present time, the salvage rate after cardiac arrest is pitifully small which motivates the exploration of primary prevention for sudden cardiac death. Before primary prevention is adopted, its efficacy, safety, and cost effectiveness must be demonstrated in controlled clinical trials. MADIT has already reported that ICD therapy improves survival better than drug therapy in patients with LVEF <0.36, unsustained VT, and inducible sustained VT. The CABG Patch Trial showed that not all high-risk groups of coronary heart disease patients benefit from prophylactic implantation of a cardiac defibrillator. It remains for the future to define additional high-risk groups that will benefit from ICD prophylaxis. The results of MUSTT will define better the identification of high-risk coronary heart disease patients and establish the role of electrophysiologically guided drug therapy for patients with left ventricular dysfunction and unsustained VT. The full-scale CATS, SCD-HeFT, and MADIT II will start recruiting in 1997 and yield new results early in the next century. As a result of these trials, we will have a steady flow of new scientific information to guide the evolution of clinical practice to control sudden cardiac death. This information should stimulate technical developments and reduce the cost of ICD therapy.[113]

References

1. National Center for Health Statistics: Advance report, final mortality statistics, 1981. Monthly Vital Statistics, Vol. 33(Suppl 3): DHHS Pub. No.(PHS)84-1120, pp 4–5.

2. Weaver WD, Cobb LA, Hallstrom AP, et al. Factors influencing survival after out-of-hospital cardiac arrest. J Am Coll Cardiol 1986;7:752–757.

3. Becker LB, Ostrander MP, Barrett J, et al. Outcome of cardiopulmonary resuscitation in a large metropolitan area: where are the survivors? Ann Emerg Med 1991;20: 355–361.

4. Lombardi G, Gallagher EJ, Gennis P. Outcome of out-of-hospital cardiac arrest in New York City. JAMA 1994;271:678–683.

5. Davies MJ, Thomas A. Thrombosis and acute coronary artery lesions in sudden cardiac ischemic death. N Engl J Med 1984;310: 1137–1140.

6. Marshall JC, Waxman HL, Sauerwein A, et al. Frequency of low-grade residual coronary stenosis after thrombolysis during acute myocardial infarction. Am J Cardiol 1990;66:773–778.

7. Fuster V, Badimon L, Badimon JJ, et al. The pathogenesis of coronary artery disease and the acute coronary syndromes. N Engl J Med 1992;326:242–250, 310–318.

8. Spaulding CM, Joly LM, Rosenberg A, et al. Immediate coronary angiography in survivors of out-of-hospital cardiac arrest. N Engl J Med 1997;336:1629–1633.

9. Gordon T, Kannel WB. Premature mortality from coronary heart disease: The Framingham Study. J Am Med Assoc 1971;215: 1617–1625.

10. Lown B. Sudden cardiac death: the major challenge confronting contemporary cardiology. Am J Cardiol 1979;43:313–328.

11. Moss AJ, Hall WJ, Cannom DS, et al, for the MADIT Investigators. Improved survival with an implantable defibrillator in coronary patients at high risk for ventricular arrhythmias. N Engl J Med 1996;335: 1933–1940.

12. Bigger JT Jr, Fleiss JL, Kleiger R, et al, and The Multicenter Post-Infarction Research Group. The relationships among ventricular arrhythmias, left ventricular dysfunction and mortality in the 2 years after myocardial infarction. Circulation 1984;69: 250–258.

13. Cripps TR, Bennett ED, Camm AJ, et al. High gain signal averaged electrocardiogram combined with 24-hour monitoring in patients early after myocardial infarction for bedside prediction of arrhythmic events. Br Heart J 1988;60:181–187.

14. Kuchar DL, Thorburn CW, Sammet NL. Late potentials detected after myocardial infarction: Natural history and prognostic significance. Circulation 1986;74:1280–1289.

15. Gomes JA, Winters SL, Stewart D, et al. A new noninvasive index to predict sustained ventricular tachycardia and sudden death in the first year after myocardial infarction: based on signal-averaged electrocardiogram, radionuclide ejection fraction and Holter monitoring. J Am Coll Cardiol 1987; 10:349–357.

16. Breithardt G, Borggrefe M. Recent advances in the identification of patients at risk of ventricular tachyarrhythmias: role of ventricular late potentials. Circulation 1987;75: 1091–1096.

17. Simson MB. Noninvasive identification of patients at high risk for sudden cardiac death: signal averaged electrocardiography. Circulation 1992;85:I–145-I–151.

18. Steinberg JS, Regan A, Sciacca RR, et al. Predicting arrhythmic events after myocardial infarction: results of a prospective study and a meta-analysis using the signal-averaged electrocardiogram. Am J Cardiol 1992; 69:13–21.

19. Odemuyiwa O, Malik M, Farrell T, et al. A comparison of the predictive characteristics of heart rate variability index and left ventricular ejection fraction for all-cause mortality, arrhythmic events and sudden death after acute myocardial infarction. Am J Cardiol 1991;68:434–439.

20. El-Sherif N, Denes P, Katz R, et al. for the Cardiac Arrhythmia Suppression Trial/ Signal-Averaged Electrocardiogram (CAST /SAECG) Substudy Investigators. Definition of the best prediction criteria of the time domain signal-averaged electrocardiogram for serious arrhythmic events in the postinfarction period. J Am Coll Cardiol 1995;25:908–914.

21. Richards DA, Cody DV, Denniss AR, et al. Ventricular electrical instability. A predictor of death after myocardial infarction. Am J Cardiol 1983;51:75–80.

22. Breithardt G, Borggrefe M, Haerten K. Role of programmed ventricular stimulation and noninvasive recording of ventricular late potentials for the identification of patients at risk of ventricular tachyarrhythmias after acute myocardial infarction. In Cardiac Electrophysiology and Arrhythmias, Zipes DP Jalife J, eds. Grune & Stratton, Inc, New York, 1985, pp 553–561.

23. Roy D, Marchand E, Theroux P, et al. Programmed ventricular stimulation in survivors of an acute myocardial infarction. Circulation 1985;72:487–494.

24. Denniss AR, Richards DA, Cody DV, et al. Prognostic significance of ventricular tachycardia and fibrillation induced at programmed stimulation and delayed potentials detected on the signal-averaged electrocardiograms of survivors of acute myocardial infarction. Circulation 1986;74: 731–745.

25. Bourke JP, Richards DAB, Ross DL, et al. Routine programmed electrical stimulation in survivors of acute myocardial infarction for prediction of spontaneous ventricular tachyarrhythmias during follow-up: results, optimal stimulation protocol, and cost-effective screening. J Am Coll Cardiol 1991;18:780–788.

26. Kleiger RE, Miller JP, Bigger JT Jr, et al, and the Multicenter Postinfarction Research Group. Decreased heart rate variability and its association with increased mortality after acute myocardial infarction. Am J Cardiol 1987;59:256–262.

27. Bigger JT Jr, Fleiss JL, Steinman RC, et al. Frequency domain measures of heart period variability and mortality after myocardial infarction. Circulation 1992;85: 164–171.

28. Farrell TG, Bashir Y, Paul V, et al. Risk stratification for arrhythmic events in postinfarction patients based on heart rate variability, ambulatory electrocardiographic variables, and the signal-averaged electrocardiogram. J Am Coll Cardiol 1991;18: 687–697.

29. Connolly SJ, Yusuf S. Evaluation of the implantable cardioverter defibrillator in survivors of cardiac arrest: the need for randomized trials. Am J Cardiol 1992;69:959–962.

30. Kuck HK, Siebels J, Schneider M, et al. The Hamburg Cardiac Arrest Study Group. Preliminary results of a randomized trial, AICD versus drugs (abstract). Rev Europ Technol Biomed 1990;12:110.

31. Siebels J, Cappato R, Ruppel R, Schneider MAE, Kuck K-H, and the CASH Investigators. ICD versus drugs in cardiac arrest survivors: preliminary results of the Cardiac Arrest Study Hamburg. PACE 1993;16: 552–558.

32. Siebels J, Kuck KH. Implantable cardioverter defibrillator compared with antiarrhythmic drug treatment in cardiac arrest survivors (the Cardiac Arrest Study Hamburg). Am Heart J 1994;127:1139–1144.

33. Connolly SJ, Gent M, Roberts RS, et al. Canadian Implantable Defibrillator Study (CIDS): study design and organization. CIDS Co-Investigators. Am J Cardiol 1993; 72:103F–108F.

34. Hinkle LE Jr, Thaler HT. Clinical classification of cardiac deaths. Circulation 1982;65: 457–464.

35. The AVID investigators. Antiarrhythmics Versus Implantable Defibrillators (AVID): rationale, design, and methods. Am J Cardiol 1995;75:470–475.

36. The Antiarrhythmics Versus Implantable Defibrillators (AVID) Investigators. Comparison of antiarrhythmic drug therapy with implantable defibrillators in patients resuscitated from near-fatal ventricular arrhythmias. N Engl J Med 1997;337: 1576–1583.

37. Epstein AE. AVID necessity. PACE 1993;16: 1773–1775.

38. Fogoros RN. An AVID dissent. PACE 1994; 17:1707–1711.

39. Mower MM. Prolongation of life with implantable cardioverter-defibrillator therapy: the proper studies are already in progress. Am J Cardiol 1994;73:419–421.

40. Singer I. AVID necessity. PACE 1994;17: 260–262.

41. Connolly SJ. An AVID dissent: commentary. PACE 1994;17:1712–1713.

42. Zipes DP. The implantable cardioverter-defibrillator: lifesaver or a device looking for a disease? Circulation 1994;89:2934–2936.

43. Greene HL, Richardson DW, Barker AH, et al, and the CAPS investigators. Classification of deaths after myocardial infarction as arrhythmic or nonarrhythmic (The Cardiac Arrhythmia Pilot Study). Am J Cardiol 1989;63:1–6.

44. Epstein AE, Carlson MD, Fogoros RN, et al. Classification of death in antiarrhythmia trials. J Am Coll Cardiol 1996;27:433–442.

45. Burkart F, Pfisterer M, Kiowski W, et al. Effect of antiarrhythmic therapy on mortality in survivors of myocardial infarction with asymptomatic complex ventricular arrhythmias: Basel Antiarrhythmic Study of Infarct Survival (BASIS). J Am Coll Cardiol 1990;16:1711–1718.

46. Ceremuzynski L, Kleczar E, Krzeminska-Pakula M, et al. Effect of amiodarone on mortality after myocardial infarction: a double-blind, placebo-controlled, pilot study. J Am Coll Cardiol 1992;20: 1056–1062.

47. Doval HC, Nul DR, Grancelli HO, et al. Randomised trial of low-dose amiodarone in severe congestive heart failure. Grupo de Estudio de la Sobrevida en la Insuficiencia Cardiaca en Argentina (GESICA). Lancet 1994;344:493–498.

48. Singh SN, Fletcher RD, Fisher SG, et al, for The Survival Trial of Antiarrhythmic Therapy in Congestive Heart Failure. Amiodarone in patients with congestive heart failure and asymptomatic ventricular arrhythmia. N Engl J Med 1995;333:77–82.

49. Connolly SJ, Cairns JA for the CAMIAT Pilot Study Group. Prevalence and predictors of ventricular premature complexes in survivors of acute myocardial infarction. Canadian Amiodarone Myocardial Infarction Arrhythmia Trial. Am J Cardiol 1992; 69:408–411.

50. Cairns JA, Connolly SJ, Roberts R, et al. Canadian Amiodarone Myocardial Infarction Arrhythmia Trial (CAMIAT): rationale and protocol. CAMIAT Investigators. Am J Cardiol 1993;72:87F–94F.

51. Camm AJ, Julian D, Janse G, Munoz A, et al. The European Myocardial Infarct Amiodarone Trial (EMIAT). EMIAT Investigators. Am J Cardiol 1993;72:95F–98F.

52. Schwartz PJ, Camm AJ, Frangin G, et al, on behalf of the EMIAT investigators. Does amiodarone reduce sudden death and cardiac mortality after myocardial infarction? The European myocardial infarction amiodarone trial (EMIAT). Eur Heart J 1994;15: 620–624.

53. Julian DG, Camm AJ, Frangin G, et al, for the European Myocardial Infarct Amiodarone Trial Investigators. Randomised trial of effect of amiodarone on mortality in patients with left-ventricular dysfunction after recent myocardial infarction: EMIAT. Lancet 1997;349:667–74.

54. Cairns JA, Connolly SJ, Roberts R, et al, for the Canadian Amiodarone Myocardial Infarction Arrhythmia Trial Investigators. Randomised trial of outcome after myocardial infarction in patients with frequent or repetitive ventricular premature depolarisations: CAMIAT. Lancet 1997;349:675–82.

55. Wever EFD, Hauer RNW. Cost-effectiveness considerations: the Dutch prospective study of the automatic implantable cardioverter defibrillator as first-choice therapy. PACE 1992;15:690–693.

56. Wever EFD, Hauer RNW, van Capelle FJL, et al. Randomized study of implantable defibrillator as first-choice therapy versus conventional strategy in postinfarct sudden death survivors. Circulation 1995;91: 2195–2203.

57. Wever EFD, Hauer RNW, Schrijvers G, et al. Cost-effectiveness of implantable defibrillator as first-choice therapy versus electrophysiologically guided, tiered therapy in postinfarct sudden death survivors:

a randomized study. Circulation 1996;93: 489–496.

58. Kuppermann M, Luce B, McGovern B, et al. An analysis of the cost effectiveness of the implantable defibrillator. Circulation 1990; 81:91–100.

59. O'Donoghue S, Platia EV, Brooks-Robinson S, et al. Automatic implantable cardioverter-defibrillator: is early implantation cost-effective. J Am Coll Cardiol 1990;16: 1258–1263.

60. Anderson MH, Camm AJ. Implications for present and future applications of the implantable cardioverter-defibrillator resulting from the use of a simple model of cost efficacy. Br Heart J 1993;69:83–92.

61. MADIT Executive Committee. Multicenter Automatic Defibrillator Implantation Trial (MADIT): design and clinical protocol. PACE 1991;14:920–927.

62. The CABG Patch Trial Investigators and Coordinators. The CABG Patch Trial. Prog Cardiovas Dis 1993;36:97–114.

63. Buxton AE, Fisher JD, Josephson ME, et al. Prevention of sudden death in patients with coronary artery disease: the Multicenter Unsustained Tachycardia Trial (MUSTT). Progr Cardiovas Dis 1993;36:215–226.

64. Mitra RL, Buxton AE. The clinical significance of nonsustained ventricular tachycardia. J Cardiovas Electrophysiol 1993;4: 490–496.

65. Buxton AE, Lee KL, DiCarlo L. Non-sustained ventricular tachycardia in coronary artery disease: relation to inducible sustained VT. MUSTT Investigators. Ann Intern Med 1996;125:35–39.

66. Bigger JT Jr, Fleiss JL, Rolnitzky LM, The Multicenter Post-Infarction Research Group. Prevalence, characteristics and significance of ventricular tachycardia detected by 24-hour continuous electrocardiographic recordings in the late hospital phase of acute myocardial infarction. Am J Cardiol 1986;58:1151–1160.

67. Kowey PR, Taylor JE, Marinchak RA, et al. Does programmed stimulation really help in the evaluation of patients with nonsustained ventricular tachycardia? Results of a meta-analysis. Am Heart J 1992;123: 481–485.

68. Wilber DJ, Olshansky B, Moran JF, et al. Electrophysiologic testing and nonsustained ventricular tachycardia: Use and limitations in patients with coronary artery disease and impaired ventricular function. Circulation 1990;82:350–358.

69. Wilber D, Olshansky B, Moran J, et al. Electrophysiological testing and nonsustained

ventricular tachycardia. Circulation 1991; 84:II–21.

70. Waxman HL, Buxton AE, Sadowski LM, et al. The response to procainamide during electrophysiologic study for sustained ventricular tachyarrhythmias predicts the response to other medications. Circulation 1983;67:30–37.

71. Kuchar DL, Rottman JN, Berger RE, et al. Prediction of successful suppression of sustained ventricular tachyarrhythmias by serial drug testing from data derived at the initial electrophysiologic study. J Am Coll Cardiol 1988;12:982–988.

72. Daubert JP, Higgins SL, Zareba W, et al. Comparative survival of MADIT-eligible but noninducible patients. J Am Coll Cardiol 1997;29(Suppl A):78A.

73. Hjalmarson A, Elmfeldt D, Herlitz J, et al. Effect on mortality of metoprolol in acute myocardial infarction. A double-blind randomized trial. Lancet 1981;iv:823–827.

74. Norwegian Multicenter Study Group. Timolol-induced reduction in mortality and reinfarction in patients surviving acute myocardial infarction. N Engl J Med 1981; 304:801–807.

75. Beta-blocker Heart Attack Trial Research Group. A randomized trial of propranolol in patients with acute myocardial infarction. I. Mortality results. JAMA 1982;247: 1707–14.

76. Yusuf S, Peto R, Lewis J, Collins R, et al. Beta blockade during and after myocardial infarction: an overview of the randomized trials. Prog Cardiovasc Dis 1985;27: 335–371.

77. The Cardiac Arrhythmia Suppression Trial (CAST) Investigators. Effect of encainide and flecainide on mortality in a randomized trial of arrhythmia suppression after myocardial infarction. N Engl J Med 1989;321: 406–412.

78. Echt DS, Liebson PR, Mitchell LB, et al, and the CAST Investigators. Mortality and morbidity in patients randomized to receive encainide, flecainide, or placebo in the Cardiac Arrhythmia Suppression Trial. N Engl J Med 1991;324:781–788.

79. The Cardiac Arrhythmia Suppression Trial II Investigators. Effect of the antiarrhythmic agent moricizine on survival after myocardial infarction. N Engl J Med 1992;327: 227–233.

80. May GS, Eberlein KA, Furberg CD, et al. Secondary prevention after myocardial infarction: a review of long-term trials. Prog Cardiovasc Dis 1982;24:331–352.

81. Furberg CD. Effect of antiarrhythmic drugs on mortality after myocardial infarction. Am J Cardiol 1983;52:32C–36C.

82. Hine L, Laird N, Hewitt P, Chalmers T. Meta-analysis of empiric chronic antiarrhythmic therapy after myocardial infarction. J Am Med Assoc 1989;262:3037–3040.

83. Coplen SE, Antman EM, Berlin JA, et al. Efficacy and safety of quinidine therapy for maintenance of sinus rhythm after cardioversion: a metaanalysis of randomized control trials. Circulation 1990;82:1106–1116.

84. Morganroth J, Goin JE. Clinical investigation: quinidine-related mortality in the short-to-medium-term treatment of ventricular arrhythmias: a meta-analysis. Circulation 1991;84:1977–1983.

85. Yusuf S, Teo KK. Approaches to prevention of sudden death: need for fundamental reevaluation. J Cardiovasc Electrophysiol 1991;2:S233–S239.

86. Teo KK, Yusuf S, Furberg CD. Effects of prophylactic antiarrhythmic drug therapy in acute myocardial infarction. An overview of results from randomized controlled trials. JAMA 1993;270:1589–1595.

87. Read RC, Murphy ML, Hultgren HN, et al. Survival of men treated for chronic stable angina pectoris: a cooperative randomized study. J Thorac Cardiovasc Surg 1978;75: 1–16.

88. European Coronary Surgery Study Group. Long-term results of prospective randomized study of coronary artery bypass surgery in stable angina pectoris. Lancet 1982; 2:1173–1180.

89. CASS Principal Investigators and Their Associates. Coronary Artery Surgery Study (CASS): a randomized trial of coronary artery bypass surgery: survival data. Circulation 1983;68:939–950.

90. Alderman EL, Fisher LD, Litwin P, et al. Results of coronary artery surgery in patients with poor left ventricular function (CASS). Circulation 1983;68:785–795.

91. Hochberg MS, Parsonnet V, Gielchinsky I, et al. Coronary artery bypass grafting in patients with ejection fractions below forty percent: early and late results in 466 patients. J Thorac Cardiovasc Surg 1983;86: 519–527.

92. Holmes DR, David K, Gersh BJ, et al, and CASS participants. Risk factor profiles of patients with sudden cardiac death and death from other cardiac causes: a report from the Coronary Artery Surgery Study (CASS). J Am Coll Cardiol 1989;13:524–530.

93. Holmes DR Jr, Davis KB, Mock MB, et al, and participants in the Coronary Artery Surgery Study. The effect of medical and surgical treatment on subsequent sudden

cardiac death in patients with coronary artery disease: a report from the Coronary Artery Surgery Study. Circulation 1986;73: 1254–1263.

94. Bolooki H. Discussion of reference 27, Hochberg, et al. Discussion of CABG in patients with ejection fractions below forty percent. J Thorac Cardiovasc Surg 1983;86: 526.

95. Tresch DD, Wetherbee JN, Siegel R, et al. Long-term follow-up of survivors of prehospital sudden cardiac death treated with coronary bypass surgery. Am Heart J 1985; 110:1139–45.

96. Gottlieb CD, Bigger JT Jr, Steinman RC, et al, for The CABG Patch Trial Investigators. Signal averaged ECG predicts death after CABG surgery. Circulation 1995;92:I-406.

97. Curtis AB, Cannom DS, Bigger JT Jr, et al, for The CABG Patch Trial Investigators. Baseline characteristics of Patients in The Coronary Artery Bypass Graft (CABG) Patch trial. Am Heart J 1997;134:787–799.

98. Bigger JT Jr, Parides MK, Levin B, et al. Changes in sample size and length of follow-up to maintain power in The CABG Patch Trial. Controlled Clinical Trials 1998; 19:1–14.

99. Bigger JT Jr, for the Coronary Artery Bypass Graft (CABG) Patch Trial Investigators. Prophylactic use of implanted cardiac defibrillators in patients at high risk for ventricular arrhythmias after coronary artery bypass graft surgery. N Engl J Med 1997;337: 1569–1575.

100. Bigger JT Jr. Why patients with congestive heart failure die: arrhythmias and sudden cardiac death. Circulation 1987;75(Suppl IV):28–35.

101. Packer M. Sudden unexpected death in patients with congestive heart failure: a second frontier. Circulation 1985;72:681–685.

102. Francis G. Should asymptomatic ventricular arrhythmias in patients with congestive heart failure be treated with antiarrhythmic drugs? J Am Coll Cardiol 1988;12:274–6.

103. Kjekshus J. Arrhythmias and mortality in congestive heart failure. Am J Cardiol 1990; 65:42I-48I.

104. DEFIBRILAT Study Group. Actuarial risk of sudden death while awaiting cardiac transplantation in patients with atherosclerotic heart disease. Am J Cardiol 1991;68: 545–546.

105. Stevenson L, Chelimsky-Fallick C, et al. Unacceptable risk of sudden death without transplantation if low ejection fraction is due to coronary artery disease. J Am Coll Cardiol 1990;15:222A.

106. Bolling S, Deeb M, Morady F, et al. AICD: a new "bridge" to transplantation. J Am Coll Cardiol 1990;15:223A.

107. Jeevanandam V, Bielefeld MR, Auteri JS, et al. The implantable defibrillator: an electronic bridge to cardiac transplantation. Circulation 1992;86:II-276-II-279.

108. Stevenson L, Fowler M, Schroeder J, et al. Poor survival of patients with idiopathic cardiomyopathy considered too well for transplantation. Am J Med 1987;83: 871–876.

109. Luu M, Stevenson WG, Stevenson LW, et al. Diverse mechanisms of unexpected cardiac arrest in advanced heart failure. Circulation 1989;80(6):1675–1680.

110. Klein H, Troster J, Haverich A. AICD as a bridge to transplant. Rev Europ Technol Biomed 1990;12:110A.

111. The German Dilated Cardiomyopathy Study Investigators. Prospective studies assessing prophylactic therapy in high risk patients: The German Dilated Cardiomyopathy Study (GDCMS)—study design. PACE 1992;15:697–700.

112. The Cardiomyopathy Trial Investigators. Cardiomyopathy trial. PACE 1993;16: 576–581.

113. Hauser RG. Attributes of a prophylactic implantable cardioverter defibrillator: how close are we? PACE 1993;16:582–585.

114. Bigger JT Jr. Primary prevention of sudden cardiac death using implantable cardioverter-defibrillators. In Singer I, ed. Implantable Cardioverter Defibrillator. Futura Publishing Co, Inc, Armonk, NY, 1994, pp 515–546.

115. Bigger JT Jr. Should defibrillators be implanted in high-risk patients without a previous sustained ventricular tachyarrhythmia? In Naccarelli GV, Veltri EP, eds. Implantable Cardioverter-Defibrillators, Blackwell Scientific Publications, Inc, 1993, pp 284–317.)

Chapter 26

The Role of Pharmacological Therapy for Ventricular Tachyarrhythmias: Where Do We Go from Here?

L. Brent Mitchell

Introduction

The patient who has experienced a sustained episode of ventricular tachycardia (VT) or ventricular fibrillation (VF) in the absence of a transient or reversible cause is at high risk of future VT/VF episodes. Accordingly, such a patient is also at high risk of sudden cardiac death. Over the past 25 years, seven therapeutic alternatives for the prevention of VT/VF and sudden cardiac death in this patient population have been proposed. Of this number, five represent pharmacological interventions—empiric standard antiarrhythmic drug therapy, individualized standard antiarrhythmic drug therapy predicted to be effective by the noninvasive (electrocardiographic monitoring) approach, individualized standard antiarrhythmic drug therapy predicted to be effective by the invasive (electrophysiological study) approach, empiric amiodarone therapy, and empiric beta-blocking drug therapy. Nevertheless, recent clinical trial evidence has indicated that a nonpharmacological approach to therapy, the implantable cardioverter-defibrillator (ICD), is superior to the best that pharmacological therapy has to offer. Where do we go from here? Of course, the answer to this question requires consideration of where we have been and where we are now.

Where Have We Been?

Natural History of Ventricular Tachycardia/Ventricular Fibrillation

Some patients have sustained VT/VF as the result of a transient or reversible cause such as electrolyte or acid-base disturbances, proarrhythmic drug effects or the acute phase of a myocardial infarction. The natural history of patients with VT/VF in these settings is normalized by removal of the cause or by the passage of a brief period of time. Other patients have sustained VT/VF in the absence of a transient or reversible cause. The natural history of these patients is dominated by recurrent episodes of VT/VF. However, accurate estimations of the probabilities of arrhythmia recurrence/sudden death in such patients are not available. Those reports[1-11] of the untreated natural history of VT/VF patients that do exist

From Singer I, Barold SS, Camm AJ (eds): Nonpharmacological Therapy of Arrhythmias for the 21st Century: The State of the Art. Futura Publishing Co, Inc., Armonk, NY, © 1998.

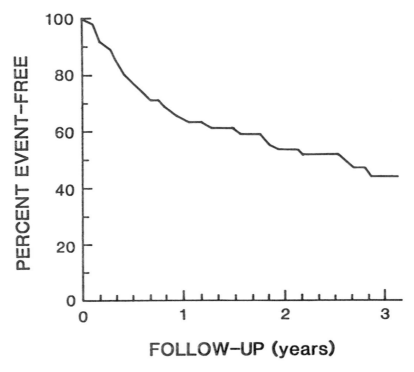

Figure 1. Actuarial probabilites of freedom from death and VF recurrence (%) over 3 years of follow-up in patients who experienced an out-of-hospital VF cardiac arrest in the absence of a transient or reversible cause, the majority of whom received no specific antiarrhythmic therapy. Redrawn with permission from Cobb LA, et al.[11]

are dated and some of the patients in each of these series received empiric standard antiarrhythmic drug therapy. The most recent of these reports, that of Cobb et al.,[11] describes the follow-up actuarial arrhythmia recurrence/death probabilities of 200 patients who had been resuscitated from an out-of-hospital VF arrest in Seattle. As shown in Figure 1, the probability of arrhythmia recurrence/death after 2 years of follow-up was approximately 50%. The best contemporary estimates of the natural history of "untreated" VT/VF patients come from those follow-up reports of patients who received an ICD without concomitant antiarrhythmic drug therapy. In such patient populations[12,13] the 2-year probabilities of arrhythmia recurrence/sudden death (as estimated by appropriate ICD therapy delivery) are not measurably different that the 50% probability forecast by the early natural history studies. An unfortu-

nate, but understandable, consequence of this very poor natural history has been a reluctance to include untreated control patient populations in subsequent assessments of therapeutic interventions.

Empiric Standard Antiarrhythmic Drug Therapy

The first therapeutic approach recommended for patients with sustained VT/VF was the empiric use of standard antiarrhythmic drug therapies.[14–16] However, early application of this approach was unable to demonstrate a beneficial effect even when using historical controls. Furthermore, more recent descriptions[17–20] of the outcomes of VT/VF patients treated with empiric standard antiarrhythmic drug therapy indicate that the prognosis may actually be worsened by such therapy. For example,

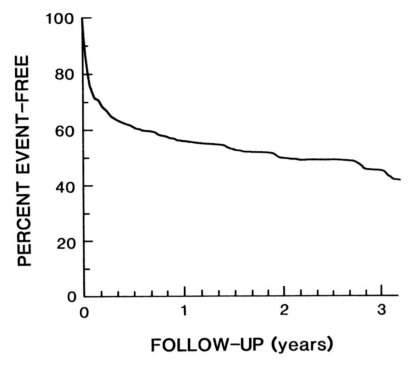

Figure 2. Actuarial probabilites of freedom from sudden death and sustained VT/VF (%) over 3 years of follow-up in patients with sustained VT/VF primarily treated with empiric standard antiarrhythmic drug therapy. Redrawn with permission from Willems AR, et al.[19]

Willems et al.[19] reported the arrhythmia recurrence/sudden death probabilities in a population of 390 patients with sustained VT or VF late (>48 hours) after myocardial infarction. Seventy-five percent of these patients were treated with empiric standard antiarrhythmic drugs alone (mostly class I agents). The 2-year arrhythmia recurrence/sudden death probability for the entire group was 49% (Figure 2), indistinguishable from that of the "untreated" control patient population previously presented by Cobb et al.[11] (Figure 1). Furthermore, the initial recurrence probabilities in the treated population were higher than those of the untreated population consistent with a proarrhythmic effect of empirically chosen standard antiarrhythmic drug therapies.

Given these observations, the use of empiric standard antiarrhythmic drug therapy for the prevention of VT/VF in high-risk patient populations has been abandoned.

Individualized Antiarrhythmic Drug Therapy

The failure of empirically chosen standard antiarrhythmic drug therapy prompted efforts to identify a reliable predictor of the ultimate efficacy of an antiarrhythmic drug regimen prior to trusting in its long-term use. Two potential approaches to the prediction of the ultimate efficacy of an antiarrhythmic drug treatment have now been described: a noninvasive (electrocardiographic monitoring) approach[21–25] and an invasive (electrophysiological study) approach.[26–30]

Each approach begins with the demonstration of an index of myocardial electrical instability in an antiarrhythmic drug-free state. Thereafter, antiarrhythmic drug therapy is predicted to be effective in long-term use by virtue of its ability to suppress the index of myocardial electrical instability.

The index of electrical instability used to guide the noninvasive approach is frequent, spontaneous ventricular premature beats. In general, an individual is considered to have sufficient ventricular ectopy to guide the noninvasive approach if 24-hour ambulatory electrocardiographic monitoring in an antiarrhythmic drug-free state demonstrates a mean of ≥30 ventricular premature beats per hour.[31,32] Thereafter, an antiarrhythmic therapy is initiated and, after steady state conditions have been reestablished, a drug assessment 24-hour ambulatory electrocardiographic examination is performed. Although the criteria used to accept a prediction of long-term antiarrhythmic drug efficacy vary, most investigators accept that the tested antiarrhythmic regimen will be effective if its use is associated with a decrease in the frequency of isolated ventricular premature beats of ≥80%, a decrease in the frequency of ventricular couplets by ≥90%, and the elimination of ventricular triplets or longer repetitive forms on both a drug assessment 24-hour ambulatory ECG and a drug assessment exercise tolerance test.[22–24,33] Therapy selected by the noninvasive approach has been demonstrated to be capable of identifying a patient-drug treatment combination with a low probability of arrhythmia recurrence/sudden death (Figure 3).[25] The index of electrical instability used to guide the invasive approach is the induction of the patient's sustained VT/VF by programmed stimulation during an electrophysiological study performed in an antiarrhythmic drug-free state. The ventricular arrhythmia that is most specific in its guidance of the invasive approach is the reproducible induction of sustained monomorphic VT.[34] Thereafter, an antiarrhythmic therapy is initiated and, after steady-state conditions have been reestablished, a drug assessment electrophysio-

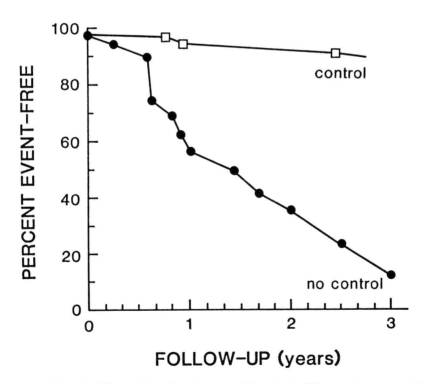

Figure 3. Actuarial probabilites of freedom from sudden death (%) over 3 years of follow-up in patients with hemodynamically compromising VT/VF treated with antiarrhythmic drugs predicted to be effective by the noninvasive approach (□ = control) or predicted to be ineffective by the noninvasive approach (• = no control). Redrawn with permission from Grayboys TB, et al.[25]

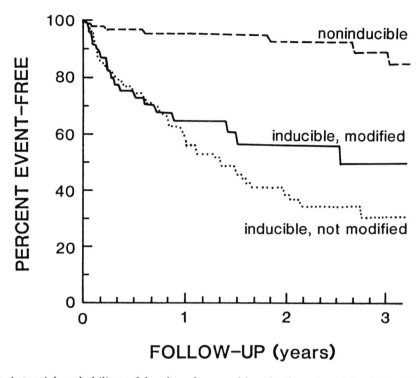

Figure 4. Actuarial probabilites of freedom from sudden death and sustained VT/VF (%) over 3 years of follow-up in patients with inducible sustained VT/VF treated with antiarrhythmic drugs predicted to be effective by the invasive approach (dashed line=noninducible) or predicted to be ineffective by the invasive approach with modification of the inducible VT/VF (solid line = inducible, modified) or without modification of the inducible VT/VF (dotted line = inducible, not modified). Redrawn with permission from Waller TJ, et al.[41]

logical study is performed. Although the criteria used to accept a prediction of long-term antiarrhythmic drug efficacy vary, most investigators accept that the tested antiarrhythmic regimen will be effective if its use is associated with the inability to induce more that four repetitive ventricular responses using up to three extrastimuli applied to the stimulation site that permitted the induction of sustained VT/VF at the baseline study.[30,35–40] Therapy selected by the invasive approach has been demonstrated to be capable of identifying a patient-drug treatment combination with a low probability of arrhythmia recurrence/sudden death (Figure 4).[41]

Empiric Amiodarone Therapy

Empiric amiodarone therapy has been used for the treatment of ventricular ar-

rhythmias since 1970.[42] Initially, this therapy was reserved for patients who had failed therapy with conventional antiarrhythmic drugs.[43–45] Nevertheless, follow-up studies of patients so treated demonstrated low arrhythmia recurrence/sudden death rates compared to historical controls (Figure 5).[43] Indeed, the antiarrhythmic effect of empiric amiodarone therapy was apparently comparable to that of an individualized standard antiarrhythmic therapy predicted to be effective by either the noninvasive or by the invasive approach. This benefit was particularly impressive given that patients subjected to empiric amiodarone therapy had already demonstrated a resistance to antiarrhythmic drug therapy. Early use of empiric amiodarone therapy was also characterized by the use of relatively high-maintenance dosages (>400 mg daily). At these dosages, amiodarone ther-

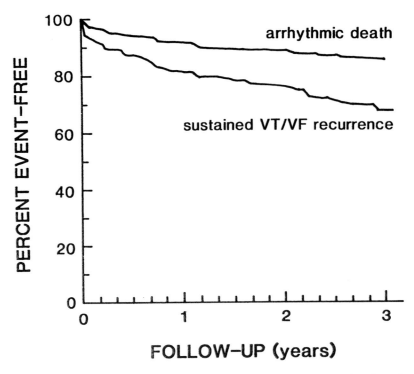

Figure 5. Actuarial probabilites of freedom from arrhythmic death and freedom from recurrent sustained VT/VF (%) over 3 years of follow-up in patients with sustained VT/VF treated with empiric amiodarone therapy. Redrawn with permission from Herre JM, et al.[43]

apy has a high probability of being associated with serious adverse effects.[46,47] Subsequent experience[48–50] with lower dosages (200–400 mg/day) has suggested that the frequency of adverse effects from amiodarone therapy can be substantially reduced without loss of the antiarrhythmic efficacy of the therapy.

Accumulated evidence supports the contention that the ultimate efficacy of amiodarone therapy in patients with VT/VF can be predicted by either the noninvasive approach[51–54] or invasive approach[51,53,55–59] to individualized antiarrhythmic drug therapy. Nevertheless, most practitioners use amiodarone empirically, a convention that began when amiodarone therapy was prescribed to VT/VF patients with no other therapeutic alternative and a prediction of therapeutic failure had no clinical value.

Empiric Beta-Blocking Drug Therapy

Isolated beta-blocking therapy for the prevention of arrhythmia recurrence/sudden death has been advocated for specific patient subgroups for many years. Those patients reported to benefit from such therapy are those with VT/VF occurring in the setting of mitral valve prolapse,[60] exercise,[61–63] acute myocardial infarction,[64–66] the long QT interval syndromes,[67] and in the absence of identifiable structural heart disease.[62,68,69]

More recently, Steinbeck et al.[70] evaluated the long-term antiarrhythmic efficacy of empiric beta-blocking drug therapy in 54 unselected patients with spontaneous VT/VF and inducible VT/VF who received metoprolol therapy as their only antiarrhythmic intervention. The metoprolol dosage was initially 25 mg twice a day and was then increased, as tolerated, to 100 mg twice a day. On follow-up, the 2-year probability of arrhythmia recurrence/sudden death in the patients so treated was approximately 45% (Figure 6), indistinguishable from that of historical, untreated patient populations. Accordingly, isolated empiric beta-blocking drug therapy is not commonly used to prevent VT/VF recurrences in this patient population. Instead, isolated beta-blocking antiarrhythmic therapy for VT/VF patients requires an efficacy prediction from either the noninvasive approach[71-73] or the invasive approach[74-76] to individualized antiarrhythmic drug therapy.

Nevertheless, there is evidence to support the ancillary use of beta-blocking drug therapy in addition to specific antiarrhythmic therapy in VT/VF patients. First, many patients with VT/VF have sustained a remote myocardial infarction and there are numerous reports of a reduction in the follow-up probability of sudden death in post-myocardial infarction patients who are prescribed empiric beta-blocking drug therapy.[77-81] Second, the electrophysiological effects and antiarrhythmic benefits afforded by individualized standard antiarrhythmic drug therapy may be overcome by sufficient beta-adrenergic stimulation.[82] Third, measurements of total and cardiac norepinephrine spillover into plasma suggest that patients with sustained ventricular tachyarrhythmias have a selective increase in arrhythmogenic cardiac sympathetic activity.[83] Thus, the efficacy of individualized standard antiarrhythmic drug therapy may be enhanced by the concomitant administration of a beta-blocking drug.[84-86] Evidence of this advantage comes from a retrospective multivariate analysis by Leclercq et al.[20] Patients with sustained VT and left ventricular ejection fractions <30% treated

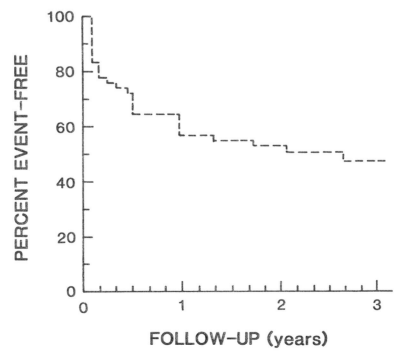

Figure 6. Actuarial probabilites of freedom from sudden death and sustained VT/VF (%) over 3 years of follow-up in patients with sustained VT/VF or syncope with inducible VT/VF treated with empiric metoprolol therapy. Redrawn with permission from Steinbeck G, et al.[70]

with a variety of empiric antiarrhythmic therapies whose therapy included a beta-blocking drug had a lower 2-year actuarial cardiac mortality probability (approximately 9%) than did those whose therapy did not include a beta-blocking drug (approximately 34%) (P<0.01).

Comparisons of Pharmacological Therapies

Empiric standard antiarrhythmic drug therapy was compared to other therapeutic approaches in the Cardiac Arrest Study Hamburg (CASH).[87] This study randomized patients who had been resuscitated from a VF cardiac arrest to receive empiric propafenone therapy, empiric beta-blocking drug therapy, empiric amiodarone therapy, or an ICD. Although CASH continues, an interim report[87] after an average follow-up of 11 months indicated that patients assigned to empiric propafenone therapy (n=56) were experiencing recurrent cardiac arrest and all-cause mortality at rates that were higher that those of patients assigned to one of the other three study therapies. Accordingly, the use of empiric propafenone in CASH was stopped and the electrophysiological community has accepted that empiric standard antiarrhythmic drug therapy for patients with VT/VF is inappropriate.

Two randomized clinical trials have now compared the long-term efficacy of therapy selected for VT/VF patients by the noninvasive and the invasive approaches to individualized standard antiarrhythmic drug therapy. The study of Mitchell et al.[39,88] randomized 57 patients with spontaneous sustained VT/VF. To participate patients must not have previously failed individualized antiarrhythmic drug therapy, had to have ≥30 ventricular premature beats per hour on a baseline antiarrhythmic drug-free 24-hour ambulatory electrocardiographic monitoring examination, and had to have sustained VT induced by programmed stimulation at a baseline antiarrhythmic

drug-free electrophysiological study. The results of an on-treatment analysis of the follow-up data of that study are shown in Figure 7.[88] The 2-year probability of arrhythmia recurrence/sudden death for patients receiving standard antiarrhythmic drug therapy predicted to be effective by the invasive approach (7%) was significantly better than was that predicted to be effective by the noninvasive approach (47%) (P=0.02). Furthermore, the 2-year probability of arrhythmia recurrence/sudden death for patients receiving therapy predicted to be effective by the noninvasive approach was indistinguishable from that of historical untreated control populations. The Electrophysiologic Study Versus Electrocardiographic Monitoring (ESVEM) study[40,89] reached a very different conclusion. The ESVEM study randomized 486 patients with spontaneous sustained VT/VF (or unexplained syncope with inducible sustained VT) who had an average of ≥10 ventricular premature beats per hour on a baseline antiarrhythmic drug-free 48-hour ambulatory electrocardiographic monitoring study and who had sustained VT (or VF if the presenting rhythm was VF) induced by programmed stimulation at a baseline antiarrhythmic drug-free electrophysiological study. The results of an on-treatment analysis of the follow-up data of the ESVEM study are shown in Figure 8.[89] The 2-year probability of arrhythmia recurrence/sudden death for patients receiving standard antiarrhythmic drug therapy predicted to be effective by the invasive approach (47%) was no different than that of patients receiving standard antiarrhythmic drug therapy predicted to be effective by the noninvasive approach (51%). Furthermore, the 2-year probabilities of arrhythmia recurrence/sudden death for both patient groups were indistinguishable from that of historical untreated control populations. The major difference between the study of Mitchell et al. and the ESVEM trial was in the outcome of patients receiving therapy that was predicted to be effective by the invasive approach. The poor performance of therapy

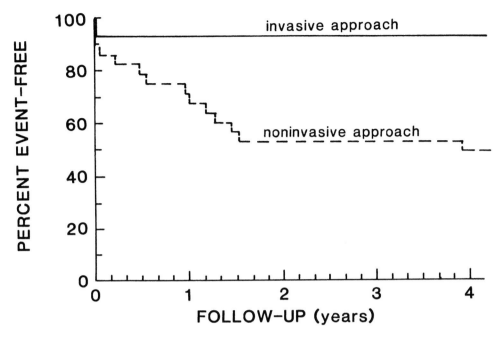

Figure 7. Actuarial probabilites of freedom from sudden death and sustained VT/VF (%) over 4 years of follow-up in patients with symptomatic VT/VF randomly assigned to antiarrhythmic drug treatment predicted to be effective by the invasive approach (solid line) or to treatment predicted to be effective by the noninvasive approach (dashed line). Redrawn with permission from Mitchell LB, et al.[88]

predicted to be effective by the invasive approach in the ESVEM study was likely the result of the combined influences of use of lax criteria for the definition of predicted effective therapy, the enrollment of a drug-resistant patient population, and the enrollment of patients with inducible VF as opposed to inducible VT. A comparative study[90] has now shown that the use of more standard criteria for the definition of predicted effective therapy than those used in the ESVEM trial are associated with more accurate efficacy predictions. Furthermore, it is now evident[91] that patients with demonstrated drug resistance have a higher probability of failure of predicted effective antiarrhythmic drug therapy than do patients without demonstrated drug resistance. These considerations support the conclusion that standard antiarrhythmic drug therapy selected by the invasive approach better prevents arrhythmia recurrence/sudden death than does that selected

by the noninvasive approach in patients who do not have demonstrated antiarrhythmic drug resistance. A substudy of the ESVEM trial randomized the order of antiarrhythmic drug trials.[92] Subsequent analysis of the combined probabilities of predicting that a specific antiarrhythmic drug would be predicted to be effective at baseline, would prove to be effective during follow-up, and would be well tolerated by the patient favored sotalol over the other standard antiarrhythmic drugs used in ESVEM (imipramine, mexiletine, pirmenol, procainamide, propafenone, and quinidine).

Steinbeck et al.[70] have compared the long-term efficacy of empiric beta-blocking drug therapy to that of individualized standard antiarrhythmic drug therapy predicted to be effective by the invasive approach. Patients were included if they had documented, sustained VT/VF or unexplained syncope. Randomization required that a baseline, antiarrhythmic drug-free electro-

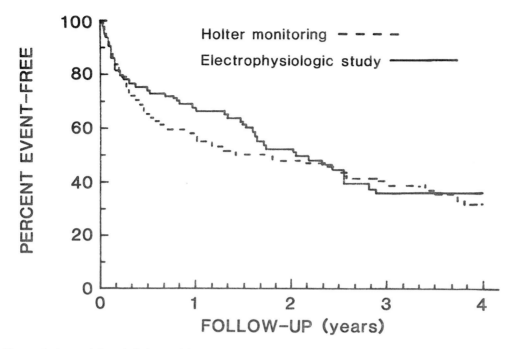

Figure 8. Actuarial probabilites of freedom from VT of >15 beats duration, VF, torsade de pointes, unmonitored syncope, cardiac arrest, or death caused by arrhythmia over 4 years of follow-up of VT/VF patients randomly assigned to antiarrhythmic drug treatment predicted to be effective by the invasive approach (solid line) or to treatment predicted to be effective by the noninvasive approach (dashed line). Redrawn with permission from Mason JW, et al.[89]

physiological study reproducibly induce at least 20 consecutive beats of VT or VF. Fifty-four patients were randomized to empiric metoprolol therapy (25 mg twice daily increased, as tolerated, to 100 mg twice daily) and 61 patients were randomized to receive standard antiarrhythmic drug therapy selected by the invasive approach. Interestingly, the most common standard antiarrhythmic drug to be predicted effective in this study was also a beta-blocking drug sotalol. An intention-to-treat analysis was presented as evidence that the follow-up probabilities of arrhythmia recurrence/sudden death were equivalent for the two randomized groups (Figure 9)[70] However, the 2-year arrhythmia recurrence/sudden death probabilities associated with empiric metoprolol therapy (52%) and associated with individualized standard antiarrhythmic drug therapy selected by the invasive approach (44%) were indistinguishable from that of historical untreated control populations. However, this result is the consequence of an inappropriate devotion to the intention-to-treat maxim. Fifty-two percent of the patients randomized to receive individualized standard antiarrhythmic drug therapy selected by the invasive approach actually received therapy that the approach predicted would be ineffective after no predicted effective therapy could be found. An on-treatment analysis reveals that the 2-year probability of arrhythmia recurrence/sudden death was lowest in patients who received standard antiarrhythmic drug therapy that the invasive approach predicted would be effective (21%), was intermediate for empiric metoprolol therapy (52%), and was highest in patients who received standard antiarrhythmic drug therapy that the invasive approach predicted would be ineffective (66%). These data lead to the conclusion that standard antiarrhythmic drug therapy predicted to be effective by the invasive approach prevents arrhythmia recurrence/ sudden death better than does empiric beta-blocking therapy.

The Cardiac Arrest in Seattle: Conventional versus Amiodarone Drug Evaluation (CASCADE) study[93,94] compared the follow-up outcomes of patients with out-of-hospital VF cardiac arrests who received empiric amiodarone therapy to those who received individualized standard antiarrhythmic drug therapy. One hundred thirteen patients were randomized to receive empiric amiodarone therapy (1,200 mg/day for up to 10 days, then 200–800 mg daily for 1 to 2 months depending on tolerance, and then a maintenance dosage of 100–400 mg daily). One hundred fifteen patients were randomized to receive standard antiarrhythmic drug therapy selected by the invasive ap-

proach or, if the invasive approach was not applicable or not successful, by the noninvasive approach. During the course of CASCADE the sudden death mortality was sufficiently high that the investigators felt the need to use an ICD in each participant. Thus, the primary outcome variable in CASCADE, termed cardiac survival, was the composite endpoint of complete syncope followed by an ICD shock, documented VT/VF, and cardiac mortality. The actuarial probabilities of this composite endpoint were lower in patients who received empiric amiodarone therapy than they were in patients treated with individualized standard antiarrhythmic drug therapy ($P = 0.007$) (Figure 10).[94] Nevertheless, these results do not support the contention that empiric amiodarone therapy is superior to properly chosen individualized standard antiarrhythmic drug

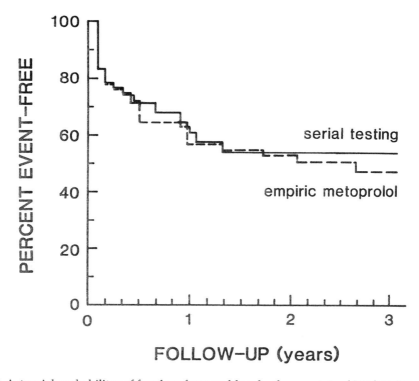

Figure 9. Actuarial probabilites of freedom from sudden death or sustained VT/VF (%) over 3 years of follow-up in patients with sustained VT/VF or syncope with inducible VT/VF randomly assigned to antiarrhythmic drug treatment selected by the invasive approach (48% on predicted effective therapy, 52% on empiric therapy after failure to find predicted effective therapy (solid line = serial testing), or to treatment with empiric metoprolol therapy (dashed line). Redrawn with permission from Steinbeck G, et al.[70]

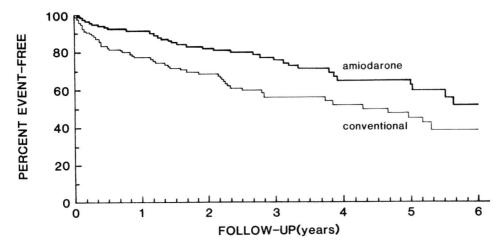

Figure 10. Actuarial probabilites of freedom from cardiac mortality, complete syncope followed by an ICD shock, or resuscitated cardiac arrest recurrence (%) over 6 years of follow-up in patients resuscitated from cardiac arrest randomly assigned to treatment with empiric amiodarone (heavy line) or to treatment with conventional antiarrhythmic drugs individualized by the invasive approach if applicable and successful or by the noninvasive approach (solid line). Redrawn with permission from The Cascade Investigators.[94]

therapy. First, individualized standard antiarrhythmic drug therapy was selected by one or the other of the invasive and noninvasive approaches. Arguments presented above have already indicated that the invasive approach selects standard antiarrhythmic drug therapy that better prevents arrhythmia recurrence/sudden death than does that selected by the noninvasive approach. More importantly, CASCADE is another example of a trial report with an inappropriate devotion to the intention-to-treat maxim. A substantial number of patients in the individualized standard antiarrhythmic drug therapy group actually received antiarrhythmic drug therapy that the last assessment approach used predicted would be ineffective—39% of patients receiving therapy selected by the invasive approach and 44% of patients receiving therapy selected by the noninvasive approach. To date, no comparison of empiric amiodarone therapy and standard antiarrhythmic therapy *predicted to be effective* by the either the invasive approach or the noninvasive approach has been reported.

Comparisons with Nonpharmacological Therapies

Nonpharmacological therapies with potential for efficacy in the treatment of patients with VT/VF include operative or transcatheter ablation/isolation of the arrhythmogenic substrate and use of an ICD.

A propensity to VT may be cured by ablation or electrical isolation of the arrhythmogenic ventricular substrate during open-heart surgery,[95,96] by catheter approaches to the direct endocardial application of destructive energy sources,[97,98] and by catheter approaches to the indirect transcoronary application of destructive materials.[99,100] To date, there have been no direct comparisons of electrosurgical or transcatheter ablative therapies to any form of pharmacological therapy. Nevertheless, the concept of cure for the patient with VT remains very attractive. Despite the absence of comparative trials, this form of therapy is already established as the preferred treatment modality for many patients with idiopathic right ventricular outflow tract VT,[101] for patients with idiopathic left septal VT,[102] and for patients with bundle branch reentrant VT.[103] Given recent developments in electrosurgical and transcatheter ablation techniques for patients with VT in patients with coronary heart disease these techniques still hold future promise of being highly effective, curative therapies in this setting.

The final treatment approach for patients with a demonstrated propensity to VT/VF is use of the ICD.[104–106] There is now substantial evidence that the ICD is the most effective form of therapy for most patients with life-threatening ventricular tachyarrhythmias. Of course, the ICD in its present form does not prevent episodes of VT/VF from occurring. Instead, it reacts to their presence with either pacing or DC shock therapies that terminate the VT/VF and restore normal heart rhythm. Accordingly, the measure of efficacy of ICD therapy is the prevention of sudden cardiac death and all-cause mortality.[107] Many early reports[104–106] of the follow-up course of VT/VF patients treated with an ICD showed actuarial probabilities of sudden death that were much better than either those of historical untreated control populations or those of pharmacologically treated patient populations, so much better as to suggest that either ICD is substantially better than pharmacological therapies[108,109] or to suggest that ICD recipients were drawn from a different patient population than previous studies.[110,111]

The initial comparative studies of pharmacological therapy and ICD therapy for patients with VT/VF used nonrandomized controls.[112–114] Fogoros et al.[112] described the outcomes of two VT/VF patient populations from the University of Pittsburgh. Patients in both groups presented with VT/VF associated with hemodynamic compromise or cardiac arrest and did not respond to treatment with standard antiarrhythmic drugs. Twenty-one patients in one group received empiric amiodarone therapy and an ICD while 29 patients in the other group received empiric amiodarone therapy alone during a time period when ICDs were tem-

porarily unavailable. The 2-year actuarial probability of sudden death was higher in those patients treated with amiodarone alone (31%) than in those patients treated with amiodarone and an ICD (0%) ($P<0.003$). Pinski et al.[113] described the outcomes of two VT/VF patient populations from the Cleveland Clinic—62 patients in one group received an ICD while 15 patients in the other group did not (having refused the recommended ICD therapy). All but one of the patients in the latter group received empiric amiodarone therapy. In this study, the 18-month actuarial probabilities of death from any cause were similar in the ICD and no ICD groups (16% and 22%, respectively). Newman et al.[114] reported the first matched case-controlled study comparing outcomes of VT/VF patients treated with empiric amiodarone therapy to those of patients treated with an ICD at Moffitt Hospital, University of California, San Francisco. Sixty VT/VF patients treated with an ICD were matched (age, left ventricular ejection fraction, type of structural heart disease, presenting arrhythmia, drug therapy status) to 120 control VT/VF patients who did not receive an ICD. The majority of patients (68%) in the latter group received empiric amiodarone therapy and the remainder (32%) received standard antiarrhythmic drugs individualized by either the noninvasive or the invasive approach. The 2-year actuarial probability of death from any cause in the patient group receiving an ICD (approximately 20%) was lower that that of the patient group not receiving an ICD (approximately 40%) ($P<0.01$). More recently, Böcker et al.[115] reported a matched case-controlled study that compared the outcomes of VT/VF patients treated with an ICD to that of patients treated with sotalol that had been predicted to be effective by the invasive approach to individualized standard antiarrhythmic drug therapy. Fifty VT/VF patients treated with an ICD after demonstrated drug resistance were matched (age, gender, left ventricular ejection fraction, extent of coronary disease, presenting arrhythmia, and year of treatment) to 50 case-control VT/VF patients who received sotalol therapy that was predicted to be effective by the invasive approach. The 2-year actuarial probability of death from any cause in the patient group receiving an ICD (11%) was lower that that of the patient group receiving individualized sotalol therapy (26%) ($P = 0.02$).

Theoretical considerations[110] suggest that, in an average group of VT/VF patients that are eligible for either ICD therapy or for pharmacological therapy, the maximum benefit from ICD therapy is unlikely to be greater than a 33% reduction in all-cause mortality. Nevertheless, these comparisons of ICD therapy and pharmacological therapy reported a much larger benefit to ICD use than should be possible. Fogoros et al.[112] reported a relative risk reduction for all-cause mortality of 87%, Newman et al.[114] reported a relative risk reduction for all-cause mortality of 56%, and Böcker et al.[115] reported a relative risk reduction for all-cause mortality of 57%. The discrepancies between these reported relative risk reductions and the theoretical maximum advantage of ICD therapy suggest that factors other than ICD use contributed to the reported benefits. The most likely explanation is that the subjects who received ICD therapy in these nonrandomized studies were drawn from a different patient population than were the subjects who received pharmacological therapy.

To study the relative efficacies of ICD therapy and pharmacological therapy in a manner free from potential bias in the distribution of patients between therapeutic approaches, randomized studies were required. Accordingly, three randomized clinical trials of ICD therapy versus pharmacological therapy were begun. The CASH[87] study started in 1987 and continues with its (now) three-way comparison of empiric amiodarone therapy, empiric beta-blocking therapy, and ICD therapy. The Canadian Implantable Defibrillator Study (CIDS)[116] started in 1990 and continues with its two-way comparison of empiric amiodarone therapy and ICD therapy. The Anti-

arrhythmics Versus Implantable Defibrillators (AVID)[117,118] trial started in 1993. In 1997, the Data and Safety Monitoring Committee recommended that the AVID trial be terminated as it had demonstrated that the ICD reduced all-cause mortality in comparison to pharmacological therapy. The AVID trial enrolled patients who had been resuscitated from VF and patients with severely symptomatic sustained VT provided the left ventricular ejection fraction was ≤0.40. VT/VF patients with class IV heart failure symptoms were excluded. At the time that the AVID trial was terminated, 1,016 patients had been randomized. Five hundred seven patients were assigned to treatment with an ICD (93% using a nonthoracotomy lead system) and 509 patients were assigned to pharmacological therapy (97% received empiric amiodarone therapy and the remainder received individualized sotalol therapy predicted to be effective by either the invasive or the noninvasive approach). The 2-year actuarial probability of death from any cause in the patient group receiving an ICD (18%) was lower than that of the patient group receiving pharmacological therapy (25%) (relative risk reduction 27%) ($P<0.02$) (Figure 11).[118] On average, ICD therapy resulted in an unadjusted survival advantage of 3.2 months after 3 years of use. Preliminary analysis indicates that this survival advantage was associated with an average incremental cost of greater than $27,500 for a cost per year of life saved of more than $100,000.[119] Unfortunately, if this preliminary analysis is correct, the cost per year of life saved by ICD therapy will be beyond the financial reach of many jurisdictions. Of course, it is probable that subgroup analyses will produce identifiable subgroups with greater advantage at lesser cost. However, the early termination of the AVID trial has reduced the population numbers available for subgroup analysis. Hopefully, this shortcoming will be rectified by the addition of patients that were enrolled in CASH and in CIDS when these studies report their findings in the near future.

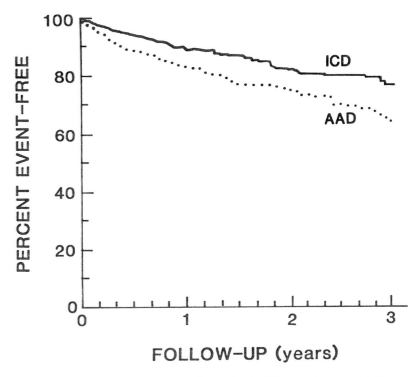

Figure 11. Actuarial probabilites of freedom from death (%) over 4 years of follow-up in patients resuscitated from VF and patients with severely symptomatic VT with a left ventricular ejection fraction <0.40 randomly assigned to receive antiarrhythmic drug treatment (97% empiric amiodarone, 3% sotalol therapy predicted to be effective by either the invasive approach or the noninvasive approach) (dotted line = AAD) or to receive an ICD (solid line = ICD). Redrawn with permission from The AVID Investigators.[118]

Meanwhile, supportive evidence that ICD therapy reduces all-cause mortality in comparison to pharmacological therapy comes from review of the prophylactic ICD trials that have been published to date. The Multicenter Automatic Defibrillator Implantation Trial (MADIT)[120–122] enrolled 196 patients with coronary heart disease, previous myocardial infarction, left ventricular ejection fraction ≤0.35, documented asymptomatic unsustained VT, and inducible sustained VT/VF at an electrophysiologic study. If sustained VT remained inducible after the intravenous administration of procainamide the subjects were randomized to receive a prophylactic ICD or to be treated in a "conventional" manner as determined by each patient's attending physician. Patients with functional class IV congestive heart failure symptoms were ex-

cluded from participation. Thirty days after randomization, most patients (74%) in the conventional therapy group were receiving amiodarone therapy. The remaining patients were receiving a class I antiarrhythmic drug (10%), a standard beta-blocking drug (8%), sotalol (8%), or no specific antiarrhythmic drug therapy (8%). By the end of the trial, 45% of the patients in the conventional therapy group were receiving amiodarone therapy. The remainder were receiving a class I antiarrhythmic drug (11%), a standard beta-blocking drug (5%), sotalol (9%) or no specific antiarrhythmic drug therapy (23%). The 2-year actuarial probability of death from any cause was lower in the 95 patients who received ICD therapy (approximately 13%) than in the 101 patients who received "conventional" therapy (32%) (P<0.009). Given that failure of procainamide therapy to prevent the induction of VT/VF predicts failure of other standard antiarrhythmic drugs,[123] the MADIT actually compared ICD therapy to antiarrhythmic drug therapy in patients known to be resistant to antiarrhythmic drug therapy. Accordingly, the results are not surprising. However, the relative risk reduction for all-cause mortality associated with ICD therapy was 59%. As discussed above, a relative risk reduction of this magnitude does not fit well with our understanding of relative cause-specific mortality rates in this sort of patient population. In MADIT the relative risk reduction for death from noncardiac or unknown causes (65%) was almost as large as the relative risk reduction for arrhythmic death (75%). Although this and other shortcomings of the MADIT have been well described,[124] most practitioners have accepted the conclusion that patients with nonsustained VT in the setting of coronary heart disease and depressed left ventricular function who have inducible sustained VT/VF and demonstrated drug resistance will benefit from ICD therapy. Indeed, the MADIT indication for ICD therapy has been accepted by the Food and Drug Administration.

The Coronary Artery Bypass Graft Patch (CABG-Patch) trial[125,126] evaluated the outcomes of patients undergoing coronary artery bypass surgery selected to be at high risk of future VT/VF episodes by virtue of left ventricular ejection fractions ≤0.35 and a positive preoperative signal-averaged ECG. The CABG-Patch trial ultimately randomized 900 patients to receive or not to receive a prophylactic epicardial patch ICD at the time of their coronary artery bypass procedure. Although the CABG-Patch trial was much larger than MADIT (coincidentally, the CABG-Patch trial had the same number of death endpoints as the MADIT had randomized patients), use of an ICD was not associated with a survival advantage. The 2-year actuarial probability of death from any cause was approximately 18% in both randomized patient groups. The very different results of the CABG-

Patch trial and of the MADIT are likely the combined result of the selection of a study population at a lesser risk of follow-up VT/VF in the CABG-Patch trial (using the signal-averaged ECG) than in the MADIT (using drug-resistant inducible sustained VT/VF) and the antiarrhythmic effect of coronary bypass graft surgery[127–130] being applied in the CABG-Patch trial but not in the MADIT. In any event, the results of the MADIT, that enrolled patients with inducible sustained VT/VF, are likely to be more relevant to the patient population with spontaneous sustained VT/VF considered in this review.

Where Are We Now?

The patient who has experienced an episode of sustained VT/VF may well require acute antiarrhythmic drug therapy for stabilization. Unless the VT/VF episode was the result of transient cause (such as that occurring in the 48 hours of an acute myocardial infarction) or was the result of a reversible cause (such as that occurring secondary to electrolyte disturbances, acid-base disturbances or proarrhythmic drug effects) a long-term specific antiarrhythmic therapy will also be required. Nevertheless, most VT/VF patients will benefit from one or more ancillary antiarrhythmic therapies such as beta-blocking drug therapy,[20,77–86] revascularization,[127–130] ASA therapy,[131] ACE inhibitor therapy,[132] or risk factor modification.[133,134]

In considering specific antiarrhythmic therapy for long-term use in these patients, arguments presented above indicate that the dominant therapies are ICD therapy, empiric amiodarone therapy, and individualized standard antiarrhythmic drug therapy (often sotalol therapy) that is predicted to be effective by the invasive approach.

When a patient's characteristics suggest a high risk of sudden cardiac death, especially in the absence of competing risks for premature death, ICD therapy has the advantage over currently available pharmacological therapies. Nevertheless, ICD therapy is expensive. Given that the major drivers of the cost of ICD therapy are the cost of the device itself and the hospital costs related to its implantation,[135,136] the cost-effectiveness of ICD therapy will be improved by reduction in the cost of the device and reduction in the duration and complexity of the hospitalization required for ICD implantation and impluse generator changes. Patients with a high probability of early death from nonarrhythmic causes are unlikely to benefit from ICD therapy in comparison to pharmacological therapy. Patients in this category may include those with functional class IV congestive heart failure symptoms and those with lethal noncardiac disorders. In such patients, the simplicity of empiric amiodarone therapy recommends its use.

When a patient's characteristics suggest a low risk of sudden death, hemodynamically stable VT without demonstrated drug resistance, ICD therapy has not been demonstrated to be superior to pharmacological therapy. A few of these patients will be amenable to cure by electrosurgery or catheter ablation of the arrhythmogenic substrate. Nevertheless, the majority of these patients will present a choice between empiric amiodarone therapy and individualized antiarrhythmic drug therapy predicted to be effective by the invasive approach. This choice is usually made by consideration of the relative advantages and disadvantages of the two therapeutic approaches. The major advantage of empiric amiodarone therapy is its initial simplicity. The major advantage of individualized standard antiarrhythmic drug therapy predicted to be effective by the invasive approach is the opportunity to avoid the adverse effect profile of long-term amiodarone therapy. Which of these two treatment alternatives is superior when both are applicable remains unknown.

Pharmacological therapy also plays an important role as an adjunct to ICD therapy in high-risk patients. Neither the routine use of empiric standard antiarrhythmic

drug therapy[137] nor the routine use of empiric amiodarone therapy[137,138] is warranted for the average patient who has received an ICD for the treatment of VT/VF. Nevertheless, patients who are experiencing frequent interactions between themselves and their device often require antiarrhythmic drug therapy either to reduce the frequency of VT/VF episodes or to prevent inappropriate ICD therapies from being delivered for sinus tachycardia or supraventricular tachyarrhythmias. Indeed, most of the early descriptive studies of the follow-up course of VT/VF patients who had received an ICD as their primary antiarrhythmic therapy reported that adjunctive antiarrhythmic drug therapy was required for more than 50% of patients.[106,139] Nevertheless, with increasing sophistication of ICD diagnostic capabilities, the frequency of use of adjunctive antiarrhythmic drug therapy in ICD patients has been decreasing.[140] The most recently proposed adjunctive pharmacological therapy for VT/VF patients who have received an ICD is that which reduces defibrillation energy requirements. Empiric sotalol therapy has been shown to decrease defibrillation energy requirements in both animal models[141] and in humans[142] and may be useful in this regard.

Where Do We Go from Here?

All other things being equal, an effective preventative therapy for VT/VF is superior to an effective reactive therapy. However, at present the best available reactive therapy for patients with VT/VF (the ICD) is more effective than are the best available preventative therapies (pharmacological therapies, electrosurgical, or transcatheter ablative/isolation therapies). However, this may not always be so. The challenge for preventative therapies is to improve to the point where their efficacy relative to the primary objective of VT/VF prevention is equal to or superior to the standard that has been set by ICD therapy relative to the secondary goal of preventing death from VT/VF when it does occur.

In the interim, pharmacological therapies still play an important role in the treatment of VT/VF patients, as acute antiarrhythmic therapy during periods of VT/VF destabilization, as primary antiarrhythmic therapy for patients at low risk of fatal VT/VF events, as primary antiarrhythmic therapy for patients with very high competing risks of death from causes unrelated to their VT/VF, and as adjunctive therapy for patients treated with an ICD who are experiencing frequent interactions between themselves and their device.

References

1. Strauss MB. Paroxysmal ventricular tachycardia. Am J Med Sci 1930;179:337.
2. Lundy CJ, McLellan LL. Paroxysmal ventricular tachycardia: an etiological study with special reference to the type. Ann Intern Med 1934;7:812.
3. Williams C, Ellis LB. Ventricular tachycardia: an analysis of thirty-six cases. Arch Intern Med 1943;71:137.
4. Trevor Cooke W, White PD. Paroxysmal ventricular tachycardia. Br Heart J 1943;5:33.
5. Herrmann GR, Hejtmancik MR. A clinical and electrocardiographic study of paroxysmal ventricular tachycardia and its management. Ann Intern Med 1948;28:989.
6. Armbrust CA Jr, Levine SA. Paroxysmal ventricular tachycardia: a study of one hundred and seven cases. Circulation 1950;1:28.
7. Herrmann GR, Park HM, Hejtmancik MR. Paroxysmal ventricular tachycardia: a clinical and electrocardiographic study. Am Heart J 1959;57:166.
8. Liberthson RR, Nagel EL, Hirschman JC, et al. Prehospital ventricular fibrillation: prognosis and follow-up course. N Engl J Med 1974;291:317.
9. Baum RS, Alvarez H III, Cobb LA. Survival after resuscitation from out-of-hospital ventricular fibrillation. Circulation 1974;50:1231.
10. Schaffer WA, Cobb LA. Recurrent ventricular fibrillation and modes of death in survivors of out-of-hospital ventricular fibrillation. N Engl J Med 1975;293:259.
11. Cobb LA, Baum RS, Alvarez H III, et al. Resuscitation from out-of-hospital ventricular fibrillation: 4 years of follow-up. Circulation 1975;52(Suppl III):III-223.
12. Leitch JW, Gillis AM, Wyse DG, et al. Reduction in defibrillator shocks with an implantable device combining antitachycardia pacing and shock delivery. J Am Coll Cardiol 1991;18:145.
13. Bardy GH, Hofer B, Johnson G, et al. Implantable transvenous cardioverter-defibrillators. Circulation 1993;87:1152.
14. Myerburg RJ, Conde C, Sheps DS, et al. Antiarrhythmic drug therapy in survivors of prehospital cardiac arrest: comparison of effects on chronic ventricular arrhythmias and recurrent cardiac arrest. Circulation 1979;59:855.
15. Myerburg RJ, Kessler KM, Estes D, et al. Long-term survival after prehospital cardiac arrest: analysis of outcomes during an 8 year study. Circulation 1984;70:538.
16. Vlay SC, Reid PR, Griffith LSC, et al. Relationship of specific coronary lesions and regional left ventricular dysfunction to prognosis in survivors of sudden cardiac death. Am Heart J 1984;108:1212.
17. Goldstein S, Landis JR, Leighton R, et al. Predictive survival models for resuscitated victims of out-of-hospital cardiac arrest with coronary heart disease. Circulation 1985;71:873.
18. Moosvi AR, Goldstein S, VanderBrug Medendorp S, et al. Effect of empiric antiarrhythmic therapy in resuscitated out-of-hospital cardiac arrest victims with coronary artery disease. Am J Cardiol 1990;65:1192.
19. Willems AR, Tijssen JGP, van Capelle FJL, et al. Determinants of prognosis in symptomatic ventricular tachycardia or ventricular fibrillation late after myocardial infarction. J Am Coll Cardiol 1990;16:521.
20. Leclercq J-F, Coumel P, Denjoy I. Long-term follow-up after sustained monomorphic ventricular tachycardia: causes, pump failure, and empiric antiarrhythmic drug therapy that modify survival. Am Heart J 1991;121:1685.
21. Winkle RA, Alderman EL, Fitzgerald JW, et al. Treatment of recurrent symptomatic ventricular tachycardia. Ann Intern Med 1976;85:1.
22. Lown B, Graboys TB. Management of patients with malignant ventricular arrhythmias. Am J Cardiol 1977;39:910.

23. Lown B. Sudden cardiac death: the major challenge confronting contemporary cardiology. Am J Cardiol 1979;43:313.

24. Lown B. Management of patients at high risk of sudden death. Am Heart J 1982;103: 689.

25. Graboys TB, Lown B, Podrid PJ, et al. Long-term survival of patients with malignant ventricular arrhythmia treated with antiarrhythmic drugs. Am J Cardiol 1982;50:437.

26. Wu D, Wyndham CR, Denes P, et al. Chronic electrophysiological study in patients with recurrent paroxysmal tachycardia: a new method for developing successful oral antiarrhythmic therapy. In Kulbertus HE, ed. Reentrant Arrhythmia: Mechanisms and Treatment. MTP Press Limited, Lancaster, PA, 1977, p 294.

27. Hartzler GO, Maloney JD. Programmed ventricular stimulation in management of recurrent ventricular tachycardia. Mayo Clin Proc 1977;152:731.

28. Fisher JD, Cohen HL, Mehra R, et al. Cardiac pacing and pacemakers II. Serial electrophysiologic-pharmacologic testing for control of recurrent tachyarrhythmias. Am Heart J 1977;93:658.

29. Horowitz LN, Josephson ME, Farshidi A, et al. Recurrent sustained ventricular tachycardia 3. Role of the electrophysiologic study in selection of antiarrhythmic regimens. Circulation 1978;58:986.

30. Mason JW, Winkle RA. Electrode-catheter arrhythmia induction in the selection and assessment of antiarrhythmic drug therapy for recurrent ventricular tachycardia. Circulation 1978;58:971.

31. Morganroth J, Michelson EL, Horowitz LN, et al. Limitations of routine long-term electrocardiographic monitoring to assess ventricular ectopic frequency. Circulation 1978;58:408.

32. Swerdlow CD, Peterson J. Prospective comparison of Holter monitoring and electrophysiologic study in patients with coronary disease and sustained ventricular tachyarrhythmias. Am J Cardiol 1985;56:577.

33. Hohnloser SH, Raeder EA, Podrid PJ, et al. Predictors of antiarrhythmic drug efficacy in patients with malignant ventricular tachyarrhythmias. Am Heart J 1987;114:1.

34. Brugada P, Green M, Abdollah H, et al. Significance of ventricular arrhythmia initiated by programmed ventricular stimulation: the importance of the type of ventricular arrhythmia induced and the number of premature stimuli required. Circulation 1984;69:87.

35. Mason JW, Winkle RA. Accuracy of the ventricular tachycardia-induction study for predicting long-term efficacy and inefficacy of antiarrhythmic drugs. N Engl J Med 1980;303:1073.

36. Swerdlow CD, Winkle RA, Mason JW. Determinants of survival in patients with ventricular tachyarrhythmias. N Engl J Med 1983;308:1436.

37. Morady F, Scheinman MM, Hess DS, et al. Electrophysiologic testing in the management of out-of-hospital cardiac arrest. Am J Cardiol 1983;51:85.

38. Ruskin JN, Schoenfeld MH, Garan H. Role of electrophysiologic techniques in the selection of antiarrhythmic drug regimens for ventricular tachyarrhythmias. Am J Cardiol 1983;52:41C.

39. Mitchell LB, Duff HJ, Manyari DE, et al. A randomized clinical trial of the noninvasive and invasive approaches to drug therapy of ventricular tachycardia. N Engl J Med 1987; 317:1681.

40. The ESVEM Investigators. The ESVEM trial: electrophysiologic study versus electrocardiographic monitoring for selection of antiarrhythmic therapy of ventricular tachyarrhythmias. Circulation 1989;79: 1354.

41. Waller TJ, Kay HR, Spielman SR, et al. Reduction in sudden death and total mortality by antiarrhythmic therapy evaluated by electrophysiologic drug testing: criteria of efficacy in patients with sustained ventricular tachyarrhythmia. J Am Coll Cardiol 1987;10:83.

42. Van Schepdael J, Solvay H. Etude clinique de l'amiodarone dans le troubles du rythme cardiaque. Presse Med 1970;78:1849.

43. Herre JM, Sauve MJ, Malone P, et al. Long-term results of amiodarone therapy in patients with recurrent sustained ventricular tachycardia or ventricular fibrillation. J Am Coll Cardiol 1989;13:442.

44. Myers M, Peter T, Weiss D, et al. Benefits and risks of long-term amiodarone therapy for sustained ventricular tachycardia/fibrillation: a minimum of three-year follow-up. Am Heart J 1990;119:8.

45. Weinberg BA, Miles WM, Klein LS, et al. Five-year follow-up of 589 patients treated with amiodarone. Am Heart J 1993;125:109.

46. Fogoros RN, Anderson KP, Winkle RA, et al. Amiodarone: clinical efficacy and toxicity in 96 patients with recurrent, drug-refractory arrhythmias. Circulation 1983;68: 88.

47. Mason JW. Drug therapy: amiodarone. N Engl J Med 1987;316:455.

48. Nicklas JM, McKenna WJ, Stewart RA, et al. Prospective, double-blind, placebo-controlled trial of low-dose amiodarone in pa-

tients with severe heart failure and asymptomatic frequent ventricular ectopy. Am Heart J 1991;122:1016.

49. Singh SN, Fletcher RD, Fisher SG, et al. Amiodarone in patients with congestive heart failure and aysmptomatic frequent ventricular ectopy. N Engl J Med 1995;333: 77.

50. Volperian VR, Havighurst TC, Miller S, et al. Adverse effects of low dose amiodarone: a meta-analysis. J Am Coll Cardiol 1997;30: 791.

51. Horowitz LN, Greenspan AM, Spielman SR, et al. Usefulness of electrophysiologic testing in evaluation of amiodarone therapy for sustained ventricular arrhythmias associated with coronary heart disease. Am J Cardiol 1985;55:367.

52. Veltri EP, Griffith LSC, Platia EV, et al. The use of ambulatory monitoring in the prognostic evaluation of patients with sustained tachycardia treated with amiodarone. Circulation 1986;74:1054.

53. Lavery D, Saksena S. Management of refractory sustained ventricular tachycardia with amiodarone: a reappraisal. Am Heart J 1987;113:49.

54. Kim S, Felder SD, Figure I, et al. Value of Holter monitoring in predicting long-term efficacy and inefficacy of amiodarone used alone and in combination with Class Ia antiarrhythmic agents in patients with ventricular tachycardia. J Am Coll Cardiol 1987;9: 169.

55. Kadish AH, Marchlinski FE, Josephson ME, et al. Amiodarone: correlation of early and late electrophysiologic studies with outcome. Am Heart J 1986;112:1134.

56. Yazaki Y, Haffajee CI, Gold RL, et al. Electrophysiologic predictors of long-term clinical outcome with amiodarone for refractory ventricular tachycardia secondary to coronary artery disease. Am J Cardiol 1987; 60:293.

57. Schmitt C, Brachmann J, Waldecker B, et al. Amiodarone in patients with recurrent sustained ventricular tachyarrhythmias: results of programmed electrical stimulation and long-term clinical outcome in chronic treatment. Am Heart J 1987;114:279.

58. Zhu J, Haines DE, Lerman BB, et al. Predictors of efficacy of amiodarone and characteristics of recurrence of arrhythmia in patients with sustained ventricular tachycardia and coronary artery disease. Circulation 1987;76:802.

59. Greenspon AJ, Volosin KJ, Breenber RM, et al. Amiodarone therapy: role of early and late electrophysiologic studies. J Am Coll Cardiol 1988;11:117.

60. Winkle RA, Lopes MG, Goodman DJ, et al. Propranolol for patients with mitral valve prolapse. Am Heart J 1977;93:422.

61. Wu D, Kou HC, Hung JS: Exercise-triggered paroxysmal ventricular tachycardia. Ann Intern Med 1981;95:410.

62. Palileo EV, Ashley WW, Swiryn S, et al. Exercise provocable right ventricular outflow tract tachycardia. Am Heart J 1982;104:185.

63. Sung RJ, Olukotun AY, Baird CL, et al. Efficacy and safety of oral nadolol for exercise-induced ventricular arrhythmias. Am J Cardiol 1987;60:15D.

64. Stock JPP, Dale N. Beta-adrenergic receptor blockade in cardiac arrhythmias. Br Med J 1963;2:1230.

65. Wasir HS, Mahapatra RK, Bhatia ML, et al. Metoprolol:- a new cardioselective beta-adrenoceptor blocking agent for treatment of tachyarrhythmias. Br Heart J 1977;39:834.

66. Rydèn L, Ariniego R, Arnman K, et al. A double-blind trial of metoprolol in acute myocardial infarction: effects on ventricular tachyarrhythmias. N Engl J Med 1983; 308:614.

67. Moss AJ, Schwartz PJ, Crampton RS, et al. The long QT syndrome: a prospective international study. Circulation 1985;71:17.

68. Buxton AE, Waxman HL, Marchlinski FE, et al. Right ventricular tachycardia: clinical and electrophysiologic characteristics. Circulation 1983;68:917.

69. Brodsky MA, Sato DA, Allen BJ, et al. Solitary beta-blocker therapy for idiopathic life-threatening ventricular tachyarrhythmias. Chest 1986;89:790.

70. Steinbeck G, Andresen D, Bach P, et al. A comparison of electrophysiologically guided antiarrhythmic drug therapy with beta-blocker therapy in patients with symptomatic, sustained ventricular tachyarrhythmias. N Engl J Med 1992;327:987.

71. Woosley RL, Kornhauser D, Smith R, et al. Suppression of chronic ventricular arrhythmias with propranolol. Circulation 1979;60: 819.

72. Podrid PJ, Lown B. Pindolol for ventricular arrhythmia. Am Heart J 1982;104:491.

73. Brodsky MA, Allen BJ, Bessen M, et al. Beta-blocker therapy in patients with ventricular tachyarrhythmias in the setting of left ventricular dysfunction. Am Heart J 1988;115: 799.

74. Duff HJ, Mitchell LB, Wyse DG. Antiarrhythmic efficacy of propranolol: comparison of low and high serum concentrations. J Am Coll Cardiol 1986;8:959.

75. Brodsky MA, Allen BJ, Luckett CR, et al. Antiarrhythmic efficacy of solitary beta-adrenergic blockade for patients with sus-

tained ventricular tachyarrhythmias. Am Heart J 1989;118:272.

76. Leclercq J-F, Leenhardt A, Lemarec H, et al. Predictive value of electrophysiologic studies during treatment with the beta-blocking agent nadolol. J Am Coll Cardiol 1990;16:413.

77. Multicenter International Study. Reduction in mortality after myocardial infarction with long-term beta-adrenergic receptor blockade. Br Med J 1977;2:419.

78. The Norwegian Multicenter Study Group. Timolol-induced reduction in mortality and reinfarction in patients surviving acute myocardial infarction. N Engl J Med 1981;304:801.

79. Julian DG, Prescott RJ, Jackson FS, et al. Controlled trial of sotalol for one year after myocardial infarction. Lancet 1982;1:1142.

80. Beta-Blocker Heart Attack Study Group. A randomized trial of propranolol in patients with acute myocardial infarction. II. Mortality results. JAMA 1982;247:1707.

81. Lichstein E, Morganroth J, Harriet R, et al. Effect of propranolol on ventricular arrhythmias. The beta-blocker heart attack trial experience. Circulation 1983;67(Suppl I):5.

82. Jazayeri MR, VanWyhe G, Avitall B, et al. Isoproterenol reversal of antiarrhythmic effects in patients with inducible sustained ventricular tachyarrhythmias. J Am Coll Cardiol 1987;14:705.

83. Meredith IT, Broughton A, Jennings GL, et al. Evidence of a selective increase in cardiac sympathetic activity in patients with sustained ventricular arrhythmias. N Engl J Med 1991;325:618.

84. Leahey EB Jr, Heissenbuttel RH, Giardina EGV, et al. Combined mexiletine and propranolol treatment of refractory ventricular tachycardia. Br Med J 1980;281:357.

85. Hirsowitz G, Podrid PJ, Lampert S, et al. The role of beta blocking agents as adjunct therapy to membrane stabilizing drugs in malignant ventricular arrhythmia. Am Heart J 1986;111:852.

86. Deedwania PC, Olukotun AY, Kupersmith J, et al. Beta blockers in combination with Class I antiarrhythmic agents. Am J Cardiol 1987;60:21D.

87. Siebels J, Cappato R, Ruppel R, et al. ICD versus drugs in cardiac arrest survivors: preliminary results of the Cardiac Arrest Study Hamburg. PACE 1993;16:552.

88. Mitchell LB, Duff HJ, Gillis AM, et al. A randomized clinical trial of the noninvasive and invasive approaches to drug therapy for ventricular tachycardia: long-term fol-

low-up of the Calgary Trial. Prog Cardiovasc Dis 1996;38:377.

89. Mason JW, and the ESVEM Investigators. A comparison of electrophysiologic testing with Holter monitoring to predict antiarrhythmic-drug efficacy for ventricular tachyarrhythmias. N Engl J Med 1993;329:445.

90. Mitchell LB, Sheldon RS, Gillis AM, et al. Definition of predicted effective antiarrhythmic drug therapy for ventricular tachyarrhythmias by the electrophysiologic study approach: randomized comparison of patient response criteria. J Am Coll Cardiol 1997;30:1346.

91. Kavanagh KM, Wyse DG, Duff HJ, et al. Drug therapy for ventricular tachyarrhythmias: how many electropharmacologic trials are appropriate? J Am Coll Cardiol 1991;17:391.

92. Mason JW, and the ESVEM Investigators. A comparison of seven antiarrhythmic drugs in patients with ventricular tachyarrhythmias. N Engl J Med 1993;329:452.

93. The Cascade Investigators. Cardiac Arrest in Seattle: Conventional versus Amiodarone Drug Evaluation (the CASCADE study). Am J Cardiol 1991;67:578.

94. The Cascade Investigators. Randomized antiarrhythmic drug therapy in survivors of cardiac arrest (the CASCADE study). Am J Cardiol 1993;72:280.

95. Guiraudon G, Fontaine G, Frank R, et al. Encircling endocardial ventriculotomy: a new surgical treatment of life-threatening ventricular tachycardias resistant to medical treatment following myocardial infarction. Ann Thorac Surg 1978;26:438.

96. Cox JL. Patient selection criteria and results of surgery for refractory ischemic ventricular tachycardia. Circulation 1989;79(Suppl I):163.

97. Klein LS, Miles WM. Ablative therapy for ventricular arrhythmias. Prog Cardiovasc Dis 1995;37:225.

98. Stevenson WG, Khan H, Sager P, et al. Identification of reentry circuit sites during catheter mapping and radiofrequency ablation of ventricular tachycardia late after myocardial infarction. Circulation 1993;88:1647.

99. Brugada P, de Swart H, Smeets J, et al. Transcoronary chemical ablation of ventricular tachycardia. Circulation 1989;79:475.

100. Nora MO, Miles WM, Klein LS, et al. Alcohol ablation of ventricular tachycardia. J Cardiovasc Electrophysiol 1991;2:456.

101. Klein LS, Shih H-T, Hackett K, et al. Radiofrequency catheter ablation of ventricular tachycardia in patients without structural heart disease. Circulation 1992;85:1666.

102. Wen M-S, Yeh S-J, Wang C-C, et al. Successful radiofrequency ablation of idiopathic left ventricular tachycardia at a site away from the tachycardia exit. J Am Coll Cardiol 1997;30:1024.

103. Miles WM. Bundle branch reentrant tachycardia: a chance to cure? J Cardiovasc Electrophysiol 1993;4:263.

104. Mirowski A. The automatic implantable cardioverter defibrillator: an overview. J Am Coll Cardiol 1985;6:461.

105. Manolis AS, Tan-Deguzman W, Lee MA, et al. Clinical experience in seventy-seven patients with the automatic implantable cardioverter defibrillator. Am Heart J 1998; 118:445.

106. Winkle RA, Mead RH, Ruder MA, et al. Long-term outcome with the automatic cardioverter defibrillator. J Am Coll Cardiol 1989;3:1353.

107. Kim SG, Fogoros RN, Furman S, et al. Standardized reporting of ICD patient outcome: the report of a North American Society of Pacing and Electrophysiology Policy Conference. PACE 1993;16:1358.

108. Fogoros R. An AVID dissent. PACE 1994; 17:1701.

109. Josephson ME, Nissam S. The AVID trial: evidence based or randomized control trials: is the AVID study too late? Am J Cardiol 1997;80:194.

110. Connolly SJ, Yusuf S. Evaluation of the implantable cardioverter defibrillator in survivors of cardiac arrest: the need for randomized trials. Am J Cardiol 1992;69:959.

111. The Antiarrhythmics Versus Implantable Defibrillators (AVID) Trial Executive Committee. Are implantable cardioverter-defibrillators or drugs more effective in prolonging life? Am J Cardiol 1997;79:661.

112. Fogoros RN, Fielder SB, Elson JJ. The automatic cardioverter defibrillator in drug-refractory ventricular arrhythmias. Ann Intern Med 1987;107:635.

113. Pinski SL, Sgarbossa EB, Maloney JD, et al. Survival in patients declining implantable cardioverter defibrillators. Am J Cardiol 1991;68:800.

114. Newman D, Sauve MJ, Herre J, et al. Survival after implantation of the cardioverter defibrillator. Am J Cardiol 1992;69:899.

115. Böcker D, Haverkamp W, Block M, et al. Comparison of d,l-sotalol and implantable defibrillators for treatment of sustained ventricular tachycardia or fibrillation in patients with coronary artery disease. Circulation 1996;94:151.

116. Connolly SJ, Gent M, Roberts RS, et al. Canadian Implantable Defibrillator Study (CIDS): study design and organization. Am J Cardiol 1993;72:103F.

117. The AVID Investigators. Antiarrhythmics Versus Implantable Defibrillators (AVID) rationale, design, and methods. Am J Cardiol 1995;75:470.

118. The AVID Investigators. A comparison of antiarrhythmic drug therapy with implantable defibrillators in patients resuscitated from near-fatal sustained ventricular arrhythmias. N Engl J Med 1997;337:1576.

119. Singh BN. Controlling cardiac arrhythmias: an overview with a historical perspective. Am J Cardiol 1997;80:4G.

120. The MADIT Executive Committee. Multicenter Automatic Defibrillator Implantation Trial (MADIT): design and clinical protocol. PACE 1991;14:920.

121. Moss AJ, Hall J, Cannom DS, et al. Improved survival with an implanted defibrillator in patients with coronary disease at high risk for ventricular arrhythmia. N Engl J Med 1996;335:1933.

122. Moss AJ. Background, outcome, and clinical implications of the Multicenter Automatic Defibrillator Implantation Trial (MADIT). Am J Cardiol 1997;80:28F.

123. Waxman HL, Buxton AE, Sadowski LM, et al. The response to procainamide during electrophysiologic study for sustained ventricular tachyarrhythmias predicts the response to other medications. Circulation 1983;67:30.

124. Friedman PL, Stevenson WG. Unsustained ventricular tachycardia: to treat or not to treat. N Engl J Med 1996;335:1984.

125. The CABG-Patch Trial Investigators and Coordinators. The Coronary Artery Bypass Graft (CABG) Patch Trial. Prog Cardiovasc Dis 1993;36:97.

126. Bigger JT Jr, and the CABG Patch Trial Investigators. A randomized trial to evaluate prophylactic use of an implanted cardiac defibrillator in patients at high risk for death after coronary artery bypass graft surgery. N Engl J Med 1997;337:1569.

127. Kron IL, Lerman BB, Haines DE, et al. Coronary artery bypass grafting in patients with ventricular fibrillation. Ann Thorac Surg 1989;48:85.

128. Kelly P, Ruskin JN, Vlahakes GJ, et al. Surgical coronary revascularization in survivors of pre-hospital cardiac arrest: its effect on inducible ventricular arrhythmias and long-term survival. J Am Coll Cardiol 1990; 15:267.

129. O'Rourke RA. Role of myocardial revascularization in sudden death. Circulation 1992;85:I-112.

130. Every NR, Fahrenbrach CE, Hallstrom AP,

et al. Influence of coronary bypass surgery on subsequent outcome of patients resuscitated from out of hospital cardiac arrest. J Am Coll Cardiol 1992;19:1435.

131. Antiplatelet Trialists' Collaboration. Secondary prevention of vascular disease by prolonged antiplatelet treatment. Br Med J 1988;296:320.

132. Pitt B. Potential role of angiotensin converting enzyme inhibitors in treatment of atherosclerosis. Eur Heart J 1995;16(Suppl K): 49.

133. Hunink MGM, Goldman L, Tosteson ANA, et al. The recent decline in mortality from coronary heart disease, 1980–1990: the effect of secular trends in risk factors and treatment. JAMA 1997;277:535.

134. Holme I. Cholesterol reduction and its impact on coronary artery disease and total mortality. Am J Cardiol 1995;76:10C.

135. Kupperman M, Luce BR, McGovern B, et al. An analysis of the cost effectiveness of the implantable cardioverter defibrillator. Circulation 1990;81:91.

136. Larsen GC, Manolis AS, Sonnenberg FA, et al. Cost-effectiveness of the implantable cardioverter-defibrillator: effect of improved battery life and comparison with amiodarone therapy. J Am Coll Cardiol 1992;19:1323.

137. Kou WH, Kirsh MM, Bolling SF, et al. Effect of antiarrhythmic drug therapy on the incidence of shocks in patients who receive an implantable cardioverter defibrillator after a single episode of sustained ventricular tachycardia/fibrillation. PACE 1991;14: 1586.

138. Huang SKS, de Guzman WLT, Chenarides JG, et al. Effects of long-term amiodarone therapy of the defibrillation threshold and the rate of shocks of the implantable cardioverter-defibrillator. Am Heart J 1991;122: 720.

139. Manz M, Jung W, Lüderitz B. Interactions between drugs and devices: experimental and clinical studies. Am Heart J 1994;127: 978.

140. Sperry RE, Stambler BS, Wood MA, et al. Reduction of antiarrhythmic drug use in patients receiving implantable cardioverter defibrillators. PACE 1996;19:61.

141. Wang M, Dorian P. dl and d sotalol decrease defibrillation energy requirements. PACE 1989;12:1522.

142. Dorian P, Newman D, Sheahan R, et al. d-sotalol decreases defibrillation energy requirements in humans: a novel indication for drug therapy. J Cardiovasc Electrophysiol 1996;7:952.

Section III

Surgical Alternatives for Arrhythmia Management

Section Editor: Igor Singer

Chapter 27

Cardiac Mapping Systems and Their Use in Treating Tachyarrhythmias

Gregory P. Walcott, Sven Reek, Helmut U. Klein, William M. Smith, Raymond E. Ideker

Introduction

For much of the twentieth century, electrodes on or in the heart have been used to map the spread of activation.[1] Hundreds of mapping studies have been performed and have supplied much information about normal and abnormal conduction and about the mechanisms of arrhythmias. Initially, recordings were made sequentially with a single electrode that was moved from point to point on the epicardium. In approximately the last 20 years, computer-assisted cardiac mapping techniques have been developed to record from many sites simultaneously.[2]

Technical Considerations in Cardiac Mapping

The fundamental tasks to map cardiac activation have remained unchanged throughout this period: the electrodes must be placed on the heart so that they are well seated to record an adequate electrogram without artifacts; the recorded potentials must be amplified; the presence and time of activation at each recording site must be determined from these recordings; the location of the recording electrodes on the heart must be ascertained; and the spread of activation throughout the mapped region must be displayed.[3]

These steps are subject to error. For example, the estimation of the activation time at an electrode site can be incorrect. Since activations may be absent because of conduction block or because of the placement of the electrode on connective tissue instead of viable myocardium, it must first be determined whether an activation even occurred at an electrode site.

Recording electrodes can be either unipolar or bipolar, but the decisions about activations can be difficult for both types of recording electrodes. With unipolar electrode recordings, one electrode is in direct contact with the heart and the return electrode is located on the body surface distant from the heart. With bipolar electrode recordings, both electrodes are placed close together on the heart. With unipolar recordings, activation is indicated by a rapid downslope in the tracing, while in bipolar recordings acti-

Supported in part by National Institutes of Health Grants HL33637, HL28429.

From Singer I, Barold SS, Camm AJ (eds): Nonpharmacological Therapy of Arrhythmias for the 21st Century: The State of the Art. Futura Publishing Co, Inc., Armonk, NY, © 1998.

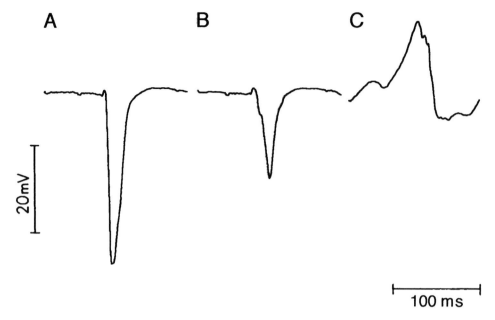

Figure 1. Examples of different types of complexes recorded at unipolar electrodes, indicating the difficulty in detecting local activation. Panel **A** shows a complex with a large amplitude and rapid downslope, representing a normal activation front passing through the tissue surrounding the electrode. Panel **B** shows a smaller complex with a less rapid downslope recorded from the center of a region of necrosis created by freezing. The nearest viable muscle is about 1.5 mm away from the recording electrode. Thus, this complex does not represent local activation but rather a distant normal activation front that at its closest point is approximately 1.5 mm from the recording site. Panel **C** also shows a small complex with a slow downslope that was generated by the passage of an activation front by a recording electrode during ventricular fibrillation. Thus, this complex does represent a local activation, albeit an abnormal one. Used with permission from Ideker RE, et al.[3]

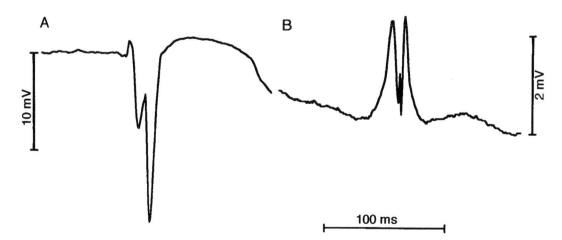

Figure 2. Examples of electrograms in which the time of activation is ambiguous. Panel **A** shows a unipolar recording with two regions of rapid downslope. Panel **B** shows a bipolar recording with more than one peak of absolute potential. Used with permission from Ideker RE, et al.[3]

vation is represented by a rapidly changing complex of almost any morphology. Figure 1 shows three unipolar complexes, each of which exhibits a distinct downslope. However, while the complexes in panels A and C of the figure represent activations, the slightly less rapid downslope in panel B does not represent an activation.

Once the presence of an activation has been identified in a recording, the time at which the activation front passes the electrode must then be determined. This time can sometimes also be ambiguous, as illustrated for both unipolar and bipolar recordings in Figure 2. Abnormal late and/or fractionated recordings (Figure 3) can arise from regions of patchy infarction or fibrosis interspersed with viable myocardium (Figure 4A) or from subendocardial regions of normal or abnormal spared myocardium

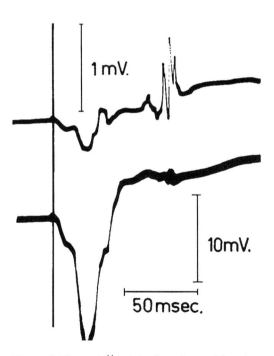

Figure 3. Durrer's[44] original tracings of fractionated electrograms over a transmural canine infarct. Multiple small amplitude deflections occur 75 ms after the beginning of the QRS complex and are recorded both in the local bipolar (top) and unipolar (bottom) electrogram. Reprinted with permission from Biermann M, et al.[43]

beneath an infarct (Figure 4B). The regions where the proper interpretation of the electrode recordings is most difficult are also the regions from which arrhythmias frequently arise.

Research and Clinical Mapping Techniques

While mapping in the animal laboratory and in the human operating room has similar goals, mapping in the animal laboratory can use more invasive techniques. For example, needles with multiple electrodes along their length can be inserted through the myocardial wall of animals to obtain multiple intramural recordings to determine the transmural activation sequence (Figure 5). In the animal laboratory, the hearts can be removed from the body at the end of the study to determine cardiac anatomy, cardiac pathology, and the location of the recording electrodes on or in the heart (Figure 6).

While plunge needles have been inserted through the wall of the heart in the human operating room on occasion,[4] most human recordings are confined to the epicardial and the endocardial surfaces of the heart. In the operating room, epicardial recordings are typically made from either electrodes embedded in plaques, in elastic socks that are pulled over the epicardium from the apex, or in parallel strips that surround the heart (Figure 7). Human or animal endocardial recordings can be obtained from: (1) an everted sock placed over a balloon that is inserted into the left ventricular cavity and then inflated so that the electrodes on the sock are in contact with the endocardium[5]; (2) a basket catheter that is closed when it is inserted into the heart chamber and is then opened so that up to eight struts, each with up to eight electrodes, contacts the endocardium (Figure 8) or (3) a balloon catheter containing up to 64 electrodes on a small balloon that is inflated in the desired ventricular or atrial cavity (Figure 9).

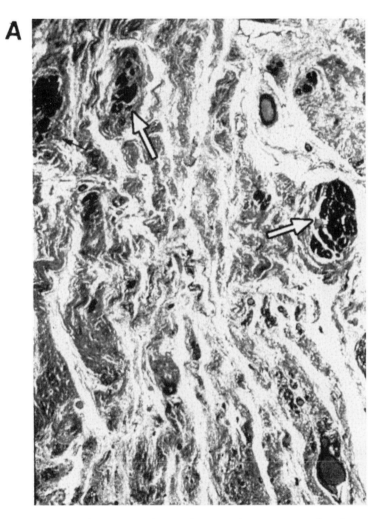

Figure 4. Photomicrographs of the types of spared myocardium associated with myocardial infarcts that may give rise to fractionated or late potentials. Panel **A** shows a photomicrograph of an old myocardial infarction scar from the left ventricle of a deceased patient. Small bundles of spared viable myocardium (arrows) traverse this scar and may serve as part of a reentrant pathway. While in this two-dimensional cross section, the surviving myocardium appears to be isolated islands of tissue, three-dimensional reconstruction of the tissue indicates that these spared regions form interconnecting strands of tissue. Therefore, the strands may activate at different times generating a fractionated, long-duration complex. Some strands may activate late because of the long, complex pathway needed to reach them, generating delayed potentials. *Continued.*

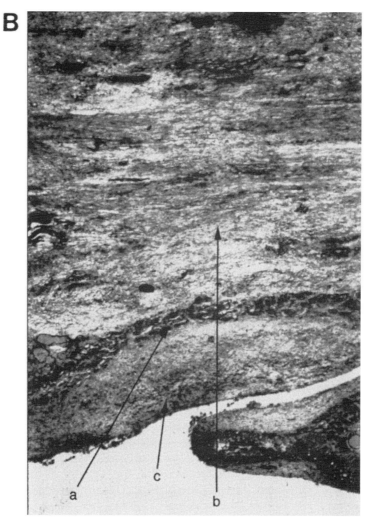

Figure 4. *(Continued)* Panel **B** demonstrates a thin rim of spared myocardium (a) between the left ventricular cavity on the bottom and an old myocardial infarct scar (b) at the top. Between the thin layer of surviving subendocardial myocardium and the endocardial cavity is a thin layer of fibroelastic connective tissue (c) that is formed in response to stretching of the infarcted wall due to aneurysmal bulging during systole in the weeks to months after the infarction occurs. The thin layer of spared myocardium is frequently an important part of the reentrant pathway of ventricular arrhythmias and is the tissue removed by endocardial resection. Abnormalities within this spared myocardial layer as well as the separation of mapping electrodes on the endocardium from this layer by the fibroelastic tissue may also be a cause for fractionated electrograms.

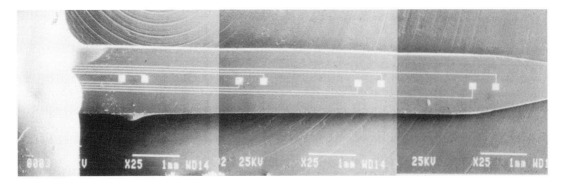

Figure 5. Scanning electron micrograph of a multi-electrode needle for mapping intramural cardiac activation. The needle is constructed using microelectronic techniques. It contains six small electrode contacts spaced 1 mm apart. Traces from each electrode can be seen running from the electrodes to the left side of the needle where wires are bonded to carry the signals to the mapping system. The needle is plunged through the ventricular wall with the right-most portion towards the endocardium and the left-most portion towards the epicardium.

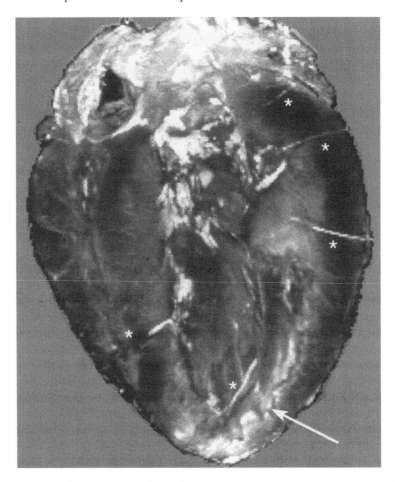

Figure 6. A longitudinal section of a three-dimensional reconstruction of a magnetic resonance image of the heart. The left and right ventricular cavities are shown. Several tracks made by plunge needles are visible (*), as is a myocardial infarct (arrow) at the apex of the left ventricle. The image is T2-weighted.

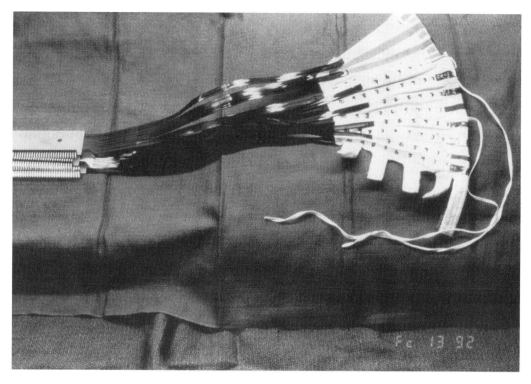

Figure 7. An electrode array for recording from the epicardium during cardiac surgery and an isochronal activation map obtained with this array. Panel **A** shows the epicardial array which consists of several polyamide strips, each of which contain 10 electrodes. The strips are held together with velcro straps and the entire array is pulled over all of the ventricular epicardium from the apex. See Figure 7, panel B, between p. 600 and p. 601.

Mapping in the Surgical Suite

Over the last several years, operative mapping has been used less frequently for surgical procedures. Many of the conditions for which it was previously used, e.g., Wolff-Parkinson-White syndrome and ventricular tachycardia, are now treated more commonly by transvenous catheter techniques than by cardiac surgery. While the maze procedure for atrial fibrillation is still primarily a surgical rather than a catheter procedure,[6] the locations of the incisions are determined primarily by anatomic landmarks instead of activation sequence data, so that operative mapping does not play a large part in this surgical procedure. It remains to be seen if thoracoscopic surgery will play a major role in the treatment of arrhythmias and whether operative mapping can contribute to this new surgical technique.

Computer-Assisted Mapping in the Clinical Electrophysiology Laboratory

While there has been a great decrease in the use of operative mapping, the development of basket catheters (Figure 8) and noncontact endocardial recording arrays (Figure 9) raise the possibility that the computer-assisted mapping techniques developed for use in the operating room can be used in the diagnosis and treatment of arrhythmias in the clinical electrophysiology laboratory using transvenous catheters introduced into the heart.

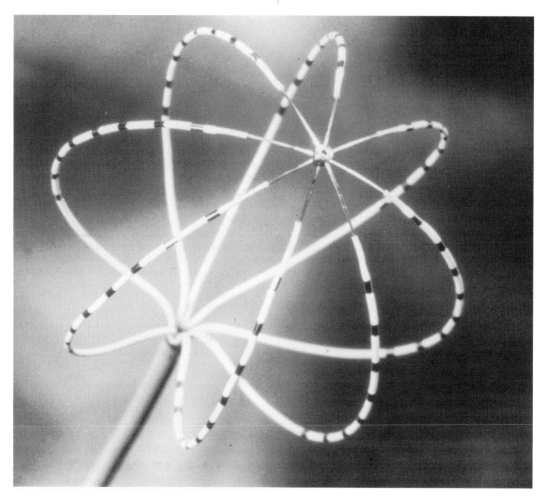

Figure 8. A basket catheter for endocardial mapping. The basket catheter is an 8F catheter that is inserted into the desired cardiac chamber with the basket in the closed position. Once the basket is in place, eight struts are distended at the distal end of the catheter as shown in the figure. Each strut contains eight electrodes that are designed to contact the endocardium when the basket is deployed. At the end of the mapping procedure, the basket is collapsed and the catheter is withdrawn. Used with permission, EP Technologies, Sunnyvale, CA.

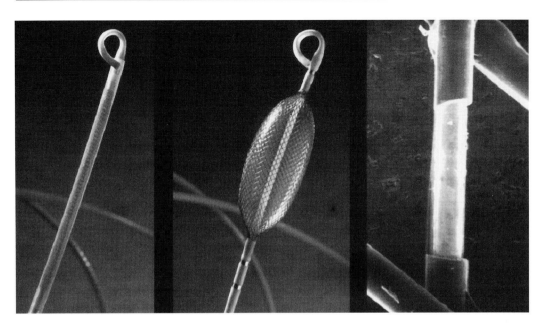

Figure 9. An endocardial balloon catheter for cardiac mapping. The catheter is 9F and is inserted into the desired cardiac cavity with the balloon deflated. Once the catheter is in place, the balloon is inflated with saline. The surface of the balloon contains 64 electrodes. While a few of these electrodes may contact the endocardium when the balloon is inflated, most do not. A mathematical inverse procedure is performed to calculate the endocardial potentials from the recorded potentials on the surface of the balloon. At the end of the mapping procedure the balloon is deflated and the catheter is removed. Used with permission from Endocardial Solutions, St. Paul, MN.

To date, catheter-based ablation for the treatment of ventricular tachyarrhythmias has focused on ventricular tachycardia.[7–10] If ventricular tachycardia is monomorphic and stable, then a single, catheter-based electrode can be moved sequentially from point to point on the endocardium to determine the activation sequence during the arrhythmia and the region to be ablated.

The ability to record from all electrodes simultaneously with an array of basket or balloon electrodes means that all recordings can be made in a single beat and raises the possibility that the site of ablation for unstable ventricular tachyarrhythmias, including ventricular fibrillation, can be determined. As recently reviewed in more detail elsewhere,[11] it may be possible to use catheter ablation to prevent ventricular fibrillation recurrence in a subset of patients who sur-

vive cardiac arrest. This subset may include those cardiac arrest survivors who meet seven prerequisites for ablation (Table 1).

The Sudden Cardiac Arrest is Caused by a Tachyarrhythmia

Except in patients with severe heart failure, Holter monitor recordings indicate that the overwhelming cause of sudden cardiac arrest is a ventricular tachyarrhythmia.[12,13] The tachyarrhythmia may be either ventricular fibrillation or ventricular tachycardia.[11]

Yet, a few patients with sudden cardiac death do not have a ventricular tachyarrhythmia. A small number have bradycardia, asystole, or electromechanical dissociation at the time the first electrocardio-

Table 1

Prerequisites for Catheter Ablation in Cardiac Arrest Survivors

- The sudden cardiac arrest is caused by a tachyarrhythmic event.
- Fibrillation starts from a localized area of organized activation.
- The fibrillation episodes arise from the same region.
- The clinical arrhythmia is inducible.
- The induced arrhythmia can be mapped.
- The localized area of origin can be ablated.
- Prevention of tachyarrhythmia recurrence by ablation can be proved.

graphic recording is obtained following the acute event. The type of arrhythmia recorded varies with the time between the cardiac arrest event and the time that the heart rhythm was recorded.[14] The incidence of asystole increases as this time interval increases. Therefore, even some of the individuals thought to have asystole might have had fibrillation that has already progressed

to electrical silence by the time the recording is made.

Fibrillation Starts from a Localized Area of Organized Activation

There is considerable evidence that the first few cycles of ventricular fibrillation arise from a small localized cardiac region.[11] During these first few cycles, all activation fronts emanate from this small region and pass outward to activate the remainder of the ventricles. This was first observed over a half century ago by Wiggers and coworkers from high-speed cinematography of contraction of the in situ canine heart during the electrical initiation of ventricular fibrillation (Figure 10).[15,16] The same finding has since been observed by several different groups of investigators[17–19] during the first few cycles of fibrillation caused by acute ischemia (Figure 11).

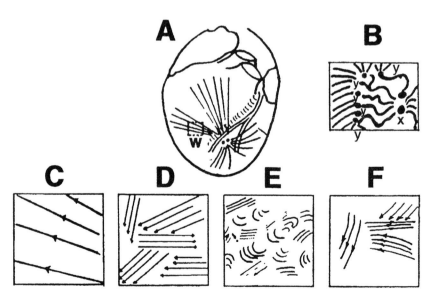

Figure 10. Diagrams indicating the spread of waves observed in analysis of moving pictures during the four stages of fibrillation described by Wiggers. Panel **A**: Spread of wavefront during initial, undulatory stage. Panel **B**: Theoretical passage of impulses from point x to form a wavefront at y. Panels **C-F**: Appearance of contraction waves in small rectangular area W, magnified: Panel **C** undulatory stage; Panel **D** convulsive stage; Panel **E** tremulous stage; and Panel **F** atonic stage. Reprinted with permission from Wiggers CJ.[15]

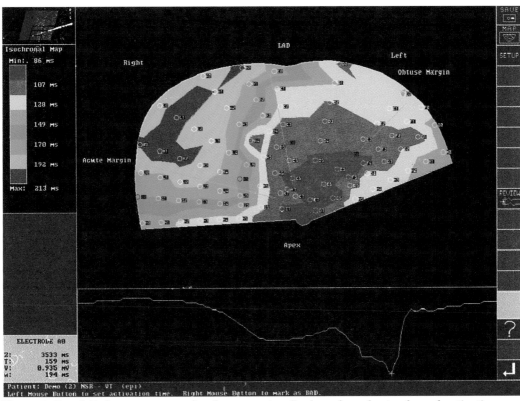

Figure 7. Panel B shows an example of a computer display of a color isochronal activation map obtained from a patient during cardiac surgery. Courtesy of Prucka Engineering Inc., Houston, TX.

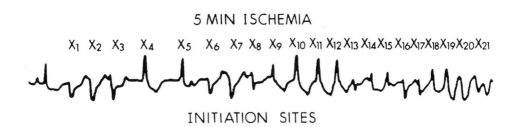

5 MIN ISCHEMIA

X_1 X_2 X_3 X_4 X_5 X_6 X_7 X_8 X_9 X_{10} X_{11} X_{12} X_{13} X_{14} X_{15} X_{16} X_{17} X_{18} X_{19} X_{20} X_{21}

INITIATION SITES

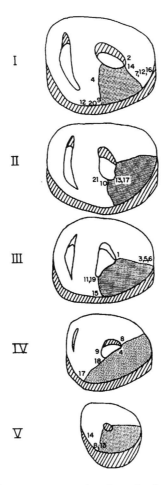

Figure 11. Sites of origin of beats at onset of tachyarrhythmia in a cat. Sections of the heart (I-V) are oriented with the base on top and apex on bottom. The surface ECG is shown above. The shaded area represents the ischemic zone after 5 min of occlusion of the left anterior descending coronary artery, defined by a pronounced decrease in amplitude and an increase in duration of bipolar recordings. Numbers represent the sites of initiation of the first 21 beats of ventricular tachycardia leading to ventricular fibrillation. Modified and used with permission from Pogwizd SM, et al.[19]

The Fibrillation Episodes Arise from the Same Region

In a subset of patients with a previous myocardial infarction and a sudden cardiac arrest caused by ventricular fibrillation, it is likely that ventricular fibrillation is initiated by a mechanism similar to that which initiates ventricular tachycardia in patients with a previous myocardial infarction.[11] In both cases, the mechanism initiating the arrhythmia is believed to be reentry (Figure 12).[20] In the patient with monomorphic ventricular tachycardia, the reentrant circuit remains stable in the spared muscle adjacent to the myocardial infarct. However, in the patient with ventricular fibrillation, it is thought that after a few cycles reentry also begins to occur in other regions leading to the less organized activation patterns of fibrillation. The reasons that activation degenerates in the latter group of patients may be that the initial reentrant cycle length is shorter; electrophysiological properties of the myocardium away from the initial reentrant pathway are more abnormal causing secondary reentrant circuits to form; or during the initial organized arrhythmia the heart is incapable of sufficient function to adequately perfuse the coronaries and thus ischemia leads to the degeneration of the arrhythmia into fibrillation.

In many patients with recurrent monomorphic ventricular tachycardia, the morphology of the tachycardia is similar for each tachycardia episode. Thus, in many of the individuals in whom the first several beats of ventricular fibrillation are an organized reentrant circuit, the location of this reentrant circuit may also be similar for different episodes of ventricular fibrillation. Even in some of the patients in whom fibrillation is caused by acute ischemia, the first few cycles of fibrillation may arise from the same region for multiple episodes of the arrhythmia if either the acute ischemia occurs repeatedly in the same region or if premature contractions arising from different sites within acutely ischemic areas serve as an initiator, but the same region of old infarction constantly functions as the arrhythmic substrate.

The Clinical Arrhythmia is Inducible

The use of programmed electrical stimulation is well established for patients with coronary artery disease and recurrent ventricular tachycardia.[21] It is possible that programmed electrical stimulation can also be used in survivors of sudden cardiac arrest to induce an arrhythmia that can be used to guide ablation therapy. Monomorphic ventricular tachycardia can be induced in many patients with coronary artery disease who have survived cardiac arrest.[22–24] If so, ablation may be guided by mapping the activation sequence during the tachycardia. In other patients fibrillation and not monomorphic tachycardia may be induced. While the induction of ventricular fibrillation during programmed electrical stimulation in patients with monomorphic ventricular tachycardia is considered to be nonspecific for ablation therapy,[25,26] the induction of ventricular fibrillation in cardiac arrest survivors with coronary artery disease is considered to be a specific endpoint that can be used to guide ablation therapy.[27–30]

The Induced Arrhythmia Can Be Mapped

In some patients in whom polymorphic ventricular tachycardia or ventricular fibrillation is induced by programmed electrical stimulation, drugs such as procainamide can be given to slow the induced arrhythmia to a more stable monomorphic ventricular tachycardia so that it can be mapped using sequential recording catheter techniques.[25,31,32] As discussed earlier in this chapter, the development of basket catheters and noncontact catheter electrode arrays suggests that it will soon be possible

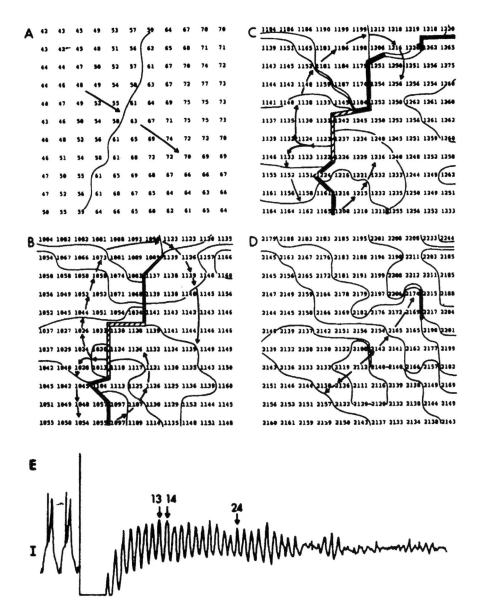

Figure 12. Activation maps during induction of ventricular fibrillation. An S_2 stimulus of 70 mA applied to the center of the mapped region at a coupling interval of 230 ms after the last beat of a basic train of S_1 stimuli (300 ms) initiated ventricular fibrillation. Numbers represent activation times in milliseconds following the stimulus at 121 epicardial recording sites. The mapped region is approximately 4x4 cm. Solid lines represent conduction block. Hashed lines represent "frame lines." Frame lines are required when the continuous activation fronts of reentry are represented by sequential isochronal maps. Activation fronts emanating from these frame lines are continuations of activation fronts from the previous map. Panel **A** shows the activation of the last beat of the train. Panels **B** and **C** demonstrate a figure-eight reentry pattern during the 13th and 14th cycles of fibrillation. By the 24th cycle, reentry can no longer be observed in the mapped region (panel **D**). The rhythm strip (panel **E**) shows a surface recording of the induced fibrillation. Arrows mark times of activation sequences depicted above. Modified and used with permission from Kavanaugh KM, et al.[20]

to map the first few cycles of ventricular fibrillation, even if these cycles of activation are too unstable and short lived to be mapped with single electrode, sequential mapping techniques. Thus, if the prerequisites previously discussed are met, these first few cycles will arise from a discrete region of the myocardium that can be identified by simultaneous recording from multiple catheter-based electrodes, and the ablation of this region will prevent recurrence of the arrhythmia.

The Localized Area of Origin Can Be Ablated

Moran et al. have shown that ventricular fibrillation can be successfully prevented by an extended endocardial resection of the spared myocardium beneath an old myocardial infarct.[33] Thus, catheter ablation could be equally successful if the ablation lesion is sufficiently large and is applied in the correct location. As just discussed, computer-assisted, multichannel, catheter-based, mapping techniques may help determine the correct location for this ablation lesion.

Advances in ablation techniques are leading to an increase in lesion size. These advances include cooling of the catheter tip for radiofrequency (RF) ablation,[34] using longer electrodes with a high-power RF generator to create larger lesions,[35] and passing RF current simultaneously through several electrodes with a shift in phase of the delivered current between the electrodes.[36] In addition, forms of energy other than RF are being investigated in an attempt to increase the size of the lesions. These alternative energy sources include lasers, microwaves, and ultrasound.[34,37–39]

The creation of larger lesions by these newer techniques may increase the efficacy of catheter ablation for sudden cardiac arrest. The larger lesions may ablate arrhythmogenic tissue that is intramural or subepicardial. In addition, if the amount of ablated tissue is larger, the required resolution of the mapping techniques will be decreased, which should make it easier to develop suitable catheter-based multi-electrode mapping techniques.

Prevention of Tachyarrhythmia Recurrence By Ablation Can Be Proved

Similar to the evaluation of the efficacy of the ablation procedure used for the treatment of monomorphic ventricular tachycardia, it is hoped that programmed electrical stimulation can be used in survivors of cardiac arrest to determine if the arrhythmogenic tissue has been successfully ablated. While the loss of ability to induce sustained ventricular arrhythmias by programmed electrical stimulation is commonly accepted as an objective endpoint for the evaluation of antiarrhythmic drug therapy, of surgery, and of catheter ablation in patients with monomorphic ventricular tachycardia, it remains to be seen if the same endpoint can be used to ascertain if ablation has successfully created a lesion that will prevent the recurrence of sudden cardiac arrest. Just as has been true in the treatment of monomorphic ventricular tachycardia, experience will determine which arrhythmias induced in treated survivors of sudden cardiac arrest are clinically meaningful and which are not.

Conclusion

In summary, the prerequisites given in Table 1 are most likely to be met in a subset of sudden cardiac arrest survivors with distinct characteristics. They will have coronary artery disease with a circumscribed old infarct scar with preserved left ventricular function and no evidence that the arrest was caused by acute ischemia. In addition, they must have arrhythmias which are inducible by programmed electrical stimulation and the site of origin of the arrhythmia must be detectable by mapping with catheter-based arrays in the ventricular cavity. These criteria probably exclude at least half of the patients who have survived a cardiac arrest.[22–24,40–42] It remains to be seen if ablation will indeed prevent sudden cardiac death in this subgroup of patients. While research is being performed to ascertain if ablation can prevent sudden cardiac death, the continued use of implantable cardioverter-defibrillators in these patients currently remains the safest course of action.

Acknowledgement: The authors gratefully acknowledge Kate Sreenan and Danielle Winkler for their assistance in preparing this manuscript.

References

1. Janse MJ. Some historical notes on the mapping of arrhythmias. In Shenasa M, Borggrefe M, Breihardt G, et al., eds. Cardiac Mapping. Futura Publishing Co, Inc, Mount Kisco, NY, 1993, pp 3–10.
2. Ideker RE, Smith WM, Wallace AG, et al. A computerized method for the rapid display of ventricular activation during the intraoperative study of arrhythmias. Circulation 1979;59:449–458.
3. Ideker RE, Smith WM, Blanchard SM, et al. The assumptions of isochronal cardiac mapping. PACE 1989;12:456–478.
4. Pogwizd SM, Hoyt RH, Saffitz JE, et al. Reentrant and focal mechanisms underlying ventricular tachycardia in the human heart. Circulation 1992;86:1872–1887.
5. Downar E, Harris L, Mickleborough LL, et al. Endocardial mapping of ventricular tachycardia in the intact human ventricle: evidence for reentrant mechanisms. J Am Coll Cardiol 1988;11:783–791.
6. Cox JL. The surgical treatment of atrial fibrillation: surgical technique. J Thorac Cardiovasc Surg 1991;101:584–592.
7. Morady F, Scheinman MM, Di Carlo LA Jr, et al. Catheter ablation of ventricular tachycardia with intracardiac shocks: results in 33 patients. Circulation 1987;75:1037–1049.
8. Evans GT Jr, Scheinman MM, Zipes DP, et al. The percutaneous cardiac mapping and ablation registry: final summary of results. PACE 1988;11:1621–1626.
9. Fitzgerald DM, Friday KJ, Wah JAYL, et al. Electrogram patterns predicting successful catheter ablation of ventricular tachycardia. Circulation 1988;77:806–814.
10. Trappe H-J, Klein H, Auricchio A, et al. Catheter ablation of ventricular tachycardia: Role of the underlying etiology and the site of energy delivery. PACE 1992;15:411–424.
11. Reek S, Klein HU, Ideker RE. Can catheter ablation in cardiac arrest survivors prevent ventricular fibrillation recurrence? PACE 1997;20:1840–1859.
12. Roelandt J, Klootwijk P, Lubsen J, et al. Sudden death during longterm ambulatory monitoring. Eur Heart J 1984;5:7–20.
13. Bayes de Luna A, Coumel P, Leclerq JF, et al. Ambulatory sudden cardiac death: mechanisms of production of fatal arrhythmia on the basis of data from 157 cases. Am Heart J 1989;117:151–159.
14. Hallstrom AP, Eisenberg MS, Bergner L. The persistence of ventricular fibrillation and its implication for evaluating EMS. Emerg Health Serv Q 1983;1:41–47.
15. Wiggers CJ. The mechanism and nature of ventricular defibrillation. Am Heart J 1940;20:399–412.
16. Wiggers CJ, Wegria R. Ventricular fibrillation due to single, localized induction and condenser shocks applied during the vulnerable phase of ventricular systole. Am J Physiol 1940;128:500–505.
17. Janse MJ, van Capelle FJL, Morsink H, et al. Flow of "injury" current and patterns of excitation during early ventricular arrhythmias in acute regional myocardial ischemia in isolated porcine and canine hearts: evidence for two different arrhythmogenic mechanisms. Circ Res 1980;47:151–165.
18. Ideker RE, Klein GJ, Harrison L, et al. The transition to ventricular fibrillation induced by reperfusion following acute ischemia in the dog: a period of organized epicardial activation. Circulation 1981;63:1371–1379.
19. Pogwizd SM, Corr PB. Mechanisms underlying the development of ventricular fibrillation during early myocardial ischemia. Circ Res 1990;66:672–695.
20. Kavanagh KM, Kabas JS, Rollins DL, et al. High-current stimuli to the spared epicardium of a large infarct induce ventricular tachycardia. Circulation 1992;85:680–698.
21. The ACC/AHA Task Force. Guidelines for clinical intracardiac electrophysiological and catheter ablation procedures. A report of the American College of Cardiology/American Heart Association task force on practice guidelines (Committee on Clinical Intracardiac Electrophysiologic and Catheter Ablation Procedures). Developed in collaboration with the North American Society of Pacing and Electrophysiology. J Cardiovasc Electrophysiol 1995;6:652–679.

22. Wilber DJ, Garan H, Finkelstein D, et al. Out-of-hospital cardiac arrest: use of electrophysiologic testing in the prediction of long-term outcome. N Engl J Med 1988;318:19–24.

23. Roy D, Waxman HL, Kienzle MG, et al. Clinical characteristics and long-term follow-up in 119 survivors of cardiac arrest: relation to inducibility at electrophysiologic testing. Am J Cardiol 1983;52:969–974.

24. Morady F, Scheinman MM, Hess DS, et al. Electrophysiologic testing in the management of survivors of out-of-hospital cardiac arrest. Am J Cardiol 1983;51:85–89.

25. Josephson ME. Recurrent ventricular tachycardia. In Clinical Cardiac Electrophysiology: Techniques and Interpretations. Lea & Febiger, Philadelphia/London, 1993, pp 417–615.

26. Wellens HJ, Brugada P, Stevenson WG. Programmed electrical stimulation of the heart in patients with life-threatening ventricular arrhythmias: what is the significance of induced arrhythmias and what is the correct stimulation protocol? Circulation 1985;72:1–7.

27. Adhar GC, Larson LW, Bardy GH, et al. Sustained ventricular arrhythmias: Differences between survivors of cardiac arrest and patients with recurrent sustained ventricular tachycardia. J Am Coll Cardiol 1988;12:159–165.

28. Swerdlow CD, Liem B, Franz MR. Summation and inhibition by ultrarapid train pacing in the human ventricle. Circulation 1987;76:1101–1109.

29. Brugada P, Green M, Abdollah H, et al. Significance of ventricular arrhythmias initiated by programmed ventricular stimulation: the importance of the type of ventricular arrhythmia induced and the number of premature stimuli required. Circulation 1984;69:87–92.

30. Morady F, DiCarlo LA Jr, Baerman JM, et al. Comparison of coupling intervals that induce clinical and nonclinical forms of ventricular tachycardia during programmed stimulation. Am J Cardiol 1986;57:1269–1273.

31. Couch OA. Cardiac aneurysm with VT and subsequent excision of aneurysm. Circulation 1959;20:251–253.

32. MADIT Executive Committee. Multicenter automatic defibrillator implantation trial (MADIT): design and clinical protocol. PACE 1991;14:920–927.

33. Moran JM, Kehoe RF, Loeb JM, et al. Extended endocardial resection for the treatment of ventricular tachycardia and ventricular fibrillation. Ann Thorac Surg 1982;34:538–552.

34. Nath S, Haines DE. Biophysics and pathology of catheter energy delivery systems. Progr Cardiovasc Dis 1995;37:185–204.

35. Langberg JJ, Gallagher M, Strickberger A, et al. Temperature-guided radiofrequency catheter ablation with very large distal electrodes. Circulation 1993;88:245–249.

36. Desai JM, Nyo H, Vera Z, et al. Two phase radiofrequency catheter ablation of isolated ventricular endomyocardium. PACE 1991;14:1179–1194.

37. Langberg JJ, Wonnell T, Chin MC, et al. Catheter ablation of the atrioventricular junction using a helical microwave antenna: a novel means of coupling energy to the endocardium. PACE 1991;14:2105–2113.

38. Chen S-A, Chiang C-E, Tai C-T, et al. Future ablation concepts of tachyarrhythmias. PACE 1995;6:852–862.

39. Saksena S. Catheter ablation of tachycardias with laser energy: issues and answers. PACE 1989;12:196–203.

40. Ruskin JN, DiMarco JP, Garan H. Out-of-hospital cardiac arrest: electrophysiologic observations and selection of long-term antiarrhythmic therapy. N Engl J Med 1980;303:607–613.

41. Skale BT, Miles WM, Heger JJ, et al. Survivors of cardiac arrest: prevention of recurrence by drug therapy as predicted by electrophysiologic testing or electrocardiographic monitoring. Am J Cardiol 1986;57:113–119.

42. Hurwitz JL, Josephson ME. Sudden cardiac death in patients with chronic coronary heart disease. Circulation 1992;85(Suppl I):I-43-I-49.

43. Biermann M, Shenasa M, Borggreffe M, et al. The interpretation of cardiac electrograms. In Shenasa M, Borggrefe M, Breithardt G, et al., eds. Cardiac Mapping. Futura Publishing Co, Inc, Mount Kisco, NY, 1993, pp 11–34.

44. Durrer D, Formijne P, van Dam RT, et al. The electrocardiogram in normal and some abnormal conditions: in revived human fetal heart and in acute and chronic coronary occlusion. Am Heart J 1961;61:303–316.

Chapter 28

Role of Electrophysiological Mapping for Ventricular Tachycardia Ablation

John M. Miller, Steven A. Rothman, Henry H. Hsia, Alfred E. Buxton

Introduction

Surgical therapy for ventricular tachycardia (VT) was the first method to offer a chance to cure individuals of this arrhythmia, while at the same time providing the opportunity to gain fundamental insights into the mechanisms of VT in man.[1–4] Both the clinical and the research outcomes of these surgical procedures initially depended heavily on mapping of VT, the process by which the location of the tissues ultimately responsible for generating the arrhythmia is determined. In the two decades since the first of these operations was performed, significant advances have been made in our understanding of VT, mapping tools have become increasingly sophisticated, and new treatment modalities (implantable cardioverter-defibrillators [ICDs] and radiofrequency [RF] catheter ablation) have been introduced and widely used. These latter therapies, which were at one time alternatives to surgery for management of VT, have now largely supplanted open heart surgery due to technological improvements. Because of this shift in types of treatment, far fewer surgical procedures are currently being performed for VT than

was the case 5 or 10 years ago, despite significant advances in mapping technology. Thus, at a time when new tools are poised to add significantly to our understanding of these arrhythmias, opportunities to apply these tools are less frequent. Consequently, relatively little new information has become available on the topic of intraoperative VT mapping in the last few years. This chapter will explore some of the history of intraoperative VT mapping, examine its current status, and suggest what the future may hold.

Surgically Treatable Ventricular Arrhythmias

The largest experience with intraoperative mapping of ventricular arrhythmias in man has been with post-myocardial infarction uniform sustained VT, dating back to the late 1970s.[1,4] Patients with a wide variety of other substrates for sustained VT have also undergone surgery, including idiopathic dilated cardiomyopathy, arrhythmogenic right ventricular dysplasia,[5] and post-tetralogy repair,[6] as well as others.[7,8] Most patients with episodes of spontaneous

From Singer I, Barold SS, Camm AJ (eds): *Nonpharmacological Therapy of Arrhythmias for the 21st Century: The State of the Art.* Futura Publishing Co, Inc., Armonk, NY, © 1998.

sustained VT (especially in the post-infarct group), will have additional VT morphologies inducible at EP study pre- or intraoperatively. Most electrophysiologists now feel that there is no fundamental distinction between a VT morphology that occurs spontaneously and one that has only been initiated in the laboratory setting; given enough time, the latter VTs often occur spontaneously.[9] Thus, all inducible VT morphologies are generally targeted for ablation at surgery.

Using currently available multi-electrode systems that can acquire mapping information from practically the entire endocardial and epicardial surface in just a few beats, even nonsustained episodes can be successfully mapped and ablated.[10] This had not been practical when the only mapping tools available were for acquisition of recordings from only single sites in a sequential fashion. At present, neither polymorphic VT nor ventricular fibrillation (VF) are considered mappable arrhythmias, although computer processing power has advanced to the point of technical feasibility. Our current understanding is that these are more global arrhythmias, rather than requiring only small portions of the ventricular mass for perpetuation, and thus mapping with intent to ablate a small critical area does not seem achievable.

Mapping Equipment

Systems for intraoperative mapping have changed dramatically in the last two decades. These range from very rudimentary systems for single-site acquisition (including equipment available in practically any electrophysiology laboratory, including a sterile recording probe of some type, strip chart recorder, and calipers) to very sophisticated multi-electrode computerized systems capable of recording and analyzing hundreds of sites simultaneously. There are advantages and disadvantages to each method. While it is apparent that multi-site systems have yielded higher overall surgical success rates,[11] it is also true that they have largely been used by groups already practiced at intraoperative mapping skills using simpler technologies. A direct comparison of the two types of systems in equally experienced hands will not likely ever be available; it is conceivable that an older, less technically advanced system in the hands of a seasoned electrophysiologist may yield more useful data than a rarely used but highly complex system used by a less-practiced operator. Different types of mapping systems and electrode configurations are discussed fully in Chapter 27.

Mapping Techniques

Of critical importance in the success of a clinical mapping procedure is the relationship between the electrophysiologist who is directing the mapping process and interpreting its results, and the surgeon who must stand by the open-chested patient doing almost nothing while the electrophysiologist seemingly wastes large amounts of precious time. There must be an understanding between these two such that the electrophysiologist is allowed the time to acquire the information he needs to direct the surgeon's ablative efforts, while he must also know when further efforts are not accomplishing this goal and the operation should proceed despite suboptimal information. Time poses a very definite limitation on the entire team; as a rule, the longer the patient is on cardiopulmonary bypass, the slower the postoperative recovery.

The vast majority of intraoperative VT mapping experience has been in the post-myocardial infarction patient. In this setting, the mechanism for VT is almost always reentry; the discussion on mapping principles that follows deals with determining the location(s) of critical portions of the circuit within which reentry takes place. In other clinical settings, automaticity or triggered activity may be the causal mechanism and the mapping principles will be different. For instance, instead of seeking mid-diastolic electrical activity, the goal of mapping is a site with a late diastolic (presystolic) electrogram preceding the QRS complex by no more than 40 ms in many cases. Since it is currently quite unusual for these cases to require surgical intervention, the following discussion will concentrate on locating essential components of a reentrant circuit in the ventricles.

Criteria for determining the location of the critical portion of the VT circuit have changed over time. In the early years of intraoperative mapping, the target tissue was that from which the earliest recording in the latter half of diastole was made. This was an operational definition arrived at largely because of technical limitations. While it was appreciated that post-infarct VT was due to reentry, early studies were unable to record electrical activity throughout the complete cardiac cycle in the majority of cases; instead, activity could be recorded during the QRS complex, slightly after its end (early diastole) and prior to its onset (late diastole, presystole). Removal of tissue from which the late diastolic recordings were made resulted in noninducibility of VT postoperatively, and thus it became standard practice to seek areas with late-diastolic electrograms during mapping procedures at surgery and in preoperative mapping. These electrogram types are now known to be recorded from exit sites for VT circuits; the fact that their surgical removal cured a high proportion of patients indicates that the resection or cryoablation damaged or removed an adjacent site containing the critical tissue from which mid-diastolic electrograms would have been recorded.

Currently, the target tissue during intraoperative mapping has the same characteristics as that during catheter mapping. Searching for a repetitive, isolated mid-diastolic potential is perhaps the most useful criterion.[12] Electrograms recorded in late diastole generally denote the exit site of a circuit, while recordings that have both a diastolic and systolic (intra-QRS) recording are from areas bridging a line of functional or anatomic block (Figure 1). Because of some of the limitations of activation mapping, some investigators have begun using isopotential mapping during VT. These maps are relatively quick to acquire and analyze and the information can be presented in several formats, including planar isopotential line or color maps and movies of isopotential loci.[13]

Confirmation of the tissue's involvement in the circuit can be accomplished in a number of ways; although useful, they are not always performed because of technical or time considerations. Included among these are pacing maneuvers such as single-beat resetting or continuous resetting (entrainment) from either a remote site (right ventricular electrode) or from the recording apparatus (Figure 2). These can be very useful but are sometimes tedious and time-consuming, and thus are not used as often intraoperatively as they are in the EP laboratory.[14–16] These techniques are as valuable when they show that the tissue being recorded is *not* within the VT circuit as when they show that the tissue *is* within the circuit. This is especially relevant when recording from very diseased tissue in which some diastolic potentials appear to be associated with the circuit but can in fact be dissociated with pacing maneuvers and thus attention directed to other areas.

In addition, physical maneuvers may be performed to alter or terminate the VT, such as application of pressure with a mapping probe or finger at the site from which the electrogram of interest was recorded, or application of a cryoprobe and cooling of the site to 0°C. In a study of 124 patients undergoing intraoperative mapping, we demonstrated that pressure applied with the mapping probe to sites suspected of being critical for continuation of tachycardia resulted in slowing and termination of VT in 79% of trials; this correlated with surgical cure of VT when this area was resected

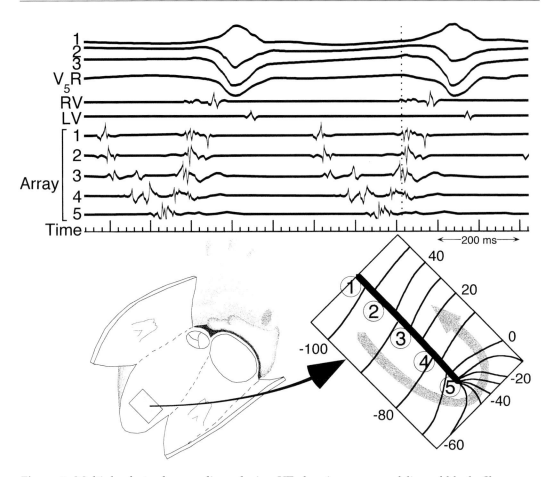

Figure 1. Multiple electrode recordings during VT showing presumed line of block. Shown are surface ECG leads 1, 2, 3 and V_5R with intracardiac recordings from right (RV) and left ventricular (LV) plunge electrodes and selected recordings from a multipolar electrode array during an intraoperative VT map. Multiple activations are recorded in several electrodes during VT (cycle length [CL] 270 ms); mid- and late diastolic components have progressively later timing from electrodes 1 to 4, while the activations around the time of the QRS onset reverse this order, "changing direction" at electrode 5. The approximate location of this section of the array is shown in the diagram at lower left, depicting the left ventricle opened along its lateral margin. At the lower right is the isochronal plot of activation times (shown in ms) of electrograms; electrode locations are shown as numbers in circles. Gray arrow indicates direction of wavefront propagation.

(Figure 3).[17] In some cases, the pressure exerted in keeping the recording electrode in good contact with the endocardium (this is especially true of relatively stiff planar electrode arrays) may be enough to either terminate VT or prevent its reinitiation. In a similar way, sites can be confirmed as being within the VT circuit by using a cryoprobe. Gallagher et al.[18] showed that cooling tissue presumed to be integral to the VT circuit to 0°C slowed and terminated VT in seven cases, and this result correlated well with surgical cure. The process is somewhat more time-consuming than exerting physical pressure, however.

The role of sinus rhythm or pacemapping in the operating room is less clear. Although the relative hemodynamic stability advantage of sinus rhythm over VT is clear during catheter endocardial mapping, this distinction is largely moot at surgery (during cardiopulmonary bypass). Sinus rhythm map-

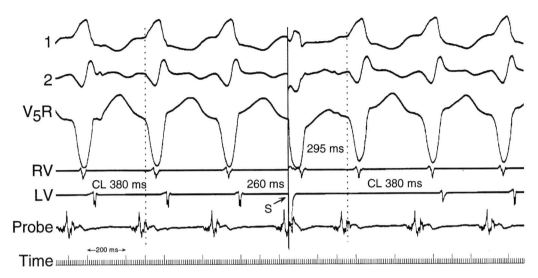

Figure 2. Resetting of ventricular tachycardia. Recordings and labels similar to Figure 1. Probe = roving bipolar probe electrode. During ventricular tachycardia, CL 380 ms, a single LV extrastimulus (S, dark arrow) is introduced 260 ms after the prior electrogram resulting in advancement of the timing of subsequent surface and intracardiac electrograms (the next VT beat occurs 60 ms earlier than expected). The probe electrogram maintains the same morphology and timing relative to the onset of the QRS after this perturbation as it does during all other VT beats; this was true over a range of coupling intervals of the extrastimulus. Dotted vertical lines denote onset of the QRS complex.

ping could still be advantageous if the information content were sufficiently sensitive and specific to guide a curative surgical procedure (Figure 4). Catheter and intraoperative studies have shown sinus rhythm mapping to be inferior to activation mapping during VT in this regard.[19-21] However, Bourke et al. have used sinus rhythm "fragmentation mapping" with reasonable success in patients with VT or VF; $^{16}/_{19}$ (84%) of operative survivors did not require anti-

arrhythmic drug therapy postoperatively, although ventricular arrhythmias were inducible in others postoperatively.[22] This technique could also be useful in patients with no inducible VT or in those with non-mappable ventricular arrhythmias (polymorphic VT or VF).

Pacemapping (pacing at a putative region within the VT circuit to replicate the 12-lead ECG during VT) has been used in the operative setting in the past.[23] Technical limita-

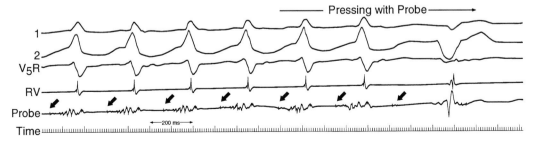

Figure 3. Pressure termination of VT. Recordings and labels as in Figure 1. During VT, the probe electrogram contains a low-amplitude mid-diastolic recording. Pressure with the mapping probe results in termination of VT after the inscription of the mid-diastolic potential.

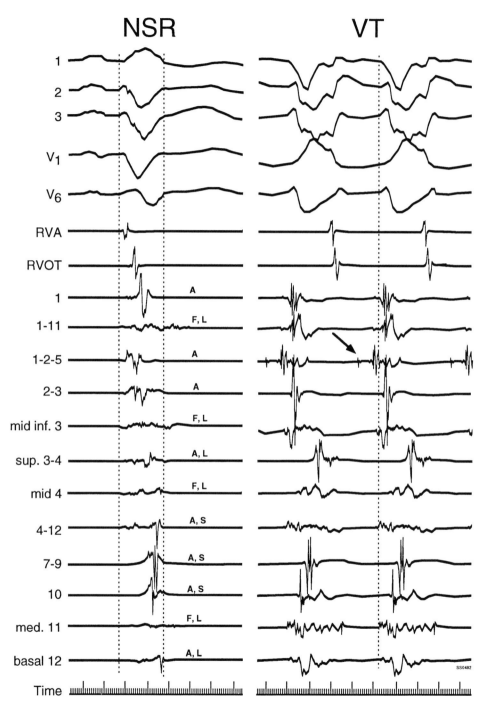

Figure 4. Comparison of sinus rhythm (NSR) and VT activation mapping. Recordings similar to Figure 1. Intracardiac recordings labeled according to a catheter endocardial mapping scheme. Sinus rhythm electrograms are characterized as abnormal (A), fractionated (F), late (L), split (S), or combinations of these. Earliest endocardial activity during VT is at site 1-2-5 (arrow); this site during NSR is abnormal, but other sites which are unimportant during VT are much more abnormal in NSR. RVA-RV apex; RVOT-RV outflow tract. Used with permission Josephson ME, et al.[63]

tions, such as alterations in chest wall configuration and surface ECG recording sites compared to the closed chest, and recording capacity, have made this technique impractical in the past. Newer mapping systems capable of recording more surface ECG leads than earlier systems have solved the latter problem, but the difficulties due to differences in recording sites remain (comparing intraoperative paced ECGs to those previously recorded on a closed chest). In addition, the time spent pacing at different locations seeking a "match" is probably better spent on activation mapping during VT. Pacemapping could be useful in unusual situations, such as if only nonsustained VT is initiated and an ECG is recorded but no activation mapping can be performed because of technical problems. Hopefully, this would be a rare circumstance.

To an extent, the mapping strategy depends on the purpose of the surgical procedure, as is discussed below; if time is felt to be critical, such as in a patient with incessant, hemodynamically unstable VT and poor ventricular function, mapping time may be budgeted to obtain only the most essential information.

Role of the Epicardium and Deeper Myocardial Layers

In the original studies of intraoperative mapping during VT, extensive mapping of both endocardium and epicardium (of both ventricles) was routinely performed. Experience showed that the earliest epicardial breakthrough was consistently later than the earliest endocardial site, and eventually epicardial mapping was abandoned as having little yield. These studies were generally performed with a roving bipolar electrode and each "site" was up to 2 cm from its nearest neighbor. In recent years, several well-executed surgical mapping papers using a higher density of mapping sites have been published in which a larger role for deeper myocardial layers and even the epicardium have been suggested. Interest in nonendocardial reentry zones has been spurred by the suboptimal cure rate of patients undergoing purely endocardial ablation for control of VT. In our older series of 353 patients undergoing intraoperative mapping and surgical ablation from 1977 to 1992, 77 patients had inducible VT postoperatively; of these, 59 were morphologies that had been observed prior to or during surgery, whereas 18 were "new" morphologies (differing in bundle branch block-type configuration or frontal plane axis by ≥90°). Of the "old" VTs that could still be induced postoperatively, intraoperative mapping data suggested endocardial critical circuit components in the vast majority. Among over 1,000 VTs during which some intraoperative mapping was performed (not all of which were completely mapped), only 21 showed conclusive evidence of essential involvement of myocardium outside the subendocardial layers (RV in 2, LV septal in 14, LV free wall intramural or epicardial in 5). These were managed with cryoablation and 86% were successfully treated surgically (i.e., no longer inducible, no spontaneous recurrences). In nearly all of these cases, mapping was performed with the single-site acquisition method, moving a probe from site to site during VT or using a multipolar plunge electrode for intramural recordings; thus the mapping was not nearly as comprehensive as can be performed currently with high-density multipolar electrode arrays. Although it is certainly possible that resection or cryoablation simply "missed" areas to which mapping had directed the surgeon's efforts, it is likely that a significant proportion of the VTs not cured by surgery had critical circuit components in nonendocardial layers. In an additional 13 patients, some VTs were mapped to areas outside the visible endocardial scar; additional resection or cryoablation of these regions resulted in noninducibility of these VTs in all cases.

More recent studies have been performed with simultaneous recordings from multipolar electrode arrays, either in sheets, inflatable balloons that conform reasonably well to the endocardial surface, or epicardial "sock" arrays (Figure 5). Some have

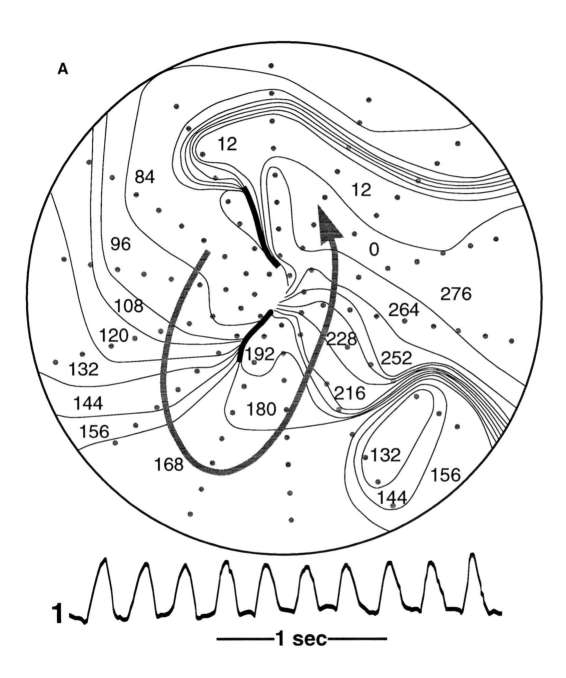

Figure 5. Isochronal maps during VT. In both panels, the endocardial surface is depicted in a polar projection with the apex at the center, septum to left, anterior wall to upper right. Small dots designate recording electrodes locations on an endocardial balloon. Isochronal maps of induced VT are displayed at 12 ms intervals; thick dark lines denote arcs of block; shaded curved arrows indicate direction of wavefront propagation. A representative ECG lead is also shown below. In **A,** the complete cardiac cycle is shown during one VT beat. Two areas of slow conduction are shown as narrowly-spaced isochrones. A second endocardial breakthrough is evident at lower right ("132"). This pattern is consistent with macroreentry around the apical infarct zone. *Continued.*

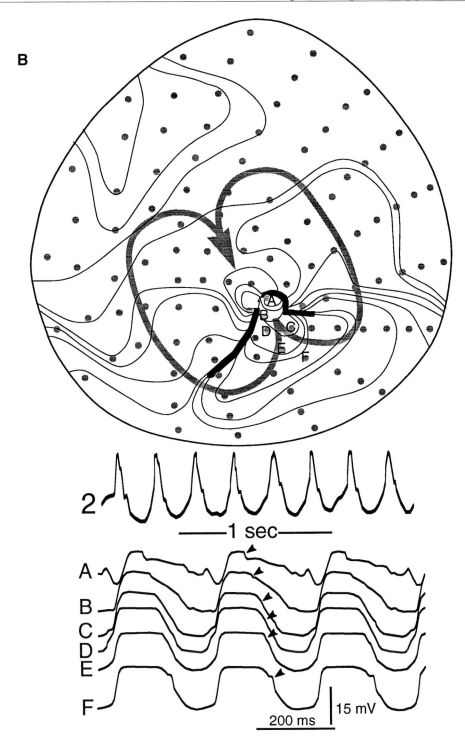

Figure 5. *(Continued)* In **B,** a complete figure-of-8 reentrant pattern is shown; mid-diastolic recordings are made from the narrow zone between arcs of block. At bottom are representative unipolar recordings from six electrodes **(A–F)** just distal to the gap in the arcs of block. Small arrowheads denote timing of local activation from each electrode. Used with permission from American College of Cardiology.[26]

also incorporated recordings from intra-mural multipolar needle electrodes. These mapping studies have shown that the pro-portion of the VT circuit (percentage of VT cycle length) that can be accounted for on the endocardium ranges from 55% to 100%, and mid-diastolic components can likewise be recorded from the endocardial surface in >80% of cases.[24-27] This would suggest a relatively limited role for extra-endocardial tissue in active participation in the VT cir-cuit. In these studies, the area from which mid-diastolic recordings can be made aver-ages approximately 1 cm.[2] Complex elec-trograms are often recorded in which multi-ple discrete activations are recorded from the same electrodes with an isoelectric inter-val between components; while these may represent activation of two bundles of tissue on opposite sides of a line of block (ana-tomic or functional) on the endocardial sur-face, it also appears that in some cases the line of block may be between the endocar-dium and deeper layers. Evidence for this comes from studies in which a multipolar recording array was used to record during VT and then during sinus rhythm pre- and immediately postresection of the endocar-dial specimen, showing that diastolic poten-tials during VT correspond to late and split potentials in sinus rhythm, which alone are eradicated by resection whereas systolic electrogram components tend to increase somewhat in amplitude (Figure 6).[28]

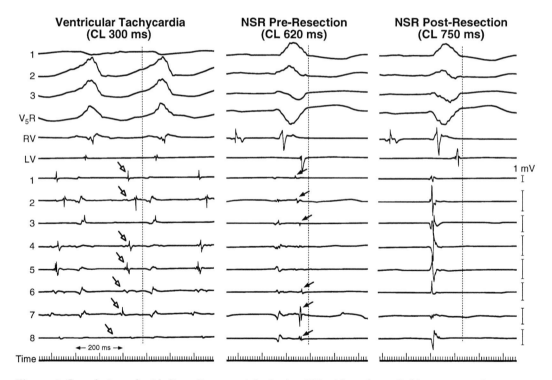

Figure 6. Correlation of mid-diastolic potentials during VT with endocardial late potentials in sinus rhythm. Recordings and labels similar to Figure 1. Electrodes 1–7 are representative recordings from a 20-electrode array. Signals were recorded from the same location during VT (left panel) and sinus rhythm prior to (center panel) and immediately following (right panel) endocardial resection. Mid-diastolic potentials are seen during VT (open arrows; line denotes QRS onset) corresponding to low-amplitude potentials (dark arrows; line denotes QRS end) that follow the end of the QRS during sinus rhythm pre-resection. These are no longer present post-resection, whereas the main component of the local electrogram has generally increased in amplitude due to removal of attenuat-ing effect of endocardial scar. At the far right are 1-mV calibration signals.

If the density of mapping electrodes is not high enough ($\leq$5 mm between electrodes), it is possible to miss recording the key mid-diastolic electrograms despite their being present on the endocardium and making recordings in the right area. We have observed several instances in which, during attempted endocardial catheter ablation of VT, no optimal target sites (electrogram criteria) could be found despite diligent searching for over an hour, resulting in several unsuccessful RF applications; yet when the catheter is moved almost imperceptibly, a typical mid-diastolic recording is observed and RF delivery at that site eradicates VT. If this particular site, which may be only a few millimeters in diameter, is not encountered, a natural (but erroneous) conclusion is that the critical portions of the responsible reentrant circuit must reside within deeper myocardial layers or the epicardium.

Some of the more recent data point more specifically to an important role for deeper myocardial layers in perpetuation of VT.[29,30] In some cases, epicardial cryoablation or laser photocoagulation have succeeded in terminating and eliminating inducibility of VT.[31] This observation in itself is not the same as proving that the epicardium has a critical role in the VT circuit, only that the epicardium contained a portion of the circuit. In other studies, epicardial ablation has terminated VT when ablation attempts at all suitable endocardial sites had failed.[32] This shows a unique role for the epicardial layers in these cases. What proportion of VTs are of this type is not clear. Certainly the success rates of 70% or more, despite very limited use of extra-endocardial ablation in the earlier surgical series suggests that a maximum of 30% of cases would potentially have unique epicardial critical circuit components (and likely less than this number, if intramural septal and free wall sites as well as "missed" endocardial sites are part of the 30%).

How can the newer data suggesting a prominent role for the epicardium or deep septal myocardium be reconciled with the older information suggesting these layers had a very limited role? One possibility is that the substrate for VT has changed over time. In the older series, we observed cases of VT following infarcts in which spontaneous or thrombolytic-induced reperfusion occurred. In such instances, the myocardial thickness in the infarct zone at surgery was much better preserved than in other cases, endocardial scar was less dense and aneurysms were infrequent. In addition, some of these patients had mapping evidence of involvement of epicardial or deep intramural layers. If a higher proportion of patients in the more recent series fit this profile, this might explain the higher reported frequency of epicardial involvement. Increased use of chemical or mechanical ("rescue angioplasty") reperfusion at the time of infarction, as well as post-infarct beta blockers and ACE inhibitors, may have altered both the prevalence of VT post-infarct as well as the anatomic location of components of the circuit.

A second potential source of discrepant results between the earlier and more recent data may be differences in the nature of the VT circuit in some cases of inferior infarction. It was noted in some early series that patients with inferior infarct-related VT had a lower surgical cure rate (56%) than those with anterior infarctions (88%).[33] Subsequent work showed that a significant proportion of VTs in patients with inferior infarction were due to circuits that incorporated a thin isthmus of surviving muscle between the basal aspect of the infarction and the mitral annulus, with macroreentry occurring around the infarct zone. Incision or cryoablation to eliminate conduction through this isthmus resulted in cure rates exceeding 90%.[34] Whether the critical portion of the circuit thus obliterated by the new surgical technique was located near the endocardial surface or in deeper layers is not clear; if it was located more toward the epicardium, this could explain some of the differences between relative frequencies of epicardial participation in older versus newer series. However, performing endocardial catheter ablation at this same basal LV isthmus in patients with apparent macroreentrant inferior infarct-related VT has yielded very good success rates; since most evidence suggests that endocardial ventricular RF lesions do not extend to the epicardial surface, these results would militate against a prominent role for the epicardial layers in these VTs.[35]

Whether these or other factors are responsible for apparent discrepancies in the degree of involvement of the epicardium and deeper myocardial layers between the earlier and more recent series is unclear. Certainly the answer to this question has implications for endocardial catheter ablation as well as surgical therapy of VT.

Preoperative Mapping Studies

Endocardial Catheter Mapping

In previous papers on intraoperative management of VT, preoperative endocardial catheter VT activation mapping played a prominent role.[36,37] This was because one could not always be certain of inducing all desired VT morphologies during surgery, and if catheter mapping information were available to guide the electrophysiologist and surgeon during surgery, the chances of a successful procedure would be increased. However, with the availability of RF catheter ablation, the likelihood is small that a patient would undergo extensive endocardial catheter mapping and yet not have an attempt at catheter ablation. Furthermore, if RF successfully eliminated inducibility of the VT, it would not be of surgical interest; if RF failed to affect the VT at all, the utility of the mapping data used to guide the RF would be suspect and of limited value at surgery. Only if RF had some effect on the VT—slowing or termination but not effecting noninducibility—would the mapping information on which it was based have adequate validity to guide surgical attack. Thus, preoperative endocardial mapping is

likely to have a lesser role now than in the past in assisting the electrophysiologist and surgeon during subsequent VT surgery.

The same can be said for preoperative *endocardial pacemapping*, a technique in which pacing is performed at various sites within the ventricle attempting to produce a 12-lead ECG exactly matching that of the targeted VT.[38] This tool has the advantage of not requiring the patient to be maintained for long periods of time in VT in order to perform detailed activation mapping. Sites need to be paced for only long enough to acquire an ECG, allowing the patient to rest between pacing attempts at different sites. Pacemapping has certain limitations, including sensitivity and specificity; that is, pacing at sites that are in fact within the VT circuit may not yield an ECG at all resembling the target VT, whereas pacing at sites remote from the critical diastolic portion of the circuit can produce nearly perfect electrocardiographic matches.[39,40]

Preoperative catheter endocardial sinus rhythm mapping has a distinct advantage over VT mapping, in that its inherent hemodynamic stability allows adequate time for a relatively dense and complete sampling of the endocardial surface. The utility of preoperative catheter sinus rhythm mapping has been debated over the years; most evidence indicates that the information derived has neither the sensitivity nor the specificity to make this technique a reliable tool to designate regions that should be specifically targeted for ablation at surgery. It may be that with additional experience, certain electrogram types or characteristics will be shown to have sufficient predictive accuracy that sinus rhythm mapping may be a primary tool in guiding ablative procedures (catheter or surgical).[19]

Morphologic Criteria (ECG During VT)

It has been known for some years that certain VT morphologies reliably "arose" from certain endocardial regions; when encountering one of these VTs, the electrophysiologist could streamline the catheter or surgical mapping procedure by focusing mapping attention on only these areas. The studies in which these criteria were developed were based primarily on mapping criteria using late diastolic activity as the indicator of VT "site of origin."[41,42] Thus, the resulting algorithms designate "exit sites" that are near but not necessarily within a critical portion of the reentrant circuit. If this limitation is kept in mind, one can still make use of the information from these studies in planning where to concentrate mapping efforts. In a relatively large study attempting to correlate 12-lead ECG morphology during VT with regions of endocardium responsible for the VT, four characteristics were identified which, when incorporated into a somewhat complex algorithm, could be used to suggest endocardial regions for focused mapping attention. These characteristics were infarct location, bundle branch block-type configuration, quadrant of frontal plane axis, and one of eight precordial R wave progression patterns. Applying this algorithm to a large series of VTs, mapping locations of up to 37% of VTs related to prior anterior infarction and 74% of VTs associated with inferior infarction could be correctly regionalized.[41] This study, as well as others using the 12-lead ECG or vectorcardiography,[43] are limited by relatively low resolution (i.e., they can only regionalize, not specify exact locations to which one should direct catheter placement), lack of applicability thus far to multisite infarction or VT unrelated to prior infarction, and their complexity. Slightly more accurate but even less easily applied is noninvasive body surface mapping during VT.[44] Using this technique, a chest array of 62 electrodes is placed on the patient and recordings made during VT. A specialized computer algorithm then constructs an isointegral map of the VT, which can then be compared to a catalog of previously mapped VTs and the responsible endocardial region identified. Although the regions thus specified are in most cases smaller in surface area than those indicated by the other algorithms based on a standard 12-lead ECG during VT, the equipment used to acquire and process the signals is specialized and its format (isointegral maps) not as familiar to most electrophysiologists as the standard ECG.

Utility of Mapping

What is the evidence that mapping, with its attendant increase in operative time and resources, adds measurably to operative success? Some have suggested that a much simpler procedure, not incorporating mapping, can provide reasonable antiarrhythmic success. For example, resection of all visible endocardial scar (including papillary muscles, if significantly scarred, with attendant mitral valve replacement) has been used with good reported success rates.[45-48] However, because of relatively small numbers of patients, short follow-up periods and variable methods of assessing antiarrhythmic efficacy, the reported postoperative VT noninducibility and spontaneous recurrence rates should be interpreted with caution. A relatively large study suggesting that mapping contributes to surgical success was performed on 100 consecutive patients who underwent intraoperative mapping and standard postoperative EP study. In this series, the completeness of mapping was closely correlated with surgical success: in patients in whom all known VTs were adequately mapped, 88% were cured surgically; in those in whom from 55% to 99% of VTs were mapped, 69% had surgical cure; and in those in whom <50% of all VTs could be mapped, only 53% were cured.[49]

Mapping also provides the only way currently available to eliminate the approximately 15% of VTs that have critical areas for reentry in deeper myocardial layers or in apparently normal endocardium (in actuality, there is almost always a layer of obvious scar tissue just beneath a rather normal-appearing endocardial sheet). In addition, those VTs occurring within the first 3–5 weeks post acute myocardial infarction (before dense endocardial scar has formed) can only be addressed by mapping.[50,51]

Unfortunately, no morphologic or other characteristics of individual VTs have yet been discovered that designate which ones require ablation of deeper myocardial layers for successful therapy. If criteria were to be developed that would reliably indicate which particular VTs would not be cured by visually guided endocardial scar excision, mapping could be reserved for only these VTs. Until such distinctions are possible, it would seem that intraoperative mapping still has a role in the surgical management of VT. Similarly, although the majority of patients with post-infarct VT have more than one morphology of VT either spontaneously or in the EP laboratory in response to programmed stimulation,[9,52] not all of these VTs represent distinct circuits. Some are clearly two different manifestations of the same circuit, either as separate exit sites, or opposite directions of wavefront propagation in the circuit.[12] As yet there are no characteristics that identify a particular VT morphology or set of VTs as members of the same circuit, such that mapping and eliminating one would obviate the need for specifically targeting others.

Problems with Mapping

Even with the best preparation, the mapping procedure can still encounter many problems that may limit its utility. The most important of these are discussed below.

1. Lack of a mappable arrhythmia. This may be either due to complete noninducibility of any ventricular arrhythmia, or initiation of either polymorphic VT/VF or only nonsustained VT. The first possibility may be caused by excessive endocardial cooling due to exposure to air (in which case warming the return from the heart-lung machine will help); it is also possible that the surgeon may have inadvertently incised the circuit

during ventriculotomy or during removal of endocardial thrombus. If nonuniform ventricular arrhythmias are repeatedly initiated, rather than stable VT, one should consider the possibility of severe active ischemia (especially in inferior infarcts, due to kinking of the left anterior descending coronary artery caused by lifting the apex to obtain adequate exposure). Nonsustained uniform VT is more readily addressed by multipolar mapping systems that can gather meaningful information during just a few cycles of VT. The endocardial activation sequence has been shown to be stable during the first few beats of VT, such as occurs in nonsustained VT, and thus the ability of modern mapping systems can largely obviate this potential problem. In any case in which no mappable arrhythmia can be initiated, sinus rhythm mapping may still be used as a reasonable indicator of regions of endocardial pathology which at least could potentially be involved in reentrant circuits.

2. Inability to determine timing of QRS complex onset (Figure 7). This is an unusual problem, characterized by very rapid VT and very wide QRS complexes in which there is no clear inflection point for the QRS onset. Lacking this, it is difficult to know whether any particular endocardial electrogram is mid-diastolic or mid-systolic. On occasion the pause following a burst of rapid pacing may allow a clear view of the QRS onset that can then be used as a "template." Otherwise, it is best to terminate the arrhythmia and try to initiate a different, mappable one rather than continuing to gather data that cannot be reliably interpreted. This problem is most typically observed in patients taking amiodarone chronically.

3. Lack of clarity as to the timing of local activation. The complex nature of many of the electrograms in the regions of interest make their interpretation complex. Bipolar recordings were favored in the earlier studies because of their resistance to offset when moving from location to location in the heart; however, unipolar recordings have

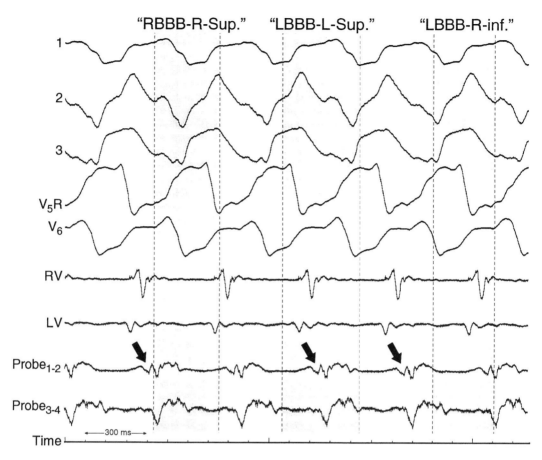

Figure 7. Rapid VT of unclear QRS morphology. Recordings and labels as in previous figures. Dotted lines denote possible onsets of QRS complexes, with resultant VT morphologies indicated below. If VT morphology is actually LBBB-R-Sup (at right), the *Probe* electrogram is presystolic indicating proximity to/location within the VT circuit; if VT morphology is actually RBBB-R-Inf (center), the *Probe* recording is from a site outside the circuit.

several advantages over bipolar, including being more specific about location and direction of wavefront propagation. Most evidence suggests that the point of maximum dV/dt in the local unipolar recording reflects local activation under the electrode, whereas peak voltage is a more reliable indicator of activation in bipolar recordings.[53-55] With less need to move electrodes in the current systems so that electrode offset artifact is less problematic, many manufacturers have configured their recording apparatus to be unipolar, and using maximum dV/dt as the timing of local activation.

4. Intermittent potentials during VT. In diseased endocardium, one can record often potentials during VT that are not present every tachycardia cycle despite stable electrode contact. This phenomenon (called "local conduction failure" or "exit block") has been observed in up to 64% of VTs and during at least one VT in 86% of patients.[56] Intermittent potentials are usually of low amplitude and typically occur on an every-other beat basis, although Wenckebach and more complex patterns are occasionally observed. Although the tissue from which these potentials are recorded is obviously not involved in the VT circuit, the timing of

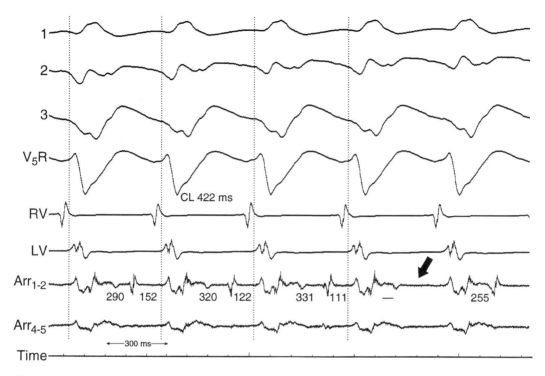

Figure 8. Intermittent conduction of mid-diastolic potentials during VT. Recordings and labels similar to Figure 1. Selected recordings made during VT from bipolar electrodes 5 mm apart on a multipolar array (Arr.) are shown. VT cycle length is constant at 422 ms. Arr$_{1-2}$ shows a mid-diastolic potential, but it exhibits Wenckebach conduction as indicated by numbers below the recording; after the 4th cycle the potential fails to conduct at all. These data indicate that the potential, despite having a morphology and timing characteristic of critical circuit components, was not essential for perpetuation of this VT.

these potentials can be mid-diastolic when they occur (Figure 8) and they can thus mislead the electrophysiologist into believing he or she is recording from within the circuit. Simply observing several cycles will reveal the true nature of these potentials. The prevalence of intermittent potentials during intraoperative mapping is far higher than that noted during catheter endocardial mapping. This may be because of the greater ease of concentrating mapping attention during surgery in areas of highly diseased endocardium that are more likely to exhibit the phenomenon, or that some condition imposed by the operation itself (endocardial cooling, stretching, or pressure or the effects of anesthetic agents) may prolong refractoriness in diseased tissue more

than is likely to occur during catheter mapping.

5. Random recording problems or interpretation errors. These may be in the form of spurious data from an electrode in poor contact or broken electrical continuity, or as inaccurate automated interpretations. In this latter category, the computer takes in very large amounts of data and assigns an activation time according to its algorithms; if one or more is incorrect, the interpretation of the results will likewise be inaccurate (Figure 9).

6. General equipment failure. The newer mapping systems are relatively more complex than the earlier less sophisticated systems; this complexity compounds being able to fix a problem that might develop

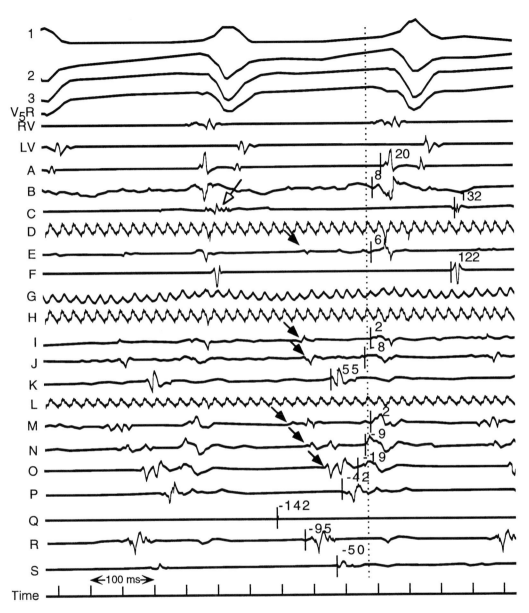

Figure 9. Example of early computerized multi-site intraoperative mapping. Recordings and labels as in previous figures, with electrograms from 19/20 electrodes on a multipolar array during VT. Dotted line is at QRS onset; short vertical lines on electrograms are computer-derived activation times (numbers relative to QRS onset). Note in **C** that an activation was marked although recording is unstable (white arrow). Dark arrows denote low-amplitude mid-diastolic potentials of significant mapping interest that were ignored by the computer algorithm. Electrodes **D, G, H, L** show 60 Hz artifact; computer-derived activations have been edited out. In **Q**, a bit-error signal was mistakenly taken by the computer as the local activation. This early effort with computerized mapping shows some of the potential problems with this technique; more recent hardware and software have largely mitigated these problems. Used with permission from Singer I, ed.[64]

during a procedure. With the older systems, a mechanically inclined electrophysiologist could fix or work around almost any equipment-related problem that arose during a mapping procedure, but this is not likely to be the case with the currently available all-electronic systems.

Intraoperative Strategies

The extent to which mapping is used during a surgical procedure for the purpose of eliminating VT depends to an extent on the ultimate purpose of the procedure. For instance, in a purely elective case, in which complete cure of VT is the goal, one should spare no effort in assuring that all VTs are adequately addressed (part of which concerns VT mapping). In another situation, a patient may have nearly incessant VT, very poor LV function, and no coronary arteries to bypass; in this type of case, one may wish to spend as little time in the operating room as possible. The portion of a surgical procedure dedicated to mapping can thus vary considerably depending on the goals, as follows:

1. If one wants to find where the critical area for a particular VT is, stimulation will be performed until that VT is initiated and careful mapping is performed along with confirmatory manuevers. Stimulation should be repeated after resection or other forms of ablation directed against the VT to ensure it has been eliminated. If not, repeated cycles of mapping, ablation, and re-stimulation are performed until VT can no longer be initiated.[57] Reproducibility of initiation in the pre-mapping stage is desirable, thereby increasing the validity of lack of inducibility post-ablation.

2. If the purpose of the procedure is to eliminate all known existing VTs and any future ones, a larger portion of the time spent on the electrophysiological portion of the procedure can be shifted to the post-ablation phase, thus spending considerable time and effort on ventricular stimulation ensuring that all inducible VT has been

eradicated. It is even reasonable in selected cases to begin the procedure by initiating and terminating VT a few times to ensure reproducible induction, then proceeding with subendocardial resection, encirclement, or cryoablation directly. This strategy leaves mapping for discerning the regions responsible for VT occurrence after a standard resection or other procedure. If no VT can be initiated after the resection (but it could be reliably induced pre-resection), no mapping is necessary; if, however, VT can be induced after the standard resection, it was obviously not completely effective and mapping to localize the residual arrhythmia's critical circuit components should be performed.

3. If mapping is primarily for research purposes (that is, other criteria such as visible scar will be used to "guide" the ablative procedure), more time can be devoted to performing detailed mapping and stimulation during VT using electrode arrays containing a large number of recording electrodes. This would be followed by the ablative procedure and a shortened post-ablative stimulation time.

Thus, based on which of these (or others) constitutes the purpose of the mapping procedure, the operative procedure will be conducted in very different ways.

Operative Outcomes

The success of a surgical procedure such as those used in treating patients with VT can be viewed as having two components: operative survival, and antiarrhythmic efficacy. It is beyond the scope of this chapter to address the factors influencing operative survival for the variety of surgical procedures that have been used to treat VT; several studies have evaluated these characteristics.[58–60] When attempting to evaluate the antiarrhythmic efficacy of surgery, one very quickly encounters difficulty in that a variety of definitions of "success" have been used in the literature. This greatly complicates making accurate comparisons between techniques and studies. Among the definitions used for a successful antiarrhythmic procedure are (roughly from least stringent to most stringent): elimination of spontaneous episodes of the so-called "clinical" VT (an ECG-documented preoperative morphology of VT); noninducibility of the "clinical" VT at postoperative EP study; elimination of spontaneous episodes of any uniform morphology VT; elimination of spontaneous episodes of any type of ventricular arrhythmia; noninducibility of any uniform morphology VT at postoperative EP study; noninducibility of any type of ventricular arrhythmia at postoperative EP study; no inducible or recurrent ventricular arrhythmia at any time postoperatively. Table 1 shows how these definitions can be applied to the very same data set and result in very different interpretations of "success."

We analyzed the long-term antiarrhythmic efficacy of subendocardial resection as a function of the results of the postoperative EP study and found that 95% of patients who had no inducible VT at this study were free from recurrent arrhythmia at 5 years postoperatively, whereas only 76% of those who had any inducible VT were similarly free from recurrences over the same time period. The vast majority of these latter patients were given either drug or defibrillator

therapy.[61] As noted above, in a small proportion of patients with inducible VT at postoperative EP study, the induced VT morphology was one that had not been observed at any prior study. In our series, this result was encountered in 6% of patients who underwent postoperative study (18/300, three of whom had subsequent spontaneous recurrent episodes of this VT). The cause of these VTs is unclear, whether they represent circuits that were present all along but not manifested due to the presence of antiarrhythmic drugs that had been stopped for the surgery, an alteration of a previous circuit (different exit site or different anatomic location of the same exit site due to surgical remodeling), or an entirely new circuit caused by the operation. Since these VTs had not been detected prior to the postoperative study, it is questionable whether even the most advanced mapping methods will be able to entirely eliminate their occasional occurrence. Finally, in some patients, very rapid uniform VT, ventricular flutter, or polymorphic VT or VF are initiated at the postoperative EP study. We and others have observed that inducibility of either very rapid uniform VT (cycle length >50 ms less than the most rapid VT known for that patient) or polymorphic VT/VF generally are not associated with a high risk of recurrent arrhythmia episodes. These re-

---

Table 1

Effect of Differing Definitions of Antiarrhythmic Efficacy on Apparent Surgical Results

Definition	Results (% Success)
Elimination of spontaneous episodes of the "clinical" VT*	96
Noninducibility of the "clinical" VT at postoperative EP study	93
Elimination of spontaneous episodes of any uniform morphology VT	91
Elimination of spontaneous episodes of any type of ventricular arrhythmia	85
Noninducibility of any uniform morphology VT at postop EP study	75
Noninducibility of any type of ventricular arrhythmia at postoperative EP study	72
No inducible or recurrent ventricular arrhythmia at any time postoperatively	68

* An ECG-documented preoperative morphology of VT.

The column at right shows percentages of patients who would meet the definitions of "surgical success" in the left column from among the authors' series of 300 patients who underwent postoperative EP study or had spontaneous VT recurrence in the perioperative period. Note that although the patients are the same in each case, the criterion used for successful outcome makes a large difference in the reported success rate.

sults were independent of mode of initial clinical presentation (stable VT or cardiac arrest).[61,62]

Based on these and other data, most electrophysiologists now believe that if uniform morphology VT can be initiated at the postoperative EP study—even if it is of a morphology not encountered previously—the patient should be treated as being at risk of recurrence of VT (antiarrhythmic medications or ICD).

The question of whether to place an ICD postoperatively in a patient who has only inducible polymorphic VT, ventricular flutter or VF is more difficult. Although the data suggest that these patients are at low risk for recurrent arrhythmia episodes,[62] the ease with which an ICD can be placed currently can understandably make one reluctant to not place one in such a situation.

Case Management Scenarios

Having set forth various strategies for intraoperative VT mapping, two case scenarios follow that illustrate these principles:

1. A 48-year-old man has a history of frequent hemodynamically well-tolerated VT recurrences, refractory to a variety of empiric antiarrhythmic agents; the majority of ATP attempts accelerate the VT requiring a shock. He has single-vessel (left anterior descending) disease on coronary arteriography, an LV apical aneurysm with overall EF 25% and preserved basal systolic function; large sessile apical thrombus overlies the distal $\frac{1}{4}$ of the LV cavity.

Analysis. This man has failed antiarrhythmic therapy, cannot be optimally managed with an ICD, and cannot safely undergo catheter ablation because of the apical thrombus; on the other hand, he has a very high likelihood of surviving a VT surgical operation and being cured of all inducible arrhythmias; since he has single-vessel disease, the procedure could be performed without needing to cool the heart or administer cardioplegia, shortening the procedure and decreasing risk; also, recurrent is-

chemia is unlikely in the near future and thus a defibrillator will not be needed.

2. A 62-year-old woman has had a recent posterolateral MI and is experiencing two or three episodes/day of rapid uniform VT refractory to lidocaine, procainamide, and intravenous amiodarone, requiring urgent cardioversion each time. Potassium, magnesium, and beta blockers result in no change. Coronary arteriography shows an occluded circumflex artery and a long 80% LAD stenosis. Intra-aortic balloon counterpulsation has no effect on arrhythmia recurrence. She is deemed too ill for transfer to an institution with more experience managing such cases.

Analysis. ICD therapy will not be satisfactory with this frequency of recurrences; catheter ablation cannot be performed with such an unstable arrhythmia; medications have failed. In such a case, taking her to the operating room and performing a relatively "blind" or visually directed endocardial resection may be adequate, although if the infarct is recent enough, there may be minimal demarcation of normal and infarcted endocardium. Options then include regular VT mapping or sinus rhythm "fragmentation" mapping, followed by resection of areas designated by mapping as being potential sites of slow conduction portions of reentrant circuits. Stimulation should be performed after this part of the procedure to ascertain if more resection or cryotherapy is needed.

Future Considerations

It can reasonably be anticipated that, with a decreasing incidence of VT in the population and further advances in ICDs and catheter ablation, there will be even less need for direct surgical therapy for VT in the future. However, as in the case with percutaneous revascularization procedures, there will almost surely be a continued role for surgery albeit less than previously. However, this is not the situation everywhere. In some economic environments—especially those with relatively rigid caps on health care expenditures and resource utilization—surgery is preferable to ICD therapy and is applied with much greater frequency than in the United States.

It can also be anticipated that continued advances in mapping technology—mainly electrode arrays, automatic interpretive algorithms, and computer hardware and processing power—will facilitate the speed and accuracy of mapping procedures and lead to still higher cure rates for this type of surgery. Additional information gathered from mapping during sinus rhythm or pacing, with systems capable of very high data recording density, may lead to criteria for determining what apparently "innocent" myocardial regions should also be ablated in order to prevent occurrence of VTs postoperatively from circuits that have yet to become manifest.

Summary and Conclusions

It is ironic that just at a time when very powerful mapping and analytical tools are becoming available to study and perhaps more effectively treat VT surgically, fewer and fewer procedures are being performed. Is there still a role for surgical therapy for VT at all? Although far more limited than a decade ago, there are still patients for whom a surgical procedure is the best option. If surgical therapy is to be undertaken, is mapping necessary to ensure a good outcome? The best chance at eliminating all inducible and spontaneous VT postoperatively depends on ablation of critical components of all VT circuits; this in turn depends to a degree on mapping since, in up to 25% of cases, these components exist outside the bounds of visible endocardial scar tissue that would ordinarily be removed or otherwise ablated. In some cases, these critical circuit components are intramural or epicardial. Because there is currently no way (aside from mapping) to determine which VTs have critical circuit components unrelated to visible scar borders, it would seem that the surgical team should be prepared to do some mapping even if the procedure is planned as being only visually directed. The investment in equipment and expertise required to obtain the best outcomes, coupled with the relatively infrequent use of surgical therapy for VT, would suggest that only a small number of centers maintain these kinds of resources and perform these procedures. A good working relationship and understanding between the surgeon and electrophysiologist is key to obtaining the best possible results from these demanding procedures.

References

1. Guiraudon G, Fontaine G, Frank R, et al. Encircling endocardial ventriculotomy: a new surgical treatment for life-threatening ventricular tachycardias resistant to medical treatment following myocardial infarction. Ann Thor Surg 1978;26:438–444.
2. Josephson ME, Horowitz LN, Farshidi A, et al. Recurrent sustained ventricular tachycardia. 1. Mechanisms. Circulation 1978;57:431–439.
3. Josephson ME, Horowitz LN, Farshidi A, et al. Recurrent sustained ventricular tachycardia. 2. Endocardial mapping. Circulation 1978;57:440–447.
4. Josephson ME, Harken AH, Horowitz LN. Endocardial excision: a new surgical technique for the treatment of recurrent ventricular tachycardia. Circulation 1979;60:1430–1439.
5. Guiraudon GM, Klein GJ, Gulamhusein SS, et al. Total disconnection of the right ventricular free wall: surgical treatment of right ventricular tachycardia associated with right ventricular dysplasia. Circulation 1983;67:463–470.
6. Harken AH, Horowitz LN, Josephson ME. Surgical correction of recurrent sustained ventricular tachycardia following complete repair of tetralogy of Fallot. J Thorac Cardiovasc Surg 1980;80:779–781.
7. Gallagher JJ, Anderson RW, Kasell J, et al. Cryoablation of drug-resistant ventricular tachycardia in a patient with a variant of scleroderma. Circulation 1978;57:190–197.

8. Graffigna A, Minzioni G, Ressia L, et al. Surgical ablation of ventricular tachycardia secondary to congenital ventricular septal aneurysm. Ann Thorac Surg 1994;57:921–924.

9. Miller JM, Kienzle MG, Harken AH, et al. Morphologically distinct sustained ventricular tachycardias in coronary artery disease: significance and surgical results. J Am Coll Cardiol 1984;4:1073–1079.

10. Branyas NA, Cain ME, Cox JL, et al. Transmural ventricular activation during consecutive cycles of sustained ventricular tachycardia associated with coronary artery disease. Am J Cardiol 1990;65:861–867.

11. Onufer JR, Cain ME: Impact of mapping and ablation of ventricular tachycardia on management strategies for the 1990s. J Cardiovascular Electrophysiol 1991;2:77–91.

12. Fitzgerald DM, Friday KJ, Yeung Lai Wah JA, et al. Electrogram patterns predicting successful catheter ablation of ventricular tachycardia. Circulation 1988;77:806–814.

13. Rokkas CK, Nitta T, Schuessler RB, et al. Human ventricular tachycardia: precise intraoperative localization with potential distribution mapping. Ann Thorac Surg 1994; 57:1628–1635.

14. Morady F, Kadish A, Rosenheck S, et al. Concealed entrainment as a guide for catheter ablation of ventricular tachycardia in patients with prior myocardial infarction. J Am Coll Cardiol 1991;17:678–689.

15. Callans DJ, Hook BG, Josephson ME. Comparison of resetting and entrainment of uniform sustained ventricular tachycardia: Further insights into the characteristics of the excitable gap. Circulation 1993;87: 1229–1238.

16. Stevenson WG, Sager PT, Friedman PL. Entrainment techniques for mapping atrial and ventricular tachycardias. JCE 1995;6: 201–216.

17. Miller JM, Ratcliffe MB, Josephson ME, et al. Response to focal pressure at site of origin of ventricular tachycardia predicts surgical result. Circulation 1992;86:570.

18. Gallagher JD, Del Rossi AJ, Fernandez J. Cryothermal mapping of recurrent ventricular tachycardia in man. Circulation 1985;71: 733–739.

19. Cassidy DM, Vassallo JA, Buxton AE, et al. The value of catheter mapping during sinus rhythm to localize site of origin of ventricular tachycardia. Circulation 1984;69: 1103–1110.

20. Kienzle MG, Miller JM, Falcone RA, et al. Intraoperative endocardial mapping during sinus rhythm: relationship to site of origin of ventricular tachycardia. Circulation 1984; 70:957–965.

21. Cassidy DM, Vassallo JA, Miller JM, et al. Endocardial catheter mapping in patients in sinus rhythm: relationship to underlying heart disease and ventricular arrhythmias. Circulation 1986;73:645–652.

22. Bourke JP, Campbell RWF, Renzulli A, et al. Surgery for ventricular tachyarrhythmias based on fragmentation mapping in sinus rhythm alone. Eur J Cardiothorac Surg 1989; 3:401–406.

23. O'Keefe DB, Curry PVL, Prior AL, et al. Surgery for ventricular tachycardia using operative pacemapping. Proc Br Coll Surg 1980; 43:116–121.

24. de Bakker JMT, Janse MJ, Van Capelle FJL, et al. Endocardial mapping by simultaneous recording of endocardial electrograms during cardiac surgery for ventricular aneurysm. J Am Coll Cardiol 1983;2:947–953.

25. Harris L, Downar E, Mickleborough L, et al. Activation sequence of ventricular tachycardia: endocardial and epicardial mapping studies in the human ventricle. J Am Coll Cardiol 1987;10:1040–1047.

26. Downar E, Harris L, Mickleborough LL, et al. Endocardial mapping of ventricular tachycardia in the intact human ventricle: evidence for reentrant mechanisms. J Am Coll Cardiol 1988;11:783–791.

27. Downar E, Saito J, Doig JC, et al. Endocardial mapping of ventricular tachycardia in the intact human ventricle. III. Evidence of multiuse reentry with spontaneous and induced block in portions of reentrant path complex. JACC 1995;25:1591–600.

28. Miller JM, Tyson GS, Hargrove WC, et al. Effect of subendocardial resection on sinus rhythm endocardial electrogram abnormalities. Circulation 1995;91:2385–2391.

29. Kaltenbrunner W, Cardinal R, Dubuc M, et al. Epicardial and endocardial mapping of ventricular tachycardia in patients with myocardial infarction. Is the origin of the tachycardia always subendocardially localized? Circulation 1991;84:1058–1071.

30. Selle JG, Svenson RH, Gallagher JJ, et al. Surgical treatment of ventricular tachycardia with Nd:YAG laser photocoagulation. PACE 1992;15:1357–1361.

31. Pfeiffer D, Moosdorf R, Svenson RH, et al. Epicardial neodymium-YAG laser photocoagulation of ventricular tachycardia without ventriculotomy in patients after myocardial infarction. Circulation 1996;94:3221–3225.

32. Svenson RH, Gallagher JJ, Selle JG, et al. Neodymium:YAG laser photocoagulation: A successful new map-guided technique for the intraoperative ablation of ventricular tachycardia. Circulation 1987;76:1319–1328.

33. Miller JM, Kienzle MG, Harken AH, et al.

Subendocardial resection for ventricular tachycardia: Predictors of surgical success. Circulation 1984;70:624–631.

34. Hargrove WC, Miller JM, Vassallo JA, et al. Improved results in the operative management of ventricular tachycardia related to inferior wall infarction: Importance of the annular isthmus. J Thorac Cardiovasc Surg 1986;92:726–732.

35. Wilber DJ, Kopp DE, Glascock DN, et al. Catheter ablation of the mitral isthmus for ventricular tachycardia associated with inferior infarction. Circulation 1995;92:3481–3489.

36. Josephson ME, Horowitz LN, Spielman SR, et al. Comparison of endocardial catheter mapping with intraoperative mapping of ventricular tachycardia. Circulation 1980;61:395–404.

37. Josephson ME, Horowitz LN, Spielman SR, et al. Role of catheter mapping in the preoperative evaluation of ventricular tachycardia. Am J Cardiol 1982;49:207–220.

38. Waxman HL, Josephson ME: Ventricular activation during ventricular endocardial pacing. I. Electrocardiographic patterns related to site of pacing. Am J Cardiol 1982;50:1–10.

39. Josephson ME, Waxman HL, Cain ME, et al. Ventricular activation during ventricular endocardial pacing. II. Role of pace-mapping to localize origin of ventricular tachycardia. Am J Cardiol 1982;50:11–22.

40. Kadish AH, Childs K, Schmaltz S, et al. Differences in QRS configuration during unipolar pacing from adjacent sites: Implications for the spatial resolution of pace-mapping. J Am Coll Cardiol 1991;17:143–151.

41. Miller JM, Marchlinski FE, Buxton AE, et al. Relationship between the 12-lead electrocardiogram during ventricular tachycardia and endocardial site of origin in patients with coronary artery disease. Circulation 1988;77:759–766.

42. Kuchar DL, Ruskin JN, Garan H. Electrocardiographic localization of the site of origin of ventricular tachycardia in patients with prior myocardial infarction. J Am Coll Cardiol 1989;13:893–900.

43. Davis LM, Byth K, Uther JB, et al. Localization of ventricular tachycardia substrates by analysis of the surface QRS recorded during ventricular tachycardia. Int J Cardiol 1995;50:131–142.

44. SippensGroenewegen A, Spekhorst H, van Hemel NM, et al. Value of body surface mapping in localizing the site of origin of ventricular tachycardia in patients with previous myocardial infarction. J Am Coll Cardiol 1994;24:1708–1724.

45. Moran JM, Kehoe RF, Loeb JM, et al. Extended endocardial resection for the treatment of ventricular tachycardia and ventricular fibrillation. Ann Thorac Surg 1982;34:538–552.

46. Moran JM, Kehoe RF, Loeb JM, et al. The role of papillary muscle resection and mitral valve replacement in the control of refractory ventricular arrhythmia. Circulation 1983;68:154–160.

47. Kron IL, Lerman BB, DiMarco JP. Extended subendocardial resection. A surgical approach to ventricular tachyarrhythmias that cannot be mapped intraoperatively. J Thorac Cardiovasc Surg 1985;90:586–591.

48. Landymore RW, Kinley CE, Gardner M. Encircling endocardial resection with complete removal of endocardial scar without intraoperative mapping for the ablation of drug-resistant ventricular tachycardia. J Thorac Cardiovasc Surg 1985;89:18–24.

49. Miller JM, Gottlieb CD, Marchlinski FE, et al. Does ventricular tachycardia mapping influence the success of antiarrhythmic surgery? J Am Coll Cardiol 1988;11:112A.

50. Miller JM, Marchlinski FE, Harken AH, et al. Subendocardial resection for sustained ventricular tachycardia in the early period after acute myocardial infarction. Am J Cardiol 1985;55:980–984.

51. DiMarco JP, Lerman BB, Kron IL, et al. Sustained ventricular tachyarrhythmias within 2 months of acute myocardial infarction: results of medical and surgical therapy in patients resuscitated from the initial episode. J Am Coll Cardiol 1985;6:759–768.

52. Waspe LE, Brodman R, Kim SG, et al. Activation mapping in patients with coronary artery disease with multiple ventricular tachycardia configurations: Occurrence and therapeutic implications of widely separate apparent sites of origin. J Am Coll Cardiol 1985;5:1075–1086.

53. Damiano RJ, Blanchard SM, Asano T, et al. The effects of distant potentials on unipolar electrograms in an animal model utilizing the right ventricular isolation procedure. J Am Coll Cardiol 1988;11:1100–1109.

54. Biermann M, Shenasa M, Borggrefe M, et al. The interpretation of cardiac electrograms. In Shenasa M, Borggrefe M, Breithardt G, eds. Cardiac Mapping. Futura Publishing Co, Mount Kisco, NY, 1991, pp 11–34.

55. Anderson KP, Walker R, Fuller M, et al. Criteria for local electrical activation: effects of electrogram characteristics. IEEE Trans Biomed Eng 1993;40:169–181.

56. Miller JM, Vassallo JA, Hargrove WC, et al. Intermittent failure of local conduction during ventricular tachycardia. Circulation 1985;72:1286–1292.

57. Haines DE, Lerman BB, Kron IL, et al. Surgical ablation of ventricular tachycardia with sequential map-guided subendocardial resection: electrophysiologic assessment and long-term follow-up. Circulation 1988;77:131–141.

58. Miller JM, Gottlieb CD, Hargrove WC, et al. Factors influencing operative mortality in surgery for ventricular tachycardias. Circulation 1988;78:44.

59. Van Hemel NM, Kingma JH, Defauw JAM, et al. Left ventricular segmental wall motion score as a criterion for selecting patients for direct surgery in the treatment of postinfarction ventricular tachycardia. Eur Heart J 1989;10:304–315.

60. Nath S, Haines DE, Kron IL, et al. Regional wall motion analysis predicts survival and functional outcome after subendocardial resection in patients with prior anterior myocardial infarction. Circulation 1993;88:70–76.

61. Hargrove WC, Josephson ME, Harken AH, et al. Endocardial resection for ventricular tachycardia in 353 patients. J Am Coll Cardiol 1994;23:480A.

62. Miller JM, Josephson ME, Hargrove WC. Significance of "nonclinical" ventricular arrhythmias induced following surgery for ventricular tachyarrhythmias. In Breithardt G, Borggrefe M, Zipes DP, eds. Nonpharmacological Therapy of Tachyarrhythmias. Futura Publishing Company, Inc., Mount Kisco, NY, 1987, pp 133–141.

63. Miller JM: Mapping of cardiac arrhythmias. In Josephson ME, Wellens HJJ, eds. Tachycardias: Mechanisms and Management. Futura Publishing Co, Inc, Mt. Kisco, 1993, pp 49–85.

64. Miller JM, Rothman SA, Addonizio VP. Surgical techniques for ventricular tachycardia ablation. In: Singer I, ed. Interventional Electrophysiology. Williams and Wilkins, Baltimore, 1997, pp 641–684.

Chapter 29

Surgical Approaches to Supraventricular Tachycardias

Gerald M. Guiraudon, George J. Klein, Colette M. Guiraudon, and Raymond Yee

Introduction

Supraventricular tachycardias are classified according to the site of their working mechanism, which is essentially reentry.[1] Atrial tachycardias include: focal atrial tachycardias, atrial flutter, and atrial fibrillation. Atrioventricular (AV) nodal tachycardias are reentrant tachycardias within the AV nodal region. Wolff-Parkinson-White syndrome requires the entire heart and a mandatory accessory AV connection for reentry. Rationale for interventions in supraventricular tachycardias is based on the arrhythmogenic anatomic substrate. The identification of the arrhythmogenic anatomic substrate is determined using preoperative EP studies and intracardiac mapping. The surgical rationale for therapy is to disable the arrhythmogenic anatomic substrate using either exclusion or ablation techniques. Ablation uses various tools: scalpel, cryoablation,[2-4] radiofrequency (RF) energy,[5-10] or other means for tissue destruction. The ways in which the targeted tissues are approached and the therapy delivered defines the type of intervention. Surgery is defined by a transparietal approach (a median sternotomy) that requires general anesthesia with endotracheal intubation, and is associated with various other adjunctive maneuvers, such as cardiopulmonary bypass, cardiotomy and aortic cross-clamping with cardioplegic myocardial preservation, before the ablative therapy can be delivered. Each of the various steps used to approach the target tissue is associated with its inherent morbidity and mortality.[11,12] The surgical risk, consequently, is associated with delivery of therapy. Catheter techniques are much less invasive than the surgical approaches. After venous and/or arterial puncture, catheters follow charted natural routes to the heart and are guided to the arrhythmogenic target. Side effects and complications are currently minimal, with dramatic progress in skill,[13] techniques, applied anatomy, and technology. Electrophysiological interventions using surgical or catheter delivery are the only curative interventions.

Currently, catheter ablation using RF electrical energy is the therapy of choice. This principle implies that patients with Wolff-Parkinson-White syndrome and atrioventricular (AV) nodal reentrant tachycardias are effectively and safely cured by catheter ablation techniques.[14] Patients with

From Singer I, Barold SS, Camm AJ (eds): Nonpharmacological Therapy of Arrhythmias for the 21st Century: The State of the Art. Futura Publishing Co, Inc., Armonk, NY, © 1998.

atrial flutter also benefit from catheter ablation techniques.[15,16] Focal atrial tachycardias may also be controlled by using catheter ablation in selected patients.[17]

Atrial fibrillation is still approached surgically in selected patients, while catheter-based and other techniques and therapeutic modalities are still being developed.[18–21]

Wolff-Parkinson-White Syndrome

The first successful surgical ablation of an accessory AV connection was performed by Sealy and colleagues in 1968.[22] Along with the development of surgical practice came a better understanding of cardiac anatomy, accessory AV connection anatomy and electrophysiology. Better understanding paved the way to more advanced surgical techniques with high efficacy and low morbidity and to catheter ablation techniques.[13]

Accessory AV connections in Wolff-Parkinson-White syndrome are distinct from the normal AV nodal-His bundle system and cross over the AV attachment. Successful techniques for ablation of accessory connection requires in-depth knowledge of the complex anatomy of the AV attachment.[23,24]

The accessory AV connections are made up of strands of working myocardium that bypass the AV attachment.[25,26] Typical accessory AV connections cross the annular attachment, most being para-annular.[27,28] Atypical accessory AV connections have been found in all parts of the nonannular attachment: within the AV myocardial septum (posterior septal or midseptal pathways), adjacent to the membranous septum (para-Hisian anterior septal pathways), within the membranous pathway (membranous pathways with aberrant preexcitation), and over the intervalvular trigone (atypical posterior septal pathways).

Two variant pathways have also been described: the posterior septal pathway with slow decremental conduction associated with the permanent form of junctional reentrant tachycardia (Coumel's tachycardias)[29,30] and the right freewall pathway (Mahaim) with anterograde decremental conduction (atriofascicular pathway associated with left bundle branch block pattern tachycardias).[31–34]

Two surgical approaches have been described: The endocardial approach was pioneered and perfected by Sealy,[22,35–37] Cox,[38] and Gallagher.[39] The epicardial approach combines epicardial exposure and cryoablation of the AV attachment.[40–42]

The heart is exposed via a median sternotomy. After extensive examination of cardiac anatomy, epicardial mapping is carried out to confirm the location of the accessory AV connection established during preoperative electrophysiological studies. Exploring electrodes are positioned along the atrial and ventricular side of the coronary sulcus at predetermined sites during atrial and/or ventricular pacing and AV reentrant tachycardias. Cardiac mapping and electrophysiological testing using pacing techniques are repeated at each step of the surgical ablation to confirm suppression of the conduction of the recognized accessory AV connection and to potentially identify a second undiagnosed connection.

The endocardial approach combines an atrial incision along the AV annulus in the region of interest and an extensive dissection of the entire region of the coronary sulcus.

The left free wall connections are approached by using a conventional exposure of the mitral valve similar to the one used for mitral valve surgery. The entire left free wall region is dissected via a semicircular atrial incision along the mitral valve annulus from the right to the left trigone. The dissection is carried out under aortic cross-clamping and cardioplegic cardiac arrest.

The posterior septal, right free wall and anterior septal regions are approached via a right atriotomy. Endocardial mapping and para-Hisian dissection can be carried out on the normothermic beating heart. However, most of the extensive dissection of the region of interest is performed under aortic cross-clamping and cold cardioplegic arrest.

The endocardial approach is associated with excellent efficacy. Surgical morbidity is associated with cold cardioplegic cardiac arrest and cardiopulmonary bypass.[38,39]

The epicardial approach combines epicardial dissection of the coronary sulcus, and exposure and cryoablation of the AV attachment (annulus).[41,42] Typical accessory AV connection can be ablated by using this approach on the beating heart without the need for cardiopulmonary bypass. The left free wall dissection is carried out by exposing the left coronary sulcus using a sling (Figure 1).[43] The AV attachment is exposed by dissection of the fat pad along the left ventricular wall. The obtuse cardiac vein is divided for better exposure, and

the coronary arteries are carefully isolated. The posterior region is well exposed by deflecting the heart upward using a right pledgeted suture. The right free wall and anterior septal regions are easily exposed. These typical accessory AV connections located within the coronary sulcus are easily ablated with the high efficacy and minimum morbidity associated with median sternotomy.[42]

Atypical accessory AV connections require an endocardial dissection carried out on the normothermic beating heart. Para-Hisian anterior septal connections are ablated by using discrete dissection of the atrial myocardium overlying the atrial membranous septum.[44] We have ablated three atypical posterior pathways located over the intervalvular trigone region using discrete cryoablation.[45]

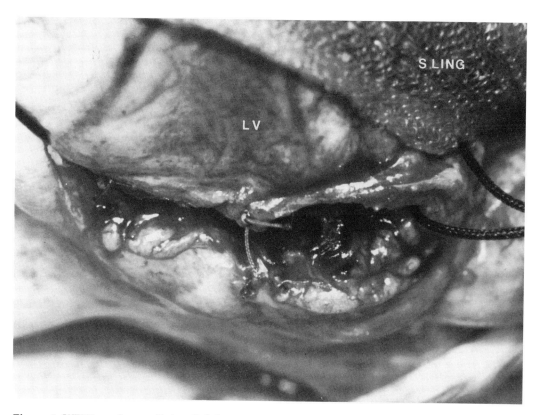

Figure 1. WPW syndrome. Epicardial dissection of left AV sulcus using the sling exposure, without using cardiopulmonary bypass.

Atypical Intramembranous Pathways

We have operated on four patients with aberrant preexcitation and surgically documented intramembranous pathways. The aberrant preexcitation was over either the right ventricular infundibulum (three patients) or the ventricular septum (one patient).[46] The pathways were ablated by discrete cryoablation of the atrial membranous septum or of the ventricular attachment. These membranous accessory pathways are characteristically located within the membranous septum, with an atrial insertion in the atrial septum and a ventricular insertion at various sites in the septum along the membranous septum attachment to the ventricular septum. The membranous pathway differs from the so-called intermediate pathways,[47] which have normal anatomic features and function and are located in the midseptal region.

Mahaim Fibers

We documented in two patients that the anatomic substrate of the so-called Mahaim's fibers associated with left bundle branch block pattern tachycardias was a right ventricular free wall accessory pathway with antegrade decremental conduction and with a His bundle-like connection lies along the right ventricular free wall (atriofascicular fiber).[31–34] Since then, both surgical and catheter ablation techniques have revealed that almost all patients with the electrophysiologically documented Mahaim entity have a right free wall accessory pathway, the site of preexcitation being either close to the AV groove or at the right ventricular apex.[48] In five patients, findings from a biopsy specimen from the right atrium documented the presence of AV nodal cells at the atrial insertion of the pathway. Our surgical experience comprises 13 patients.[49] The surgical technique that is used in this setting is identical to that used for right free wall accessory pathway dissection combined with endocardial cryoablation.

The Permanent Form of Junctional Reciprocating Tachycardia (Coumel's Tachycardia)

Surgical dissection of the posterior septal region has documented that the permanent form of junctional reciprocating tachycardia is associated with a posterior septal accessory pathway, with decremental retrograde conduction only. A conventional posterior septal dissection using the epicardial approach uniformly ablates the pathway.[30]

Coronary Sinus Diverticulum

Coronary sinus diverticulum is associated with posterior septal pathways that exhibit maximal preexcitation and a short antegrade refractory period.[50,51] At surgery the coronary sinus diverticulum is readily visible (Figure 2). Diverticulum is composed of a pouch and a neck that opens into the coronary sinus proximal to the midcardiac vein. The neck diameter ranges from 5 to 10 mm. Accessory pathway conduction is usually interrupted when the neck of the diverticulum is divided. This represents evidence suggesting that the accessory pathway is part of the diverticulum.

Multiple Accessory Pathways

We defined multiple accessory pathways as widely separated sites of preexcitation in distinct regions.[52] Preoperative electrophysiological studies identify the presence of multiple pathways in about 7% of the patients.[53] A second pathway can become apparent only after ablation of the dominant accessory pathway. Most unexpected pathways that are detected intraoperatively are posterior septal pathways capable of only retrograde AV conduction. Multiple accessory pathways are ablated in sequence. If possible, the accessory pathway that does not require cardiopulmonary bypass is ablated first.

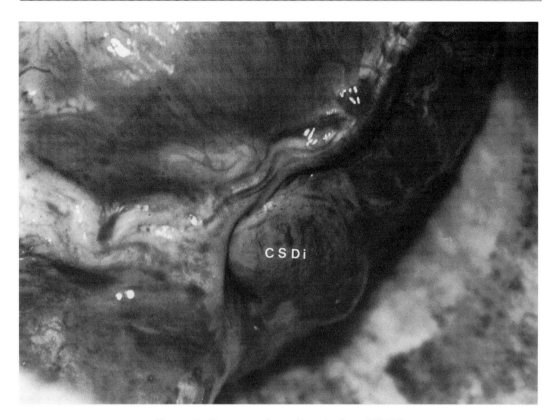

Figure 2. Coronary sinus diverticulum (CS Di).

Associated Cardiac Lesions

Two congenital cardiac abnormalities are associated with the preexcitation syndrome: Ebstein's anomaly and the coronary sinus diverticulum. Symptomatic Wolff-Parkinson-White syndrome associated with Ebstein's anomaly does not necessarily require anatomic repair, but all such surgical repairs of Ebstein's anomaly should be combined with ablation of the associated preexcitation syndrome. Our current surgical strategy for concomitant cardiac procedures (coronary artery bypass grafting and valve replacement) is to ablate the accessory pathway first as an independent procedure and then to proceed with performing the associated cardiac surgical procedure.

Results

Before the era of catheter ablation, we reported on 502 patients who were operated on before August 1990. In all, 500 patients were cured without any mortality and with low morbidity (mean follow-up, 4 years). These results were similar to those from other reported series.[28] The number of patients referred to surgery abruptly decreased after the fast development of catheter ablation in 1990.[54] Catheter ablation has replaced surgery as the primary therapy. We recently reviewed our experience over the last 2 years. We operated on four patients with the Wolff-Parkinson-White syndrome referred from Canada or the US.

Atrioventricular Nodal Reentrant Tachycardias

Atrioventricular nodal reentrant tachycardia is a very common type of supraventricular tachycardia. It was long accepted knowledge that the reentrant mechanism

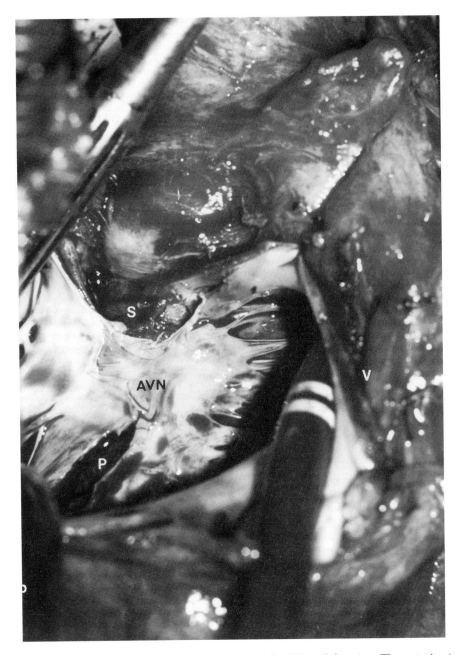

Figure 3. AV nodal reentrant tachycardia. Dissection of the AV nodal region. The anterior (superior) input (S) has been dissected by extensive approach to the right coronary fossa. The posterior (inferior) input (P) has been dissected as well. The node is still covered by the atrial wall (AVN).

was within the compact AV node.[55] Because this concept precluded a direct surgical approach to disable the reentrant mechanism, His bundle ablation was the electrophysiological intervention that was used in severe resistant cases. However, an inadvertent cure of a patient with AV nodal reentrant tachycardia after attempted surgical ablation of the AV node suggested that discrete lesions of the AV node could interrupt the tachycardia.[56] Marques-Montes and colleagues[57] and Johnson and colleagues[58] were the first to report effective surgical approaches to the AV nodal region to interrupt AV nodal reentrant tachycardias.

The rationale of surgical approaches was consistent with AV nodal physiology as described by basic scientists[59] and with AV nodal anatomy.[60] To reconcile data from various disciplines, the concept of the greater AV nodal area that encompasses the AV node as well as its atrial input was described.[61] The reentrant mechanism may include the greater AV nodal area and use atrial inputs as part of the reentrant circuit.

Surgical approaches suggested that either modification or ablation of at least one atrial input was associated with disabling of the reentrant mechanism. Johnston and colleagues were the first to report two sites of atrial retrograde activation over the coronary sinus os and at the apex of the triangle of Koch, consistent with the posterior atrial inputs and the superficial atrial input (currently labeled anterior, referring to the anterior septal position), respectively.

Direct surgical approaches to the AV node for AV nodal reentrant tachycardia used sharp dissection of the AV nodal atrial inputs guided by endocardial mapping[58] or not[61,62] or cryomodification (perinodal cryoablation) (Figure 3).[63] Currently, surgical techniques for AV nodal reentrant tachycardias are no longer used. Ablation using catheter delivery is associated with excellent control of the tachycardia and with more discrete electrophysiological changes.[64]

Atrial Tachycardias

Focal atrial tachycardias are classified into two subgroups: Ectopic atrial tachycardias originate from outside the sinus node area, and sinus node tachycardias originate from within the sinus node area.

Ectopic atrial tachycardias are rare in the adult population (0.5–1%) and most frequent in children (10% of supraventricular tachycardias).[65] At electrophysiological studies, they have the characteristics of automatic focus tachycardias. During tachycardia the P-wave morphology significantly differs from that of sinus node P-waves. The side of origin is mostly within the right atrial wall (68%) along the crista terminalis, the left atrial free wall (26%), and the interatrial septum (6%). The tachycardia is frequently incessant. These characteristics explain why tachycardia-induced dilated cardiomyopathy is frequently present (60% of cases). Ectopic atrial tachycardias are potentially severe arrhythmias. Surgical techniques are considered only after attempted catheter ablation. Because ectopic atrial tachycardias are not inducible, preoperative catheter mapping must be obtained to precisely localize the site of origin.

Surgical techniques use resection, cryoablation, and exclusion, singly or in combination. Resection applies to right atrial free wall and right and left appendage locations. Appendectomies may not require cardiopulmonary bypass. Right atrial excision is repaired by using an autologous pericardial patch. Cryoablation can be combined with resection but is particularly convenient for septal locations. Exclusion is used essentially for the left atrial locations.

Our experience comprises five patients; none of them had incessant tachycardia associated with tachycardia-induced dilated cardiomyopathy.[66] Three patients had a right free wall tachycardia localized over the inferior segment of the crista terminalis and underwent extensive right free wall resection combined with autologous pericardial patch reconstruction. One patient had a right atrial appendage tachycardia. The right atrial appendage was resected without using cardiopulmonary bypass. One patient had a left atrial tachycardia. Because the location of the tachycardia was not accurately determined, a left atrial exclusion was carried out. There were no surgical complications. No patient had recurrence of tachycardia. The patient with left atrial exclusion developed AV nodal conduction disturbances associated with syncopal ventricular pauses during long-term follow-up. A permanent pacemaker was implanted.

Lowe and colleagues[65] published a review of the literature. One hundred twenty-five patients with ectopic atrial tachycardia were reviewed. Fifty-two patients were treated with antiarrhythmic drugs; 46 (89%) of them were controlled. Seventy-three patients were treated with surgical techniques; 56 (77%) were controlled.

Sinus node tachycardias comprise inappropriate sinus node tachycardias and reentrant sinus node tachycardias. Surgical experience with inappropriate sinus tachycardias documented that surgical ablation was associated with good short-term results[66] but poor long-term results[67] complicated with AF and AV conduction disturbances. These surgical results suggest that catheter ablation[68] and other ablative techniques[69] are only palliative. Catheter ablation in patients with reentrant sinus node tachycardias[70] attain good results, consistent with those obtained by surgical ablation.

Atrial Flutter

Atrial flutter was first characterized by its electrocardiographic pattern[71] as a rapid, regular atrial tachycardia associated with a typical sawtooth configuration of the atrial electrogram on the surface electrocardiogram. Atrial flutter in humans has been classified as *common* if negative flutter waves are present in leads II, III, and aVF and as *uncommon* if flutter waves are positive in these same leads.[72] More recently, the common flutter was labeled type 1, and the uncommon flutter was labeled type 2.[73]

Currently, there is a large body of experimental[74–77] and clinical[78–84] evidence that documents that atrial flutter is associated with a macroreentry mechanism associated with a large excitable gap in the right atrium and an area of slow conduction in the triangle of Koch. Recent studies showed that the common and uncommon types may share the same mechanism and location.[85,86]

The reentrant circuit is determined by the functional anatomy of the right atrium. The area of slow conduction at the base of the triangle of Koch in the area of the coronary sinus os occupies a segment (isthmus) between the inferior vena cava and the tricuspid valve orifices (Figure 4). The reentrant activation exits the area of slow conduction and propagates rapidly via the anterior and middle internodal pathways, which are anterior to the fossa ovalis. The reentrant activation then circulates through the sinus node area, travels caudally within the crista terminalis, and returns to the base of the triangle of Koch where the slow-conducting isthmus slows down the activation before it exits again. In addition, the fossa ovale and transversal relative slow conduction (anisotrope) contribute to the presence of a zone of septal block.[87]

We reported the first successful surgical correction of atrial flutter.[79] The current accepted rationale is to ablate the slow-conducting isthmus between the inferior vena cava orifice and the tricuspid valve annulus at the base of the triangle of Koch, using cryoablation.[88] We used a different rationale in our first case: a right atrial transection was carried out to interrupt the two limbs of the circuit (internodal pathways and crista terminalis). We obtained four intraoperative mappings at surgery. Epicardial maps in two patients confirmed the slow conduction over the isthmus and circular activation of the right atrium, while the left atrium received collateral activation from the circuit. Endocardial cardiac mapping was obtained in two patients. Circular activation around the tricuspid annulus and an area of slow conduction in the isthmus was present in one patient. In the other patient, circular activation within the isthmus and triangle of Koch was present.

Surgical technique used extensive epicardial cryoablation of the area between the tricuspid annulus, the coronary sinus os, and the orifice of the inferior vena cava. In four patients, endocardial cryoablation was used with extensive ablation of the base of the triangle of Koch.

Our experience comprises seven male patients (age 33 to 63) with problematic symptoms (duration 4–20 years). No patient had associated structural heart disease. All patients had the common form. Preoperative electrophysiological studies confirmed the typical characteristics of the flutter with an area of slow fragmented conduction in the

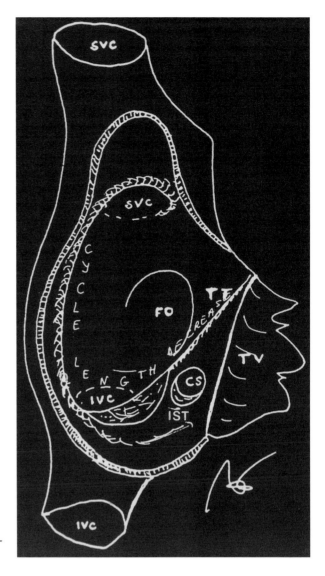

Figure 4. Atrial flutter. Schematic depiction of isthmus (IST).

coronary sinus os region and a large excitable gap within the right atrium.

Postoperatively, there were no complications. At predischarge electrophysiological studies, atrial flutter was not inducible. During long-term follow-up, one patient had recurrence of AF and underwent a corridor operation 1 year later. The six other patients were free of arrhythmia without taking antiarrhythmic drugs with follow-ups of 16, 9, 8, 3, 2, and 2 years, respectively.

Successful surgical ablation combined with intraoperative mapping gave insight into the potential mechanism of atrial flutter.

Atrial Fibrillation

Atrial fibrillation has been defined by its electrocardiographic pattern. It has long been considered an elusive target for electrophysiological interventions until recently, when the first successful direct approach was developed.[89] Since then, during the last 10 years, new interventions were designed using surgical or catheter delivery. Rationales for intervention are based on multiple premises, namely atrial anatomy and function, atrial pathology, and mechanism of atrial fibrillation.

Atrial Anatomy

Atria are two compliant pouches between the continuous venous flow return and the intermittent ventricular flow output. The anatomy of atria may appear simple at first, but is in fact very complex.[90] Atria are made of a grossly spherical wall which is on the endocardial side, irregular and rugged. The myocardial cells are in total disarray on histological sections. The myocardium is perforated by many large orifices or interrupted by absence of myocardial cells. Atria constitute a complex heterogenous tridimensional structure.

Atrial Function

Atria harbor the heart's chronotropic function which is located within the sinus node and the AV node areas. Cardiac chronotropic function is the main determinant of increased cardiac output during exercise combined with increased ventricular contractility.[91] Atrial contraction is critical to maintain cardiac output of the failing heart by increasing the ventricular end-diastolic pressure and/or volume (Starling's law).[92] The respective roles of chronotropic function and atrial contraction (normal sinus rhythm versus normal ventricular chronotropic function without concomitant atrial contraction) have not been elucidated as yet.

Prevention of intra-atrial thrombus formation is the major function of atria. The normal atrial anatomy, especially the left atrial appendage, is prone to intracavitary thrombus. The causes of thrombus formation include: alteration of atrial geometry (increased left atrial dimension), pathological alteration of the atrial wall (endothelium), loss of contraction and concomitant loss of the left atrial appendage washout. But overall, the left atrial appendage is the main site of left atrial intracavitary thrombus.[93–95]

Atrial Pathology

Atrial fibrillation is commonly associated with structural heart disease: rheumatic heart disease: mitral valve disease; dilated cardiomyopathy; and chronic pericarditis. Lone AF occurred in patients without evidence of structural heart disease and known causes of AF.

Histology of AF associated with structural heart disease has been well reported.[96,97] Recent work has focused on "lone atrial fibrillation," which seems to occur in the absence of structural heart disease.[98,99] We have reported atrial pathology in 12 patients with lone AF who had a corridor operation.[100,101] Atrial pathology of lone AF documented the following striking features: (1) some atria presented with evidence of primary atrial cardiomyopathy; (2) some atria showed only myocardial hypertrophy consistent with tachycardia-induced cardiomyopathy (remodeling); (3) significant pathology of sinus node tissue, even in the absence of sinus node dysfunction; and (4) a dramatic decrease in nerve endings, confirming the critical role of the autonomous nervous system, albeit these findings appeared paradoxical.

The incidence of intracavitary thrombus depends on associated heart disease and history of AF. Thrombi are essentially found in the left atrial appendage and the left atrial posterior wall (mitral valve disease).

Mechanism

Atrial fibrillation was long considered due to rapid, chaotic atrial activation associated with irregular fast ventricular contraction. Moe speculated that AF was associated with concomitant multiple wavelets of activation. Allessie et al. confirmed Moe's hypothesis on an animal model.[102] Currently, the accepted mechanism for "common" AF is random reentry.[103,104] Atrial propensity to sustain AF (atrial vulnerability) is determined by atrial size, wall structure, and the spatial distribution of electrophysiological characteristics (dispersion). These conditions vary over time depending on the underlying mechanism and duration of AF. The longer the atria fibrillate, the more sustained the fibrillation (atrial remodeling); *atrial fibrillation begets atrial fibrillation.*[105] Moreover, this currently accepted mechanism of AF may not be the only one.

Mapping provides insights into initiation and perpetuation of AF.[106] A rapid sustained stationary reentry circuit may be identified as the perpetuating mechanism.[107,108] Mapping of human AF, albeit less extensive, has documented both types: reentry circuit perpetuating the AF[109,110] or a self-sustained multi-wavelet mechanism.

Recently, Jalife and his group have studied the mechanism of initiation of AF.[111] A reentry circuit (rotor) may transform into a drifting spiral that may bifurcate and produce sustained AF.

To conclude, AF can be focal in nature in terms of initiation and perpetuation. Consequently, its interventional therapy could be focal as well.

Clinical Presentation

Patients with AF have multiple clinical presentations.[112] The presenting symptoms can be associated with the arrhythmia itself, the associated structural heart disease, or the left atrial thrombosis.

Interventional Rationales

Surgical rationales are aimed at disabling random reentry which include the following: exclusion, reduction, fragmentation, and channeling (Figure 5).[113]

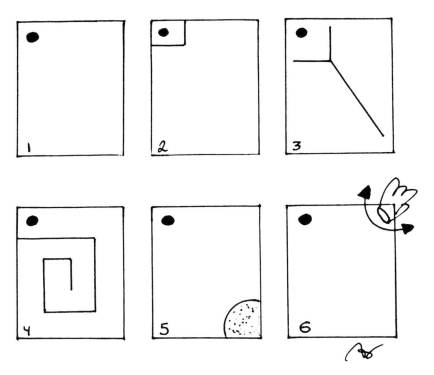

Figure 5. Atrial fibrillation. Schematic depiction of rationales aimed at disabling random reentry. #1. The two-dimensional atrial walls are depicted as a rectangle with the solid circle representing the sinus node. #2. Exclusion/reduction. The sinus node is isolated from fibrillating atrial tissue. #3. Fragmentation/atriotomies. #4. Channeling transforms two dimensional atria into unidimentional structure. #5. Focal ablation to neutralize focal (discrete) initiating/perpetuation tachycardia. #6. Left atrial appendectomy aimed at decreasing intraatrial clot formation and systemic emboli.

Exclusion/reduction is aimed at excluding the fibrillating atrium, while reducing the surface area in the rest of the atria and preventing AF.

Fragmentation uses atriotomies to construct semi-excluded atrial segments where random reentry cannot sustain while they all can contract in harmony.

Channeling transforms atria in one-dimensional structure by construction of narrow strips of atria tissue where random reentry cannot sustain.

Focal discrete interventions are not used as yet because intraoperative comprehensive atrial mapping is not developed as yet. The second concern is that vicarious perpetuating reentrant circuits can occur at other sites. In another perspective, focal ablation of tachycardia associated with the Wolff-Parkinson-White syndrome, AV nodal reentrant tachycardia, or other focal atrial tachycardia may prevent AF from occurring.

Cardiac denervation or modification of the autonomic nervous system has not been developed thus far. We failed in the mid-1970s to achieve adequate cardiac denervation in humans and failed to prevent vagal-induced AF.

Cardiac autotransplantation used by Batista et al.[114] to allow easier ex vivo mitral valve repair is associated with restoration of sinus rhythm function. Cardiac denervation, albeit combined with subtotal resection of the left atrium, could be the effective mechanism. Atriotomies per se alter the atrial autonomic innervation.[115]

Other interventional rationales should be developed to make the intervention easier and simpler.

Interventional Endpoints

Three *primary endpoints* are paramount: stroke prevention, maintenance of cardiac function, and symptom relief.

Stroke Prevention: No study to date has documented that any surgical technique significantly decreased risk of stroke more than long-term warfarin therapy.

Improved cardiac function should be associated with increased exercise capacity and potentially prolonged life expectancy. Some studies have demonstrated improved cardiac index[116] and/or improved left ventricular ejection fraction.[117] No study has specifically addressed the issue of exercise tolerance.

Symptom Relief: All surgical techniques provide adequate relief of symptoms. However, the least invasive intervention such as RF ablation of the AV node combined with pacemaker implantation provides excellent control of symptoms.

Secondary endpoints are essentially a way to assess the effect of the intervention rather than its efficacy: i.e., interruption of AF, restoration of sinus rhythm, restoration of adequate chronotropic function, and evidence of atrial contraction.

Other endpoints are cessation of antiarrhythmic drug therapy and absence of pacemaker implantation.

A large number of endpoints suggests that the criteria for success, as far as electrophysiological interventions are concerned, are multiple and controversial. The same ambiguity exists for goals of the medical therapy: heart rate control, maintenance of sinus rhythm, stroke prevention, and symptom relief.

Indications for surgical EP interventions are far from being well-defined. Patient selection is based on associated heart disease, duration of AF, drug efficacy, and associated structural heart disease. Currently, selected patients requiring mitral valve repair seem to be the best candidates for concomitant surgery for AF.

Cardiac Surgical Techniques

The following surgical techniques have been reported: (1) the corridor operation based on an excluded channel that houses the sinus node and the AV node; (2) the left atrial exclusion, which isolates the fi brillating left atrium; (3) the maze operation, which combines exclusion/reduction with the subtotal exclusion of the left atrium, and channeling and fragmentation; (4) the compartment operation, which fragments the atria in two or three segments; (5) the spiral, which "channels" the left and right atria; (6) cardiac autotransplantation, which combines cardiac denervation with subtotal exclusion and remodeling of the left atrium.

The Case for the Left Atrial Appendectomy

Although all reported surgical approaches for AF do not include a left atrial appendectomy, we strongly believe that the *left atrial appendage* should be excluded in all patients operated on for or with AF, as well as all patients having cardiac surgery, for the following reasons.

The *left atrial appendage* is the site of left atrial thrombi in 50% of patients with rheumatic AF[118] and in 90% of patients with nonrheumatic atrial AF.[119] Resection of the left atrial appendage should decrease dramatically the incidence of stroke by more than 50%.[120] Resection of the left atrial appendage has no known side effects and/or complications. Although its function is not known, its presence acts as a potential source for left atrial thrombus even in patients in sinus rhythm. Left atrial appendectomy is not associated with any specific complications, is well documented to be safe by the worldwide experience of left atrial ligation after closed mitral valve repair carried out via the left atrial appendage.[121]

Left atrial appendectomy should be a routine fixture of all cardiac surgery considering the life expectancy of the population and the increased prevalence of AF as the population focus gets older.

The Corridor Operation

A strip (channel) of atrial tissue (corridor) is isolated to restore sinus node function.[122–124] The strip of atrial tissue has a small surface area and should be able to sustain AF. The corridor operation is performed under cardiopulmonary bypass and cold cardioplegic cardiac arrest (Figure 6). The surgical technique comprised exclusion of the left atrial free wall by using a horseshoe incision along the attachment of the left atrial wall onto the atrial septum. Construction of the corridor itself uses a horseshoe incision attaching onto the tricuspid annulus delineating the corridor, which includes a cuff of right atrium that harbors the sinus node region, the AV node region, and a strip of atrial septum bridging the two nodes.

We have reported our experience with nine patients[122] with drug refractory AF. Initial results demonstrate that the corridor operation can maintain sinus rhythm in patients with AF. Since then five additional patients have had a corridor operation. Improved selection criteria allowed normal sinus node function after surgery in all.

Gursoy et al. reported five patients with the corridor operation for "lone atrial fibrillation." Sinus node chronotropic function was normal postoperatively with good exercise tolerance.[125]

Van Hemel et al. reported 36 patients with the corridor operation for paroxysmal lone AF.[126] The follow-up period was 41 ± 16 months. Thirty-one patients had successful construction of the corridor. Twenty-five patients were arrhythmia-free without medication (4-year actuarial freedom, 72 ± 9%). Twenty-six patients had normal sinus node function at rest and during exercise (4-year actuarial freedom of sinus node dysfunction, 81 ± 7%). Five patients had pacemaker implantation.

Overall, the corridor operation gave good control of the arrhythmia, restored sinus rhythm, with a good functional capacity; one patient from Utrecht (The Netherlands) ran a marathon.

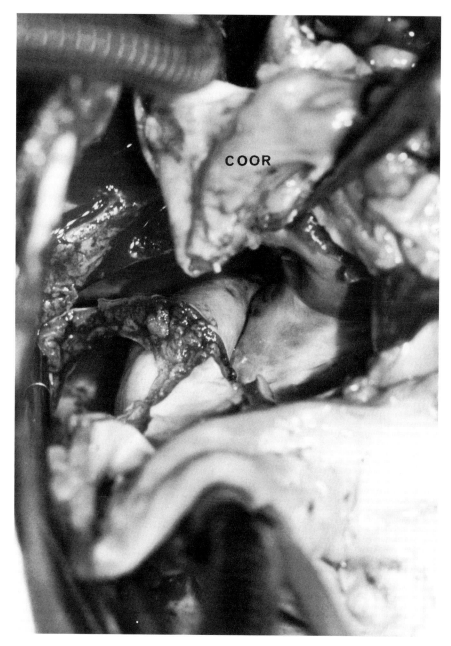

Figure 6. Corridor operation, operative view, COOR = corridor.

The Maze Operation

Since the first report,[127] the maze operation has undergone many modifications and alterations by its designer and others.[128–131] The master plan comprises a subtotal left atrial exclusion and multiple atriotomies combined with cryoablation. One left atriotomy divides the circular cuff of the left atrium around the mitral valve. Multiple right and septal atriotomies fragment and channel the right atrium and septum (maze III).

Cox et al. reported 87 patients with the maze procedure for the treatment of atrial flutter and/or fibrillation. Three patients died during surgery. Two patients had postoperative transient ischemic attacks. In the first 3 months after surgery, 47% of patients had recurrence of AF or atrial flutter. Of the 78 patients with more than 3 months of follow-up, 32 required permanent pacing (AAI). Some patients had sinus node dysfunction before surgery. All patients were assessed in terms of exercise tolerance, arrhythmia (Holter), and cardiac function (atrial contraction). Overall, atrial fibrillation/flutter has been controlled by surgery alone in 71 of 78 patients, whereas 32 patients (41%) required a pacemaker implantation. Since then, Cox has presented his continuing experience with 90 patients, confirming good results with the maze III procedure.

Morris et al.[117] reported their experience with the maze operation in 19 patients with nonvalvular AF. There was no mortality and all patients were in sinus rhythm 6 months after surgery with documented right and left atrial contraction. Other authors reported results with restoration of sinus rhythm in about 80% of cases.[132]

Left Atrial Isolation

Graffigna et al. have reported left atrial isolation in 184 patients with concomitant mitral valve surgery.[116] Seventy-one percent of patients returned to sinus rhythm after surgery, whereas 19% of patients with only mitral valve surgery returned to sinus rhythm (no controlled trial; $P < .001$). Patients with restored sinus rhythm had significantly greater cardiac index at discharge.

Boriani et al. recently reported a comparative study in patients with left atrial isolation combined with mitral valve surgery.[133] At 6 months, the mVO$_2$ was not significantly different than in the control group, 23.3 ± 7.25 versus 22 ± 5.6.

Fragmentation or Compartment Operation (Open Corridor)

Shyu et al.[134] reported their experience with the compartment operation in 22 patients. All patients had concomitant mitral valve surgery. The compartment operation is best described as an *open corridor* operation, the atriotomy which "normally" isolates the left atrium and the corridor itself are left incomplete and allow persistent connections between the three constructed segments of atria.

The compartment operation was not associated with increased surgical morbidity. Fourteen patients (64%) were in sinus rhythm at 6 months of follow-up. Atrial mechanical function, as assessed by echo Doppler studies, was not always present after restoration of sinus rhythm.

Cardiac Autotransplantation

Recently, Batista et al. advocated, at the 9th annual meeting of the EACTS in Paris, France, the use of cardiac autotransplantation[114] for in vitro repair of complex cardiac lesions. Their experience included 84 patients. Sixty-two were female and 22 were male (age 18 to 75 years). Eighty-three patients were in chronic AF and one presented with the long QT syndrome. The left atrial diameter was greater than 6 cm, in 68 patients, and between 6 and 4 cm in 16 patients. All patients were in sinus rhythm in the early postoperative period. Thirteen patients died in perioperative period. At 6-month follow-up, 5 of 71 survivors were in AF. All patients with a left atrial dimension smaller than 4 cm postoperatively were in sinus rhythm.

These remarkable results remind us that the role of the autonomic nervous system has been underestimated or neglected by EP interventionists.

Comments

Although surgical techniques are associated with good surgical results, surgical successes are not evidence that the surgical rationales are true.

Surgical techniques may fail to interrupt AF, to reestablish sinus node function with adequate chronotropic response to exercise, and to restore atrial contraction.

Failure to interrupt AF: The identical AF mechanism could be present postoperatively because: (1) the surgical rationale is inappropriate, (2) the working mechanism is a variant of the one currently accepted (focal mechanism?), or (3) the surgery was not adequately executed. Failure to interrupt AF may be an illusion because new atrial tachycardia, such as multifocal atrial tachycardia, which can mimic the clinical presentation of AF are present after surgery. Current catheter electrophysiological studies have inherent limitations in distinguishing among these various mechanisms. These postoperative arrhythmias may be transitory, but are disturbing evidence that our understanding of AF is rudimentary and that there might be more than one working mechanism.

Failure to restore sinus node function: Sinus node dysfunction may be present before surgery, or can be induced surgically because of the site of atriotomies and/or associated ischemic changes. Although pacemaker implantation can restore atrial contraction and chronotropic function, sinus dysfunction is a significant setback.

Atrial contraction: Loss of atrial contraction can be part of surgical design (corridor or left atrial exclusion) or because of irreversible myocardial damage. Underlying cardiac pathology has been overlooked in most studies.

Surgical Indications

Surgical indications remain controversial. Other nonpharmacological electrophysiological interventions provide excellent control of arrhythmia with fewer side effects and/or risks. Patients with mitral valve disease who require concomitant mitral valve surgery seem to be an acceptable indication and is currently used by some surgical teams.[135-138] Concomitant surgery for AF seems a benign adjunct to mitral valve surgery although it may increase surgical risk in various ways: atriotomies, prolongation of aortic cross-clamping, and/or cardiopulmonary bypass time. Mitral valve disease associated with AF is a complex entity with multiple components: valvular anatomy, left ventricular function, left atrial dimension, duration of symptoms, age, sex, etc. Recent studies show that left ventricular function is the main independent prognostic marker. A recent review[139] of long-term follow-up of patients after mitral valve repair shows no difference between patients with or without AF in terms of survival and even morbidity at 5 years. Despite the large number of reported patients with combined surgery for AF, no comparative randomized series has been published in terms of outcome. Atrial fibrillation might share the same fate as ventricular arrhythmia in patients with coronary artery disease. The premier prognostic marker is cardiac function, which dwarfs all other markers or symptoms, even when those symptoms are the primary clinical presentation.

Further Directions

If electrophysiological assessment of AF becomes more precise, new rationales may develop guided by atrial mapping. Atrial fibrillation may be associated with a focal perpetuating site that could be ablated.

Recently, catheter ablation techniques have been used to control AF. First, Haissaguerre et al. used catheter ablation techniques for unusual forms of AF.[18] These developments suggest that catheter ablation of AF may be common practice in the foreseeable future.[19,21]

Recent studies have presented three new concepts: (1) catheter techniques can safely produce linear transmural ablation (such as incisions),[140,141] (2) segmental linear ablation can prevent atrial fibrillation to either initiate,[142] or perpetuate,[143,144] and (3) the initiating/perpetuating mechanism might be "focal" reentry within the pulmonary vein (left superior).[145] Current surgical techniques may "overkill" without added benefit.

The Case for Video-Assisted Surgery for Atrial Fibrillation

Video-assisted thoracic surgery (VATS) can provide excellent approach to[146] (1) the left lateral wall of the left atrium, and the left atrial appendage, and (2) the wall of the right atrial free wall. VATS can also provide access to the posterior wall of the left atrium and the roof of the left atrium. Via these accesses, the atrial wall can be mapped using multi-electrode plaques as well "neutralized" using various tools and energies (RF, cryoablation, etc.). VATS can be associated with good control of the arrhythmia and with minimal side effects.

VATS allows the surgeon to carry out a left atrial appendectomy, which may prove to be the most beneficial intervention for AF.

References

1. Guiraudon GM, Klein GJ, Yee R. Surgery for cardiac tachyarrhythmias. Highlights 1990;6:5–10.
2. Guiraudon GM. Cryoablation, a versatile tool in arrhythmia surgery [Editorial]. Ann Thorac Surg 1987;43:129–130.
3. Harrison L, Gallagher JJ, Kasell J, et al. Cryosurgical ablation of the AV node–His bundle: a new method for producing AV block. Circulation 1977;55:463.
4. Klein GJ, Harrison L, Ideker RF, et al. Reaction of the myocardium to cryosurgery: electrophysiology and arrhythmogenic potential. Circulation 1979;59:364.
5. Warin JF. Catheter ablation of accessory atrioventricular connections. In Touboul P, Waldo AL, eds. Atrial Arrhythmias: Current Concepts and Management. St. Louis Mosby Year Book, 1990, pp 476–487.
6. Warin JF, Haissaguerre M, Lemetayer P, et al. Catheter ablation of accessory pathways with a direct approach: results in 35 patients. Circulation 1988;78:800–815.
7. Brugada P, Wellens HJJ. Where to fulgurate in supraventricular tachycardia. In Fontaine G, Scheinman MM, eds. Ablation in Cardiac Arrhythmias. Futura Publishing Co. Inc, Mount Kisco, NY, 1987, pp 141–149.
8. Jackman WM, Wang X, Friday KJ, et al. Catheter ablation of accessory atrioventricular pathways (Wolff-Parkinson-White syndrome) by radiofrequency current. N Engl J Med 1991;324:1605–1611.
9. Calkins H, Sousa J, El-Atassi R, et al. Diagnosis and cure of the Wolff-Parkinson-White syndrome or paroxysmal supraventricular tachycardias during a single electrophysiologic test. N Engl J Med 1991;324:1612–1662.
10. Leather RA, Leitch JW, Klein GJ, et al. Radiofrequency catheter ablation of accessory pathways: a learning experience. Am J Cardiol 1991;68:1651–1655.
11. Kirklin JW. The science of cardiac surgery. Eur J Cardiothorac Surg 1990;4:63–71.
12. Buckberg GD. Myocardial protection: an overview. Semin Thorac Cardiovasc Surg 1993;5,2:98–106.
13. Scheinman MM. North American Society of Pacing and Electrophysiology (NASPE) survey on radiofrequency catheter ablation: implications for clinicians, third party insurers, and government regulatory agencies. PACE 1992;15:2228–2231.
14. Scheinman MM. Catheter ablation: present role and projected impact on health care for

patients with cardiac arrhythmia. Circulation 1991;83:1489–1498.

15. Kirkorian G, Moncada E, Chevalier P, et al. Radiofrequency ablation of atrial flutter: efficacy of an anatomically guided approach. Circulation 1994;90:2804–2814.

16. Olshansky B, Okumura K, Henthron R, et al. Atrial mapping of human atrial flutter demonstrates reentry in the right atrium. J Am Coll Cardiol 1988;7:194A.

17. Chen SA, Chiang CE, Yang CJ, et al. Radiofrequency catheter ablation of sustained intraatrial reentrant tachycardia in adult patients. Circulation 1993;88:578–587.

18. Haissaguerre M, Marcus FI, Fischer B, Clementy J. Radiofrequency catheter ablation in unusual mechanisms of atrial fibrillation: report of 3 cases. J Cardiovasc Electrophysiol 1994;5:743–751.

19. Haissaguerre M, Gencel L, Fischer B, et al. Successful catheter ablation of atrial fibrillation. J Cardiovasc Electrophysiol 1994;5:1045–1052.

20. Elvan A, Pride HP, Eble JN, Zipes DP. Radiofrequency catheter ablation of the atria reduces the inducibility and duration of atrial fibrillation in dogs. Circulation 1995;91:2235–2244.

21. Swarz J, Pellersels G, Silvers J, et al. A catheter-based approach to atrial fibrillation in humans. Circulation 1994;90(Suppl 4):I-335.

22. Sealy WC, Hattler BG, Blumennschein SD, et al. Surgical treatment of Wolff-Parkinson-White syndrome. Ann Thorac Surg 1969;8:1–11.

23. Guiraudon GM. Anatomy of atrioventricular attachments, connections and junction: in medio stat virtus [Editorial Comment]. JACC 1994;24:1732–1734.

24. McAlpine WA. Heart and Coronary Arteries: An Anatomical Atlas for Clinical Diagnosis, Radiological Investigation, and Surgical Treatment. Springer-Verlag, New York, 1975.

25. Wood FC, Wolferth CC, Geckeler GD. Histologic demonstration of accessory muscular connections between auricle and ventricle in a case of short PR interval and prolonged QRS complex. Am Heart J 1943;25:454–462.

26. Hackel DB. Anatomic basis for preexcitation syndromes. In Benditt DG, Benson DW, eds. Cardiac Preexcitation Syndromes: Origins, Evaluation and Treatment. Martinus Nijhoff, Boston, 1986, pp 31–40.

27. Guiraudon G, Klein G, Sharma A, Yee R. Regional subclassification of accessory pathways in the Wolff-Parkinson-White syndrome based on dissection and electrophysiology. PACE 1989;12(Suppl 1):653A.

28. Guiraudon GM, Klein GJ, Yee R. Surgery for Wolff-Parkinson-White syndrome and supraventricular tachycardias. In Josephson ME, Wellens HJJ, eds. Tachycardias: mechanisms and management. Futura Publishing Co, Inc, Mount Kisco, NY, 1993, pp 479–504.

29. Coumel P, Cabrol C, Fabiato A, et al. Tachycardie permanente par rythme reciproque. 1. Preuves du diagnostic par stimulation auriculaire et ventriculaire. Arch Mal Coeur 1967;60:1830.

30. O'Neill BJ, Klein GJ, Guiraudon GM, et al. Results of operative therapy in the permanent form of junctional reciprocating tachycardia. Am J Cardiol 1989;63:1074–1079.

31. Klein GJ, Guiraudon GM, Kerr CR, et al. "Nodoventricular" accessory pathway: evidence for a distinct accessory atrioventricular pathway with atrioventricular node-like properties. J Am Coll Cardiol 1988;11:1035–1040.

32. Gallagher JJ. Variations of preexcitation: update 1984. In Zipes DP, Jalife J, eds. Cardiac Electrophysiology and Arrhythmias. Grune & Stratton, Orlando, FL, 1984, pp 419–433.

33. Cappato R, Schluter M, Weib C, et al. Catheter-induced mechanical conduction block of right-sided accessory fibers with Mahaim-type preexcitation to guide radiofrequency ablation. Circulation 1994;90:282–290.

34. Grogin HR, Lee RJ, Kwasman M, et al. Radiofrequency catheter ablation of atriofascicular and nodoventricular Mahaim tracts. Circulation 1994;90:272–281.

35. Sealy WC. Kent bundles in the anterior septal space. Ann Thorac Surg 1983;36:180–186.

36. Sealy WC. The evolution of the surgical methods for interruption of right free wall Kent bundles. Ann Thorac Surg 1983;36:29–36.

37. Sealy WC, Gallagher JJ. The surgical approach to the septal area of the heart based on experiences with 45 patients with Kent bundles. J Thorac Cardiovasc Surg 1980;79:542–551.

38. Cox JL, Gallagher JJ, Cain ME. Experience with 118 consecutive patients undergoing operation for the Wolff-Parkinson-White syndrome. J Thorac Cardiovasc Surg 1985;90:490–501.

39. Gallagher JJ, Sealy WC, Cox JL, et al. Results of surgery for preexcitation in 200 cases. Circulation 1981;64(Suppl IV):146.

40. Guiraudon GM, Klein GJ, Gulamhusein S, et al. Surgical repair of Wolff-Parkinson-

White syndrome: a new closed-heart technique. Ann Thorac Surg 1984;37:67–71.

41. Guiraudon GM, Klein GJ, Sharma AD, et al. Closed heart technique for Wolff-Parkinson-White syndrome: further experience and potential limitations. Ann Thorac Surg 1986;42:651–657.

42. Guiraudon GM, Klein GJ, Sharma AD, et al. Surgery for the Wolff-Parkinson-White syndrome: the epicardial approach. Semin Thorac Cardiovasc Surg 1989;1:21–33.

43. Guiraudon GM, Klein GJ, Yee R, et al. Surgical epicardial ablation of left ventricular pathway using sling exposure. Ann Thorac Surg 1990;50:968–971.

44. Guiraudon GM, Klein GJ, Sharma AD, et al. Surgical approach to anterior septal accessory pathways in 20 patients with the Wolff-Parkinson-White syndrome. Eur J Cardiothorac Surg 1988;2:201–206.

45. Guiraudon GM, Klein GJ, Sharma AD, et al. "Atypical" posterior septal accessory pathway in the Wolff-Parkinson-White syndrome. J Am Coll Cardiol 1988;12:1605–1608.

46. Teo WS, Guiraudon GM, Klein GJ, et al. A unique preexcitation pattern related to an atypical anteroseptal accessory pathway. PACE 1992;15(Pt 1):1696–1701.

47. Gallagher JJ, Selle JG, Sealy WC, et al. Intermediate septal accessory pathways (IS-AP): a subset of preexcitation at risk for complete heart block/failure during WPW surgery. Circulation 1986;74(Suppl 2):387.

48. Murdock CJ, Klein GJ, Guiraudon GM, et al. Epicardial mapping in patients with "nodoventricular" accessory pathways. Am J Cardiol 1991;68:208–214.

49. Guiraudon CM, Guiraudon GM, Klein GJ, "Nodal ventricular" Mahaim pathway histologic evidence for an accessory atrioventricular pathway with AV node-like morphology. Circulation (Suppl II) 1988;78(4):II-40.

50. Guiraudon GM, Guiraudon CM, Klein GJ, et al. The coronary sinus diverticulum: a pathological entity associated with the Wolff-Parkinson-White syndrome. Am J Cardiol 1988;62:733–735.

51. Arruda MS, Beckman KJ, McClelland JH, et al. Coronary sinus anatomy and anomalies in patients with posteroseptal accessory pathway requiring ablation within a venous branch of the coronary sinus. J Am Coll Cardiol 1994;23:224A.

52. Guiraudon GM, Klein GJ, Sharma AD, et al. Multiple accessory pathways—the elusive posterior septal pathways: experience with 17 patients. PACE 1988;11(Suppl):935A.

53. Gallagher JJ, Sealy WC, Kasell J, et al. Multiple accessory pathways in patients with the preexcitation syndrome. Circulation 1976;54:571–590.

54. Guiraudon GM, Guiraudon CM, Klein GJ, et al. Operation for the Wolff-Parkinson-White syndrome in the catheter ablation era. Ann Thorac Surg 1994;57:1084–1088.

55. Sharma AD, Yee R, Guiraudon GM, Klein GJ. AV nodal reentry: current concepts and surgical treatment. In Zipes DP, Rowlands DJ, eds. Progress in Cardiology. Lea & Febiger, Philadephia, 1988, pp 129–145.

56. Pritchett ELC, Anderson RW, Benditt DG, et al. Reentry within the atrioventricular node: surgical cure with preservation of atrioventricular conduction. Circulation 1979;60:440–446.

57. Marquez-Montes J, Rufilanchas JJ, Esteve JJ, et al. Paroxysmal nodal reentrant tachycardia, surgical cure with preservation of atrioventricular conduction. Chest 1983;83:690–694.

58. Ross DL, Johnson DC, Denniss AR, et al. Curative surgery for atrio-ventricular junctional ("AV nodal") reentrant tachycardia. J Am Coll Cardiol 1985;6:1282–1392.

59. Meijler FL, Janse MJ. Morphology and electrophysiology of the mammalian atrioventricular node. Physiol Rev 1988;68:608–647.

60. Anderson RH, Becker AF, Brechenmacher C, et al. The human atrioventricular junctional area: a morphological study of the A-V node and bundle. Eur J Cardiol 1975;3:11–25.

61. Guiraudon GM, Klein GJ, van Hemel N, et al. Anatomically guided surgery to the AV node. AV nodal skeletonization: experience in 46 patients with AV nodal reentrant tachycardia. Eur J Cardiothorac Surg 1990.

62. Guiraudon GM, Klein GJ, Sharma AD, et al. Skeletonization of the atrioventricular node surgical alternative for AV nodal reentrant tachycardia: experience with 32 patients. Ann Thorac Surg 1990;49:565.

63. Cox JL, Holman WL, Cain ME. Cryosurgical treatment of atrioventricular node reentrant tachycardia. Circulation 1987;76:1329–1336.

64. Natale A, Wathen M, Wolfe K, et al. Comparative atrioventricular node properties after radiofrequency ablation and operative therapy of AV node reentry. PACE 1993;16(Pt I):971–977.

65. Lowe JE, Hendry PJ, Packer DL, Tang AS. Surgical management of chronic ectopic atrial tachycardia. Sem Thorac Cardiovasc Surg 1989;1:58–66.

66. Guiraudon GM, Klein GJ, Yee R. Supraventricular tachycardias: the role of surgery. PACE 1993;16(Pt II):658–670.

67. Sharma AD, Klein GJ, Guiraudon GM, et

al. Paroxysmal sinus tachycardia: further experience with subtotal right atrial exclusion suggesting diffuse atrial disease. J Am Coll Cardiol 1986;7:128A.

68. Morillo CA, Klein GJ, Thakur RK, et al. Mechanism of "inappropriate" sinus tachycardia: role of sympathovagal balance. Circulation 1994;90:873–877.

69. Gomes A, Mehta D, Langan MN. Sinus node reentrant tachycardia. PACE 1995; 18(Pt I):1045–1057.

70. Sanders WE, Sorrentino RA, Greenfield RA, et al. Catheter ablation of sinoatrial node reentrant tachycardia. JACC 1994;23: 926–934.

71. Jolly WA, Ritchie WT. Auricular flutter and fibrillation. Heart 1910;2:177.

72. Prinzmetal M, et al. The auricular arrhythmias. Charles C. Thomas, Springfield, IL, 1952.

73. Wells JL, MacLean WAH, James TN, Waldo AL. Characterization of atrial flutter: studies in man after open heart surgery using fixed atrial electrodes. Circulation 1979;60: 665–673.

74. Lewis T, Freil HS, Stroud WD. Observations upon flutter and fibrillation. II. The nature of auricular flutter. Heart 1920;7:191.

75. Boineau JP, et al. Natural and evoked atrial flutter due to circus movement in dogs. Am J Cardiol 1980;45:1167.

76. Allessie MA, et al. Intraatrial reentry as a mechanism for atrial flutter induced by acetylcholine in rapid pacing in the dog. Circulation 1984;70:123.

77. Page P, et al. A new model of atrial flutter. J Am Coll Cardiol 1986;8:872.

78. Puech P, Latour H, Grolleau R. Le flutter et ses limites. Arch Mal Coeur 1970;63:116.

79. Klein GJ, Guiraudon GM, Sharma AD, et al. Demonstration of macro-reentry and feasibility of operative therapy in the common type of atrial flutter. Am J Cardiol 1986;57:587–591.

80. Disertori M, et al. Evidence of a reentry circuit in the common type of atrial flutter in man. Circulation 1983;67:434.

81. Waldo AL, et al. Entrainment and interruption of atrial flutter with atrial pacing: studies in man following open heart surgery. Circulation 1977;56:737.

82. Waldo AL, Carlson MD, Biblo LA, et al. The role of transient entrainment in atrial flutter. In Touboul P, Waldo AL, eds. Atrial Arrhythmias: Current Concepts and Management. Mosby Year Book, St. Louis, 1990, p 210.

83. Cosio FG. Endocardial mapping of atrial flutter. In Touboul P, Waldo AL, eds. Atrial arrhythmias: current concepts and manage-

ment. Mosby Year Book, St. Louis, 1990, p 229.

84. Chauvin M, Brechenmacher C, Voegltin JR. Applications de la cartographie endocavitaire a l'etude du flutter auriculaire. Arch Mal Coeur 1983;76:1020.

85. Cosio FG, Goicolea A, Lopez-Gil M, et al. Atrial endocardial mapping in the rare form of atrial flutter. Am J Cardiol 1990;66: 715.

86. Puech P, Gallay P, Grolleau R. Mechanism of atrial flutter in humans. In Touboul P, Waldo AL, eds. Atrial arrhythmias: current concepts and management. Mosby Year Book, St. Louis, 1990, p 190.

87. Allessie MA, Rensma W, Brugada J, et al. Modes of atrial reentry. In Touboul P, Waldo AL, eds. Atrial Arrhythmias: Current Concepts and Management. Mosby Year Book, St. Louis, 1990, p 112.

88. Guiraudon, GM, Klein GJ, van Hemel N, et al. Atrial flutter: lessons from surgical interventions (musing on atrial flutter mechanism). PACE 1996;19(Pt II):1933–1938.

89. Guiraudon GM, Campbell CS, Jones DL, et al. Combined sino-atrial node atrioventricular isolation: A surgical alternative to His bundle ablation in patients with atrial fibrillation. Circulation 1985;72(Suppl 2):III–220.

90. Guiraudon GM, Guiraudon CM. Atrial functional anatomy. In Kingma JH, van Hemel NM, Lie KI, eds. Atrial Fibrillation: A Treatable Disease? Kluwer Academic Publisher, Boston, 1992, p 23.

91. Lamas GA. Physiological consequences of normal atrioventricular conduction: applicability to modern cardiac pacing. J Cardiac Surg 1989;4:89.

92. Robinson TF, Factor SM, Sonnenblick EH. The heart as a suction pump. Sci Am 1986; 254;6:84.

93. Aberg H. Atrial fibrillation: I. A study of atrial thrombosis and systemic embolism in a necropsy material. Acta Med Scand 1969; 185:373–379.

94. Acar J, Cormier D, Grimberg G, et al. Diagnosis of left atrial thrombi in mitral stenosis: Usefulness of ultrasound techniques compared with other methods. Eur J Cardial 1991:12(Suppl B):70–76.

95. Cormier B, Serafini D, Grimberg D, et al. Detection of thrombosis of the left atrium in mitral valve stenosis. Arch Maladies Coeur Vaisseaux 1991;84:1321–1326.

96. James TN. Diversity of histopathologic correlates of atrial fibrillation. In Kulbertus HE, Olson SB, Schlepper M, eds. Atrial Fibrillation. Astra Publishers, Modudal, Sweden, 1982, p 13.

97. Bharati S, Lev M. Histology of the normal

and diseased atrium. In Falk RH, Podrid PJ. Atrial Fibrillation, Mechanisms and Management. Raven Press, New York, 1992, p 15.

98. Frustaci A, Caldarulo M, Buffon A, et al. Cardiac biopsy in patients with "primary" atrial fibrillation: histologic evidence of occult myocardial diseases. Chest 1991;2:303.

99. Sekiguchi M, Hiroe M, Kasanuki H, et al. Experience of 100 atrial endomyocardial biopsies and the concept of atrial cardiomyopathy [abstract]. Circulation 1984; 70(Suppl)2:118.

100. Guiraudon CM, Ernst NM, Guiraudon GM, et al. The pathology of drug resistant lone atrial fibrillation in eleven surgically treated patients. In Kingma JH, van Hemel NM, Lie KI, eds. Atrial Fibrillation: A Treatable Disease? Kluwer Academic Publishers, Boston, 1992, p 41.

101. Guiraudon CM, Ernst NM, Klein GJ, et al. The pathology of intractable "primary" atrial fibrillation. Circulation 1992;86(Suppl I)4:I–662.

102. Moe GK. On the multiple wavelet hypothesis of atrial fibrillation. Arch Int Pharmacodyn 1962;140:183.

103. Allessie MA, Lammers WJEP, Bonke FIM. Experimental evaluation of Moe's multiple wavelet hypothesis of atrial fibrillation. In Zipes DP, Jalife J, eds. Cardiac Electrophysiology and Arrhythmias. Grune & Stratton, Inc., New York, 1985, p 265.

104. Allessie M, Kirchhof C. Termination of atrial fibrillation by class IC antiarrhythmic drugs, a paradox? In Kingma JH, van Hemel NM, Lie KI, eds. Atrial Fibrillation: A Treatable Disease? Kluwer Academic Publishers, Boston, 1992, p 265.

105. Wijffels M, Kirchhof C, Frederiks J, et al. Atrial fibrillation begets atrial fibrillation. Circulation 1993;86(Suppl I):I–18.

106. Allessie MA. Reentrant mechanisms underlying atrial fibrillation. In Zipes DP, Jalife J, eds. Cardiac Electrophysiology: From Cell to Bedside, 2nd edition. W.B. Saunders Company, Toronto, Ontario, 1995, pp 562–566.

107. Schuessler RB, Grayson TM, Bromberg BI, et al. Cholinergically mediated tachyarrhythmias induced by a single extrastimulus in the isolated canine right atrium. Circ Res 1992;71,5:1254–1267.

108. Morillo CA, Klein GJ, Jones DL, et al. Chronic rapid atrial pacing: structural, functional, and electrophysiological characteristics of a new model of sustained atrial fibrillation. Circulation 1995;91:1588–1595.

109. Harada A, Sasaki K, Fukushima T, et al. Atrial activation during chronic atrial fibrillation in patients with isolated mitral valve disease. Ann Thorac Surg 1996;61:104–112.

110. Cox JL, Canavan TE, Schuessler RB. The surgical treatment of atrial fibrillation: II. Intra-operative electrophysiologic mapping and description of the electrophysiologic basis of atrial flutter and atrial fibrillation. J Thorac Cardiovasc Surg 1991;101: 406–426.

111. Pertsov AM, Davidenko JM, Salomonsz R, et al. Spiral waves of excitation underlie reentrant activity in isolated cardiac muscle. Circ Res 1993;631–650.

112. Stanton MS, Miles WM, Zipes DP. Atrial Fibrillation and Flutter. In Zipes DP, Jalife J, eds. Cardiac Electrophysiology From Cell to Bedside. W.B. Saunders Company, Toronto, 1990, pp 734–742.

113. Guiraudon GM, Guiraudon CM, Klein GJ, et al. Atrial fibrillation: functional anatomy and surgical rationales. In Farré J, Moro C, eds. Ten Years of Radiofrequency Catheter Ablation. Futura Publishing Co., Inc., Armonk, NY, 1998, pp 289–310.

114. Batista RJV, Cunha MA, Takeshita N, et al. Cardiac autotransplantation: A new approach for the treatment of complex cardiac problems. In Programme Book, 9th Annual Meeting. The European Association for Cardio-Thoracic Surgery, Paris France, September 24–27, 1995, p 248.

115. Elvan A, Pride HP, Eble JN, et al. Radiofrequency catheter ablation of the atria reduces the inducibility and duration of atrial fibrillation in dogs. Circulation 1995;91: 2235–2244.

116. Graffigna A, Ressia L, Pagnani F, et al. Left atrial isolation for the treatment of atrial fibrillation due to mitral valve disease: hemodynamic evaluation. N Trend Arrhyth IX 1993;4:1069.

117. Morris JJ, Stanton MS, Hammil SC. The maze procedure: A reproducibly safe and effective cure for refractory nonvalvular atrial fibrillation. Circulation (Suppl I) 1995; 92:I–264.

118. Shrestha NK, Moreno FL, Narciso GV, et al. Two-dimensional echocardiographic diagnosis of left atrial thrombus in rheumatic heart disease: a clinicopathologic study. Circulation 1983;67:341–347.

119. Leung DYC, Black IW, Crannery GB, et al. Prognostic implications of left atrial spontaneous echo contrast in nonvalvular atrial fibrillation. J Am Coll Cardiol 1994;24: 755–62.

120. Blackshear JL, Odell JA. Appendage obliteration to reduce stroke in cardiac surgical patients with atrial fibrillation. Ann Thorac Surg 1996;61:755–759.

121. Christides C, Cabrol C, Cabrol A, et al. Reinterventions sur protheses valvulaires mitrales: a propose de 16 malades. Coeur 1974; 515–523.

122. Leitch JW, Klein G, Yee R, et al. Sinus node-atrioventricular node isolation: long-term results with the corridor operation for atrial fibrillation. J Am Coll Cardiol 1991;17,4:970.

123. Guiraudon GM, Klein GJ, Yee R. Supraventricular tachycardias: the role of surgery. PACE 1993;I,16,1:658–670.

124. Guiraudon GM, Klein GJ, Guiraudon CM, Yee R. Treatment of atrial fibrillation: preservation of sinoventricular impulse conduction (the corridor operation). In: Olsson SB, Allessie MA, Campbell RWF. Atrial Fibrillation: Mechanisms and Therapeutic Strategies. Futura Publishing, Co, Inc, Armonk, NY, 1994, p 349.

125. Gursoy S, de Bruyne B, Atie J, et al. Interatrial dissociation following the corridor operation: Role of atrial contraction in thrombogenesis. Eur Heart J 1991; 12(Suppl):337.

126. van Hemel NM, Defaux JJAMT, Kingma JH, et al. Long-term results of the "corridor" operation for atrial fibrillation. Br Heart J 1994;71:170.

127. Cox JL. Evolving applications of the maze procedure for atrial fibrillation. Ann Thorac Surg 1993;55:578–580.

128. Cox JL, Boineau JP, Schuessler RB, et al. Successful surgical treatment of atrial fibrillation: review and clinical update. JAMA 1991;266:1976–1980.

129. Cox JL, Boineau JP, Schuessler RB, et al. Five-year experience with the maze procedure for atrial fibrillation. Ann Thorac Surg 1993;56:814–824.

130. Cox JL, Boineau JP, Schuessler RB, et al. Surgical interruption of atrial reentry as a cure for atrial fibrillation. In Olsson SB, Allessie MA, Campbell RWF, eds. Atrial Fibrillation: Mechanisms and Therapeutic Strategies. Armonk, NY, Futura Publishing Company, Inc, 1994, pp 373–404.

131. Cox JL, Schuessler RB, Cain ME, et al. Surgery for atrial fibrillation. Sem Thorac Cardiovasc Surg 1989;1:67–73.

132. Kim Y-J, Sohn D-W, Park Y-B, et al. Restoration of atrial mechanical function after maze operation: Is it affected by the same factors as the restoration of sinus rhythm? JACC 1996;27(Suppl A):261A.

133. Boriani G, Capucci A, Marinelli G, Biffi M, et al. Left atrial isolation combined with mitral valve surgery: Hemodynamic evaluation during cardiopulmonary exercise test. JACC 1996;27(Suppl A):260A.

134. Shyu K-G, Cheng J-J, Chen J-J, et al. Recovery of atrial function after atrial compartment operation for chronic atrial fibrillation in mitral valve disease. JACC 1994;24: 392–398.

135. Brodman RF, Frame R, Fisher JD, et al. Combined treatment of mitral stenosis and atrial fibrillation with valvuloplasty and left atrial maze procedure. J Thorac Cardiovasc Surg 1994;107:622.

136. Hioki M, Ikeshita M, Iedokoro Y, et al. Successful combined operation for mitral stenosis and atrial fibrillation. Ann Thorac Surg 1993;55:776–778.

137. McCarthy PM, Cosgrove DM, Castle LW, et al. Combined treatment of mitral regurgitation and atrial fibrillation with valvuloplasty and the maze procedure. Am J Cardiol 1993;71:483–486.

138. Kosakai Y, Kawaguchi AT, Isobe F, et al. Cox maze procedure for chronic atrial fibrillation associated with mitral valve disease. J Thorac Cardiovasc Surg 1994;108: 1049–1055.

139. Chua YL, Schaff HV, Orszulak TA, Morris JJ. Outcome of mitral valve repair in patients with preoperative atrial fibrillation. J Thorac Cardiovasc Surg 1994;107:408–415.

140. He DS, Mackey S, Marcus FI, Graham A, et al. Radiofrequency energy for cardiac ablation using a multipolar catheter in sheep. Circulation (Suppl I);92:I–265.

141. Nakagawa H, Yamanashi WS, Pitha JV, et al. Creation of long linear transmural radiofrequency lesions in atrium using a novel spiral ribbon: saline irrigated electrode catheter. JACC 1996;27(Suppl A):188A.

142. Avitall B, Helms RW, Chianng W, et al. Nonlinear atrial radiofrequency lesions are arrhythmogenic: a study of skipped lesions in the normal atria. Circulation 1995;92: I–265.

143. Tondo C, Otomo K, Antz M, et al. Successful radiofrequency catheter ablation of atrial fibrillation by a single lesion to the interatrial septum. Circulation 1995;(Suppl I);92:1–265.

144. Haines DE, McRury IA. Primary atrial fibrillation ablation (PAFA) in a chronic atrial fibrillation model. Circulation 1995;(Suppl I);92,8:I–265.

145. Haissaguerre M, Jais P, Shah DC, et al. Radiofrequency catheter ablation for paroxysmal atrial fibrillation in humans: elaboration of a procedure-based on electrophysiological data. In Murgatroyd FD, Camm AJ, eds. Nonpharmacological Management of Atrial Fibrillation. Futura Publishing Co., Inc, Armonk, NY, 1997, pp 257–279.

146. Inderbitzi R. Surgical Thoracoscopy. Springer-Verlag, Berlin, Germany, 1994.

Chapter 30

Modifications to the Maze Procedure for Surgical Ablation of Atrial Fibrillation

T. Bruce Ferguson, Jr.

Introduction

Atrial fibrillation (AF) is a common arrhythmia that is associated with significant symptoms and morbidity. The symptoms of palpitations, presyncope, dyspnea, and exertional intolerance may be caused by poorly controlled ventricular response rates at rest or with exercise, or the irregular ventricular response to the rapid atrial rhythm which results in beat-to-beat variability of ventricular filling.[1,2] A minority of patients, such as those with dilated or ischemic cardiomyopathy, will also have exacerbation of congestive heart failure due to the loss of atrial contribution to ventricular filling, so-called loss of atrial transport function. The major morbidity of AF is attributable to left atrial thrombus formation and subsequent thromboembolic events, especially embolic stroke.[3,4] Although the risk of stroke may be reduced with warfarin anticoagulant therapy, it is still higher than observed in the general population.[4] The goals of ablation therapy in AF, therefore, must be to either improve symptoms or decrease atrial thrombus formation and subsequent embolic events. This chapter will discuss the maze III and modifications to the maze III surgical therapy for this arrhythmia.

Ablative Therapy for Atrial Fibrillation

When medical therapy fails to control the ventricular response associated with rapid AF, the initial interventional approach has been to surgically ablate the His bundle and implant a VVI pacemaker. In many series, however, patients with VVI pacing and congestive heart failure experienced a 50% 3-year mortality. Moreover, this approach still doesn't address the problems of thromboembolism or loss of transport function that remain in these patients.[4]

An "ideal" ablative procedure for AF would accomplish five goals: (1) elimination of AF as a clinical arrhythmia; (2) restoration of sinus rhythm; (3) maintenance of AV synchrony; (4) restore atrial transport function; and (5) by virtue of goals 1–4, decrease or eliminate the risk of thromboembolism by eliminating passive stasis of blood in either or both atria.[5] The appropriateness of any intervention, then, needs to be judged against these five criteria; to the degree that one or more are not successfully achieved, the ablative therapy may be considered less than optimal.

From a technical standpoint, any ablative therapy designed to eliminate AF should

From Singer I, Barold SS, Camm AJ (eds): Nonpharmacological Therapy of Arrhythmias for the 21st Century: The State of the Art. Futura Publishing Co, Inc., Armonk, NY, © 1998.

theoretically (1) reduce the critical number of reentrant circuits available to maintain the fibrillatory process; (2) reduce the surface area of the atrium available to maintain the fibrillatory process; or (3) accomplish a combination of 1 and 2, above. The current surgical approaches discussed below have in general been directed in one of these three areas.

Technical Evolution of the Maze III Procedure

The first maze procedure was performed by James L. Cox, MD in September 1987. That patient was followed for 6 months, and then the second procedure was performed. This observation process was repeated until the safety and efficacy of the initial operative approach was documented.[6]

As is the case with most new techniques, information obtained during the early experience is used to modify the approach(es) utilized. These modifications led to the development of the maze III procedure.[4,7,8]

The reasons for these modifications were:

1. inability to achieve maximal heart rates with exercise (blunted sinus node response), corrected by moving the atrial septal incision in a posterocaudal direction and the right atrial free wall incisions away from the sinus nodal area;
2. inability to document left atrial transport function in approximately 30% of patients with obvious right atrial transport function, corrected by preserving Bachmann's bundle which facilitates conduction across the dome of the atria; and
3. a requirement for new pacemaker placement in approximately 40% of patients, "controlled" by recognizing that in these patients elimination of the AF unmasked clinically apparent sick sinus disease.[9] With

one exception, these pacemakers have been for *atrial* and not ventricular conduction support.

The Maze III Procedure

The surgical goal of the maze III procedure[4,7,8,10] is to: (1) reduce the critical number of reentrant circuits available to maintain the fibrillatory process; and (2) reduce the surface area of the atrium available to maintain the fibrillatory process. Importantly, the success of the operation depends on the newly created anatomic relationships between the surgical incisions and the fixed anatomic obstacles in the atria: the superior and inferior cavae and tricuspid valve anulus on the right side, and the pulmonary veins and mitral valve anulus on the left side.

The surgical technique has been extensively described, and is beyond the scope of this chapter.[5,8,11] A schematic of the maze III procedure is shown in Figure 1.

After completion of the maze procedure, reentrant circuits cannot form because the distances between the incisions, the nonconducting fibrous skeleton of the heart, and the fixed anatomic obstacles of the right and left atrium are such that reentrant circuits cannot form; this is because the circuit becomes extinguished by one of these excisions or obstacles before a reentrant loop can be established. The only sustained conduction pathway originates from the sinus nodal area, proceeds anteriorly around the right atrial tissue, enters the atrial septum anteriorly, and depolarizes the AV nodal tissue; this anterior atrial depolarization carries across to the anterior left atrium and then around posteriorly to depolarize the tissue beneath the pulmonary veins. Conduction down the atrial fibers contained within the coronary sinus is interrupted, however, by placement of a cryolesion on the left atrial side of the sinus. The remainder of the posterior atrial free walls are de-

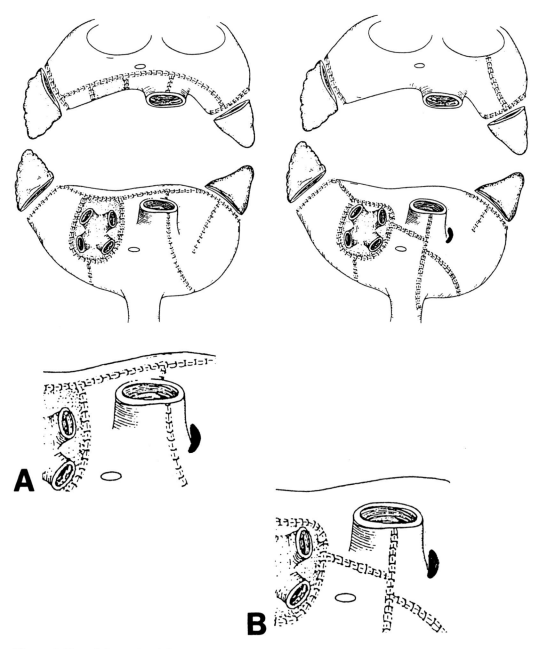

Figure 1. Top: Schematic of the maze I **(A)** and the maze III **(B)** procedure. The top of each figure shows the anterior aspect of the atria; the bottom shows the posterior atria. Note the absence of the incision across the top of the atrium. The sinus node is depicted as the black kidney-bean shaped structure on (B), and the AV node as the open oval circle. The actual sinus node complex encompasses the tissue anterior and lateral (to the right in the lower panel) to the superior vena cava, between the suture lines. Note the rearrangement of incisions to remove the incision across Bachmann's bundle and away from the sinus node area. **Bottom:** Closeup of the superior vena cava region of the heart, depicting the maze I incisions (left) and their proximity to Bachmann's bundle anteriorly and the sinus node complex anterolaterally. The right panel shows the same depiction for the maze III procedure. Modified and used with permission from Singer I, ed.[5]

polarized from the wavefront exiting the atrial septum posteriorly. Thus, normal AV conduction is maintained and the entire atrium is depolarized in sequential fashion after this operative procedure.

Current Results with the Maze III Procedure

A total of 139 patients underwent surgical intervention between 1987 and January 1995 at Washington University.[12] The following analysis will compare the results with the maze I and II procedures with those from the currently performed maze III procedure.[7,10] The maze II procedure was an intermediate modification between I and III utilized in only 15 patients. This was technically more complicated to perform, and was further modified into the technically straightforward maze III procedure.

The mean age of the overall population was 52 ± 11.5 years; 55% of patients had paroxysmal fibrillation or flutter, while 45% had chronic AF at the time of surgery. Arrhythmia intolerance was the indication for surgical intervention in 65% of cases, while drug intolerance was present in 11%. A previous thromboembolic event was present as the symptom for surgery in the remaining 24%. Only a small percentage of patients had abnormal ventricular function preoperatively. Thirty-one percent of patients underwent a concomitant cardiac surgical operation at the time of the maze procedure.

There were three perioperative deaths in the overall series (2.2%), one in the I/II group and two in the III group. There was one late death, at 4 years.

Forty-seven patients underwent the I/II procedure, while the remaining 92 have undergone the maze III procedure. Except for the difference in patients undergoing reoperation, the patient demographics are similar in both groups. With the exception of the reoperative patients, the patient demographics for all patients, regardless of operative procedure, were the same (Table 1).

Table 1
Demographics

	Maze I/II		Maze III	
	#	%	#	%
Patients	47		92	
Mean age (years)	51 ± 12		54 ± 11	
Males	33	77	64	70
Preoperative arrhythmia				
paroxysmal	25	53	53	58
chronic	22	47	39	42
Prior surgery	13	27	4	4
Concomitant surgery	15	32	39	42

Modified and used with permission from Singer I, ed.[5]

Perioperative complications for the two groups are listed in Table 2. The incidence of atrial arrhythmias is similar. These are thought to be related to shortening of atrial refractoriness as a result of surgical intervention; as the atrium heals, refractoriness returns to normal and the reentrant circuits responsible for the perioperative arrhythmias become extinguished against the surgical suture lines and the fixed anatomic obstacles of the left and right atria.

The incidence of the remaining complications in each group is low, and similar be-

Table 2
Perioperative Complications

	Maze I/II		Maze III	
	#	%	#	%
Deaths	1	2.1	2	2.2
Atrial Arrhythmias	19	40.4	38	41.3
Fluid Retention	7	14.8	6	6.5
Bleeding	3	6.4	2	2.2
Stroke	1	2.1	0	
TIA	1	2.1	1	1.1
MI	0		1	1.1

TIA = transient ischemic attack; MI = perioperative myocardial infarction.
Modified and used with permission from Singer I, ed.[5]

Table 3
Long-Term Follow-Up

		Maze I/II		Maze III	
		#	%	#	%
Total Patients		47		92	
Procedural Survivors		46		90	
Pacemakers	Total	25	54.3	25	27.8
	New	20		17	
Preop SSS		18		15	
	% of PM		72.0		60.0
Preop PM		5		8	
	% of PM		20.0		32.0
Iatrogenic Injury		1	4.5	1	1.2
Pts > 3 Months F/U		46		78	
Transient Ischemic Attack		1	2.2	1	1.3
Blunted Sinus Response		31	67.4	6	7.7
Arrhythmia Recurrence		9	19.6	0	
Atrial Flutter		6	13.1	0	
Atrial Fibrillation		3	6.5	0	
Atrial Transport Function					
Patients Analyzed		43		53	
Left Atrium		30	69.8	48	90.5
Right Atrium		43	100	52	98.1

SSS = sick sinus syndrome; PM = pacemaker.
Modified and used with permission from Singer I, ed.[5]

tween the two groups, and similar to those for other open heart antiarrhythmia procedures.[11]

Table 3 illustrates the follow-up data for these patients. All operative survivors were "at risk" for the requirement for pacemaker implantation; this requirement was reduced from 54.3% (25 of 46) in the I/II group to 27.8% (25 of 90) in the maze III group. The vast majority of patients requiring pacemaker implantation continue to have evidence of sick sinus syndrome preoperatively, or had already undergone implantation of a pacemaker system for conduction system disease. Only two pacemaker patients overall have sustained an iatrogenic injury, one patient in the first group with devascularization of the sinus node and one patient in the maze III group with an anomalous coronary sinus repair and postoperative complete heart block. This patient is the only patient in the entire series requiring ventricular pacing (Table 4).

Table 4
Results of Preoperative Clinical and Electrophysiological Evaluation of Sinus Node Function (9/87–12/93) (N = 103)

	Pacemaker		No Pacemaker	
	N	%	N	%
Total Patients	43		60	
EPS +	13	30.2	2	3.3
Holter +	12	27.9	2	3.3
Clinical Assessment +	6	13.9	1	1.6
Evaluation −	12	27.9	55	91.7
Prior PM Placement	10			
SSS	6			
His Ablation	3			
HOCM	1			
New Postoperative Implant	33			
sinus bradycardia	20			
junctional rhythm	11			

Modified and used with permission from Singer I, ed.[5]

Late follow-up (>3 months) is available for all but one patient in I/II, and in 78 of 92 patients in the maze III group (Table 3).

Transient ischemic attacks have occurred in 3% of the first group, and in 1% of the maze III group.

The incidence of a blunted response to exercise has been reduced from 65% to 8%, most likely for the reasons outlined above. The remaining incidence of chronotropic abnormality is probably related to underlying sinoatrial nodal disease.

Nine of 46 patients had a late recurrence of fibrillation (n = 3) or flutter (n = 6) in the maze I/II group. All have been effectively controlled with medication. There have been no recurrences in late follow-up following the maze III procedure.

Postoperative atrial transport function has been documented in the majority of patients by any one of five tests: intraoperative visualization, transesophageal echocardiography, transthoracic echocardiography, three-dimensional MRI scanning, and hemodynamic assessment of AV pacing compared with ventricular pacing. A positive study with any evaluation has constituted demonstration of transport function.

Forty-three of 46 group I/II patients underwent postoperative evaluation for transport function; 53 of 98 group III patients were evaluated. Right atrial transport function was present in all 43 group I/II patients. Of the 53 patients receiving follow-up for transport function in the III group, 52 (98%) had right atrial transport present.

In the I/II group, 30 of 43 (70%) patients had left atrial transport, while 48 of 53 (90%) patients in the III group had documented left-sided atrial function present. Thus, with the maze III modification, both right and left-sided transport is present in 98% and 90% of patients, respectively. The mechanism whereby this small remaining group of patients cannot generate left-sided atrial systole remains uncertain.

Finally, whether long-term freedom from fibrillation will in fact decrease the theoretical risk of thromboembolism compared to a control population is unclear and will be difficult to demonstrate, due to the low incidence of events in patients this age with "lone" fibrillation.[10] Clearly, however, the procedure does not increase the incidence of thromboembolism.

Modifications to the Concept of the Maze Procedure

As outlined above, the original maze concept was based on the following premises:

1. that AF was a microreentrant or small (in size) cycle-length macroreentrant arrhythmia;
2. that multiple reentrant circuits could exist at the same time in the atrium;
3. that initiation and termination of these multiple reentrant circuits occurred spontaneously during the arrhythmia;
4. that these reentrant circuits were transient in both time and location;
5. that the circuits could be interfered with by the normal physiological and anatomic barriers in the heart.

These premises were derived from intraoperative mapping studies of AF. The majority of the patients undergoing mapping had associated electrophysiological disease at the time of surgery, and because of the risk of thromboembolism with manipulation of the heart, very few had valvular disease associated with chronic AF. The results of these intraoperative mapping studies have been well-described.[4,12,13] In these patients, the mapping data demonstrated that unlike all other forms of clinical arrhythmias amenable to surgical correction, no discrete anatomic foci could be discerned for these transient reentrant circuits.

These studies led Jim Cox, John Boineau, Rick Schuessler, and co-workers[4] to conclude that intraoperative electrophysiological mapping could not be used for AF ablation surgery, because the mapping data acquired a time t_0 would not correspond electrophysiologically to the conditions present at time $t_{>0}$, when the ablation was applied. Thus electrophysiological criteria could not be used to perform the procedure and importantly, to confirm the intraoperative success of the ablation.

Concomitantly, clinical experience and follow-up studies with Guiraudon and De-Fauw's corridor procedure[14,15] demonstrated that although this operation failed to eliminate AF, it did document that in the fibrillating heart, atrial tissue could be excluded from the fibrillating tissue and conduct electrical impulses in a normal fashion. The corollary was that the isolated areas of the left and right atrium remained large enough in size, surface area, and/or mass to sustain the reentrant circuits of the fibrillation. This was corroborated from the data obtained experimentally and clinically with the left atrial isolation procedure (described below), designed for left-sided ectopic atrial tachycardias.[16] Thus, on the right side of the atrium the normal anatomic boundaries were utilized to decrease the areas of contiguous atrial tissue, including the orifices of the inferior and superior vena cavae and the tricuspid annulus. On the left side, the veins were eliminated as a circumferential patch. On both sides the appendages were removed. As discussed below, these basic principles of a narrow pathway of conduction between the two nodal tissues and "compartmentalization" of the atrial free wall and septal tissues have been adhered to in the majority of the eventual surgical modifications to the maze III procedure.

The "gold standard" of the maze III was established over a 4-year time interval. During this time, several factors dampened the enthusiasm for altering the "standard technique" that had been developed. Early experimental attempts to interrupt atrial flutter with simple incisions were unsuccessful. Likewise, some lesser procedures (e.g., fewer atrial incisions) were for the most part unsuccessful in effectively eliminating AF. In patients with prior surgery, the operation was noted to be more difficult and the recurrence rate of atrial arrhythmias was higher. This led to the conclusion that the previous surgical incisions forced alteration of the "standard" technique, and this was thought to be contributing to the less succesful outcome in this group.

Despite its excellent success as an antiarrhythmic procedure, there are conceptually several reasons to alter the maze III procedure. These include: (1) decreasing the technical complexity of the procedure; (2) decreasing the time required to perform the procedure; and (3) permitting application of the simpler procedure to a larger group of patients.

These conceptual technical alterations to the procedure could include: (1) reduction in overall atrial mass; (2) elimination of one or more incisions; (3) change in relative placement of one or more incisions; (4) substitution of one or more surgical incisions by an alternative ablation technique; and (5) addition to the surgical approach a pharmacologic or neuropharmacological ablation mechanism. Procedures falling within these general categories are discussed below. For the reasons outlined above, however, purely electrophysiologic-based modification of the procedure has not proven possible.

Reduction in Atrial Mass

Massive atrial size, not typically seen in this country, has been more commonly seen in Japan, Korea, and the Pacific Rim. Since reduction of mass alone cannot be accomplished without multiple incisions, a number of abstracts delineating removal of excessively large amounts of atrial tissue at the time of the maze III or some modification to the procedure have been reported.[10,12,17]

Elimination of Incision(s) and/or Change in Incision Placement

The Arrhythmogenicity of Surgical Approaches to the Left Atrium

There are three surgical approaches to the left atrium used for access to the mitral valve apparatus. The traditional right lateral approach (an incision only involving left atrial tissue) through Waterston's groove is the same as the right side of the pulmonary vein encircling incision.[18] The two additional approaches are the transseptal approach,[19] which is similar to the maze III septal incision, and the superior septal incision,[20] which divides surgically Bachmann's bundle.

Utley and colleagues[18] retrospectively reviewed a series of 149 patients undergoing mitral procedures through one of these surgical approaches. In patients in sinus rhythm preoperatively, a surgical incision across Bachmann's bundle was more arrhythmogenic (sustained postoperative AF or junctional rhythm requiring a permanent pacemaker) than the transseptal incision. The standard left-sided only incision was associated with the highest rate of return of sinus rhythm (80%) and the lowest requirement for permanent pacemaker implantation (9%). Finally, in the patients with preoperative AF, the left-sided-only incision resulted in a 19% conversion to sinus rhythm, as compared to 5% and 6%, respectively for the approaches involving the septum. From an arrhythmia ablation perspective, this retrospective analysis suggests that right-sided therapy, if incomplete (e.g., fewer right-sided incisions) or mislocated (e.g., across Bachmann's bundle) might in fact be arrhythmogenic in this valve-associated patient population.

Left Atrial Isolation Procedure

The left atrial isolation procedure was originally designed for ectopic atrial tachycardias originating on the left side of the atrium that could not be localized at the time of intraoperative mapping.[16] In this procedure, the free wall of the left atrium was surgically isolated from the atrial septum and the remainder of the heart. The isolated left atrium continued to be subject to the ectopic focus, while the remainder of the atrium was restored to sinus rhythm. As applied to AF, the left atrium continues fibrill-

ating while the right side is restored to normal sinus rhythm.

Investigators in Italy have performed a left isolation procedure in 100 patients with AF secondary to mitral valve disease undergoing operative intervention, with 70% of patients maintaining sinus rhythm at follow-up.[21] Duration of fibrillation preoperatively longer than 6 months was a risk factor for recurrence. It was not anticipated that the risk of thromboembolism would be decreased by isolation of the left atrium, which could continue to fibrillate, and therefore the left atrial isolation technique does not meet the criteria for an "ideal" ablative procedure. Sinoatrial function was satisfactory in all patients who maintained persistence of sinus rhythm; during the same time interval in their institution, a nonrandomized group of patients with AF undergoing mitral procedures without the left atrial isolation had persistent fibrillation postoperatively in 80% of patients.

Modifications to the Left Side

Brodman and colleagues[22] described a case in which only the left-sided portion of the maze was performed in a patient undergoing mitral commissurotomy. Atrial flutter, not fibrillation, was inducible at late electrophysiological study. Hioki[23] reported altering the pulmonary vein encircling incision by dividing instead the left pulmonary veins from the right pulmonary veins. No recurrence of AF occurred in this case, but Cox has argued against both of these modifications.[24,25]

These surgical experiences generated additional considerations regarding the electroanatomic origin of atrial flutter and fibrillation in these patients with primary idiopathic disease: (1) the local effective refractory periods (ERPs) of the left atrium appear to be shorter than those of the right atrium; (2) due to the longer ERPs (and therefore longer reentrant circuits) on the right side, atrial flutter is more likely to occur on the basis of reentry in the right atrium; and (3) due to the shorter ERPs (and therefore shorter reentrant circuits) on the left side, AF is more likely to occur on the basis of reentry in the left atrium. To eliminate the recurrence of both flutter and fibrillation, therefore, a procedure that involves both sides appears to be necessary in this setting.

Simplification Based on Intraoperative Mapping Studies: Valvular Disease

Sueda and colleagues from Hiroshima[26] have used intraoperative mapping studies to document a difference in electrophysiological characteristic between the mean left

and right AF cycle lengths in patients with concomitant mitral valve disease. In (perhaps) distinction to idiopathic AF in the absence of valvular disease, activation patterns of AF in conjunction with mitral valve disease were postulated by Harada[27] to be driven electrically by the left atrium. Sueda's data demonstrated that chronic fibrillation in conjunction with mitral disease was associated with the shortened refractory period of the distended left atrium (range 129–169 ms in the right atrium versus 114–139 ms in the left atrium). A simple left-sided atrial procedure was devised (Figure 2) using cryosurgery, left atrial ap-

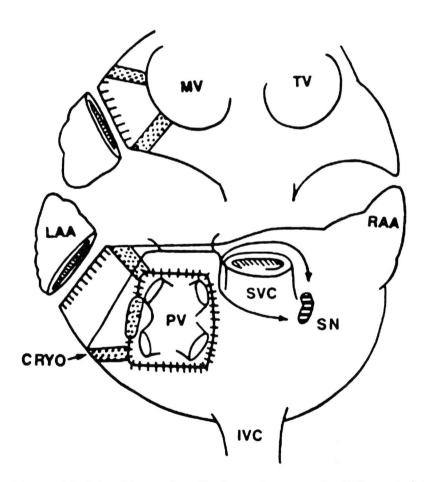

Figure 2. Schema of the left atrial procedure. The four pulmonary veins (PV) were isolated and the left atrial appendage (LAA) was excised. Cryoablation (CRYO) was delivered to the posterior wall of the left atrium, between the superior and posterior edges of the LAA. (IVC = inferior vena cava; MV = mitral valve; RAA = right atrial appendage; SN = sinus node; SVC = superior vena cava; TV = tricuspid valve). Used with permission from Sueda T, et al.[26]

pendectomy, and the pulmonary vein encircling incision to eliminate AF in 91% of this subset of patients at a mean of 11 months of follow-up. Left atrial size decreased postoperatively significantly as well, with atrial transport demonstrated in 100% of the right atria and 80% of the left atria of the patients in sinus rhythm postoperatively. Moreover, their intraoperative mapping data in patients with concomitant valvular disease suggest that there may be differences electrophysiologically between this form of AF and the idiopathic form predominant in the Washington University experience.

Substitution of One or More Incisions by an Alternative Ablation Technique

Perhaps the most interesting work in modification of the maze procedure has been done in this area in the last few years. Fortunately or unfortunately, most of these alterations have been performed in patients with concomitant valvular (principally mitral) heart disease.

Initially, several centers simply "added" the maze III procedure onto valve repair or replacement surgery, with excellent results.[7,17] In general, patients with concomitant disease were thought to be better candidates for the combined procedure if they were less than 70 years of age, had normal ventricular function, had had embolic events related to long-standing (greater than 1 year duration) fibrillation, were medically refractory and severely symptomatic, had a left atrial dimension greater than 60 mm, and finally, had an easily reparable valve lesion.

Over the past 5 years, Kosakai's group at Osaka have been much more aggressive in (1) modifying and simplifying the maze III technique and (2) applying it to patients with concomitant valvular disease, including patients with prior valve replacements.[28–30] Their recent report[29] consisted of data on 101 AF patients operated on electively by combining a modified maze III procedure with repair of valvular, congenital, and other anomalies; 24 patients underwent a repeat open-heart procedure. Operative mortality was 2%, postoperative sinus rhythm was present in 82%, junctional in 4%, and persistent AF in 14%. All of these recurrent AF patients had mitral valve disease; 73% of patients had a normal-sized transmitral A wave and 88% had a normal sized transtricuspid A wave detected postoperatively.

Their modification of the maze III procedure is shown in Figure 3, along side a similarly depicted maze III schematic. Extensive use of cryoablation is used to save intraoperative procedure time. The location of the incisions on the right side are different as well; in the modified procedure, none of the three (posterior, left, and right) sinus nodal arteries are incised. However, all three are cryoablated along their length at some point.

An additional report delineated delayed but ultimately sustained exercise capacity with restoration of sinus node response in a subset of these same patients.[30] Of the 25 patients studied postoperatively, 18 had valve surgery and seven had septal defects closed. Sinus conversion was obtained in 23 of 25 patients by 1 month after surgery. Sinoatrial response to exercise was attenuated by surgery up to 6 months postoperatively. Exercise capacity was improved in the late phase after surgery, and this improvement was related to the extent of restoration in the sinoatrial nodal response.

Thus, these studies document the highly successful surgical ablation of AF even in a population of patients with associated valvular heart disease, where the factors contributing to the genesis of the AF may be different that in idiopathic disease. Moreover, they demonstrate an overall improvement in exercise capacity in these patients that is largely dependent on the recovery of the sinus node response to exercise, further documenting the importance of restoration of sinus rhythm if safe and feasible.

These studies raise additional interesting questions, however, about the assessment of results following ablative procedures for AF. In the setting of idiopathic disease, complete cure of the arrhythmia was the "gold standard" that the operation (the maze III)

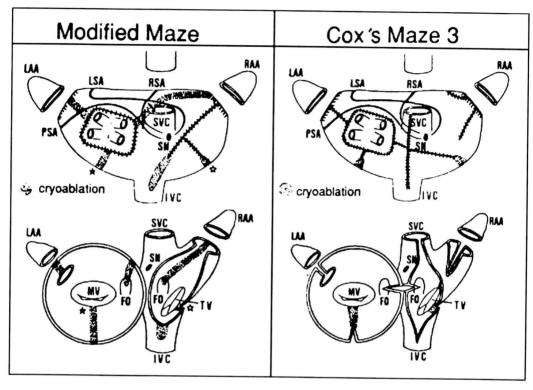

Figure 3. Surgical techniques. Atriotomies (solid line with cross bars) and cryoablation (dotted area) with variations of sinus node artery for the current modification **(left)** and the maze III **(right). Top:** posterior views of the cardiac base. **Bottom:** endocardial views of the atria. Areas of cryoablation at valvular annuli were close to the circumflex artery (closed asterisk) and the right coronary artery (open asterisk). LAA = left atrial appendage; RAA = right atrial appendage; SN = sinus node; LSA = left sinus node artery; RSA = right sinus node artery; PSA = posterior sinus node artery; SVC = superior vena cava; IVC inferior vena cava; MV = mitral valve; TV = tricuspid valve; FO = fossa ovalis. Used with permission Kosakai Y, et al.[29]

was effectively designed to achieve. In the setting of concomitant mitral valve disease, particularly of rheumatic origin, it is unclear at this point if these (or any) modifications of the maze technique can be as effective as an arrhythmia-ablative procedure as the maze III procedure itself. In this more complex patient population, however, if the antiarrhythmic portion of the procedure is only 80% successful is that a "failure?" Alternatively, it is unclear that now with these therapies available and well-tested it is justified to accept the presence of preoperative AF postoperatively in order to minimize overall operative mortality and morbidity in this setting of combined procedures for mitral valve disease. Further complicating this dilemma is the fact that a significant

number of patients with rheumatic mitral disease have impaired ventricular function at the time of surgery. From a functional point of view, it is precisely this group of patients in whom restoration of sinus rhythm and atrial transport would be expected to be of greatest benefit.[10] Similar arguments apply to prospective or prophylactic maze procedure(s) in other cardiac disease states.[31,32]

Pharmacological and/or Neuropharmacological Ablation Mechanisms Plus Surgery

Zipes et al, in a recently published series of epicardial fat pad ablations in dogs, were able to eliminate AF by altering the innervation pattern to the atrial tissue.[33] These data show, as have data from Boineau and Schuessler,[34,35] that a combination of surgical or ablative therapy and innervation ablation might result in a simplified procedure that would be equally effective in selected patients as the maze III.

Conclusions

The maze III procedure continues to be the "gold standard" of therapy for elimination of AF and restoration of normal sinus rhythm, and is the standard against all other less invasive or modified therapies should be judged. It is legitimate to question whether there may be differences electrophysiologically and anatomically between idiopathic AF and fibrillation associated with left-sided valvular disease. The continued development and evaluation of techniques based on the anatomic and electrophysiological components of this arrhythmia will challenge investigators for a number of years to come.

References

1. Barbier P, Alioto G, Buazzi MD. Left atrial and ventricular filling in hypertensive patients with paroxysmal atrial fibrillation. J Am Coll Cardiol 1994;24:165–170.
2. Ortiz J, Niwano S, Abe H, Rudy Y, et al. Mapping the conversion of atrial flutter to atrial fibrillation and atrial fibrillation to atrial flutter. Circulation Res 1994;74:882–894.
3. Peterson P, Kastrup J, Brinch K, et al. Relation between left atrial diameters and duration of atrial fibrillation. Am J Cardiol 1987;60:382–384.
4. Cox JL, Boineau JP, Schuessler RB, et al. Electrophysiologic basis, surgical development and clinical results of the Maze procedure for atrial flutter and fibrillation. In Karp RB, Wechsler AS, eds. Advances in Cardiac Surgery. Vol 6. Mosby-Year Book Inc. St. Louis, 1995, pp 1–67.
5. Ferguson TB Jr. Surgical approach to atrial flutter and fibrillation. In Singer I, ed. Interventional Electrophysiology. Williams and Wilkins, Baltimore, 1997.
6. Cox JL, Boineau JP, Schuessler RB, et al. Five year experience with the maze procedure for atrial fibrillation. Ann Thorac Surg 1993;56:814–824.
7. Cox JL, Boineau JP, Schuessler RB, et al. Modification of the Maze procedure for atrial flutter and atrial fibrillation. I. Rationale and surgical results. J Thorac Cardiovasc Surg 1995;110:473–484.
8. Cox JL, Boineau JP, Schuessler RB, et al. Modification of the Maze procedure for atrial flutter and atrial fibrillation. II. Surgical technique of the maze III procedure. J Thorac Cardiovasc Surg 1995;110:485–495.
9. Ferguson TB Jr, Kater KM, Boineau JP, et al. The requirement for permanent pacemaker therapy following the Maze procedure for atrial fibrillation: incidence and therapeutic indications. PACE 1994;17:862A.
10. Ferguson TB Jr. The future of arrhythmia surgery. J Cardiovasc Electrophysiol 1994;5:621–634.
11. Cox JL. The maze III procedure for treatment of atrial fibrillation. In Sabiston DC, cd. Atlas of Cardiothoracic Surgery. W.B. Saunders Inc., Philadelphia, 1995, pp 460–475.
12. Ferguson TB Jr, Cox JL. Surgical Treatment of Arrhythmias. In Edmunds FH, ed. Cardiac Surgery. 1996.
13. Ferguson TB Jr, Schuessler RB, Hand DE, et al. Lessons learned from computerized mapping of the atrium. J Electrophysiol 1993;26:210–219.
14. Guiraudon GM, Campbell CS, Jones DL, et al. Combined sino-atrial node atrio-ventricular isolation: a surgical alternative to His bundle ablation in patients with atrial fibrillation. Circulation 1985;72:220A.
15. Defauw JJ, Guiraudon GM, van Hemel NM, et al. Surgical therapy of paroxysmal atrial fibrillation with the "corridor" operation. Ann Thorac Surg 1992;53:564–571.
16. Williams JM, Ungerleider RM, Lofland GK, et al. Left atrial isolation: new technique for the treatment of supraventricular arrhythmias. J Thorac Cardiovasc Surg 1980;80:373–380.
17. McCarthy PM, Castle LW, Maloney JD, et al. Initial experience with the maze procedure for atrial fibrillation. J Thorac Cardiovasc Surg 1993;105:1077–1087.
18. Utley JR, Leyland SA, Nguyenduy T. Comparisons of outcomes with three atrial incisions for mitral valve operations: Right lateral, superior septal and transeptal. J Thorac Cardiovasc Surg 1995;109:582–587.

19. Barner HB. 1992 update (1985: combined superior and right lateral left atriotomy with division of the superior vena cava for exposure to the mitral valve). Ann Thorac Surg 1992;54:594.

20. McGrath LB, Levett JM, Gonzalez-Levin L. Safety of the right atrial approach for combined mitral and tricuspid valve procedures. J Thorac Cardiovasc Surg 1988;96:756–759.

21. Graffigna A, Pagani F, Minzioni G. Left atrial isolation associated with mitral valve operations. Ann Thorac Surg 1992;54:1093–1098.

22. Brodman RF, Frame R, Fisher JD, et al. Combined treatment of mitral stenosis and atrial fibrillation with valvuloplasty and a left atrial maze procedure. J Thorac Cardiovasc Surg 1994;107:622.

23. Hioki M, Ikeshita M, Iedokoro Y, et al. Successful combined operation for mitral stenosis and atrial fibrillation. Ann Thorac Surg 1993;55:776–778.

24. Cox JL. Surgical treatment of atrial fibrillation. J Thorac Cardiovasc Surg 1992;104:1492–1494.

25. Cox JL. Combined treatment of mitral stenosis and atrial fibrillation with valvuloplasty and a left atrial maze procedure. J Thorac Cardiovasc Surg 1994;107:622–624.

26. Sueda T, Nagata H, Shikata H, et al. Simple left atrial procedure for chronic atrial fibrillation associated with mitral valve disease. Ann Thorac Surg 1996;62:1796–1800.

27. Harada A, Sasaki K, Fukushima T, et al. Atrial activation during chronic atrial fibrillation in patients with isolated mitral valve disease. Ann Thorac Surg 1996;61:104–112.

28. Kosakai Y, Kawaguchi AT, Isobe F, et al. Cox maze procedure for chronic atrial fibrillation associated with mitral valve disease. J Thorac Cardiovasc Surg 1994;108:1049–1055.

29. Kosakai Y, Kawaguchi AT, Isobe F, et al. Modified Maze procedure for patients with atrial fibrillation undergoing simultaneous open heart surgery. Circulation 1995; 92(Suppl II):II-359–II-364.

30. Tamai J, Kosakai Y, Yoshioka T, et al. Delayed improvement in exercise capacity with restoration of sinoatrial node response in patients after combined treatment with surgical repair for organic heart disease and the Maze procedure for atrial fibrillation. Circulation 1995;91:2392–2399.

31. Bonchek LI, Burlingame MW, Worley SJ, et al. Cox/maze procedure for atrial septal defect with atrial fibrillation: Management strategies. Ann Thorac Surg 1993;55:607–610.

32. Cox JL. Evolving applications of the maze procedure for atrial fibrillation. Ann Thorac Surg 1993;55:578–580.

33. Randall WC, Ardell JL. Nervous control of the heart: anatomy and pathophysiology. In Zipes DP, Jalife J. eds. Cardiac Electrophysiology: From Cell to Bedside. W.B. Saunders and Co., Philadelphia, 1990, pp 291–299.

34. Schuessler RB, Grayson TM, Bromberg BI, et al. Cholinergically mediated tachyarrhythmias induced by a single extrastimulus in the isolated canine right atrium. Circ Res 1992;71:1254–1267.

35. Schuessler RB, Kawamoto T, Hand DE, et al. Simultaneous epicardial and endocardial activation sequence mapping in the isolated canine right atrium. Circulation 1993;88:250–263.

Chapter 31

Surgical Treatment of Ventricular Tachycardias

Gerard M. Guiraudon, George J. Klein, Raymond Yee, Donald Switzer

Introduction

Surgery for ventricular tachycardias (VTs) developed in the mid-1970s. The first surgical attempts were aimed at VTs not associated with coronary artery disease.[1–3] Shortly thereafter, VTs associated with coronary artery disease (left ventricular LV aneurysm) were approached,[4,5] after simple aneurysmectomy was proved ineffective.[6]

Despite its success, surgery for ventricular arrhythmias never reached maturity. A very minute segment of a huge patients' population was operated on, even in the golden years of electrophysiological surgical intervention. The reasons for the poor showing were twofold: (1) surgery for VTs is associated with significant risk because of associated LV dysfunction, and (2) patients with severe LV dysfunction are more susceptible to malignant VT. On the other hand, surgical therapy is associated with an excessive risk in this patient subgroup.[7] In other words, surgery is denied because of excessive risk to patients who need it the most. Patients with good LV function have a low risk of arrhythmia death, but also have low risk (and low benefit) surgery. Consequently, surgery is often carried out on low- risk patients, who are the ones who benefit less from arrhythmia control.

During the same period, other electrophysiological interventions were developing: the implantable cardioverter-defibrillator (ICD),[8–10] catheter ablation,[11–13] and new antiarrhythmic drugs. These less invasive interventions proved effective with minimal morbidity and mortality.

Surgery for VT has made two major contributions: (1) it documented that VT can be permanently suppressed by ablating a critical segment of the reentrant circuit, the location of which can be determined by intraoperative mapping, and (2) intraoperative mapping contributed greatly to the understanding of mechanism and critical segment of myocardium (arrhythmogenic anatomic substrate).

Surgical rationale for VT is based on mechanism, pathophysiology, definition of target (arrhythmogenic anatomic substrate), mapping (localization of substrate), and surgical techniques.

Arrhythmogenic Anatomic Substrate

The *concept* of arrhythmogenic anatomic substrate was developed at the beginning

From Singer I, Barold SS, Camm AJ (eds): Nonpharmacological Therapy of Arrhythmias for the 21st Century: The State of the Art. Futura Publishing Co., Inc., Armonk, NY, © 1998.

of surgery for ventricular arrhythmia.[1–3,14] This concept was derived from the pathophysiology of the Wolff-Parkinson-White syndrome, where the accessory atrioventricular (AV) pathway is the obligatory segment that loops the loop of the reentry circuit.

The *definition* of the arrhythmogenic anatomic substrate can be formulated as follows: the arrhythmogenic anatomic substrate is a segment of ventricular myocardium, the presence of which is necessary but insufficient for the tachycardia to initiate and sustain. This capsule definition requires further elaboration. Ventricular tachycardia may include not only the observed VT morphologies, but also the tachycardias that can occur after suppression of the observed (clinical) tachycardias. One tachycardia morphology may use as "the necessary link" more than one myocardial segment. A patient may have undocumented VT morphologies. The definition of the arrhythmogenic substrate can be either restrictive or comprehensive. According to the latter concept, all actually arrhythmogenic and potentially arrhythmogenic substrates are incorporated into the "expanded substrate" definition.

Pathology of the Arrhythmogenic Anatomic Substrate

The "necessary link" is very rarely anatomically delineated (as a bundle) but is usually functionally defined.[15] The link may have complex morphology, with ramifications associated with either dead-end pathways, or multiple vicarious pathways. These so-called "necessary links" associated with slow conduction are found mostly in pathological myocardium which exhibits a nonhomogenous structure with excess of fibrosis or other connective tissue and a disarray of myocardial cells and/or bundles. The anatomy of the substrate can be viewed at the micro- and macro-levels. At the micro-level, the anatomic substrate appear complex and small. At the macro-level, two major considerations can be made: (1) the slow conduction pathway appears unique and has the form of a simple channel (figure-of-eight model[15–18]), and (2) the greater the mass of pathological tissue, the greater the arrhythmogenicity.[19] This is particularly true for the infarct scar and for arrhythmogenic right ventricular dysplasia.

Time Dependency

Arrhythmogenicity varies over time. The pathology can be progressive and/or is modified by other factors. These other factors, which are included into the nonsufficient characteristics, may involve the rest of the ventricles, the autonomic nervous system, the blood supply (coronary artery disease), and other factors. These other factors can be actually major determinants in setting the condition for arrhythmias to initiate and/or sustain. Arrhythmogenicity, in other words, is not confined to the substrate as defined above.[20,21]

Identification and Localization of the Substrate

Identification and localization of the substrate can be achieved by using either electrophysiological testing and/or anatomic landmarks.

Electrophysiological Testing

Preoperative electrophysiological studies can provide two important clues: (1) the endocardial site of the earliest activation of the QRS during VT,[3] and (2) diastolic potentials, which may be in close proximity to the origin of QRS activation during VT.[3,22] If these potentials are chronologically or sequentially dependent, they may represent the electrical activation of the slow conducting segment (arrhythmogenic anatomic substrate) of the reentry loop.[23,24]

Intraoperative Cardiac Mapping

The actual technique of cardiac mapping is described later. Cardiac mapping provides three critical guides to help localize the anatomic substrate: (1) the site of origin or the earliest site of ventricular activation during VT can be localized to the epicardial, endocardial, or intramural structures; (2) the endocardial area where abnormal diastolic activation is recorded (delayed potential, fractionation, etc.); and (3) the actual reentrant activation can be recorded in its entirety as well as the actual site of the slowly conduction segment.

Cardiac mapping, except in rare cases, does not delineate the arrhythmogenic substrate. It is assumed that the earliest activation during VT is near the exit of the slow conduction pathway.[1–3,5,25] Consequently, the entire area surrounding the site within a radius of 2.5 to 3.0 cm is deemed arrhythmogenic and qualifies as arrhythmogenic substrate.[3] Even when the actual circuit is delineated, clinical experience showed that a larger area than the current slow conducting segment should be described as the arrhythmogenic anatomic substrate for improved outcomes.[26] Mapping during sinus rhythm is associated with similar limitations. Areas where no abnormal electrical activation are recorded cannot be ruled out as being nonarrhythmogenic because of inherent limitations of the technique. To conclude, cardiac mapping is a help more than a guide to delineate the arrhythmogenic anatomic substrate in the operating room setting.

Anatomic Landmarks

Morphological boundaries have been developed based on the associated pathology. Electrophysiological testing and intraoperative cardiac mapping have greatly contributed to our understanding of the pathology. It has been established that the arrhythmogenic anatomic substrate is localized within the pathological tissue or at the transitional area between normal and abnormal myocardial tissues when the pathology is discrete. Endocardial fibrosis and the subjacent myocardial layer are the most common site of the arrhythmogenic anatomic substrate for VTs associated with an infarct scar.[4,5] Anatomic landmarks are very reliable when the pathology is discrete and nonprogressive. Anatomic landmarks are either absent and/or nonreliable when pathology is diffuse, poorly demarcated, and/or progressive.

The *target* for surgery and other electrophysiological interventions is the arrhythmogenic anatomic substrate. This simply defined goal matches well the clear and simple definition of the substrate, but requires further elaboration to be operative. The above considerations about the arrhythmogenic substrate showed that the delineation of the substrate is "operator-dependent" and is influenced by the following factors:

1. Is the aim of surgery to suppress current and future arrhythmias? The latter goal implies that all potentially arrhythmogenic areas of myocardium are included within the substrate.
2. The bullet/target principle: instead of matching the "bullet" (therapy) with the "target" (arrhythmogenic substrate), interventionists have a strong tendency to do the opposite, i.e., to match the target with the bullet for various reasons. The best example of this might be illustrated by the example of radiofrequency catheter ablation. Because radiofrequency energy, when delivered via an intravascular catheter, can produce only discrete, small lesions, interventionists are looking for discrete small targets as the actual small myocardial bundle which is the site of the necessary slow conduction link. These small discrete targets are not always detectable.

Furthermore, their neutralization may not interrupt the tachycardia and their long-term results are uncertain.[27]

3. The "size" factor is illustrated by two correlated pieces of evidence: the greater the mass of abnormal myocardial tissue, the greater the chance that arrhythmia will recur.[19] The larger the area of arrhythmogenic tissue neutralized, the greater the chances of permanently suppressing the arrhythmia.

4. Preservation of LV function is the most dramatic limiting factor to extensive neutralization of arrhythmogenic myocardium. Surgical technique is therefore a compromise between extensive neutralization of arrhythmogenic myocardium and preservation of ventricular function. Failure to suppress arrhythmia may not be associated with failure of technique, but with inability to carry it out because of unacceptable impact on function, i.e., critical locations, involvement of valvular structures, and other considerations.[28]

5. It is critical to determine before the planned surgery what the anticipated results and acceptable limitations and shortfalls of the surgical intervention are in order to assess the potential for good surgical outcome.[29]

Cardiac mapping, anatomic landmarks, and cardiac function and anatomy are therefore used to delineate and select the target (arrhythmogenic anatomic substrate) and to formulate a surgical plan. This last consideration explains the ongoing controversy about the role and value of cardiac mapping for VT.

Intraoperative Cardiac Mapping

Cardiac mapping is a technique used to record electrical activity of the heart and to display the timing and sequence of activation spatially in an integrated manner.[30] The site of recording may be epicardial, endocardial, or intramural. The recording mode may be unipolar or bipolar, or both. The method of display involves activation time (isochronic map), potential amplitude (isopotential map), or potential morphology (postexcitation or fractionation map). Maps are obtained during sinus rhythm or induced ventricular arrhythmia.

A critical issue is the way the recordings are obtained from the various cardiac sites. A hand-held roving probe can be used. However, point-by-point technique is feasible only if the cardiac activation is stable and each QRS complex is identical to the preceding complex during the exploration. The hand-held probe must be moved from one site to the other after a sufficient number of complexes have been recorded at each site. The technique is appropriate for mapping during sinus rhythm or sustained monomorphic VT.

Multi-electrode systems allow simultaneous recording of a large number of sites.[31-33] The epicardial electrodes may be affixed on a mesh that encompasses the heart like a sock. An endocardial electrode array can be attached on an inflatable balloon introduced into the left ventricle via a left ventriculotomy, the aortic root,[33] or the left atrium. Epicardial and endocardial mapping can be carried out simultaneously. Computerized mapping is of particular interest when the VT is poorly tolerated, and when the tachycardia is nonsustained, polymorphic, or has multiple morphologies. Normothermic cardiopulmonary bypass cardiac assist is used whenever necessary.

Cardiac mapping identifies critical sites: (1) The site of "origin" of the tachycardia, or the site of the earliest activation of the QRS complex during VT. The onset of the QRS as well the activation time at various sites can be difficult to determine. (2) The areas where "abnormal" electrical activity is recorded: arrhythmogenic areas. These areas can be endocardial or epicardial. (3)

In a few patients, the actual macroreentrant circuit can be identified.

Most of the online information is crude and can be misleading even after it is corroborated by thermal mapping or pacemapping. The reliability of the information depends on the site of recording (RV free wall, septum, LV free wall), associated structural disease, and preoperative endocardial mapping. Cardiac mapping allows spatial correlation of the site of the tachycardia(s) and the arrhythmogenic area(s) with a segment of the anatomic lesions. However, that does not imply that the rest of the lesion is not potentially arrhythmogenic.

Intraoperative mapping has proved to be a valuable source of information for research. Its role in the operating room to give instantaneous guidance to the surgical technique is less than adequate for several reasons. Cardiac mapping is not feasible in all patients (between 15% and 50%) and when feasible is frequently incomplete.[34,35] Promoters of intraoperative mapping explain surgical failure to control the arrhythmia by incomplete or misleading mapping.[36] Others did not observe any improvement in arrhythmia control after starting to use a better sophisticated mapping system.[37] Rokkas et al. reported a new way to map VT using multiplexed electrodes with epicardial sock and/or endocardial balloon using potential distribution mapping which be available to the surgical team almost online.[38] They suggest that better results are associated with extensive comprehensive mapping when multiple tachycardia morphologies associated with multiple sites of origin are identified, and extensive ablation of arrhythmogenic scar is performed accordingly.[39] This supports the tenet: "the more ablation the better." All potentially arrhythmogenic tissues should be ablated as long as it is done without damaging normal myocardium, whatever the results of cardiac mapping suggest. This concept has been successfully used at our institution[35–40] and many others.[41,42] This approach is used successfully when mapping is not feasible or deemed incomplete.[43–46]

Surgical and Preoperative Plan

Surgical indication is only considered after thorough assessment of the patient, including cardiac anatomy and function, and extensive electrophysiological studies to estimate the location and size of the arrhythmogenic substrate. Patient co-morbidity is taken into account. Surgical technique is indicated when it brings very significant advantages compared to other electrophysiological interventions, i.e., ICD implant, catheter ablation, or antiarrhythmic drugs. Surgical indication should comply with the *no/no* principle to be acceptable: no failure/ no complication. In other words, surgery must be expected to suppress the VT with minimum associated morbidity.

An operative plan should be carefully designed before surgery. This plan is to be followed if intraoperative mapping is not feasible for whatever reason. The plan is modified only when very strong counter-evidence is obtained intraoperatively, either pertaining to cardiac pathology and/or the results of intraoperative cardiac mapping. Surgical rationale is a compromise between the preservation of the cardiac function and the neutralization of the current and/or potentially arrhythmogenic lesions. It is based on two surgical concepts: *exclusion and ablation.* The concept of exclusion is aimed at confining the arrhythmogenic mechanism from involving the rest of the heart and producing ventricular arrhythmia.[4] The best model of exclusion is the right ventricular free wall disconnection.[47] The concept of ablation is aimed at neutralizing the arrhythmogenic lesion(s).[1–3,5] There are a large number of ablative techniques available to accomplish this goal: transmural resection, endocardial resection, ventriculotomy, cryoablation, and laser photocoagulation.

Surgical rationales can be implemented using various "tools," including the scalpel, cryoablation, laser, and caustic chemicals such as lugol solution. The choice of the tool is based on the assessment of its specific advantages and disadvantages. Cryosurgery and laser photocoagulation produce a well-demarcated mass of neutralized tissue that does not require further surgical intervention and does not impair normal surrounding myocardium. Cryosurgery is enhanced by concomitant cold cardioplegic cardiac arrest, whereas laser photocoagulation can be used on the normothermic beating heart.

Ventricular Tachycardias Associated with Coronary Artery Disease

Ventricular arrhythmias associated with coronary artery disease are the leading cause of death in North America.[48] Exten-sive coronary artery disease is the most prevalent finding in patients with sudden cardiac death.

The infarct scar is the site of the arrhyth-mogenic substrate, in most patients. The infarct scar (LV aneurysm or discrete segmental wall motion abnormality) develops in the chronic phase after acute myocardial infarction.[49] Typically it comprises a central fibrotic zone that is thin walled and was formerly the site of transmural necrosis (Figure 1). The central fibrotic zone is circumscribed by a border made of a fibrotic tissue and normal or abnormal myocardial cells in dis-array (Figure 2). Ischemic lesions are lo-cated in the subendocardium. Endocardial

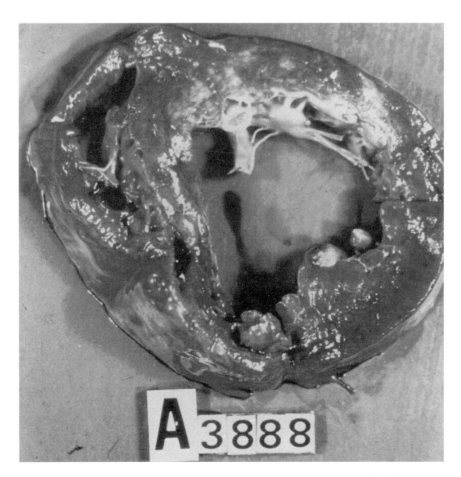

Figure 1. Coronary artery disease. LV infarct scar at the macroscopic level. There is a small scar over the septum and the inferior wall with mild LV dilation and low arrhythmogenicity.

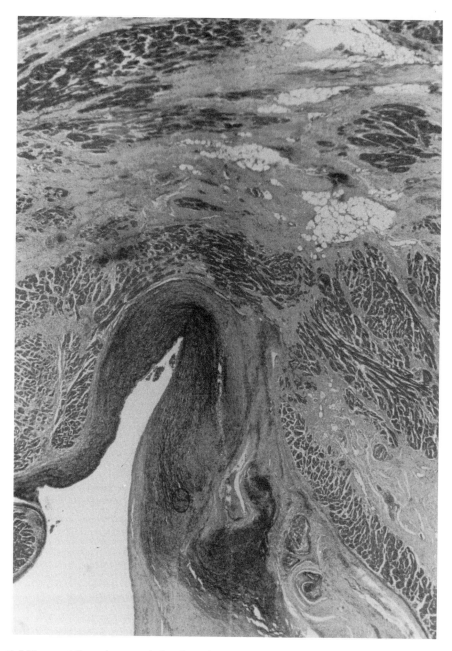

Figure 2. LV scar at the microscopic level: endocardial segment of the border zone. The endocardial fibrosis is manifest. There are many myocardial "bundles" isolated by fibrotic or fatty tissue. Each bundle is a potential arrhythmogenic substrate.

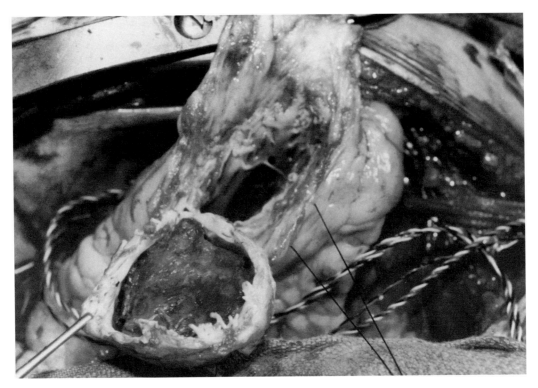

Figure 3. Operative view of a LV aneurysm. There was a discrete aneurysm with extensive clot which has been resected en bloc with a clear limit. Cryoablation was used to complete ablation of arrhythmogenic tissue. Patient was free of arrhythmia for 15 years.

fibrosis develops opposite the subendocardial ischemic myocardium and is a reliable anatomic landmark to delineate the extent of the infarct scar (Figure 3). However, the infarct scar is rarely consistent with the preceding description. The necrosis may not be transmural, the scar may not be discrete, and the endocardial fibrosis may not be manifest. An associated ischemic cardiomyopathy usually masks discrete limits of an infarct scar. Large patches of chronic ischemic lesions may be present at a distance from the infarct scar and be arrhythmogenic, making identification and ablation of such area difficult.

Prognosis of VTs associated with coronary artery disease is essentially determined by the extent of LV dysfunction. Left ventricular ejection fraction is the most powerful independent marker of risk for subsequent sudden death.[7]

Surgical Techniques

Encircling Endocardial Ventriculotomy

Because of the poor results associated with LV aneurysmectomy (Figure 3), even after epicardial mapping, we developed the first direct surgical approach for VT: encircling endocardial ventriculotomy.[4] The first patient was operated on November 12, 1975. In 1981, we reported our experience with 29 patients who underwent an encircling endocardial ventriculotomy for sustained recurrent VT after myocardial infarction.[50] The results of the initial clinical experience documented that the surgical rationale based on the electrophysiological concept was effective. However, further experience based on experimental studies[51] and clinical studies[52] suggested that the extensive ventriculotomy was associated with

LV dysfunction. Consequently, Ostermeyer et al. modified the surgical technique while keeping the same rationale: they described a partial endocardial encircling incision guided by intraoperative endocardial mapping with excellent short- and long-term results.[53]

Encircling Endocardial Cryoablation

Based on the same concept as the encircling endocardial ventriculotomy,[40] encircling endocardial cryoablation is designed to "neutralize" as much noncontractile, potentially arrhythmogenic tissue, without impairing the normally contracting surrounding myocardium. Cryosurgery was first used in cardiac surgery for His bundle ablation[54] and subsequently applied to the treatment of VTs.[55] Cryosurgical lesions are discrete and sharply demarcated from adjacent tissue. They are homogeneous and nonarrhythmogenic.[56] Cryoablation induces necrosis of myocardial fibers but spares the collagenous framework. The chronic scar is made of dense fibrotic tissue, which has no tendency to rupture or dilate.

We reported our experience with 33 patients.[40] At surgery the entire visible scar was cryoablated using large cryoprobes (1.5 cm, $-60°C$ during 2 min) applied endocardially and epicardially when deemed necessary. Intraoperative mapping was informative in 14 patients. The preoperative plan was modified based on intraoperative mapping evidences in two patients.

Thirty-two patients were discharged; one died postoperatively. Postoperative electrophysiological testing was associated with inducible VTs in two patients (one was discharged on amiodarone and the other had an ICD implanted via a left subdiaphragmatic approach).[57] The mean follow-up was 5 years. All patients free of arrhythmias at discharge remained arrhythmia- free. One patient on amiodarone required ICD implant after out-of-hospital cardiac arrest. A patient with an ICD had frequent episodes of tachycardia with frequent shock; requested the ICD to be deactivated and died 2 years after surgery. Nine patients had evidence of heart failure during follow-up; four died of cardiac failure and two had heart transplants. Three patients died of cancer. The actuarial survival at 5 years was 82% (Figure 4).

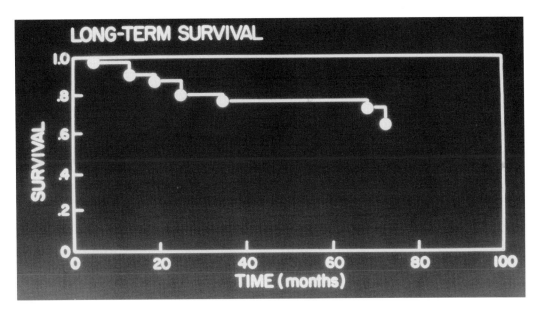

Figure 4. Five-year actuarial survival of 33 patients with encircling endocardial cryoablation.

Subendocardial Resection

Josephson et al. described subendocardial resection (SER).[5] This operation entailed pre- and/or intraoperative mapping of a tachycardia "site of origin" and then a limited endocardial excision of the surrounding arrhythmogenic area. The piece of tissue excised was approximately 5 cm². Approximately 70% of patients had no inducible tachycardia at postoperative electrophysiological study, and most of the remainder were rendered noninducible with the addition of antiarrhythmic medications that had been ineffective preoperatively. Ventricular function was well preserved after operation, and LV ejection fraction improved in some patients, presumably because of aneurysm resection.

Several important modifications of these procedures were subsequently described. The current technique[58] is carried out as follows: cardiopulmonary bypass is instituted at 37°C, and the left ventricle is vented through the left atrium. The ventricle is opened through the anterior or inferior scar or aneurysm. In 90% of cases, VT can be induced by programmed electrical stimulation and mapped. All tachycardias are mapped, whether or not they have appeared clinically. In patients with anterior wall aneurysms, subendocardial resection and adjunctive cryoablation are performed at 37°C with the heart beating. Ablation of the tachycardias is confirmed by repeat stimulation studies. Most of the endocardial scar is resected, but papillary muscles are spared. Concomitant coronary bypass grafts are constructed after the ventricle is closed, and cardioplegia is instilled. Because of more difficult exposure, cardioplegia is used for SER after completion of mapping for inferior wall tachycardias.

A total of 269 patients have been reported.[58] All had a previous myocardial infarction and sustained VT. Twenty percent presented with cardiac arrest, and 80% had palpitations, angina, or presyncope. Seventy-five percent had a LV aneurysm with a mean ejection fraction of 28%.

Ventricular tachycardias could not be induced postoperatively using programmed electrical stimulation in two-thirds of the patients. With antiarrhythmic drug therapy, more than 90% of patients were free of ventricular arrhythmias. Better control of arrhythmias was possible as more morphologies of ventricular arrhythmia were mapped at surgery. Forty patients died postoperatively (15%). An ejection fraction less than 20%, emergency operation, and history of prior heart surgery significantly increased operative mortality. Amiodarone did not affect operative outcome. Five-year actuarial survival was approximately 60%; heart failure was the most prominent cause of death.

Other Approaches

The ablative technique does not seem critical: excision, incision, cryoablation, and laser photocoagulation seem to accomplish similar goals and could be used selectively or in combination. Recently Moosdorf et al. documented that laser photocoagulation can be applied successfully epicardially on the closed beating heart.[59] If confirmed, these results can encourage epicardial laser ablation of VTs using minimally invasive techniques.

It should be noted that control of ventricular arrhythmia is only one side of the coin. The associated LV dysfunction remains the most common cause of death in all surgical series. The extent of impairment of the LV function is the most powerful independent variable of risk for sudden cardiac death. Determinants of LV function are multifactorial: new ischemic events, progression of coronary artery disease, and progression of cardiomyopathy are factors independent of surgical ablation and/or LV aneurysmectomy.

Patient Selection

Since the dramatic development of the ICD,[8] the role of surgical ablation has been

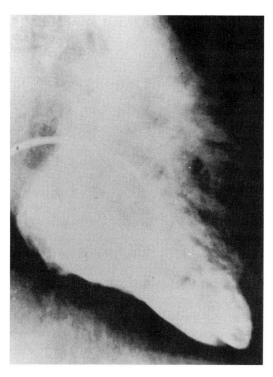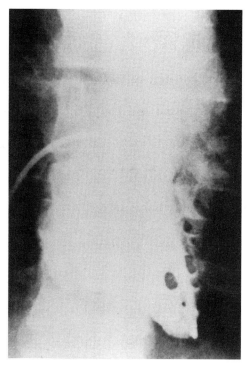

Figure 5. Right ventriculogram of a patient with arrhythmogenic right ventricular dysplasia. Right panel shows well the three areas of dilation (infundibulum, apex, and base). The left panel shows the septal trabeculations.

revisited without definite answers based on clinical trial. Because surgical ablation may provide the best long-term quality of life, surgery is still contemplated when feasible, with relatively low surgical risk. Patient selection has been emphasized as an important factor in minimizing surgical mortality by van Hemel et al.[60,61] Using the LV score system of the CASS study, they were able to operate on more than 100 patients without a mortality. Arrhythmia surgery can be safely carried out if three or more of the nine segments identified on the LAO and RAO views (Figure 5) are contracting normally. Other authors have successfully selected patients using similar methods.[44] This patient population with preserved LV function has a low surgical risk and good long-term survival, regardless of the surgical therapy.[61] Other criteria, as described by the Philadelphia group,[58] are valuable guides,

but strategies in EP intervention for VT are still essentially empirical.[62]

Surgical Technique

Surgical techniques are concerned mainly with two issues: (1) the value of intraoperative mapping, and (2) the best ablative techniques associated with minimal damage to the contracting myocardium.

The University of Pennsylvania series, using map-guided segmental endocardial resection with or without the adjunct of cryoablation, is a monumental series that has been a model and a great reference resource for many years. All series must be compared with that standard.[63,64]

Other groups used cryoablation[65] or laser photocoagulation.[66–68] Sequential ablation based on repeated sequential mapping has been advocated. Cardiac mapping has given some clue to unexplained failure associated with inferior LV aneurysm.[69] Unfortunately, there are no scientific grounds to compare these variant approaches validly.[70]

Prognostic markers for successful surgical ablation of arrhythmias are not well defined and vary from one series to the other. Monomorphic sustained VT of one of two morphologies associated with a discrete arrhythmogenic scar (aneurysm) are ideal indicators. The site of origin of the tachycardia and/or the location of the infarct scar are associated with inconsistent results. Septal origin is either reported to be difficult[46] or easy[43] to ablate. The inferior wall location is reported either a risk for failure[46] or not.[43] Amiodarone has been suggested as a risk factor. In a recent retrospective study, Mickleborough et al. reported that amiodarone was the only cause of death.[71] Although consistent with other experience, these results remained questionable because large surgical series using amiodarone preoperatively in large doses did not report any morbidity or mortality.[58,61]

Intraoperative Mapping

Intraoperative mapping has two roles: (1) as a guide for surgical ablation, and (2) as a research tool to retrospectively analyze surgical failures or explore pathophysiology of the scar. As a research tool, comprehensive intraoperative mapping has dramatically contributed to basic as well as applied science. For example, the identification of epicardial breakthrough in inferior scars,[69] or the understanding of activation of deep septal origins of the tachycardias,[32] or subendocardial arrhythmogenic pathways has been clarified by operative mapping techniques.[72]

It is an open question whether specific refinement in patient selection improves results of surgical ablation. All surgical series are cohort descriptive studies. However, a 5-year survival and freedom from arrhyth-

mia does not seem dramatically better than with other interventions. van Hemel et al. have recently published a randomized study comparing antiarrhythmic drug and surgical therapies.[73] They could not document any advantage to the surgical technique, which was associated with a higher risk of total cardiac death. Despite inherent limitations, this remarkable study by a well-experienced center shows that surgical ablation in a very selected patient population with preserved LV function is not the first choice, but an alternative option.

Our current approach is as follows: patients with ventricular arrhythmia associated with coronary artery disease must have complete assessment of cardiac functional anatomy and full electrophysiological assessment. When indicated, myocardial revascularization must be performed and has been documented to decrease arrhythmia death,[74] especially in patients with ischemia-induced arrhythmia.[75] In a small group of patients, concomitant ablation of ventricular arrhythmia can be carried out if it is associated with no additional risk and if it is also deemed highly effective. After successful revascularization, patients are reassessed and the appropriate nonsurgical EP intervention is selected. Surgical ablation of arrhythmia in patients who do not require CABG is indicated in very few patients.

Future developments are determined by the current philosophy in cardiac surgery, exemplified by minimally invasive ablation of AV accessory pathways. To paraphrase Lucan, the "medium is the message." The future is in a better delivery (medium), i.e., catheter techniques, minimally invasive approaches. Although surgical techniques are currently more successful because surgical ablation is extensive, future catheter techniques are likely to neutralize the arrhythmogenic target with minimal collateral damage.

Arrhythmogenic Right Ventricular Dysplasia

Although surgery for control of VT associated with arrhythmogenic right ventricu-

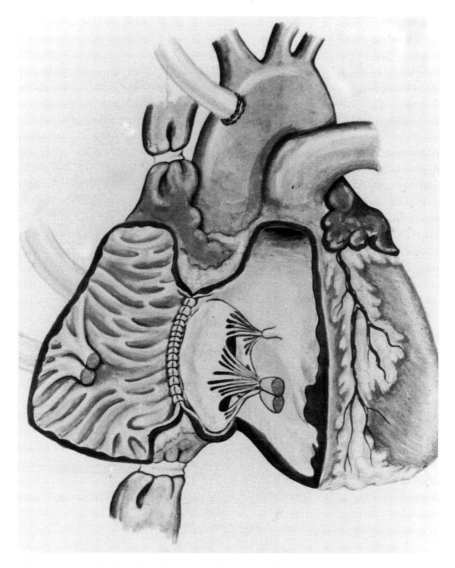

Figure 6. Schematic depiction of right ventricular free wall disconnection, which isolates the entire right free wall.

lar dysplasia has only involved a very small number of patients, it is still indicated today in a very select, small group of patients. The surgical experience with arrhythmogenic right ventricular dysplasia has made dramatic contributions to the understanding of VT mechanism and the associated substrate. The rationale for surgical "ablation" and/ or exclusion were initially developed for and applied to patients with arrhythmogenic right ventricular dysplasia.

Arrhythmogenic right ventricular dysplasia is a recently identified clinical entity.[76] The lesions involve essentially the right ventricular free wall and, to a lesser extent, the left ventricle. The right ventricular free wall is dilated and presents with large dome-shaped bulges over the infundibulum, apex, and basal portion of the inferior right ventricular wall. These bulging areas are akinetic or dyskinetic. The right ventricular trabeculation is increased in size and number. The subepicardial fat is abundant, and the myocardium is infiltrated or replaced by fat. This fatty infiltration gives the myocardium its characteristic appearance. Microscopic examination shows fatty infiltration and hypertrophy or degeneration of myocardial cells. Patchy subendocardial fibrosis may be present.

Clinical characteristics are now well recognized and identification of disease is easy. Surgery for arrhythmogenic right ventricular dysplasia has evolved over time. During the 1973–1981 period, we operated on 12 patients with problematic drug-resistant tachycardias.[3] A discrete ventriculotomy/resection at the site of epicardial breakthrough (origin) of ventricular activation during VT and/or at the site of late diastolic activation during sinus rhythm (arrhythmogenic area) were performed. There were no intraoperative complications. All patients were discharged free of tachycardia. During long-term follow-up (mean 36 months), five patients had recurrences. In two patients, tachycardias were not problematic and were not treated. Long-term recurrence of tachycardia was likely associated with the large amount of adipose right ventricular wall left intact. Consequently, the entire right ventricular wall was isolated after 1981. Since then we carried out a right ventricular free wall disconnection in 10 patients.[77,78] Surgical indication was based on failure of nonsurgical electrophysiological interventions. One patient died perioperatively of malignant hyperthermia. One pa-

tient had early recurrence of left VT. During long-term follow-up, three patients with a low LV ejection fraction preoperatively (0.44, 0.35, 0.30) died of congestive heart failure 5 months, 3 years, and 11 years postoperatively. The six other patients with good LV function had excellent control of arrhythmia with preserved cardiac function.[78]

Right ventricular free wall disconnection (Figure 6) for arrhythmogenic right ventricular dysplasia is feasible and associated with long-term good results in selected patients,[79,80] as corroborated by others' experience. Our experience suggests that patient selection is essentially based on LV function. A normal LV ejection fraction implies that the left ventricle is not involved in the pathological process and that good cardiac function can be anticipated postoperatively, as well as arrhythmia control.

Because right ventricular free wall disconnection is a major cardiac procedure, it should be confined to a small number of patients with preserved LV function after well-documented failure of nonsurgical electrophysiological interventions.

Conclusion

Surgical experience with VT not only contributed to the well-being of patients with no other efficient alternative therapies at that time, but also provided an irreplaceable wealth of data that has dramatically contributed to the knowledge and understanding of mechanisms and substrate of VT.

References

1. Guiraudon G, Frank R, Fontaine G. Interet des cartographies dans le traitement chirurgical des tachycardies ventriculaires rebelles recidivantes. Nouv Presse Med 1974;3:321.
2. Fontaine G, Guiraudon G, Frank R, et al. La cartographie epicardique et le traitement chirurgical par simple ventriculotomie de certaines tachycardies ventriculaires rebelles par reentree. Arch Mal Coeur 1975;68: 113–124.
3. Guiraudon G, Fontaine G, Frank R, et al. Sur-

gical treatment of ventricular tachycardia guided by ventricular mapping in 23 patients without coronary artery disease. Ann Thorac Surg 1981;32:439–450.
4. Guiraudon G, Fontaine G, Frank R, et al. Encircling endocardial ventriculotomy: a new surgical treatment for life-threatening ventricular tachycardias resistant to medical treatment following myocardial infarction. Ann Thorac Surg 1978;26:438–444.
5. Josephson ME, Harken AH, Horowitz LN.

Endocardial excision: a new surgical technique for the treatment of recurrent ventricular tachycardia. Circulation 1979;60:1430–1439.

6. Couch OA. Cardiac aneurysm with ventricular tachycardia and subsequent excision of aneurysm. Circulation 1959;20:251–253.

7. DiMarco JP, Haines DE. Sudden cardiac death. Curr Prob Cardiol 1990;15:185–232.

8. Mirowski M, Reid PR, et al. Termination of malignant ventricular arrhythmias with an implanted automatic defibrillator in human beings. N Engl J Med 1980;303:322–324.

9. Moss AJ, Hall WJ, Cannon DS, et al. for The Multicenter Automatic Defibrillator Implantation Trial Investigators. Improved Survival with an implanted defibrillator in patients with coronary disease at high risk for ventricular arrhythmia. N Engl J Med 1996;335:1933–1940.

10. The Antiarrhythmics Versus Implantable Defibrillators (AVID) Investigators. A comparison of antiarrhythmic-drug therapy with implantable defibrillators in patients resuscitated from near-fatal ventricular arrhythmias. N Engl J Med 1997;337:1576–1583.

11. Tchou P, Jazayeri M, Denker S, et al. Transcatheter electrical ablation of right bundle branch: a method of treating macroreentrant ventricular tachycardia attributed to bundle branch reentry. Circulation 1988;78:246–257.

12. Okumura K, Olshansky B, Henthorn RW, et al. Demonstration of the presence of slow conduction during sustained ventricular tachycardia in man: use of transient entrainment of the tachycardia. Circulation 1987;75:369–378.

13. Budde T, Breithardt G, Borggrefe M. Catheter ablation for ventricular tachycardia. In Saksena S, Goldschlager N, eds. Electrical Therapy For Cardiac Arrhythmias: Pacing Antitachycardia Devices, Catheter Ablation. W.B. Saunders Co., Philadelphia, 1990, pp 651–663.

14. Morady F, Frank R, Kou WH, et al. Identification and catheter ablation of a zone of slow conduction in the reentrant circuit of ventricular tachycardia in humans. J Am Coll Cardiol 1988;11:775–782.

15. Klein GJ, Ideker RE, Smith WM, et al. Epicardial mapping of the onset of ventricular tachycardia initiated by programmed stimulation in the canine heart with chronic infarction. Circulation 1979;60:1375–1384.

16. de Bakker JMT, Janse MJ, van Capelle FJL, et al. Endocardial mapping by simultaneous recording of endocardial electrograms during cardiac surgery for ventricular aneurysm. J Am Coll Cardiol 1983;2:947–953.

17. Tyagi S, Sharma A, Guiraudon G, et al. Intra-

operative cardiac mapping of preexcitation syndromes and ventricular tachycardia. J Electrophysiol 1989;3(1):47–64.

18. El Sherif N, Mehra R, Gough WB, et al. Ventricular activation pattern of spontaneous and induced ventricular rhythms in canine one-day-old myocardial infarction: evidence for focal and reentrant mechanisms. Circ Res 1982;51:152–166.

19. Blanchard SM, Walcott GP, Wharton JM, et al. Why is catheter ablation less successful than surgery for treating ventricular tachycardia that results from coronary artery disease? PACE 1994;17(Pt I):2315–2335.

20. Schwartz PJ, La Rovere MT, Vanoli E. Autonomic nervous system and sudden cardiac death: experimental basis and clinical observation for post-myocardial infarction risk stratification. Circulation 1992;85(Suppl I):1–77.

21. Coumel P. Cardiac arrhythmias and the autonomic nervous system. J Cardiovasc Electrophysiol 1993;4(3):338.

22. Klein H, Karp RB, Kouchoukos NT, et al. Intraoperative electrophysiologic mapping of the ventricles during sinus rhythm in patients with a previous myocardial infarction. Circulation 1982;66:847–853.

23. Brugada P, Hoshiar, Abdollah H, et al. Continuous electrical activity during sustained monomorphic ventricular tachycardia: observations on its dynamic behavior during the arrhythmia. Am J Cardiol 1985;55:402–411.

24. Waldo AL, Henthorn RW. Use of transient entrainment during ventricular tachycardia to localize a critical area in the reentry circuit for ablation. PACE 1989;12:231–244.

25. Stevenson WG, Hassan H, Sager P, et al. Targeting endocardial sites for catheter ablation of ventricular tachycardia after myocardial infarction. Circulation 1992;86:I–519.

26. Miller JM, Ratcliffe MB, Josephson ME, et al. Response to focal pressure at site of origin of ventricular tachycardia predicts surgical result. Circulation 1992;86:570.

27. Gürsit S, Schlüter M, Chiladakis I, et al. Radiofrequency current ablation of ventricular tachycardia at the area of slow conduction. Circulation 1992;86:I–520.

28. Miller JM, Kienzle MG, Harken AH, et al. Subendocardial resection for ventricular tachycardia: predictors of surgical success. Circulation 1984;70:624–631.

29. Spiker B. Guide To Clinical Trials. Lippincott-Raven, New York, 1996.

30. Gallagher JJ, Kasell JH, Cox JL, et al. Techniques of intraoperative electrophysiologic mapping. Am J Cardiol 1982;49:221–240.

31. Downer E, Parson ID, Mickleborough LL, et

al. On-line epicardial mapping of intraoperative ventricular arrhythmias: initial clinical experience. J Am Coll Cardiol 1984;4: 703–714.

32. Kawamura Y, Page PL, Cardinal R, et al. Mapping of septal ventricular tachycardia: clinical and experimental correlations. J Thorac Cardiovasc Surg 1996;112:914–925.

33. Vermeulen FEE, van Hemel NM, Guiraudon GM, et al. Cryosurgery for ventricular bigeminy using a transaortic closed ventricular approach. Eur Heart J 1988;9:979–990.

34. Page PL, Cardinal R, Shenasa M, et al. Surgical treatment of ventricular tachycardia: regional cryoablation guided by computerized epicardial and endocardial mapping. Circulation 1989;80:1124–1134.

35. Thakur RK, Guiraudon GM, Klein GJ, et al. Intraoperative mapping is not necessary for VT surgery. PACE 1994;17(Pt II):2156–2162.

36. Kron IL, Lerman BB, DiMarco JP. Extended subendocardial resection: a surgical approach to ventricular tachyarrhythmias that cannot be mapped intraoperatively. J Thorac Cardiovasc Surg 1984;90:586–591.

37. Lawrie GM, Pacifico A, Kaushik R, et al. Factors predictive of results of direct ablative operations for drug-refractory ventricular tachycardia: analysis of 80 patients. J Thorac Cardiovasc Surg 1991;101:44–45.

38. Rokkas CK, Nitta T, Schuessler RB, et al. Human ventricular tachycardia: precise intraoperative localization with potential distribution mapping. Ann Thorac Surg 1994; 57:1628–1635.

39. Miller JM, Gottlieb CD, Marchlinski FE, et al. Does ventricular tachycardia mapping influence the success of antiarrhythmic surgery? J Am Coll Cardiol 1988;11:112A.

40. Guiraudon GM, Thakur RK, Klein GJ, et al. Encircling endocardial cryoablation for ventricular tachycardia after myocardial infarction: experience with 33 patients. Am Heart J 1994;128:982–989.

41. Ostermeyer J, Gorggrefe M, Breithardt G, et al. Direct, electrophysiology guided operations for malignant ischemic ventricular tachycardia. PACE 1994;17(Pt II):550–551.

42. Niebauer MJ, Kirsh M, Kadish A, et al. Outcome of endocardial resection in 33 patients with coronary artery disease: correlation with ventricular tachycardia morphology. Am Heart J 1992;124:1500–1506.

43. Lee R, Mitchell JD, Garan H, et al. Operation for recurrent ventricular tachycardia. J Thorac Cardiovasc Surg 1994;107:732–742.

44. Nath S, Haines DE, Kron IL, et al. Regional wall motion analysis predicts survival and functional outcome after subendocardial re-section in patients with prior anterior myocardial infarction. Circulation 1993;88:70–76.

45. Willems AR, Tijssen JGP, van Capelle FJL, et al. Determinants of prognosis in symptomatic ventricular tachycardia or ventricular fibrillation late after myocardial infarction. J Am Coll Cardiol 1990;16:521–530.

46. Selle JG, Svenson RH, Gallagher JJ, et al. Surgical treatment of ventricular tachycardia with Nd:YAG laser photocoagulation. PACE 1992;15:1357–1361.

47. Guiraudon GM, Klein GJ, Gulamhusein SS, et al. Total disconnection of the right ventricular free wall: surgical treatment of right ventricular tachycardia associated with right ventricular dysplasia. Circulation 1983;67: 463–470.

48. Gillum RF. Sudden coronary death in the United States. Circulation 1989;79:756–765.

49. Mallory CK, White PD, Salgedo-Salgar J. The speed of healing of myocardial infarction. Am Heart J 1989;18:647A.

50. Guiraudon, G, Fontaine G, Frank R, et al. Apport de la ventriculotomie circulaire d'exclusion dans le traitement de la tachycardie ventriculaire recidivante apres infarctus du myocarde. Arch Mal Coeur 1982;75: 1013–1021.

51. Ungerleider RM, Holman WL, Stanley TE III, et al. Encircling endocardial ventriculotomy (EVV) for refractory ischemia ventricular tachycardia II. Effects on regional myocardial blood flow. J Thorac Cardiovasc Surg 1982;83:850.

52. Ostermeyer J, Breithardt G, Borggrefe M, et al. Surgical treatment of ventricular tachycardias. Complete versus partial encircling endocardial ventriculotomy. J Thorac Cardiovasc Surg 1984;87:517–525.

53. Ostermeyer J, Borggrefe M, Breithardt G, et al. Direct operations for the management of life-threatening ischemic ventricular tachycardia. J Thorac Cardiovasc Surg 1987;94: 848–865.

54. Harrison L, Gallagher JJ, Kasell J, et al. Cryosurgical ablation of the AV node-His bundle: a new method for producing AV block. Circulation 1977;55:463.

55. Gallagher JJ, Anderson RW, Kasell J, et al. Cryoablation of drug-resistant ventricular tachycardia in a patient with a variant of scleroderma. Circulation 1978;57:190.

56. Klein GJ, Harrison L, Ideker RF, et al. Reaction of the myocardium to cryosurgery: electrophysiology and arrhythmogenic potential. Circulation 1979;59:364–368.

57. Guiraudon GM, Klein GJ, Sharma AD, et al. Surgery for Wolff-Parkinson-White syndrome: further experience with an epicardial approach. Circulation 1986;74:525–529.

58. Hargrove WC, Miller JM. Risk stratification and management of patients with recurrent ventricular tachycardia and other malignant ventricular arrhythmias. Circulation 1989;79:1–178–1–181.

59. Moosdorf R, Pfeiffer D, Schneider C, et al. Intraoperative laser photocoagulation of ventricular tachycardia. Am Heart J 1994;127:1133–1138.

60. van Hemel NM, Kingma JH, Defauw JAM, et al. Left ventricular segmental wall motion score as a criterion for selecting patients for direct surgery in the treatment of post-infarction ventricular tachycardia. Eur Heart J 1989;10:304–315.

61. Hemel NM van, Defauw JAM, Kingma JH, et al. Risk factors of map-guided surgery for postinfarction ventricular tachycardia, a 12 year experience. Eur Heart J 1992;13:1662A.

62. Elefteriades JA, Biblo LA, Batsford WP, et al. Evolving patterns in the surgical treatment of malignant ventricular tachyarrhythmias. Ann Thorac Surg 1990;49:94–100.

63. Hargrove WC, Josephson ME, Marchlinski FE, et al. Surgical decisions in the management of sudden cardiac death and malignant ventricular arrhythmias: subendocardial resection, the automatic internal defibrillator, or both. J Thorac Cardiovasc Surg 1989;97:923–928.

64. Hargrove WC. Surgery for ischemic ventricular tachycardia—operative techniques and long-term results. Semin Thorac Cardiovasc Surg 1989;1:83–87.

65. Caceres J, Werner P, Jazayeri M, et al. Efficacy of cryosurgery alone for refractory monomorphic sustained ventricular tachycardia due to inferior wall infarction. J Am Coll Cardiol 1988;11:1254–1259.

66. Selle JG, Svenson RH, Sealy WC, et al. Successful clinical laser ablation of ventricular tachycardia: a promising new therapeutic method. Ann Thorac Surg 1986;42:38–384.

67. Svenson RH, Gallagher JJ, Selle JG, et al. Neodymium:YAG laser photocoagulation: a successful new map-guided technique for the intraoperative ablation of ventricular tachycardia. Circulation 1987;76:1319–1328.

68. Saksena S, Hussain M, Gielchinsky I, et al. Intraoperative mapping-guided argon laser ablation of malignant ventricular tachycardia. Am J Cardiol 1987;59:78–83.

69. Svenson RH, Littmann L, Gallagher JJ, et al. Termination of ventricular tachycardia with epicardial laser photocoagulation: a clinical comparison with patients undergoing successful endocardial photocoagulation alone. J Am Coll Cardiol 1990;15:163–170.

70. Bailar JC III, Mosteller F, eds. Medical Uses of Statistics. New England Journal of Medicine Books, Waltham MA, 1986.

71. Mickleborough LL, Maruyama H, Mohamed S, et al. Are patients receiving amiodarone at increased risk for cardiac operations? Ann Thorac Surg 1994;58:622–629.

72. de Bakker JMT, van Capelle FJL, Jansen MJ, et al. Macroreentry in the infarcted human heart: the mechanism of ventricular tachycardia with a "focal" activation pattern. J Am Coll Cardiol 1991;18:1005–1014.

73. van Hemel NM, Kingma JH, Defauw JJAM, et al. Continuation of antiarrhythmic drugs, or arrhythmia surgery after multiple drug failures. A randomized trial in the treatment of postinfarction ventricular tachycardia. Eur Heart J 1996;17:564–573.

74. Kelly P, Ruskin JN, Vlahakes GJ, et al. Surgical coronary revascularization in survivors of prehospital cardiac arrest: its effect on inducible ventricular arrhythmias and long-term survival. J Am Coll Cardiol 1990;15:267–273.

75. Berntsen RF, Gunnes P, Liet M, et al. Surgical revascularization in the treatment of ventricular tachycardia and fibrillation exposed by exercise-induced ischaemia. Eur Heart J 1993;14:1297–1303.

76. Marcus FI, Fontaine GH, Guiraudon G, et al. Right ventricular dysplasia. A report of 24 cases. Circulation 1982;65:384A.

77. Guiraudon GM, Klein GJ, Gulamhusein SS, et al. Total disconnection of right ventricular free wall: surgical treatment of right ventricular tachycardia associated with right ventricular dysplasia. Circulation 1983;67:463–470.

78. Guiraudon GM, Klein G, Guiraudon C, et al. Long term prognosis of patients with right ventricular free wall disconnection for arrhythmogenic right ventricular dysplasia: left ventricular ejection fractions as a marker of outcome. PACE 1996;19(Pt II):628.

79. Misaki T, Watanabe G, Iwa T, Tsubota M, et al. Surgical treatment of arrhythmogenic right ventricular dysplasia: long-term outcome. Ann Thorac Surg 1994;58:1380–1385.

80. Doig C, Nimkhedkar K, Bourke JP, et al. Acute and chronic hemodynamic impact of total right ventricular disarticulation. PACE 1991;14(pt II):1971–1975.

Section IV

Advances in Cardiac Pacing

Section Editor: S. Serge Barold

Chapter 32

Pacemaker Implantation:
The Old and New

Peter Belott

Introduction

Historically, the 1950s mark the beginning of modern artificial pacing.[1] In 1958, Drs. Seymour Furman and J.B. Schwedel passed the first transvenous endocardial electrode for prolonged cardiac pacing.[2] Almost simultaneously, Drs. Rune Elmqvist and A.K.E. Senning developed a totally implantable pacemaker system with an epigastric pocket and the electrodes connected subcutaneously to the heart.[3] These two events introduced both the transvenous and epicardial approaches to cardiac pacing. To this day, these two fundamentally different anatomic approaches have stood the test of time, as safe and reliable methods for pacemaker implantation. Initially, the majority of pacemaker implantations were performed via the cardiothoracic surgeon using the epicardial approach under general anesthesia. This was largely due to the fact that many pacemaker implantations were associated with open cardiac procedures such as valve replacements and repair of congenital defects. The pacemakers were large and more easily placed in a subcutaneous abdominal pocket. This approach was further reinforced by the lack of a truly reliable endocardial lead system. With the development of reliable endocardial lead systems, the transvenous endocardial approach by cutdown soon replaced an open-chest procedure. This approach precluded the use of anesthesia but required some form of imaging for appropriate electrode placement. As pacing technology advanced, the electrode systems became extremely reliable. The development of a fixation mechanism all but eradicated the complication of lead dislodgement. In addition, the pulse generators have become greatly reduced in size. At the same time, integrated circuitry technology and modern battery technology radically reduced the pacemaker size and the required surgery. What once required a major open-chest procedure under general anesthesia could be carried out via a simple cutdown and relatively minor surgery. In the late 1970s, Littleford and Spector introduced the percutaneous sheath-set technique for venous access via the subclavian vein.[4] This technique and variations on its theme revolutionized pacemaker implantation. This percutaneous technique also generated controversy with respect to its safety. Subsequently, the implantation procedure, previously the exclusive domain of the cardiovascular surgeon, has become the purview of the invasive cardiologist.

From Singer I, Barold SS, Camm AJ (eds): Nonpharmacological Therapy of Arrhythmias for the 21st Century: The State of the Art. Futura Publishing Co, Inc., Armonk, NY, © 1998.

Similarly, the procedure has undergone a transition from the operating room to the cardiac catheterization laboratory or special procedures room. The luxury of an anesthesiologist, except in special circumstances, has disappeared with the implanting physician assuming these additional responsibilities. In addition, the procedure that once required a rather protracted hospital stay could now be performed on an ambulatory basis. More recently, the subclavian crush phenomenon has resulted in a rethinking of the percutaneous subclavian approach. There has been a shift back to the cephalic vein cutdown and the development of percutaneous techniques for access of the axillary vein.

The transmyocardial or epicardial approach has seen little change over the years. A transthoracic endocardial lead placement technique by atriotomy and limited thoracotomy for unusual pathophysiological and congenital anomalies has been developed. In addition, more recently, thoracoscopy has been used for the placement of epicardial electrodes.

Thus, over the past 40 years, modern cardiac pacing has seen radical changes in anatomic approach, preoperative planning, implanting personnel, and implant facility. The discipline that was once exclusively that of the cardiac surgeon has been passed on to the invasive cardiologist and electrophysiologist. The procedure, initially preserved for the operating room, is now performed in a special studies or catheterization laboratory. General anesthesia has been replaced by simple conscious sedation and the procedure that once required a lengthy hospital stay is now carried out on an ambulatory basis. This chapter reviews pacemaker implantation techniques, both old and new, from a historical perspective. The techniques are reviewed with respect to anatomic approach, concerns over safety, special applications, and potential complications. Solutions and alternatives are also discussed. Suggested management of complex implant situations and the ambulatory approach to permanent pacemaker implantation are also explored.

Anatomic Approach

There are two basic anatomic approaches to permanent cardiac pacing.[5,6] The first is the epicardial which requires general anesthesia and surgical access to the epicardial surface of the heart. The second is the transvenous approach which involves passage of electrodes through a vein to the endocardial surface of the heart. This approach is performed under local anesthesia with conscious sedation. Electrodes can be placed on the epicardium by a variety of techniques. This involves a subxiphoid incision, a limited thoracotomy, or a direct application of electrodes on the exposed heart. More recently, mediastinoscopy and/or thoracoscopy have been used to apply permanent epicardial electrodes. The transvenous approach can be performed by venous cutdown, percutaneous venous access, or a combination of the two.

A thorough understanding of the venous anatomic structures of the head, neck, and upper extremities is imperative for safe venous access.[7,8] Byrd had demonstrated this concept with his description of anterior and posterior displaced clavicles[9] (Figures 1–3). The posterior displaced clavicle, as seen in chronic obstructive pulmonary disease, can make venous access extremely hazardous. Similarly, the anteriorly displaced clavicle that is found in the elderly kyphoscoliotic patient with anteriorly bowed clavicles renders percutaneous access next to impossible. An appreciation of these anatomic variations is essential if one is to avoid the complications of pneumothorax, hemopneumothorax, and unsuccessful venipuncture. It should also be appreciated that the right ventricle is an anterior structure, the apex of which is usually located anteriorly and to the left (Figure 4). Although the normal location is distinctly to the left of the midline, occasionally it can be rotated anteriorly and to the right. In extreme circum-

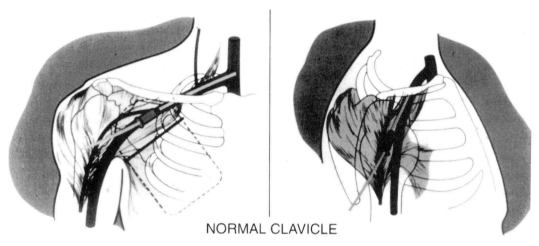

Figure 1. The normal anatomic position of the clavicle as seen in the anterior and lateral projection. Used with permission from Byrd CL.[9]

stances, this displacement will rotate the right ventricular apex to the right of the midline. If this is not appreciated, lead placement can be extremely difficult if not impossible.

Transvenous Pacemaker Placement

Historically, the venous cutdown technique has been the primary means of venous access for pacemaker electrode insertion. The cephalic vein has been commonly used in this approach either from the right or left side. Occasionally, the more experienced surgeon has cannulated the internal jugular and the deeper axillary vein via this approach. Little departure from this pacemaker implantation technique had occurred until the late 1970s when Littleford and Spector introduced the percutaneous sheath-set technique for venous access via the subclavian vein.[10] This technique and

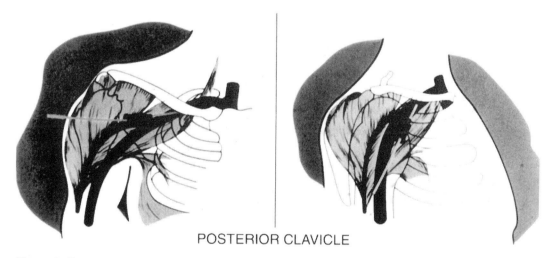

Figure 2. Posterior displacement of the clavicle, recognized by the horizontal position of the deltopectoral groove. Used with permission from Byrd CL.[9]

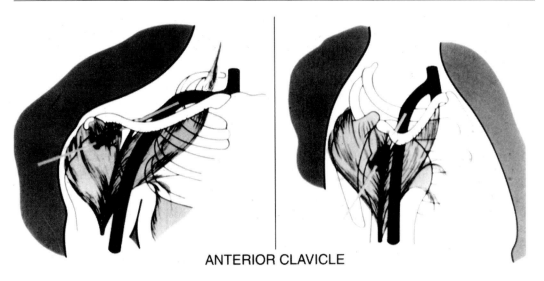

ANTERIOR CLAVICLE

Figure 3. Anterior displaced clavicle, recognized by nearly vertical deltopectoral groove. Used with permission from Byrd CL.[9]

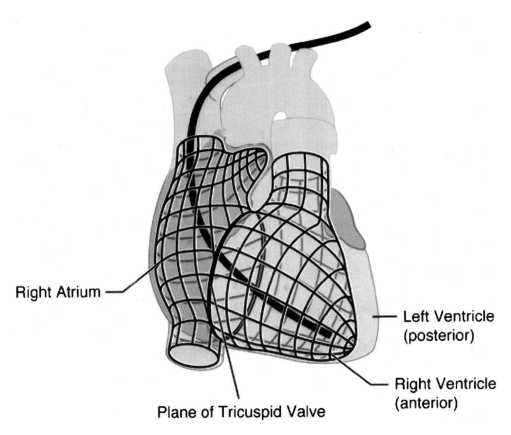

Right Atrium

Left Ventricle (posterior)

Right Ventricle (anterior)

Plane of Tricuspid Valve

Figure 4. The anterior orientation of the right ventricle. Used with permission from Belott PH, et al.[73]

Table 1
Venous Strictures for Pacemaker Lead Insertion

Cephalic vein
Axillary vein
Subclavian vein
Internal jugular vein
External jugular vein
Femoral vein
Inferior vena cava

variations on its themes have revolutionized pacemaker implantation. The percutaneous technique, however, has generated considerable controversy with respect to its safety. The percutaneous sheath-set technique has proven to be especially efficacious for dual chambered pacing. With the development of peel-away sheath, the problems of sheath removal from the permanent electrode were resolved. All that remained was skill in puncturing the desired venous structure. Once again, a thorough knowledge of both normal and abnormal anatomy was obviously essential. In more recent times, a combination of the cutdown and percutaneous techniques has been used to successfully access a venous structure. This involves a cutdown on the vein for vascular control and subsequent direct percutaneous access of the vessel via the Seldinger technique. Common venous structures for pacemaker placement are listed in Table 1.

Venous Cutdown of the Cephalic Vein - Cephalic Venous Access

The cephalic vein is found in the deltopectoral groove. This is a groove defined by the lateral border of the pectoralis muscle and the medial border of the deltoid muscle, at the level of the coracoid process. At the level of the coracoid process, a 1½ to 2 inch incision is made along the deltopectoral groove. The incision is carried directly through the dermis.

The skin incision should be carried out in a single stroke. Multiple strokes will generally result in irregular skin margins. Of course, the skin should be generously infiltrated with local anesthesia. Once the initial incision has been made, a Weitlaner self-retaining retractor can then be applied for exposure.

Using gentle strokes with scalpel, the incision is carried down to the surface of the pectoralis muscle. The Weitlaner is continuously reapplied as the subcutaneous tissue falls away and tension is released. Along the way, with the Weitlaner retractor holding the tissue edge with support, the deltopectoral groove can clearly be identified.

The deltopectoral groove is then opened using Metzenbaum scissors. Further reapplication of the Weitlaner self-retaining retractor to the medial head of the deltoid and lateral head if the pectoralis muscle will afford excellent exposure. Careful dissection of the deltopectoral groove will eventually expose the cephalic vein. At times, this vessel is extremely diminutive and atretic.

If the cephalic vein is too small, further dissection may be carried proximally. In rare instances, dissection will actually be carried to the axillary vein. Once exposed, the cephalic vein is freed from its fibrous attachments and 0 silk ligatures are applied proximally and distally (Figure 5A). Once adequate venous control has been obtained, a horizontal venotomy is made with an iris scissor and an 11 scalpel blade (Figure 5B). The vein should be supported at all times with smooth forceps. Using mosquito clamps, forceps, or vein pick, the venotomy is opened and the electrode(s) introduced (Figure 5C). Once venous access has been achieved, the electrodes are positioned in the appropriate chambers using standard techniques.

Percutaneous Access of the Subclavian Vein

Percutaneous vascular access has been used for many years by the cardiologist with the Seldinger technique. In this tech-

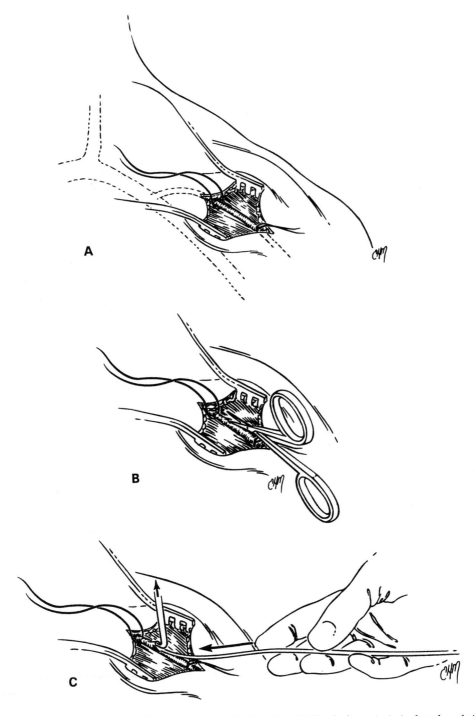

Figure 5. (A) Introduction of a lead into the cephalic vein. **(B)** Cephalic vein is isolated and tied off distally. Venotomy performed with iris scissor. **(C)** Lead inserted while venotomy is held open with vein pick. Used with permission from Belott PH, et al.[73]

nique, a large-bore needle is used to percutaneously puncture the vascular structure. A wire is introduced through the needle into the vessel and the needle is removed over the wire and exchanged for a catheter or sheath. Today, prepackaged introducer sets are used for this purpose (Figure 6A).

Once again, it is important that the operator be completely familiar with normal anatomy and anatomic landmarks. The traditional subclavian puncture is carried out in the middle third of the clavicle. This location is frequently associated with an increased risk of vascular trauma, pneumothorax, and lack of success. An alternative approach calls for the puncture at the apex formed by the clavicle and first rib (Figure 6B).[11] This location is remote from the apex of the lung and the venous structure is more easily accessed because it is much larger.

If the operator chooses to use the conventional approach with a medial stick, the area is initially infiltrated with local anesthesia. Puncture is carried out with the needle aimed in a medial and cephalic direction. It is important to maintain the patient in an anatomic position. Maneuvers that artificially open the costoclavicular and infraclavicular spaces should be avoided. The common practice of placing towels between the scapula or extending the line may result in undesirable puncture of the costoclavicular ligament or subclavius muscle. The medial venous puncture clearly increases the success rate as well as dramatically reducing the risk of pneumothorax and vascular injury.

An 18-gauge thin-wall needle is used for the percutaneous venipuncture. Once the vessel has been entered, the guidewire is inserted and the tip positioned in the midright atrium (Figure 7A,B). Fluoroscopy should always be used to check position of the wire. The wire should never be forced; if any resistance is encountered, readvancement is advised.

When the wire is observed to coil in the needle tip, it is probably extravascular. In this case, it is advisable to remove the guidewire and needle as a unit and perform a new venous stick. In certain instances, the extravascular guidewire may create a hematoma that will collapse the venous structure and preclude subsequent successful venous reentry. In this case it is advisable to proceed to an alternate venous access site by either cutdown or move to the opposite side. It is important to note that the risk of pneumothorax increases with the number of unsuccessful percutaneous punctures. One of the more frustrating experiences occurs when the guidewire tracks into the internal jugular vein. Once venous access is achieved, every effort should be made to retain it. If the guidewire tracks into the internal jugular vein, a subtle change in the needle angle should be effected and the guidewire retracted into the needle while the needle is still in the vascular structure. The advancement will usually result in passage of the guidewire through the innominate vein to the superior vena cava. This maneuver may have to be repeated several times to effect passage. If this problem persists, one may use a small 5F or 6F rubber dilator to act as a catheter to steer the guidewire into its proper trajectory. The rubber dilator may also be used for the injection of contrast to define the venous anatomy.

After successful venous access and positioning of the guidewire, the skin incision is created. The incision should be directed along anatomic lines. The area is generously infiltrated with local anesthesia. Once again, the incision is created with a single stroke initiated from the needle, carried through the skin, through the dermis, medially and inferiorly for approximately 2 inches. Once the incision has been carried out, the Weitlaner self-retaining retractor is applied similar to that described in the venous cutdown. The Weitlaner retractor holds the tissue under tension, broad strokes with the scalpel are carried from wound corner to wound corner. The incision is carried down to the surface of the pectoralis muscle. Care is taken to avoid violating the pectoralis fascia. The Weitlaner retractor is continually reapplied to effect tissue tension.

A

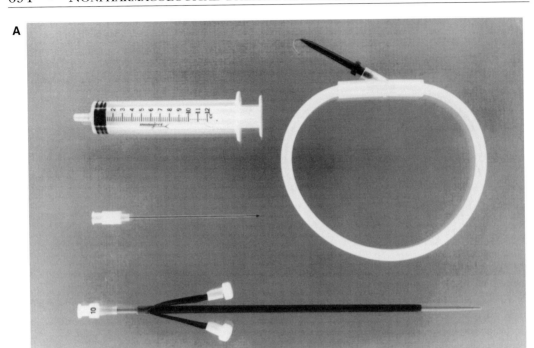

B

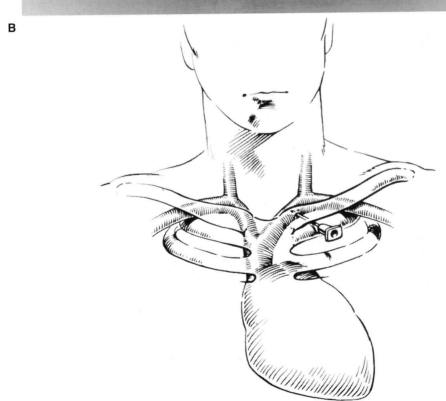

Figure 6. (A) Percutaneous introducer set, prepackaged with rubber dilator, sheath, guidewire, 18-gauge needle, and 10-cc syringe. Used with permission from Belott PH, et al.[73] **(B)** Extreme medial and cephalad needle trajectory in the "subclavian window." Used with permission from Belott PH, et al.[11]

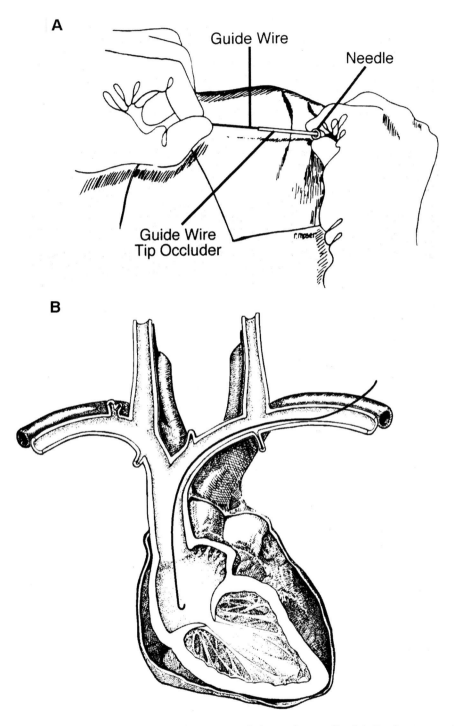

Figure 7. (A) Guidewire with tip-occluder is passed down the needle. **(B)** Guidewire is advanced to the mid-right atrium. Used with permission from Belott PH, et al.[75]

The lateral aspect of the incision is opened by the Metzenbaum scissors, maintaining a plane directly on top of the pectoralis muscle. Once the incision has been carried to the surface of the pectoralis muscle and there is good exposure of the puncture site, a figure-of-eight suture stitch is applied about the needle (Figure 8).[12] This stitch will serve for hemostasis throughout the procedure. Once the initial preparations of the wound are completed, the needle may be removed from the guidewire and a sheath set applied. The dilator and sheath are advanced over the guidewire with a continuous forward motion (Figure 9). It is important to avoid twisting or rotating the dilator sheath, as this motion may result in tearing of the sheath's leading edge at the sheath-dilator transition. This will also result in sheath buckling that can preclude introduc-

tion. After successful passage of the sheath set, the dilator is removed and the electrode passed down the sheath (Figure 10). It is recommended that when the dilator is removed, the guidewire be retained and the electrode passed alongside the guidewire. The sheath is then retracted and peeled away. Positioning of the electrode within the lead in situ is unwise because it may result in air embolism or unnecessary blood loss. With the sheath removed, hemostasis is achieved by applying tension to the figure-of-eight stitch (Figure 11). The retention of the guidewire is a variation of the standard introducer technique. The retained guidewire may provide unlimited venous access and the ability to exchange and introduce additional electrodes by simply applying another sheath set to the guidewire. The retained guidewire should be held to the

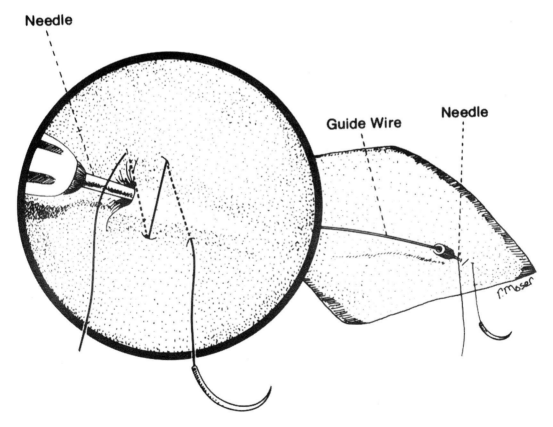

Figure 8. Initial dissection complete, figure-of-eight stitch is placed about the needle. Used with permission from Belott PH, et al.[75]

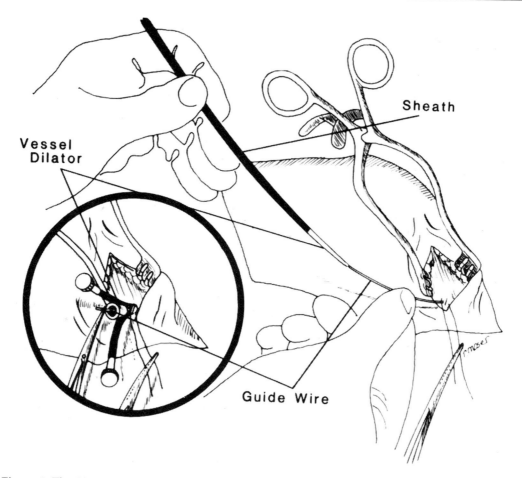

Figure 9. The 18-gauge thin-walled needle removed, the sheath set is applied to the guidewire and advanced into the venous system. Used with permission from Belott PH, et al.[75]

drape with a clamp to avoid inadvertent dislodgement. The retained guidewire can serve as a ground for the unipolar threshold analysis instead of the grounding plate. It can also be used as an intracardiac lead for the recording of atrial electrograms or as an electrode for emergency pacing. The guidewire should be retained in both single and dual chamber procedures until satisfactory lead position is attained.

Blind Subclavian Puncture

There has been an ongoing debate with respect to the safety and efficacy of the blind subclavian puncture. Parsonnet et al. and Furman have compared the complications of the percutaneous approach with the safety of the cephalic cutdown.[13–15] Parsonnet, in analyzing the pacemaker implantation complication rates with respect to contributing factors, reviewed 632 consecutive implants over a 5-year period performed by 29 different implanting physicians at a single institution. There were 37 perioperative complications. The complications were analyzed together with experience of the implanting physicians. Percutaneous venous access was associated with the highest complication rate and contributed significantly to a 5.7% overall complication rate. If the complications related to the percutaneous approach were excluded,

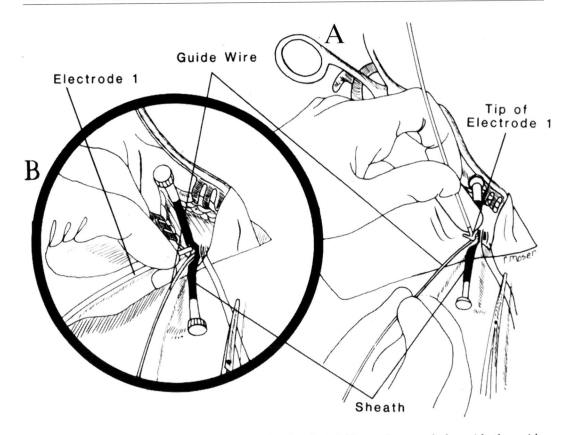

Figure 10. (A) Pacemaker electrode entering the sheath. **(B)** Electrode passed alongside the guide-wire. Used with permission from Belott PH, et al.[75]

the complication rate dropped to a more acceptable 3.5%. The highest complication rate was among physicians implanting less than 12 pacemakers per year with the least pacing experience. Because of the high incidence of complications associated with percutaneous venous access, Parsonnet et al. recommend that this approach be reserved as a second choice to unsuccessful cutdowns. Parsonnet et al. did not analyze the complications as a function of the precise percutaneous technique used. There was no mention of the subclavian window or the safe zone described by Byrd. Indeed, experience and meticulous attention to technique are essential for save subclavian access.

Similarly, Furman has demonstrated a remarkable efficiency of the cutdown approach for dual chambered pacing, particularly with unipolar leads. The cutdown technique was less useful for bipolar leads via a single cephalic vein. Furman reported no vascular or pleural complications in a series of 3,500 cases using the cutdown approach for single or dual chamber pacemaker implants. Furman has emphasized that the complication rate of a blind subclavian puncture technique has probably been underestimated. A list of the common complications associated with the percutaneous approach are listed in Table 2.

Air Embolization

Air embolization is a well-known complication of the percutaneous approach. To avoid this problem, it has been recommended that the patient should be well hydrated and placed in the Trendelenburg

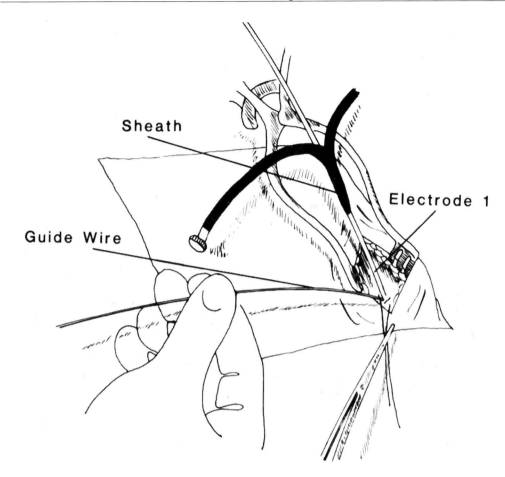

Figure 11. The sheath is retracted, tension applied to the figure-of-eight stitch. The guidewire is retained and clamped to the drape. Used with permission from Belott PH, et al.[75]

Table 2
Percutaneous Complications

1. Pneumothorax
2. Hemothorax
3. Hemopneumothorax
4. Laceration, subclavian artery
5. Arteriovenous fistula
6. Nerve injury
7. Thoracic duct injury
8. Cheilothorax
9. Lymphatic fistula

position. Unfortunately, the cardiac catheterization laboratory precludes this approach. The most important step in prevention is awareness on the part of the implanting physician for the risks of embolization. There are many steps that may be taken to avoid this complication[16] (Table 3).

The time of greatest risk is when the dilator is removed from the sheath set. In a patient with complete heart block or a state of overhydration, there is generally little or no risk. On the other hand, an elderly, dehydrated patient who has been n.p.o. for many hours is at risk for a serious air embolization. It is recommended that prior to the procedure, any pacemaker patient approached from the percutaneous point of view be maintained in a mild state of over-hydration. The patient's state of hydration should be assessed just prior to removal of the dilator.

By careful withdrawal of the dilator from the sheath, one can assess the patient's state of hydration and venous pressure with the cycles of respiration. In a patient who is well hydrated or with high venous pressure, there is a continuous flash of blood from the sheath despite the cycles of respiration. On the other hand, a dehydrated patient will manifest with no blood meniscus or flash of blood and, with each inspiration, retraction of the meniscus. If the blood meniscus is observed to move inward, the dilator is rap-idly readvanced back into the sheath to avoid air embolism during this assessment. If the patient is deemed to be at high risk for air embolization, several precautions should be instituted. First, the lower ex-tremities can be elevated to increase venous return. This is carried out by the insertion of a wedge. Second, if the patient is sleeping or oversedated, it is important to arouse the patient and achieve total patient coopera-tion with respect to the cycles of respiration.

Table 3
Prevention of Air Embolism During Permanent Pacemaker Procedures

---

 I. Awareness of the potential problem
 II. Well-hydrated patient, avoiding long periods of N.P.O.
 III. Awareness of when patient is at greatest risk—open sheath in vein
 IV. Assess hydration: (take a peak)
 V. High-risk patient
   a) Increased hydration/wide-open IVs
   b) An awake, cooperative patient
   c) Elevate lower extremities/wedge
   d) Trendelenburg position (if available)
   e) Expeditious lead placement and sheath re-moval
   f) Check for introduction of air
   g) Continuous monitoring (vital signs, oxygen saturation, blood pressure)
 VI. In an extremely high-risk, uncooperative pa-tient, intubation and temporary loss of con-sciousness may be required

---

In addition, increased hydration can be ini-tiated by increasing the administration of intravenous fluids. Measures such as pinch-ing the sheath with the lead have proven to be completely ineffective. Expeditious lead insertion is extremely important. The lead should be inserted rapidly and the sheath totally removed. The practice of slowly peeling the sheath in situ should be totally avoided. A pacemaker electrode should never be positioned with the sheath set in place. More recently, a peel-away sheath with a hemostatic valve has been developed that completely avoids the problem of air embolization (Figure 12).

Contrast Venography

Contrast venography has been used to fa-cilitate subclavian puncture. This technique was first described by Hayes and col-leagues.[17] In this technique, a venous line is established on the side of planned venous access. It is advisable to use a large-gauge needle. Contrast material (10–20 mL) is in-jected rapidly into the intravenous line fol-lowed by a saline flush. Occasionally, this is facilitated by a nonsterile assistant mas-saging the contrast material through the pe-ripheral venous system underneath a sterile drape. Fluoroscopy is then used to direct the needle to the site of venous access as defined by the contrast material (Figure 13). In the cardiac catheterization laboratory or special studies room, a mask or map may be obtained for guidance after the contrast material has dissipated. This technique has been extremely helpful in locating the sub-clavian vein and has also been applied to other venous structures.

Percutaneous Approach
for Dual Chambered Pacing

Dual chambered pacing calls for the in-troduction of an atrial and ventricular elec-trode. The cutdown technique is less suited for this approach as all too often the ce-

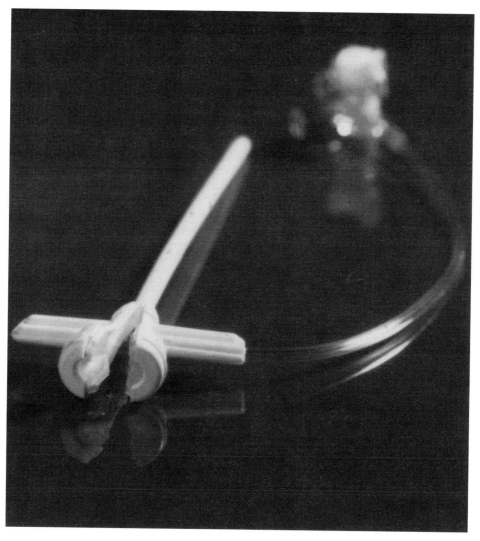

Figure 12. Pacemaker peel-away sheath with hemostatic valve. Courtesy of Pressure Products, Inc., Rancho Palos Verdes, CA.

phalic vein can hardly accommodate one electrode, and even less two. The percutaneous approach appears ideally suited for dual chambered pacing as there is potential for unlimited access to the venous circulation. Various options for dual chambered pacing venous access are listed in Table 4. There are five percutaneous approaches for dual chambered pacing.

1. The first approach uses two separate percutaneous sticks and the application of two separate sheaths.[18] This approach increases the risk of complications related to the venipuncture process in addition to possibly not finding the vessel a second time. There is also increased risk of pneumothorax, air embolism, bleeding, and vascular trauma.

2. The second technique utilizes one percutaneous stick and the use of a large sheath set that will accommodate the passage of both atrial and ventricular electrodes.[19,20] The passage of two electrodes down one

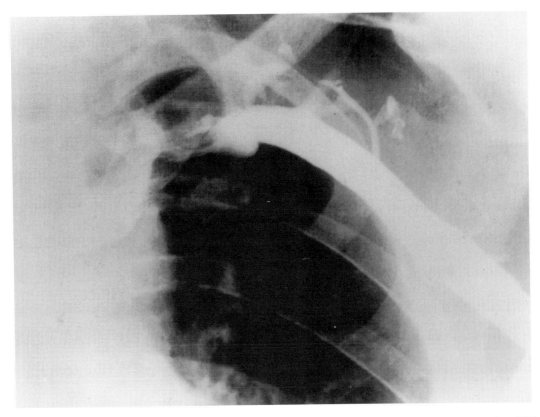

Figure 13. Venipuncture guided by contrast venography. Used with permission from Belott PH, et al.[74]

Table 4
Venous Access for Dual Chambered Pacing

I. Venous cutdown: Isolate one or two veins
II. Percutaneous: Two separate sticks and sheath applications
III. Percutaneous: Two electrodes down one large sheath
IV. Percutaneous: Retained guidewire (Belott technique)
V. Cutdown with cephalic vein guidewire (Ong-Barold technique)

sheath is less desirable because the large sheath may increase the risk of air embolization and blood loss. In addition, there is increased frustration from electrode dislodgement and entanglement.

3. The retained guidewire technique appears to be the most desirable approach as it provides unlimited access to the central circulation.[21–23] One is never committed or compromised. There is less risk of bleeding, pneumothorax, and air embolization. This author prefers the retained guidewire technique. The ventricular electrode should be positioned first. This is both safe and practical. It is safe since, once positioned, there is always electrical support of the ventricles should asystole occur. It is also preferred, since the initially placed ventricular electrode is less susceptible to dislodgement during positioning of the second electrode. Once the ventricular electrode is in position, it is stabilized by leaving the stylet in the vicinity of the lower right atrium. The electrode is also secured by use of a suture sleeve at the

puncture site. After the ventricular electrode is stabilized, a second sheath set is applied to the retained guidewire (Figures 14, 15). The atrial electrode is introduced, positioned, and secured. The retained guidewire is only removed after one is completely satisfied with both electrode positions and there is no need to exchange. Hemostasis is effected by the figure-of-eight suture stitch.

4. A fourth approach uses the combination of the sheath-set technique and a venous cutdown approach. Ong et al. have described the cephalic guidewire technique.[24] This technique involves the cutdown and isolation of the cephalic vein (Figure 16). Instead of performing a venotomy, the vein is punctured percutaneously and a guidewire and sheath set applied. Unlike the cutdown technique, the cephalic vein is completely sacrificed. If the guidewire is retained, multiple sheath set exchanges and lead placements can be carried out (Figure 17). Once again, hemostasis is effected by compression and/or the application of a figure-of-eight suture stitch. Despite sacrificing the cephalic vein, there have been no reports of venous complications.

Upgrading Techniques for Dual Chambered Pacing

It is now appreciated that when approaching a patient for permanent transvenous pacemaker, every effort should be made to preserve atrial and ventricular rela-

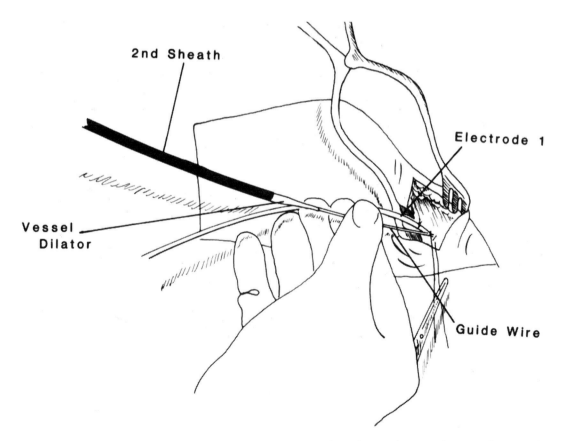

Figure 14. Application of second sheath set to the retained guidewire for introduction of a second electrode. Used with permission from Belott PH, et al.[75]

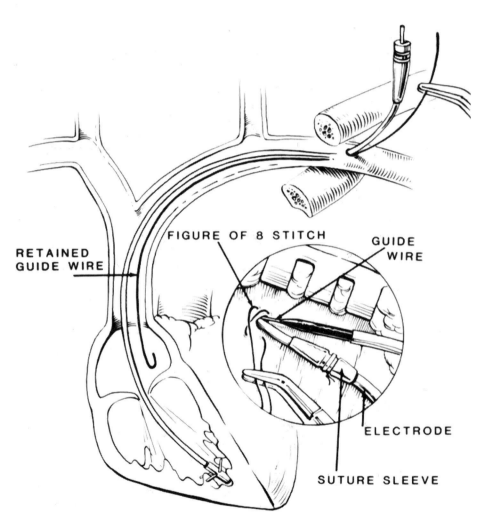

Figure 15. The retained guidewire technique. The insert shows the secured ventricular electrode and suture sleeve, figure-of-eight stitch held by a clamp, and a second sheath set applied to the retained guidewire. Used with permission from Belott PH, et al.[11]

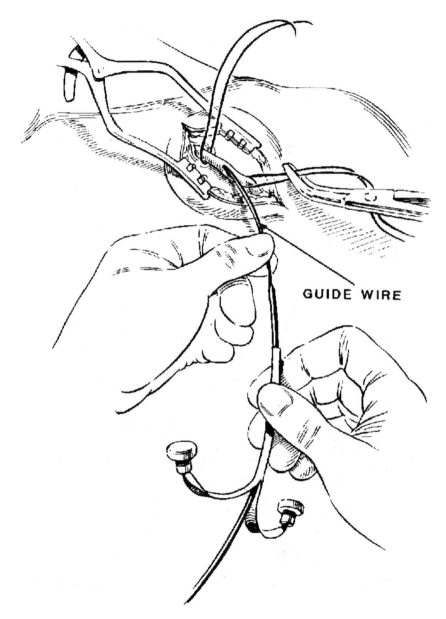

GUIDE WIRE

Figure 16. The Ong-Barold technique. For discussion, see text. Used with permission from Belott PH, et al.[11]

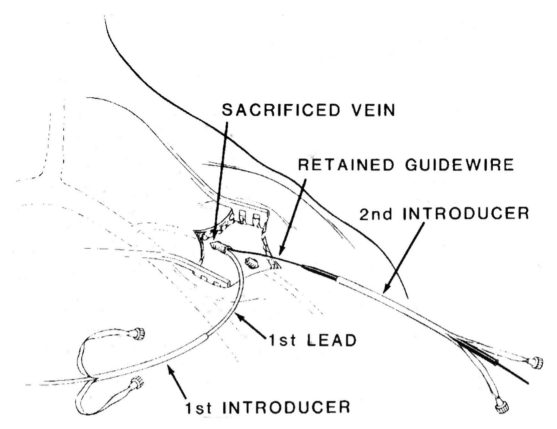

SACRIFICED VEIN

RETAINED GUIDEWIRE

2nd INTRODUCER

1st LEAD

1st INTRODUCER

Figure 17. The Ong-Barold technique in combination with the retained- guidewire technique for introduction of a second electrode. Used with permission from Belott PH, et al.[11]

tionships. Sensitive to this concept, the majority of the patients today receive dual chamber pacing systems. There is, however, a large group of patients who have previously received single chamber, ventricular demand pacing systems. There is also an even smaller group of patients who have previously received single chamber atrial pacing systems. Many of the patients with the VVI systems are symptomatic with the "pacemaker syndrome." In addition, the smaller group of atrially paced patients who have previously received single chamber atrial pacing systems are symptomatic with the development of AV block.

Many of the symptomatic patients with the VVI system required pacemaker system upgrade with the addition of an atrial electrode. In addition, the smaller group of atrially paced patients who are symptomatic

with AV block will require ventricular support with the addition of a ventricular electrode. Both groups of patients require pacemaker system upgrades with the addition of a second electrode.

The conventional pacemaker system upgrade technique involves placement of a second electrode. In addition, this procedure is also combined with a pulse generator change. The dilemma with pacemaker system upgrade is the required supplemental venous access for placement of a second lead.

Venous access can be carried out by either cutdown or the percutaneous approach. If the initial electrode has been placed via cutdown, the isolation of a second vein for venous access will prove extremely difficult. In this case, the percutaneous approach should be attempted. Conversely, if the initial electrode has been placed percutaneously, then a second percutaneous approach or a cutdown is possible. The second percutaneous puncture is usually carried out just lateral to the initial venous entry site. If any difficulty is encountered, fluoroscopy is used to guide the lead using the chronic ventricular electrode for reference.[25,26] There is potential risk of damaging the initial electrode and care should be taken to avoid its direct puncture. The use of radiographic materials can help define the venous structure as well as its patency.

Contralateral Subclavian Vein Access

Occasionally, the vessel to be recannulated is thrombosed or obstructed precluding venous access on the same side. In this case, contralateral venous access should be considered (Figure 18A-C).[27] In this instance, the desired electrode is passed via the contralateral subclavian vein, positioned, and subsequently tunneled back to the original pocket (Figure 19). The contralateral puncture site requires a limited skin incision of about 1.5 cm. It is carried down to the surface of the pectoralis muscle and used for anchoring the electrode with its suture sleeve. Once the electrode has been positioned, it is anchored and secured. The proximal end of the electrode is then tunneled back to the original pocket.

Pacemaker Lead Compression and Alternate Percutaneous Techniques

Frequently, the solution to one problem merely creates another. Case in point is the extreme medial subclavian percutaneous technique. Although this approach is safe and avoids the complication of pneumothorax and expedites venous access, it has been implicated in the cause of premature pacemaker lead failure by a conductor fracture and insulation damage. Electrode failure as a result of an extreme medial approach has been called "the subclavian crush phenomenon." Fyke was first to report insulation failure of two leads placed side by side by the percutaneous approach to the subclavian vein where there was a tight costoclavicular space.[28] This phenomenon has now been extensively reported in the literature.[29-34] There are a number of proposed mechanisms and potential solutions. The electrodes of a more complex design, such as bipolar coaxial construction are most susceptible to this phenomenon. A more lateral percutaneous approach has been suggested to avoid the crush phenomenon. More recently, the axillary vein has been suggested as an alternate site of venous access to avoid the crush phenomenon. This was first suggested by Dr. Byrd in his proposed "safe introducer technique."[35] Byrd defines a safety zone for percutaneous venous access very similar to the subclavian window (Figure 20). In addition, several conditions must be fulfilled. An essential condition of puncture is adequate ease of needle insertion that avoids friction, puncture of bone, cartilage, or tendon (Figure 21). If a puncture cannot be safely conducted within a safety zone, the axillary vein is then percutaneously cannulated.

The axillary vein is actually a continuation of the subclavian vein after it exits the superior mediastinum and crosses the first rib. It is frequently called the extrathoracic portion of the subclavian vein. This vein is usually quite large. The axillary vein traverses the anterolateral chest wall into the axilla (Figure 22). It crosses the deltopectoral groove at approximately the level of the coracoid process. At the level of the teres major and latissimus dorsi muscles, it becomes the basilic vein. The axillary vein is covered by both pectoralis major and minor muscles. It runs medial and parallel to the deltopectoral groove for approximately 1–2 cm (Figure 23). The cephalic vein, a common venous access site for pacemaker implantation, drains directly into the axillary vein just superior to the pectoralis minor. The axillary vein is an excellent site for

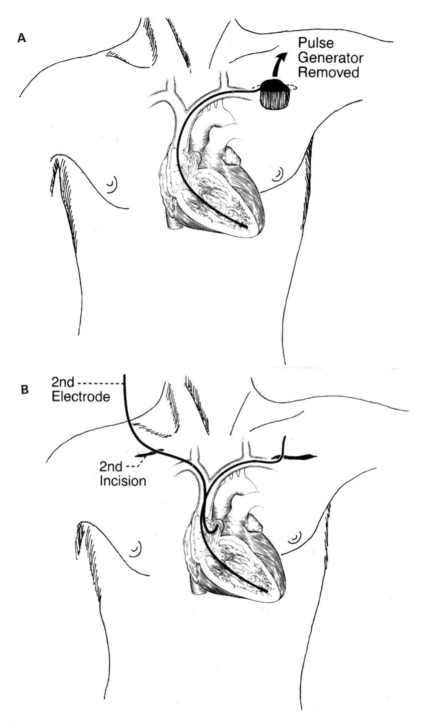

Figure 18. Pacemaker system upgrade using contralateral subclavian vein. **(A)** The pacemaker pocket is opened and the old pulse generator and lead are dissected free, externalized, and disconnected. **(B)** A second lead is inserted via the contralateral subclavian vein. Used with permission from Belott PH, et al.[74]

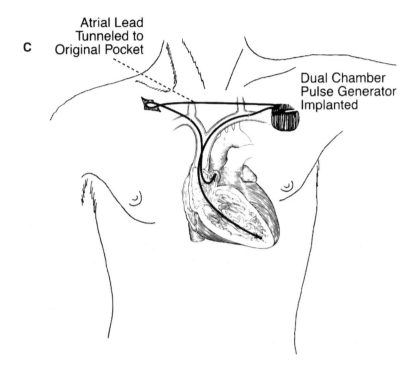

Figure 18. *(Continued)* **(C)** The second lead is tunneled back to the initial pocket. Used with permission from Belott PH, et al.[74]

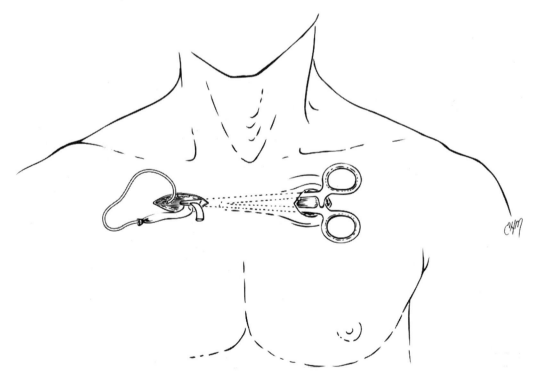

Figure 19. Lead in Penrose drain is grasped by a clamp and pulled from donor site to recipient wound. Used with permission from Belott PH, et al.[73]

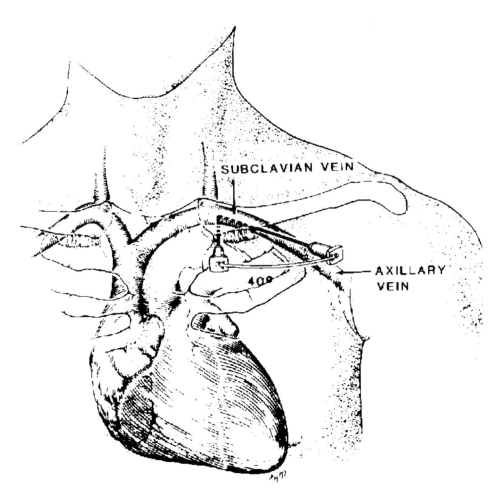

Figure 20. Anatomic orientation of the "safety zone." Used with permission from Belott PH, et al.[11]

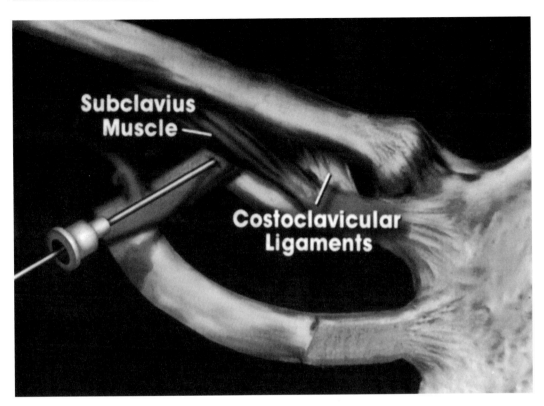

Figure 21. Access of the extrathoracic portion of the subclavian vein. Used with permission from Byrd CL, et al.[64]

venous access, but is never considered as it is a rather deep structure. The surface landmarks of note are the infraclavicular space, deltopectoral groove, and the coracoid process.

The axillary venous approach is actually not new. It was initially reported in 1987 by Nichalls as an alternate site route of venous access for large central lines.[36] Nichalls developed a technique from cadaver dissection by which he established reliable landmarks. He described the axillary vein as infraclavicular. The needle is always anterior to the thoracic cavity, generally tangential to the chest wall to avoid pneumothorax and hemopneumothorax. The landmarks used by Nichalls for axillary vein puncture are described as follows (Figure 24):

The vein starts medial at a point below the medial aspect of the clavicle where the space between the clavicle and first rib be-

come palpable. The vein extends laterally to a point three fingerbreadths below the inferior aspect of the coracoid process. The skin is punctured along the medial border of the pectoralis minor muscle at a point above the vein as it is defined by the surface landmarks. The axillary vein is punctured by passing the needle anterior to the first rib, maneuvering posteriorly to medially, corresponding to the lateral to medial course of the axillary vein. The needle passes between the first rib and clavicle. It is also recommended that the arm be adducted 45°.

The Nichalls' experience was further reinforced by Taylor and Yellowlees, who reported an experience with this technique in 102 consecutive patients with only four failures and one pneumothorax.[37] In the technique described by Byrd, an 18-gauge thin-wall needle is guided by fluoroscopy and

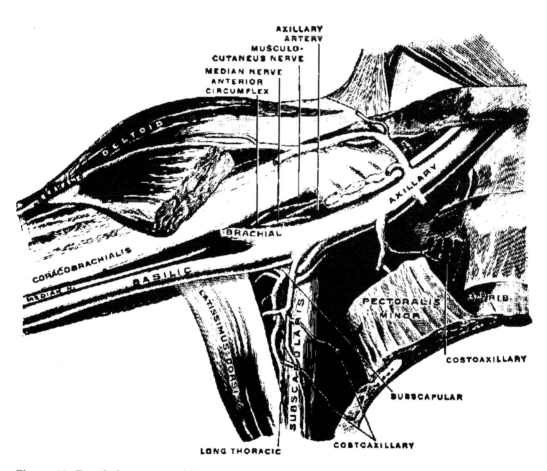

Figure 22. Detailed anatomy of the anterolateral chest demonstrating the axillary vein with the pectoralis major and minor muscles removed. Used with permission from Belott PH, et al.[74]

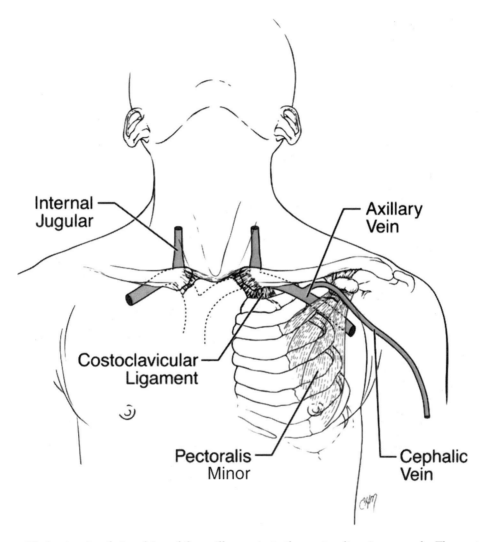

Figure 23. Anatomic relationships of the axillary vein to the pectoralis minor muscle. The pectoralis major has been removed. Note the cephalic vein draining directly into the axillary vein at approximately the first intercostal space. Used with permission from Belott PH, et al.[74]

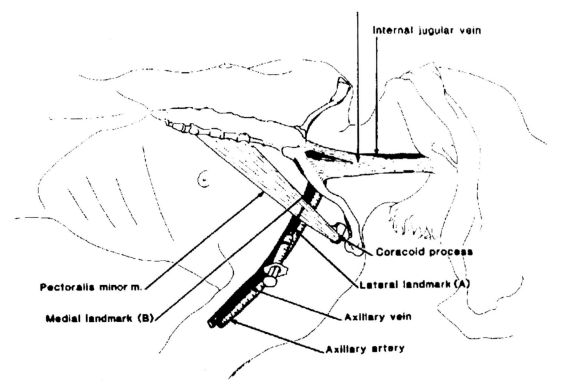

Internal jugular vein

Coracoid process

Lateral landmark (A)

Pectoralis minor m.

Medial landmark (B)

Axillary vein

Axillary artery

Figure 24. Nichalls' landmarks for axillary vein puncture. Used with permission from Belott PH, et al.[11]

directed to the medial portion of the first rib. With the needle perpendicular to the first rib, it is walked laterally until the axillary vein is punctured.[35] This is indicated by the aspiration of venous blood (Figure 25). The guidewire is inserted and the introducer is subsequently applied per standard technique. It is important to note that the needle path is always directed anterior to the thoracic cavity to avoid the risk of pneumothorax. Byrd has subsequently reported success in a series of 213 consecutive cases where the extrathoracic portion of the subclavian vein (axillary vein) was successfully cannulated as a primary approach.[38]

Subsequently, Magney et al. reported a new approach to percutaneous subclavian venipuncture to avoid lead fracture.[39] This technique is similar to Byrd's, only uses extensive surface landmarks for venipuncture (Figure 26). The technique involves puncture of the extrathoracic portion of the sub-

clavian vein or axillary vein. The location of the axillary vein is defined as the intersection with a line drawn between the middle of the sternal angle and the tip of the coracoid process. This was generally near the lateral border of the first rib. Since January 1996, this author has used a primary axillary venous puncture approach with considerable success. This technique uses a modification of both Byrd and Magney's recommendations. The deltopectoral groove is used as a primary landmark. In the relatively asthenic individual, the deltopectoral groove is defined by palpation and the curvature of the chest wall noted. An incision is made inferomedially from the deltopectoral groove at the level of the coracoid process for approximately 2 inches (4 cm). The incision is carried down to the level of the pectoralis muscle and the deltopectoral groove is visualized. The pectoralis muscle is then directly punctured. The needle tract is tan-

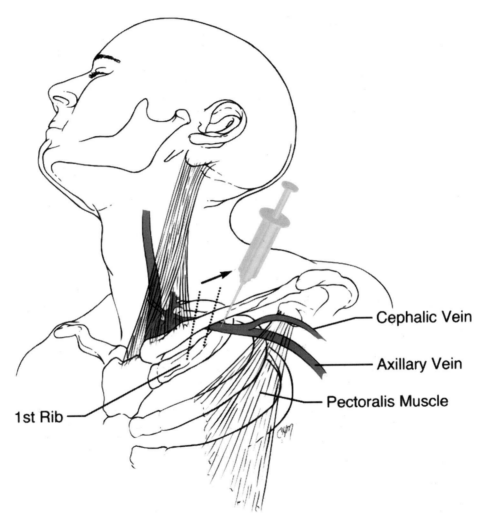

Figure 25. Byrd's technique for access of the extrathoracic portion of the subclavian vein. Sequential needle punctures are walked posterolateral along the first rib. Used with permission from Belott PH, et al.[73]

A

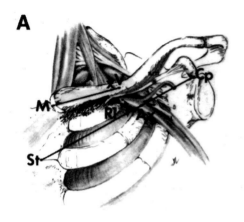

B

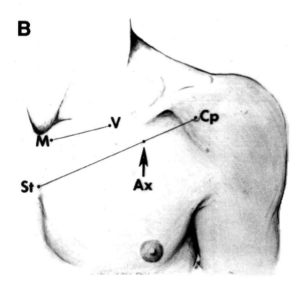

Figure 26. Deep (**A**) and superficial (**B**) anatomic relationships of the Magney approach to subclavian venipuncture. Point M indicates the medial end of the clavicle. X defines a point on the clavicle directly above the lateral edges of the clavicular/subclavius muscle (tendon complex) R1. Point V overlies the center of the subclavian vein as it crosses the first rib. St = center of the sternal angle; Cp = coracoid process: Ax = axillary vein; Star = costoclavicular ligament; Open circle with closed circle inside = costoclavicular ligament; sm = subclavius muscle. The arrow points to Magney's ideal point for venous entry. Used with permission from Magney JE, et al.[39]

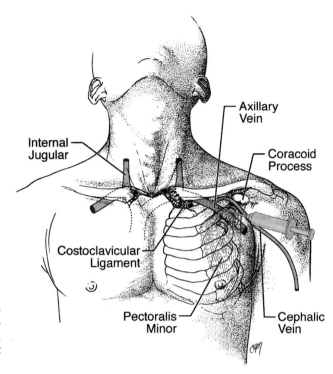

Internal Jugular

Axillary Vein

Coracoid Process

Costoclavicular Ligament

Pectoralis Minor

Cephalic Vein

Figure 27. Needle trajectory for direct axillary vein puncture in relationship to the deltopectoral groove. Used with permission from Belott PH, et al.[74]

gential to the chest wall and parallel to the visualized deltopectoral groove, 1–2 cm medial (Figure 27). If the vein is not entered, fluoroscopy is used to define the first rib (Figures 28, 29). The needle is advanced and touches the first rib and sequential needle punctures are walked laterally and posteriorly until the venous structure is entered.

The axillary vein may also be isolated via direct cutdown (Figure 30). Using Metzenbaum scissors, the fibers of the pectoralis major muscle are separated adjacent to the deltopectoral groove at the level of the coracoid process. This will be just above the level of the superior border of the pectoralis minor. The pectoralis major is split in this area and the fibers are gently teased apart. In an access parallel to the muscle bundles, the axillary vein will be found directly underneath the pectoralis major. A pursestring stitch is applied about the vein and it can be cannulated via either the percutaneous or cutdown approach. A purse-string

stitch will serve for hemostasis and ultimately assist in anchoring the electrode after positioning.

A number of techniques have been developed to assist access for the axillary vein. Varnagy et al. have described a technique for isolating the cephalic and/or axillary vein.[40] This technique consists of introducing a J-ended Teflon guidewire through the vein in the antecubital fossa under fluoroscopic control. The metal guidewire is then palpated in the deltopectoral groove or identified by fluoroscopy (Figure 31). This guides subsequent cutdown or puncture of the vessel by fluoroscopy. The cutdown can be performed on the vein and the intravascular guidewire pulled out of the venotomy to allow application of an introducer. It is felt that this technique offers the benefits of rapid venous access while avoiding the hazards of pneumothorax associated with the percutaneous approach. If the percutaneous approach is used, the puncture can always

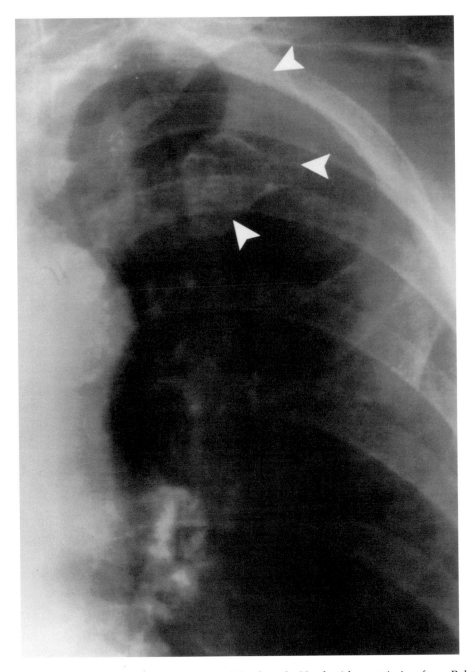

Figure 28. X-ray demonstrating the location of the fist rib. Used with permission from Belott PH, et al.[74]

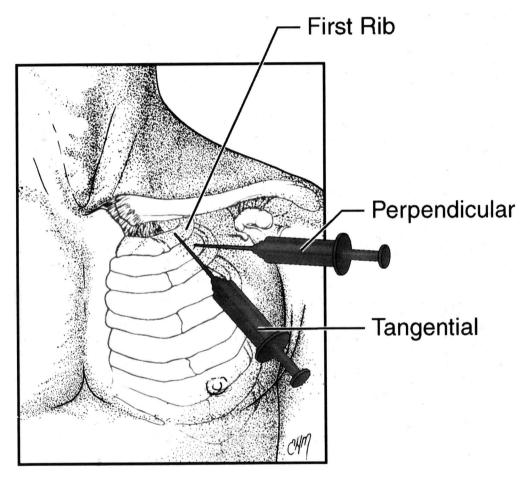

Figure 29. Needle trajectory in relationship to the first rib for axillary vein puncture. Note that when the needle is held tangential, there is little risk of pneumothorax and little risk of entering the intercostal space. Used with permission from Belott PH, et al.[74]

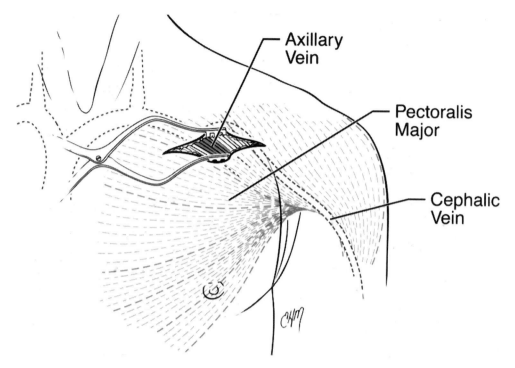

Figure 30. Cutdown on the axillary vein through the pectoralis major and minor muscles. Used with permission from Belott PH, et al.[74]

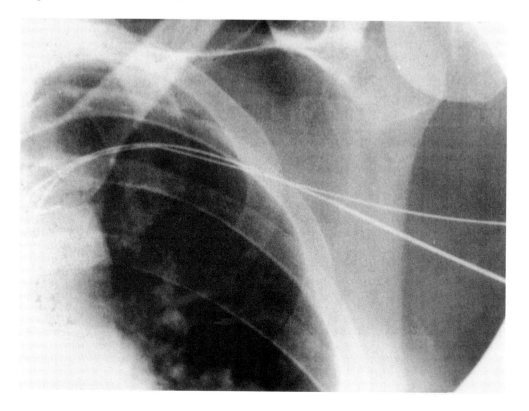

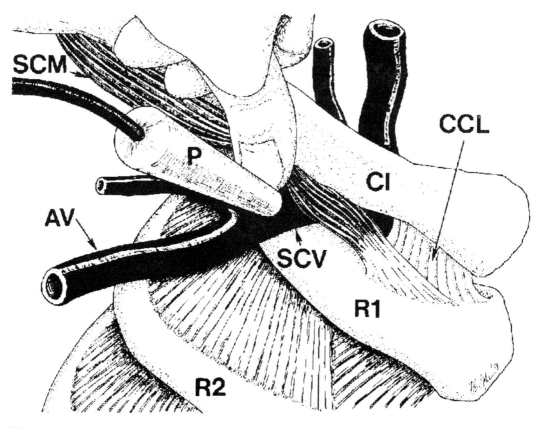

Figure 32. Doppler location of the axillary vein crossing the first rib. AV = axillary vein; CCL = costoclavicular ligament; Cl = clavicle; P = Doppler probe; R1 = first rib; R2 = second rib; SMC = subclavius muscle; SCD = subclavian vein. Used with permission from Fyke FE.[42]

be extrathoracic using fluoroscopy to guide the needle to the guidewire. As previously mentioned, axillary puncture can be facilitated by the use of contrast venography. The venous anatomy can be observed by fluoroscopy in the pectoral area and, if possible, recorded for repeat viewing. The needle trajectory and venipuncture are guided by the contrast material in the axillary vein.[17] Once again, laboratories with sophisticated imaging capabilities can create a mask. Spencer et al. have reported the use of contrast venography for localizing the axillary vein in 22 consecutive patients.[41] More recently, venous access of the axillary vein has been guided by the use of both Doppler and ultrasound. Fyke has described a Doppler-guided extrathoracic introducer insertion technique in 59 consecutive patients with a simple Doppler flow detector.[42] A total of 100 leads were placed by this technique. A sterile Doppler flow detector is moved along the clavicle once the vein is entered, the location and angulation of the probe are noted, and a venipuncture carried out (Figure 32). Care is taken to

Figure 31. Percutaneous access of the axillary vein using a J wire for reference when introduced via the antecubital vein. Used with permission from Belott PH, et al.[74]

avoid directing the beam beneath the clavicle. In this technique, the Doppler probe directs the needle to the venous structure, in this case the axillary vein.

Gayle et al. have developed an ultrasound technique that directly visualizes the needle puncture of the axillary vein.[43] A portable ultrasound device with sterile sleeve and needle holder are used. The ultrasound head is placed over the skin surface in the vicinity of the axillary vein. Once identified, the puncture is directly visualized and the Seldinger guidewire technique used. Since this technique directly visualizes the axillary vein, it has been used with considerable success for both pacing and defibrillator electrodes (Figure 33). There have been no pneumothoraces. The technique can be carried out transcutaneously or through the incision on the surface of the pectoralis muscle (Figure 34).

The axillary vein is becoming a common venous access site for pacemaker and defibrillator implantation, given the concerns of the subclavian crush phenomenon and the requirement for insertion of multiple elec-

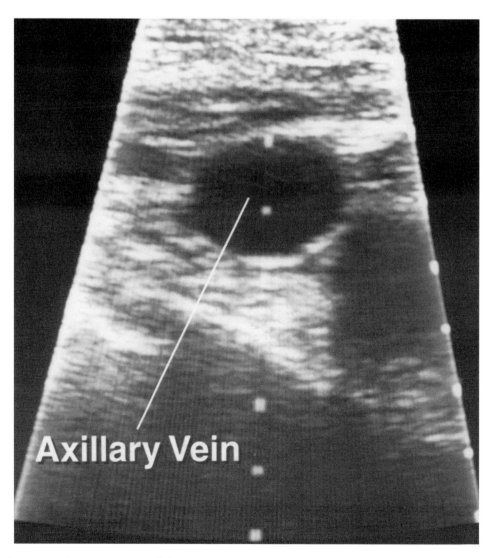

Figure 33. Ultrasonic image of the axillary vein. Used with permission from Gayle DD, et al.[43]

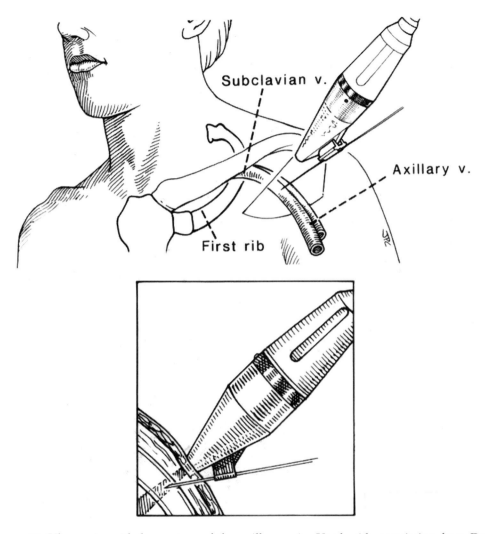

Figure 34. Ultrasonic-guided puncture of the axillary vein. Used with permission from Dymax Corporation, Pittsburgh, PA.

trodes for dual chambered pacing and the large complex electrodes for transvenous defibrillation. There are now a number of reliable techniques for axillary venous access (Table 5). Given the recent interest in the axillary vein, it is recommended that the implanting physician be thoroughly familiar with the anatomy of the anterior thoracic wall, shoulder, and axilla. It is imperative that an interested implanting physician visit the anatomic laboratory to refresh and review the regional anatomy and surface landmarks.

Table 5
Techniques for Axillary Venous Access

I. Blind percutaneous puncture using surface landmarks
II. Blind puncture through pectoralis major muscle using deep landmarks
III. Direct cutdown on the axillary vein
IV. Fluoroscopy: Needle walked along first rib
V. Contrast venography
VI. Doppler-guided
VII. Ultrasound-guided

Jugular Venous Access

The jugular vein has been used for permanent pacemaker implantation as an alternate cutdown site.[44] This is a large venous structure that lies in the cervical triangle defined by the lateral border of the omohyoid muscle, inferior border of the digastric muscle, and the medial border of the sternocleidomastoid (Figure 35). It is covered by the superficial cervical fascia and platysma muscle. It is easily identified because it is just lateral to the external carotid, which is easily palpable. Many authors have described exotic, sophisticated landmarks to define its location, when in reality simple

palpation of the carotid pulse defines the jugular vein. Punctures immediately lateral to the carotid pulse are frequently rewarded with success. Historically, jugular venous access has been considered when the traditional venous cutdown of the cephalic vein has been unsuccessful. This approach is less desirable than the subclavian, axillary, and cephalic vein placement because of the increased risk of lead fracture and potential erosion. The acute angle that is created in the lead after it exits the venous structure as it is brought down over the clavicle to the pacemaker pocket creates circumstances for this problem. Also, this procedure is somewhat more involved as tunneling is re-

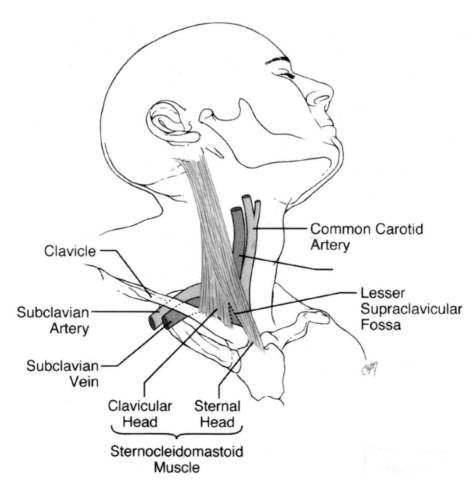

Figure 35. Anatomic relationships of the right internal jugular vein and common carotid artery. Used with permission from Belott PH, et al.[73]

quired to bring the lead to the pacemaker pocket. If tunneling is performed under the clavicle, there is increased risk of vascular injury and pneumothorax. If the lead is tunneled over the clavicle, the tissue is typically thin and there is greater chance for erosion. As a rule, the right internal jugular approach is preferred. However, both right and left internal and external jugular veins have been used. The jugular venous approach usually involves two separate incisions, one above and one below the clavicle.

Initially, the jugular venous approach was by cutdown. An alternative percutaneous technique has been proposed that requires little attention to anatomic landmarks and dissection. Additionally, an initial supraclavicular incision is not required. This approach involves percutaneous access of the right internal jugular vein. Access to the internal jugular vein is best obtained with the patient in a normal anatomic position with the head facing anterior. Rotating the head to the left should be avoided because this distorts the anatomy. The carotid artery is palpated in the lower third of the neck. The internal jugular vein is lateral to the common carotid artery. The two structures are parallel and lie side by side. Addressing the patient on the right side with the right internal jugular approach, the implanting physician places the middle finger along the course of the common carotid artery. The course of the internal jugular will be under the index finger. In fact, the index and middle fingers side by side are generally analogous to the size and orientation on the surface of the skin to the deeper internal jugular vein and common carotid artery, as they run side by side underneath the skin. The venous puncture anywhere along the course should enter the internal jugular vein. Pneumothoraces are usually totally avoided if the puncture is made above the clavicle. The needle is held perpendicular to the plane of the neck rather than angled. This helps avoid infraclavicular puncture and potential pneumothorax. Once the needle has entered the vein, it can be gently angled inferiorly for

passage of the guidewire. If the internal carotid artery is inadvertently punctured, the needle is simply removed and pressure held over the puncture site. A repeat attempt at venipuncture is then made a bit lateral to the initial stick.

Once the guidewire is in place, the technique is essentially identical to the standard procedure. A small incision is carried laterally down the shaft of the needle to the surface of the sternocleidomastoid muscle. If more tissue depth is required, the muscle can be split and the incision carried directly down over the vein. A small Weitlaner retractor is used for more adequate exposure. It is important to place a figure-of-eight suture for vascular control, hemostasis, and anchoring (Figure 36A). The retained guidewire technique may be used for placement of both atrial and ventricular electrodes.

After lead placement, a hemostatic suture is applied and the lead is anchored to the muscle body using the suture sleeves. A second incision for pocket formation is made infraclavicularly. The leads are then tunneled to the pocket by standard tunneling technique (Figure 36B). When the electrodes are tunneled under the clavicle, care must be taken to avoid vascular trauma. Conversely, when tunneling over the clavicle, every effort should be made to ensure optimal tissue depth to avoid potential erosion. The tunneling technique described by Roelke et al. for submammary pacemaker implantation may also be used for infraclavicular tunneling.[59] A long 18-gauge spinal needle can be passed from the infraclavicular incision to the supraclavicular incision. The guidewire is passed, the sheath set applied and tunneled to the supraclavicular incision. The rubber dilator is removed. The lead to be used is inserted in the distal end of the sheath and tied. Once secured, the lead and sheath are pulled through to the infraclavicular incision (see Figure 41). The external jugular vein is less frequently used for venous access as it is more inferiorly located and there is a high risk of pneumothorax and vascular complications. Its location

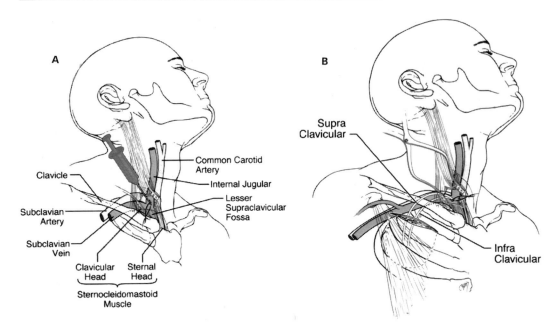

Figure 36. (A) Percutaneous venous access of the right internal jugular vein. Weitlaner retractor placed demonstrating the figure-of-eight stitch. Used with permission from Belott PH, et al.[73] **(B)** Lead(s) tunneled over and under the clavicle to the infraclavicular pocket. Used with permission from Belott PH, et al.[74]

is less precise and successful cannulation more frustrating.

Femoral Venous Access

Venous access in the inguinal area has been reported as an alternate site for pacemaker implantation. If one punctures the venous structure above Poupart's ligament, it is anatomically the iliac vein; below Poupart's ligament, it is designated as the femoral vein. Iliac vein puncture has been reported as an alternate source for single and dual chambered implantation.[45,46] Ellestad and French[45] have reported a 90-patient experience using the iliac vein as an alternative source. This vein can be used for transvenous lead placement when an abdominal pocket is desired. It is usually reserved for patients with little pectoral tissue, such as in the case of bilateral mastectomy, extensive pectoral radiation damage, or for a variety of other cosmetic reasons.

A small incision is made above the inguinal ligament above the vein, just medial to palpable femoral artery (Figure 37). The incision is carried down to the fascia above the vein. The vein is then punctured via the Seldinger sheath-set technique with the guidewire retained for dual chambered implants. A figure-of-eight stitch or purse-string suture is placed for hemostasis. The suture is placed through the fascia, around the lead as it enters the vein. Special long (85 cm) leads are positioned in a conventional manner and secured to the fascia by use of a tie around the suture sleeve and lead. A horizontal incision is made at the second site just lateral to the umbilicus. This is carried down to the surface of the rectus sheath. A pacemaker pocket is created in a conventional manner.

Preparations are then made for tunneling of the leads from the initial incision to the newly created pocket by use of one of the various standard tunneling techniques. Active fixation electrodes are recommended for both atrial and ventricular lead placement. In the Ellestad experience, lead dislodgements have been reported as a major weakness in this approach with 9 of 42, or 21% of atrial, and 5 of 67, or 7% of ventricular leads in the Ellestad-French experience requiring lead repositioning. Venous thrombosis and lead fracture do not appear to be a problem, although the published experience with this approach is relatively small and the latter is difficult to discern. Obviously, the complication of pneumothorax associated with the percutaneous approach does not exist. Similarly, the complication of air embolization is not a problem.

Use of the Coronary Sinus for Cardiac Pacing

The coronary sinus has historically been used for pacing both by design and inadvertently.[47] More recently, the coronary sinus has been used for multi-site pacing. In the past, this has proven to be an extremely

unreliable site for ventricular pacing and has been avoided. In the case of desired atrial pacing, the coronary sinus has proven to be an ideal location. The major problem with coronary sinus pacing has been access and lead stability. Prior to the development of reliable atrial electrodes, the coronary sinus was a popular site for lead placement for atrial pacing. The best position for atrial pacing is the proximal coronary sinus. This is also the least stable position. Special coronary sinus leads have been developed to enhance position stability. These leads generally consist of a flexible elongated tip that reaches deep into the coronary sinus, wedging it into the great cardiac vein for stability. When simultaneous right and left atrial pacing is desired, a distal coronary sinus location has been used. Primary coronary sinus catheterization requires experience. With the growing number of implanting electrophysiologists who use the coronary sinus routinely for their diagnostic studies, this experience has become somewhat of a

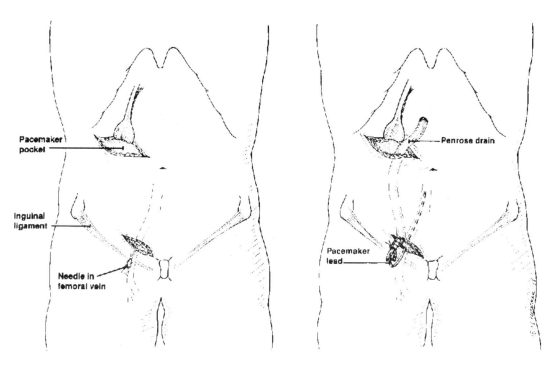

Figure 37. Use of the right iliac vein for placement of pacemaker leads. Used with permission from Ellestad MH, et al.[45]

moot point. In addition, as more pacemaker implantations are performed in the cardiac catheterization laboratory equipped with sophisticated x-ray equipment, including biplane, the required beneficial fluoroscopic projections for placement are more easily achieved. As a rule, placement of a coronary sinus lead is much easier from the left. A generous curve is required on the lead. Coronary sinus placement is confirmed by a posterior lead position on fluoroscopy in the lateral or the left anterior oblique projections. In addition, lead placement will not be associated with ventricular ectopy. As a popular approach to atrial pacing, the coronary sinus is used infrequently today. As bi-atrial pacing becomes more important for control of atrial arrhythmias and four-chamber pacing desirable for the management of cardiomyopathy, there has been a resurgence in the use of the coronary sinus.

Electrode Placement via Anomalous Venous Structures

Occasionally, one encounters a persistent left superior vena cava. Embryonologically, the normal left superior vena cava becomes atretic. There is, however, a 0.5% incidence of structural persistence of patency connected with the coronary sinus. Persistence of the left superior vena cava actually represents failure in the development of the left innominate vein. This vein normally forms by communication of the right and left anterior cardinal veins. In this situation, the left anterior cardinal vein persists and continues to drain into the brachiocephalic veins and sinus venosus. This ultimately develops into a left superior vena cava which empties directly into the coronary sinus (Figure 38A). Normally, the left innominate vein develops as an anastomosis between the left and right anterior cardinal veins. It should be noted that frequently with persistent left superior vena cava, there is an associated atresia and complete absence of the right superior vena caval system (Figure

38B). In 10%–15% of patients, one will encounter a totally absent right superior vena cava. In this situation, venous access for pacing from the right is virtually impossible. Despite the fact that there are reported classic physical and radiographic findings, the diagnosis is generally discovered unexpectedly at the time of pacemaker or ICD implantation.

Placement of electrodes via a persistent left superior vena cava can prove extremely challenging if not impossible.[48-53] A fair knowledge of anatomy and radiographic orientation is essential. If one proceeds from the left and is confronted with a persistent left superior vena cava, it must be appreciated that lead or leads are actually advanced into the coronary sinus and out its ostium into the right atrium. If the right ventricular apical positions are to be achieved, the lead must then be negotiated at an acute angle to cross the tricuspid valve. This is best accomplished by having the lead form a large loop on itself using the lateral right atrial wall for support (Figure 38C). This maneuver can prove to be extremely challenging. Depending on anatomy, occasionally such efforts will prove unsuccessful, and changing the sites of venous access must be considered. At this point, it is prudent to assess the patency of the right venous system with contrast and angiographic techniques.[54] If one encounters a persistent left superior vena cava, an assessment of the right superior vena cava via contrast injection may prove helpful. This can be carried out by advancing a standard end-hole catheter from the left superior vena cava to the vicinity of the right superior vena cava. Occasionally, such communication does not exist. If the right superior vena cava is absent, the iliac vein approach, as previously described by Ellestad, or one of the epicardial approaches is recommended.

In the case of a persistent left vena cava where an atrial electrode is required, a positive fixation screw-in electrode is recommended (Figure 38C).[55,56] The use of a preformed atrial J will prove difficult if not

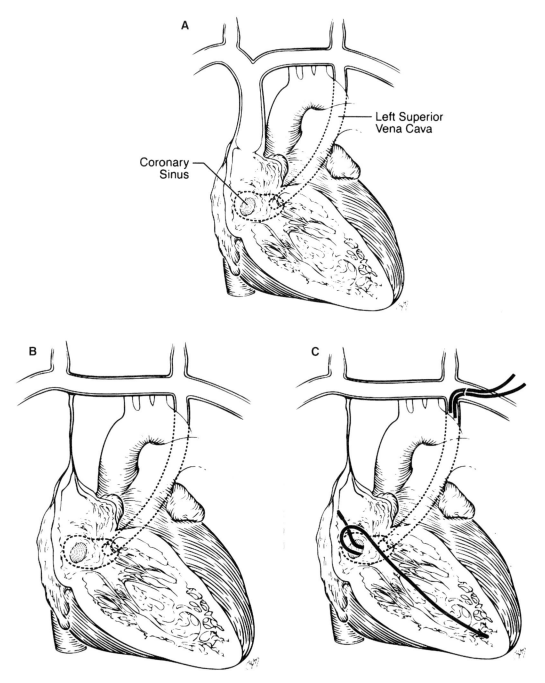

Figure 38. (A) Persistent left superior vena cava. **(B)** Persistent left superior vena cava with absent right superior vena cava. **(C)** Placement of atrial and ventricular electrodes via persistent left superior vena cava and absent right superior vena cava. Used with permission from Belott PH, et al.[74]

impossible. Dislodgement of the preformed J is also a concern. When using a positive fixation electrode, careful mapping and high-output studies should be carried out to avoid pacing of the right phrenic nerve. As a rule, the anterior right atrial position is preferred. An absent right superior vena cava from a right- sided approach will also require changing approach sites. In this case, the expected venous tortuosity of the persistent left superior vena cava should alert one to request longer electrodes; at times an 85-cm lead will be required. Again, it is advisable to use positive fixation leads in anticipation of dislodgement problems.

Permanent pacemakers have also been implanted using the inferior vena cava via a retroperitoneal approach. West et al. reported the case of a 48-year-old male with congenital heart disease.[57] The patient had undergone multiple procedures to correct transposition of the great vessels with a functional single ventricle and subvalvular pulmonic stenosis. The patient had multiple surgical procedures, including a palliative Blalock shunt and Glenn procedure. At age 47, the patient developed complete AV block. Given the complex congenital anomalies and subsequent corrective procedures, venous access to the right atrium and ventricle was complicated by loss of continuity between the right atrium and the superior vena cava. This precluded a standard transvenous access. An epicardial approach was also less desirable, given the patient's multiple surgical procedures. It was elected to perform a retroperitoneal approach via a transvenous right flank incision. The inferior vena cava was infiltrated and cannulated retroperitoneally (Figure 39). Bipolar active fixation screw-in electrodes were used in both the atrium and the ventricle. The venous insertion site was secured and hemostasis effected by purse-sting sutures. The pulse generator was implanted and the subcutaneous pocket formed in the anterior abdominal wall.

In a similar approach, pacemaker leads have been placed via transhepatic cannulation. Fischberger et al. have reported percu-taneous transhepatic cannulation via fluo-roscopic guidance. Once venous access has been achieved percutaneously with the guidewire transhepatically, a sheath set is applied, allowing the subsequent introduction of a permanent pacing electrode. This procedure has been reserved for complex congenital anomalies that preclude venous access via a superior vein and avoids an unnecessary thoracotomy.

Inframammary Implantation for Optimal Cosmetic Effect

The use of the principles of plastic surgery for standard pacemaker implantation can be adapted for optimal cosmetic effect.[58] This is of particular value in young women. The technique involves more surgery and is best performed under modified or complete general anesthesia. Because of more postoperative wound pain, an overnight stay is also advised. The procedure lends itself well to the percutaneous approach for both single and dual chambered pacing. After the subclavian vein has been accessed, a limited 1–2 cm initial incision is made. This incision is carried to the surface of the pectoralis muscle, allowing enough room to secure the electrode with the suture sleeves. A second incision is then made under the breast along the breast fold. A standard pacemaker pocket is created under the breast (Figure 40). Care is taken to stay on top of the pectoralis fascia. The pocket is carefully inspected for hemostasis. A tract from the pacemaker pocket to the initial incision is infiltrated with local anesthesia. The proximal connector pin is then brought to the inframammary pocket using standard tunneling techniques. The proximal connector pin can be placed in a Penrose drain and tied. A long clamp is then passed from the inframammary pocket to the initial incision. The Penrose drain with electrode is then grasped and pulled to the pacemaker pocket. The pulse generator and electrodes are connected and the incision closed. It is recommended that a Parsonnet (C.R. Bard,

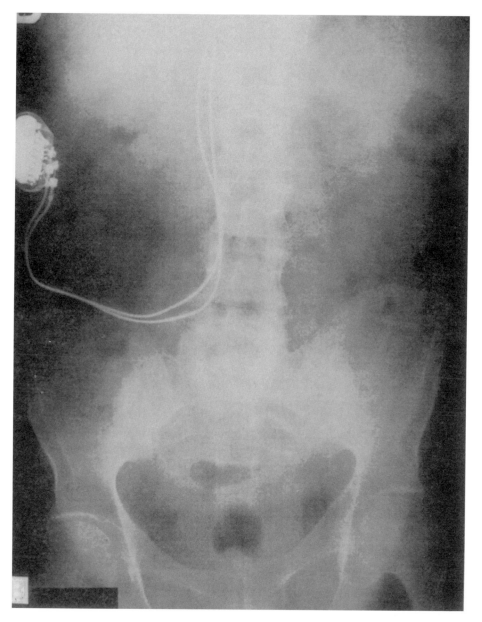

Figure 39. Posterior-anterior abdominal x-ray showing the position of the pacemaker and the generator lead inserted into the inferior vena cava. Used with permission from West JNW, et al.[57]

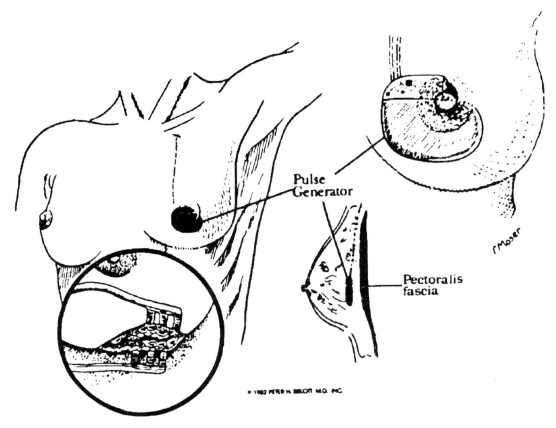

Figure 40. Inframammary incision and placement of pulse generator with tunneled electrodes. Used with permission from Belott PH, et al.[11]

Inc., Billerica, NE) pouch be used to avoid rotation of the pulse generator and leads under the breast tissue. In addition, a bipolar pacing system is essential to avoid pectoralis muscle stimulation.

An alternate approach calls for a second incision made in the axilla with the arm in abduction. The incision is carried to a depth that exposes the muscular fascia. In this case, the pulse generator is placed subpectorally. Roelke et al. have described a submammary pacemaker implantation technique that uses unique tunneling.[59] In this technique, a 1-cm horizontal incision is made over the deltopectoral groove 1 cm inferior to the clavicle. A percutaneous subclavian puncture for cephalic vein cutdown for venous access is then carried out. The electrodes are positioned and anchored. A

2–3 cm horizontal incision is made under the medial third of the inframammary crease. The incision is carried down to the level of the pectoralis fascia and blunt dissection is used to create a pocket superficial to the pectoralis fascia behind the breast. A 20-cm, 18-gauge pericardiocentesis needle is directed from the inframammary pocket to the infraclavicular incision. A J guidewire is then passed from the submammary pocket through the needle and infraclavicular incision. The needle is removed, and using the retained guidewire technique, two 10F introducer dilators are passed consecutively over the guidewire. The free ends of the atrial and ventricular electrodes from the infraclavicular incision are placed in the sheaths and secured with a tie (Figure 41). The sheath sets are then withdrawn to the inframammary pocket. This innovative tunneling technique has been extremely successful and well tolerated.

Shefer et al. have described a retropectoral transaxillary percutaneous technique for optimal cosmetic effect.[60] This technique is performed under local anesthesia and conscious sedation. Venography is used to confirm the relationship of the axillary vein to surface anatomy. A marker is then placed in the axillary vein via the antecubital fossa (Figure 42A). This usually consists of temporary transvenous pacing wire or a 0.032 mm guidewire. The patient is then prepped and draped about the ipsilateral axilla. Under local anesthesia and fluoroscopic control, a 16-gauge thin-walled needle is inserted and guided medially in a cranial and anterior direction to meet and cross the temporary pacing wire marker in the axillary vein (Figure 42B). The axillary vein is punctured when the tip of the needle touches and moves the marker wire. Venipuncture is confirmed by aspiration of venous blood. A 0.038 guidewire is then introduced and the needle discarded. A longitudinal incision is made along the posterior border of the pectoralis muscle in the axilla (Figure 43A). The pectoralis fascia is then exposed by blunt dissection and the retropectoral space opened. One or two pacing electrodes can then be placed by conventional techniques. The electrodes are secured by their suture sleeve to the pectoralis fascia. The

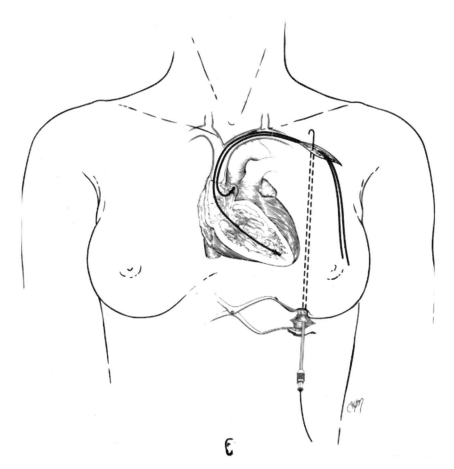

Figure 41. Subcutaneous tunneling with guidewire and sheath. Redrawn and used with permission from Roelke M, et al.[59]

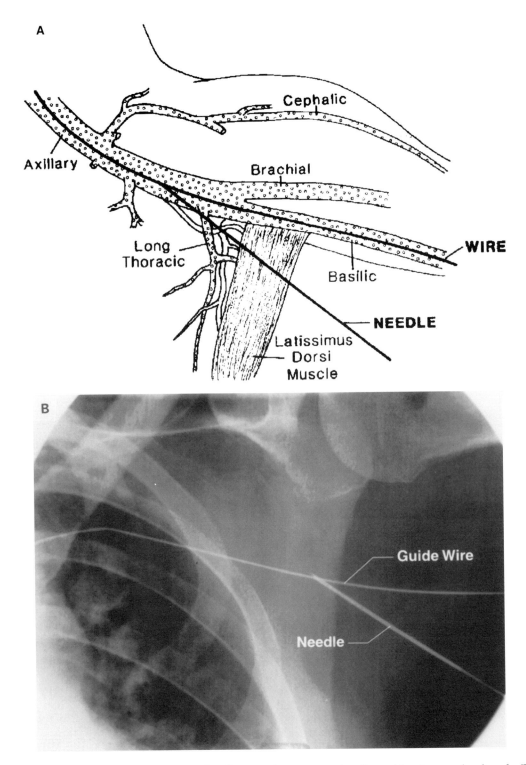

Figure 42. (A) Stylized illustration of axillary venipuncture using the guidewire as a landmark. **(B)** X-ray of needle accessing the axillary vein using the guidewire as a landmark. Used with permission from Shefer A, et al.[60]

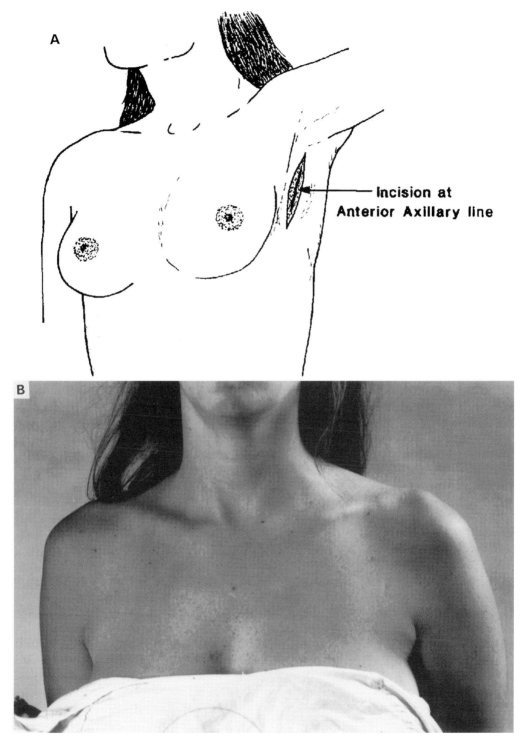

Figure 43. (A) Anterior axillary incision. **(B)** Frontal view of patient after transaxillary retropectoral pacemaker implantation. There are no visible scars. Used with permission from Shefer A, et al.[60]

leads are then connected to the pacemaker and inserted in the retropectoral pocket. At completion of the case, the temporary pacing lead and guidewire marker are removed. This technique offers optimal cosmetic result (Figure 43B), and there has been no restriction in physical activity or movement of the shoulder joint.

Epicardial Electrode Placement

At one time, epicardial pacemaker electrode placement was the implant technique of choice. It required extensive surgery and general anesthesia. In recent times, transvenous implantation techniques have replaced this approach. Today, epicardial lead placement is reserved for those patients undergoing cardiac surgery. This is largely due to the safety and efficacy of the transvenous approach. Epicardial systems are also frequently associated with patient discomfort from the abdominal location of the pacemaker pulse generator. Today, only rare and unusual circumstances result in an epicardial implant. These include patients undergoing cardiac surgery, patients with recurrent transvenous dislodgings, and patients with a prosthetic tricuspid valve or a congenital anomaly such as tricuspid atresia.

Epicardial approach does offer the advantage of mapping for ideal pacing thresholds and other electrophysiological parameters. The electrodes are directly attached to epicardium and pulled to a subcutaneous pocket, usually in the upper abdomen. There are three distinct epicardial approaches (Figure 44): the subxiphoid, the left subcostal, and the left anterolateral thoracotomy.[61] The subxiphoid and the left subcostal preclude a thoracotomy. The subxiphoid approach exposes the diaphragmatic surface of the heart and right ventricle. At times, the right ventricle is extremely thin and care should be taken to avoid laceration that may require a more extensive tho-

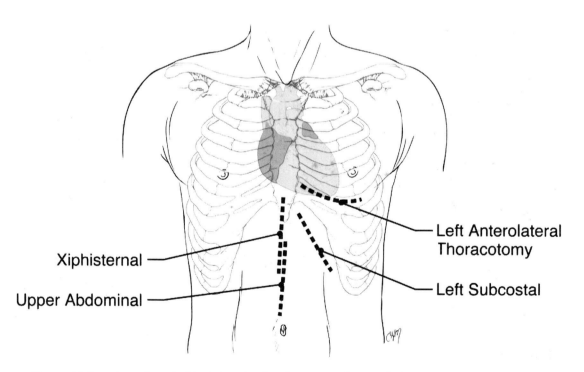

Figure 44. Location of surgical incisions for the placement of epicardial systems. Used with permission from Belott PH, et al.[73]

racotomy and even cardiopulmonary by-pass. The left subcostal and anterolateral thoracotomy utilize the left ventricle for electrode placement. General anesthesia is required for all epicardial pacemaker implantation techniques. In addition, these procedures are performed in the operating room by the cardiothoracic surgeon.

Transthoracic Endocardial Lead Placement

Transvenous endocardial lead placement is occasionally impractical, impossible, or contraindicated. Westerman and van der Vanter have described a transthoracic technique requiring general anesthesia and a limited thoracotomy for electrode placement.[62] The pacemaker electrodes are passed and positioned transatrially through the sixth intercostal space. The right atrium is identified and the electrode is passed transatrially through an incision or by using a sheath set. Hemostasis is effected by a purse-string suture about the entry site. Fluoroscopy can be used for ventricular placement of a tined or screw-in electrode. All electrodes are then secured to the endocardial surface. Sutures placed under the tines secure the electrode. The electrodes are then driven through an atriotomy into the atrial cavity and out the atrial muscles at a point of desired endocardial fixation. The electrodes are pulled through the incision and snugged to the endocardium by pulling and tying the double-ended suture (Figure 45). This approach has been recommended over the epicardial approach as better thresholds may be achieved. Once again, this approach is extremely useful in the pediatric population with complex congenital anomalies.

Hayes et al. have described a similar technique of endocardial atrial electrode placement at the time of corrective cardiac surgery.[63] In this procedure, epicardial pacing was avoided because of poor pacing and sensing thresholds. Traditionally, at the time of cardiac surgery, the patient requiring a dual chamber system would receive epicardial ventricular electrodes. The atrial electrode was placed transvenously later in hospitalization. In the postoperative period, a dual chamber system appeared crucial for optimal hemodynamics. In the Hayes et al. technique, a dual chamber pacemaker patient with severe tricuspid regurgitation and chronic endocardial electrodes required removal of all endocardial electrodes and placement of a prosthetic tricuspid valve. New epicardial electrodes were placed on the ventricle. Stable atrial pacing and sensing was achieved by transatrial endocardial placement in the atrial appendage (Figure 46). In the Hayes case, the lead was secured by purse-string ligatures about the incision.

Byrd has described an alternate technique to the standard epicardial approach in five patients.[64] This technique allows for conventional transvenous electrodes to be implanted in patients requiring an epicardial approach. It has been used in patients with superior vena cava syndrome, anomalous pulmonary venous drainage, or in younger patients with innominate vein thrombosis. The technique involves a limited surgical approach under general anesthesia. A small 4–5 cm incision is made in the third or fourth intercostal space. The third and fourth costal cartilages are excised and the right atrial appendage exposed. An atriotomy is performed and the introducer placed inside an atrial purse-string suture and secured in a vertical position. The atrial and ventricular electrodes are passed down a standard sheath set into the atrium (Figure 47). Using standard techniques, including fluoroscopy, the electrodes are positioned. Once the electrodes are positioned, the introducer is removed and the purse-string suture used to close the atriotomy and secure the electrodes. The pacemaker is placed in a pocket created adjacent to the incision on the right anterior chest wall. This technique offers the advantage of implantation of a conventional system with minimal morbidity, compared to the standard epicardial implantation. The chest is never entered and the time required for such a procedure is similar to the transvenous approach. The technique, however, requires general anesthesia, violation of the epicardium, and an obligatory right-sided approach.

Recently, Schaerf et al. have described a thoracoscopic approach for implantation of cardioverter-defibrillator epicardial patches as well as myocardial pacing electrodes.[65] Thoracoscopy is generally used for pulmonary procedures and thoracoscopic pericardiotomy and drainage of pericardial spaces.

The technique uses small intercostal incisions and hollowed trocars that are placed at entry sites in the chest cavity. When compared to a thoracotomy, thoracoscopy is less invasive and the postoperative recovery time is generally swift. It can be performed easily on an outpatient basis. Schaerf et al. have demonstrated that implantable cardioverter-defibrillator epicardial patches and sutureless myocardial pacing electrodes can safely be implanted via the thoracoscopic approach. The electrodes and patches are

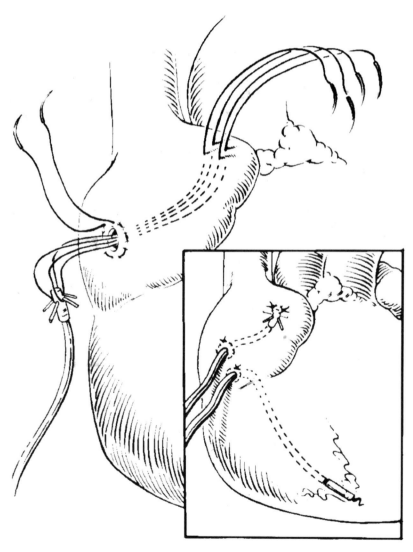

Figure 45. Atrial lead placement through atriotomy and purse-string suture. Atrial and ventricular electrodes positioned and atriotomies secured. Used with permission from Belott PH, et al.[11]

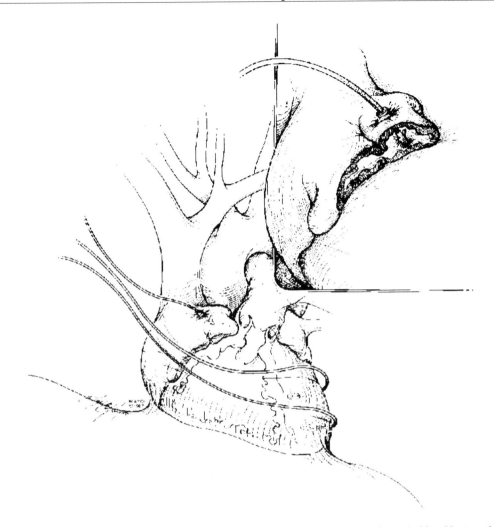

Figure 46. Atrial lead placement. Inset: In the upper right shows atrial endocardial lead being placed through the wall of the right atrial appendage with the tip of the pacemaker lead abutting endocardial surface. A purse- string suture is placed around the lead at the point of entry. Relationship atrial leads is also shown. Used with permission from The Mayo Foundation, Hayes DL, et al.[63]

not damaged when placed through the required trocars. The approach appears to reduce morbidity because it does not entail retraction of the ribs, subxiphoid, or sternum. The incisions are small and there is minimal associated pain. When compared to a subxiphoid approach, there is excellent exposure and visibility. Compared to transvenous implants, long subcutaneous tunneling is unnecessary. This approach, with its limited surgery, also offers potential patient benefit with shorter operating times, lower hospital costs, and an outpatient ap-

plication. More recently, since thoracoscopy is much less invasive than thoracotomy, it is an ideal technique for biventricular pacing and end-stage dilated cardiomyopathy that requires the placement of a left ventricular lead.

Ambulatory Pacemaker Procedures

In the early days of cardiac pacing, the pulse generators were large, surgery more

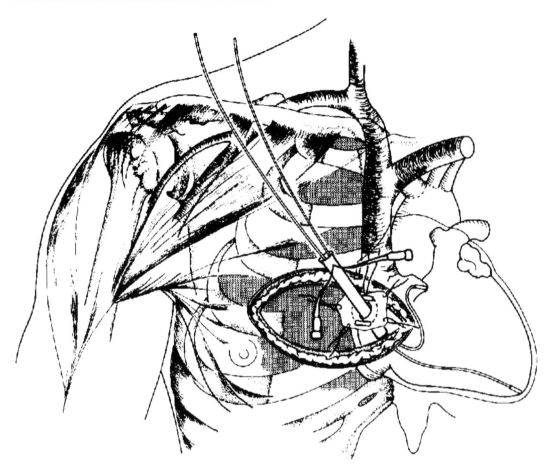

Figure 47. This limited surgical approach consists of the resection of the third costal cartilage through a small incision, reflection of the pleura, and opening of the pericardium. An introducer and transvenous leads are inserted through a right atrial purse-string suture. The leads are positioned in the right ventricle and right atrium using standard fluoroscopic techniques. Through the incision, the subcutaneous pocket is constructed over the pectoralis muscle on the right anterior chest wall in its normal position. The leads are connected to the pacemaker without the need for an adapter or tunneling. Used with permission from Byrd CL, et al.[64]

Table 6
Ambulatory Pacemaker Procedure Analysis 1983–1995

														Total
Year	83	84	85	86	87	88	89	90	91	92	93	94	95	
TP	99	102	112	110	112	123	100	107	135	119	145	113	97	1474
TA	34	34	56	60	78	87	70	87	124	94	128	104	87	1043
TRUE	8	16	44	56	78	86	68	83	124	90	125	102	87	967
<24	26	18	12	4	0	1	2	4	0	4	3	2	0	76
% AMB	34	34	50	60	69	70	70	77	91	78	88	92	88	69

TP = total procedures (all procedures performed); TA = total ambulatory (true ambulatory plus those discharged <24 hours); TRUE = true ambulatory (admitted and discharged on the same day); <24 = <24-hour (admitted and discharged the following morning); % AMB = percent ambulatory per year.

involved, and catastrophic complications, such as lead dislodgement, perforation, and wound infection, and frequent hospitalizations were usually prolonged. The prospect of a brief hospital stay appeared heretic and unthinkable. Today, where experience is high and surgery is limited, complications are rare. Most importantly, the major concerns over lead dislodgement and potential asystole are virtually nonexistent with positive fixation electrode systems and reliable pulse generators. If one actually reflects on the current pacemaker populations, truly pacemaker-dependent patients are few and far between. The patients are generally worked up on an ambulatory basis with symptoms of presyncope and syncope that are detected by outpatient ambulatory monitoring. They are subsequently admitted to the hospital for permanent pacemaker placement. If this procedure were performed on an ambulatory basis and one experienced total failure, the worst that would occur is a patient who is no better off than prior to the procedure. Today, where the issues of cost containment are at their highest, the prospects of an ambulatory pacemaker procedure are very attractive.

The safety and efficacy of this approach have been demonstrated both in Europe and in the United States.[66–68] Recently, Belott has reported a 13-year experience with ambulatory pacemaker procedures.[69] The original concerns over pacemaker complications clearly are unfounded.[70–73] In the United States today, despite the obvious potential financial benefits, these issues have yet to be clearly sorted out. In the United States, financial incentives would continue to support an inpatient admission for optimal hospital reimbursement. At the same time, the third-party carrier, more specifically Medicare, benefits the least. In addition, when forced to perform procedures on an ambulatory basis, the current situation requires the patient to contribute a 20% co-pay of the overall bill. This clearly further supports the inpatient approach to permanent pacemaker procedures.

As previously mentioned, the Belott experience now stands over 13 years with over 1,474 pacemaker procedures, of which 1,043 have been performed on an ambulatory basis (Table 6). Of these procedures, 967 were performed on a true ambulatory basis with the patient admitted and discharged on the same day. It would appear that over the 13-year period, 69% of all pacemaker procedures were ambulatory. From 1990 to 1995, 85% of procedures were ambulatory. There were no pacemaker deaths or emergencies. There are two axioms that have been borne out from this experience. First, if there are any doubts or concerns, any patient's hospitalization can be extended; and second, it is felt that any operator is always truly aware of the problem patient, and for such a patient who has potentially sustained a complication, their hospitalization can always be extended. Given the gratifying results of this 13-year experience, all elective permanent pacemaker procedures at our pacemaker center are performed on an ambulatory basis. This includes new implants, electrode repositions, upgrade procedures, electrode extractions, and pulse generator changes.

References

1. Schecter DC. Modern era of artificial cardiac pacemakers. In Schecter DC. Electrical Cardiac Stimulation. Medtronic Inc, Minneapolis, 1983, pp 110–134.
2. Furman S, Schwedel JB. An intracardiac pacemaker for Stokes-Adams seizures. N Engl J Med 1959;261:948.
3. Senning A. Discussion of a paper by Stephenson SE Jr, et al. Physiologic patient-wave stimulator. J Thorac Cardiovasc Surg 1959;38:639.
4. Littleford PO, Spector SD. Device for the rapid insertion of permanent endocardial pacing electrode through the subclavian vein: preliminary report. Ann Thorac Surg 1979;27:265.
5. Smyth NPD. Techniques of implantation. Atrial and ventricular thoracotomy and

transvenous. Progr Cardiovasc Dis 1981;23: 435.

6. Smyth NPD. Pacemaker implantation. Surgical techniques. Cardiovasc Clin 1983;14:31.

7. Netter FH. Atlas of Human Anatomy, fifth printing. Ciba Geigy Medical Education, West Caldwell, 1992, pp 174–176, 186, 200, 201.

8. Netter FH. The Ciba Collection of Medical Illustrations, volume 5, Heart, Ciba Medical Education Division, Summit, 1981, pp 22–26.

9. Byrd C. Current clinical applications of dual chamber pacing. In Zipes DP, ed. Proceedings of a Symposium. Medtronics, Inc, Minneapolis, 1981, p 71.

10. Littleford PO, Spector SD. Device for the rapid insertion of permanent endocardial pacing electrodes through the subclavian vein. Preliminary report. Ann Thorac Surg 1979;27:265.

11. Belott PH, Byrd CL. Recent developments in pacemaker implantation and lead retrieval. In Barold SS, Mugica J, eds. New Perspectives in Cardiac Pacing, 2. Futura Publishing Co Inc, Mount Kisco, NY, 1991, pp 105–131.

12. Belott PH. Implantation techniques: new developments. In Barold SS, Mugica J, eds. New Perspectives in Cardiac Pacing. Futura Publishing Co. Inc, Mount Kisco, NY, 1988, pp 258–259.

13. Parsonnet V, Bernstein AD, Lindsay B. Pacemaker implantation complication rates. An analysis of some contributing factors. J Am Coll Cardiol 1989;13:917.

14. Furman S. Venous cutdown for pacemaker implantation. Ann Thorac Surg 1986;41:438.

15. Furman S. Subclavian puncture for pacemaker lead placement. PACE 1986;9:467.

16. Belott PH. A Practical Approach to Permanent Pacemaker Implantation. Futura Publishing Co, Inc, Mount Kisco, NY, 1995, pp 59–63.

17. Higano ST, Hayes DS, Spittell PC. Facilitation of the subclavian introducer technique with contrast venography. PACE 1992;15:731.

18. Parsonnet V, Werres R, Atherly T, et al. Transvenous insertion of double sets of permanent electrodes. JAMA 1980;243:62.

19. Bognolo PA, Vijayanagar RR, Eckstein PR, et al. Two leads in one introducer technique for A-V sequential implantation. PACE 1982;5: 217.

20. Vandersalm TJ, Haffajee CI, Okike ON. Transvenous insertion of double sets of permanent electrodes through a single introducer: clinical application. Ann Thorac Surg 1981;32:307.

21. Belott PH. A variation on the introducer

technique for unlimited access to the subclavian vein. PACE 1981;4:43.

22. Gessman LJ, Gallagher JD, Mac Millan, et al. Emergency guidewire pacing: new methods for rapid conversion of a cardiac catheter into a pacemaker. PACE 1984;7:917.

23. Belott PH. Retained guidewire introducer technique, for unlimited access to the central circulation: a review. Clin Prog Electrophysiol Pacing 1981;1:59.

24. Ong LS, Barold S, Lederman M, et al. Cephalic vein guidewire technique for implantation of permanent pacemakers. Am Heart J 1987;114:753.

25. Bognolo DA, Vijaranagar RR, Eckstein PF. Method for reintroduction of permanent endocardial pacing electrodes. PACE 1982;5: 546.

26. Bognolo DA, Vijay R, Eckstein P, et al. Technical aspects of pacemaker system upgrading procedures. Clin Prog Electrophysiol Pacing 1983;1:269.

27. Belott PH. Use of the contralateral subclavian vein for placement of atrial electrodes in chronically VVI paced patients. PACE 1983;6:781.

28. Fyke FE III. Simultaneous insulation deterioration associated with side- by-side subclavian placement of two polyurethane leads. PACE 1988;11:1971.

29. Stokes K, Staffeson D, Lessar J, et al. A possible new complication of the subclavian stick: conductor fracture. PACE 1987;10:748.

30. Subclavian venipuncture reconsidered as a means of implanting endocardial pacing leads. Issues Intermedics, Inc. December 1987, pp 1–2.

31. Subclavian puncture may result in lead conductor fracture. Medtronic News XVI:27, 1986/87.

32. Fyke FE III. Infraclavicular lead failure. Tarnish on a golden route, editorial comment. PACE 1993;16:445.

33. Jacobs DM, Fink AS, Miller RP, et al. Anatomical and morphological evaluation of pacemaker lead compression. PACE 1993;16: 373.

34. Magney JE, Flynn DM, Parsons JA, et al. Anatomical mechanisms explaining damage to pacemaker leads, defibrillator leads, and failure of central venous catheters adjacent to the sternoclavicular joint. PACE 1993;16:445.

35. Byrd CL. Safe introducer technique for pacemaker lead implantation. PACE 1992;15:262.

36. Nichalls RWD. A new percutaneous infraclavicular approach to the axillary vein. Anesthesia 1987;42:151.

37. Taylor Yellowlees I. Central venous cannulation using the infraclavicular axillary vein. Anesthesiology 1990;72:55.

38. Byrd CL. Clinical experience with the extrathoracic introducer insertion technique. PACE 1993;16:1781.

39. Magney JE, Staplin DH, Flynn DM, et al. A new approach to percutaneous subclavian venipuncture to avoid lead fracture or central venous catheter occlusion. PACE 1993; 16:2133.

40. Varnagy G, Vasquez R, Navarro D. New technique for the cephalic vein approach in pacemaker implants. PACE 1995;18:1807A.

41. Spencer W, III, Kirkpatrick C, Zhu DWX. The value of venogram-guided percutaneous extrathoracic subclavian venipuncture for lead implantation. PACE 1996;19:700A.

42. Fyke FE III. Doppler-guided extrathoracic introducer insertion. PACE 1995;18:1017.

43. Gayle DD, Bailey JR, Haistey WK, et al. A novel ultrasound-guided approach to the puncture of the extrathoracic subclavian vein for surgical lead placement. PACE 1996; 19:700.

44. Said SA, Bucx JJ, Stassen CM. Failure of subclavian venipuncture: the internal jugular vein as a useful alternative. Int J Cardiol 1992;35:275.

45. Ellestad MH, French J. Iliac vein approach to permanent pacemaker implantation. PACE 1986;12:1030.

46. Antonelli D, Freedberg NA, Rosenfeld T. Transiliac vein approach to a rate-responsive permanent pacemaker implantation. PACE 1993;16:1751.

47. Bai Y, Strathmore N, Mond H, et al. Permanent ventricular pacing via the great cardiac vein. PACE 1994;17.

48. Dosios T, Gorgogiannis D, Sakorafas G, et al. Persistent left superior vena cava. A problem in transvenous pacing of the heart. PACE 1991;14:389.

49. Hussaine SA, Chalcravarty S, Chaikhouni A. Congenital absence of superior vena cava: unusual anomaly of superior systemic veins complicating pacemaker placement. PACE 1981;4:328.

50. Ronnevik PK, Abrahamsen AM, Tollefsen J. Transvenous pacemaker implantation via a unilateral left superior vena cava. PACE 1982;5:808.

51. Cha EM, Khoury GH. Persistent left superior vena cava. Radiology 1972;103:375.

52. Colman AL. Diagnosis of left superior vena cava by clinical inspection: a new physical sign. Am Heart J 1967;73:115.

53. Dirix LY, Kersscochot IE, Fiernens H, et al. Implantation of a dual chambered pacemaker in a patient with persistent left superior vena cava. PACE 1988;11:343.

54. Giovanni QV, Piepoli M, Pietro Q, et al. Cardiac pacing in unilateral left superior vena cava: evaluation by digital angiography. PACE 1991;14:1567.

55. Robbens EJ, Ruiter JH. Atrial pacing via unilateral persistent left superior vena cava. PACE 1986;9:594.

56. Hellestrand KJ, Ward DE, Bexton RS, et al. The use of active fixation electrodes for permanent endocardial pacing via a persistent left superior vena cava. PACE 1982;5:180.

57. West JNW, Shearmann CP, Gammange MD. Permanent pacemaker positioning via the inferior vena cava in a case of single ventricle with loss of right atrial-vena cava continuity. PACE 1993;16:1753.

58. Belott PH, Bucko D. Inframammary pulse generator placement for maximizing optimal cosmetic effect. PACE 1983;6:1241.

59. Roelke M, Jackson G, Hawthorne JW. Submammary pacemaker implantation. A unique tunneling technique. PACE 1994;17: 1793.

60. Shefer A, Lewis SB, Gang ES. The retropectoral transaxillary permanent pacemaker: description of a technique for percutaneous implantation of an invisible device. PACE 1996;16:1646.

61. Hayes DL, Holmes R Jr, Furman S, eds. A Practice of Cardiac Pacing. 3rd ed. Futura Publishing Co, Inc, Mount Kisco, NY, 1993, pp 271–274.

62. Westerman GR, Van Dervanter SH. Transthoracic transatrial endocardial lead placement for permanent pacing. Ann Thorac Surg 1987;43:445.

63. Hayes DL, Vliestra RE, Puga FJ, et al. A novel approach to atrial endocardial pacing. PACE 1989;12:125.

64. Byrd CL. Transatrial implantation of transvenous pacing leads as an alternative to implantation of epicardial leads. RBM 1990; 12:60.

65. Schaerf R, Biderman P, Weigel RB. Thoracoscopic implantation of ICD epicardial patches and myocardial pacing leads: potential alternative to major thoracic procedures. Medtronic News 21,46.

66. Zegelman M, Kreyzer J, Wagner R. Ambulatory pacemaker surgery: medical and economical advantages. PACE 1986;9:1299.

67. Belott PH. Outpatient pacemaker procedures. Int J Cardiol 1987;17:169.

68. Belott PH. Ambulatory pacemaker procedures: editorial. Mayo Clin Proc 1988;63:301.

69. Belott PH. Ambulatory pacemaker procedures: a 13-year experience. PACE 1996;19: 699.

70. Hayes DL, Vliestra RE, Trusty JM, et al. Can pacemaker implantation be done as an outpatient? J Am Coll Cardiol 1986;7:199.

71. Hayes DL, Vliestra RE, Trusty JM, et al. A

shorter hospital stay after cardiac pacemaker implantation. Mayo Clin Proc 1988;63:236.

72. Haywood GA, Jones SM, Camm AJ, et al. Day case permanent pacing. PACE 1991;14:773.

73. Belott PH, Reynolds CW. Permanent pacemaker implantation. In Ellenbogen K, Wilkoff B, et al, eds. Clinical Cardiac Pacing. WB Saunders, Philadelphia, 1995, pp 460–483.

74. Belott PH. Unusual access sites for permanent cardiac pacing. In Barold SS, Mujica J, eds. Recent Advances in Cardiac Pacing: Goals for the 21st Century, Vol. 4. Futura Publishing Co., Inc, Armonk, NY, 1998, pp 137–180.

75. Belott PH. A Practical Approach to Permanent Pacemaker Implantation. A videotape and manual. Futura Publishing Co., Inc, Armonk, NY, 1995.

Chapter 33

The Technique of Transvenous Lead Extraction

Bruce L. Wilkoff, Ayman S. Al-Khadra

Introduction

The need for extraction of chronically implanted transvenous pacemaker and defibrillator leads was unrealized until recently. Although the development and implantation of these leads represented a significant milestone in arrhythmia management, reducing morbidity and cost, and increasing reliability, it created certain problems that are specific to this type of instrumentation. In contrast to the ease of implanting these leads by the transvenous route, scar tissue and fibrosis that accumulate with time makes their safe extraction a challenge.

Three basic conceptual issues dominate the transvenous removal of leads. The first is the endovascular reaction to the transvenous implantation of the lead. Fibrotic scar tissue and thrombosis form at areas of endothelial contact (Figure 1). The scar tissue progresses as a function of time in thickness, tenacity, and calcification as it engulfs the lead.[1] Certain patients react more strongly than others do. Sometimes the mechanical obstruction to venous flow or fibrotic response results in complete thrombosis of the implantation vein or the venous structures leading to the heart. The scar holds onto the lead and resists explantation.

The second major issue is the physical characteristics of the transvenous lead, in particular, its basic construction, tensile strength, and its fixation mechanism. These properties affect the development of thrombus and/or scar tissue, and handling characteristics when the lead is subjected to unusual forces during extraction. The tensile strength of the conductor, the connections along the lead, and insulators all influence the removability of the lead. The lead that has poor tensile properties will be removed in pieces, if at all. On the other hand, if a lead is very strong and refuses to be withdrawn from the heart, the inability of the lead to break up into pieces may produce myocardial damage and potentially fatal complications. The fixation mechanism influences the degree of attachment of the lead to the heart. Active fixation leads usually permit smoother removal than passive fixation leads, although both have been associated with consistent removal. Under some circumstances, there are issues that require specific care in lead removal with a particular lead. An example would be the retaining J wire found in many leads designed by Cordis Pacemaker Corporation and sold by both Cordis and Telectronics Inc. (Table 1).

The third major issue or hurdle to transvenous lead extraction is that the con-

From Singer I, Barold SS, Camm AJ (eds): Nonpharmacological Therapy of Arrhythmias for the 21st Century: The State of the Art. Futura Publishing Co, Inc., Armonk, NY, © 1998.

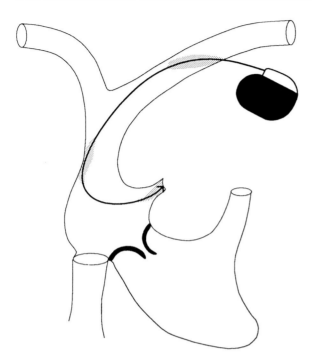

Figure 1. Fibrotic attachments of transvenous leads. Thrombotic and fibrotic tissue form along the length of the lead at sites of contact between the lead and the endovascular structures. Typical locations include vein entry site, the SVC wall, and at the electrode–endocardium interface. The strongest fibrosis is often found not at the lead tip but along the brachiocephalic vein or in contact with the other leads. This fibrotic tissue thickens and frequently becomes calcified with time. Reproduced with permission from Singer I, ed.[16]

trol of the tools during extraction is indirect. There is no direct visualization or ability to intervene along the implantation vein all the way to the endocardial surface. Thus, if there is an untoward disruption of a vascular structure, the situation may remain unperceived and delay a potentially life-saving intervention. Nothing substitutes for familiarity and experience with the tools and the techniques, and good judgment. Anyone who intends to use these techniques is strongly urged both to view the videotape produced by Cook Pacemaker Corporation and to observe extractions performed by an experienced extractor.[2] Plans are being made by NASPE to formalize the process of training and credentialing physicians involved with lead extraction.[3]

Indications

Indications for lead removal can be divided into two categories: infectious and noninfectious. Pacemaker system infection can present as wound dehiscence, migration, erosion, pain, sepsis, fever, chills, or bacteremia. Regardless of the presentation, the only consistently effective approach to resolving the infection is total removal of the pacemaker and leads. This is not a very aggressive approach if one considers the consequences of partially treated foreign body-associated infections. Physical examination is often very unimpressive and frequently a patient will have a fever of unknown etiology or positive blood cultures and an otherwise completely normal physical examination. Even so, delaying the removal of the pacemaker when there is no other clear cause to explain the symptoms will ultimately produce a prolonged course for the patient. Temporizing by burying the pacemaker deeper or by incomplete lead removal will rarely be effective and frequently cause more extensive scar tissue formation that is more difficult to approach.

Noninfectious indications for lead extraction relate to the inability to use the presently implanted leads or the potential for producing direct harm to the patient. These indications include mechanical problems, such as a conductor or insulation failure, patient response issues such as poor sensing or pacing, or a change in the diagnosis such as the need for an implantable cardioverter-defibrillator (ICD) in a patient with a unipolar ventricular pacemaker lead in the right ventricular apex. Depending on the age and health of the patient, the potential for future problems, and the risk of the extraction procedure, it may or may not be advisable to remove leads for some of these indications. There are some instances where the physical presence of pacing or defibrillation leads left in place could cause harm to the patient,

and their removal is clearly indicated. Examples of potentially harmful circumstances include subclavian or superior vena cava thrombosis, extreme clavicular pain, and the potential for producing cardiac laceration with tamponade.

Indications for removing pacemaker leads can also be divided into *mandatory indications* (potentially life-threatening conditions), *necessary indications* (conditions that would produce significant morbidity), and *discretionary indications* (conditions that pro-

Table 1
Telectronics Lead Models with Shape Retaining J Wire

Model Name	Model Number	J Wire Location	J Wire Distal Tip Location	Polarity	Fixation
Accufix™	033-802ξ	Outside Outer Coil	Ring Electrode	Bipolar	Retractable screw
Accufix DEC™	033-812ξ	Outside Outer Coil	Ring Electrode	Bipolar	Retractable screw
Accufix™	329-701*	Outside Outer Coil	Ring Electrode	Bipolar	Retractable screw
Accufix™	330-801*	Outside Outer Coil	Ring Electrode	Bipolar	Retractable screw
Encor DEC™	033-856ξ	Inside Inner Coil	Tip Electrode	Bipolar	Tines
Encor™	327-747*	Inside Inner Coil	Tip Electrode	Bipolar	Tines
Encor™	327-754*	Inside Inner Coil	Tip Electrode	Bipolar	Tines
Encor™	329-749*	Inside Inner Coil	Tip Electrode	Bipolar	Tines
Encor™	329-754*	Inside Inner Coil	Tip Electrode	Bipolar	Tines
Encor™	330-848ξ	Inside Inner Coil	Tip Electrode	Bipolar	Tines
Encor™	330-854*	Inside Inner Coil	Tip Electrode	Bipolar	Tines
Encor DEC™	033-757ξ	Inside Only Coil	Tip Electrode	Unipolar	Tines
Encor™	327-745*	Inside Only Coil	Tip Electrode	Unipolar	Tines
Encor™	327-745P*	Inside Only Coil	Tip Electrode	Unipolar	Tines
Encor™	327-752*	Inside Only Coil	Tip Electrode	Unipolar	Tines
Encor™	327-752P*	Inside Only Coil	Tip Electrode	Unipolar	Tines
Encor™	328-752*	Inside Only Coil	Tip Electrode	Unipolar	Tines
Encor™	328-752P*	Inside Only Coil	Tip Electrode	Unipolar	Tines
Encor™	329-748*	Inside Only Coil	Tip Electrode	Unipolar	Tines
Encor™	329-748A*	Inside Only Coil	Tip Electrode	Unipolar	Tines
Encor™	329-748P*	Inside Only Coil	Tip Electrode	Unipolar	Tines
Encor™	329-755A*	Inside Only Coil	Tip Electrode	Unipolar	Tines
Encor™	330-748*	Inside Only Coil	Tip Electrode	Unipolar	Tines
Encor™	330-755*	Inside Only Coil	Tip Electrode	Unipolar	Tines
EnGuard/Atrial DF™	040-022 Ψξ	Inside Inner Coil	Tip Electrode	ICD	Tines
EnGuard/Atrial DF™	040-069ξ	Inside Inner Coil	Tip Electrode	ICD	Tines
EnGuard/Atrial DF™	040-112 Ψξ	Inside Inner Coil	Tip Electrode	ICD	Tines

* US and worldwide marketing; Ψ US investigational device; ξ Non-US distribution.
Data from Cook Vascular Incorporated multi-center lead extraction registry. Presented at the annual scientific sessions of the North American Society for Pacing and Electrophysiology (NASPE), May 7, 1997, New Orleans, LA. Data based on attempted extraction of 3040 leads from 1895 patients by 23 physicians who verified complete reporting of procedures from January 1994 through February 1997.[10]

duce no immediate harm, but where extraction might improve future care).[4] In general, infectious conditions are considered mandatory indications to extract pacemaker and defibrillator leads, as are conditions that reduce the effectiveness of continued pacemaker or defibrillation support for the patient or that can create a potentially fatal complication. All other conditions involve the removal of leads for the prevention of future problems. No matter how the indications for lead extraction are categorized, it is essential that the risks of keeping the pacemaker or defibrillator lead in place are weighed against the risks of removal. As the tools for and the experience with extraction increases, the potential morbidity is reduced, the likelihood of success increases, and the appropriateness of intervention increases.

Outcome

The results of transvenous extraction have been reported and analyzed by the voluntary registry coordinated through Cook Pacemaker, Inc.,[5] data reported through Dr. Charles Byrd,[6] data reported through The Cleveland Clinic Foundation,[7] and recent experience with the Telectronics J lead extraction.[8,9] (Tables 2 and 3). Percutaneous extraction of leads is safer and more successful in experienced hands. According to recent results from the national registry, complete or partial removal was achieved in 98% of patients, with less than 1% risk of major complications in experienced centers.[10]

Key Principles

There are three important principles to understand in lead extraction: control of the pacemaker lead body, controlled disruption of fibrotic tissue (counterpressure), and countertraction at the endocardial surface. Paying attention to these three principles will allow the extractor to predict problem-

Table 2
Lead Extraction Success Rates

Clinical Characteristics	Complete (%)	Partial (%)	Failed (%)
Implant Duration			
1 year	98.9	0.8	0.3
2–4 years	97.8	1.9	0.3
5–7 years	94.1	5.1	0.9
8–24 years	83.6	12.6	3.8
Fixation			
Active	94.5	4.2	1.2
Passive	93.0	5.8	1.2
Placement			
Atrial	96.2	3.1	0.7
Ventricular	91.4	6.8	1.8
Total	93.8	4.9	1.2

Data from Cook Vascular Incorporated multi-center lead extraction registry. Presented at the annual scientific sessions of the North American Society for Pacing and Electrophysiology (NASPE), May 7, 1997, New Orleans, LA. Data based on attempted extraction of 3040 leads from 1895 patients by 23 physicians who verified complete reporting of procedures from January 1994 through February 1997.[10]

atic leads that will require specialized instruments to assist in extraction.

Control of the pacemaker lead body includes binding of its elements, and applying uniform forces on the entire length of the lead, so that it can be removed in one piece without distortion or elongation. This control not only facilitates complete lead removal, but also more controlled disruption of the fibrotic tissue along the lead. The second principle is the controlled disruption of the fibrotic tissue through intravascular counterpressure. Not all of the fibrosis is disrupted at once. Early experience with nontelescoping sheaths was neither safe nor as effective as telescoping sheaths.[11] Telescoping sheaths (Table 4) have been used to effectuate a controlled disruption of the fibrotic tissue. These cylindrical tools are made of two metal or polymer sheaths with beveled edges. Their use allows the operator to disrupt the fibrotic attachments a few millimeters at a time. The inner sheath peels the lead away from the fibrotic attachments.

Table 3
Complications by Intervention*

Complication	Deaths (percentage)	Total (percentage)
Thoracotomy repair (tamponade or hemothorax)	2 (0.11%)	14 (0.74%)
Drainage - pericardiocentesis (hemopericardium or tamponade)	0	7 (0.37%)
Drainage - chest tube (hemothorax and pneumothorax)	0	4 (0.21%)
Transfusions	0	5 (0.26%)
Pulmonary embolism	0	1 (0.05%)
Subclavian AV fistula	1 (0.05%)	2 (0.11%)
Total	3 (0.16%)	28 (1.48%)

* Some patients have multiple events.

Data from Cook Vascular Incorporated multi-center lead extraction registry. Presented at the annual scientific sessions of the North American Society for Pacing and Electrophysiology (NASPE), May 7, 1997, New Orleans, LA. Data based on attempted extraction of 3040 leads from 1895 patients by 23 physicians who verified complete reporting of procedures from January 1994 through February 1997.[10]

The second outer sheath, which is just slightly larger than the inner sheath, shields it from the fibrotic tissue and reduces friction. The outer sheath also would not buckle because it is reinforced by the inner sheath. This technique of slowly dissecting away the fibrotic tissue with the telescoping sheaths is known as *counterpressure*. The force is applied tangentially to the vessel wall and adhering fibrous tissue. Counterpressure is therefore associated with potentially higher risk of vascular injury than other steps during lead extraction. By slowly advancing the sheaths over the electrode, only a modest degree of tensile integrity is required by the lead and by the vein

Table 4
Countertraction Sheath Characteristics

Material	Color	Inner Sheath Length	Inner Sheath Inner/Outer	Outer Sheath Length	Outer Sheath Inner/Outer
Polypropylene	Yellow	15" & 18"	8.4 F/10.7 F	13" & 16"	11.6 F/13.9 F
Teflon™ B	Black	15" & 18"	8.5 F/12.0 F	13" & 16"	12.8 F/16.0 F
Teflon™-Femoral	Black	36"	8.5 F/12.0 F	27.4"	12.8 F/16.0 F
Teflon™ C	Black	15" & 18"	9.5 F/13.0 F	13" & 16"	14.3 F/18.0 F
Polypropylene	White-Special	15" & 18"	9.7 F/12.3 F	13" & 16"	13.3 F/15.6 F
Polypropylene	Green	15" & 18"	10.0 F/12.1 F	13" & 16"	13.1 F/15.2 F
Steel	Silver	10"	10.4 F/11.9 F	7.75"	12.7 F/13.7 F
Polypropylene	White-Regular	15" & 18"	11.4 F/13.6 F	13" & 16"	14.1 F/16.1 F
Laser 12F	Blue	15.7"	8.3 F/12.4 F	12.6"	13.4 F/17.0 F
Laser 14F	Grey	15.7"	10.2 F/14.5 F	12.6"	15.5 F/19.3 F
Laser 16F	Black	15.7"	12.5 F/16.7 F	12.6"	18.2 F/22.6 F

Countertraction sheath pairs can be used singly, together, mixed and/or exchanged to influence the strength, sharpness, flexibility, stiffness and rotational torque of the system. An example of mixing two types of sheaths includes the use of an outer steel sheath to hold open the space between the clavicle and the first rib while an inner Teflon™ B sheath slides down to cover a protruding J wire of an Accufix™ lead. If the outer Teflon™ B sheath had been used, the clavicle and first rib would have pinched the sheaths preventing advancement. If a polypropylene inner or if both inner and outer sheaths were used, too much counterpressure would be required to redirect the sheaths from the brachiocephalic vein to the SVC. This would have retracted the lead and potentially lacerated the venous structures.

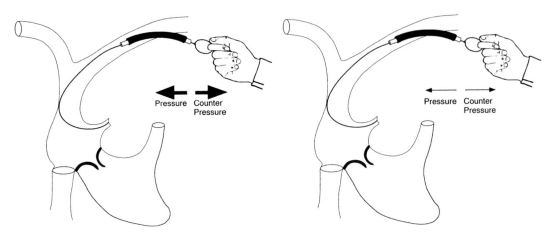

Figure 2. Appropriate counterpressure. The withdrawal force exerted on the looped end of the locking stylet should be minimal but equal to that necessary to prevent the force exerted on the sheaths from altering the course of the lead. Since the location and tenacity of the fibrotic tissue is unknown, a moment to moment adjustment of the opposing forces and comparison with the high magnification fluoroscopic image is required. If the locking stylet slips then withdrawal force on the looped end of the stylet fails to counter the advancement force. It is safe to advance the sheaths only around a change in direction (e.g., from the left brachiocephalic vein to the SVC) when the end is tethered by fibrosis and there is control of the lead body. In the two drawings, note that the pressure arrows are equal in size to the counterpressure arrows. Reproduced with permission from Singer I, ed.[16]

leading to the heart. As such, the risk of lead fragmentation and cardiovascular disruption is greatly reduced (Figure 2).

The third major principle is intravascular *countertraction.* One of the major sites for fibrosis is the lead–myocardium interface. After the lead has been peeled away from all of its endovascular contacts except the lead tip, most of the force applied to the end of the lead is now transferred to the endocardial surface. This withdrawal force can invaginate the ventricular or atrial myocardium and cause hemodynamic compromise and/or cardiac laceration. However, by bracing the large sheath against the endocardial surface, the heart cannot invaginate when firm and nonsudden traction is applied. Instead, the lead is released from its endocardial entrapment. The force of countertraction is perpendicular to the endocardial surface, and as such is associated with lower risk of endovascular trauma than counterpressure.

The above principles of control of the lead body, controlled counterpressure, and controlled countertraction are good only as long as certain assumptions are met. The basic assumption is that the lead travels through a normal venous route to the heart and remains intracardiac. Certainly, the incidence of patent foramen ovale, atrial septal defects, and ventricular septal defects should make us aware that the lead may not be on the venous side of the heart. Prior to the procedure, careful examination of the paced ECG should suggest this possibility to the clinician. In addition, leads passing into the coronary sinus are associated with significant scar tissue and produce a particular hazard to the advancement of telescoping sheaths. Sometimes a lead will migrate across the myocardium into the pericardial space. This can happen in the atrium, at the AV ring, or in the right ventricle. If one of these leads is extracted, tamponade can result. As long as the lead traverses the normal venous structures to the heart and as long as the chest x-ray, ECG, and other data support a diagnosis of normal lead positioning, then it is appropriate to apply the tools described below.

Preoperative Evaluation

The history and physical examination should focus on the original indication and surgical details of the pacemaker implantation. There may have been multiple operations and significant clues as to what might be encountered during the extraction procedure. A radiographic examination of the chest including an overpenetrated PA and lateral chest x-ray should be obtained. Fluoroscopic views and/or venography of the leads and the superior veins may be necessary. The pacemaker should be fully evaluated with pacing and sensing thresholds, unipolar and bipolar if possible, and determination made as to the necessity of replacing the electrodes. The urgency of intervention and the potential need for a temporary pacemaker is vital.

The vast majority of lead extractions at the Cleveland Clinic Foundation are performed under local anesthesia with deep intravenous sedation as needed. However, when there are multiple leads to be extracted, when there is a large amount of debridement required, or if the patient is excessively anxious, it is entirely appropriate to use general anesthesia. It is mandatory to ensure echocardiographic and surgical backup support in case there is urgent need for pericardiocentesis or thoracotomy.

The Operation

The operation can take place wherever the best environment exists for the extracting physician. Often fluoroscopy is far superior in the cardiac catheterization laboratories or electrophysiology laboratories while anesthesia and surgical support are better in the operating room. In either case, a comfortable environment with excellent fluoroscopy including higher magnification fluoroscopy and anesthesia support must exist. Echocardiography, pericardiocentesis, and thoracotomy should be available if necessary. Almost all of the procedures at The Cleveland Clinic Foundation are performed in the Electrophysiology Laboratories where all of these conditions exist. Two large-bore intravenous lines and an arterial line are placed. It is also entirely appropriate to have a central venous line. If a patient has demonstrated pacemaker dependency, even if the ventricular lead is not to be removed, a temporary pacemaker is appropriate. The temporary pacing wire is placed and located in a stable position in the heart away from the destination of the soon-to-be extracted ventricular lead. This will allow for tugging on the lead to be extracted without the risk of dislodgment or perforation of the right ventricle with the temporary wire at the same time. Sometimes it is appropriate to place the ventricular pacing lead in the coronary sinus, which is conveniently located far away from the ventricular leads. A wide surgical preparation from the neck down to the abdomen including the femoral area is appropriate.

The Superior Venous Approach

The approach to extraction from the vein of implantation has been revolutionized by the advent of the Excimer laser. However, the technique depends on the skilled application of the traditional approach of counterpressure and countertraction. Therefore, first the traditional techniques will be described in detail and then modifications for the laser technique will be discussed.

The incision is made to optimize linear access to the vein of insertion (Figure 3) and the generator is delivered through that incision. Particularly in infected cases, separate incisions may be necessary for debridement of the pocket and removal of the electrodes from the vein. Dissection is carried down to the suture sleeves, which are identified and removed. The generator is then removed from the pocket and the terminal pin cut from the lead. Traction is applied to the lead from the suture tie-down site in order to draw the cut end of the lead through the scar tissue. This prevents the need for dissecting the lead free from the tissue. It is essential that all leads are dissected free of fibrotic tissue to as close as possible to the

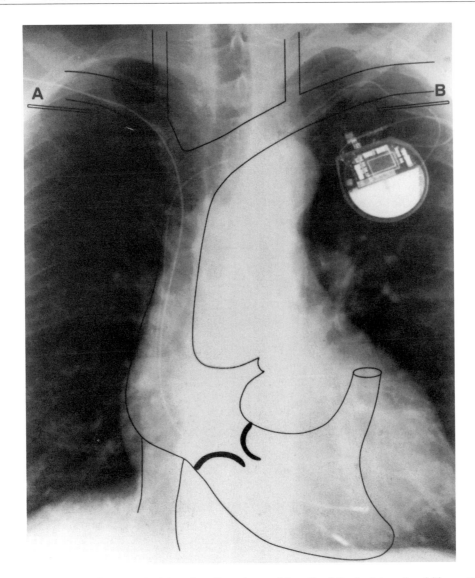

Figure 3. Chest x-ray locating incision sites. Location and length of the incision should be optimized to permit linear access to the venous entry site. Particularly for the entry of the nonflexible steel sheaths, the incision should radiate from the venous entry site laterally in order to enable the sheath to be oriented in all three axes to follow the course of the lead into the vein. The linear overlay drawings labeled A and B represent reasonable locations for incisions for this patient. Reproduced with permission from Singer I, ed.[16]

leads' insertion into the vein. This extravascular fibrous tissue is frequently responsible for damage to the telescoping sheaths.

Testing of the leads that are not to be removed is important before and after the extraction procedure. Although it is rare to damage the conductor or insulation of the other leads if attention is paid to their pro-tection, these leads are at risk, particularly during the introduction of the steel sheaths at the level of the clavicle. Another troublesome area is when the two leads are intertwined or wrapped around each other. When the sheaths are advanced under these circumstances, rotation of the outer sheath in both directions and withdrawal of the sheath after the lead is removed can dislodge the remaining lead. Finally, fibrotic attachments between the atrial and ventricular leads at the RA-SVC junction can significantly bind the leads and prevent extraction or unintentionally dislodge the other lead.

After all leads have been dissected free, the proximal ends of the leads are prepared. Preparation consists of incising the insulation circumferentially about the lead (Figure 4). For co-axial bipolar leads, the outer conductor is then stretched and cut off, leaving the inner insulation and the inner conductor. The inner insulation is then incised allowing there to be a stair-step progression from outer insulation to the outer coil to

inner insulation to the inner coil. The conical coil expander is then used to expand the slightly crushed most proximal tip of the inner lead conductor (Figure 5). A standard pacemaker stylet is passed through the electrode to its distal tip to ascertain the distance that the locking stylet must travel and to clear the lumen of potential debris. The conductor coil is then sized with gauge pins (Figure 6), and the gauge of the largest gauge pin that snugly but freely enters the conductor coil lumen to its fullest extent corresponds to the gauge of the locking stylet to be used. It is necessary to size leads of the same make and model because there may be a difference of one or two sizes. The appropriate locking stylet (Figure 7) is then

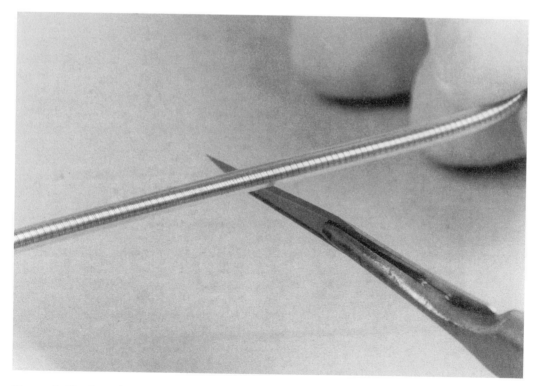

Figure 4. Cutting of insulation. When cutting the inner or outer insulation, the lead is grasped between the thumb and forefinger of both hands while the assistant positions the cutting edge of the #11 scalpel blade underneath the lead. The lead is rotated while dragging the lead over the sharp edge of the scalpel. The circumscribed fragment of insulation is removed from the lead, the outer conductor is stretched over the cut end and trimmed off with the suture scissors. The inner insulation is then removed using a similar technique. It is important not to damage the remaining outer insulation and the inner coil since they will be used to control the lead body with the locking stylet and suture. Reproduced with permission from Singer I, ed.[16]

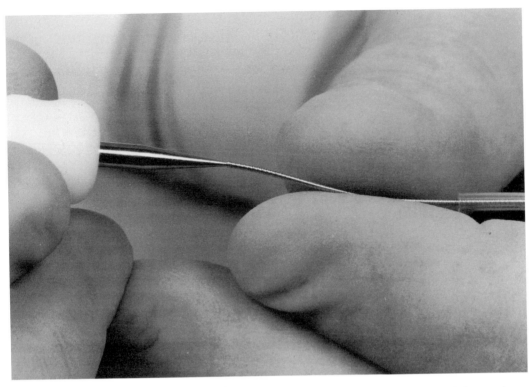

Figure 5. Coil expander. The conical coil expander is used to enlarge the cut tip of the conductor coil. The conductor coil is often distorted when it is cut. If not expanded, the gauge pins may undersize the coil and the locking stylet may not grasp the lead strongly. Sometimes the filament on the locking stylet will become hung up on the partially crimped end or the damaged conductor coil. Reproduced with permission from Singer I, ed.[16]

passed all the way to the farthest reaches of the lead, optimally to the distal electrode. When the stylet locks further down the lead, it produces shorter segments of the lead to elongate. The locking stylet is then locked by turning it counterclockwise four to ten times. A gentle tug is given and then a repeat of the counterclockwise rotation is performed. The most common reason that a locking stylet does not lock is undersizing, which is a consequence of damage to the proximal segment of electrode, or failure to use the coil expander prior to sizing with gauge pins. After the locking stylet has been secured, a strong suture, usually 0-gauge, is securely tied around the outer insulation compressing the insulation and the outer coil and inner coil as much as possible with a tight square knot. The long end of the suture is tied tautly between its attachment on the insulation to the looped end of the locking stylet, providing for parallel and simultaneous traction on the outer insulation and on the conductor coil (Figure 8). This latter step is performed on all leads except for the Telectronics ''J'' lead extractions.

A new and more easily used locking stylet is now available. This side-locking Wilkoff stylet is manufactured in three sizes to fit conductor coils from .019 to .023, .024 to .027, and .028 to .030 inches (Figure 9). The stylet has a barb at its distal tip that is angled to lock when the cylinder of the stylet is advanced. The stylet is used in the same fashion as the traditional locking stylets but does not need to be sized as carefully, locks more strongly, and is usually reversible. Rotation of this stylet will brake the locking mechanism, but a new stylet can still be introduced and securely locked.

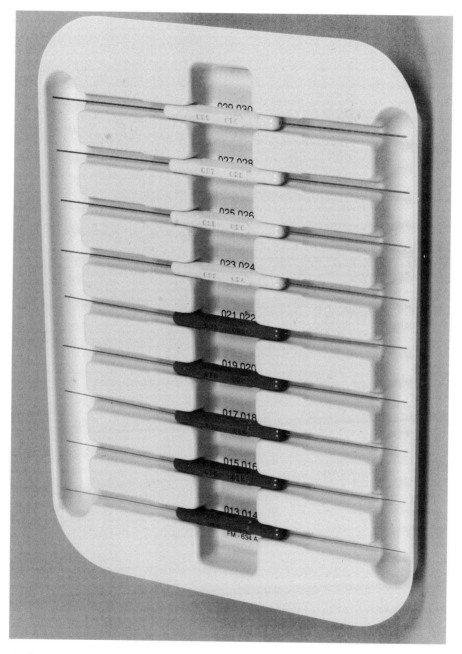

Figure 6. Gauge pin set. The gauge pins are manufactured from diameters of 0.013″ to 0.030″ to measure the internal diameter of the conductor coil. The corresponding locking stylet should fit snugly within the properly sized conductor coil. Reproduced with permission from Singer I, ed.[16]

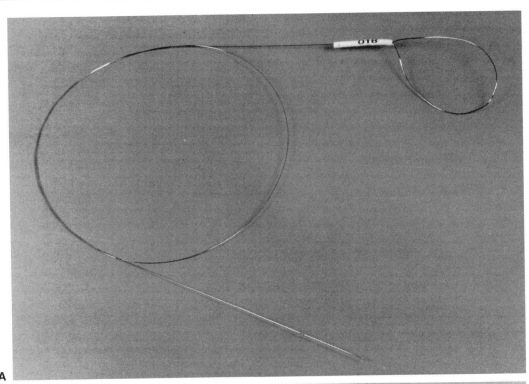

A

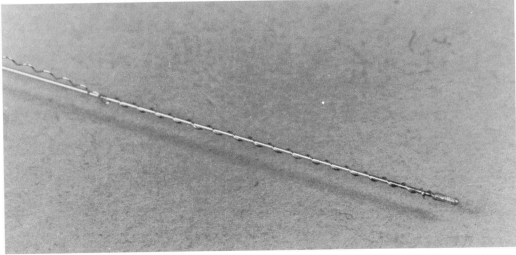

B

Figure 7. Locking stylet. **(A)** The locking stylet is slightly thinner than the corresponding gauge pin. The filament braised to the tip of the locking stylet rubs against the conductor coil. When advancing the stylet down the lead, the stylet should be withdrawn slightly to roughen up the filament. If it is hard to advance the stylet after the slight withdrawal, then this should be done less frequently, but if the stylet does not seem to be locking well then it should be done more frequently. **(B)** Locking stylet tip. The tip of the locking stylet has a thin flattened filamentous wire braised to the tip. When properly sized, the filament will uncoil when the locking stylet is rotated counterclockwise. Often the locking stylet must be rotated clockwise to permit passage to the lead tip. Once the locking stylet is advanced to its farthest extent, the stylet must be rotated counterclockwise to activate the locking mechanism. The wire then becomes a strong fastener to the lead tip and compresses the conductor coil and prevents stretching of the lead during extraction efforts. Reproduced with permission from Singer I, ed.[16]

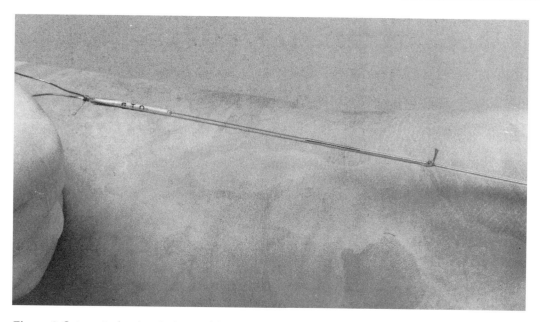

Figure 8. Suture tied to insulation and locking stylet. A strong suture is tied tightly to the insulation and also to the looped end of the locking stylet to enhance the control of the lead body. If multiple conductor coils are available, then a locking stylet should be introduced into each coil. Pulling on the insulation, with the help of the suture, facilitates the advancement of the sheaths by minimizing the tendency of the insulation and attached fibrotic debris to bunch up and bind on the sheaths. This is particularly important for ICD leads. Reproduced with permission from Singer I, ed.[16]

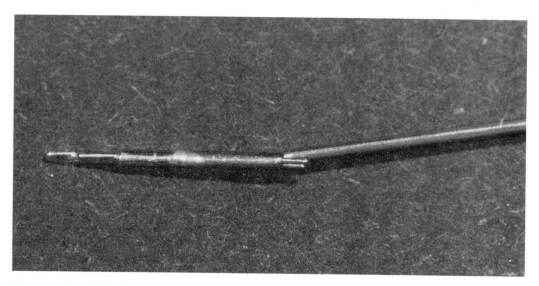

Figure 9. The Wilkoff stylet. This stylet has a reversible side-locking mechanism, obviating the need for precise measurement of the inner diameter of the inner coil. It is manufactured in three sizes to fit conductor coils from .019 to .023, .024 to .027, and .028 to .030 inches. The stylet has a barb at its distal tip that is angled to lock when the cylinder of the stylet is advanced.

When determining which lead should be removed first, all of the available information regarding the number of leads in each vein, duration of implantation, the intrinsic tensile strength of the leads, the security of the locking stylet, and venous access are utilized. All factors that favor easy extraction point to the lead that should be removed first. The reasoning behind this is that whichever lead is removed first, much of the interlead fibrosis is disrupted during that extraction. Consequently, the more difficult lead to remove becomes easier to remove only after the first lead is removed.

Vessel entry is one of the key elements of lead extraction. The use of the straight telescoping stainless steel sheaths greatly facilitates this step (Figure 10). The intent of these sheaths is to penetrate the fibrosis that is generally dense near the lead insertion into the vein. These sheaths should not be advanced into the superior vena cava and should be advanced only during high-magnification fluoroscopy (Figure 11), looking for evidence of damage to the lead or the sheaths. It is not necessary to pull on the leads to any extent during this phase. All that is required is alignment of the sheaths in a triaxial plane so that the sheaths will slide over the monorail-like lead. It will often be necessary to rotate the inner and outer sheaths to disrupt the fibrosis surrounding the lead, as well as change trajectory of the steel sheaths as the sheaths are advanced over the lead. These sheaths should be rotated and advanced slowly.

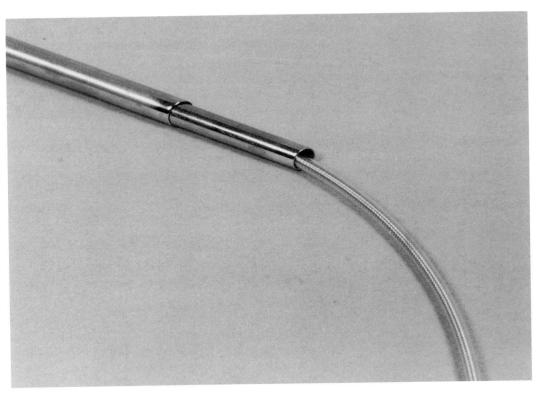

Figure 10. Steel sheaths. The steel sheaths are not sharp, but are thinner and stronger than the Teflon™ or polypropylene sheaths. They prevent the use of excessive force during vein entry, especially if the lead enters through a narrow space under the clavicle or through fibrotic or calcified tissue. They can be safely passed as long as they can be maneuvered to follow the course of the lead. The steel sheaths are extremely useful in separating leads from each other during their course through the left brachiocephalic vein. Reproduced with permission from Singer I, ed.[16]

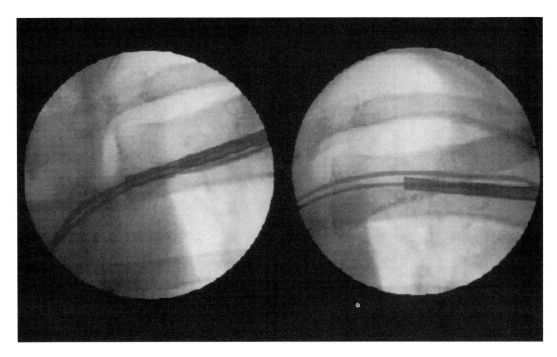

Figure 11. Triaxial positioning. The steel sheaths, in particular, are safe and effective only if they are oriented in the x, y, and z planes as they are advanced over the lead. Any lateral force is ineffective in producing sheath advancement and increases the likelihood of binding on the lead or produces an acute bend or crimp in the sheath. Comparison of the fluoroscopic image with the manipulation of the locking stylet and the sheaths is essential to effective lead extraction. The two fluoroscopic images demonstrate the reorientation of the steel telescoping sheaths as they are passed into the subclavian vein on the right and down the brachiocephalic vein on the left. Reproduced with permission from Singer I, ed.[16]

Once the steel sheaths have been passed to the level where the lead starts to bend around a corner, the steel sheaths need to be exchanged for either Teflon™ or polypropylene sheaths (Figure 12). This exchange should be performed quickly and while obstructing the outer sheath with the operator's fingertip to avoid air embolism. It is preferable to use relatively stiffer sheaths as long as there is strong control of the lead. These relatively stiffer high barium content or special polypropylene sheaths, labeled "WIL," allow for greater strength along the lead as they are advanced. They tend to kink less and transfer the torque to the counter pressure site. Flexible and soft sheaths that are not strong enough to peel away the fibrosis are less safe than the more rigid sheaths. Again, the retraction force on the looped end of the locking stylet should not be excessive. The force should be equal to that which allows advancement of the sheaths while holding the lead away from the outer arc of the insertion vein and into the heart (Figures 2 and 13). These sheaths should not be advanced directly against the vessel wall but rather the leads should be peeled away from the wall of the vessel, bringing the lead into the center of the vascular lumen. Failure to advance the sheaths after initial progress is likely to be due to damage to their leading edge and requires their replacement. The use of the pin vise is extremely advantageous in improving control of the sheaths and limiting fatigue while manipulating the relatively thin and frequently bloody and slippery telescoping sheaths (Figure 14). The ability to rotate the

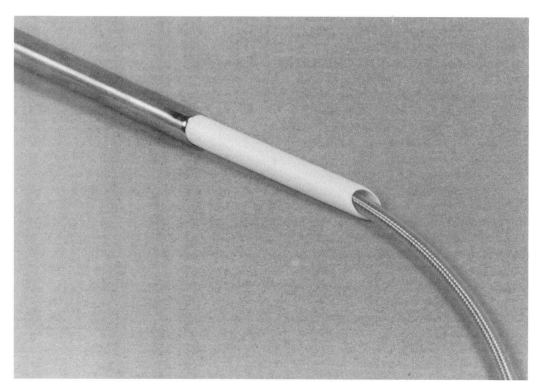

Figure 12. Exchange of sheaths. It is better to exchange one sheath at a time to maintain the progress produced with the previous sheaths. If the sheaths fail to progress it may be due to damage to the tip of the sheath. **(A)** The steel inner sheath has been replaced by an inner polypropylene special high-barium sheath to maintain good strength and increase flexibility to advance the sheath into the SVC. Reproduced with permission from Singer I, ed.[16]

sheaths often allows the sheaths to be advanced when simple pushing or advancement fails.

Sometimes during the counterpressure technique, the locking stylet will slip, but depending on the lead the insulation and/ or the conductor coil may be sufficient to control the lead during advancement of the sheaths. As long as you hold on to part of the lead it should be possible to advance the sheaths. However, the extractor should be very sensitive to the fact that it is possible to uncover bare wire in the vascular space, which if retracted upon could slice through the cardiac or venous structures or cut through the sheaths. Caution should be taken to locate the segment of the sheath from which the lead emerges. It is sometimes possible to see the pacing wire exiting the sheath a few millimeters to a centimeter

behind the tip, which indicates damage to the telescoping sheaths. The sheaths then will need to be removed and possibly replaced from above or from below with the femoral technique. It is not unusual for the lead to come free after the fibrosis in the subclavian vein is freed up or as soon as the attachments between the leads all the way down to the atrial lead are freed up.

The most significant fibrotic attachments do not usually occur at the endocardial surface. At this level, patience and slow steady pressure are required. If the locking stylet is still locked and the control of the lead is strong, then the sheath will keep the cavity of the right heart from invaginating. No sudden or ripping actions should be applied. Sometimes the lead will release from the myocardium but the fibrosis will be too large to enter the sheath. It is therefore help-

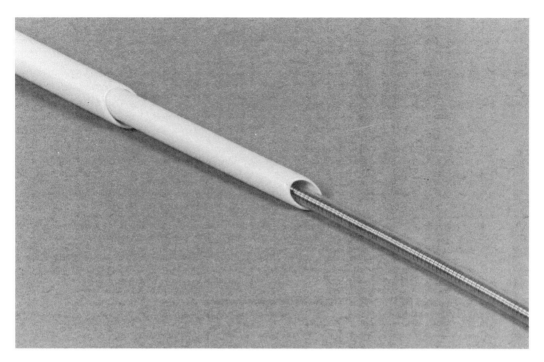

Figure 12. *(Continued)* **(B)** The steel outer sheath has been replace by the matching outer polypropylene special high-barium sheath to continue counterpressure along the lead down to the endocardial surface for countertraction. Reproduced with permission from Singer I, ed.[16]

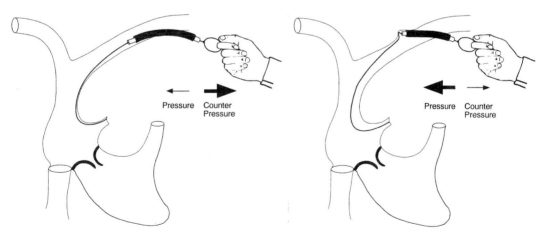

Figure 13. Pitfalls of counterpressure. There are two types of errors made during counterpressure. When insufficient counterpressure is exerted on the locking stylet, the lead loses its properties that guide the sheaths safely down the center of the venous structures to the heart. Since the sheaths (even the softest) are relatively stiff and perfectly straight, the sheaths will tend to scrape against the venous walls and increase the risk of laceration (right panel). If excessive counterpressure applied, the lead will be withdrawn from the vein and from the heart without peeling of the fibrotic material from the lead. The opportunity for countertraction is lost which increases the risk of myocardial avulsion and cardiac laceration and tamponade (left panel). Reproduced with permission from Singer I, ed.[16]

ful to periodically gently retract the lead and sheaths together to see if the job is completed. Since the relatively large diameter fibrosis may inhibit its withdrawal from the subclavian vein, once withdrawn from the heart and into the SVC additional attempts at retraction of the inner sheath and lead into the outer sheath are usually successful. This will limit the irritation and trauma to the subclavian, cephalic, or jugular veins as the lead is withdrawn. After removal of the telescoping sheaths, bleeding can be controlled in the majority of patients with simple pressure. Occasionally a purse-string or figure-of-eight suture will be required to control bleeding. Placement of the purse-string suture after lead preparation and prior to the use of the sheaths is advisable. If there is little or no bleeding, the suture can be removed.

If the indication for lead removal is mechanical failure, there is no evidence of infection, and the patient continues to require arrhythmia therapy, pacemaker or defibrillator leads can be placed at the same time after completion of the extraction part. Vascular access can be maintained by inserting a long J-shaped guidewire into the inferior vena cava through the outer sheath, which is left in the superior veins after lead removal. Extreme care needs to be exercised to avoid air embolism while this exchange is taking place. The outer sheath is then removed and a long introducer is guided along the wire to the level of the right atrium. Insertion of short introducers that end in the superior veins will increase the risk of extravascular lead insertion. The new permanent lead should be positioned in an area that is distant from the site that was occupied by the extracted leads.

Superior Venous Approach Utilizing Laser Sheaths

The recent introduction of Excimer laser sheaths (Spectranetics Corporation, Colo-

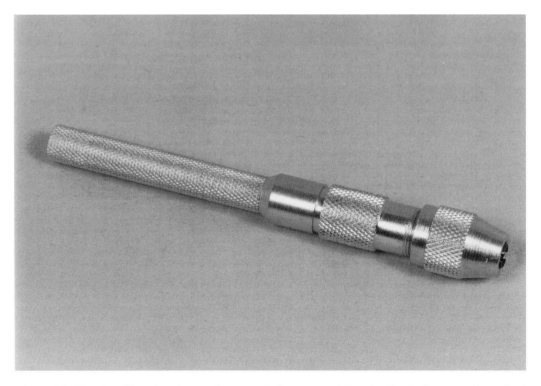

Figure 14. Pin vise. The pin vise can be mounted on any of the sheaths to improve the grip for rotational torque. This is particularly useful with the steel and special high-barium content polypropylene sheaths since these sheaths are able to transmit the rotational torque to the sheath tip. Reproduced with permission from Singer I, ed.[16]

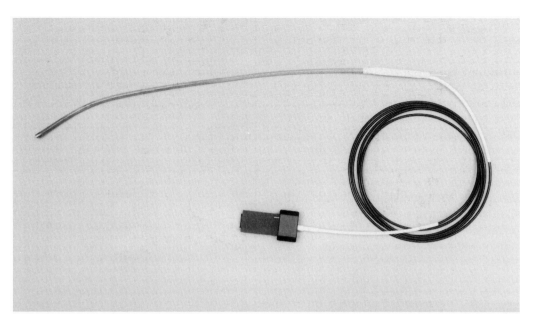

Figure 15. The laser extraction sheath. Excimer laser sheaths, made by Spectranetics Corporation, are used in conjunction with an outer Teflon™ sheath. They emit circumferential laser between the two stainless steel rings at the tip. Currently, these catheters come in three sizes (12F, 14F, 16F) and can therefore also be used to extract ICD leads.

rado Springs, CO) represents an important addition to the available tools that are used in extraction of pacemaker leads (Figure 15). These sheaths replace the inner telescoping sheaths and are used in conjunction with an outer Teflon sheath, during the counterpressure phase of the extraction. By ablating fibrous tissue directly in contact, and within a few millimeters of the tip of the laser sheath, the amount of counterpressure necessary to cut through adhesions is greatly minimized. Because counterpressure is associated with the highest risk during lead extraction, it is reasonable to expect that using the laser will reduce morbidity and increase the likelihood of uncomplicated and complete lead extraction.

The laser sheath design is based on concepts similar to those used to devise laser coronary angioplasty systems. The catheters, which come in sizes ranging from 12F to 16F, are made of inner and outer polymer tubing. A single layer of optical fibers runs spirally between both layers of the tubing. At the distal end of the catheter the tubings terminate in two stainless steel bands with beveled edges. In addition to protecting the catheter tip and the optical fibers, they serve as a radiopaque marker at the catheter tip. Between the two rings exits a single circumferential ring of laser light. The CVX-300 Excimer XeCl system emits 135-ns pulses at a repetition rate of 25–40 Hz.

The steps involved in extraction of leads using laser sheaths are very similar to the standard techniques. The leads are dissected and prepared as described above. The use of metal sheath is advisable when there are excessive calcifications or very dense fibrosis under the clavicles and at the vein entry site. Before using the laser sheath, the system is calibrated. The ablation rate is determined both by fluence (energy density per pulse) and repetition rate (pulses per sec). The fluence and repetition rate for this procedure are 60 mJ/mm^2 and 40 Hz, respectively. The maximum recommended laser firing time is 10,000 pulses (25 sec at 40 Hz).

The laser catheter is used in conjunction with an outer sheath. Using a "fish tape" device, the handle of the locking stylet is threaded through the inner lumen of the laser catheter, and the proximal end of the lead is pulled into the catheter. Using the same counterpressure technique described above, the laser catheter and the outer sheath are advanced until an obstruction is met. The laser catheter is then activated. While it is firing, gentle pressure is used to advance it by about 1 mm per second. As soon as the catheter passes through the obstruction, the laser is stopped. Then, the outer sheath is advanced over the laser catheter until the next obstruction is met. The laser is advanced from venous entry to within 0.5 to 1 cm of the myocardium. The laser should not be applied to the myocardium to free the lead tip. Countertraction may be applied, however, utilizing the outer sheath. As expected, the laser may not be successful in areas where there is dense calcification. Unless this area can be freed using the outer sheath and then passed into the laser catheter, progress is unlikely and could cause vascular laceration. Resorting to larger laser or nonlaser sheath may be necessary.

The results using laser-assisted lead extraction has been very promising. Recent data from the Pacing Lead Explant with the Excimer Sheath (PLEXES) trial showed a success rate of 94% in patients randomized to laser extraction compared to 64% in those randomized to the standard approach. Total removal of 88% of the leads not removed using the standard approach was successfully completed with the addition of laser techniques.[12] Of the 244 patients who had laser extraction, three had complications including one death. This complication rate is consistent with the rate observed in the Cook extraction registry.[10]

The Transfemoral Approach

Transfemoral techniques are important adjuncts to the superior venous approach but may increase the risk of deep venous thrombosis and pulmonary thromboembolism. At the Cleveland Clinic, usage of the stiffer polypropylene sheaths and the pin vise has permitted the removal of 94.7% of pacemaker leads by the superior vein approach. Since a prepectoral incision is almost always required for the removal of the pulse generator and preparation of the lead for removal, we prefer to complete the job without resorting to the femoral technique. However, skill with the femoral technique is necessary to consistently and safely remove all leads.

The femoral approach is required when there is failure to progress with the telescoping sheaths or when the lead has been cut or retracted into the vein. Some operators may feel more comfortable with manipulating catheters from the femoral vein. The tools for femoral extraction have markedly improved as more femoral cases have been performed. The lead is prepared for extraction in a fashion similar to that described in the superior venous approach. The lead is freed, the suture sleeve is removed, and the lead is cut near the insertion of the subclavian vein. Then, the femoral workstation is introduced from the femoral vein, preferably on the right side.

The original Byrd femoral workstation is a 16F Teflon sheath with venous check flow valve and a side port. Through this sheath, several tools can be passed to snare and retrieve the lead or lead fragment. Options include but are not restricted to the traditional Byrd workstation countertraction sheath preloaded with a tip-deflecting guidewire and a Dotter basket in either the straight or curved configuration or the needle's-eye snare with a straight or curved sheath (Figure 16). If the tip-deflecting wire and Dotter basket are used, the guidewire is looped around the lead so that the tip of the wire can be caught in the Dotter basket. The lead is then gently pulled down from the superior veins. The reversible nature of the loop formed by the tip-deflecting guidewire and Dotter basket around the lead allows the lead to be grasped at several levels and be progressively pulled down. Pulling the lead down out of the subclavian vein is facilitated by the fact that the mediastinum re-

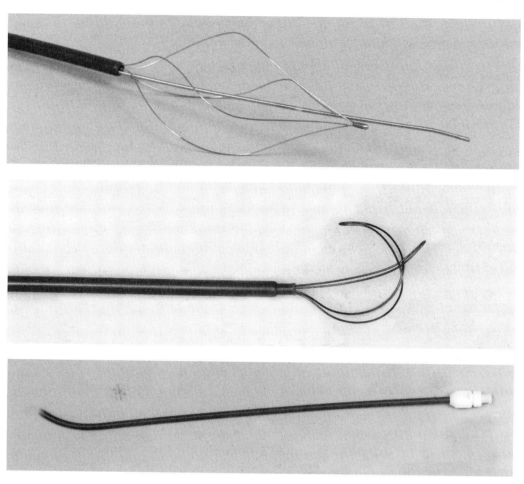

Figure 16. Femoral extraction tools. Extraction of leads using the femoral approach is more versatile, but demands specially designed tools. An important first step is to be able to securely grasp the lead at particular points that will give mechanical advantage during countertraction. This can be accomplished using Dotter basket snare and Cook deflection catheter (top panel). The deflection catheter encircles the lead and then the Dotter snare grasps the tip of the deflection catheter. The loop is then pulled into the workstation catheter. A more recently introduced tool, the needle's eye (middle panel), also enables the operator to grasp and release the lead multiple times with ease and precision. Using this instrument, the lead is entrapped between the hook of the system and the needle. Advancing the inner sheath traps the lead so that the outer sheath can be used for countertraction. The recent introduction of curved femoral sheaths increases maneuverability and increases the ease of grasping the lead fragments (bottom panel).

sists downward movement. The lead is then pulled further into the countertraction sheath and the sheath is advanced over the lead down to the endocardial surface for a countertraction procedure as described above. Sometimes the outer 16F sheath of the Byrd femoral workstation can be advanced over the countertraction sheath and can be used in conjunction with the inner sheath for countertraction.

As an alternative to the Dotter basket, the Amplatz gooseneck snare and tip-deflecting guidewire can be advanced through the Byrd femoral workstation without an inner sheath. The guidewire is looped over the lead and grasped by the snare. In the same way previously described, the lead can be sequentially grasped, pulled down, and regrasped so that the lead can be pulled out of the superior venous structures. Countertraction is used to remove the lead. The Amplatz gooseneck snare is also good for removing leads that have retracted into the venous structures by loosening the free tip of the lead. Since there is no locking stylet, the lead often stretches and breaks before the lead is removed. It is then necessary to regrasp the lead and try again.

The needle's-eye is easier to use than the tip-deflecting guidewire and the Dotter basket if a significant loop is formed by the lead in the atrium. Once the hook of the system is over the loop of the lead, the needle is advanced. Advancing the inner sheath traps the lead so that the outer sheath can be used for countertraction. Combining these newer tools with the new curved femoral sheaths allows better control over the lead all the way to the distal electrode and increases the rate of complete lead extraction from the femoral route.

The largest problem with the femoral techniques is that the tools are not easily steered in three dimensions. Except for the newer extraction devices, it is difficult to grasp the lead in a way that the lead can be released if the grasping does not produce an advantageous hold on the lead. In addition, soft Teflon sheaths, used with the femoral tools, provide little power in breaking up fibrotic tissue and have been particularly frustrating in the removal of defibrillator leads. The curved Teflon inner femoral sheaths improve the steering of the various grasping tools such as the tip-deflecting guidewire, Amplatz gooseneck snare, Dotter basket, and needle's-eye snare (Figure 16).

After lead removal using the femoral technique, it is advisable to allow slight back-bleeding to remove whatever clot might have formed around the 16F insertion site. Afterwards continuous pressure needs to be held for 10 min to prevent further bleeding. Care should be taken to watch the patient for deep venous thrombosis and/or pulmonary embolism. The inner and outer sheath system needs to be thoroughly flushed whenever the femoral countertraction sheath is removed and replaced to change or adjust the tools.

Postoperative care involves control of pain and looking for signs of bleeding and infection. In the absence of infection, recovery is comparable to any other pacemaker procedure. The patient usually stays overnight and goes home the next day. Vigorous activities are limited for approximately 2 weeks. At 6 weeks the patient returns for reprogramming of their new permanent pacemaker system for optimal efficiency of capture and sensing and to ensure that the situation has been resolved without complications. Late complications are extremely rare, and in our experience have involved the subacute development of a modest hemothorax over a 3-week period of time, subclavian vein thrombosis, and poor function of the replacement pacemaker leads.

Implantable Defibrillator Leads

Several aspects about the design and components of defibrillator leads distinguish them from pacemaker leads. There are also significant differences among different defibrillator leads. These reflect inherent differences in the approaches to defibrillation adopted by different companies (e.g., presence of two shocking electrodes, integrated and dedicated sensing circuits, and the requirement for additional superior vena cava lead). This results in each lead having its own characteristics in terms of tensile strength, insulator, number of conductors, diameter, propensity toward marked fibrosis, and support during extraction. In comparison with pacemaker leads, ICD leads are larger in diameter with multiple conductors increasing the rate of mechanical failure. A recent study from our institution showed that defibrillator lead extractions were performed earlier after implantation than pacemaker leads,[13] and a greater percentage of those leads were extracted for lead failure. Defibrillator leads have rough, large surface area electrodes that promote fibrosis. Each of these factors works against easy removability.

When extracting transvenous defibrillator systems' leads, it is advisable to remove the superior vena cava lead before removing the ventricular lead. The advantage is related to the relative ease of removal and that breaking up the fibrotic tissue between the leads facilitates the removal of the ventricular lead. The steps that are required during removal of these leads are very similar in principle to removal of pacemaker leads. The ventricular Medtronic Transvene™ leads and the CPI Endotak™ leads have been implanted for a longer time compared to other models. We will discuss the approach to extraction of both of these leads, as well as other defibrillator leads separately.[14,15]

The Endotak™ lead comes in several model series from the original 50 series to the 120 series. Most of the presently implanted leads are 60 or 70 series leads. The following comments are pertinent only to these two lead model series. Endotak™ leads are Silastic insulated, slightly more than 12F tripolar leads. Two of the electrodes are shocking springs and the third is a sensing and pacing tip electrode. There are two Teflon-coated wires that allow for substantial pulling power to be placed on the lead. These Teflon-coated wires go to the shocking electrodes. There is a standard pacing conductor coil, which can be sized and instrumented with a locking stylet similar to pacing electrodes. In order to take advantage of the two extra Teflon-coated wires to control the lead body, the pulse generator is removed from the pocket and the lead cut just distal to the Y branch in the lead.

A second incision in the prepectoral area is necessary in patients with abdominal implants to facilitate release of the two suture sleeves and for passage of sheaths into the subclavian or cephalic vein. If there is no infection, the lead is pulled through the tissues to the pectoral incision. The insulation is circumscribed around the three conductors 6–8 cm from the venous insertion and removed from the lead. If there is an abdominal pocket infection, the lead is cut, leaving as much lead in the pectoral pocket. The lead remnant is removed from the abdominal incision. The locking stylet is secured via the standard approach. However, both Teflon wires are tied back to the looped end of the locking stylet and secured firmly and tautly to the locking stylet. In addition, the suture is tied around the existing insulation and back to the looped end of the locking stylet as with pacemaker leads. Now control of the lead body is maintained by traction on all four elements: the locking stylet, two Teflon-coated wires, and the suture. The diameter of the Endotak™ lead is great enough so that only the larger diameter steel telescoping sheath and the larger diameter high-barium content telescoping polypropylene sheath can be advanced over the lead. When the steel sheath is advanced into the subclavian vein, the lead usually will stretch so that the proximal coil pulls back into the brachiocephalic vein. Often the steel sheath will, with some encouragement, slide over the proximal spring and due to the elastic nature of this lead, the spring will exit the vein. The steel sheath must follow the course of the lead and change the trajectory of its insertion according to the path of the lead. It is necessary to rotate the sheath and align the lead in order to encourage the lead to pass through the steel sheath. Often the coil is roughened up and difficult to pass into the steel sheath.

After this has been accomplished, the steel sheath is removed and the larger diameter or outer high-barium sheath is advanced over the lead. The high-barium sheath passes relatively easily to the middle brachiocephalic vein and down toward the superior vena cava. Use of the pin vise is helpful in order to advance the sheath over the distal spring. The lead usually disengages when the distal spring is peeled away from the inferior wall of the right ventricle. If there is failure to progress with the sheaths from above, then the lead needs to be cut and snared via the transfemoral approach. Transfemoral countertraction is often a time-consuming approach since the femoral sheaths are softer and more malleable, requiring time and patience to pass through the fibrotic attachments.

Extraction of the Transvene™ lead as well as other triaxial leads is different mainly because of the lack of Teflon-coated high-voltage wires. The lead is prepared in a fashion similar to bipolar coaxial leads. It is then cut with sufficient length in the prepectoral pocket to allow the insertion of the locking stylet and suture as with bipolar coaxial leads. Locking stylets are placed not only in the coaxial bipolar lead but also in the superior vena cava lead (if applicable). As stated above, it is advisable to remove the smaller diameter superior vena cava lead before removing the right ventricular lead. Telescoping steel and polypropylene sheaths are required to remove the superior vena cava lead due to the considerable fibrosis that usually forms between the roughened surface of the superior vena cava lead, the ventricular lead, and the brachiocephalic vein. After the superior vena cava lead is removed, the ventricular lead is removed in a relatively standard fashion. The Transvene™ lead is an active fixation electrode and it is possible to unscrew the electrode by rotating the locking

stylet and the inner conductor coil. This can be observed under fluoroscopy with separation of the radiopaque marker at the lead tip. Compared to the Endotak™ lead there appears to be more fibrosis with the proximal shocking electrode of the Transvene™ lead. However, there is much less fibrosis around the ventricular shocking electrode. Once the proximal electrode is removed, removal of the ventricular portion is generally less complicated.

Several adaptations to pacemaker lead extraction tools have been produced for the removal of ICD leads. Tangerine-colored telescoping polypropylene sheaths are sized so that they are both long enough and large enough to be advanced over ICD leads as telescoping sheaths. These sheaths are relatively thin and kink easily. However, it is useful to be able to use the flexibility and strength of the telescoping mechanism in the removal of these leads. A second useful tool is the flexible steel sheath (Figure 17). This instrument provides the strength of cutting and flexibility, but increases the risk of cutting the lead. If repeatedly rotated, the sheath can fracture during the extraction process. The third tool is the 16F Excimer laser sheath used with the 22F outer Teflon sheath. This sheath appears to be a major advantage in the removal of ICD leads. Its large diameter and relative inflexibility hamper it. Use of lubrication between the

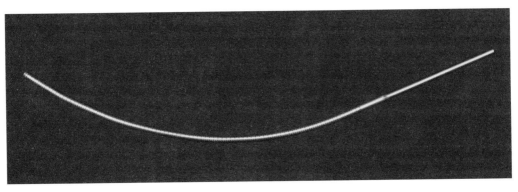

Figure 17. The flexible steel sheath. This sheath is very similar in composition to the stiff metal sheaths except for having numerous discontinuous slots arranged radially that allow for lateral flexibility without significantly decreasing their strength. This enables these sheaths to be used to tear fibrous tissue beyond the subclavian vessels.

laser and the outer sheath and on the outer surface of the outer sheath helps to reduce the friction that sometimes impedes progress. In our experience, use of these tools permitted complete removal of 52 of 54 ventricular ICD leads and there was a failed extraction in only one patient (1.9%). No significant complications have occurred but these extractions are significantly more difficult than pacemaker leads implanted for the same duration.

Table 5
Classification of Accufix™ J Lead Fractures

Class I	**No fracture** suspected
Class II	**Fracture** suspected, No protrusion
Class III	Fracture suspected, with **Protrusion**
Class IV	Fracture with **Migration**

Classification of J lead fracture severity as identified via chest x-ray, digital fluoroscopy or direct visualization. Classification was proposed by the Telectronics Physician Advisory Committee for the Multi-Center Study.

Telectronics J Leads

There are three series of Telectronics J leads. Most of the publicity and problems have been directed toward the active fixation models: Accufix™ #330-801, #329-701, #033-802, and Accufix DEC™ #033-812. However, there are some passive fixation J leads: Encor™ #330-854, #330-755, and #329-755A, the Encor DEC™ #033-856 and #033-757, and atrial ICD leads: EnGuard/Atrial DF™ #040-112, #040-069, and #040-022. In addition, there are a number of older passive fixation Cordis leads that also used this construction and have not been identified with any reported injuries.

The original passive fixation leads have a reinforcing J wire inserted within the inner conductor in the lumen usually reserved for the pacemaker stylets. The wire continues past the ring electrode and is connected to the distal electrode (see Table 1). Therefore, the lead is protected from J wire protrusion by the inner and outer conductors, as well as the outer insulation until it passes the ring electrode, and by the inner conductor and outer insulation between the ring and tip electrodes. The active fixation or Accufix™ leads were redesigned to have the J reinforcing wire moved from inside of the inner coil to outside of the outer conductor coil just internal to the outer insulation. The J wire is braised or crimped to the proximal edge of the ring electrode and travels under the outer insulation up to the straighter portion of the lead. Therefore, there is less protection from protrusion and potential pa-

tient injury with the Accufix™ than with the passive fixation Telectronics J leads (Table 5). The estimated actual prevalence of J wire fracture is 24.5% based on the results of the fluoroscopic examinations within the multicenter study and the known false negative detection rate. Special considerations for removal of both active and passive fixation versions of the leads depend on the condition of the J wire (Figure 18). The most important principle in removing the Accufix™ lead is to keep the J wire shielded from the vascular space by the lead's insulation and/or extraction sheaths. In order to accomplish this task, care is taken not to pull on the lead prior to advancing the sheaths over the ring electrode. Digital fluoroscopy is only about 50% sensitive and is highly dependent on the skill and experience of the observer.[8]

Since even a small protrusion or a fracture without protrusion can be dangerous if the outer insulator is retracted or removed, all leads, when being removed, should be treated as though there is a frank protrusion (Table 6). A small protrusion can produce big problems if the edge of the sheath catches and lifts up the J wire without ensheathing it. During the extraction procedure, especially when the sheaths are not easily advanced, consideration of the condition of the lead, the J wire, and the sheaths need to be evaluated. If protrusion is seen on chest x-ray or fluoroscopy, extra care needs to be taken not to withdraw the J portion out of the atrium into the smaller diameter superior or inferior vena cava. Do not

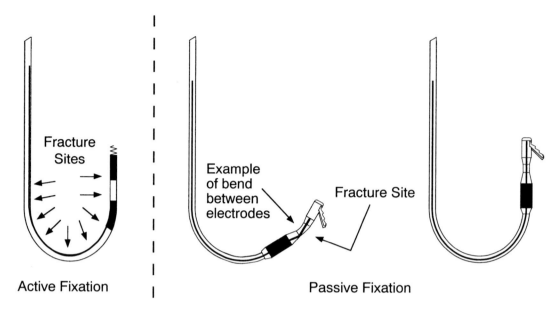

Figure 18. Telectronics J leads. The flattened J shaped wire is located external to the outer conductor and connected to the proximal end of the ring electrode in the active fixation J leads and internal to the outer conductor and continues to the distal electrode in both the bradycardia and ICD passive fixation J leads. Fractures and protrusion of the J wire usually occur at positions indicated by the arrows. Reproduced with permission from Singer I, ed.[16]

forget that while dissecting the lead free in the pacemaker pocket and untying the suture sleeve, inadvertent but significant withdrawal force can be placed on the lead placing the patient at risk for J lead trauma.

There are two technical obstacles to extracting the Accufix™ lead. The first is the very strong corkscrew active fixation mechanism, and the second is the J wire. After dissection of the lead down to its insertion vein, the slotted stylet is advanced down to the lead tip. The atrial version of the slotted stylet promotes advancement around the J curvature of the lead. However, it is somewhat flimsy and it is often easier to advance the ventricular version that is much stiffer. Considerable care is sometimes required to retract the screw mechanism. If the screw-in mechanism is not retracted, then it is doubly important that retraction of the lead does not occur until after the sheaths are advanced. If a protrusion exists and the lead is rotated in order to unscrew the screw, it is possible that the J wire will lacerate the circumference of the atrium. Since the screw is very strong, when unretracted, it is likely to tear a hole in the atrium. Often, the use of an oblique fluoroscopic view is helpful in determining whether the screw has been retracted. After the screw is retracted, the locking stylet, (0.026″ or side-locking Wilkoff) is inserted and locked. A suture is tied around the outer insulation, binding the

Table 6
Fracture Detection Rate by Fluoroscopy

Fracture Class	Population %	95% Confidence Interval
I	82.0%	80.1–83.8
II	13.5%	11.9–15.2
III	4.1%	3.2–5.1
IV	0.4%	0.2–0.9

Data from the Multi-Center Study based on 1,679 fluoroscopic screenings performed as of April 8, 1996. Physicians performed the evaluations with the aid of a teaching videotape but with various degrees of experience and different equipment.

Reference: Telectronics Incorporated. Personnel communication on July 1, 1996.

outer insulation and the outer coil with the J wire sandwiched in-between. The suture is cut and *not extended* up to the looped end of the locking stylet. If traction is exerted on the outer insulation by pulling on the suture, it is not uncommon to disassemble the lead at the level of the ring electrode (Figure 18). The outer insulation, which was formerly acting as a sheath to the J wire, now exposes the J wire to the atrium. A formerly controlled protrusion then becomes an overt protrusion and could potentially embolize. Taking care not to pull on the lead, the steel sheaths are advanced over the lead peeling it away from the ventricular lead and the vascular space.

It is often possible to pass the sheath several centimeters down the subclavian vein and into the brachiocephalic vein. These sheaths are then withdrawn and Teflon B sheaths are used to pass over the lead. Teflon B sheaths are used since they are more flexible and permit little or no withdrawal force on the lead when rounding the corner at the superior vena cava. If the fibrosis succumbs to the Teflon sheaths and encases the lead to the level of the ring electrode then the J wire is within the sheaths and the lead can be removed. Often there is significant fibrotic attachment of the distal electrode porous tip to the atrium. Care should be taken in peeling the lead away from the atrial wall. There is often significant fibrosis to the ventricular lead.

If the Teflon sheaths cannot be passed without retracting the lead into the superior vena cava, then a femoral approach is required. The lead must be grasped within the atrium and pulled into the femoral countertraction sheaths before withdrawing the lead into the inferior vena cava. The gooseneck Amplatz snare has proven to be particularly useful in this process. It is still necessary to retract the screw-in mechanism. The snare can then be used either to grasp and withdraw just the protruded J wire or to grasp the protruded J wire and the lead proximal to the ring electrode and withdraw the entire lead into the Byrd femoral workstation sheath. It is important that the distal portion of the lead is not snared since this will promote disassembly of the lead. What is likely to happen is that the fibrosis will hold onto the outer insulation in the superior veins while the distal electrode and inner insulation and ring electrode slide out of the outer conductor and insulation. This could produce an embolization of the J wire. There is much less room for error with extraction of these J leads and constant observation of the relationship of the sheaths, J wire, the lead, the vascular space, and the heart must be maintained. The 12F laser sheath has been extremely effective in the removal of J wire leads and is the tool of choice for these leads. The principles required for removing the passive fixation version of this lead are similar except for the retraction of the active fixation mechanism. However, it is less likely that the J wire will escape since it is within the confines of the outer conductor. Early reports suggest that distal tip deformation (distortion of the segment of the lead between the ring and tip electrodes) have been observed in a few leads. Distal tip deformation is more frequently seen with implantation techniques that use right subclavian vein introducer implantation due to the acute angle and potential kinking of the introducer. If the lead is advanced against the kinked introducer, damage can be produced. Once bent, the J wire is more vulnerable. It is possible that a fractured J wire could protrude into the path of any stylet advanced through the inner conductor coil and force the J wire out of the lead and directly into the atrial wall. Although the experience is much more limited with this lead, and the precise indications for removal not worked out, wisdom dictates that similar precautions should be used as with the Accufix™ lead.

Lead Replacement after Lead Removal

If there is no evidence of infection and a new pacemaker lead is required, it is often possible to reuse the previous vascular access. This is true whether the access is through the cephalic or the subclavian vein. Once the sheaths are intravascular and the lead is removed, the sheaths can be used as access for a J tip guidewire. Subsequently, a lead dilator with a long peel-away introducer is advanced over the J tip guidewire. The only particular risk associated with this approach is that the guidewire can be advanced through a false lumen. If there is any resistance to the reinsertion of the guidewire or the subsequent introduction of the pacing lead, this approach should be abandoned and a separate venous insertion planned. Long introducers permit access of the lead directly to the cardiac structures without catching on the stenotic, weakened, or torn fibrotic tissue in the subclavian, brachiocephalic, and superior vena cava structures. A large percentage of complications associated with lead extraction have been produced during the reintroduction of a lead through the standard (short) introducer sheath or the outer extraction sheath when the tip of the sheath is left in the brachiocephalic vein. Use of the long peel-away sheaths and avoiding the reintroduction of leads through the outer extraction sheath prevents this complication. This is a great time saver and can be an extremely safe way of recapturing the insertion vein.

Conclusion

With the demonstrated safety and efficacy of current pacemaker and implantable defibrillator systems, criteria for implanting these devices became less stringent. The marked increase in the number and complexity of implanted systems uncovered the potential need for the development of technique and skills to remove these systems in many situations. Extraction of transvenous pacemaker and implantable defibrillator leads thus became a distinct clinical procedure, requiring specialized tools, techniques, and training. In experienced hands, this procedure not only improves outcome by preventing and treating potentially life-threatening situations, but it also increases the number of options available to the treating physician. This is achieved with minimal risk to the patient during and after the procedure. The need for extracting defibrillator leads has added to the level of complexity of the procedure and has required introduction of newer specialized instruments. Recent introduction of laser extraction sheaths and other specially designed tools will lead to further improvement in success rates and reduction in the risk of complications. It needs to be emphasized, however, that judgment, adequate training, and careful patient selection are the most important factors in ensuring the success and safety of this procedure.

References

1. Stokes KB, Anderson J, McVenes R, et al. The encapsulation of polyurethane-insulated transvenous cardiac pacemaker leads. Cardiovasc Pathol 1995;4(3):163–171.
2. Interventional Lead Extraction: Concepts, Tools, and Techniques. Video tape by Cook Pacemaker Corporation, 1992.
3. NASPE Lead Extraction Policy Conference: 18th annual session of the North American Society of Pacing and Electrophysiology, New Orleans, May 1997. (In Review)
4. Byrd CL, Schwartz SJ, Hedin N. Intravascular techniques for extraction of permanent pacemaker leads. J Thorac Cardiovasc Surg 1991;101:989.
5. Smith HG, Fearnot NE, Byrd CL, et al, for the U.S. Lead Extraction Database. Five-years experience with intravascular lead extraction. PACE 1994;17:II;2016–2020.
6. Byrd CL. Management of implant complications. In Clinical Cardiac Pacing. Ellenbogen KA, Kay GN, Wilkoff BL, eds. WB Saunders, Philadelphia. 1995, pp 519–520.
7. Brodell GK, Castle LW, Maloney JD, et al. Chronic transvenous pacemaker lead removal using a unique, sequential transvenous system. Am J Cardiol 1990;66(12):964–966.
8. Telectronics Pacing Systems. Accufix™ Atrial J Leads (Models 329-701, 330-801 and 033-812) J Retention Wire Fracture. Technology Memo, August 1995.

9. Lloyd MA, Hayes DL, Holmes DR Jr, et al. Extraction of the Telectronics Accufix 330-801 atrial lead: the Mayo Clinic experience. Mayo Clin Proc 1996;71:230–234.

10. Data from Cook Vascular Incorporated Multicenter Lead Extraction Registry. Presented in part at the annual scientific sessions of the North American Society for Pacing and Electrophysiology (NASPE), May 7, 1997, New Orleans, LA.

11. Brodell GK, Wilkoff BL. A novel approach to determining the cause of pacemaker lead failure. Cleve Clin J Med 1992;59(1):91–92.

12. Byrd C, Wilkoff BL, Love C, et al. Clinical study of the laser sheath: results of the PLEXES trial. PACE 1997;20:(Pt II)1053.

13. Niebauer MJ, Wilkoff BL, Van Zandt H, et al. Nonthoracotomy defibrillator lead extraction: comparison with ventricular pacing leads. PACE 1997;20:(Pt II)1071.

14. Wilkoff BL, Smith HJ, Goode LB. Transvenous extraction of nonthoracotomy defibrillator leads: an emerging technical challenge. Eur JCPE 1994;4(2):132.

15. Maloney JD, Wilkoff BL, Smith HJ, et al. Feasibility of percutaneous extraction of defibrillator leads. Circulation 1995;92:8, I–151.

16. Singer I, ed. Interventional Electrophysiology. Williams and Wilkins Medical Publishers, Baltimore, 1997, pp 1055–1084.

Chapter 34

New Indications for Cardiac Pacing

S. Serge Barold

Introduction

Over the last 10 years, several new indications for pacing have emerged. In patients without conduction system disease, these include obstructive hypertrophic cardiomyopathy (OHCM), end-stage dilated cardiomyopathy with congestive heart failure (CHF), and orthostatic hypotension. In the presence of organic or functional conduction system disease, a very long PR interval (with unfavorable hemodynamic consequences) and neurally mediated (malignant vasovagal) syncope also constitute new indications for pacing. Pacing for malignant vasovagal syncope is discussed in Chapter 38.

Obstructive Hypertrophic Cardiomyopathy

Many studies have shown that dual chamber pacing can be effective therapy for symptomatic relief in patients with OHCM[1–20] (Table 1). Single chamber right ventricular (RV) pacing should not be considered because loss of atrioventricular (AV) synchrony coupled with left ventricular (LV) diastolic dysfunction results in hemodynamic compromise with decreased ventricular filling and increased left atrial

and pulmonary capillary wedge pressures (PCWP).[21]

Acute Studies

Acute hemodynamic studies have shown that most patients develop a significant drop in the resting LV outflow tract (LVOT) gradient during DDD pacing with an optimal (short) AV delay.[2,3,11,13,22,23] The acute hemodynamic response during pacing studies does not reliably predict which patients will benefit from DDD pacing and such studies are generally no longer recommended.[24] A few patients in most series demonstrated no hemodynamic improvement with temporary pacing.[3,22,23,25,26] Yet, some will improve on a long-term basis[23] suggesting that factors other than paradoxical septal motion, e.g., cellular and molecular modification of the myocardium, account for the hemodynamic changes. In some cases, lack of acute hemodynamic benefit may be caused by failure to achieve ventricular depolarization because of a short spontaneous PR interval.

Permanent Pacing

Long-term pacing is beneficial in patients with drug-refractory OHMC with a resting

From Singer I, Barold SS, Camm AJ (eds): Nonpharmacological Therapy of Arrhythmias for the 21st Century: The State of the Art. Futura Publishing Co, Inc., Armonk, NY, © 1998.

Table 1
World-Wide Results of Dual Chamber (DDD) Pacing in 401 Patients with Obstructive Hypertrophic Cardiomyopathy

Authors	Center	No	NYHA Before	NYHA After	LV Outflow Gradient Before	LV Outflow Gradient After	Exercise Duration (min) Pre	Exercise Duration (min) Post	Follow-up (Mo)
McDonald et al.[1]	Ireland	11	3	1.5	43	?	7.7	10.1	24
Jeanrenaud et al.[3]	Switzerland	7	—	—	67 ± 42	17 ± 10	—	—	44 ± 11
Fananapazir et al.[6]	NIH, Bethesda	84*	3.2 ± 0.5	1.6 ± 0.6	96 ± 41**	27 ± 31	5.3 ± 2.7	7.2 ± 2.8	26 ± 9
Gras et al.[8]	France	30	3.2 ± 0.5	1.4 ± 0.5	112 ± 31	19 ± 12	—	—	34 ± 14
Yusvinkevich et al.[9]	Russia	17	3.3 ± 0.9	1.6 ± 1.1	73 ± 39	38 ± 34	10.9 ± 4.4	12.9 ± 3.6	3.0
Umman et al.[10]	Turkey	5	2.6 ± 0.5	1.6 ± 0.5	78 ± 20	42 ± 17	—	—	2.2 ± 3
Nishimura et al.[12]	Mayo Clinic	19	2.9 ± 0.4	2.4 ± 0.7	76 ± 61	55 ± 38	5.7 ± 2.7	6.9 ± 2.2	3.0
Gambhir et al.[11]	India	12	3.0	?	94 ± 29	39 ± 15	—	—	?
Slade et al.[13]	England/ France/ Poland	56†	2.8 ± 0.5	1.7 ± 0.7	78 ± 31	36 ± 25	—	—	11 ± 11
Gadler et al.[14]	Sweden	19	2.8 ± 0.4	1.8 ± 0.5	22 ± 6 (98 ± 31)*†	(42 ± 26)*†	—	—	12 ± 9
Gadler et al.[14]	Sweden	22	3.0 ± 0.6	1.9 ± 0.5	86 ± 40	36 ± 24	—	—	12 ± 9
Sadoul et al.[15]	France	16	—	—	79 ± 21	24 ± 17	—	—	18.7 ± 9.5
Kappenberger et al.[17]††	Switzerland (PIC Study)	83	angina 1.4 dyspnea 2.4	0.7 1.0	71 ± 62	28 ± 23	—	—	12
Sakai et al.[19]	Japan	9	—	—	96	17	—	—	6.0
Iliou et al.[20]	France	11	3.0 ± 0.4	2.3 ± 0.3	39 ± 19	14 ± 7	—	—	12

NYHA = New York heart Association; * = 74 patients with rest obstruction and 10 patients with provocable obstruction only; ** = gradients in patients with rest obstruction only.

*† All patients had a provocable left ventricular outflow tract gradient shown in parentheses, † 2 patients had only provocable obstruction.

†† Double blind study with pacemaker turned off for 3 months. Adapted from Fananapazir L, et al.[18] with permission.

gradient >30 mm Hg or provocable gradient ≥30–50 mm Hg due to prominent basal septal hypertrophy.[14,17,18] Reliable evaluation of pacemaker treatment is difficult because of the dynamic nature and variability of the LVOT gradient that occur independently of the way it is measured. In most patients (80%–85%) with drug-refractory OHCM, permanent DDD pacing with a short AV interval (50–150 ms and often less than 100 ms) reduces symptoms (angina, dyspnea, presyncope, syncope, and palpitations) and results in improved functional status (demonstrable by treadmill testing) long-term exercise capacity, quality of life and reduction of pharmacotherapy.[13,17] In most patients, the resting LVOT gradient diminishes by about 50% during DDD pacing without significant alteration in blood pressure or cardiac output while mitral regurgitation decreases,[27–29] yet there is no correlation between the magnitude of reduction of LVOT gradient and functional improvement.[13,17]

All drug-refractory patients should be considered for a trial of permanent pacing. Further fine tuning of the pacemaker (AV interval, etc.) can then be carried out in patients who initially exhibit suboptimal or no benefit. In rare cases, if truly unsuccessful, the pacing system could eventually be taken out.

Long-Term Pacing: Clinical Studies

Fananapazir et al.[2] (from NIH) first reported in 1992 the benefit of dual chamber pacing in 44 patients with OHCM refractory to verapamil and beta adrenergic blocking drugs, and in 1994, they presented follow-up data on 84 patients (74 patients had resting LVOT gradients >30 mm Hg and 10 patients had LVOT gradients >55 mm Hg with provocation only).[6] At a mean follow-up of 2.3 ± 0.8 years (maximum 3.5 years), the New York Heart Association (NYHA) functional class improved (Table 1, $P<.00001$). Symptoms were eliminated in 28 patients (33%), improved in 47 patients (56%), but remained unchanged in seven patients (8%). Table 1 shows that pacing produced a significant drop in the mean LVOT gradient ($P<.00001$). In the patients with resting LVOT obstruction, the LVOT gradient was eliminated or insignificant in 65% and unchanged in 8%. Two patients died suddenly (97% cumulative 3-year survival rate). In both patients, symptoms and LVOT gradient had improved before sudden death. Symptoms and provocable LVOT gradient were also reduced in all 10 patients without significant resting, but provocable LVOT gradient. In the 84 patients, persistence of the LVOT gradient and symptoms were mostly related to inability to preexcite the interventricular septum and the onset of atrial fibrillation[6] (Table 2).

As documented in their 1992 report,[2] Fananapazir et al.[6] also demonstrated in follow-up cardiac catheterization studies a progressive reduction of the LVOT gradient during sinus rhythm (compared to baseline study in sinus rhythm) when the pacemaker was turned off.

Jeanrenaud et al.[3] also studied the chronic effects of pacing in OHCM in seven patients who received verapamil and beta blockers and DDD pacemakers with an AV interval of 50–90 ms programmed to its optimal value (mean, 63 ± 18 ms) (Table 1). Observations were made at midterm (11 ± 10 months) and long-term (after 44 ± 11 months) follow-up. In all seven patients there was striking improvement, particularly with respect to angina. Dyspnea also improved, and two patients with previous syncope reported no further episodes. At the midterm assessment, the mean resting

LVOT gradient during DDD pacing was 40 ± 31 mm Hg, rising to 65 ± 34 mm Hg when the pacemakers were switched off. The latter values in sinus rhythm were similar to those obtained during the acute baseline study. In contrast, Fananapazir et al.[2] observed a reduction of the resting LVOT gradient as early as 6 weeks after pacemaker implantation during sinus rhythm when the pacemakers were switched off. However, in the study of Jeanrenaud et al.,[3] at long-term follow-up, the mean resting LVOT gradient dropped to 17 ± 10 mm Hg during DDD pacing, significantly lower than at the midterm follow-up. When the pacemakers were switched off the mean resting LVOT gradient rose to 31 ± 36 mm Hg, significantly lower than at the start of the study or the midterm follow-up.[3]

Fananapazir et al.[30] recently evaluated the long-term (5.0 ± 0.7 years) results of DDD pacing therapy in 48 patients with OHCM and symptoms refractory to verapamil and beta blockers (mean age: 48 ± 15 years). The results are shown in Table 3.

Table 2

Possible Explanations for Failure of DDD Pacing to Improve Symptoms or to Relieve LVOT Obstruction

Inappropriate Pacemaker Programming:
- Inadequate ventricular pre-excitation: Programmed AV delay too long.
- Interference with left atrial emptying: Programmed AV delay too short.

Inadequate Pacemaker Trial Period

Other Associated Abnormalities:
- Proximal or high septal ventricular lead position
- Aberrant papillary muscle obstructing LV outflow
- Primary mitral valve regurgitation*
- Mid-cavity LV obstruction**
- Atrial and/or ventricular tachyarrhythmias
- LV diastolic dysfunction
- Inappropriate drug therapy

---

* The mitral valve regurgitation in OHCM may be primary, and difficult to distinguish from severe mitral regurgitation due to systolic anterior motion of the mitral valve when the outflow obstruction is relieved.

** Pacing may relieve mid-cavity obstruction.

Reproduced with permission from Fananapazir L, et al.[18]

Table 3
Five-Year Results of Dual Chamber Pacing in Obstructive Hypertrophic Cardiomyopathy (NIH Data-48 Patients—Mean age 48 ± 15 years)

Evaluation	NYHA	Sinus Rhythm			DDD Pacing		
		CO	PCW	LVG	CO	PCW	LVG
Baseline	3.1 ± 0.4	5.0 ± 1.1	15 ± 7	88 ± 51			
5-Year	1.7 ± 0.7	4.9 ± 1.0	13 ± 5	34 ± 39*	4.6 ± 1.1	13 ± 5	24 ± 30*
DDD Pacing Switched Off for 6 Months At 5-Year Follow-up (6 Patients)							
Baseline	3.2 ± 0.4	5.0 ± 1.5	10 ± 4	71 ± 40			
5-Year	1.5 ± 0.6	4.9 ± 0.8	14 ± 4	14 ± 24**	5.0 ± 0.8	11 ± 3	12 ± 20**
6 Months	1.7 ± 0.8	4.7 ± 0.4	12 ± 3	18 ± 24**			

All pressures in mm Hg.
NYHA = New York Heart Association; CO = cardiac output L/min; PCW = capillary wedge pressure; LVG = left ventricular outflow tract gradient.
* P < 0.0001 compared to baseline.
** P < 0.05 compared to baseline.
Reproduced with permission from Fananapazir et al.[30]

DDD pacing was switched off in six patients in whom the LVOT gradient had been reduced by >50% in sinus rhythm at the 5-year follow-up study. Table 3, bottom, shows the results after a further 6-month period without pacing during this period. It appears that LV obstruction does not return in some patients after the pacemaker is switched off for a long time. This finding and the reduction in LVOT gradient recorded in sinus rhythm at the 5-year evaluation provide further evidence of pacing-induced cardiac remodeling.[30]

A European double-blind randomized study of DDD versus placebo AAI pacing (30 ppm) involving 83 patients with a resting LVOT gradient >30 mm Hg clearly showed the benefit of DDD pacing.[17] After 12 weeks, the pacing modes were inverted (crossover) for another 12 weeks. Seventeen of 83 patients (20%) required early reprogramming from AAI to DDD because of persistent symptoms or deterioration. DDD significantly improved symptoms, quality of life, and exercise tolerance. The LVOT gradient fell from 59 ± 36 mm Hg to 30 ± 25 mm Hg (P<0.001) with DDD pacing. Seventy-nine of the 83 patients (95%) preferred DDD pacing. Subsequent follow-up of patients for 1 year showed that pacing was beneficial on pressure gradient and symptoms in 72 patients (87%).[31]

Indications for Pacing

The implantation of a dual chamber pacemaker is relatively simple and seems to offer the same benefits as septal myectomy at lower cost and risk. Indeed, permanent pacing could soon become first-line therapy for OHCM. Often patients can discontinue drug therapy because pacing alone can produce striking clinical improvement.[2] Elderly patients[32] as well as children[33,34] with OHCM can also benefit from DDD pacing. However, about 10% of the patients with OHCM do not respond favorably to pacing and a few actually deteriorate.[12]

The 1998 ACC/AHA guidelines for implantation of pacemakers list medically refractory symptomatic hypertrophic cardiomyopathy with significant resting or provoked LV outflow obstruction as a class IIb indication.[35] Many believe that a class IIa designation would have been more appropriate.

Importance of Pacemaker Function and Programmability

Most patients improve clinically to a degree comparable to that achieved with myectomy and the favorable response to pacing is closely tied to optimization of the AV interval.[36]

1. *Site of Ventricular Pacing.* The ventricular lead must be positioned in the most distal part of the RV apex. Pacing the proximal septum just beneath the tricuspid valve or high septal area produces no significant fall in the gradient.[37,38] Lack of improvement may require repositioning of the RV pacing lead with the aid of echocardiographic imaging to ensure a distal apical position because fluoroscopy and QRS morphology are imprecise markers of lead position.

2. *AV Interval.* Dual chamber pacemakers must be programmed with a short AV interval (occasionally as short as 50 ms) to avoid spontaneous ventricular depolarization and to ensure ventricular capture at all times to provide apical preexcitation. The AV interval must therefore be carefully individualized. The optimal AV interval varies widely and has to be determined for each individual patient on the basis of Doppler echocardiographic measurements, LVOT gradient, stroke volume, and parameters of the LV filling such as transmitral flow and blood pressure.[39,40] The atrial contribution to ventricular filling is crucial and AV intervals that are too short may be deleterious.[36,41,42] When the AV delay is too short, LV diastolic filling becomes impaired despite a drop in the LVOT gradient. The left atrial pressure will rise and the cardiac output will decrease.

a. The optimal paced AV delay may be significantly longer than the sensed AV delay.[13]

b. The optimal AV delay may occasionally vary with the passage of time and should be reevaluated at each follow-up visit.

c. The AV delay must be optimized at rest (and at several faster rates) and on effort. Patients must undergo a treadmill stress test to determine the optimal AV delay on exercise and whether they can maintain a paced ventricular rhythm at all times.

d. An auto-adaptive AV interval that shortens automatically with exercise and acceleration of the atrial rate is an important feature.

e. *Negative AV Interval Hysteresis.* This capability is designed to maintain full ventricular capture. The degree of shortening of AV nodal conduction during physiological stress is not predictable. If the pacemaker senses spontaneous ventricular depolarization within the AV interval, it will automatically shorten the AV delay (by a programmable value) so that the AV delay becomes shorter than the Ap-Vs or As-Vs interval.[43] A search function will ultimately restore the original AV delay if circumstances are appropriate.

f. When the PR interval is short, prolongation of AV conduction by drugs or AV nodal radiofrequency (RF) catheter ablation may be useful to achieve the optimal AV interval to ensure pacemaker-controlled ventricular depolarization in the absence of ventricular fusion.[45,46] Ablation permits exclusive pacemaker activation of the LV and longer AV intervals to promote optimal LV filling.[7,39] Such an approach can produce significant improvement in patients who fail to benefit from pacing alone, even at short AV intervals.

Alternatively, simultaneous right and left atrial pacing can be performed. Daubert et al.[47] used biatrial pacing (right atrial appendage and coronary sinus for left atrial stimulation) in conjunction with a DDD pacemaker in patients with OHCM with or without intra- or interatrial conduction delay. This arrangement (triple chamber pacemaker) permits optimization of the mechanical AV delay on the left side of the heart. Shortening of the effective AV delay avoids RF ablation to produce an optimal AV delay and ensures continual pacemaker-controlled ventricular depolarization.

3. *Atrial Sensing.* Atrial sensing is extremely important and meticulous care must be taken at the time of implantation to ensure a good atrial signal. Atrial sensing should also be evaluated on exercise.

4. *Polarity.* Because these patients can also develop life-threatening ventricular tachyarrhythmias, a bipolar dual chamber pacemaker should be implanted in case an ICD is required in the future. Such a dual chamber device should be a dedicated bipolar unit in that reset to the VVI or VOO mode secondary to electrical interference or battery depletion occurs in the bipolar and not the unipolar mode because the latter may interfere with detection of ventricular tachyarrhythmias by an ICD.

5. *Rate-Adaptive Function.* Patients should be evaluated for atrial chronotropic incompetence estimated to occur in about 30% of OHCM patients.[48] Such patients would benefit from DDDR rather than DDD pacing.[48] Ideally, all patients should receive a DDDR device because concurrent medications may blunt the atrial chronotropic response.

6. *Automatic Mode Switching.* This function is important because it prevents tracking of rapid atrial rates from atrial tachyarrhythmias a common complication of OHCM.

7. *Optimal Upper Rate*

a. *Myocardial Ischemia.* Myocardial ischemia can occur in OHCM in the absence of coronary artery disease. Patients may develop angina and electrocardiographic abnormalities consistent with ischemia and infarction and frequently show replacement scarring at autopsy.[49,50] Patients (especially those with previous cardiac arrest and syncope) may show exercise-induced reversible defects with thallium scintigraphy indistinguishable from those in patients with ischemia caused by coronary artery disease.[51,52] Improvement of the scintigraphic abnormalities occur after surgical relief of LVOT obstruction.[53] Preliminary studies suggest that dual chamber pacing improves coronary blood flow and reduces myocardial ischemia.[54–57] The mechanisms of myocardial ischemia in the absence of epicardial coronary artery disease include:

(1) Excessive myocardial O_2 demand that exceeds the capacity of the coronary system to deliver oxygen. Atrial pacing can precipitate myocardial ischemia and abnormalities in lactate metabolism in susceptible patients with reduced coronary vasodilator response.[58,59]

(2) Abnormal (narrowed) intramural coronary arteries (which are components of the thickened myopathic ventricle) and inadequacy of capillary density with respect to the greatly increased LV muscle mass.[49,50]

(3) Systolic compression of large coronary arteries by myocardial bridges.

(4) Diastolic occlusion of intramyocardial coronary arteries secondary to marked elevations of LV diastolic pressure.

Brinker[60] advocates establishing an upper rate limit that avoids ischemia during pacing. Thus myocardial scintigraphy on exercise should be considered in many if not all OHCM patients considered for cardiac pacing. Such evaluation is particularly important in patients with atrial chronotropic incompetence in whom excessive pacing rates during DDDR pacing should be avoided. Concomitant anti-ischemic therapy with beta blockers and verapamil may reduce or eliminate myocardial ischemia.[52]

  b. *Wenckebach Upper Rate Response with Long AV Intervals.* The pacemaker should be programmed with a relatively high maximum rate and relatively short postventricular atrial refractory period (PVARP) to avoid a Wenckebach upper rate response. In some patients with retrograde ventriculoatrial conduction, a short PVARP requires an effective algorithm for the termination of endless loop tachycardia almost as soon as it starts. A fast upper rate must be avoided in patients with demonstrable cardiac ischemia. Ideally, the maximum allowable sinus rate that avoids ischemia should be determined with a radionuclide stress test. When using beta blockers to prevent ischemia program the upper rate should be programmed accordingly.

8. Dual Chamber Defibrillator vs. Pacemaker. Now that the implantation procedure of a dual chamber defibrillator is similar to that of a dual chamber pacemaker, the question arises as to whether it would be preferable to implant a dual chamber defibrillator (with DDDR pacing capability) because of OHCM patients are at risk of malignant ventricular tachyarrhythmias and sudden death as well as atrial tachyarrhythmia often associated with serious hemodynamic consequences. The main issue is cost.

Possible Mechanism of Beneficial Effect

The effect of DDD pacing is optimal only when RV apical stimulation is synchronized to atrial systole, producing optimal filling and activation of LV apex before septal contraction, a mechanism called inversion of ventricular contraction[13] or apical preexcitation.[43] The beneficial response may be related to altered or paradoxical motion of the ventricular septum with widening of the LVOT and reduction of LVOT gradient associated with diminished mitral regurgitation (provided there is no primary abnormality of the mitral valve), increase in LV filling and eventually reduced contractility as a result of pacing. Jeanrenaud and Kappenberger[61] observed a 12% reduction in septal motion (particularly the midportion) with AV pacing (without reduction in global EF) and paradoxical septal motion in only one of nine patients, while Betocchi et al.[62] showed a decrease in septal EF.

Acute pacing may cause deterioration of LV diastolic function and increase in filling pressures.[62,64] On a chronic basis, this does not seem to translate into a clinical problem despite the deterioration of certain indices of LV diastolic function reported by some workers.[30,63,65–68]

There is a progressive reduction in the LVOT gradient with time.[69] When the pacemaker is switched off during follow-up of more than a few months, the original LVOT gradient in normal sinus rhythm remains reduced on a short-term basis,[2,3] possibly weeks, though little data exist about this finding. This suggests that there is a pacing-induced remodeling of the myocardial resulting in LV dilatation, permanent hemodynamic and possibly morphological changes,[70] or a mechanical memory effect.[71,72]

In some studies, serial echocardiographic evaluation suggests localized thinning of the LV wall and increase in the end-systolic volume.[6,20,68,69] Therefore, changes in hypertrophy and LV systolic function may explain the progressive and sustained effect on the LVOT gradient.[69]

In summary, the beneficial effects of pacing are due to a reduction of LVOT gradient, reduction of mitral regurgitation, depression of LV systolic function, possible regression of LV hypertrophy, and remodeling.[40]

Unresolved Questions About the Benefit of Pacing

The use of pacing in OHCM raises a number of questions.

1. How does long-term pacing affect the degree of mitral regurgitation, which contributes substantially to symptoms of dyspnea in many patients?
2. Do the patients continue to benefit long-term? Is there some unrecognized harmful adaptation with dual chamber pacing? Will LV enlargement and depression of systolic and diastolic function[73] be detrimental long-term and contribute to eventual heart failure?.
3. What are the cellular and biochemical changes in the myocardium? How does pacing influence ventricular remodeling and myocardial structure?
4. How can we identify noninvasively patients unsuitable for pacing? Obstruction other than subaortic or patients with anatomic abnormalities of the mitral valve may not respond to pacing. However, preliminary data suggest that patients with mid-cavity obstruction may also respond.[18]
5. Is a combination of pacing with drugs better than pacing alone?
6. Can conventional or two-site biatrial pacing prevent atrial fibrillation?
7. Changes in the natural history and prevention of sudden death with pacing have not been determined.

Nonobstructive Hypertrophic Cardiomyopathy

Cannon et al.[74] reported the results of permanent dual chamber pacing in 12 patients with symptomatic nonobstructive HCM (no resting LVOT gradient and no LVOT gradient >30 mm Hg during Valsalva maneuver, amyl nitrite inhalation, or isoproterenol infusion). DDD pacing was associated with improvement in symptoms and effort tolerance, but there was a need for reinitiation of medical therapy and no objective evidence of hemodynamic benefit was demonstrated. On this basis, Cannon et al.[74] concluded that chronic DDD pacing cannot as yet be recommended for routine use in the management of patients with nonobstructive HCM who are symptomatic despite medical therapy.

Congestive Heart Failure

Hochleitner et al.[75] in 1990 reported the beneficial effects of DDD pacing (short AV interval of 100 ms) in the treatment of end-stage idiopathic dilated cardiomyopathy (DMC) in 16 patients without AV block in whom conventional therapy had failed. There was striking improvement of dyspnea at rest and pulmonary edema, as well as a significant decrease in NYHA functional class, left atrial and RV dimensions, and reduced cardiothoracic ratio. The short AV interval appeared to reduce mitral regurgitation and improve LV filling.

Hochleitner et al.[76] then reported the long-term efficacy of dual chamber (DDD) pacing in the treatment of end-stage idiopathic dilated cardiomyopathy in a longitudinal study of up to 5 years in 17 patients. The considerable clinical improvement achieved after implantation of a DDD pacemaker with an AV delay of 100 ms was maintained throughout the follow-up period or until death. Improvement was associated with a consistent decrease in NYHA class and an increase in LVEF. Cardiothoracic ratio, resting heart rate, and echocardiographic dimensions progressively decreased, and systolic and diastolic blood pressure increased except in the four patients who underwent heart transplantation. The median survival time from pacemaker implantation was 22 months. Three patients refused cardiac transplantation because of the dramatic clinical improvement in response to DDD pacing. Nine died suddenly (undefined or after a thromboembolic event) and one died from carcinoma. No patient required rehospitalization owing to worsening heart failure. Three patients were evaluated after interruption of pacing for 2–4 hours (000 mode). Within the first 2 weeks after pacemaker implantation and, to a smaller extent, after 6 and 12 months, cardiac function decreased after pacing withdrawal. The LVEF upon acute interruption of DDD pacing decreased from 32% ± 3% to 18% ± 3% and from 30% ± 4% to 23% ± 5% at 2 weeks and 1 year, respectively, after the initiation of DDD pacing (n = 9), whereas after 5 years the response to DDD withdrawal was not significant (40% ± 2% to 39% ± 2%) (n = 3). However, the decreases in diastolic blood pressure and the increase in heart rate after pacing withdrawal persisted through the observation period. The considerable deterioration in cardiac function after short-term removal of DDD pacing in the early stages eventually disappeared, suggesting that DDD pacing may have a beneficial impact on damaged myocardium.

Soon after Hochleitner et al.[75] reported their long-term results, others used this therapy in another seven cases (six with coronary artery disease) with success.[77–79] Since then, acute[80–87] and long-term[88–92] studies with conventional DDD pacing in patients with CHF of various etiologies have yielded conflicting results (Tables 4 and 5). Acute improvement even in selected patients has been inconsistent.[80–87] Two major long-term studies[88,89] have been disappointing, though the long-term study of Brecker et al.[90] suggests improvement is possible in highly selected patients.

Mechanism of Beneficial Effect

Brecker et al.[84] studied the acute effect of DDD pacing with a short AV interval on

Table 4
Dual Chamber Pacing in Congestive Heart Failure and LV Dysfunction: Acute Studies

Authors	Year	Etiology	CHF	# of Patients	LVEF	AV Interval (ms)	Benefit
Brecker et al.[84]	1992	3 CAD, 9 DCM	?	12	?	Optimized	CO and exercise duration increased. All pts had MR and/or TR
Feliciano et al.[86]	1994	?	Yes	17	21 ± 6%	100, 125, 150, 175, 200	No
Paul et al.[87]	1994	8 CAD, 4 DCM	Yes	12	?	6–150	CO increased in 8 pts. Those with highest LVEDP showed the greatest CO increase
Innes et al.[80]	1994	4 CAD, 8 DCM	Yes	12	21 ± 2.5%	60, 100	Stroke and cardiac index declined
Nishimura et al.[81]	1995	7 CAD, 8 DCM	?	15	19%	60, 100, 120, 140, 180, 240	CO increased only in 8 pt group with PR > 200 ms not in pts with normal PR
Scanu et al.[82]	1996	8 CAD, 10 DCM	Yes	18	26 ± 6.5%	20 ms decrements	CO increased in pts with first degree AV block and/or short ventricular filling time
Shibane et al.[83]	1997	5 CAD, 4 DCM	Yes	9	28 ± 8%	50, 75, 100, 150, 200	No
Mathew et al.[85]	1997	— 3 ACM	Yes	3	Normal	60, 100, 120, 140, etc.	No

CAD = coronary artery disease; CHF = congestive heart failure; CO = cardiac output; AV = atrioventricular; DCM = dilated cardiomyopathy; LV = left ventricular; EDP = end-diastolic pressure; TR = tricuspid regurgitation; ACM = amyloid cardiomyopathy; MR = mitral regurgitation; pt = patient; EF = ejection fraction.

Table 5
Conventional Dual Chamber Pacing in Congestive Heart Failure: Long-Term Studies

Authors	Year	Etiology	CHF	# of Pts.	LVEF	AV Interval (msec)	Follow-up	Benefit
Auricchio et al.[78]	1993	CAD	Yes	2	21%	100	6–52 wk	Both patients improved. One died 6 weeks later of CHF related to refractory atrial fibrillation
Hochleitner et al.[79]	1993	CAD	Yes	4	13%	100	12 mo	Clinical improvement. LVEF increased to 26%
Linde et al.[88]	1995	7 CAD	Yes	10	21 ± 9%	70–120 optimal	6 mo	3 pts improved in NYHA Class. Only 1 pt showed consistent improvement in SV, CO, LVEF and NYHA Class
Gold et al.[89]	1995	8 CAD	Yes	12	20 ± 6%	100	4–6 wk	No improvement in NYHA Class or LVEF
Brecker et al.[90]	1995	ESCM PR = 215 ± 70 ms QRS = 170 ± 30 ms MR and/or TR	?	12	SF = 13 ± 5%	Optimal	12 mo	All pts improved, but 5 died. Improvement was sustained during follow-up
Greco et al.[91]	1997	CM	?	21	16 ± 4%	100–120	2.4 ± 0.6 yr	LVEF rose to 23 ± 4%. NYHA increased from 2.2 ± 0.4 to 3.7 ± 0.5
Ansalone et al.[92]	1997	5 CAD PR ≥ 0.24 sec LBBB. Moderate to severe MR	?	12	20%	100–120	22 ± 4 mo	No increase in CO or LVEF. Effect on quality of life and prognosis was uncertain

CAD = coronary artery disease; CHF = congestive heart failure; CO = cardiac output; SF = shortening fraction; NYHA = New York Heart Association; CM = dilated cardiomyopathy; LV = left ventricular; EDP = end-diastolic pressure; SV = stroke volume; LBBB = left bundle branch block; ES = end-stage; LVEF = left ventricular ejection fraction; MR = mitral regurgitation; TR = tricuspid regurgitation; pt = patients.

ventricular filling time and exercise capacity in 12 patients with dilated cardiomyopathy (three with ischemic etiology) and functional mitral or tricuspid regurgitation. Their report did not indicate whether the patients were in CHF failure at the time of the study.[84] The duration of both mitral and tricuspid regurgitation were shorter with brief AV intervals and both LV and RV filling times were longer. In patients with presystolic (diastolic) mitral regurgitation (known to occur in patients with complete or first degree AV block and those with severe LV disease even when the PR interval is normal), DDD pacing abolished presystolic mitral regurgitation and increased the time available for forward flow. Short AV delays were associated with greater cardiac output at rest and striking improvement in exercise duration. All patients with QRS ≥0.12 sec improved.

The role of mitral regurgitation was demonstrated by Rossi et al.[93] in a series of 20 patients with third degree AV block and isolated mitral regurgitation. An optimally short AV delay (98 ± 7 ms) produced a significant reduction in the severity of mitral regurgitation and increase in stroke volume.[93]

Causes of Divergent Results

Many factors are responsible for the widely divergent results of conventional DDD pacing for CHF.[94]

1. Different NYHA classes.
2. Varying duration of CHF.
3. Varying incidence of right-sided failure and pulmonary hypertension.

4. Heterogeneous patient population: coronary artery disease versus idiopathic dilated cardiomyopathy.
5. Varying degrees of mitral and/or tricuspid regurgitation.
6. Different severity of CHF. With markedly elevated pulmonary capillary wedge pressures, atrial contribution may be negligible.
7. No separation of patients with normal and long PR intervals and those with interatrial and/or interventricular conduction abnormalities.
8. Uncontrolled studies and varying protocols.
9. Varying duration of follow-up.
10. Varying methods of evaluation: invasive versus noninvasive.
11. AV interval was fixed in many studies and not optimized.
12. Chronic effect of therapy is not predictable from the acute response.
13. No standardized drug therapy.
14. Effect on survival is unknown. Sudden death is common.

Identification of Patients with Severe CHF Regardless of Etiology Who May Benefit from Conventional DDD Pacing with a Short AV Interval

It does not make sense at this juncture to consider conventional DDD pacing in nonselected patients. The following recommendations are based on the work of Brecker and Gibson[95] and those of the Mayo Clinic workers.[40] They should be considered as preliminary in the absence of substantial experience.

1. Long PR interval in the resting ECG. However, not all patients with long PR intervals will respond. As emphasized by Glickson et al.[40] in some patients a long interatrial conduction time with a long PR interval produces appropriately timed mechanical AV synchrony, while oth-

ers may have poor or absent atrial contraction.
2. Substantial intraventricular conduction delay: QRS >140 ms.[95]
3. Prolonged functional mitral regurgitation of at least 450 ms and a short ventricular filling time <200 ms. According to The Mayo Clinic workers[40] patients who respond best exhibit early cessation of transmitral flow and diastolic mitral regurgitation. Abolition or diminution of mitral regurgitation may be an important factor in the beneficial effect of pacing.
4. A temporary pacing study should demonstrate hemodynamic benefit. According to The Mayo Clinic workers, during temporary pacing "responders" will show an increase in systolic blood pressure and an increase in peak mitral regurgitation velocity reflecting a higher LV systolic pressure and lower left atrial pressure.[40] Favorable acute data do not guarantee a beneficial long-term outcome.

Patients should understand that subsequent benefit is not predictable with certainty.[40,96] In this respect, Linde et al.[88] noted that initial hemodynamic changes correlated poorly with long-term outcome. Of seven patients who had an improvement in stroke volume after 1 day of pacing, only two were subsequently improved. Of the three patients without an initial change in stroke volume, only one improved during long-term follow-up. However, selection criteria were different from those advocated by Brecker and Gibson,[95] i.e., PR = 0.18 ± 0.04 sec (two patients with first degree block) QRS = 0.11 ± 0.02 sec (one patient with left bundle branch block); number of patients with mitral regurgitation unspecified).

Biventricular Pacing

In 1994, Cazeau et al.[97] reported the benefit of four chamber pacing in a single patient with refractory heart failure and dilated cardiomyopathy. Simultaneous RV and LV pacing was used to restore a more physiological activation sequence, a process known as resynchronization. In this patient, biatrial pacing was also undertaken to optimize AV synchrony because of interatrial conduction delay. This initial success has generated a number of acute studies showing hemodynamic improvement with biventricular or LV pacing in patients with severe LV systolic dysfunction.[98–104] Although preliminary long-term experience in a relatively small number of patients with heart failure and major intraventricular conduction disturbances seems promising,[105–110] biventricular or LV pacing (with or without biatrial pacing) is presently investigational. Technology and patient selection remain problematic.

First Degree Atrioventricular Block

Schüller and Brandt defined the pacemaker syndrome in terms of "symptoms and signs present in the pacemaker patient which are caused by inadequate timing of atrial and ventricular contractions."[111] This characterization also applies to patients without an implanted pacemaker when "inadequate timing of atrial and ventricular contractions" causes a similar hemodynamic derangement.[112,113] In this regard, Chirife et al.[114] have called the hemodynamic disturbance produced by marked first degree AV block as the "pacemaker syndrome without a pacemaker" and other workers have referred to this entity as the "pseudopacemaker syndrome."[115–117]

Several reports have now documented the benefit of dual chamber pacing in patients with symptomatic marked first degree AV block and normal LV function[114–119] (Table 6). A number of the reported patients developed the problem secondary to ablation of the fast pathway for the treatment of AV nodal reentry tachycardia.[115–117]

Chirife et al.[114] reported a 40-year-old patient with first degree AV block (PR = 400 ms) at a rate of 74 bpm who complained of dyspnea with minimal household chores. Clinical and noninvasive evaluation revealed no evidence of organic heart disease. The patient became asymptomatic after implantation of a DDD pacemaker (Table 6). Subsequently, Mabo et al.[118] also indicated that very long PR intervals can cause severe hemodynamic impairment. They reported

Table 6
Pacing for Long PR Interval

Author	Year	# of Pts.	PR at Rest	Effect of Exercise or Faster Rate	Benefit of Pacing
Chirife et al.[114]	1990	1	400	NS	Improved
Zornosa et al.[115]	1992	3	365, 380, 270	PR intervals lengthened progressively at rates >100 bpm	All improved
Mabo et al.[118]	1993	8	410 ± 45	No shortening of PR interval	All improved. Exercise duration ↑ 44%, cardiac output on exercise ↑ 29%, mean PCWP ↓ 33%
Kim et al.[116]	1993	1	360*/ 160–180	NS	Improved

NS = not stated; PCWP = pulmonary capillary wedge pressure.
* Intermittent and sudden prolongation of PR interval associated with "pacemaker syndrome."

data on eight patients with very long PR intervals (410 ± 45 ms) and severe symptoms on exercise (pacemaker syndrome without a pacemaker).[118,119] No "A" wave was seen on the echo Doppler transmitral flow imaging. During exercise, there was no adaptation (shortening) of the PR interval so that sinus P waves occurred immediately after or within the QRS complex of the preceding cycle. The patients improved remarkably after implantation of a DDD pacemaker. The duration of exercise increased by 44%, cardiac output on exercise increased by 29%, and the mean PCWP decreased by 33%, all statistically significant changes.

Zornosa et al.[115] described a complication of RF ablation of the AV junction in three patients who developed long PR intervals (365, 380, and 270 ms) with progressive PR prolongation at faster rates. The long PR intervals during low levels of activity were associated with inappropriate sinus tachycardia and fatigue. In all three patients, symptoms resolved after placement of a dual chamber pacemaker. Kim et al.[116] also reported a patient with AV nodal reentry tachycardia in whom attempted slow pathway ablation (by RF) cause intermittent failure of fast pathway conduction resulting in highly symptomatic first degree AV block and hypotension (drop from 110 to 90 mm Hg systolic). Symptoms were intermittent (lightheadedness, chest fullness, and weakness) and correlated with the sudden shift from a PR interval of 160–180 ms to 360 ms without any intermediate values. A permanent dual chamber pacemaker provided symptomatic relief.

During markedly prolonged anterograde AV conduction, the close proximity of atrial systole to the preceding ventricular systole produces the same hemodynamic consequences as continual retrograde ventriculoatrial conduction.[115–118] Patients with a markedly prolonged PR interval may or may not be symptomatic at rest. They are, of course, more likely to become symptomatic with mild to moderate levels of exercise when the PR interval does not shorten ap-

propriately and atrial systole moves progressively closer to the previous ventricular systole.[115–119] Thus, the hemodynamic disorder caused by a very long PR interval on exercise resembles the exercise-induced pacemaker syndrome produced by AAIR pacing when for a variety of reasons, a paced AV interval lengthens disproportionately relatively early during exercise.[120]

First Degree Atrioventricular Block and Diastolic Mitral Regurgitation

PR prolongation often causes hemodynamically inconsequential diastolic mitral regurgitation in patients with preserved LV function.[121–126] In a normal heart, abrupt termination of forward flow at the end of atrial systole initiates a closing motion of the mitral valve. The "atriogenic" closure is incomplete and the mitral valve can reopen if atrial systole is not followed by properly timed ventricular systole. In patients with a prolonged PR interval, atrial contraction with premature and incomplete "atriogenic" closure of the mitral valve causes reversal of the LV-left atrial pressure gradient (in the absence of ventricular systole), and can result in varying degrees of end-diastolic mitral regurgitation in mid or late diastole. Although inconsequential in the normal heart, diastolic mitral regurgitation may contribute to some extent to the unfavorable hemodynamic circumstances present in patients with severe LV systolic dysfunction and first degree AV block. Elimination of diastolic mitral regurgitation plays as yet an undefined role in overall hemodynamic benefit of dual chamber pacing in selected patients with severe LV dysfunction, CHF, and first degree AV block. In such patients, abolition of diastolic mitral regurgitation may result in more optimal hemodynamics because of a lower left atrial pressure and higher LV preload at the onset of LV systole.[40]

Indication for Pacing

Wharton and Ellenbogen[127] have argued that "symptomatic first degree AV block with symptoms suggestive of pacemaker syndrome" should be a class I indication for permanent pacing. They emphasized that "symptoms can be subtle in some patients or may be of sufficiently long duration that temporary pacing may be indicated to document improvement or reversal of long-standing problems." However, the 1998 ACC/AHA guidelines for pacemaker implantation state that "first degree AV block with symptoms suggestive of pacemaker syndrome and documented alleviation of symptoms with temporary pacing" constitutes a class IIA indication.[35]

Levine[128] has also emphasized that certain investigations are required to make the diagnosis of "pacemaker syndrome without a pacemaker" and justify the implantation of a permanent pacemaker. These include:

1. Temporary DDD pacing (with more physiological AV interval) in a hospital setting with ambulation and treadmill exercise testing to demonstrate improvement of symptoms and exercise tolerance;
2. Temporary DDD pacing with either invasive hemodynamic monitoring (Swan-Ganz catheter, arterial line, etc.) or echo Doppler studies to demonstrate improved hemodynamics with a more physiological AV interval.

However, such investigations should not be mandatory before pacemaker implantation if the diagnosis is obvious and the long PR interval does not shorten on exercise.

Pacemaker Syndrome with Pacemaker as a Bystander

The implantation of a pacemaker with an appropriate AV interval in patients with markedly prolonged PR interval can cause the pacemaker syndrome with the pacemaker itself as a bystander. In other words, the pacemaker can initiate a pacemaker syn-drome, but the device is not necessary for its perpetuation. In such patients, P wave undersensing can occur in the presence of an adequate atrial electrogram if the PVARP is excessively long so that a relatively fast sinus rate pushes the P wave closer and closer to the preceding PVARP.[129–132] A similar problem can occur with a relatively short programmed PVARP whenever a sensed ventricular extrasystole (VPC) activates an automatic PVARP extension.[130] If a subsequent sinus P wave falls within the extended PVARP, it will be unsensed. The unsensed P wave in the PVARP then gives rise to a conducted spontaneous QRS complex which the pacemaker interprets as a VPC (no preceding sensed atrial activity), whereupon it generates another automatic PVARP extension. Thus, when the atrial rate remains relatively fast and AV conduction is markedly delayed, P waves will continually occur within the extended PVARP. In other words, the excessively long PVARP is perpetuated from cycle to cycle because the pacemaker continually interprets the spontaneous conducted QRS complex as a VPC. A long PVARP can therefore recreate the original hemodynamic disturbance for which the pacemaker was implanted.

Prevention of the above potential problems requires:

1. a relatively short PVARP;
2. capability of programming "off" the automatic post ventricular extrasystole PVARP extension;
3. elimination of the post-VPC PVARP extension whenever a P wave is detected within the extended PVARP immediately before the next ventricular sensed event; and
4. ablation of the AV junction. Kuniyashi et al.[117] used such an innovative approach with a resultant complete AV block, a procedure conceptually similar to AV nodal ablation for the prevention of endless loop tachycardia where a P wave

also occurs close to the preceding QRS complex.[133]

Orthostatic Hypotension

The use of atrial tachypacing (100/min) for the treatment of orthostatic hypotension was first proposed by Moss et al.[134] in 1980, but it never became popular (Table 7). Soon afterwards, Goldberg et al.[135] described the unsuccessful use of temporary atrial pacing alone in a single patient. From 1980 to 1992, only three additional cases were reported. Kristinsson.[136] reported two cases of drug refractory orthostatic hypotension treated with permanent AAI pacing at a rate of 95 ppm during the day and 55 ppm at night (programming was done by the patient). The patients improved with virtual disappearance of orthostatic hypotension for about 2 years except when they forgot to program their pacemaker to 95/min in the morning.[136] Both patients continued taking fludrocortisone acetate after pacemaker implantation. Cunha et al.[137] also reported in 1990 the marked improvement over a period of 9 months of a patient with drug refractory orthostatic hypotension who re-

ceived an atrial pacemaker also designed to pace at 60 ppm at night and 96 ppm during the day with rate programming performed by the patient.

Weissman et al.[138] renewed interest in the use of atrial tachypacing in a 1992 report of five cases of drug refractory orthostatic hypotension treated with permanent pacemakers (three AAI, one DDD and one DDDR) with a follow-up of 1 year (Table 7). After pacemaker implantation, all patients received fludrocortisone and three also received propranolol. Three patients were able to lead a nearly normal life with virtually no orthostatic hypotension. One patient showed moderate improvement, but another one did not. The lower rate of the pacemakers varied from 90/min to 100/ min.

It seems that most patients with idiopathic orthostatic hypotension have a markedly attenuated heart rate response to hypotension associated with the upright posture. The impaired chronotropic response may further accentuate the orthostatic hypotension by allowing a longer peripheral runoff during diastole.[138] Tachypacing by reducing the duration of diastole augments the diastolic and mean blood pressure in pa-

Table 7
Pacing for Orthostatic Hypotension

Authors	Year	#	Pacemaker	Rate (ppm)	Drug Therapy	Follow-Up	Benefit
Moss et al.[135]	1980	1	AAI	100	?	10 mths	Yes
Goldberg et al.[136]	1980	1	Temporary atrial	90–100	No	No	No
Kristinsson et al.[137]	1983	2	AAI	95 (day) 55 (night)	Yes (all)*	2 years	Yes
Cunha et al.[138]	1990	1	AAI	96 (day) 60 (night)	?	9 mths	Yes
Weissman et al.[139]	1992	5	3 AAI, DDD, DDDR	90–100 (95)	Yes (all)*	1 year	4 improved
Grubb et al.[140]	1993	1	DDDR	RVPEP (sensor controlled)	?	4 mths	Yes

RVPEP = right ventricular preejection period.
* All on fludrocortisone.

tients with residual adrenergic activity. Weissman et al.[138] suggested that patients without adrenergic tone would probably not derive any benefit from tachypacing. A pacemaker for tachypacing should not be used as sole therapy for orthostatic hypotension. Adjunctive drug therapy with fludrocortisone seems essential and should be supplemented by beta blockers, added salt intake, and other measures.[138]

Grubb et al.[139] recently reported the use of DDDR pacing with a sensor system controlled by the RV preejection period (systolic time interval from the onset of electrical ventricular depolarization to the onset of RV ejection) for the treatment of severe refractory orthostatic hypotension. The system adequately sensed the patient's fall in blood pressure when sitting or standing by a fall in the RV filling causing shortening of the preejection interval. Consequently, the pacemaker augmented its rate (from 60

ppm to 110–120 ppm) accordingly, thereby preventing syncope. No further orthostatic or syncopal episodes occurred over a 9-month follow-up period. (The report did not mention whether additional drug therapy was used.) This novel approach avoids continuous tachypacing and its potential harmful effects on the heart. This experience suggests that developments in sensor technology may allow earlier and more appropriate response to alterations in blood pressure and posture and greater applicability of this form of therapy.

All patients considered for atrial pacing should undergo repeated testing in the supine and upright positions with or without pacing (90–100 ppm) by a temporary atrial or AV sequential pacing system. The procedure is best done on a tilt table so the patient is always supported. If rapid atrial pacing blunts the degree of hypotension, pacing therapy is likely to be helpful.

References

1. McDonald K, McWilliams E, O'Keefe B, et al. Functional assessment of patients treated with permanent dual chamber pacing as primary treatment for hypertrophic cardiomyopathy. Eur Heart J 1988;9: 893–898.
2. Fananapazir L, Cannon RO III, Tripodi D, et al. Impact of dual chamber permanent pacing in patients with obstructive hypertrophic cardiomyopathy with symptoms refractory to verapamil and β-adrenergic blocker therapy. Circulation 1992;85: 2149–2161.
3. Jeanrenaud X, Goy JJ, Kappenberger L. Effects of dual chamber pacing in hypertrophic obstructive cardiomyopathy. Lancet 1992;339:1318–1323.
4. McDonald KM, Maurer B. Permanent pacing as treatment for hypertrophic cardiomyopathy. Am J Cardiol 1991;68:108–110.
5. Richter T, Cserhalmi M, Lengyel M, et al. Changes in left ventricular hemodynamics of hypertrophic obstructive cardiomyopathy (HOCM) patients treated with VAT pacing. In Baroldi G, Camerini F, Goodwin JF, eds. Advances in Cardiomyopathies. Springer-Verlag, New York, 1990, pp 168–174.
6. Fananapazir L, Epstein ND, Curiel RV, et al.

Long-term results of dual chamber (DDD) pacing in obstructive hypertrophic cardiomyopathy. Evidence for progressive symptomatic and hemodynamic improvement and reduction of left ventricular hypertrophy. Circulation 1994;90:2731–2742.
7. Gras D, Daubert C, Mabo P. Value of cardiac pacing in hypertrophic obstructive cardiomyopathy refractory to medical treatment. Arch Mal Coeur 1995;88:577–583.
8. Gras D, Pavin D, De Place C, et al. What is the status of patients with hypertrophic obstructive cardiomyopathy treated by DDD pacing for more than 1 year? Circulation 1995;92(Suppl I):I–780.
9. Yusvinkevich SA, Khirmanov VN, Domashenko AA, et al. Treatment of HOCM by short AV-delay DDD pacing. PACE 1995; 18:1807A.
10. Umman S, Oncul A, Umman B, et al. Dual chamber pacemaker implantation in patients with hypertrophic obstructive cardiomyopathy. PACE 1995;18:1813A.
11. Gamhir DS, Arora R, Khalilullah M. Dual chamber pacing in hypertrophic obstructive cardiomyopathy. PACE 1993;16:1525A.
12. Nishimura RA, Trusty JM, Hayes DL, et al. Dual chamber pacing for hypertrophic cardiomyopathy: a randomized, double-blind,

crossover trial. J Am Coll Cardiol 1997;29: 435–441.

13. Slade AKB, Sadoul N, Shapiro L, et al. DDD pacing in hypertrophic cardiomyopathy: a multicenter clinical experience. Heart 1996; 75:44–49.

14. Gadler F, Linde C, Juhlin-Dannfelt A, et al. Long-term effects of dual chamber pacing in patients with hypertrophic cardiomyopathy without outflow tract obstruction at rest. Eur Heart J 1997;18:636–642.

15. Sadoul N, Simon JP, de Chillou C, et al. Interets de la stimulation cardiaque permanente dans les myocardiopathies hypertrophiques et obstructives rebelles au traitement medical. Arch Mal Coeur 1994;87: 1315–1323.

16. Sadoul N, Slade AKB, Simon JP, et al. Dual chamber pacing in refractory hypertrophic obstructive cardiomyopathy: a two-centre European experience in 34 consecutive patients. J Am Coll Cardiol 1995;25:233A.

17. Kappenberger L, Linde C, Daubert C, et al. Pacing in hypertrophic obstructive cardiomyopathy: a randomized crossover trial. Eur Heart J 1997;18:1249–1256.

18. Fananapazir L, Atiga W, Tripodi D, et al. Therapy in obstructive hypertrophic cardiomyopathy: the role of dual chamber (DDD) pacing. In Barold SS, Mugica J, eds. Recent Advances in Cardiac Pacing. Goals for the 21st Century. Futura Publishing Co, Armonk, NY, 1998, pp 35–50.

19. Sakai Y, Kawakami Y, Shimada S, et al. AV sequential pacing in hypertrophic obstructive cardiomyopathy, comparison between acute and chronic effects. Circulation 1996; 94:I–502.

20. Iliou MC, Lavergne TL, Hernigou A, et al. Left ventricular remodeling by long-term dual chamber pacing in hypertrophic obstructive cardiomyopathy. Circulation 1996;94:I–361.

21. Gross JN, Keltz TN, Cooper JA, et al. Profound "pacemaker syndrome" in hypertrophic cardiomyopathy. Am J Cardiol 1992; 70:1507–1511.

22. Sadoul N, Simon JP, Chillon C, et al. Usefulness of temporary dual chamber pacing to determine indication for pacemaker implantation in patients with drug- resistant obstructive hypertrophic cardiomyopathy. PACE 1993;16:1120A.

23. McAreavey D, Fananapazir L. Acute pacing studies are not valuable in predicting long term benefits of DDD pacing for LV outflow obstruction in hypertrophic cardiomyopathy. J Am Coll Cardiol 1994;23:10A.

24. Daubert JC. Pacing and hypertrophic ob-

structive cardiomyopathy. PACE 1996;19: 1141–1142.

25. Jeanrenaud X, Kappenberger L. The optimal patient for pacemaker treatment of hypertrophic obstructive cardiomyopathy. PACE 1993;16:1120A.

26. Gross JN, Ben-Zur UM, Greenberg MA, et al. Acute hemodynamic assessment fails to identify hypertrophic cardiomyopathy patients responsive to DDD pacing. J Am Coll Cardiol 1994;23:324A.

27. Gras D, Mabo P, De Place C, et al. Outcome of mitral regurgitation in obstructive hypertrophic cardiomyopathy treated by DDD pacing. Circulation 1994;90(Suppl):I–443.

28. Gras D, Mabo P, de Place C, et al. Regression of mitral regurgitation with DDD pacing in obstructive hypertrophic cardiomyopathy. PACE 1995;18:1784A.

29. Pavin D, de Place C, Matali P, et al. Chronic DDD pacing reduces mitral regurgitation in hypertrophic obstructive cardiomyopathy. PACE 1997;20:1601A.

30. Fananapazir L, Tripodi D, McAreavey D. Five-year results of dual chamber pacing in obstructive hypertrophic cardiomyopathy patients with severe symptoms. PACE 1998;21:791A.

31. Jeanrenaud X. Rate of adverse cardiac events after one-year of dual chamber pacing in hypertrophic obstructive cardiomyopathy (HOCM): results of the PIC study group. Circulation 1997;96:I–95.

32. McAreavey D, Fananapazir L. Ventricular pre-excitation is highly effective for elderly patients with obstructive hypertrophic cardiomyopathy and symptoms refractory to medication. J Am Coll Cardiol 1993;21: 354A.

33. McAveavey D, Atiga W, Tripodi D, et al. Permanent dual chamber pacing is an effective therapy for relief of LV outflow obstruction in children with hypertrophic cardiomyopathy. PACE 1994;17:746A.

34. Rishi F, Hulse JE, Auld DO, et al. Effects of dual chamber pacing for pediatric patients with hypertrophic obstructive cardiomyopathy. J Am Coll Cardiol 1997;29:734–740.

35. Gregoratos G, Cheitlin MD, Freedman RA, et al. ACC/AHA guidelines for implantation of cardiac pacemakers and antiarrhythmia devices: a report of the American College of Cardiology/American Heart Association task force on practice guidelines (Committee on pacemaker implantation). J Am Coll Cardiol 1998;31:1175–1209.

36. Gras D, Daubert C, Leclercq C, et al. Obstructive hypertrophic cardiomyopathy treated by DDD pacing: the major impor-

tance of AV synchrony. J Am Coll Cardiol 1994;23:11A.

37. Matsumato K, Saitou J, Mukosaka K, et al. Influences of changing the pacing site on the hemodynamic improvement by DDD pacing in patients with hypertrophic obstructive cardiomyopathy. Circulation 1993;88(Suppl 1):I–210.

38. Gadler F, Linde C, Juhlin-Dannfeldt A, et al. Influence of right ventricular pacing site on left ventricular outflow tract obstruction in patients with hypertrophic obstructive cardiomyopathy. J Am Coll Cardiol 1996; 27:1219–1224.

39. Glickson M, Espinosa RE, Hayes DL. Expanding indications for permanent pacemakers. Ann Intern Med 1995;123:443–451.

40. Glickson M, Hayes DL, Nishimura RA. Newer clinical applications of pacing. J Cardiovasc Electrophysiol 1997;8:1190–1203.

41. Gras D, de Place C, LeBreton H, et al. Importance of atrioventricular synchrony in hypertrophic obstructive cardiomyopathy treated by cardiac pacing. Arch Mal Coeur 1995;88:215–223.

42. Jeanrenaud X, Aebischer N, for the PIC Study Group. Importance of the AV interval during dual chamber pacing in hypertrophic obstructive cardiomyopathy: Results from the PIC study group. J Am Coll Cardiol 1997;29(Suppl A):111A.

43. Mayumi H, Kohno H, Yasui H, et al. Use of automatic mode change between DDD and AAI to facilitate native atrioventricular conduction in patients with sick sinus syndrome or transient atrioventricular block. PACE 1996;19:1740–1747.

44. Chang AC, McAreavey D, Tripodi D, et al. Radiofrequency catheter atrioventricular node ablation in patients with permanent cardiac pacing systems. PACE 1994;17: 65–69.

45. Jeanrenaud X, Schlapfer J, Fromer M, et al. Dual chamber pacing in hypertrophic obstructive cardiomyopathy: beneficial effect of atrioventricular junction ablation for optimal left ventricular capture and filling. PACE 1997;20:293–300.

46. Gadler F, Linde C, Darpo B. Modification of atrioventricular conduction as adjunct therapy for pacemaker-treatment with hypertrophic obstructive cardiomyopathy. Eur Heart J 1998;19:132–138.

47. Daubert C, Gras D, Pavin D, et al. Biatrial synchronous pacing to optimize hemodynamic benefit of DDD pacing in hypertrophic obstructive cardiomyopathy. Circulation 1995;92:I–780.

48. Slade AKB, Keeling PJ, Prasad K, et al. Acute evaluation of DDD versus DDDR mode predicts additional benefit of rate adaptive pacing in hypertrophic cardiomyopathy. J Am Coll Cardiol 1994;23:10A.

49. Louie EK, Edwards LC III. Hypertrophic cardiomyopathy. Progr Cardiovasc Dis 1994;36:275–308.

50. Maron BJ, Bonow RO, Cannon RO III, et al. Hypertrophic cardiomyopathy. Interrelations of clinical manifestations, pathophysiology and therapy. N Engl J Med 1987;316: 780–789.

51. O'Gara PT, Bonow RO, Maron BJ, et al. Myocardial perfusion abnormalities in patients with hypertrophic cardiomyopathy: assessment with thallium 201 emission computer tomography. Circulation 1987;76: 1214–1223.

52. Dilsizian V, Bonow RO, Epstein SE, et al. Myocardial ischemia detected by thallium scintigraphy is frequently related to cardiac arrest and syncope in young patients with hypertrophic cardiomyopathy. J Am Coll Cardiol 1993;22:796–804.

53. Cannon RO III, Dilsizian V, O'Gara PT. Impact of surgical relief of outflow obstruction on thallium perfusion abnormalities in hypertrophic cardiomyopathy. Circulation 1992;85:1039–1045.

54. Thomson H, Fong W, Stafford W, et al. Reversible ischemia in hypertrophic cardiomyopathy. Br Heart J 1995;74:220–223.

55. Takeuchi M, Abe H, Kuroiwa A. Effect of dual chamber atrioventricular sequential pacing on coronary flow velocity in a patient with hypertrophic obstructive cardiomyopathy. PACE 1996;19:2153–2155.

56. Posma JL, Banksman PK, Van Der Wall EE, et al. Effects of permanent dual chamber pacing on myocardial perfusion in symptomatic hypertrophic cardiomyopathy. Heart 1996;76:358–362.

57. Le Helloco A, Gras D, Devillers A, et al. Influence of DDD pacing on myocardial perfusion in patients with hypertrophic cardiomyopathy. PACE 1997;20:1592A.

58. Cannon RO III, Rosing DR, Maron BJ, et al. Myocardial ischemia in patients with hypertrophic cardiomyopathy: contribution of inadequate vasodilator reserve and elevated left ventricular filling pressures. Circulation 1985;71:234–243.

59. Cannon RO III, Schenke WH, Maron BJ, et al. Differences in coronary flow and myocardial metabolism in rest and during pacing between patients with obstructive and patients with non-obstructive hypertrophic cardiomyopathy. J Am Coll Cardiol 1987; 10:53–62.

60. Brinker JA. Permanent pacemakers: optimal choices for specific clinical scenarios,

Intelligence Reports in Cardiac Pacing and Electrophysiology II 1992, (No. 2) 1.

61. Jeanrenaud X, Kappenberger L. Regional wall motion during pacing for hypertrophic cardiomyopathy. PACE 1997;20:1673–1681.

62. Betocchi S, Losi MA, Piscione F, et al. Effects of dual chamber pacing in hypertrophic cardiomyopathy on left ventricular outflow tract obstruction and on diastolic function. Am J Cardiol 1996;77:498–502.

63. Betocchi S, Losi MA, Briguori C, et al. Long-term dual chamber pacing reduces left ventricular outflow tract obstruction but impairs diastolic function in hypertrophic cardiomyopathy. Circulation 1997;96(Suppl I):I–645.

64. Nishimura RA, Hayes DL, Ilstrup DM, et al. Effect of dual chamber pacing on systolic and diastolic function in patients with hypertrophic cardiomyopathy: acute Doppler echocardiographic and catheterization hemodynamic study. J Am Coll Cardiol 1996;27:421–430.

65. Erwin J, McWilliams E, Gearty G, et al. Hemodynamic assessment of dual chamber pacing in hypertrophic cardiomyopathy using radionuclide angiography. Br Heart J 1986;55:507A.

66. McDonald K, O'Sullivan JJ, King C, et al. Dual chamber pacing improves left ventricular filling in patients with hypertrophic cardiomyopathy. Eur Heart J 1989;10(Suppl):401.

67. Pavin D, Llirbat ML, de Place C, et al. Optimized pacing therapy may prevent deterioration of left ventricular diastolic function in hypertrophic obstructive cardiomyopathy. PACE 1998;21:792A.

68. Fananapazir L, McAreavey D. Therapeutic options in patients with obstructive cardiomyopathy and severe drug-refractory symptoms. J Am Coll Cardiol 1998;31:259–264.

69. Pavin D, de Place C, le Breton H, et al. Long-term effects of DDD pacing on hypertrophic obstructive cardiomyopathy. J Am Coll Cardiol 1997;29(Suppl A):388A.

70. Tavel ME, Fananapazir L, Goldshlager NF. Hypertrophic obstructive cardiomyopathy. Problems in management. Chest 1997;112:262–264.

71. Wigle ED, Rakowski H, Kimball BP, et al. Hypertrophic cardiomyopathy. Clinical spectrum and treatment. Circulation 1995;92:1680–1692.

72. Nishimura RA, Symanski JD, Hurrell DG, et al. Dual chamber pacing for cardiomyopathies: a 1996 clinical perspective. Mayo Clinic Proc 1996;71:1077–1087.

73. Symanski JD, Nishimura RA. The use of pacemakers in the treatment of cardiomyopathies. Curr Probl Cardiol 1996; 21:385–444.

74. Cannon RO III, Tripodi D, Dilsizian V, et al. Results of permanent dual chamber pacing in symptomatic nonobstructive hypertrophic cardiomyopathy. Am J Cardiol 1994;23:571–576.

75. Hochleitner M, Hortnagl H, Ng CK, et al. Usefulness of physiologic dual chamber pacing in drug-resistant idiopathic dilated cardiomyopathy. Am J Cardiol 1990;66:198–202.

76. Hochleitner M, Hortnagl H, Hortnagel H, et al. Long term efficacy of physiologic dual chamber pacing in the treatment of end-stage idiopathic dilated cardiomyopathy. Am J Cardiol 1992;70:1320–1325.

77. Kataoka H. Hemodynamic effect of physiologic dual chamber pacing in a patient with end-stage dilated cardiomyopathy: a case report. PACE 1991;14:1330–1335.

78. Auricchio A, Sommariva L, Salo RW, et al. Improvement of cardiac function in patients with severe congestive failure and coronary artery disease by dual chamber pacing with shortened AV delay. PACE 1993;16:2034–2043.

79. Hochleitner M, Hortnagl H, Gschnitzer F. Dual chamber pacing in patients with end-stage ischemic cardiomyopathy. Lancet 1993;345:1543.

80. Innes D, Leitch J, Fletcher P. VDD pacing at short atrioventricular intervals does not improve cardiac output in patients with dilated heart failure. PACE 1994;17:959–965.

81. Nishimura RA, Hayes DL, Holmes DR Jr, et al. Mechanism of hemodynamic improvement by dual chamber pacing for severe left ventricular dysfunction: an acute Doppler and catheterization hemodynamic study. J Am Coll Cardiol 1995;25:281–288.

82. Scanu P, Lecluse E, Michel L, et al. Effets de la stimulation cardiaque double chambre temporaire dans l'insuffisance cardiaque refractaire. Arch Mal Coeur 1994;89:1643–1649.

83. Shinbane J, Chu E, De Marco T, et al. Evaluation of acute dual chamber pacing with a range of atrioventricular delays on cardiac performance in refractory heart failure. J Am Coll Cardiol 1997;30:1295–1300.

84. Brecker SJD, Xiao HB, Sparrow J, et al. Effects of dual chamber pacing with short atrioventricular delay in dilated cardiomyopathy. Lancet 1992;340:1308–1312.

85. Mathew V, Chaliki H, Nishimura RA. Atrioventricular sequential pacing in cardiac amyloidosis: an acute Doppler echocardiographic and catheterization hemodynamic study. Clin Cardiol 1997;20:723–725.

86. Feliciano Z, Fisher ML, Corretti MC, et al. Acute hemodynamic effect of A-V delay in patients with congestive heart failure. J Am Coll Cardiol 1994;23:349A.

87. Paul V, Morris-Thurgood J, Cowell R, et al. Impaired ventricles: is short AV delay pacing beneficial and can we predict in whom? PACE 1994;17:776A.

88. Linde C, Gadler F, Edner M, et al. Results of atrioventricular synchronous pacing with optimized delay in patients with severe congestive heart failure. Am J Cardiol 1995;75:919–923.

89. Gold MR, Feliciano Z, Gottlieb SS, et al. Dual chamber pacing with a short atrioventricular delay and congestive heart failure: a randomized study. J Am Coll Cardiol 1995;26:967–973.

90. Brecker SJ, Kelly PA, Chua TP, et al. Effects of permanent dual chamber pacing in end-stage dilated cardiomyopathy. Circulation 1995;92(Suppl I):I–7.

91. Greco O, Brofmann P, Khirmanov V, et al. Dilative cardiomyopathy and dual chamber pacing with shortened AV delay: long-term results. PACE 1997;20:1574A.

92. Ansalone G, Auriti A, Giannantoni P, et al. Physiological pacing with a short AV delay in patients with dilated cardiomyopathy, baseline first degree AV block and LBBB. PACE 1997;20:1575A.

93. Rossi R, Muia N Jr, Turco V, et al. Short atrioventricular delay reduces the degree of mitral regurgitation in patients with a sequential dual chamber pacemaker. Am J Cardiol 1997;80:901–905.

94. Auricchio A, Salo RW, Klein H, et al. Problems and pitfalls in evaluating studies for pacing in heart failure. G Ital Cardiol 1997; 27:593–599.

95. Brecker SJ, Gibson DG. What is the role of pacing in dilated cardiomyopathy? Eur Heart J 1996;17:819–824.

96. Paul V, Cowell R, Thurgood-Morris J, et al. Short atrioventricular delay pacing in heart failure: acute hemodynamic improvements do not predict long-term results. PACE 1995;18:847A.

97. Cazeau S, Ritter P, Bakdach S, et al. Four chamber pacing in dilated cardiomyopathy. PACE 1994;17:1974–1979.

98. Kerwin WF, Botvinick EH, O'Connell JW, et al. Biventricular pacing in dilated cardiomyopathy: acute improvements in biventricular ejection fraction correspond with measures of improved RV/LV synchrony. PACE 1998;21:837A.

99. Kass DA, Chen CH, Fetics M, et al. Ventricular function in patients with dilated cardiomyopathy is improved by VDD pacing at left, but not right ventricular sites. J Am Coll Cardiol 1998;31:31A.

100. Leclercq C, LeBreton H, Pavin D, et al. Acute hemodynamic response to biventricular DDD pacing in patients with severe congestive heart failure and without conventional indication for permanent pacemaker. Circulation 1997;96:I–95.

101. Gilard M, Etienne Y, Mansourati J, et al. Acute hemodynamic study during pacing at different sites in patients with end-stage cardiac failure. Is biventricular pacing the optimum? PACE 1997;20:1129A.

102. Cazeau S, Ritter P, Lazarus A, et al. Heart failure: acute hemodynamic improvement provided by multisite acute biventricular pacing. J Am Coll Cardiol 1997;29(Suppl A): IIIA.

103. Brockman RG, Olsovsky MR, Shorofsky SR, et al. The acute hemodynamic effects of pacing site and mode in congestive heart failure. J Am Coll Cardiol 1998;31(Suppl A): 389A.

104. Blanc JJ, Etienne Y, Gilard M, et al. Evaluation of different ventricular pacing sites in patients with severe heart failure: results of an acute hemodynamic study. Circulation 1997;96:3273–3277.

105. Cazeau S, Ritter P, Lazarus A, et al. Multisite pacing for end-stage heart failure: early experience. PACE 1996;19:1748–1757.

106. Leclercq C, Cazeau S, Ritter P, et al. Permanent biventricular pacing: a new alternative to treat end-stage congestive heart failure? Circulation 1997;96:I–95.

107. Auricchio A, Stellbrink C, Block M, et al. Clinical and objective improvements in severe congestive heart failure patients using univentricular and biventricular pacing: preliminary results of a randomized prospective study. J Am Coll Cardiol 1998; 31(Suppl A):31A.

108. Cazeau S, Leclercq C, Gras D, et al. Four-year experience of biventricular pacing in congestive heart failure. PACE 1998;21: 791A.

109. Daubert C, Cazeau S, Leclercq C, et al. Outcome of patients chronically implanted with biventricular pacing systems for end-stage congestive heart failure. PACE 1997; 20:1103A.

110. Leclercq C, Cazeau S, Victor F, et al. Comparative effects of permanent biventricular pacing in Class III and Class IV patients. PACE 1998;21:911A.

111. Schuller H, Brandt J. The pacemaker syndrome: old and new causes. Clin Cardiol 1991;14:336–340.

112. Brinker JA. Pursuing the perfect pacemaker. Mayo Clin Proc 1989;64:587–591.

113. Ellenbogen KA, Gilligan DM, Wood MA, et al. The pacemaker syndrome: a matter of definition. Am J Cardiol 1997;79:1226–1229.

114. Chirife R, Ortega DF, Salazar AL. "Pacemaker syndrome" without a pacemaker. Deleterious effects of first-degree AV block. RBM 1990;12:22A.

115. Zornosa JP, Crossley GH, Haisty WK Jr, et al. Pseudopacemaker syndrome: a complication of radiofrequency ablation of the AV junction. PACE 1992;15:590A.

116. Kim YH, O'Nunain S, Trouton T, et al. Pseudo-pacemaker syndrome following inadvertent fast pathway ablation for atrioventricular nodal reentrant tachycardia. J Cardiovasc Electrophysiol 1993; 4:178–182.

117. Kuniyashi R, Sosa E, Scanavacca M, et al. Pseudo-sindrome de marcapasso. Arq Bras Cardiol 1994;62:111–115.

118. Mabo P, Cazeau S, Forrer A, et al. Isolated long PR interval as only indication of permanent DDD pacing. J Am Coll Cardiol 1992;19:66A.

119. Mabo P, Varin C, Vauthier M, et al. Deleterious hemodynamic consequences of isolated long PR intervals: correction by DDD pacing. Eur Heart J 1992;13(Suppl):225A.

120. den Dulk K, Lindemans F, Brugada P, et al. Pacemaker syndrome with AAI rate-variable pacing: importance of atrioventricular conduction properties, medication and pacemaker programmability. PACE 1988; 11:1226–1230.

121. Rutishauser W, Wirz P, Gander M, et al. Atriogenic diastolic reflux in patients with atrioventricular block. Circulation 1966;34: 807–817.

122. Schnittger I, Appleton CP, Hatle LK, et al. Diastolic mitral and tricuspid regurgitation by Doppler echocardiography in patients with atrioventricular block: new insight into the mechanism of atrioventricular valve closure. J Am Coll Cardiol 1988;11: 83–88.

123. Appleton CP, Basnight MA, Gonzalez MS, et al. Diastolic mitral regurgitation with atrioventricular conduction abnormalities: relation of mitral flow velocity to transmitral pressure gradients in conscious dogs. J Am Coll Cardiol 1991;18:843–849.

124. Panidis IP, Ross J, Munley B, et al. Diastolic mitral regurgitation in patients with atrioventricular conduction abnormalities: a common finding by Doppler echocardiography. J Am Coll Cardiol 1986;7:768–774.

125. Ishikawa T, Kimura K, Miyazaki N, et al. Diastolic mitral regurgitation in patients with first-degree atrioventricular block. PACE 1992;15:1927–1931.

126. Ishikawa T, Sumica S, Kimura K, et al. Critical PQ interval for the appearance of diastolic mitral regurgitation and optimal PQ interval in patients implanted with DDD pacemakers. PACE 1994;17:1989–1994.

127. Wharton JM, Ellenbogen KA. Atrioventricular conduction system disease. In Ellenbogen KA, Kay GN, Wilkoff BL, eds. Clinical Cardiac Pacing. WB Saunders, Philadelphia, 1995, pp 304–320.

128. Levine PA. Uncommon applications for pacing therapy and minimizing reimbursement hassles. Siemens-Pacesetter Sylmar, CA, 1992.

129. Greenspon AJ, Volasin KJ. "Pseudo" loss of atrial sensing by a DDD pacemaker. PACE 1987;10:943–948.

130. Wilson JH, Lattner S. Undersensing of P waves in the presence of adequate P wave due to automatic postventricular atrial refractory period extension. PACE 1989;12: 1729–1732.

131. van Gelder BM, van Mechelen R, den Dulk K, et al. Apparent P wave undersensing in a DDD pacemaker post exercise. PACE 1992;15:1651–1656.

132. Dodinot B, Beurrier D, Simon JP, et al. "Functional" loss of atrial sensing causing sustained first to high-degree AV block in patients with dual chamber pacemakers. PACE 1993;16:1189A.

133. Pitney M, Davis M. Catheter ablation of ventriculoatrial conduction in the treatment of pacemaker mediated tachycardia. PACE 1991;14:1013–1017.

134. Moss AJ, Glaser W, Topol E. Atrial tachypacing in the treatment of a patient with primary orthostatic hypotension. N Engl J Med 1980;302:1456–1457.

135. Goldberg MR, Robertson RM, Robertson D. Atrial tachypacing for primary orthostatic hypotension. N Engl J Med 1980;303: 885–886.

136. Kristinsson A. Programmed atrial pacing for orthostatic hypotension. Acta Med Scand 1983;214:79–83.

137. Cunha UG, Machado EL, Santana LA. Programmed atrial pacing in the treatment of neurogenic orthostatic hypotension in the elderly. Arquivos Brasil Cardiol 1990;55: 47–49.

138. Weissman P, Chin MT, Moss AJ. Cardiac tachypacing for severe refractory orthostatic hypotension. Ann Intern Med 1992; 116:650–651.

139. Grubb BP, Wolfe DA, Samoil D, et al. Adaptive rate pacing controlled by right ventricular preejection interval for severe refractory orthostatic hypotension. PACE 1993; 16:801–805.

Chapter 35

Newest Developments in Rate-Adaptive Pacing

David L. Hayes, MD

Introduction

When rate-adaptive pacing was introduced in the mid-1980s, it was embraced rapidly by the pacemaker community. In the United States it is estimated that more than 70% of pacemakers currently implanted have rate-adaptive pacing capability.

In the early single chamber (AAIR, VVIR) rate-adaptive pacemaker era, investigators were quick to demonstrate hemodynamic advantages of rate-adaptive modes, i.e., VVIR versus VVI, AAIR versus AAI.[1] Similarly, when dual chamber rate-adaptive pacing was introduced later in the 1980s, literature emerged demonstrating hemodynamic superiority of DDDR over DDD in the chronotropically incompetent patient.[2] Although there are other benefits of rate-adaptive pacing, correcting the chronotropic response remains the most important.[3]

There are multiple issues that must be covered when considering "newest developments in rate-adaptive pacing." By necessity, currently available sensors must be reviewed to place potential and/or investigational sensors into perspective. Although the field of rate-adaptive pacing has been relatively static in the first half of the 1990s with the exception of its increasing acceptance, there is now exciting literature emerging regarding newer sensors as well as dual sensor technology.

Indications for Rate-Adaptive Pacing

The indications for rate-adaptive pacing are relatively straightforward. VVIR is indicated primarily for the patient with chronic atrial fibrillation and a slow ventricular response that requires bradycardia support. AAIR, not widely utilized, is appropriate for the patient with sinus node dysfunction and intact atrioventricular (AV) node conduction. Even though sinus node dysfunction comprises a significant number of all patients requiring permanent pacing,[4] many clinicians remain uncomfortable with a system that does not provide ventricular pacing support.

Chronotropic incompetence also remains the primary indication for DDDR pacing. However, DDDR has been advocated for any patient requiring dual chamber pacing given the future clinical flexibility that is provided. For example, should a patient

From Singer I, Barold SS, Camm AJ (eds): Nonpharmacological Therapy of Arrhythmias for the 21st Century: The State of the Art. Futura Publishing Co, Inc., Armonk, NY, © 1998.

with a DDDR pacemaker develop atrial fibrillation, the pacemaker can be programmed to VVIR. If the patient is symptomatic with traditional DDD upper rate response, i.e. symptomatic 2:1 AV block, optimal programming of sensor response in a DDDR pacemaker may provide "sensor-driven rate-smoothing."[5]

In analyzing 269 patients receiving a total of 274 DDDR pacemakers only 51% were dismissed from the hospital programmed to a rate-adaptive mode.[6] However, during follow-up 18% required programming to a different pacing mode and the DDDR pacemaker provided the necessary programmable flexibility to meet the patient's changing clinical needs.

Prescribing practices for rate-adaptive pacemakers appear to vary with the level of the implanter's experience. Utilization of rate-adaptive pacemakers is shown in Figure 1. This figure, taken from the *World Survey on Cardiac Pacing: United States 1993* by Bernstein and Parsonnet,[4] contrast two sources of information. Industry estimates of rate-adaptive pacemaker utilization is less than that of survey respondents. This suggests that survey respondents, generally felt to have a greater interest and level of experience in cardiac pacing, tended to use rate-adaptive pacemakers more frequently.

Sensors Available for Rate-Adaptive Pacing

In an effort to classify sensors on the basis of their response to physiological variables, Rossi[7] divided sensors into five orders (Table 1). Sensors can also be classified as

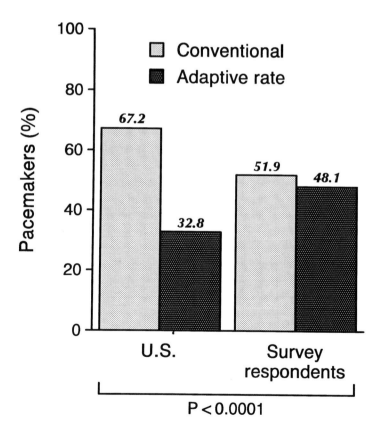

Figure 1. 1993 data of United States use of rate-adaptive versus non-rate-adaptive (conventional) pacemakers. The bars labeled "US" represent industry-based data of total pacemakers distributed in 1993. This differs significantly from the type of pacemaker used by the physicians responding to the 1993 US survey.[4] Used with permission from Bernstein AD, et al.[4]

Table 1
Potential Sensor Interactions

Pacemaker rate will:
- Only respond to the rate of change of sensor #1 and to the absolute value of sensor #2.
- Only respond to sensor #1 to a certain level of exertion and thereafter responds to sensor #2.
- Only respond to sensor #1 when sensor #2 also indicates a rate change.
- Only respond to sensor #1 when sensor #2 is above or below a certain value.

Adapted from T. Nappholz, personal communication, 1989.

open or closed loop. All commercially available sensors are "open-loop" sensors in that the parameter being sensed requires input externally to optimize sensor response and the sensor is unable to react appropriately to stimuli that do not affect the specific sensor. Rate-adaptive sensors that respond to noncardiac signals generally have a reduced response to emotional or psychological stress. Conversely, a closed-loop system would

ideally not require external input or manipulation because intrinsic feedback to the sensor would self-regulate its response. The ideal closed-loop sensor would respond to emotional as well as physical stress.

A variety of sensors appropriate for rate-adaptive pacing have subsequently been developed and are displayed in Figure 2 as endpoints of some physiological response. Some of these sensors are clinically avail-

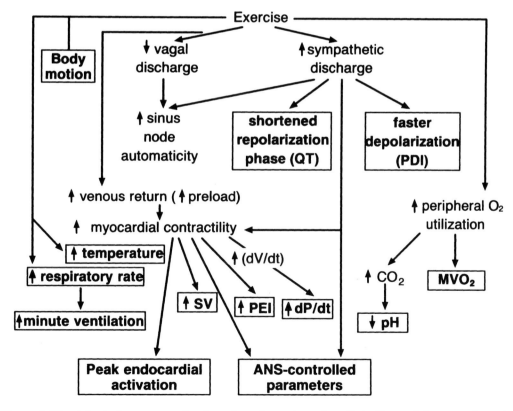

Figure 2. Physiological responses that have been investigated or clinically used for rate-adaptation of permanent pacemakers. The "boxed" terms represent the endpoints used for rate adaptation.

able, others undergoing clinical investigation and/or market available outside the United States and others have previously been investigated and subsequently abandoned. Sensor availability varies because even though some sensors may have never been clinically released as single sensor rate-adaptive pacing systems, e.g., ventricular depolarization gradient (VDG) and dP/dt, it is possible that such sensors will eventually be used as part of a multi-sensor pacing system.

Three varieties of sensors account for the vast majority of rate-adaptive pacing systems worldwide. Activity sensing and minute ventilation have been the primary rate-adaptive pacing systems in the United States, but have also been widely used throughout the world. In Europe, stimulus-T or "QT" sensing pacemakers have been used extensively as well. This sensor has only recently been introduced in the United States and is currently available only as part of an investigational dual sensor pacemaker protocol.

A brief description of clinically relevant sensor technology follows. It is not the purpose of this chapter to discuss specific products. Other excellent sources of such information exist.[8] In addition, the technical manual of each rate-adaptive pacemaker is a good source of information regarding sensor capabilities within a specific device.

Activity Sensors

Activity-controlled pacing with vibration detection (piezoelectric crystal or accelerometer) is currently the most widely used form of rate adaptation because it is simple, easy to apply clinically, and rapid in onset of rate response.[9,10]

The main difference between the piezoelectric crystal sensor and the accelerometer is that the former senses vibration from "up and down" motion and the accelerometer also senses anterior and posterior motion. Accelerometer-based systems may respond more appropriately to specific activities

such as cycling. For example, the typical cyclist may not generate much vibratory sensation above the trunk level. Therefore, a piezoelectric-crystal based rate-adaptive pacemaker may have a limited response to bike riding. However, since the accelerometer senses anterior/posterior motion, it may be more responsive for an activity such as cycling.

Other than a specific circumstance such as cycling, the debate continues as to whether there is, in general, any significant and demonstrable advantage of accelerometer-based activity sensing over piezoelectric crystal-based activity sensing.

On balance, the literature suggests a slight advantage of accelerometer-based activity sensing.[11,12] The potential accelerometer advantages are largely twofold. The first is in improving the specificity of sensor response, i.e., avoiding inappropriate sensor response. For example, investigators[9,10] have shown a tendency to a more physiological heart rate response and lesser response to local pressure and tapping with accelerometer-based pacemakers than with piezoelectric crystal-based pacemakers. Alt et al.[13] have described rhythmic body motion such as walking or bike riding to typically be in the range of 1–8 Hz. Nonexercise-related vibrations that arise from such sources as riding in a car or nonspecific skeletal muscle noise are often greater than 10 Hz. The accelerometer, which limits analysis of signals to the 1–10 Hz range, should be more specific in its response to activity.

A study by Matula et al.[14] compared first generation piezoelectric crystal-based activity sensing pacemakers to a second generation accelerometer-based activity sensing pacemaker. At the lowest of three controlled walking speeds (92 steps/min) the accelerometer-based system increased rates from 107 ± 8 bpm during walking on a level plane to 124 ± 8 bpm with stair climbing. When descending stairs the heart rate was 105 ± 12 bpm. The piezoelectric crystal-based system responded with a lower pacing rate with stair climbing, 97 ± 9 bpm, than when descending stairs, 113 ± 7 bpm.

At faster walking speeds, the difference between the activity sensors was not appreciated.

Investigators from the same institution believe that the accelerometer response to activity can be even more physiologically appropriate if additional morphological criteria are applied to analysis of the signal's amplitude in the positive and negative directions.[15]

Attempts have been made to demonstrate measurable hemodynamic advantage with accelerometer versus piezoelectric crystal-based rate-adaptive pacemakers. The difficulty in this comparison is that no pacemaker incorporates both types of activity sensors. The comparison must therefore be between populations of patients or by assessing the patients with devices externally strapped onto the patient's chest. Both methods are less than perfect and so is the subsequent data.

There have been subsequent variations of activity sensors including a gravitational sensor able to discriminate changes in vertical gravitational acceleration[16] and measurement of electrical signals from a moving magnetic ball.[17]

Minute Ventilation Sensors

Minute volume (respiratory rate times tidal volume) has an excellent correlation with metabolic demand. In a rate-adaptive pacing system, measurement of minute volume is accomplished by emitting a small charge of known current (1 mA every 15 ms) from the pacemaker and measuring the resulting voltage at the lead tip.[18] When both current and voltage are known, transthoracic impedance can be measured between the ring electrode and the pacemaker can. Because transthoracic impedance varies with respiration and its amplitude varies with tidal volume, the impedance measurement can be used to determine respiratory rate and tidal volume. A pacing algorithm uses the minute volume measurements to alter pacing rate.[19] Long-term reliability of the minute volume sensor has been excellent.[20]

Minute ventilation was introduced by Telectronics Pacing Systems, Inc. (Englewood, CO). Telectronics Pacing Systems, Inc. is no longer in existence as a pacemaker manufacturer but minute ventilation sensor technology has been acquired by others. This sensor will undoubtedly continue to have a significant role in the field of rate-adaptive pacing.

Stimulus-T or QT Sensing Pacemaker

The interval from the onset of a paced QRS complex to the end of the T wave has been used for rate adaptation for many years.[21] This *stimulus-T interval* is affected by autonomic activity and heart rate. This relationship allows measurement of the stimulus-T interval to be used for rate adaptation. The QT-sensing rate-adaptive pacing system has been very successful clinically.

Temperature Sensors

Because central venous temperature increases with exercise, it is reasonable to consider this parameter as the basis for a physiological sensor. The rise in temperature can be measured by a thermistor contained within the right ventricular portion of the pacing lead.[22] At the onset of exercise, core body temperature decreases as cooler peripheral blood is returned to the central circulation. Temperature-sensing rate-adaptive pacemakers have been available for many years but have never gained widespread acceptance, in part because a special pacing lead is required and also because rate response is less adequate at low workloads because of the relatively slow response of central venous temperature.[23]

Other Sensors

The *preejection interval* is the systolic time interval from the onset of electrical ventricular depolarization to the onset of ventricular ejection. In terms of ventricular pacing, the preejection interval is the interval between a right ventricular pacing stimulus and the onset of contraction determined by an impedance catheter.[24,25] The preejection interval shortens as exercise workload increases and can be used as a signal to increase the pacing rate. An increase in heart rate does not appreciably affect the preejection interval; that is, no significant positive feedback occurs. *Stroke volume*, also measured by an impedance catheter in the right ventricle, can be used for rate-adaptive pacing by incorporation of a pacing algorithm that alters the pacing rate to keep the right ventricular stroke volume relatively constant and within physiological values.[25]

Change in right ventricular pressure, dP/dt, has been used for rate-adaptive pacing. dP/dt is measured by incorporating a pressure transducer in the right ventricular portion of the pacing lead.[26,27] In clinical investigations and in follow-up, the sensor has performed very well. However, a rate-adaptive pacing system utilizing this sensor has never been market released.

Mixed venous oxygen saturation, measured with hemoreflectance oximetry, varies with physical activity and changes rapidly with the onset of exercise. In a study of 81 patients with cardiovascular pathology and 27 normal subjects, McElroy et al. demonstrated the potential efficacy of mixed venous oxygen saturation as a sensor for rate-adaptive pacing. They demonstrated:

"(1) A highly linear heart rate-VO₂ relation in each subject (the average slope of this relation was greater P less than 0.05 in patients with more severe failure); (2) VE was highly correlated with exercise heart rate, and its slope was not different between normal subjects and patients; and (3) Mixed venous temperature and pH were poor predictors of exercise heart rate, particularly at low or moderate levels of work; however, SVO₂ was highly correlated with heart rate for all levels of work."[28]

For a rate-adaptive pacing system, the oximeter is incorporated in the right ventricular portion of the pacing lead. The greatest

challenge has been to find a stable sensor. Initial studies in animals and humans are encouraging.[29]

Fourteen patients with a chronically implanted mixed venous oxygen saturation rate-adaptive pacing system were followed for a mean of 44 months (2–63 months).[30] During follow-up, there was excellent correlation between central venous oxygen saturation derived from the pacing system and that obtained by invasive measurements. Success with oxygen saturation rate-adaptation in a dual chamber pacemaker has also been described.[31]

Paced depolarization integral (PDI) is a less well known physiological sensor.[32,33] The concept of PDI refers to the vector integral of the paced QRS, or ventricular depolarization gradient, which has been investigated as a single sensor system but never market released.[34] The concept of PDI is somewhat complex and refers to the vector integral of the paced QRS or ventricular depolarization gradient (VDG).[35] Lau[36] explains the clinical response of the VDG as follows. During fixed-rate ventricular pacing, exercise and the effect of circulating catecholamines will decrease the VDG. An increase in pacing rate will increase the VDG. Therefore, in a normal heart the VDG should remain relatively unchanged during exercise and other forms of stress and represents a "closed loop" rate-adaptive pacing system.

PDI responds relatively rapidly, similar to the rate response of an activity sensor. The disadvantages of this sensor had been the potential for rate response to decrease after the initial rate response despite an increase in the workload. In addition, a paradoxical response to posture has been seen resulting in a lower pacing rate when the patient is upright during a head-up tilt.[36]

Newer Sensors

Of significant interest is monitoring of autonomic activity and utilization of this information as the basis for a rate-adaptive pacing system. Some aspects of autonomic monitoring are a part of stimulus-T sensing pacemakers as well as pacemakers incorporating paced depolarization integral (ventricular depolarization gradient), both of which have been previously described.

The basis for the *autonomic nervous system (ANS)* sensor developed by Schaldach[37] is best described from a passage from one of his descriptive manuscripts[38]:

". . . the depolarization and repolarization behaviour of the myocardial cell, which is also subject to autonomic influences, can be utilized by two kinds of intracardiac potential measurements to quantify ANS activity. The ventricular evoked response (VER) reflecting the heart's electrical activity after a pacing stimulus has a close relationship to the monophasic action potential (MAP), which reproduces very closely the action potential of a myocardial cell. Upon sympathetic stimulation, the plateau potential is raised to a certain degree due to increased Ca2+ currents, and the repolarization starts earlier and with a steeper slope as a consequence of an increased K+ outward current. As clinical measurements show, these effects are visible in both VER and MAP signals, being therefore suitable sensor signals for monitoring of ANS activity.

. . . recent advances in electrode technology and biomedical research have led to new concepts of physiological rate-adaptive pacing which utilize the electrode at the same time as a biosensor to monitor ANS activity and thus, avoid the use of a large number of artificial sensors."

A 1996 publication[39] described a multicenter experience with ANS-controlled pacemakers. A total of 262 patients had received the ANS-controlled pacemaker in with an average patient age of 62 ± 7 years of which 178 were single chamber and 84 were dual chamber. Patients underwent bicycle ergometry, ambulatory monitoring, and psychological stress studies to determine the clinical response of the ANS-controlled pacemaker (Figure 3). The authors concluded that ANS-controlled closed-loop rate-adaptive pacing could be successfully accomplished and that the sensor responds appropriately both to physical and psychological stress.

Another new rate-adaptive pacing system incorporates a microaccelerometer in the tip of a normal endocardial pacing lead. The microaccelerometer is inside a rigid, hermetically sealed capsule and an associated electronic circuit pre-processes the signal to allow transmission through the catheter.[40] The capsule is insensitive to ventricular pressures and fibrosis at the lead tip and sen-

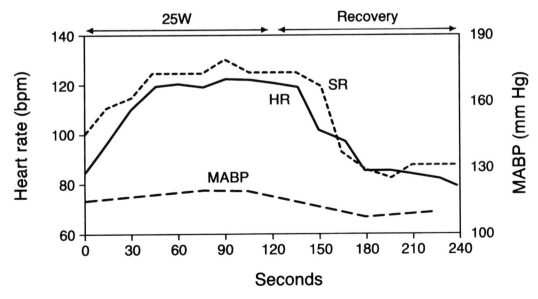

Figure 3. Comparison of sinus rate and ANS-controlled sensor-driven VVIR pacing as a patient performs bicycle ergometry. Used with permission from Schaldach M.[38]

sitive only to internal forces generated by myocardial movement. The peak endocardial acceleration (PEA) is represented by the peak-to-peak value of the endocardial acceleration signal measured inside a time window containing the isovolumic contraction phase. The PEA can be correlated with dP/dt max and should therefore represent the heart's contractile function (Figure 4).

A temporary pacing study was performed in six patients with the patients being studied at rest, during physical exer-

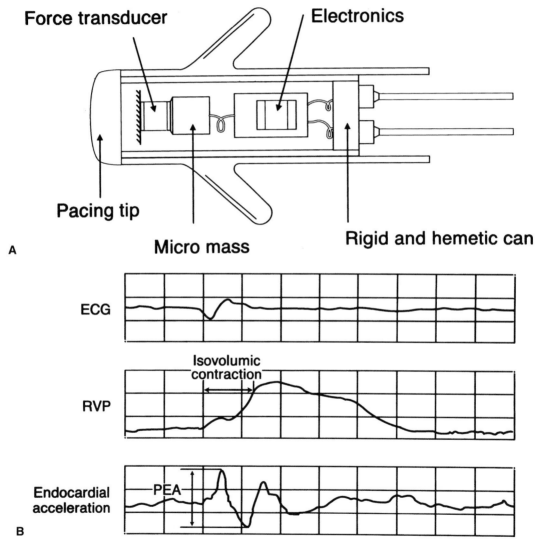

Figure 4. A: The sensor is described as a microaccelerometer that is housed inside a rigid, perfectly hermetic capsule within the distal portion of the lead. An associated electronic circuit pre-processes the signal to ensure its correct transmission through the catheter. The rigidity of the capsule allegedly makes the sensor totally insensitive to ventricular pressures and to fibrosis on the lead tip, leaving the sensor sensitive only to the inertial forces generated by myocardial movement. Used with permission from Sorin Biomedica. **B:** Simultaneous ECG and RVP (right ventricular pressure curve) as well as the Peak Endocardial Acceleration (PEA) waveform. The PEA is represented by the peak-to-peak value of the endocardial acceleration signal measured inside a time window containing the isovolumic contraction phase. Used with permission from Sorin Biomedica.

cise, and during dobutamine infusion.[40] During exercise, paced heart rate increased from 68 ± 13 bpm to 131 ± 16 bpm and dobutamine infusion at 10 mg/kg/min increased the paced ventricular rate to 120 ± 11 bpm. The authors concluded that PEA increases during adrenergic stimulation and follows changes in heart rate.

Early clinical results with the PEA sensor as part of a chronically implanted system are available. In a series of 24 patients who received the microaccelerometer system that senses myocardial contractility, ambulatory monitoring and bicycle ergometry were performed during follow-up.[41] During these activities the PEA values increased two- to threefold at exercise, except in two cases where they were unable to document a significant increase in PEA. One patient demonstrated false positive PEA which resulted in short-term erroneous upper rate behavior. The remainder of the patients demonstrated appropriate rate response.

Success has also been demonstrated in a 1-year follow-up of a multicenter collection of 79 patients receiving a PEA sensor in a dual chamber pacing system. [42]

PEA is of potential value in certain clinical circumstances. Its utility was shown in three patients undergoing cardiac surgery.[43] In all three patients the PEA roughly paralleled the corresponding cardiac index and changed consistently during administration of cardioactive drugs.

French investigators have used PEA pacing systems in patients with malignant neurally mediated syncope.[44,45] They postulated that detection of the initial increase in sympathetic activity that is felt to precede the symptomatic hypotension could theoretically be detected by the PEA. Detection of this early increase in inotropic activity could then allow early pacing intervention. Success was demonstrated in both temporary[44] and permanent pacing studies.[45]

Dual Sensor Rate-Adaptive Pacing

The overall performance of market-approved single sensor rate-adaptive systems has been excellent. However, the perfect sensor would mimic the response of the normal sinus node at all levels of activity and during emotional stress.

Clinical problems with available rate-adaptive pacing systems have been minimal. Both activity-sensing and minute ventilation devices may respond to nonphysiological stimuli. For example, with activity sensing systems, rate acceleration may occur when tapping the pulse generator or rolling over on the pacemaker. A paradoxical rate response has also been shown in that a faster sensor-driven rate response is often seen when a patient descends stairs than when ascending stairs.[46] Minute ventilation rate response may be interrupted if the patient is talking during exercise, and arm movement may result in a rate increase even if minute ventilation remains unchanged. These changes occur because minute ventilation is an impedance-based measurement and may be affected by any movement that alters thoracic impedance. Although response to nonphysiological stimuli represents less than perfect specificity of the sensor response, activity, minute ventilation, and stimulus-T sensors have served patients very well.

The perfect sensor would be resistant to these nonphysiological stimuli. Although some "closed-loop" physiological sensors could potentially be at or near 100% specificity, none are available clinically.

Even before excellent clinical results had been achieved with several single sensor rate-adaptive pacing systems, the concept of multi-sensor systems was raised. A multisensor rate-adaptive pacing system could improve specificity by having one sensor verify or cross-check the other. For example, a dual sensor pacemaker could be designed such that if sensor #1 reacted to a stimulus with a rate response but sensor #2 indicated that a rate increase was inappropriate, no rate increase would occur. Both sensors would have to indicate a rate increase before it would be allowed.

Several basic concerns had to be addressed in developing a dual sensor pacemaker including sensor interaction and programming. Sensor interaction could potentially be designed in several ways (Table 1). The method of programming the rate-adaptive response and sensor interaction was also critical. Early concerns were raised about the potential complexity of programming two or more sensors, especially if programming of the sensors was done independently of one another.

Because some sensors perform in a more physiological manner at low levels of exercise and others perform in a more physiological manner at high levels of exercise, combination of two or more sensors could better simulate the normal sinus node response.[47]

A multi-sensor study that was ahead of its time was performed by Stangl et al. [48] In their temporary pacing study, they compared seven different sensors in 12 control patients with normal sinus rhythm. The system was designed as a transvenous temporary pacing system and the patients were exercised using bicycle ergometry. They described several potential sensor combinations after analyzing rate response at low and high workloads to find complementary combinations that could mimic normal sinus rhythm better than any single sensor. They found the best combination of sensors to be mixed venous oxygen saturation and temperature. (This study did not include activity sensing which has been the most widely used sensor clinically.)

It took years to clinically implement the early observations of dual or multi-sensor systems. A significant body of literature detailing clinical results with dual sensor rate-adaptive pacing systems has now emerged. Sensor combinations that are available in certain world markets as well as dual sensors undergoing investigation are listed in Table 2.

Devices using dual sensors are available in the United States, as of the writing of this chapter, only as clinically investigational devices. Most of the existing literature has come from Europe and Asia.

The first VVIR dual sensor pacemaker, the Vitatron-Topaz, began clinical investigation in August 1991 and was clinically released in Europe in January 1992. This device combines activity and QT interval sensing.

The Topaz (Model 515, Vitatron Medical, Dieren, the Netherlands) VVIR pacemaker incorporates QT interval sensing and activity sensing (vibration sensing via a piezoelectric crystal). The pacemaker can be programmed to operate as a single sensor, QT interval or activity, or dual sensor. If dual sensor is chosen the relative contribution of each sensor is determined by programming Sensor Blending™ as QT < activity, QT = activity, or QT > activity. Automatic in dual sensor modes in this pacemaker is a feature dubbed "sensor cross-checking" (Figure 5). If there is disagreement between the two sensors, this feature prevents an inappropriately high pacing rate from being maintained. The QT and activity slopes, i.e., the

---

Table 2
Available Sensor Combinations and Dual Sensors Under Investigation

Sensors	Company	Modes
Minute Ventilation and Activity (Piezoelectric crystal)	Medtronic	DDDR, DVIR, DDIR, VDIR, VVIR, AAIR, ADIR
QT Interval and Activity (Piezoelectric crystal)	Vitatron	DDDR, DDIR, VDDR, VVIR, AAIR
Gravitational accelerometer and microaccelerometer (PEA)	Sorin Biomedica	DDDR, VDDR, DDIR, DVIR, VVIR, VVTR, AAIR, AATR
PDI and Minute Ventilation	Telectronics[1]	VVIR

[1] This device is not currently available and unclear if it will be further investigated or marketed in the future.

QT interval

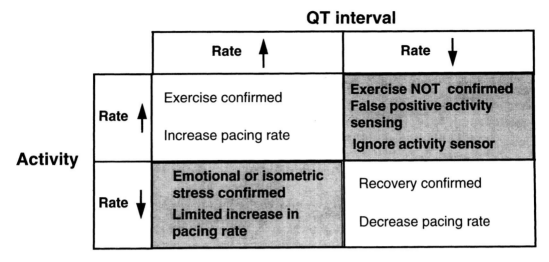

Figure 5. Diagram demonstrating logic involved in sensor cross-checking. Sensors must be in agreement regarding the appropriateness of a rate increase for any change in the paced rate to occur. Modified and used with permission from Vitatron, Inc.

change in pacing rate for a given change in QT interval or activity threshold, are automatically measured and adapted whenever the pacing rate achieves the programmed upper rate limit. Van Krieken et al. have investigated this algorithm and found it to be effective requiring 2–5 weeks to reach full rate response.[49]

There are many follow-up studies available detailing the safety, reliability, and perceived superiority of a dual sensor.[50–55] The study from the Topaz Study Group includes the first 90 implants of this pacemaker. Sensor blending was determined from an initial exercise test. The majority of the patients were programmed to QT = activity. A much smaller subset were programmed to QT < activity, and an even smaller group to QT > activity. Three patients were programmed to activity as a single sensor. Activity sensing alone was used only if T wave sensing was unsatisfactory. QT interval sensing alone was not an option in the study. Sensor Cross-Checking[TM] was tested by tapping on the pacemaker, application of massage equipment over the pacemaker, mental stress, and staircase walking. In the tests used to simulate false positive activity sensing, the pacemaker initially increased

the pacing rate but when exercise was not confirmed by the cross-checking mechanism, i.e., there was absence of significant QT interval shortening, the pacing rate gradually declined toward the lower rate limit.

Sulke et al. compared performance values from 10 patients with Medtronic Legend Plus (VVIR) to 20 normal subjects.[56] Patients subjective preference of exercise capacity and functional status was lower in VVI, $P < 0.05$, versus VVIR. When assessed for sensor preference, 40% preferred the activity sensor alone, 30% preferred the dual sensor, and no preference was noted by the remaining 30%. When asked to declare the least acceptable sensor, 30% preferred dual sensor the least, 30% minute ventilation alone, one patient (10%) equally disliking dual sensor and minute ventilation, and the remainder without a preference. Interestingly, no patient noted activity sensing alone to be the least acceptable. The authors concluded that there is no distinct clinical advantage of dual sensor rate-adaptive pacing over activity sensing pacing but potential disadvantages of increased size, complexity, cost, and compromised longevity.

Of the complications reported by Con-

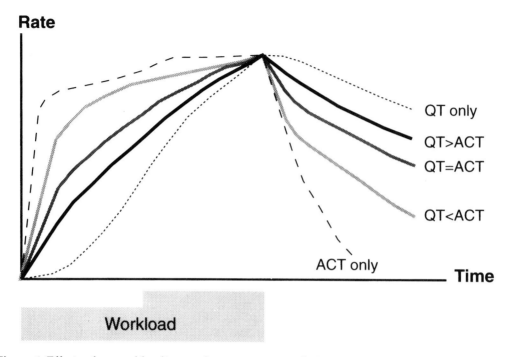

Figure 6. Effects of sensor blending on the rate response of a Vitatron dual sensor, QT and activity, pacemaker. Used with permission from Vitatron, Inc.

nelly et al.[50] only two were related to rate-adaptive function. These patients had T wave undersensing requiring programming to activity sensing only.

The authors concluded that the pacemaker functions satisfactorily in terms of Sensor-Blending™ and Sensor Cross-Checking™ and therefore offers advantages over single sensor pacemakers (Figure 6). In a study of only eight patients with the Topaz dual sensor pacing system, Cowell et al.[57] reached the conclusion that this sensor combination resulted in an attenuated initial rate response compared to activity alone and an inappropriately prolonged recovery time after burst activity. However, the subsequent larger series by Connelly et al.[50] does not substantiate these concerns.

The Legend Plus (Medtronic Inc, Minneapolis, MN) VVIR pacemaker combines activity sensing and minute ventilation. The activity sensor responds to body vibrations via a piezoelectric crystal.

In this pacemaker the rate is determined by the faster of the two sensors. The wisdom of this combination rests in the fact that activity is capable of giving a rapid early rate response to exercise and the more physiologically driven minute ventilation maintaining rate response during more prolonged exercise. In the dual sensor mode, the sensors are programmed independently although during programming the programmer provides suggested rate-response settings for activity and minute ventilation via an "exercise test" that is an interactive feature of the system. Wahlstrand et al.,[58] in a series of 11 patients, felt that the exercise test provided an accurate and simple means of programming the dual sensor response. Conversely, in a study of 11 patients with the Legend Plus, another group of investigators felt that the rate-response parameters that were automatically chosen by the programmer were not accurate enough.[59]

In a study of 52 patients with the Legend Plus, Crossley et al.[60] compared activity sensing and minute ventilation as single sensors to the combination of the two. They concluded that the combination of sensors may provide a metabolic advantage because it resulted in a higher heart rate at anerobic threshold and a higher VO_2 max. In a metabolic study performed by Alt et al.,[61] this sensor combination provided a more appropriate physiological pacing response than activity alone as shown by a better correlation to VE/VO_2 and peak heart rates obtained. Other studies of the Legend Plus performance have shown fewer false positive responses to minute ventilation pacing when programmed to the dual sensor mode,[62] and appropriate peak heart rate response to ascending and descending stairs when compared to activity sensing alone.[63]

A VVIR pacemaker combining minute ventilation and paced depolarization integral (PDI) has also been investigated but is not currently available.

The combination of PDI with minute ventilation should provide initial rate response via PDI and rate response during later stages of exercise via minute ventilation. There is limited information available regarding clinical results with this dual sensor pacemaker and with the subsequent demise of Telectronics Pacing System Inc., it is unclear if this particular dual sensor pacemaker will be pursued.

In one study, five patients with the minute ventilation/PDI pacemaker were reported by Slade et al.[64] They found the initial rate response to be best with PDI alone or dual sensor response compared to minute ventilation alone. The paradoxical response of PDI sensing to posture was minimized in the dual sensor mode and the interference with minute ventilation that can be seen if the patient is talking during exercise was minimized in the dual sensor mode. Cowell et al.[65] assessed four patients with the Sentri system and also found that false negative responses with minute ventilation were reduced in the dual sensor mode. The paradoxical posture response was observed in the dual sensor mode.[65]

The first dual chamber dual sensor rate-adaptive pacemaker (Diamond Model 800, Vitatron Medical, Dieren, the Netherlands)

combined activity sensing with QT interval sensing. Connelly and colleagues[66] reported use of this pacemaker in 23 patients followed for a mean of 6 months. Their experience was favorable and they did not find follow-up or initial programming to be unduly time-consuming or complex. The device includes automatic slope adaptation for both QT interval and activity thresholds. They activated this feature in all patients and found it helpful in initial programming of rate-adaptive features.

Stangl[67] considered possible sensor combinations in terms of whether a special "sensor" lead would be required. Combinations that can be accomplished with a standard lead include the previously described activity/QT interval, activity/minute ventilation, and minute ventilation/PDI. He also included stroke volume as a fast-reacting impedance-derived parameter that could potentially be combined with minute ventilation or QT interval.

Of systems that would require a "special lead," combinations of oxygen saturation/temperature, temperature/activity, and oxygen saturation/intracardiac pressure/stroke volume were suggested as being potentially complementary.

Proving the Clinical Benefit of Two or More Sensors

During initial clinical evaluation of single sensor rate-adaptive pacemakers, the clinical advantages of rate adaptation over fixed-rate pacing in the chronotropically incompetent patient was easily and repeatedly demonstrated. It may be more difficult to demonstrate objective clinical gains with a dual sensor rate-adaptive pacemaker over a single sensor.

From the initial studies with dual sensor pacemakers the advantage of one sensor verifying the rate response of the other sensor and preventing a rate response to a nonphysiological event seems evident. What has not yet clearly emerged is if dual sensors will impart any improvement in exercise tolerance either objectively or subjectively. Several investigators have used metabolic exercise testing to compare single and dual sensor systems. Benditt et al.[68] performed maximal cardiopulmonary exercise testing in 14 chronotropically incompetent patients receiving an activity/minute ventilation dual sensor system. Although VO_2 max and maximum heart rate were comparable whether the patient was in the activity mode, minute ventilation mode, or dual sensor mode, there was a smaller O_2 deficit and shorter mean response time with activity and dual sensor than with minute ventilation. Based on these findings the authors concluded that O_2 uptake kinetic analysis will provide a potentially useful means to discern subtle differences among sensors and advantages of dual sensors.

In a similar study involving six patients with a QT interval/activity dual sensor system, Leung and colleagues[69] compared the single sensors to the combination. They found a lower O_2 debt with activity than with QT interval sensing or dual sensor and concluded that dual sensors may not result in objective metabolic improvement even though the dual sensor rate profile may be more normal than that of either single sensor.

Using a dual sensor DDDR pacemaker (minute ventilation and activity) Leung et al. demonstrated a shorter sensor delay time and time to 50% and 90% rate response with the dual sensor versus minute ventilation alone.[70] In addition, the sensor blending and cross-checking algorithm was shown to be relatively immune to false triggering, i.e., tapping on the pacemaker and/or arm swinging.

Lau and colleagues[71] also demonstrated that sensor cross-checking at rest in a dual sensor, activity/QT, pacemaker appropriately limited rate response in the overprogrammed dual sensor VVIR mode.

In a 1995 study using an activity/minute ventilation pacemaker, patients underwent metabolic exercise testing and compared dual sensor response to a "strapped-on" activity sensing-only pacemaker.[72] The investigators found the dual sensor rate-adaptive pacing system resulted in pacing rates more proportional to metabolic indicators than did the "strapped-on" activity sensing-only mode.

Applicability of dual sensor single chamber pacing systems to the pediatric population has been described by Celiker et al.[73] A dual sensor, activity, and QT sensor pacing system was evaluated in 15 children with a mean age of 5.9 ± 3.9 years. They felt that dual sensor pacing may offer distinct advantages, specifically in terms of sensor cross-checking and avoidance of inappropriate sensor rate response.

Lau has raised several potential concerns with dual sensor pacing systems including more complex programming and greater battery consumption as two or more sensors are monitored and activated.[74]

Taborsky et al. attempted to compare time and technological components necessary for follow-up of a dual sensor system.[75] In the limited assessment of 10 patients they concluded that the dual sensor system did not prolong the time required for regular follow-up of single sensor pacemakers, in part because of the "automatic" features available on the dual sensor pacemaker.

On balance, no definite statements can be made regarding clinical superiority of dual sensor rate-adaptive pacing systems. Although the studies summarized have, in general, shown some objective advantage of dual sensor systems in small populations of patients, subjective improvement is less obvious. In a recent editorial, Barold and Clementy state that "programming of rate adaptive parameters need not be precise for clinical benefit. It is therefore questionable whether patients will feel better with a dual-sensor device compared with a correctly programmed single sensor system with a well-designed algorithm."[76]

What can be stated definitively about dual sensor rate-adaptive pacing systems? It does seem clear that sensor cross-checking will prevent inappropriate false positive rate response if complementary sensors are utilized.[76–79] It also seems likely that a dual sensor pacemaker will be more expensive than a single sensor pacemaker. Coupled with another disadvantage of probable increased current drain to accomplish dual sensor activities, battery longevity may be compromised.

Other Potential Sensor Benefits

Another potential application of sensors is for the detection of tachyarrhythmias. Cohen and Liem[80] designed a dual sensor algorithm using mean right atrial pressure sensor and mixed venous O_2 saturation. Using this combination of sensors there was 100% sensitivity and 73% specificity in the detection of tachyarrhythmias.

Use of physiological sensors could theoretically provide clinical information that could be helpful in managing various cardiopulmonary disorders. Whether part of a single or dual sensor system, sensors that collect physiological data, i.e., stroke volume, preejection interval, mixed venous oxygen saturation,[31] ANS parameters,[37,38] could be used in managing nonbradyarrhythmic disorders such as left ventricular dysfunction, pulmonary disease, autonomic dysfunction, etc.

In summary, dual sensor rate-adaptive pacing systems will undoubtedly become commonplace clinically in the near future. Although some limited objective advantages of these systems have been demonstrated, whether they offer significant objective advantages or subjective improvement for the patient is not yet well established. Such benefits will need to be determined and considered along with the probable incremental cost of dual sensor systems over available single sensor systems.

Improving Sensor Automaticity

With the earliest activity-sensing pacemakers it was noted that the sensor would at times need to be reprogrammed at a later date due to pocket maturation and improvement in the patient's exercise capabilities after chronotropic response was restored.[81,82] Minute ventilation sensor-driven pacemakers also required reprogramming in some patients as conditioning improved.

The current generation of rate-adaptive pacemakers, both single and dual sensor systems, use an increasing degree of automaticity to assist in programming and optimization of sensor function.[82,83]

Many rate-adaptive pacemakers provide histograms of achieved sensor-driven paced rates to assist in reprogramming of the sensor variables in an effort to optimize chronotropic response[84] (Figure 7). Some pacemakers will display sinus-achieved heart rates as well as raw or passive sensor data, i.e., how the sensor would have responded had it been activated (Figure 8). Still others provide autocalibration of their slope, adjusting slope against patient activity levels as determined by maximum and minimum sensor values over a given period of time[85] (Figure 9). The efficacy of an automatically optimized dual sensor rate-adaptive pacing system was assessed by Lau et al.[82] Twelve patients with complete heart block and a pacemaker with automatically adaptive activity and QT sensors were exercised with collection of sinus and sensor-indicated rates. During exercise testing there was an excellent correlation ($r = 0.96 \pm 0.02$, $P < 0.001$) between sinus and sensor-indicated rates. Although correlation at the most vigorous levels of exercise was less satisfactory, most of the sensor-indicated rates were within the normal sinus rhythm variation of 15 beats/minute.

Summary and Future Predictions

Rate-adaptive pacing has rapidly become an integral part of pacemaker prescribing practices. Utilization rates of rate-adaptive pacing will only continue to increase. Only healthcare economics pro-

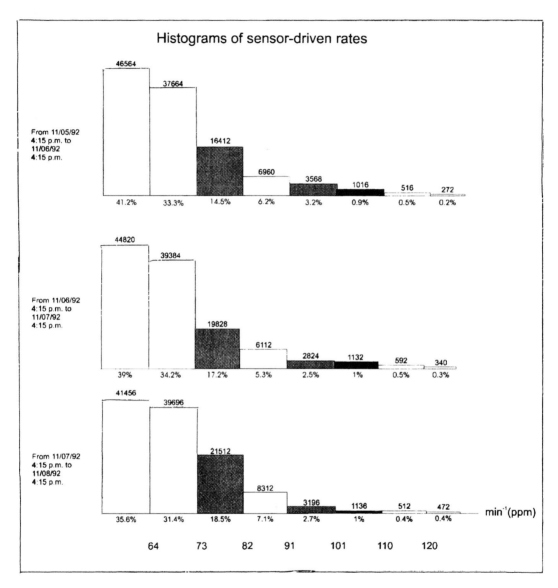

Figure 7. Histograms from a DDDR pacemaker of sensor-driven rates over the 3 days prior to pacemaker interrogation. The pacemaker collects every rate calculated and records them in three successive histograms of 24 hours each. Each histogram is divided into eight rate bins divided equally between the programmed lower rate and the programmed maximum sensor-driven rate. Used with permission of ELA Medical, Paris, France.

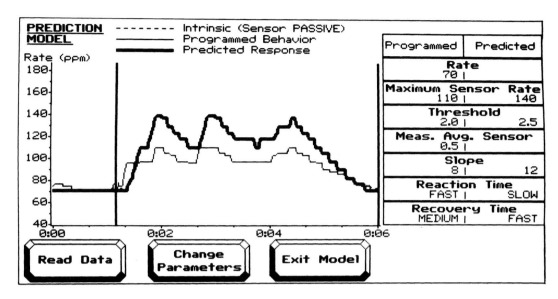

Figure 8. Example of telemetry from a pacemaker that allows the clinician to predict rate response at different sensor parameters. This Rate-Response Prediction Model example is from a Trilogy™ DR+ by Pacesetter, Inc. This model allows the clinician to assess a variety of rate-modulated parameters without requiring the patient to repeatedly exercise. Used with permission from Pacesetter Systems, Inc. a St. Jude Medical Company.

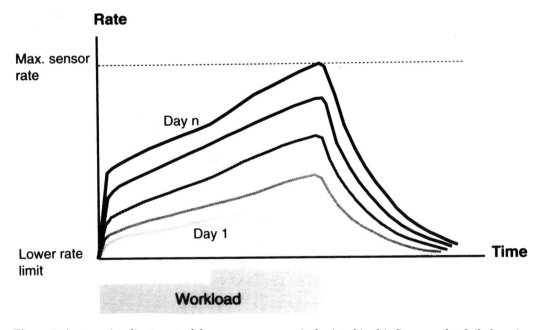

Figure 9. Automatic adjustment of the sensor response is depicted in this figure as the daily learning process in a Vitatron dual sensor pacemaker. The QT interval and activity slopes are automatically adjusted at the lower and upper rate limits by this process. Once activated, the pacemaker requires approximately 14 days for the slopes to be optimized, after which only minor variations occur. Used with permission from Vitatron, Inc.

hibits using rate-adaptive pacemakers 100% of the time. A simplified pacing mode selection algorithm that limits choices to VVIR for patients with chronic atrial fibrillation and DDDR for all other patients would provide the greatest future flexibility for all patients.

The near future will also bring increased use of dual sensor pacemakers. Even if the objective benefit is no better defined, the introduction of additional sensor combinations, especially a combination that would allow accurate sensor cross-checking and at the same time provide appropriate rate response to psychological as well as physical stress, will drive the pacing community toward dual sensor pacemakers. Although rate-adaptive pacing systems that are truly "closed loop" have been in the development stages much longer, some are now in clinical use. Mixed venous oxygen saturation, PEA and ANS-controlled rate-adaptive pacing systems all hold promise. In addition, even though PDI and dP/dt were never market released as single sensor pacing systems, the sensors have clinical merit and will hopefully reemerge as part of a multi-sensor pacing device.

References

1. Silverman BG, Gross TP, Kaczmarek RG, et al. The epidemiology of pacemaker implantation in the United States. Public Health Rep Jan.-Feb. 1995;110(1):42–46.
2. Janosik DL, Labovitz AJ. Basic physiology of cardiac pacing. In Ellenbogen KA, Kay GN, Wilkoff BL, eds. Clinical Cardiac Pacing. WB Saunders, Philadelphia, 1995, pp 167–186.
3. Camm AJ, Fei L. Chronotropic incompetence. Part II: Clinical implications. Clin Cardiol 1996;19:503–508.
4. Bernstein AD, Parsonnet V. Survey of cardiac pacing and defibrillation in the United States in 1993. AJC 1996;78:187–196.
5. Higano ST, Hayes DL, Eisinger G. Sensor-driven rate smoothing in a DDDR pacemaker. PACE 1989;12:922–929.
6. Hayes DL, Von Feldt L. Utilization of rate-adaptive pacing modes in a DDDR pacemaker. PACE 1993;16:873A.
7. Rossi P. Rate-responsive pacing: biosensor reliability and physiological sensitivity. PACE 1987;10:454–466.
8. Manz M, Jung W, Lewalter T, et al. Single and Multisensor pacemaker systems. In Saksena S, Luderitz B, eds. Interventional Electrophysiology: A Textbook. Second edition. Futura Publishing Company, Inc, Armonk, NY, 1996, pp 91–103.
9. Alt E, Millerhagen JO, Heemels J-P. Accelerometers. In Ellenbogen KA, Kay GN, Wilkoff BL, eds. Clinical Cardiac Pacing. WB Saunders, Philadelphia, 1995, pp 267–276.
10. Benditt DG, Duncan JL. Activity-sensing, rate-adaptive pacemakers. In Ellenbogen KA, Kay GN, Wilkoff BL, eds. Clinical Cardiac Pacing. WB Saunders, Philadelphia, 1995, pp 167–186.
11. Lazarus A, Mitchell K, for the Dromos DR Investigators Group. A prospective multicenter study demonstrating clinical benefit with a new accelerometer-based DDDR pacemaker. PACE 1996;19:1694–1697.
12. Matula M, Holzer K, Zitzmann E, et al. Behavior of various activity-based pacing systems under treadmill exercise testing with variable slopes. Z Kardiol 1993;82:108–115.
13. Alt E, Matula M, Theres H, et al. The basis for activity controlled rate variable cardiac pacemakers: an analysis of mechanical forces on the human body induced by exercise and environment. PACE 1989;12:1667–1680.
14. Matula M, Schlegl M, Alt E. Activity controlled cardiac pacemakers during stairwalking: a comparison of accelerometer with vibration guided devices and with sinus rate. PACE 1996;19:1036–1041.
15. Schmidt M, Ammer R, Evans F, et al. Improving accelerometer-based rate adaptive pacing by means of second generation processing. PACE 1996;19:1698–1703.
16. Bongiorni M, Soldati E, Arena G, et al. Multicenter clinical evaluation of a new SSIR pacemaker. PACE 1992;15(Pt II):1798–1803.
17. Faerestrand S, Ohm OJ. Clinical study of a new activity sensor for rate adaptive pacing controlled by electrical signals generated by the kinetic energy of a moving magnetic ball. PACE 1994;17:1944–1949.
18. Nappholtz T, Valenta H, Maloney J, et al. Electrode configurations for a respiratory impedance measurement suitable for rate responsive pacing. PACE 1986;9:960–964.
19. Slade AK, Pee S, Jones S, et al. New algorithms to increase the initial rate response in a minute volume rate adaptive pacemaker. PACE 1994;17(Pt II):1960–1965.

20. Li H, Neubauer SA, Hayes DL. Follow-up of a minute ventilation rate adaptive pacemaker. PACE 1992;15(Pt II):1826–1829.

21. Connelly DT, Rickards AF. The evoked QT interval. In Ellenbogen KA, Kay GN, Wilkoff BL, eds. Clinical Cardiac Pacing. WB Saunders, Philadelphia, 1995, pp 250–257.

22. Jolgren D, Fearnot N, Geddes L. A rate-responsive pacemaker controlled by right ventricular blood temperature. PACE 1984;7: 794–801.

23. Benditt DG, Mianulli M, Lurie K, et al. Multiple-sensor systems for physiologic cardiac pacing. Ann Intern Med 1994;121(12): 960–968.

24. Chirife R. Physiological principles of a new method for rate responsive pacing using the pre-ejection interval. PACE 1988;11(Pt I): 1545–1554.

25. Salo R, O'Donoghue S, Platia EV. The use of intracardiac impedance-based indicators to optimize pacing rate. In Ellenbogen KA, Kay GN, Wilkoff BL, eds. Clinical Cardiac Pacing. WB Saunders, Philadelphia, 1995, pp 234–249.

26. Kay GN, Philippon F, Bubien RS, et al. Rate modulated pacing based on right ventricular dP/dt: quantitative analysis of chronotropic response. PACE 1994;17:1344–1354.

27. Yee R, Bennett TD. Rate-adaptive pacing controlled by dynamic right ventricular pressure (dP/dt max). In Ellenbogen KA, Kay GN, Wilkoff BL, eds. Clinical Cardiac Pacing. WB Saunders, Philadelphia, 1995, pp 212–218.

28. McElroy PA, Janicki JS, Weber KT. Physiologic correlates of the heart rate response to upright isotonic exercise: relevance to rate-responsive pacemakers. JACC 1988;11: 94–99.

29. Kay GN, Bornzin GA. Rate-modulated pacing controlled by mixed venous oxygen saturation. In Ellenbogen KA, Kay GN, Wilkoff BL, eds. Clinical Cardiac Pacing. WB Saunders, Philadelphia, 1995, pp 187–200.

30. Faerestrand S, Ohm OJ, Stangeland L, et al. Long-term clinical performance of a central venous oxygen saturation sensor for rate adaptive cardiac pacing. PACE 1994;17: 1355–1372.

31. Lau CP, Tai YT, Lee IS, et al. Utility of an implantable right ventricular oxygen saturation-sensing pacemaker for ambulatory cardiopulmonary monitoring. Chest 1995;107: 1089–1094.

32. Callaghan F, Vollmann W, Livingston A, et al. The ventricular depolarization gradient: effects of exercise, pacing rate, epinephrine, and intrinsic heart rate control on the right

ventricular evoked response. PACE 1989; 12(Pt II):1115–1130.

33. Singer I, Callaghan FJ. Evoked potentials as a sensor for rate-adaptive pacing. In Ellenbogen KA, Kay GN, Wilkoff BL, eds. Clinical Cardiac Pacing. WB Saunders, Philadelphia, 1995, pp 258–266.

34. Singer I, Olash J, Brennan F, et al. Initial clinical experience with a rate responsive pacemaker. PACE 1989;12:1458–1464.

35. Callaghan F, Vollmann W, Livingston A, et al. The ventricular depolarization gradient: effects of exercise, pacing rate, epinephrine, and intrinsic heart rate control on the right ventricular evoked response. PACE 1990;12: 1115–1130.

36. Lau CP. Ventricular depolarization gradient and output pulse parameters. In Lau CP, ed. Rate Adaptive Cardiac Pacing: Single and Dual Chamber. Futura Publishing Co, Inc., Armonk, NY, 1993, pp 137–146.

37. Schaldach M. New aspects in electrosimulation of the heart. Med Progr Technol 1995; 21:1–16.

38. Schaldach M. Various methods of monitoring the autonomic nervous system using the pacing lead as a sensor: clinical results and prospectives. In Oto Am, ed. Practice and Progress in Cardiac Pacing and Electrophysiology. Kluwer Academic Publishers, Netherlands, 1996, pp 209–238.

39. Witte J, Reibis R, Pichlmaier AM, et al. ANS-controlled rate-adaptive pacing: a clinical evaluation. Eur JCPE 1996;6:53–59.

40. Occhetta E, Perucca A, Rognoni G, et al. Experience with a new myocardial acceleration sensor during dobutamine infusion and exercise test. Eur JCPE 1995;5:204–209.

41. Timmermans AJM and the Dutch Sorin Best Living Investigators. First experiences with the Biomechanical Endocardial Sorin Transducer (BEST) and the BEST Living DDDR pacing system. PACE 1997;20:1532A.

42. Adornato E, Gaggini G, Garberoglio B, et al. One year follow-up of the new Peak Endocardial Acceleration (PEA) based pacemaker (BEST-Living System). PACE 1997;20:1544A.

43. Colella A, Vaccari G, Dovelini E, et al. Pea endocardial accelerometer in critical settings. PACE 1997;20:1568A.

44. Deharo J-C, Peyre J-P, Ritter P, et al. A sensor-based evaluation of heart contractility in patients with head-up tilt induced neurally mediated syncope. PACE 1997;20:1568A.

45. Deharo J-C, Peyre J-P, Ritter P, et al. Adaptive rate pacing controlled by a myocardial contractility index for treatment of malignant neurally mediated syncope. PACE 1997;20:1568A.

46. Soberman J, McAlister H, Klementowicz, et

al. Paradoxical responses in activity-sensing pacemakers. PACE 1988;11:507A.

47. Lau CP. The combination of sensors and algorithms. In Lau CP, ed. Rate Adaptive Cardiac Pacing: Single and Dual Chamber. Futura Publishing Co, Inc, Armonk, NY, 1993, pp 213–227.

48. Stangl K, Wirtzfeld A, Heinze R, et al. A new multisensor pacing system using stroke volume, respiratory rate, mixed venous oxygen saturation, and temperature, right atrial pressure, right ventricular pressure, and dP/dt. PACE 1988;11:712–724.

49. Van Krieken FM, Perrins JP, Sigmund M. Clinical results of automatic slope adaptation in a dual sensor VVIR pacemaker. PACE 1992;15:1815–1820.

50. Connelly DT and the Topaz study group. Initial experience with a new single chamber, dual sensor rate responsive pacemaker. PACE 1993;16:1833–1841.

51. Sermasi S, Marconi M, Scazzinz L, et al. Multisensor rate-response pacemaker, clinical-technical analysis on the self-control of the sensors. PACE 1993;16:1935A.

52. Landman MAJ, Senden PJ, Buys EM. Sensor cross checking in a dual sensor pacemaker during activity artifacts and emotional stress. Eur JCPE 1992;2:A23.

53. Binner L, Brummer T, Kochs M, et al. Single and dual chamber rate responsive pacing using a new dual sensor pacemaker. PACE 1993;16:1205A.

54. Nzayinambaho K, Aubert A, Roels P, et al. Clinical experience with the Sensor Cross-Checking™ feature from a rate response pacemaker using a dual sensor. PACE 1993; 16:1205A.

55. El Allaf D, Beckers J, Demeure B, et al. One year experience with 21 patients implanted with a rate responsive pacemaker using a dual sensor. PACE 1993;16:1205A.

56. Sulke N, Tan K, Kamalvand K, et al. Dual sensor VVIR mode pacing: is it worth it? PACE 1996;19:1560–1567.

57. Cowell R, Paul V, Ilsley C. Dual sensors: twice the benefit for double the problems? Cardiostimolazione 1992;10:239.

58. Wahlstrand J, Alt E, Fotuhi P, et al. Initial experience with Legend Plus exercise test as a means of rate response optimization. PACE 1993;16:1939A.

59. Ovsychcher I, Guldal M, Karaoguz R, et al. Clinical evaluation of automatic programming of rate-adaptive ventricular pacemakers controlled by double sensors. Eur JCPE 1994;4:114A.

60. Crossley G, Greenberg S, Benditt D, et al. Dual sensor rate response with activity and minute ventilation. Eur JCPE 1994 4:38A.

61. Alt E, Combs W, Fotuhi P, et al. Initial experience with a new dual sensor SSIR pacemaker controlled by body activity and minute ventilation. PACE 1995;18:1487–1495.

62. Danilovic D, Pavlovic S, Vilimirovic D, et al. Minute ventilation sensor: evaluation of MV range and MV acceleration time for preventing false positive pacing with Legend Plus (SSIR dual sensor) pacemaker. PACE 1993; 16:1917A.

63. Combs W, Alt E, Fotuhi P, et al. Response of Legend Plus a dual sensor pacing system to ascending and descending stairs. PACE 1993;16:1916A.

64. Slade AKB, Pee S, Jones S, et al. Patterns of response with 3 dual-sensor single chamber rate adaptive pacemakers. Eur JCPE 1994;4: 38A.

65. Cowell R, Morris-Thurgood J, Cornu E, et al. Initial experience of a prototype dual sensor rate-adaptive pacemaker that utilizes MV and the PDI. Cardiostimolazione 1992;10: 275–276.

66. Connelly DT, Aggarwal RK, Ray GS, et al. Initial experience with a dual sensor, dual chamber rate adaptive pacemaker. PACE 1994;17:805A.

67. Stangl K, Laule M. Combinations of parameters. In Alt E, Barold SS, Stangl K, eds. Rate-Adaptive Cardiac Pacing. Springer-Verlag, NY, 1993, pp 314–317.

68. Benditt DG, Mianulli M, Curtis A, et al. Oxygen uptake kinetic analysis for evaluation of a dual sensor rate-adaptive pacemaker: a multi-center study. Eur JCPE 1994:4;38A.

69. Leung SK, Lau CP, Wu CW, et al. Quantitative comparison of different sensor modes in multi sensor rate-adaptive pacing. Eur JCPE 1994;4:37A.

70. Leung SK, Lau CP, Tang MO, et al. New integrated sensor pacemaker: comparison of rate responses between an integrated minute ventilation and activity sensor and single sensor modes during exercise and daily activities and nonphysiological interference. PACE 1996;19:1664–1671.

71. Lau CP, Leung SK, Lee IS. Delayed exercise rate response kinetics due to sensor cross-checking in a dual sensor rate adaptive pacing system: the importance of individual sensor programming. PACE 1996;19: 1021–1025.

72. Alt E, Combs W, Fotuhi P, et al. Initial clinical experience with a new dual sensor SSIR pacemaker controlled by body activity and minute ventilation. PACE 1995;18: 1487–1495.

73. Celiker A, Alehan D, Tokel NK, et al. Initial experience with dual-sensor rate-responsive

pacemakers in children. Eur Heart J 1996;17: 1251–1255.

74. Lau CP. The combination of sensors and algorithms. In Lau CP, ed. Rate Adaptive Cardiac Pacing: Single and Dual Chamber. Futura Publishing Co. Inc., Armonk, NY, 1993, pp 213–227.

75. Taborsky M, Neuzil P, Vopalka R. Follow-up of patients with dual sensor pacemakers place more demand on time and technology? PACE 1993;16:1205A.

76. Barold SS, Clementy J. The promise of improved exercise performance by dual sensor rate adaptive pacemakers. PACE 1997;20: 607–609.

77. Sinha S, Shilling RJ, Kaye GC, et al. Clinical evaluation of a dual sensor rate responsive pacemaker. PACE 1994;17:1950–1954.

78. Cowell R, Morris-Thurgood J, Paul V, et al. Are we being driven to two sensors? Clinical benefits of sensor cross-checking. PACE 1993;16:1441–1444.

79. Gencel L, Garrigue S, Guerin P, et al. Inappropriate acceleration of minute ventilation and QT interval sensing rate-responsive pacemakers in sleep apnea syndrome. Eur JCPE 1996;6:185A.

80. Cohen TJ, Liem B. A combined oxygen-pressure sensing algorithm improves tachyarrhythmia detection. PACE 1993;16:857A.

81. Hayes DL, Christiansen JR, Vlietstra RE, et al. Follow-up of an activity-sensing, rate-modulated pacing device, including transtelephonic exercise assessment. Mayo Clin Proc 1989;64:503–508.

82. Lau CP, Leung SK, Guerola M, et al. Comparison of continuously recorded sensor and sinus rates during daily life activities and standardized exercise testing: efficacy of automatically optimized rate adaptive dual sensor pacing to simulate sinus rhythm. PACE 1996;19:1672–1677.

83. Cazeau S, Ritter P, Lazarus A, et al. Diagnostic functions in implantable cardiac pacemakers. In Daubert JC, Prystowsky EN, Ripart A, eds. Prevention of Tachyarrhythmias with Cardiac Pacing. Futura Publishing Co, Inc, Armonk, NY, 1997, pp 179–187.

84. Hayes DL, Higano ST, Eisinger G. Utility of rate histograms in programming and follow-up of a DDDR pacemaker. Mayo Clin Proc 1989;64:495–502.

85. Gentzler RD, Lucas EH. Automatic sensor adjustment in a rate modulated pacemaker. North American Trilogy DR+ Phase I clinical investigators. PACE 1996;19:1809–1812.

86. Wilkoff B. Intravascular lead extraction: details and keys to success. In Singer I, ed. Interventional Electrophysiology. Williams and Wilkins, Baltimore, 1997.

Chapter 36

Clinical Applications of Mode-Switching for Dual Chamber Pacemakers

Kenneth A. Ellenbogen, Mark A. Wood, Harry G. Mond, S. Serge Barold

Introduction

Almost 50% of patients undergoing pacemaker implantation in some registries have sick sinus syndrome.[1,2] Many of these patients also have paroxysmal supraventricular tachycardia, especially atrial flutter and atrial fibrillation (AF).[2,3] Patients with paroxysmal AF or atrial flutter who have undergone radiofrequency (RF) ablation of the atrioventricular (AV) junction make up an increasingly large percentage of patients with the "tachy-brady" syndrome. Ideally, dual chamber pacemakers provide patients with the optimal hemodynamic and functional status.[4] Such patients pose a challenge because dual chamber pacing may result in tracking of supraventricular tachyarrhythmias leading to a rapid paced ventricular response (Figure 1).

This large group of patients with bradycardia-tachycardia syndrome undergoing pacemaker implantation represents a challenge to dual chamber pacing with conventional pulse generators. We will discuss the management of such patients with conventional pulse generators and then review the use of automatic mode switching in detail.

Management of Patients with Conventional Pulse Generators

There are a variety of approaches that clinicians have relied on to manage patients with bradycardia-tachycardia syndrome. These have been reviewed in detail elsewhere.[5–7] An early approach was to implant a single chamber VVI pacemaker. This avoided the problems caused by intermittent tracking of supraventricular tachyarrhythmias associated with dual chamber pacing but deprived patients of AV synchrony. Another option for patients with intact AV nodal conduction is single chamber AAI or AAIR pacing. In these patients, appropriate bradycardia support is provided during sinus rhythm and the pacemaker is inhibited or delivers ineffective atrial pacing stimuli during AF. This approach to patients with AF and intact AV nodal conduction is rarely used today, primarily because of concern about the development of AV block over time and the potential need for RF ablation of the AV junction for control of symptoms sometime in the future.

A simple approach that was sometimes

From Singer I, Barold SS, Camm AJ (eds): Nonpharmacological Therapy of Arrhythmias for the 21st Century: The State of the Art. Futura Publishing Co, Inc., Armonk, NY, © 1998.

used in the past was to implant a DDD or DDDR pulse generator and program the upper rate to a relatively low heart rate close to the programmed lower rate. The disadvantage of this approach is that if the sinus rate is faster than the upper rate, pacing resembles the DDI (DDIR) pacing mode. The lower upper rate also severely limits exercise, by causing AV dyssynchrony when the sinus rate increases above the upper rate.

Another popular approach in the 1980s to the management of these patients was to implant a pulse generator that had separately programmable atrial- driven and sensor-driven upper rates.[8] This feature is not available in all DDDR pulse generators, but when available allowed the clinician to program a lower atrial-tracked upper rate (e.g., 110 bpm) and a higher sensor-driven upper rate (e.g., 140 bpm). This approach has obvious limitations, including the occurrence of sinus tachycardia which is not tracked because the sensor does not indicate a sufficient level of exertion. Careful programming of the sensor slope and threshold is necessary to allow appropriate atrial pacing during exercise.

A DDD pulse generator with a retriggerable atrial refractory period will switch itself automatically to the DVI mode when it senses a fast atrial rate. In this situation, referred to as dual demand pacing, any atrial signals sensed during the noise sampling period (generally the last 100 or 150 ms of the postventricular atrial refractory period [PVARP]) do not start a new AV interval, but reinitiate an entirely new total atrial refractory period (Figure 2). The atrial pacing is of no use and wastes energy. Short runs of atrial tachycardia or even frequent atrial ectopic beats can induce DVI pacing. The dual demand functions on a beat-to-beat basis and thus variable sensing during AF may result in an erratic rate response. This is a technique sometimes used for pacemaker response to electromagnetic interference. This feature is available in a few pulse generators, including Biotronik Gemnos, Siemens DDD 674, and some Telectronics dual chamber models. The feature

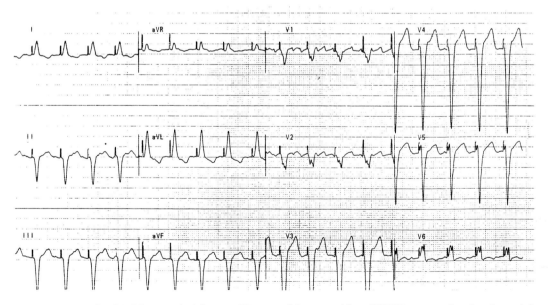

Figure 1. A 12-lead ECG recorded from a 77-year-old man with a DDDR pacemaker implanted 3 years earlier for sick sinus syndrome, AV block, and intermittent AF. This tracing shows ventricular tracking of atrial flutter- fibrillation at the upper rate limit. The patient had an ischemic cardiomyopathy and presented to the emergency room in pulmonary edema after a 2-day history of palpitations resulting in chest pain and progressive shortness of breath.

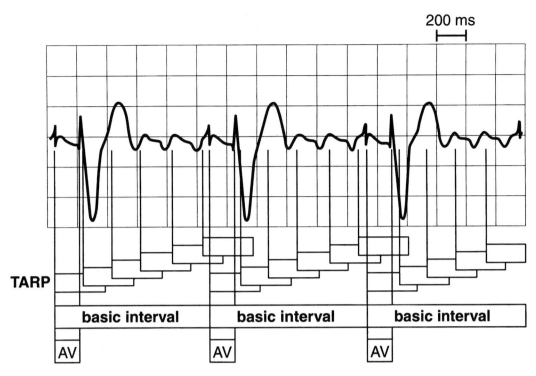

Figure 2. Diagrammatic representation of the retriggerable refractory period of the Biotronik Gemnos. Continual retriggering of the atrial refractory period causes the DDD pulse generator to operate in the atrial asynchronous mode at the lower rate, i.e., DVI mode when the P-P interval is shorter than the atrial refractory period. The first 125 ms of the PVARP represent the atrial blanking period during which signals cannot be sensed. The next 60 ms of the PVARP comprise a noise sampling period. If a P wave falls in this noise sampling period, it will not trigger an AV inteval, but instead retrigger a full atrial refractory period.

may or may not be a programmable function.

DDI and DDIR Pacing

The DDI and DDIR modes were initially conceived to handle patients with sick sinus syndrome, AV block, and paroxysmal supraventricular tachycardia. This pacing mode was used widely in the 1980s but has fallen out of use with the widespread availability of mode-switching pacemakers. In patients with older pulse generators where mode switching is not present, this pacing mode may be useful. The functional characteristics, limitations, and adverse effects have been recently reviewed by Barold and Irwin et al. [9–11] DDI pacing results in AV synchrony only in two situations when the patient's atrial rate is lower than the programmed lower rate or during intact or *relatively normal AV conduction* if the spontaneous atrial rate exceeds the programmed lower rate (Figure 3). Importantly, with DDI or DDIR pacing AV synchrony is lost in patients with AV block and a sinus rate above the programmed lower rate or the sensor-determined atrial rate. In this case, the P waves sensed by the atrial channel will march through the pacing cycle, moving closer and closer to the preceding paced ventricular beat. The pacemaker is functioning in the VVI or VVIR mode with AV dissociation, as long as the sinus rate is greater than the programmed lower rate. The patient's intrinsic atrial activity does not affect the timing of the atrial output pulse and the

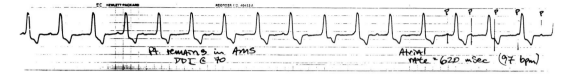

Figure 3. Rhythm strip from a patient demonstrating DDI pacing. This patient was initially programmed to DDD pacing with mode switching programmed to a rate of 170 bpm. During exercise, "double sensing" of both the atrial signal and the farfield ventricular paced QRS lead to inappropriate AMS. The pacing mode switched from DDD to the DDI mode. Loss of AV synchrony resulted. The atrial rate was 97 bpm and P waves can be seen marching through the tracing with no relationship to the paced QRS (courtesy of John Griffin, MD).

pulse generator will deliver an atrial stimulus at the termination of the atrial escape interval. AV dissociation also occurs in the DDIR mode in patients with AV block when the sinus rate is faster than the sensor-driven rate. Thus, DDI and DDIR pacing frequently results in effective VVI pacing when patients have retrograde VA conduction, VVI pacing when the sinus rate is above the lower programmed rate, and long periods of functional undersensing with long postventricular atrial blanking periods. As a result, patients with heart block paced DDI or DDIR may not derive the hemodynamic benefits of AV synchrony when in sinus rhythm.

On the basis of these arguments, the DDI or DDIR mode cannot be recommended as first-line therapy in patients with AV block, spontaneous or induced, or in patients with paroxysmal supraventricular tachyarrhythmias and AV block. Patients with AV block and a normal sinus mechanism are better served by appropriately programmed DDDR devices designed with a protective algorithm for the recognition of SVT and automatic mode switching. Patients with the bradycardia-tachycardia syndrome and intact AV conduction are generally placed on AV nodal blocking drugs to slow their ventricular response during atrial tachyarrhythmias. As a result, these patients may now demonstrate varying degrees of AV block during tachycardia. If there is little or no sinus slowing on these negative dromotropic agents, patients will be disadvan-

taged during sinus rhythm during the DDI(R) mode.

Fallback Mechanisms

Traditional fallback mechanisms were introduced over 10 years ago in some dual chamber pacemakers and were designed to provide a degree of protection against rapid ventricular paced rates during supraventricular tachyarrhythmias. In the traditional fallback concept, when the atrial rate exceeds the programmed upper rate or tachycardia detection rate for a given duration, the pulse generator activates an algorithm that produces a slower ventricular pacing rate, with or without maintaining the same pacing mode.[12,13] During traditional fallback, a dual chamber pulse generator either functions in the VVI mode with uncoupling of atrial activity from the ventricular paced complexes or remains in its programmed mode. The ventricular pacing rate then gradually decreases or falls back to the programmed fallback rate. If the DDD (VDD) mode is maintained during fallback, the device provides automatic gradual lengthening of the upper rate interval from cycle to cycle. In this way, progressive slowing of the programmed upper rate occurs until the fallback rate is obtained. The pulse generator automatically returns to its previous dual chamber mode with 1:1 AV synchrony when the sensed atrial rate drops below the tachycardia detection rate.

Certain features of the fallback mode are

worth emphasizing. Programmable features of fallback algorithms are similar to programmable features of most automatic mode-switching algorithms and are described below. The type of fallback response is often programmable as well. The response to a tachycardia can consist of: maintaining the same pacing mode by slowing the ventricular paced rate, or conversion to another pacing mode with resultant control of the ventricular paced rate by virtue of the new pacing mode. This latter response is called automatic mode switching (AMS™, a trademark of Telectronics). Henceforth, the term "AMS" or automatic mode conversion will be used in a generic sense only to describe an algorithm that provides for a change from an atrial tracking mode to a nonatrial tracking mode upon sensing a supraventricular tachyarrhythmia. Atrial monitoring is retained during the nonatrial tracking pacing mode. Finally, there is automatic restoration of the atrial tracking mode upon cessation of the supraventricular tachyarrhythmia. Automatic mode switching is a form of fallback.

Automatic Mode Switching

The Telectronics Meta DDDR 1250 first popularized mode switching. This pulse generator is a minute ventilation rate-adaptive pacemaker that responded to supraventricular tachyarrhythmia with automatic and immediate switching to the VVIR mode.[14] The device was designed with an algorithm that would initiate mode switching in response to a single sensed signal in the PVARP beyond the first 100-ms atrial blanking period.[15] The PVARP automatically shortened in response to the sensor-indicated heart rate. The initiation of mode switching could occur in response to a single atrial extrasystole, but could also occur and lead to "inappropriate" mode switching in response to a premature ventricular extrasystole with retrograde VA conduction or upon sensing a farfield paced QRS complex in the atrial channel. Instances of mode switching could also occur after the abrupt

onset of exercise if a sinus P wave fell in the PVARP early during exercise before the PVARP shortened. Conversion to the VVIR allowed for an appropriate heart rate as determined by the sensor input. The AMS mode should be considered VDI or VDIR in all devices because of monitoring of the atrial rate during supraventricular tachycardia. The pacing mode reverts to dual chamber pacing when no atrial electrical events occur in the PVARP for up to three cycles.

This algorithm of this first generation mode-switching device was refined in subsequent devices to provide for less abrupt and "inappropriate" mode switching. The algorithm in the second generation device (Meta DDDR 1254, 1256) resulted in improved specificity for the detection of supraventricular tachyarrhythmias.[16] In these devices, the mode-switching algorithm is programmable on/off, the number of atrial events is programmable, and the atrial rate at which automatic mode switching occurs is also programmable. The atrial blanking periods have been extended to the first 150 ms of the PVARP and the first 120 ms of the AV delay.

General Features of Automatic Mode Switching and Fallback

Contemporary pulse generators that have automatic mode-switching or fallback algorithms should have a number of programmable parameters to provide clinicians with the flexibility that is needed to adequately program these devices. These features include:

1. The fallback rate should be programmable. Optimally, the fallback rate can be programmable to an intermediate rate or an appropriate physiological rate in a rate-adaptive pacing mode so the heart rate does not abruptly decrease to the lower rate limit. With AMS, fallback is determined by the mode to which the pacemaker switches. This is generally a nonatrial tracking mode, and

can be rate adaptive according to design or programmability. Mode switching should be available in other modes than DDDR, including DDD or VDD(R) modes. In nonrate-adaptive pacing modes, the fallback mode is usually VVI and the fallback rate is usually the lower rate limit. Some pulse generators switch to the DDI or DDIR pacing mode. These modes are also effectively nonatrial tracking modes (e.g., the DDI mode functions like the VVI mode and the DDIR mode functions like the VVIR mode).

2. The number of atrial events above the tachycardia detection rate (interval) required to initiate automatic mode switching or the fallback mechanism and the tachycardia detection rate (interval) should be programmable. The number of atrial events and the rate at which automatic mode switching occurs should be a programmable parameter. Different companies have incorporated different algorithms for counting the number of atrial events.[17,18] The two major classes of algorithms utilized include those that count to a certain number of events before initiating mode switching (Telectronics Meta 1250, 1254, and 1256) or those that are constantly calculating a matching

atrial interval corresponding to an increasing or decreasing atrial rate (Medtronic Thera DR 7940, 7960, and Pacesetter Trilogy DR +). These algorithms do not calculate a mean or average atrial rate, but an interval that is gradually diminished until it is less than the tachycardia detection interval whereupon AMS is activated. The tachycardia detection rate (interval) should be separately programmable from the upper rate limit. This provides maximal flexibility and allows the clinician to discriminate between high atrial rates during exercise or inappropriate mode switching that may occur due to double sensing (see below).

The first widely available commercial device for AMS, the Telectronics Meta DDDR 1250, 1254, and 1256 utilized an algorithm that had a counter (called the atrial rate monitor or ARM) to keep track of the number of beats above the tachycardia detection interval. If the number of beats prior to mode switch was programmed to 5, then the counter would start at 0 and increment by 1 every time an atrial signal is sensed faster than the tachycardia detection interval. Every time the interval from the first sensed event to the next sensed event is slower (longer) than the programmed AMS criteria, the ARM decrements by 1. When the ARM reaches the programmed value, AMS occurs (Figure 4A,B).

Figure 4. A: A schematic representation of a patient with and without failure to mode switch during atrial flutter that illustrates how the algorithms for the Telectronics Meta DDDR 1254 works. In this figure, the top tracing shows the pacemaker timing cycles. AVD = AV delay; PVARP = postventricular atrial refractory period; API = atrial protection interval. The atrial blanking periods during the AV delay and PVARP are shown below in black. The idealized patient's P waves during atrial flutter are shown below. A_{st} = atrial sensed P wave; A_{ns} = atrial P wave not sensed because it lands during one of the atrial blanking periods. The ARM is the atrial high rate monitor. ARM = 0 indicates that the pacemaker has not yet sensed a P wave above the atrial tachycardia detection rate. In the META DDDR 1254, the ARM counts from 0 upward to the programmed number of tachycardia detection beats for each atrial signal it senses during the AV interval or PVARP, but not in an atrial blanking period. It counts down by 1 each time there is an atrial signal absent. Mode switching will not occur because of alternate P waves falling into the atrial blanking periods. **B:** AMS to the VVIR mode occurs during atrial flutter. The device is reprogrammed from an AV delay of 200 ms to an AV delay of 120 ms. Following reprogramming, atrial signals land in the "sensing" or nonatrial blanking portion of the PVARP. The atrial tachyarrhythmia monitor (or ARM) counts up to 5, and then mode switch to VVIR occurs.

META DDDR 1254

Flutter 240 bpm (250 ms)
2:1 Block, Rate 120

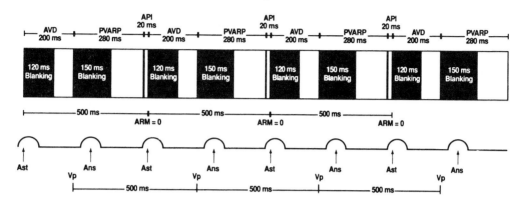

AVD = 200 ms PVARP = 280 ms

Lower Rate 60, Max Rate 120, AMS Rate 150 bpm (400 ms)
AMS Count 5, Sensor Rate 60 ppm (rest)

A

META DDDR 1254

Flutter 240 bpm (250 ms)
2:1 Block, Rate 120, then AMS to VVIR, Rate 60

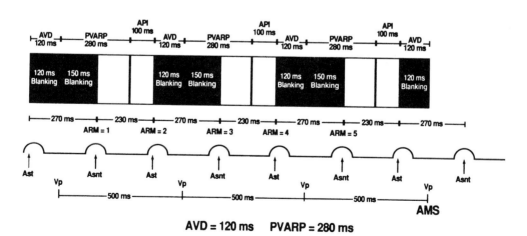

AVD = 120 ms PVARP = 280 ms

Lower Rate 60, Max Rate 120, AMS Rate 150 bpm (400 ms)
AMS Count 5, Sensor Rate 60 ppm (rest)

B

The Medtronic Thera DR 7940 and 7960 and the Pacesetter Trilogy DR 2360 use a "matching" atrial interval.[17,18] The Pacesetter device measures a filtered atrial rate interval. If the P-P interval is shorter than the filtered atrial rate interval (FARI), the FARI is decreased by 38 ms. If the P-P interval is longer than the FARI, the FARI is increased by up to 25 ms. Shortening or lengthening of the FARI interval occurs depending on each atrial rate interval. Once the FARI is below the maximal tracking interval, pacing returns to the DDDR or DDD mode. The Medtronic device works in a similar fashion, incrementing the mean or "matched" atrial interval by 8 ms if the PP interval is greater than the mean atrial interval and decrementing by 23 ms every time the PP

interval is shorter than the mean atrial interval (Figure 5).

An initial experience with a unique mode switching algorithm has been reported by den Dulk et al.[19] These investigators described their experiences with a mode-switching algorithm that works on a beat-to-beat basis (Vitatron Diamond DDDR 800). This mode-switching algorithm is incorporated into a unipolar, dual sensor, dual chamber rate-adaptive pacemaker. Atrial events occurring within a physiological range calculated from a running average of the atrial rate are tracked. This physiological range is defined as being 15 beats/min (bpm) greater or lesser than the running average. When the atrial rate exceeds an average paced or sensed atrial physiological rate

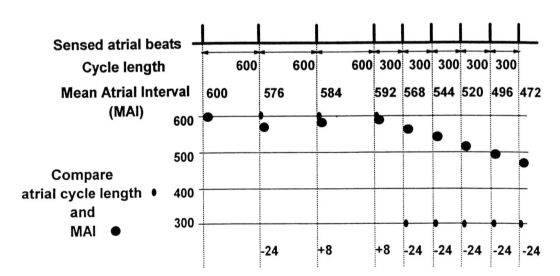

then, . . . , if P-P<=MAI -24 ms, and, if P-P>MAI +8ms

Figure 5. Schematic depiction of how the algorithm for AMS in the Medtronic Thera DR 7940i works. Note that this algorithm is based on a running average of the atrial rate and may be less susceptible to AMS after a short episode of atrial tachycardia or AF, however, may take longer to restore AV pacing after the atrial arrhythmia has teminated. In this example, the mean atrial interval is calculated and the value is increased by 8 ms or decreased by 24 ms based on whether the atrial cycle length is slower or faster than the preceding mean atrial interval. In this example an atrial tachycardia at 300 ms occurs after the first three beats. The weighting of the MAI favors AMS despite intermittent signal dropout.

Table 1
Atrial Sensitivity Programming

Atrial Sensitivity (mV)		Failure of AMS	Intermittent Track AF	Oversense of Noise	Undersense of AF	
					Episodes	Duration(s)
High	0.35	0%*	17%*	57%*	6%*	2.2 ± 1.6*
Nominal	0.77	0%*	27%	34%*	19%*	8.3 ± 2.8*
Half PWA	2.1	9%*	50%*	10%*	36%*	47 ± 1.9*
Half AF	1.5	0%*	48%*	20%*	17%*	7 ± 3.5*

Used with permission from Leung S-K, et al.[27]
Data derived from bipolar atrial electrograms recorded during sinus rhythm and atrial fibrillation.
Half PWA = half of the atrial EGM amplitude measured in sinus rhythm.
Half AF = half of the mean atrial EGM in atrial fibrillation.
Ineffective AMS = when ventricular pacing occurred at ≥100 bpm ≥1/3 of time during atrial fibrillation.
* P < 0.05 by chi square.

by 15 bpm or the atrial rate abruptly exceeds the maximum tracking rate, the system will switch modes. To avoid frequent episodes of AV dyssynchrony that may occur with premature atrial contractions, this device delivers atrial synchronization pulses a safe interval from the sensed prior atrial premature event. Table 1 reviews the different detection algorithms, atrial blanking periods, and diagnostics of selected devices from different manufacturers.

A recent preliminary report from Kay and colleagues suggested that different mode-switching algorithms may provide optimal patient acceptance depending on the speed of mode switching.[20] This group downloaded software in patients with the Medtronic Thera DR and compared three different mode-switching algorithms in 18 patients programmed to one of three different mode-switching algorithms for 1 month. These algorithms either provided mode switching after one beat (instantaneous), four to seven beats (2–3 sec), and after 5–10 sec using the standard algorithm (MAI). The patients were then asked to choose which algorithm was associated with the fewest symptoms. Three methods were used to assess mode-switching algorithms: symptom frequency, symptom severity, and subjective preference. The patients preferred the mode-switching

algorithm that was intermediate in speed—the mode-switching algorithm that resulted in mode switching in four to seven beats over the ones that switched faster or slower.

Leung and colleagues have reported preliminary results comparing the latency for AMS, the number of beats tracked at >100 bpm during AF, and the latency for AV resynchronization once AF ceases with three different pulse generators.[21] They found that devices that used a rate and number of beats cutoff for mode switching tended to have a fast onset and recovery from AMS, but a fluctuating ventricular response during AF. Devices that use a mean atrial rate gave a stable and smooth decrease in pacing rate during AF-induced AMS, but some may result in a delay in AMS response and prolong the duration of time before resumption of AV synchrony after AF terminated.

3. The pulse generator should have programmable atrial sensitivity that allows for sensing of low-amplitude atrial signals during AF. In general, this may require programming atrial sensitivity to values of 0.15–1.0 mV. The potential problems involved in sensing low-amplitude atrial signals are further discussed below.

4. Atrial blanking periods may be programmable or nonprogrammable and represent portions of the timing cycle where atrial activity is not sensed. The role of atrial blanking periods in leading to misdiagnosis and failure to diagnose atrial arrhythmias is discussed extensively below.

5. A device should incorporate diagnostic data, histograms, storage of intracardiac electrogram that provide information about the frequency, duration, total time, and other relevant clinical information about AMS events. This is essential for confirming appropriate or inappropriate function of the AMS algorithm. This information needs to be examined carefully because superficial perusal of this information can result in making inappropriate clinical decisions. An example of this is illustrated by Figure 6A-C.

Complexity of Atrial Sensing and Detection of Atrial Tachyarrhythmias

Reliable sensing of atrial depolarization is essential for appropriate function of AMS.

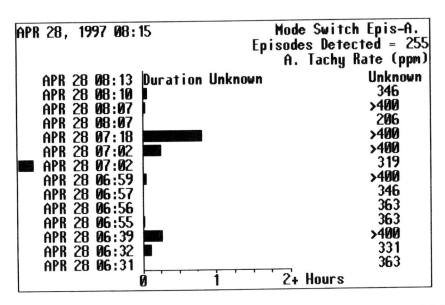

Figure 6. A: Examples of diagnostic data telemetered from a Medtronic Thera DR 7960i is shown in the top panel. This summary diagostic shows the date and time of the most recent 14 episodes of mode switching as well as the measured atrial rate and the AMS duration. In this patient, AF had recently become persistent several months prior to the patient's pacemaker evaluation. The patient complained of intermittent palpitations. A 24-hour Holter monitor demonstrated persistent AF and frequent episodes of high rate pacing. Intermittent undersensing during AF resulted in the mode- switching oscillations shown here. The mean atrial electrogram amplitude in sinus rhythm was 1.5 mV. The atrial sensitivity was programmed to 0.5 mV.

B

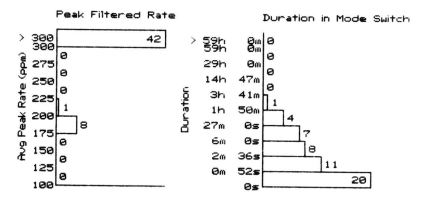

Figure 6. (Continued) B: This shows interrogated data from a Pacesetter Trilogy DR⁺. The telemetered data shows duration of time in mode switch for a variety of atrial rates in bins of 24 bpm. Individual episodes are not date and time stamped.

C

294-09 SN 001011   MAY 30, 97 02:23 PM
            OTHER DIAGNOSTIC COUNTERS   DDD-R

NUMBER OF TIMES THE PACEMAKER-MEDIATED
TACHYCARDIA TERMINATION ALGORITHM WAS
ACTIVATED 0
NUMBER OF HIGH RATE EPISODES 3
THE LONGEST HIGH RATE EPISODE
        BEGAN AT: MAY 10,   02:14 PM
        DURATION: 0   HRS   1   MIN
        NUMBER OF CYCLES IN EPISODE: 75
        HIGHEST RATE: 202   MIN-1   (297   MS)

        DATA COLLECTED SINCE: MAY 01,   02:13 PM

Figure 6. *(Continued)* **C:** This shows interrogated data from an Intermedics Marathon. The teleme-tered data gives information on the percent of atrial activity in different rate ranges. Information about the longest high rate episodes including the duration can be obtained.

Sensing of atrial flutter and AF presents challenges in terms of both atrial over- and undersensing. Wood et al. used conventional quadripolar electrophysiology catheters to measure atrial electrogram amplitude during sinus rhythm, atrial flutter, and AF.[22] We measured mean peak-to-peak bipolar atrial electrogram amplitude during sinus rhythm and either AF or atrial flutter in 69 patients. The coefficient of variation of individual electrogram amplitudes during both atrial fibrillation and flutter was also analyzed and the 20th percentile of electrogram amplitudes in AF and atrial flutter were compared to the mean sinus rhythm amplitudes. We found an excellent correlation between mean amplitude of the atrial electrogram during sinus rhythm and atrial flutter (R = 0.94) and a somewhat poorer relationship between mean atrial electrogram amplitude in sinus rhythm and AF (R = 0.79). The coefficient of variance of in-dividual electrogram amplitudes was much greater in AF than in atrial flutter or sinus rhythm (sinus rhythm: 18.8 ± 12.7; atrial fibrillation: 41.6 ± 9.2; and atrial flutter: 22.3 ± 13.1). By determining 20th percentile electrogram amplitudes in AF and atrial flutter to mean sinus rhythm amplitudes, intermittent very low electrogram amplitude values (<0.3 mV) were often seen despite large electrogram amplitudes during sinus rhythm. For example, during AF 11 of 17 patients (65%) with sinus rhythm electrogram amplitudes ≤1.5 mV had a 20th percentile of fibrillation electrograms <0.3 mV.

Additional Sensing Considerations

There are several additional practical and theoretical considerations for rapid and specific detection of AF other than atrial electrogram amplitude as discussed above. Several groups have studied atrial electrogram morphology during AF in animals and in man. These investigators have demonstrated a remarkably wide variation in amplitude and morphology of unipolar atrial signals in patients during and between different episodes of AF. These different types of AF have been correlated with the number of propagating waves in the right atrium by Allessie and his colleagues.[23] The average median AF interval was correlated with the type of AF and the rate of AF. As the median AF interval was shorter, the variation in AF intervals was larger. Waldo and colleagues described the morphology of a single bipolar atrial electrogram during postoperative AF, and classified four types of AF.[24] Like Allessie's findings, these investigators found that as the rate of AF increased, the electrograms became more fragmented. Waldo used the temporal fragmentation of a single bipolar electrogram to characterize the different types of AF and Allessie used the spatial fragmentation of AF wavefronts in the right atrium. The major point that these investigators make is that any algorithm for detecting AF must be robust, and somehow account for the widely varying amplitudes and morphology of signals during AF in an individual patient, and somehow discriminate between these low-amplitude signals and farfield sensed intracardiac signals as well as pacing polarization artifacts.

In addition to having an amplifier with high sensitivity and an appropriate frequency response, preliminary reports have suggested shorter interelectrode distances may be more ideal for sensing atrial signals. For example, Baerman et al. have recorded atrial electrograms from a custom designed decapolar catheter to assess the effects of different bipolar lead configurations on the atrial rate, electrogram amplitude, electrogram morphology, atrial amplitude probability density function, and atrial electrogram frequency spectrum in the 2–9 Hz band.[25] With closer bipolar spacing, the recorded rate was lower than that measured

with more widely spaced bipolar pairs. Electrode position closer to the atrial wall and more closely spaced bipolar pairs resulted in atrial electrograms that were more "organized and discrete." In contrast to amplitude measurements, frequency analysis of atrial electrograms was more robust and was relatively unchanged by electrode spacing.

The ability of unipolar sensing to discriminate between AF and myopotential sensing was examined by Lewalter et al.[26] They found that appropriate atrial sensing was programmable in 50% of patients allowing the pacemaker to appropriately respond to atrial flutter or AF without myopotential triggering during sinus rhythm. Appropriate discrimination between atrial flutter and myopotentials was possible in three of three patients. As a general rule, the authors do not advocate unipolar atrial sensing in patients whom mode switching will be programmed on because of the high incidence of inappropriate mode switching due to sensing of myopotentials and farfield sensing of ventricular electrograms.

The difficulty in selecting optimal atrial sensitivity is highlighted by a preliminary report from Leung et al.[27] These investigators stored bipolar atrial electrograms on tape from 15 patients with 780 episodes of AF. This information was replayed into three dual chamber devices with AMS algorithms. Various sensitivities were programmed and the patients were evaluated at each atrial sensitivity for failure of automatic mode switching, ineffective automatic mode switching (ventricular pacing $\geq$100 bpm for $\geq$1/3 of time during AMS) response to AF, intermittent tracking of AF, oversensing of noise, and number and duration of undersensing of AF (Table 2). The investigators concluded that AMS function was limited depending on the programmed atrial sensitivity.

Atrial undersensing is an issue in patients with both paroxysmal and chronic AF. With intermittent undersensing or "signal dropout" patients with chronic AF will be treated as if they have paroxysmal AF (Figure 6A). The recorded data logs or episode

Table 2
Atrial Blanking Periods in Automatic Mode Switching Algorithms from Various Devices

Device	Tachycardia Detection	Atrial Blanking Period(s)	Mode Switch/ Fallback	Diagnostics
Meta 1256 (Teletronics)	Programmable rate, Number of beats	120 ms during AV interval + 150 ms in PVARP	DDDR → VVIR DDD → VVI	Number of episodes
THERA 7960i (Medtronic)	Mean or matched atrial interval, programmable rate	50–100 during AV delay + ≤150 ms during PVARP	DDDR → DDIR DDD → DDI	Number of episodes, date/ time stamp, duration of 14 last episodes, atrial rate, ± atrial EGMs
TRILOGY DR+ 2860 (Pacesetter)	Mean or matched atrial filtered interval, programmable rate	Programmable from 50–200 ms in 25 ms Δ + 100 ms during AV delay	DDDR → DDIR DDD → DDI	Rate, duration and total number of episodes
MARATHON DR (Intermedics)	Programmable rate, number of beats	60 ms of the AV interval + 100 ms of PVARP	DDDR → DDIR DDD → VVI	Total number of episodes, time, date, duration of last episode
VIGOR DR (CPI)	Programmable rate, fixed number of beats (8 of 10)	Entire AV delay + 80 ms of PVARP	DDDR → VVIR DDD → VVI	Total number of episodes
CHORUS RM 7034 (ELA Medical)	Upper rate limit	Entire AV delay + up to 359 ms of PVARP programmable in 30 ms Δ	DDD → VDI DDDR → VVIR DDD → VVI	Total number of episodes (time, date and duration from histogram)
DIAMOND II (VITATRON)	Band around physiologic rate; non-programmable number of beats (=1), rate (±15 bpm) above physiological rate	AV delay + programmable PVARP from 50–300 ms in 25 ms Δ	DDDR → DDIR DDD → DDI Flywheel down to lower rate	Total duration of episodes, time stamp

PVARP = postventricular atrial refractory period.

histograms will reveal frequent episodes of AF occurring over a very short time frame. There may be multiple episodes of mode switching occurring every hour (Figure 7). Patients with chronic AF may experience intermittent palpitations and may have frequent spells of upper rate pacing. In patients with paroxysmal AF, episodes of AF or portions of episodes of AF may occur when the atrial electrogram amplitude falls below the programmed sensitivity and once again intermittent upper rate tracking may occur (Figure 8). To avoid this problem, newer more dynamic sensing algorithms for AF are needed to optimize the variability in atrial electrogram amplitude. Similar sensing algorithms have been used in implantable cardioverter-defibrillators. A

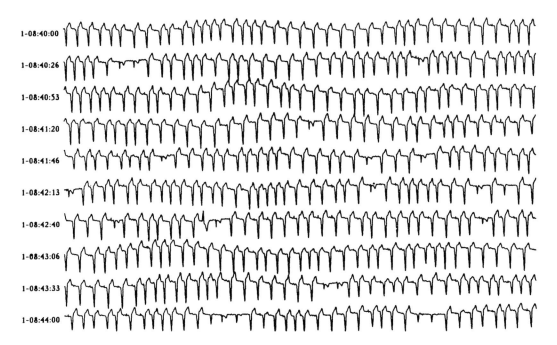

Figure 7. Rhythm strips from a 24-hour Holter monitor showing intermittent episodes of upper rate pacing due to intermittent mode switching in a patient with atrial flutter.

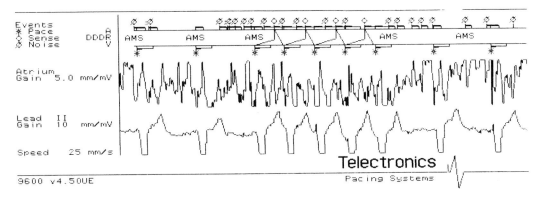

Figure 8. Example of intermittent AMS due to atrial signal dropout during AF. This and subsequent figures from the Telectronics Meta DDDR 1256 use a similar format. The Telectronics 9600 programmer printout demonstrates from top to bottom simultaneous recordings of timing events in ladder diagram fashion and atrial electrograms followed by rhythm strips. Atrial and ventricular pacing are denoted by (*) and sensing by open diamonds (◇). On the timing events channel, the solid filled rectangles are the atrial and ventricular blanking periods, and the open rectangles are the AV delay, PVARP, and refractory periods. The PVARP is shown above and the ventricular refractory period below. Inspection of the atrial electrograms during AF reveals a short period of signal dropout associated with upper rate tracking during reversion from AMS before AMS is reinitiated.

recently described algorithm to allow for AMS despite some atrial undersensing has been proposed by Bonnet et al.[28] These investigators proposed "high" and "low" criteria that allow for intermittent atrial undersensing. The high criteria is satisfied if more than 28 of 32 cycles are abnormally "accelerated," and the low criteria is satisfied if more than 36 of 64 cycles are "accelerated." The sensitivity of the algorithms to diagnose AF approached 100% for atrial sensitivities programmed to 0.4–1.0 mV. The mean time to diagnose AF was 28 ± 26 sec with the high criteria and 68 ± 27 sec with the low criteria.[29] Sensing of less than 23% of AF events resulted in failure to diagnose the arrhythmias by both algorithms. Such an algorithm would be useful because of its high sensitivity, but no information is provided about its specificity at various programmed sensitivities. A major disadvantage of this algorithm would be the long time required until AMS occurs.

Atrial Blanking Periods and Atrial Sensing

Pacemakers with automatic mode switching have certain periods of the pacemaker timing cycle where atrial activity is not sensed. These periods of the timing cycle are called the atrial blanking periods. A paced or sensed atrial event initiates an atrial blanking period that takes up part or all of the AV delay. A ventricular paced or sensed event initiates the PVARP and another atrial blanking interval called the postventricular atrial blanking period which is initiated after the sensed or paced ventricular event and extends through a portion of the PVARP. In some devices, the duration of the postventricular atrial blanking period may be programmable. The purpose of the atrial blanking period after an atrial sensed or paced event is to avoid sensing of a portion of the atrial electrogram or atrial polarization artifact that could result in double sensing or false

counting of nonatrial events. This may be termed "nearfield" oversensing. The purpose of the atrial blanking period after a paced or sensed ventricular event is to avoid farfield oversensing of the ventricular event by the atrial channel or the ventricular polarization artifact that could result once again in double or false counting of nonatrial events.[30,31]

Failure of Automatic Mode Switching

We and others have reported failure of automatic mode switching in response to a variety of atrial tachyarrhythmias.[32,33] AMS may fail to occur under a variety of circumstances. These include if the amplitude of the atrial electrogram is intermittently or consistently too small to be sensed or if the atrial signal is intermittently or consistently occurring during the atrial blanking period. A variety of factors may affect whether AMS occurs (Table 3).

In paroxysmal atrial flutter or atrial tachycardia where the atrial rate may vary between 150 bpm and 350 bpm, alternate P

Table 3

Factors Affecting Occurrence of Automatic Mode Switching (AMS)

Amplitude of Atrial Electrogram
  Timing of signal dropout
  Variation in signal amplitude
Frequency Content of Atrial Signal
Atrial Cycle Length
Atrial Blanking Periods
Type of Atrial Lead
  Bipolar vs. unipolar
  Spacing of electrodes
  Lead position (relative to anulus or coronary sinus)
Specific Type of AMS Algorithm: Advantages vs. Disadvantages
  Specificity vs. sensitivity
  Specificity vs. speed of AMS
  Failure to maintain AMS
  Frequency of intermittent AMS

waves occurring during an atrial blanking period may not be uncommon. This can lead to a variety of clinical symptoms, and may be detected incidentally by Holter monitoring, or after patient complaints of intermittent palpitations or breathlessness. This situation arises because the duration of the postventricular atrial blanking period imposes mathematical limits on the detection of atrial arrhythmias for AMS. For example, if the AV delay = 150 ms and the postventricular atrial blanking period = 150 ms, then the pacemaker will not be able to sense atrial flutter that occurs at a rate of 240 bpm (cycle length = 250 ms) on a 1:1 basis because sensing of alternate P waves will occur and the patient will track the arrhythmia at the upper rate limit. Restoration of appropriate mode switching would require programming the AV delay to 50 ms. If the postventricular atrial blanking period measures 150 ms, this would result in 150 + 50 ms = 200 ms which is shorter than the atrial flutter cycle length (250 ms) and AMS is activated because each atrial signal is sensed. This behavior may be less common with algorithms that utilize a mean atrial rate, but can still occur. This is illustrated in Figure 10B. As a result of every second or third beat falling into an atrial blanking period, patients will have several short intervals (lowering the matching atrial interval) followed by a long interval (increasing the matched atrial interval) which tends to drive the matched atrial interval back toward the baseline. Patients with devices that utilize a "matched" atrial rate algorithm may demonstrate variable times of AMS onset depending on the atrial flutter rate. These devices do not allow programming of the number of intervals to activate AMS. In a computer simulation (of the Medtronic Thera DR 7960i) using standard pacing intervals and outputs, atrial rates from 200 bpm to 400 bpm resulted in mode switch delays at a detection rate of 175 bpm ranging from 4.5 sec to 13 sec. The programming suggestions described below can be helpful, but greater programming flexibility

of atrial blanking periods may not completely solve the problem.

Other steps can be taken to enhance the specificity and sensitivity of AMS algorithms and avoid cases where AMS fails to occur. These include programming the AMS algorithm to the most sensitive setting (e.g., the least number of beats and the lowest detection rate) to diminish the chances of atrial undersensing contributing to this problem. Lengthening of the total atrial refractory period is another solution to this problem because the atrial blanking periods remain constant and thus occupy less of the timing cycle. Atrial activity has more chance to be sensed during the total atrial refractory period. Some devices are blanked for the entire duration of the AV interval while others are not. Shortening the AV delay so that the AV delay plus the postventricular atrial blanking period is shorter than the tachycardia cycle length will promote AMS occurring. With this approach, suboptimal AV synchrony may result, however. Alternatively, lengthening the AV delay to a value longer than the atrial cycle length will force at least one more P wave beyond the atrial blanking period and into the AV interval. This also will likely result in loss of AV synchrony. Another solution to this problem is to have programmable atrial blanking periods that allow the physician to adjust this parameter to avoid every other atrial signal falling during this portion of the timing cycle. Programming an increase in atrial sensitivity may help to reduce intermittent atrial undersensing of a low-amplitude signal.

We have noted that AMS failure in patients with atrial flutter typically presents as intermittent mode switching, which we call "mode-switching oscillations." An example of this is shown in Figures 9A-C and 10. Typically, patients are going in and out of mode switching for variable periods of time. These oscillations may tend to be particularly annoying to patients because of the return of intermittent rapid palpitations

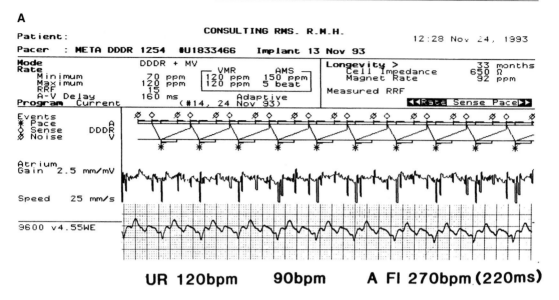

A

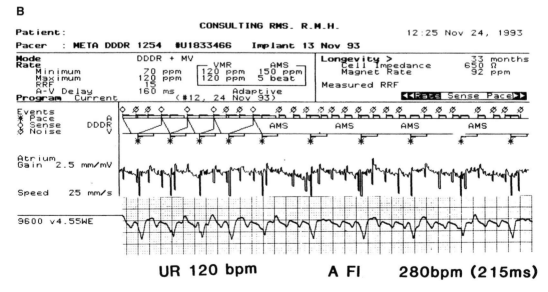

Figure 9. Example of failure of automatic mode switching in a patient with atrial flutter (Telectronics Meta DDDR 1254). The patient is an 86-year-old male with sick sinus syndrome and paroxysmal atrial flutter taking 160 mg/day of sotalol. A P wave at implant was 5 mV and the device was programmed to an upper rate of 120 bpm, atrial sensitivity = 0.3 mV, and AV delay = 160 ms. The Telectronics 9600 programmer printout demonstrates simultaneous recordings (from top to bottom) of events and calibrated atrial and ventricular electrogram, with rhythms strip below (not recorded simultaneously). Inspection of the atrial electrogram reveals atrial flutter waves, most landing in the postventricular atrial blanking period. **A:** There is no mode switching with ventricular pacing and tracking at the upper rate limit. *continued.*

Figure 9. B: The atrial rate during atrial flutter is shown to vary slightly in this patient. The atrial rate is increased from Figure 9A and this results in more consistent AMS occurring. *continued.*

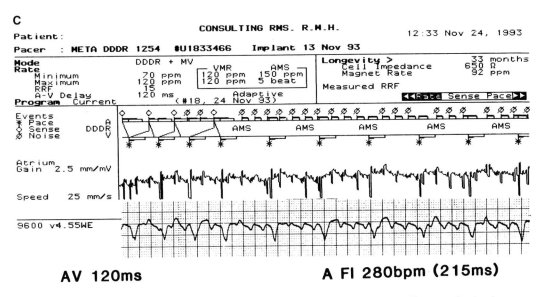

AV 120ms   **A Fl 280bpm (215ms)**

Figure 9. C: The AV interval is reprogrammed from 120 ms to 160 ms. This results in the most consistent AMS occurring.

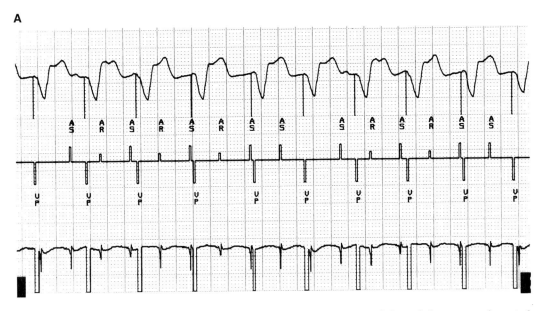

Figure 10. A schematized illustration of a printout from a patient with how failure to mode switch may occur in a patient with a Medtronic Thera DRi during atrial flutter. In this example, in **A** (from top to bottom) is shown a simultaneous surface ECG, Marker Channel® (Medtronic), and intracardiac atrial electrograms. The patient is in atrial flutter and about every second or third atrial electrogram falls into an atrial blanking period. The Thera uses a calculated mean atrial interval. *Continued.*

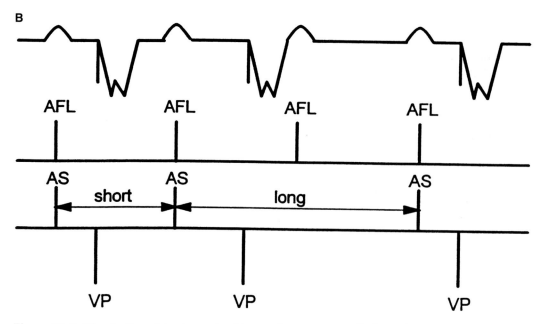

Figure 10. B: The rhythm strip shows tracking at the upper rate. Failure of AMS occurs because of short-long alternating cycle lengths as shown below which result in the MAI being below the cutoff rate.

which may occur frequently, sometimes several times a minute.

Pacemaker Diagnosis of Atrial Arrhythmias Using a Nonatrial Sensor

Some pacemakers combine information from a nonatrial sensor for diagnosis of atrial arrhythmias. For example, sensing of a rapid atrial rate by the atrial lead without corresponding nonatrial sensor activity indicates an unphysiological atrial arrhythmia. Under these circumstances, fallback or AMS would be activated. The advantages of such devices is increased specificity, with the disadvantage being more complex algorithms and probably increased time duration before AMS would occur.

The Intermedics Marathon DDDR pacemakers incorporates a new SmarTracking™ algorithm.[34] This device uses an accelerometer to define a physiological band whose upper limit is defined by the SmarTracking rate. In the absence of sensor input, the paced ventricular rate is limited to the SmarTracking rate. An earlier version of this algorithm was nonprogrammable and limited the ventricular tracking rate to 35 bpm above the lower rate limit when activity was not detected. Limitations to SmarTracking include an irregular paced ventricular rate during AF at rest, and a rapid and irregular ventricular paced rate with AF during exercise because the algorithm is disabled. The SmarTracking algorithm allows the ventricular tracking rate to vary with the level of physical activity based on the sensor indicated rate (Figure 11). In one study, patients with pacemakers that utilized the algorithm during AF had a paced ventricular rate during strenuous activity such as a fast walk or climbing stairs which was similar to what was found with the conditional ventricular tracking limit algorithm, and found to be excessively fast. SmarTracking, however, was associated with a slower ventricular rate during AF at rest and with low levels of exercise, such as a slow walk. Secondly, the ventricular rate was still highly irregular during AF using this algorithm. Most patients were aware of the irregular ventricular response and two of six patients requested early termination of this pacing mode. These investigators suggested that SmarTracking may limit the ventricular rate at the onset of a supraventricular tachycardia until the mode-switching algorithm is activated. Fahreaus and Brüls have confirmed these findings, showing the use of a sensor-based "protection" mechanism can lead to less variation and oscillation of ventricular rate due to intermittent undersensing of atrial signals during AF.[35]

Clinical Implications of AMS

With increasing use of DDDR pacing and AMS algorithms, it is clear we need to understand more about the sensitivity, specificity, and usefulness of these algorithms.[36] The value of the diagnostic and telemetered information on mode-switching episodes needs further clarification.

Clinical Trials

A recent randomized study compared three pacing modalities: DDDR with AMS, DDDR with conventional upper rate behavior, and VVIR pacing in 48 patients with a history of atrial tachyarrhythmias.[37] Pacemakers were programmed to each modality for 4 weeks in a randomized crossover design. All patients completed three different symptom questionnaires at the end of each pacing period. At the end of the study patients were asked to choose their preferred

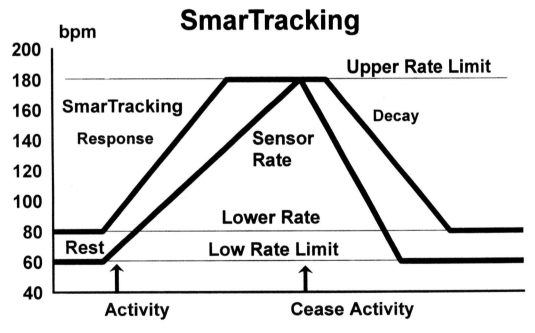

Figure 11. Schematic diagram of Intermedics Marathon SmarTracking™ algorithm. This algorithm is described in the text. The SmarTracking algorithm results in a continuously changing ventricular tracking limit based on sensor input. For example, if an atrial tachyarrhythmia occurs at a rate of 110 bpm (below the programmed automatic mode-switching rate), the SmarTracking algorithm will limit the ventricular tracking rate to a rate that the sensor determines is appropriate for that level of activity. If SmarTracking determines the rate of 110 is "inappropriate" for that level of activity, it won't track the ventricular rate. This algorithm limits ventricular tracking of atrial rates not due to exercise, particularly those below the upper rate limit. The SmarTracking algorithm has a programmable lower rate, response curve, and decay curve.

pacing mode. DDDR with mode switching was significantly better than both VVIR and conventional DDDR pacing. Early termination of DDDR pacing with mode switching occurred in only 3% of patients, 33% of patients with VVIR pacing had early termination, and 19% of patients with DDDR pacing had early termination. All patients with rapid mode-switching devices and no evidence of inappropriate mode switching preferred the DDDR pacing mode with mode switching over VVIR pacing, and 14% of patients with slower mode-switching devices preferred the VVIR pacing mode. Patients were also able to exercise longer and were less symptomatic during DDDR pacing and mode switching than with VVIR pacing.

Specificity

A major concern in the interpretation of mode-switching diagnostics is the specific-

ity of episodes characterized as "atrial fibrillation." We and several other groups have used the episodes of tachycardia classified as "ventricular tachycardia" by ICDs to analyze the circadian periodicity of ventricular tachycardia as well as to describe clustering and nonlinear modeling of episodes of tachycardia.[38] Before data logs from patients with mode-switching episodes can be used for mathematical modeling, verification of the specificity of these episodes must be assured. This could be a powerful tool for characterizing patients with vagally mediated or adrenergically mediated AF and targeting pharmacological or other therapies based on the pattern of episodes. Additionally, patients with large numbers of episodes of AF or particularly long episodes may require anticoagulation, or need changes in antiarrhythmic drug therapy based on this information.

Concerns about the specificity of mode

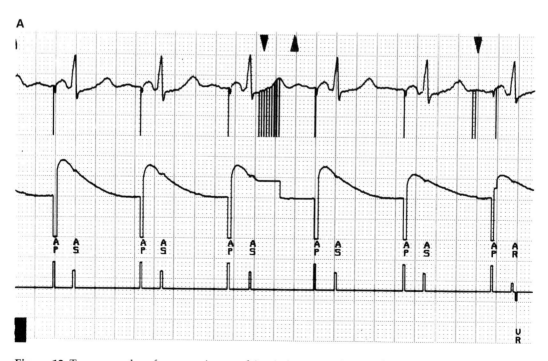

Figure 12. Two examples of oversensing resulting in inappropriate mode switching. These examples both illustrate the lack of specificity in general that mode switching may demonstrate. **A:** A patient with sick sinus syndrome is being atrially paced at 70–80 bpm. The atrial output is set to 3.5 V, 0.4 ms. The atrial sensitivity is programmed to 0.35 mV. At this atrial sensitivity, there is evidence of double sensing which resulted in mode switching with the AMS rate programmed to 150 bpm (not shown).

B

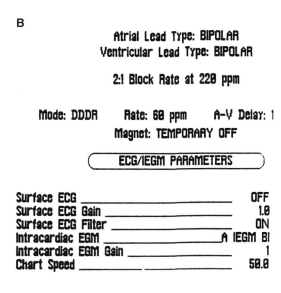

Atrial Lead Type: BIPOLAR
Ventricular Lead Type: BIPOLAR

2:1 Block Rate at 220 ppm

Mode: DDDR   Rate: 60 ppm   A-V Delay: 1
Magnet: TEMPORARY OFF

⟨   ECG/IEGM PARAMETERS   ⟩

Surface ECG _____ OFF
Surface ECG Gain _____ 1.0
Surface ECG Filter _____ ON
Intracardiac EGM _____A IEGM BI
Intracardiac EGM Gain _____ 1
Chart Speed _____ 50.0

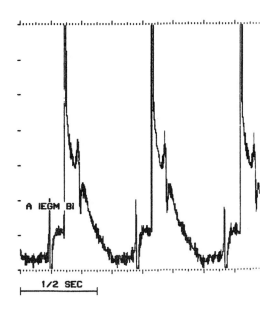

A IEGM BI

1/2 SEC

Figure 12. *(Continued)* **B:** Another example of inappropriate mode switching is shown. This patient has evidence of farfield sensing of an R wave on the atrial channel during exercise. In this patient, during high levels of exercise, the AMS algorithm was activated and resulted in loss of AV synchrony with mode switch to the DDI pacing mode (courtesy of John Griffin, MD).

switching have been raised by a number of investigators.[39,40] For example, we are troubled by the observations of Love et al. reporting an incidence of 66% of patients with mode switching enabled having episodes of AF.[41] In patients *without* a prior history of atrial arrhythmias, they reported 55% of patients having episodes of AF. These investigators feel that these data demonstrate a high incidence of AF even in patients without a prior history of AF. An alternative explanation, and one that we believe is likely responsible, is that many of these episodes represent "inappropriate mode switches" due to oversensing. Johnson et al. reported inappropriate mode-switching episodes in patients with the Medtronic Thera DR pacemakers programmed to nominal settings (atrial and ventricular outputs at 3.5 V, 0.4 ms, and atrial sensitivity = 0.5 mV) in 12% of patients.[39] The majority of episodes were believed to be due to farfield "R" wave sensing, with the rest due to nearfield "A" wave sensing.

In another study, Frohlig et al. studied 62 patients with the Medtronic Thera DR and found 40% of patients with mode-switching episodes that were not attributed to AF (Figure 12).[40] The majority of inappropriate mode-switching episodes were due to atrial sensing of atrial paced beats. This generally occurred 62–211 ms after atrial pacing. This was believed to be the most common cause of inappropriate mode switching. Mode switching due to atrial oversensing of farfield ventricular signals, either within the AV interval prior to signal detection on the ventricular channel or in the PVARP was less commonly seen. Reprogramming of atrial sensitivity or of the atrial blanking period generally abolished ventricular farfield sensing. Specific patterns of oscillations in atrial rate that are consistent with atrial oversensing were described. In our experience, many patients with episodes of mode switching classified in the range of 175–250 bpm represent double sensing of either farfield or nearfield events, and episodes where the atrial rate is reported as greater than 400 bpm likely represent AF. Clearly, devices with electrogram storage would help greatly in reviewing the data logs and confirming the etiology of the arrhythmia.[42] This lack of specificity of mode-switching algorithms may lead to significant symptomology of palpitations and a less improved quality of life.

Sensitivity

Additionally, optimizing the amplitude of the atrial electrogram during sinus rhythm will improve AMS reliability and make programming of atrial sensitivity to ensure AMS easier.[43] New algorithms, such as automatic atrial sensitivity adjustment, may enhance the specificity of AMS during AF without increasing the incidence of oversensing. Another problem that will need to be solved by newer AMS algorithms and devices is the effect of biatrial pacing or newer atrial pacing sites on detection of AF. The effect of sensing from two widely dispersed sites or from near the AV valve ring will lead to problems with oversensing of ventricular farfield potentials and inappropriate mode switches. Diagnostics that store atrial electrograms may be necessary for interpretation of these episodes. Pacemakers may benefit from development from highly specific AF algorithms of atrial defibrillators.

Summary

Optimal pacing in patients with intermittent tachycardias consists of dual chamber pacing with a programmable mode-switching algorithm. This algorithm should be robust and allow programming of atrial sensitivity and a variety of mode-switching parameters, including atrial blanking periods. Mode-switching diagnostics must be carefully reviewed before important clinical decisions are made.

References

1. Lamas GA, Pashos CL, Normand SLT, et al. Permanent pacemaker selection and subsequent survival in elderly Medicare pacemaker recipients. Circulation 1995;91: 1062–1063.
2. Ellenbogen KA, Peters RW. Indication for permanent and temporary cardiac pacing. In Ellenbogen KA, ed. Cardiac Pacing. Blackwell Scientific, Cambridge, MA, 1996, pp 1–36.
3. Sgarbossa EB, Pinski SL, Maloney JD, et al. Chronic atrial fibrillation and stroke in paced patients with sick sinus syndrome: prevalence of clinical characteristics and pacing modalities. Circulation 1993;88:1045–1053.
4. Clarke M, Sutton R, Ward D, et al. Recommendations for pacemaker prescription for symptomatic bradycardia. Br Heart J 1991;6: 185–191.
5. Mond HG, Barold SS. Dual chamber, rate adaptive pacing in patients with paroxysmal supraventricular tachyarrhythmias: protective measures for rate control. PACE 1993; 16:2168–2185.
6. Barold SS, Mond HG. Optimal antibradycardia pacing in patients with paroxysmal supraventricular tachyarrhythmias: role of fallback and automatic mode switching mechanisms. In Barold SS, Mugica J, eds. New Perspectives in Cardiac Pacing 3. Futura Publishing Co, Inc., Mt. Kisco, NY, 1993, pp 483–518.
7. Sutton R. Mode switching in DDDR pacing. In Aubert AE, Ector H, Stroobandt R, eds. Cardiac Pacing and Electrophysiology. Kluwer Academic Publishers, Dordrecht, The Netherlands, 1994, pp 363–370.
8. Higano ST, Hayes D, Eisinger G. Advantage of discrepant upper rate limits in a DDDR pacemaker. Mayo Clin Proc 1989;64:932–939.
9. Barold SS. The DDI mode of cardiac pacing. PACE 1987;10:480–484.
10. Irwin M, Harris L, Cameron D, Louis C, et al. DDI pacing: indications, expectations, and follow-up. PACE 1994;17:274–279.
11. Barold SS. Optimal pacing in the brady-tachy syndrome. Cardiol Rev, in press.
12. Barold SS, Mond HG. Fallback responses of dual chamber (DDD and DDDR) pacemakers. PACE 1994;17:1160–1165.
13. Mayumi H, Uchida T, Shinozaki K, et al. Use of a dual chamber pacemaker with a novel fallback algorithm as an effective treatment for sick sinus syndrome associated with a transient supraventricular tachyarrhythmia. PACE 1993;16:992–1000.

14. Lau CP, Tai YT, Fong PC, et al. Atrial arrhythmia management with sensor controlled atrial refractory period and automatic mode swithching in patients with minute ventilation sensing dual chamber rate adaptive pacemakers. PACE 1992;15:1504–1514.

15. Meta DDDR Model 1250 multiprogrammable minute ventilation volume rate responsive pulse generator with telemetry. Physician's Manual, Telectronics, Englewood, Colorado, 1990.

16. Meta DDDR Model 1254 multiprogrammable minute ventilation volume rate responsive pulse generator with telemtry. Physician's Manual, Telectronics, Englewood, Colorado, 1994.

17. Ovsycher IC, Katz A, Bondy C. Initial experience with a new algorithm for automatic modes switching from DDDR to DDIR. PACE 1994;18:1908–1912.

18. Levine PA, Bornzin GA, Barlow J, et al. A new automode switch algorithm for supraventricular tachycardias. PACE 1994;17(Pt II):1900–1907.

19. den Dulk K, Dijkman B, Pieterse M, et al. Initial experience with mode switching in a dual sensor, dual chamber pacemaker in patients with paroxysmal atrial tachyarrhythmias PACE 1994;17(Pt II):1900–1907.

20. Kay GN, Hess M, Marshall H, et al. Effect of mode switching algorithm in patient symptoms. PACE 1997;20:1064A.

21. Leung S-K, Lam T-F, Tse H-F, et al. Different responses to atrial fibrillation in three automatic mode switching algorithms. PACE 1997;20(Pt II):1497A.

22. Wood MA, Moskovljevic P, Stambler BS, et al. Comparison of bipolar atrial electrogram amplitude in sinus rhythm, atrial fibrillation, and atrial flutter. PACE 1996;19:150–156.

23. Konings K, Kirchhof CJHJ, Smeets JRLM, et al. High-density mapping of electrically induced atrial fibrillation in humans. Circulation 1994;89:1665–1680.

24. Wells JL, Karp RB, Kouchoukos NT, et al. Characterization of atrial fibrillation in man: studies following open heart surgery. PACE 1978;1:426–438.

25. Baerman JM, Ropella KM, Sahakian AAV, et al. Effect of bipole configuration on atrial electrograms during atrial fibrillation. PACE 1990;13:78–87.

26. Lewalter T, Schimpf R, Jung W, et al. Prospective evaluation of mode switch behavior in patients with dual chamber pacing and unipolar atrial leads: relevance of atrial fibrillation/flutter potentials and myopotential triggering. PACE 1996;19(Pt II):642A.

27. Leung S-K, Lau C-P, Lam C, et al. How should atrial sensitivity be programmed for optimal automatic mode switching? J Am Coll Cardiol 1997;29(Suppl A):149A.

28. Bonnet J-L, Brusseau E, Limousin M, et al. Mode switch despite undersensing of atrial fibrillation in DDD pacing. PACE 1996;19(Pt II):1724–1728.

29. Gencel L, Geroux L, Clementy J, et al. Ventricular protection against atrial arrhythmias in DDD pacing based on a statistical approach: clinical results. PACE 1996;19(Pt II):1729–1733.

30. Schüller H, Reuter J, Clausson E, et al. Far field R wave sensing: an old problem reappearing. PACE 1996;19(Pt II):631A.

31. Sweesy M, Mayotte M, Erickson S, et al. Mode switching and far field R wave sensing. PACE 1997;20(Pt II):1229A.

32. Ellenbogen KA, Mond HG, Wood MA, et al. Failure of automatic mode switching: recognition and management. PACE 1997;20 (Pt I):268–275.

33. Palma EC, Kedarnath V, Vankwalla V, et al. Effect of varying atrial sensitivity, AV interval, and detection algorithm on automatic mode switching. PACE 1996;19(Pt II):1734–1739.

34. Kamalvand K, Kotsakis A, Tan K, et al. Evaluation of a new pacing algorithm to prevent rapid tracking of atrial tachyarrhythmias. PACE 1996;19(Pt II):1714–1718.

35. Fahreaus T, Brüls A. A new dual protection mechanism against high rate ventricular pacing during atrial tachyarrhythmias. PACE 1997;20(Pt II):1534A.

36. Ritter P, Cazeau S, Kojoukharov Y, et al. Critical analysis of the different algorithms designed to protect the paced patient against atrial tachyarrhythmias in dual chamber pacing. In Aubert AE, Ector H, Stroobandt R, eds. Cardiac Pacing and Electrophysiology. Kluwer Academic Publishers, Dordecht, The Netherlands, 1994, pp 355–362.

37. Kamalvand K, Tau K, Kotsakis A, et al. Is mode switching beneficial? A randomized study in patients with paroxysmal atrial tachyarrhythmias. J Am Coll Cardiol, in press.

38. Wood MA, Simpson PM, Liebovitch LS, et al. Temporal patterns of venticular tachyarrhythmias: insights form the implantable cardioverter defibrillator. In Dunbar S, Ellenbogen KA, Epstein AE, eds. Sudden Cardiac Death. Futura Publishing Co, Inc, Mt. Kisco, NY, 1997.

39. Johnson BW, Bailin SJ, Solinger B, et al. Frequency of inappropriate automatic pacemaker mode switching as assessd 6 to 8 weeks post implantation. PACE 1996;19(Pt II):II–720.

40. Fröhlig G, Kindermann M, Heisel A, et al. Mode switch without atrial tachyarrhythmia. PACE 1996;19(Pt II):II–592.

41. Love CJ, Wilkoff BL, Heggs S. Incidence of mode switch in a general pacemaker population. PACE 1997;20(Pt II):II–1131.

42. Mabo P, Daubert C, Limousin M, et al. Atrial electrogram storage: a new tool for atrial arrhythmia diagnosis in pacemaker patients. PACE 1996;19(Pt II):II–721A.

43. Ricci R, Puglisi A, Azzolini P, et al. How should atrial sensitivity be programmed in automated mode switching pacemakers? PACE 1997;20(Pt II):II–1063.

Chapter 37

Pacemaker Automaticity:
Enabled by a Multiplicity of New Algorithms

Paul A. Levine, S. Serge Barold

Introduction

The history of pacing has been one of progressive efforts to fine tune the capabilities of the implanted system to restore the normal or near-normal physiological status of patients. In the past few years, the number of algorithms and other pacemaker functions have grown exponentially facilitated by a change in the basic device design. Originally, pacemakers were hardware based while now they are, to an increasing degree, software based.[1,2] Only the exceptional patient requires all of the new algorithms. In many cases, a number of algorithms, modes, and other capabilities are mutually incompatible. The manufacturers, via software, disallow inappropriate combinations, although in some cases, what is apparently inappropriate occasionally turns out to be of clinical benefit as our knowledge base expands. A prime example is the use of rate hysteresis in dual chamber pacing for the treatment of neurocardiogenic syncope. While many of these new algorithms are beneficial to individual patients, they have the potential for compromising the effectiveness of therapy when applied inappropriately. Thus one must understand both

their indications and their contraindications. Further, the relative incremental benefit of many of these algorithms is small for the majority of the paced population, particularly in contrast to the earlier generation of devices. The original VOO pacemaker, while the least sophisticated pacemaker, probably had the greatest benefit because it was used for patients with recurrent ventricular asystole.

New algorithms have greatly increased the automaticity of the implanted pacemaker. They allow automatic adjustments of its various parameters optimizing pacemaker function while minimizing the need for physician intervention. The fully automatic pacemaker is a goal that is being progressively realized, although not yet fully achieved in any single device (Table 1).

Heart Rate

Rate Modulation

The normal sinoatrial node is the heart's primary pacemaker. It automatically modulates the rate to match the physiological requirements. At rest, the heart rate tends to

From Singer I, Barold SS, Camm AJ (eds): Nonpharmacological Therapy of Arrhythmias for the 21st Century: The State of the Art. Futura Publishing Co, Inc, Armonk, NY, © 1998.

Table 1
Algorithms Contributing to Pacemaker
Automaticity

Rate Control
  Rate Modulation
    Automatic Sensor Functions
      Auto Threshold
      AutoSlope
      Sensor Cross-checking
      Sensor Blending
    Sleep or Rest Mode
  Neurocardiogenic Syncope
    Rate hysteresis
    Sudden Rate Drop Response
  Pathological atrial tachyarrhythmias
    Automatic Mode Switch
    Independently programmable MTR and MSR
  Pacemaker-Mediated Tachycardias
    PMT identification and termination algo-
      rithms
Atrioventricular Conduction
  Protection against paroxysmal AV block-AV/PV
    Hysteresis
    AutoIntrinsic Conduction Search-sensed and
      paced AV hysteresis
    DDD/Automatic Mode Change
  Rate Responsive sensed or paced AV delay
  Maintenance of ventricular pacing
    Negative sensed and paced AV hysteresis
Sensitivity
  Autosensitivity
Capture
  AutoCapture Pacing System
Lead Supervision

slow while it increases during periods of stress such as exercise, emotion, fever, or congestive heart failure. In the presence of high-grade AV block in conjunction with a normal sinus node, a properly functioning DDD pacemaker provides rate modulation by tracking the intrinsic atrial depolarization.[3,4] This is the most physiological of any of the rate-adaptive systems.

In sinus node dysfunction, the intrinsic atrial rate may not increase in proportion to physiological stress. In the early 1980s, it was shown that a faster paced ventricular rate during a period of physical exertion produced a beneficial increase in cardiac output, even without 1:1 AV synchrony.[5-7] In chronotropic incompetence, a sensor-

based pacemaker can detect signals other than the P wave to reflect the need for an increased rate. Initially, sensor-driven systems were restricted to single chamber pacemakers but since the late 1980s, these sensors have also been incorporated in dual chamber pacing systems.

The most commonly utilized signal is physical motion including vibration and acceleration.[8-10] Other commercially available signals include minute ventilation[11,12] as detected by transthoracic impedance changes, central venous temperature,[13,14] and the QT (stimulus-T) interval.[15,16] Sensors that have been studied include right ventricular pressure (dP/dT),[17] ventricular depolarization gradient,[18,19] a variety of intracardiac intervals (LV ejection time, preejection period) based on impedance changes measured by injection of an electrical signal into the cardiac cycle,[20-22] central venous oxygen saturation,[23,24] partial pressure of oxygen, and myocardial contractility.[25,26] Most recently, two sensors have been combined to allow the strengths of one to balance the weaknesses of the other.[27-31]

While sensor-based devices allow for *automatic modulation of the pacemaker-controlled heart rate*, the available systems are primarily open loop and must be set by the physician. They will function within those parameters but will not further modulate the responsiveness of the sensor settings based on the patient's general level of activity. More intelligent systems that can automatically adjust the sensor-based parameters have now been introduced.

Sensor threshold is the system's ability to detect the sensor input signal. In some systems, the pacemaker will automatically monitor and report this signal. The "threshold" can also be set to "AUTO," which means that the responsiveness of the pacemaker will automatically adjust to the relative changes in the amplitude of the sensor signal. This modulation, as in St. Jude's Synchrony and Trilogy family of pacemakers, is based on a running average developed over the preceding 18 hours and is continuously updated. After a period of inactivity, i.e., bed rest, the system will automatically become more responsive to incoming sensor signals whereas after a period of activity, it becomes progressively less responsive. This is similar to the normal diurnal or circadian modulation of rate where the degree of rate increase is greater early in the day shortly after arising as compared to the evening.

The *sensor slope* or *rate response factor* defines the degree of rate change that will result in response to a given sensor-input signal. In some recent devices such as the Trilogy DR+® pacemaker, slope can also be set to automatically adjust itself. In the early clinical experience reported in abstract form, the pacemaker's response has correlated very closely with detailed testing performed at the time of routine follow-up.[32] Similar capabilities are being incorporated in other devices via selection of the patient's relative lifestyle (sedentary, normal, active) through the programmer.[33,34]

It is generally acknowledged that no single sensor can totally mimic the rate-modulated capabilities of the normally functioning sinus. The activity sensors including the piezo-electric crystal bonded to the housing of the pulse generator or the various accelerometers provide a very rapid response to the onset of activity but the degree of heart rate response is not proportional to the degree of sustained levels of physical exertion, and this sensor will not respond to nonactivity-based physiological stress. Minute ventilation provides a proportional response to sustained levels of activity and is considered more physiological. The algorithms are improving, and St. Jude Medical has introduced a fifth generation minute ventilation algorithm in it's Tempo® family of pacemakers, which now provides a dual slope response more closely mimicking the normal heart rate response to physical activity. This was not the case with the earlier generation algorithms or the first generation algorithms from other manufacturers in which the response to the onset of physical activity is blunted. The QT sensor could respond to physiological stress other than

activity but was also delayed in its onset. To balance the strengths of one sensor against the weaknesses of different sensors, manufacturers are beginning to combine sensors in the same device. Two new capabilities have been introduced. One is *sensor cross-checking* where there can be an initial increase in heart rate with respect to activity, but this response is blunted unless there is a concomitant response by the other sensor. Sensors that have been combined include activity and minute ventilation, activity and central venous temperature, and activity and the QT interval. Sensor cross-checking with a single sensor has also been used in some devices to increase the specificity of the automatic mode switching algorithm, allowing it to respond to presumably pathological atrial tachycardias that are below the programmed maximum tracking rate if they occur when the patient is at rest with minimal sensor-input (Table 2).

The second new capability is *sensor blending* or allowing the physician to adjust the degree to which each sensor will contribute to an increase in the heart rate during a period of activity. Two sensors will, theoretically, improve the specificity of the sensor response, and although it is not yet a closed-loop system, will further refine the system's ability to automatically set its own parameters over a period of time.

Sleep Mode

Another aspect of the heart rate is the normal circadian or diurnal variation.[35–37] As a third of an individual's life is spent sleeping and the mean heart rate during sleep is lower than the resting heart rate when awake, modeling the pacemaker's response to mimic this circadian rate pattern seems to be a reasonable goal. Based on the heart rate variability literature, the lowest resting heart rates occur while asleep (early morning hours) and the highest resting heart rates occur in the early afternoon hours. Although there are not a large number of pacing studies evaluating the hemodynamic effects and clinical benefits of diurnal variations in heart rates, Chew et al.[38] have shown subtle changes in diastolic function after only 3 weeks of pacing where the base rate never falls below 80 bpm.

There are multiple potential beneficial effects of incorporating the technological equivalent of diurnal variation in a permanent pacemaker. These include modeling the natural rhythm of the resting normal heart rate, improved patient comfort with slower rates at night, provision of a physiological recovery period for the heart with greater rest being allowed at the slower rates and possible reduced battery current drain and increased system longevity. For the single lead VDD pacing systems, sleep mode will minimize the likelihood of pacemaker syndrome because the effective pacing mode during physiological sinus node slowing will be VVI.

The indications for sleep mode include sinus node dysfunction without paroxysmal supraventricular tachycardias and with or without AV block. Sleep mode may also be helpful, depending on the algorithm design, when rate hysteresis is enabled in the management of neurocardiogenic syncope by preventing the abrupt increase in the paced rate that would otherwise occur with physiological sinus node slowing during sleep.

The relative contraindications to this al-gorithm or clinical settings where it would not be expected to be required include complete heart block with normal sinus node function where a low base rate should be selected to allow control of the ventricular paced rate by the sinus mechanism. Bradycardia-dependent tachyarrhythmias would also be a contraindication to sleep mode.

There are two algorithmic approaches to sleep mode that may be characterized as *static sleep mode* and *dynamic sleep mode*. In static sleep mode, the physician programs two specific times in the pacemaker—the time when the individual normally goes to sleep and the time usually associated with waking.[39,40] The fact that most paced patients are elderly and often sleep fitfully and frequently wake during the night limits the effectiveness of this first generation algorithm. This problem becomes exacerbated when traveling even if not changing time zones. During static sleep mode, the base rate is decreased during the fixed programmed hours of sleep and any sensor drive must start from this lower rate which may be too low if the patient is up and about. With dynamic sleep mode, the adjustment to the lower resting rate is based on the sensor-input to pacemaker microprocessor via a parameter termed the activity variance,[41-43] although changes in the QT interval have also been proposed as a means of differentiating periods of rest from activ-

Table 2
Interactions of Atrial and Sensor Activity During DDDR Pacing

Atrial Rate	Slow	Slow	Fast	Fast
Sensor 1 Response	Slow	Fast	Slow	Fast
Sensor 2 Response	Fast	Fast	Slow	Fast
Pacemaker Interpretation	Sinus bradycardia, Patient at rest	Sinus bradycardia, Patient active	Pathologic atrial tachycardia	Sinus tachycardia
Pacemaker Response	Pace or sense according to lower rate timing or blunted sensor response	Pace in accord with sensor response	Place cap on Maximum Tracking Rate, Mode Switch to nontracking mode	Rate controlled by either sinus or sensor depending on programmed parameters

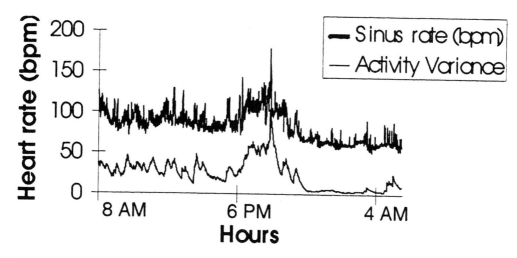

Figure 1. Twenty-four hour plot of heart rate variability with respect to time as recorded with a modified Holter monitor. One channel recorded heart rate data while the second channel was connected to a pacemaker to record the activity variance, which is automatically calculated by the microprocessor within the pacemaker based on an averaging technique from the raw sensor signal. The bpm scale only refers to the heart rate, not the activity variance.

ity.[44] An activity variance below a preset minimum will trigger sleep mode response (Figure 1). Not only can the rate slow during sleep with time zone changes as with travel, but also during daytime naps. Basing the sleep response on the relative sensor input, the base rate will not decrease if the individual stays up late at night or wakens during the night to go to the bathroom. If sleep mode had been engaged, the sensor input will cancel the sleep rate, immediately restoring the paced rate to the higher daytime resting rate. Any further increase in sensor-driven rate will start from this higher rate level. Thus, dynamic sleep mode uses the sensor mechanism to better modulate the rate throughout the entire 24 hours, not just in response to increased activity. Having enabled this algorithm, it becomes essential that the clinician be able to assess the effectiveness of the pacing system's behavior. This is accomplished with a variety of diagnostic event counters made possible by the microprocessor combined with significant random access memory (RAM) used to acquire the data (Figure 2).

Work is in progress to further modulate the base rate to mimic the normal circadian variation in base rate during the course of the day.[45]

Neurocardiogenic Syncope

The primary therapy for neurocardiogenic syncope is pharmacological (salt, mineralocorticoids, beta blockade, negative inotropic agents, vagolytic agents, or serotonin reuptake inhibitors). The syndrome is comprised of two major components—vasodepression and cardioinhibition.[46–48] If cardioinhibition were the sole component, then standard pacing would be very effective in preventing these episodes. However, in cases where vasodepression is the sole component, pacing will be ineffective. Most commonly, both vasodepression and cardioinhibition are present and when pharmacological therapy proves to be either ineffective or not tolerated, pacing has been helpful in ameliorating the symptoms but it may not totally eliminate either the syncope or presyncope and accompanying symptoms.

Over the years, a multiplicity of pacing algorithms have been utilized to treat the

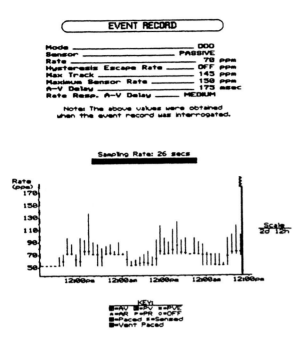

Figure 2. Event record, which is a time-based total system performance counter from a Trilogy DR + ® with sleep mode enabled implanted in a patient with sinus node dysfunction and marked chronotropic incompetence. At a sampling interval of 26 sec, the behavior of the pacing system over the preceding 60 hours is documented. The top and bottom of the vertical lines represent the peak and minimal heart rates achieved during the time period represented by each line. The crossbar represents the mean heart rate. Diurnal variation in heart rate performance is readily documented along with periods of heart rate slowing during the middle of the day. On questioning, these episodes correlated with an afternoon and evening nap.

cardioinhibitory component of this syndrome in highly selected patients. The results have been mixed because the pathophysiological mechanism involves varying degrees of vasodilation and bradycardia manifested as either sinus arrest with or without AV block. It is now known that when pacing is required, atrial transport is essential because these individuals are relatively hypovolemic during the episode. Thus, single chamber ventricular pacing is not likely to help.[49] As AV block may occur, single chamber atrial pacing would be ineffective, thus mandating dual chamber pacing support for the infrequent spells.

There are two options with respect to conventional dual chamber pacing. One is to program a low base rate, but when pacing is required, the rate is likely to be too low. The other is to program a high base rate, but then pacing will often occur when the patient does not require pacing support. In the mid-1980s, a standard dual chamber pacemaker was modified to provide dual chamber pacing support (DDI mode) at a high base rate but allowing the native rate to fall to a significantly lower rate before pacing would begin by using rate hyster-

esis.[50,51] Thus, when pacing was not required, the pacemaker would remain inhibited. When pacing was initiated by the first cycle of low-rate AV or ventricular pacing at the hysteresis escape rate, the system would then stimulate the heart at the higher programmed base rate. One of the limitations of this first generation algorithm was heart rate slowing during sleep would also trigger periods of rapid pacing. Since then, a number of algorithms have been introduced to enhance the specificity of the response. These include the sudden rate drop response where one programs the escape rate, the rapidity with which the sinus rate must fall to the escape rate, the number of cycles that the system remains at the lower rate before a rate increase will occur and then the higher rate at which a sustained period of dual chamber pacing will occur (Figure 3). A refinement to the original DDI mode with rate hysteresis is an addition of a search function such that after a period of time at the higher rate, the system automatically slows the rate to look for return of a native rhythm.

An algorithmic capability that has not yet been systematically tested is that of the

DDD mode with rate hysteresis combined with AV/PV delay hysteresis and dynamic sleep mode. This will allow the system to respond to pure AV block by P wave tracking, pure sinus node dysfunction with intact AV conduction with functional single chamber atrial pacing at a high rate after a single escape cycle. Should there be both sinus arrest and AV block, AV pacing at a high rate but with a physiologically optimal shorter AV delay. In St. Jude Medical's Trilogy DR + ®, the specificity of this algorithm can be further enhanced by enabling its dynamic sleep mode capability as both algorithms are controlled by the microprocessor in the pacemaker. Sleep mode, being based on the level of sensor activity and not preset times, will disable the high rate response during physiological sinus node slowing when sleeping. At these times, there will be pacing support at the escape rate to prevent the heart rate from falling below this level

while the individual is resting but it will preclude pacing at the higher rate. When the individual is up and about, the sensor input to the pacemaker will disable the sleep mode and a decrease in the intrinsic rate to the hysteresis escape rate will trigger pacing at the higher rate.

A study by Petersen and colleagues[51] reported their experience with 32 patients with documented cardioinhibition in association with neurocardiogenic syncope who were treated with pacing therapy. Most patients had their pacemaker programmed to DDI with hysteresis and although syncope was not absolutely prevented, the incidence was markedly reduced. Anecdotal reports as to the sudden rate drop response of the Medtronic Thera[52] and a similar capability in the Vitatron Diamond[53] have shown positive results. The results of the North American Vasovagal Pacing study (NAVPAC)[54] were presented at the 1997 meeting of

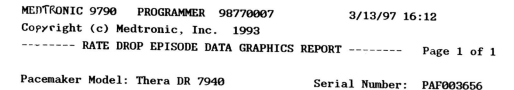

```
MEDTRONIC 9790    PROGRAMMER  98770007         3/13/97 16:12
Copyright (c) Medtronic, Inc.  1993
-------- RATE DROP EPISODE DATA GRAPHICS REPORT --------   Page 1 of 1

Pacemaker Model: Thera DR 7940              Serial Number:  PAF003656
```

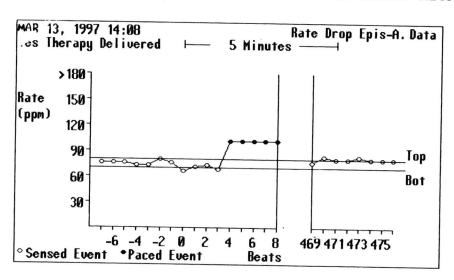

Figure 3. Rate drop episode data graphic from a patient with a Medtronic Thera DR® demonstrating the programmed rate range through which the rate must decrease before pacing will be initiated at a higher rate in a patient with neurally mediated syncope.

NASPE. This study showed a dramatically positive impact of pacing using the sudden rate drop response compared to conventional pharmacological therapy in delaying the time to first recurrence of syncope in a selected series of 56 patients with a high incidence of recurrent syncope.

Related to malignant vasovagal syncope is hypersensitive carotid sinus syndrome. It tends to occur in the older individual and when it induces recurrent syncope, there is a greater tendency to use dual chamber pacing with some form of rate hysteresis as these patients also benefit from a higher rate during their spells (Figure 4) but between episodes, they do not require pacing.[55-57]

Pathological Atrial Tachyarrhythmias

In the early experience with DDD pacing, patients with high-grade AV block and paroxysmal atrial tachyarrhythmias (most common being atrial fibrillation) were difficult to manage. This group of patients either received a VVI(R) or DVI pacemaker which, between episodes of the arrhythmia, resulted in the loss of coordinated atrial transport. The benefit of atrial transport associated with normal sinus node activity between episodes of the atrial arrhythmias was sacrificed to avoid the adverse consequences of tracking a pathological atrial tachyarrhythmia at relatively high rates. For those patients with relatively normal AV nodal conduction and sinus node dysfunction, DDI(R)[58,59] was an effective solution in that this mode would not track any atrial activity and, unlike the DVI mode, would not compete with intrinsic atrial rhythm. Rate modulation allowed the DDI mode to provide for rate increases during physical activity in the presence of atrial chronotropic incompetence. In recent years, RF ablation of the AV node or His bundle has become an increasingly popular method for managing patients with paroxysmal atrial fibrillation who cannot be stabilized or controlled pharmacologically.[60-64] While this induces complete heart block mandating a

pacemaker, it only became an effective mode of therapy, particularly in young individuals, with the development of automatic mode switching (AMS).[65-70] AMS is an algorithm within the DDD(R) modes that recognizes a pathological atrial tachyarrhythmia and automatically converts from a tracking to a nontracking mode, either VVI(R) or DDI(R) (Figure 5). The system continues to monitor the atrial rhythm and with the return of sinus rhythm, reverts to the atrial tracking [DDD(R)] mode.

The diagnosis of a pathological atrial arrhythmia is usually based on the sensed atrial rate which is either equal to the MTR and MSR or a programmable parameter independent of these two upper rate limits. This parameter has been labeled the *mode switch rate* or *atrial tachycardia detection rate* and may be recognized by the system either counting a given number of short cycles that exceed that defined rate or calculating a running average until the average atrial rate exceeds the programmed detection rate. The purpose of these special detection algorithms is to balance specificity and sensitivity. The clinical community learned from the experience with the first generation of AMS algorithm introduced in the Telectronics' Meta DDDR pulse generator that while a very sensitive system will rapidly detect every tachyarrhythmia, it will also respond to isolated premature beats and retrograde P waves.

Initiation of AMS involved solving a number of challenges. The standard PVARP would limit sensing of very rapid atrial rates, but for AMS, sensing is allowed during the terminal portion of this timing cycle. The PVARP is divided into two segments. Absolutely no sensing is allowed in the early portion of the PVARP termed the postventricular atrial blanking period (PVAB). It is intended to minimize sensing of farfield R waves, and if these are not present, can be as short as possible. In some devices, such as the St. Jude Medical Trilogy DR + ®, this is a programmable parameter. The second portion serves as both a noise-sampling window as well as an atrial tachyarrhyth-

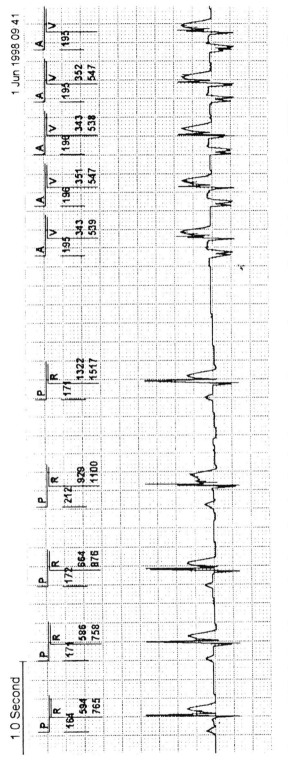

Figure 4. ECG obtained from a simulator showing the simultaneous telemetry of event markers during activation of DDD pacing with rate hysteresis. The escape rate was set to 40 ppm and the base rate set to 110 ppm.

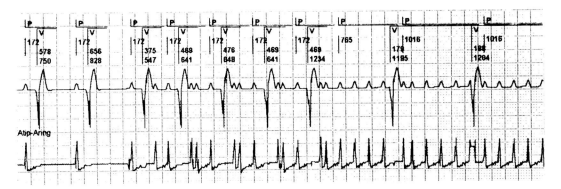

Figure 5. Simultaneous ECG and atrial electrogram generated by a heart rate simulator interfaced with a DDDR pacemaker demonstrating the development of an atrial tachycardia and activation of automatic mode switch. The first three cycles on the tracing represent normal P wave tracking. The pacemaker is functioning in the DDI mode during the last three cycles with a brief intervening period where the algorithm identifies and confirms a sustained supraventricular tachycardia that exceeds the atrial tachycardia detection rate.

mia-sensing window allowing the pacemaker to detect atrial rates that exceed the 2:1 block rate associated with upper rate behavior.

If the amplitude of the intrinsic deflection of the pathological atrial arrhythmia is intermittently too low (Figure 6), the rhythm may not be consistently sensed or if the atrial arrhythmia is slower than the mode switch or atrial tachycardia detection rate, the system will remain in a tracking mode. In an effort to enhance the specificity of the response, some systems, such as the Vitatron Diamond®, utilize cross-checking between the sensed atrial rate and the sensor input to the pacemaker in an effort to discriminate between relatively slow pathological atrial rhythms from sinus tachycardia. A sensed high atrial rate with significant sensor input being defined as an appropriate match thus maintaining tracking, even in the presence of an atrial arrhythmia whereas an even minimally elevated atrial rate with virtually no sensor input would suggest that the individual is at rest and hence, the faster atrial rate would be interpreted as pathologic. In these systems, mode switching may occur at rates that are below the maximum tracking rate. A limitation of this algorithm is that mode switching may occur in response to physiological

sinus tachycardias which occur at rest in response to a physiological stress other than physical exertion.

In an effort to further enhance the specificity of the AMS response, requirements that the fast atrial rhythm be present for a programmable duration or start abruptly in a manner analogous to sudden onset criteria utilized in ICDs for ventricular tachyarrhythmias have been implemented in some devices.

While the majority of pacemaker patients are elderly, in which case programming a low upper rate limit would not be physiologically limiting, this would be inappropriate for the young patient who remains active and whose sinus rate can be pushed to very high limits. The otherwise normal individual who underwent AV nodal ablation for paroxysmal atrial fibrillation is the ideal candidate for a DDD(R) pacemaker with AMS capability. The ability to set the mode switch rate below the atrial tachyarrhythmia rate (so that it will recognize the pathological rhythm), but well above the potential sinus tachycardia rates to preclude switching during appropriate pacemaker upper rate behavior would provide the best results. It has been recommended that the atrial channel be programmed to a very sensitive setting to facilitate recogni-

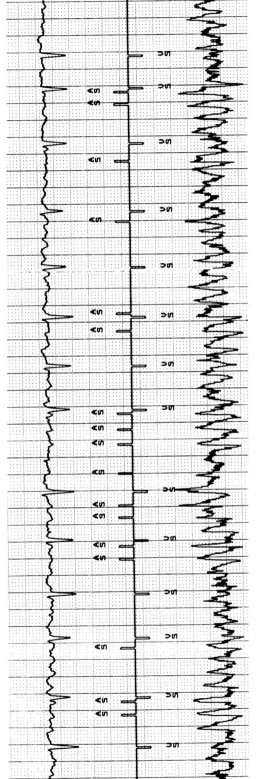

Figure 6. Simultaneous surface ECG, event markers, and atrial electrogram from a patient with a Medtronic Prodigy DR® recorded at the time of an office evaluation. The patient was in atrial fibrillation. The mode switch graphic indicated very frequent episodes all within a short period of time but occurring the day previously. This suggested mode switch oscillation. The pacemaker had been programmed to the DDI mode at the time this recording was obtained. The present episode was not recognized as an atrial tachyarrhythmia due to the low amplitude and low frequency components of the atrial fibrillatory signals. Thus, there was intermittent tracking.

tion of the pathological rhythm as there may be marked variation in the amplitude of the intrinsic atrial signal.

Since most contemporary DDDR pacemakers have some form of mode switching capability, one needs to look carefully at the specifications of the algorithm, the atrial tachyarrhythmias that have been either documented or are anticipated, and the clinical status of the patient in selecting the device. Some of the features that need to be considered include the ability to independently program the maximum tracking, maximum sensor, and mode switch or atrial tachycardia detection rates. Another feature would be the ability to program a sufficiently long sensed AV delay (PV delay) so as to eliminate fusion beats in the presence of intact AV conduction. The increased atrial sensitivity combined with the ability to sense atrial activity during the PVARP increases the likelihood of sensing the farfield R wave or ventricular evoked potential, predisposing to an inappropriate diagnosis of an atrial tachyarrhythmia. Although most farfield R waves will occur within 100 ms of the ventricular output pulse, there are occasions when longer intervals are present in which case one wants the ability to program the PVAB, which is allowed in some devices. By the same token, if there is no farfield R wave, programming the PVAB as short as possible will maximize the system's ability to recognize rapid atrial rates.

Independent of the specific algorithm, there needs to be a variety of diagnostic counters that will report the number of mode switching episodes that have occurred since the previous evaluation along with some information as to the duration of these episodes and atrial rates that triggered each episode (Figure 7). Such counters will allow the physician to track the evolution of the patient's arrhythmia and its response to other interventions over time. Without this additional information, the clinician's ability to monitor the effectiveness of this algorithm is significantly limited.

PMT Detection and Termination Algorithms

The usual pacemaker-mediated or endless loop tachycardia (PMT) is a macroreentrant tachycardia where ventricular pacing is associated with retrograde VA conduction to the atria, the retrograde P wave is sensed by the pacemaker which then triggers another ventricular output. If retrograde VA conduction can be sustained, the PMT will continue as the faster rate is likely to cause overdrive suppression of the sinus mechanism. It is estimated that 60%–70% of patients with sinus node dysfunction and 30% of patients pacemakers for AV block have intact retrograde VA conduction.[81-86] PMTs were relatively common in the early days of DDD pacing when PVARP programmability was virtually nonexistent.[87-90]

A PMT may be initiated by any event that induces AV dissociation allowing the atrium to physiologically recover so that a ventricular extrasystole (VE) or paced ventricular beat is able to conduct in a retrograde direction. While VEs are the most common initiator of a PMT, other causes include atrial undersensing and oversensing and atrial noncapture. Once initiated, the PMT may run at the programmed maximum tracking rate or at a rate below the MTR if there is a long VA conduction interval. The latter has been called a balanced endless loop tachycardia.

A number of approaches have been used to prevent a PMT or recognize it and then automatically terminate it.[91] Apart from programming the standard PVARP,[92] the most common preventive algorithms involve automatic extension of the PVARP in association with a VE.[93,94] A VE, according to the pacemaker, is a sensed R wave not preceded by a pacemaker recognized atrial event. The lengthened PVARP will preclude atrial sensing during this time but this may simply postpone the PMT by one cycle if the subsequent atrial output pulse occurs at a time when the atrial myocardium is still

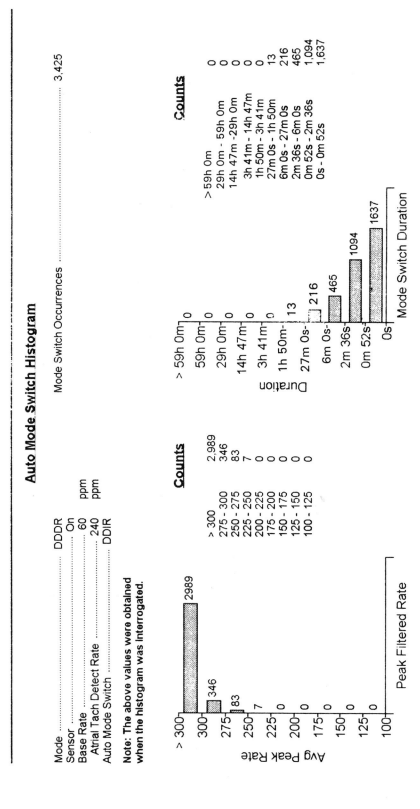

Figure 7. Automatic mode switch histogram from a St. Jude Medical Trilogy DR+® pulse generator. A total of 3,425 mode switch episodes had been recorded, the majority with filtered atrial rates above 300 ppm consistent with atrial fibrillation and most lasting under 2.5 min. These data will be helpful to evaluate the response to either pharmacological therapy or adjustments in the pacing system parameters when the patient returns for the next evaluation.

physiologically refractory secondary to the retrograde atrial depolarization contained in the extended PVARP. When the ventricular output pulse is released, retrograde conduction to the atrial myocardium then becomes possible. In the presence of intact conduction with a first degree AV block, sustained pacemaker inhibition may occur in association with the PVARP extension[91,95] (Figure 8). In an effort to avoid both of these possibilities, a further refinement is an algorithm called + PVARP on PVC. In this algorithm, the PVARP is increased to 480 ms following a VE, but to assure atrial capture, there is an additional 350 ms alert period before an atrial output will be delivered. The atrial escape interval for this one cycle becomes 830 ms independent of the programmed lower rate or DDDR mode. If a P wave occurs just prior to the end of the extended PVARP, the delay in the delivery of the atrial output would assure atrial capture. However, the fixed length of the post-VE atrial escape interval results in a shorter effective escape cycle if the programmed lower rate limit is very long. If the lower rate interval was relatively high due to either programming or sensor drive, the post-VE escape cycle would be slower. In a patient with bradycardia-dependent tachyarrhythmias such as torsade de pointes, this algorithm might allow the development of an intrinsic tachyarrhythmia.[96–99] Hence, in such a situation, one would not use the + PVARP on PVC feature.

A recent enhancement to the PVC detection algorithm includes identification of intrinsic atrial activity within the terminal portion of the PVARP. While a P wave occurring within the PVARP will not be tracked, a native R wave occurring shortly after completion of the PVARP will be labeled a conducted R wave rather than a VE thereby enhancing the diagnostic specificity of the PVC detector and precluding an inappropriate extension of the PVARP following this native ventricular complex.

In the present era of DDDR pacing, a long PVARP has an additional potential problem. As the lower rate (AV pacing) is increased under sensor drive, the longer PVARP will predispose to undersensing of native atrial beats and competition. Even if the retrograde P wave is not sensed because it coincides with the PVARP thus preventing a PMT, the native atrial depolarization may render the atrium physiologically refractory to the subsequent atrial output pulse delivered shortly after the native P wave when the atrial escape interval has been shortened in response to sensor drive. This may allow the system to develop a sustained period of retrograde VA conduction, functional undersensing of the retrograde P wave (because it coincides with the PVARP), and functional atrial noncapture (because it coincides with the physiological refractory period of the atrial myocardium)[100] (Figure 9). The result is a rhythm that has been called repetitive non-reentrant VA synchrony and is a potential cause of pacemaker syndrome during sensor drive.[101] Prevention requires a PVARP as short as possible. A rate-responsive PVARP that shortens as the rate increases incorporated in several devices provides a solution to this problem. A feature called noncompetitive atrial pacing can also prevent this disturbance (discussed later).

As a shortened PVARP will predispose to PMTs in patients with intact retrograde conduction, algorithms are needed to recognize a PMT and then intervene to terminate it. In the first generation algorithm, a PMT was defined as atrial sensed ventricular pacing (PV or As-Vp) at or above a programmable rate for a preset number of cycles ranging from 6 to 16. When this criteria was fulfilled, the system either withheld a ventricular output[102] or extends the PVARP[103] for one cycle. This resulted in a pause in the rhythm and termination of the PMT. However, these first generation algorithms were unable to differentiate a PMT from an intrinsic atrial or sinus tachycardia that was being tracked by the pacemaker. When the definition of the PMT required that the rate be at the maximum tracking rate, a balanced endless loop tachycardia running at a rate below the MTR would not initiate a PMT response and the

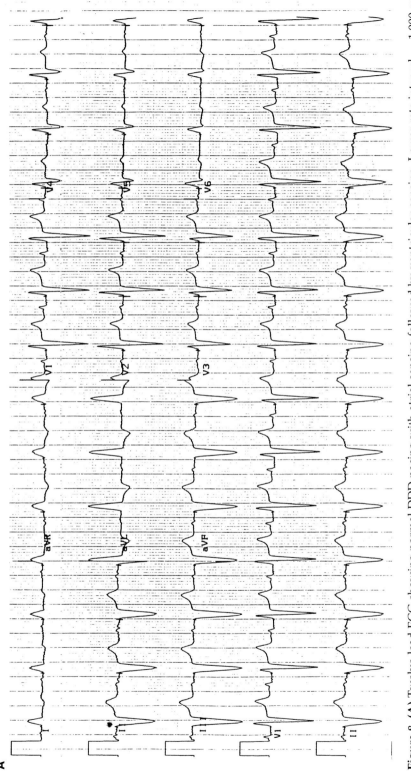

Figure 8. (A) Twelve-lead ECG showing normal DDD pacing with atrial sensing followed by ventricular sensing. Lower rate interval = 1,000 ms; AV = 150 ms; postventricular atrial refractory period (PVARP) = 200 ms; post PVC PVARP extension = 400 ms.

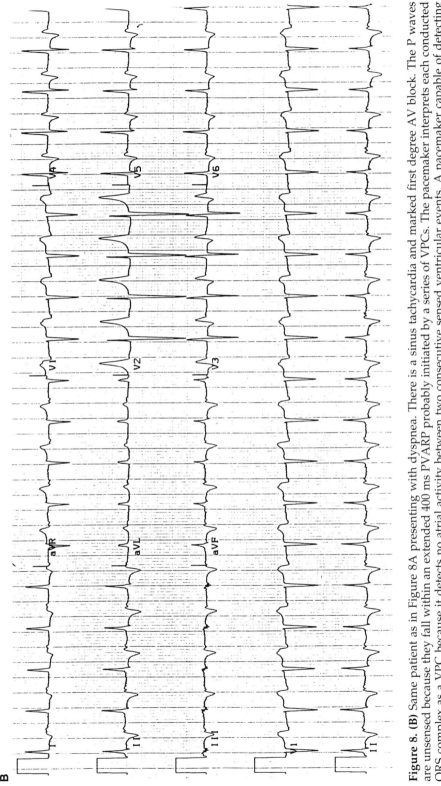

Figure 8. (B) Same patient as in Figure 8A presenting with dyspnea. There is a sinus tachycardia and marked first degree AV block. The P waves are unsensed because they fall within an extended 400 ms PVARP probably initiated by a series of VPCs. The pacemaker interprets each conducted QRS complex as a VPC because it detects no atrial activity between two consecutive sensed ventricular events. A pacemaker capable of detecting the P wave within the PVARP could automatically terminate this situation by canceling the PVARP extension or by the delivery of a noncompetitive atrial stimulus as discussed in the text. In this case the PVARP extension was programmed off because it was not needed in the presence of VA conduction block. The sinus tachycardia was probably secondary to the hemodynamic derangement.

patient might be locked into this rhythm for sustained periods of time. An enhancement of the algorithm allowed the clinician to select a rate less than the MTR for patients with balanced endless loop tachycardias.[103] In the presence of physiological atrial tachyarrhythmias, these algorithms would induce repetitive pauses when the paced rate equaled or exceeded the PMT defined rate.

A second generation PMT detection and termination algorithm used the stability of the VP interval as a diagnostic parameter any time the P sensed V paced rhythm exceeds a preset or programmable rate. Once a stable VP interval is identified, the PV interval is either shortened as in ELA Chorus®[104] or extended as in the St. Jude Trilogy DR+®[105] and the VP interval associated with this cycle is monitored. An intrinsic atrial rhythm would be associated with a change of the ensuing VP interval whereas the VP interval is usually stable in the presence of a PMT. If the rhythm is labeled sinus, no further intervention is initiated thus avoiding all pauses. If the rhythm is labeled a PMT, the system either extends the PVARP on the next cycle which will result in a relative pause in the rhythm or delivers an atrial output pulse 330 ms after the sensed P wave (Figure 10). In the vast majority of patients, 330 ms would be sufficient time for the atrial myocardium to physiologically recover to allow atrial capture. The induced atrial depolarization renders the atrium physiologically refractory to retrograde conduction that might otherwise follow the paced ventricular output. The PMT is terminated without the pauses associated with the earlier algorithms while avoiding the false positive responses to intrinsic atrial tachyarrhyth-

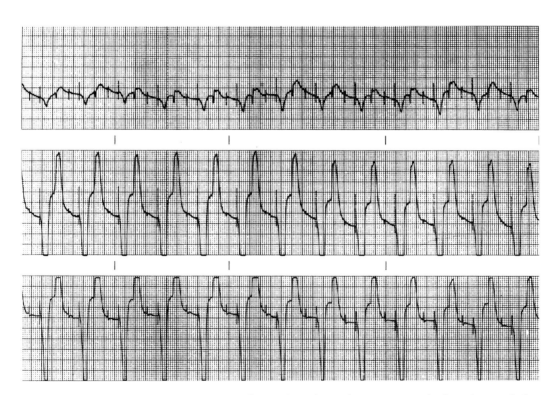

Figure 9. Repetitive nonreentrant VA synchrony (AV desynchronization arrhythmia), recorded in a three-lead compound surface and esophageal electrocardiogram to enhance atrial activity as shown in the upper strip. There is retrograde VA conduction with the P wave falling in the PVARP. The succeeding atrial stimulus is ineffectual because it occurs within the atrial myocardial refractory period generated by the preceding unsensed retrograde P wave.

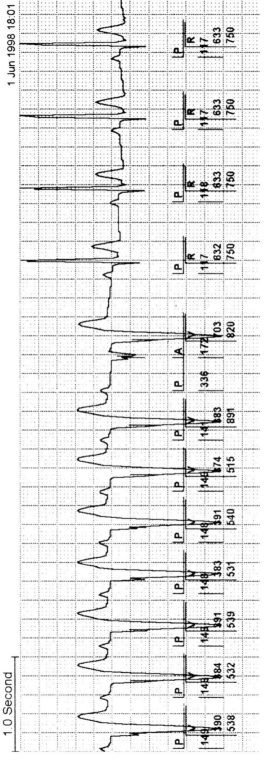

Figure 10. Termination of a "PMT" demonstrated with an ECG simulator using a second generation PMT detection and termination algorithm. After identifying a relatively stable VP interval, the system withholds a ventricular output after the ninth sensed P wave, delivers an atrial output 330 ms after the sensed P wave and this is followed by release of a ventricular output at the AV delay. This minimizes the pause associated with previous PMT termination algorithms.

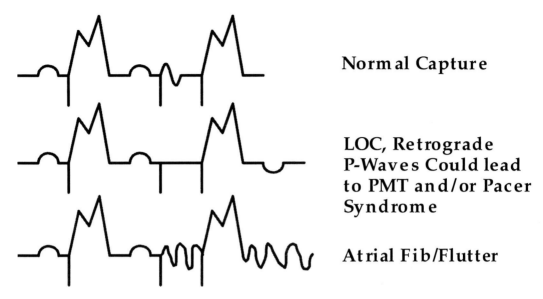

Normal Capture

LOC, Retrograde P-Waves Could lead to PMT and/or Pacer Syndrome

Atrial Fib/Flutter

Figure 11. Competitive atrial pacing. Middle panel: Lack of capture (LOC) by an atrial stimulus falling in the atrial myocardial refractory period generated by a preceding atrial depolarization may cause retrograde VA conduction with pacemaker-mediated tachycardia (PMT or endless loop tachycardia) or repetitive nonentrant VA synchrony (Figure 9) that may cause pacemaker syndrome. Bottom panel: An atrial stimulus falling in the vulnerable period of the atrium may precipitate atrial fibrillation or flutter. The vulnerable zone is <300 ms. Courtesy of Medtronic Inc.

mias. This is expected to become a very valuable capability as physicians begin to program shorter PVARP and devices are delivered to the market with automatic shortening of the PVARP (and ventricular refractory period) as the rate increases under sensor drive.

Noncompetitive Atrial Pacing

In the Medtronic Thera and Kappa DDDR pacemakers, noncompetitive atrial pacing (NCAP) is a programmable feature to prevent atrial pacing from being closely coupled to atrial activity within the PVARP (Figure 11). NCAP is available only in the DDDR mode. Even if it is not programmed NACP is automatically enabled for one beat following endless loop tachycardia termination or a PVC response, both of which use an extended PVARP of 400 ms. A refractory sensed atrial event falling in the PVARP starts a 300 ms NCAP period during which

no atrial pacing may occur (Figure 12). If an atrial stimulus is scheduled to occur during the NCAP period, the atrial escape interval is extended until the NCAP period expires. If no pacing stimulus is scheduled to occur during the NCAP period, timing of the atrial escape interval is unaffected. When an atrial stimulus is delayed by NCAP, the pacemaker attempts to maintain a stable ventricular rate by shortening the paced AV interval (to no less than 30 ms in the Kappa device). When a relatively short lower rate interval and long PVARP are programmed, NACP operation may cause ventricular pacing with an interval slightly longer than the lower rate interval.

Atrioventricular Conduction

The first algorithms to automatically shorten the AV interval were relatively limited to reflect enhanced conduction through the AV node associated with elevated levels

NCAP Operation

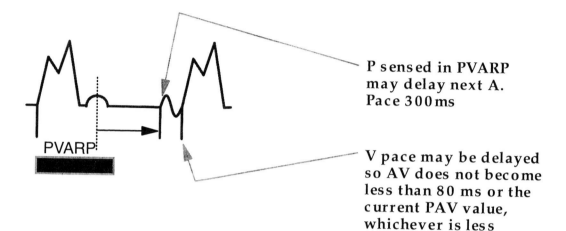

P sensed in PVARP may delay next A. Pace 300 ms

V pace may be delayed so AV does not become less than 80 ms or the current PAV value, whichever is less

Figure 12. Operation of the Medtronic noncompetitive atrial pacing (NCAP) feature. The atrial pacing stimulus is delayed if necessary and the AV interval is compressed to compensate for the delayed atrial stimulus. In the Thera series the paced AV interval is maintained at 80 ms (or the programmed value if less) and in the Kappa 400 device the paced AV interval does not shorten to less than 30 ms. Courtesy of Medtronic.

of catecholamines. DDD with rate-responsive or adaptive AV delays were shown to be superior to either DDD pacing with a fixed AV delay or VVIR pacing in clinical studies using a within-patient cross-over design.[106-108] The algorithms have been progressively refined such that both paced (AV) and sensed (PV) atrioventricular delays will progressively shorten as the rate increases. Further, the degree of shortening is programmable in some pacing systems along with the ability to independently limit the degree of AV delay shortening (Figure 13).

Rate-responsive AV delay, also called rate-adaptive AV delay or an adaptive AV interval, automatically shortens the AV interval in response to either sensor drive or the sensed atrial rhythm allowing the physician to program the optimal AV delay at rest and provide an effective AV interval at higher rates.

Positive AV/PV Hysteresis

Positive AV interval hysteresis allows a long AV interval which will be the domi-nant interval when AV conduction is relatively intact and a shorter AV interval when there is AV block.

A number of studies have demonstrated that for a patient without AV block, with normal left ventricular function, and a narrow QRS complex, AAI(R) pacing provides optimal hemodynamics.[109,110] However, many physicians are uncomfortable with single chamber atrial pacing and prefer the back-up ventricular protection provided by a dual chamber pacing system. Until recently, there were two methods for managing these patients. One was to program the dual chamber system to the single chamber AAI(R) mode and reprogram to a dual chamber mode if AV block develops. This leaves the patient unprotected if AV block develops. The second option was to program a long AV delay (i.e., 300 ms). While this will provide protection against AV block, the very long AV delay combined with a disordered ventricular activation sequence as the need arises will not result in optimal hemodynamics.[111-113]

The new algorithm allows for both a long AV delay when AV nodal conduction is intact and a shorter, more physiological AV delay when there is AV block and ventricular pacing is required.[114–116] The result is functional single chamber atrial pacing when conduction is intact and appropriate dual chamber pacing in the presence of even first degree AV block. With these new algorithms, after the first cycle of AV pacing (Ap-Vp or As-Vp) at the long AV interval, the subsequent AV interval is delivered at a shorter and more physiological duration (Figure 14). Since the paced or sensed AV delay may be shorter than the intrinsic conduction, it will lock the device into pacing at the shorter AV delay unless the system can automatically determine whether or not intrinsic AV nodal conduction has returned. This capability is termed *search*. After either a set number of cycles or a programmable

period of time, the system automatically extends the AV interval to the longer base interval. If a native R wave occurs within this extended interval, the longer base AV interval is again engaged thus inhibiting the ventricular output and reestablishing functional single chamber atrial pacing with more physiologically appropriate back-up ventricular support (Figure 15).

Two new algorithms have been introduced to address this subset of patients. In the ELA Chorum®[114] device, the algorithm is DDD/AMC® where AMC means "automatic mode change." The system functions in the AAI(R) mode, but learns the AR interval. If the AR interval + 31 ms expires without a sensed R wave, AV pacing is initiated with a search performed every 100 cycles if spontaneous AV nodal conduction is not

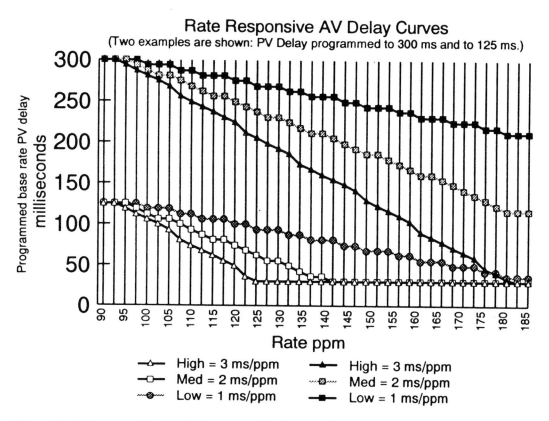

Figure 13. Rate responsive AV delay curves. The degree of RRAVD is programmable in terms of the rate of decline. In addition, it can start from the programmed AV delay, either paced or sensed, and there is a programmable minimal AV delay that will limit the further decrease in AV delay should the rate continue to increase. Two sets of curves are shown, one staring at an AV delay of 120 ms and the other at an AV delay of 300 ms.

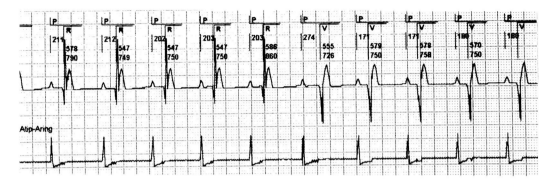

Figure 14. Positive AV/PV hysteresis. As demonstrated with an ECG simulator connected to the pacemaker, the pacemaker is inhibited by an intrinsic rhythm. In the middle of the tracing, there is a single cycle of PV pacing at a long AV delay (274 ms), presumably due to the transient development of AV block. This is followed by atrial sensed ventricular pacing at a PV delay of 171 ms which is shorter than the PR interval identified by the pacemaker of 200–210 ms.

previously identified. In St. Jude Medical's Trilogy DR + ®,[115] there is positive AV/PV hysteresis termed autointrinsic conduction search® available in the DDD(R) modes. The basic paced or sensed AV delay is selected by the physician and then an additional hysteresis interval is added to this to facilitate functional single chamber atrial pacing. If AV block develops, there will be one cycle of AV or PV pacing at the long interval followed by pacing at the shorter AV/PV interval until either intact conduction spontaneously resumes or after 255 cycles have been completed, a search is performed where the AV/PV interval is lengthened looking for resumption of conduction.

The primary indications for this algorithm include sinus node dysfunction with intact AV nodal conduction, Stokes-Adams syncope due to paroxysmal AV block and, depending on the other capabilities of the pulse generator, neurocardiogenic syncope including both malignant vasovagal syncope and hypersensitive carotid sinus syndrome.

Negative AV Interval Hysteresis

Negative AV interval hysteresis is a capability unique to the St. Jude Medical Tril-

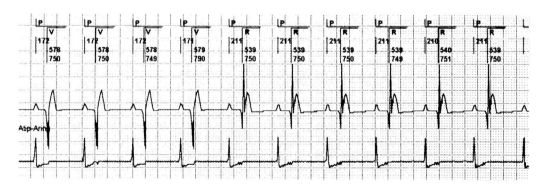

Figure 15. After a period of pacing, a search mechanism is initiated where the system automatically extends the paced or sensed AV delay. If a native R wave occurs within the extended AV delay, the longer AV delay is maintained, restoring intact AV nodal conduction and allowing for a normal ventricular activation sequence.

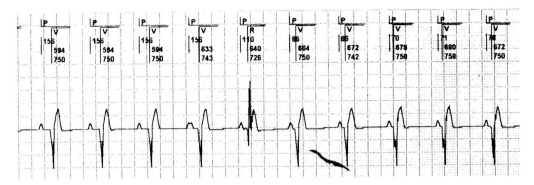

Figure 16. Negative AV/PV hysteresis demonstrated using an ECG simulator. Stable PV pacing is interrupted by one PR cycle at a shorter As-Vs interval than the PV interval. This causes the As-Vp (PV) interval to shorten by the programmed delta. After a period of pacing, the system will extend the AV/PV interval to determine if intact conduction is still present or will allow the longer interval to remain in effect.

ogy DR+® pacemaker. The intent is to maintain full ventricular capture for patients who are being paced for hypertrophic obstructive cardiomyopathy (HOCM). A short AV delay usurps control of ventricular activation from the normal conduction system. The resultant activation contributes to a reduction in LV outflow tract obstruction. However, these patients also have non-compliant or stiff ventricles and require maintenance of atrial transport. Effectively, they require the longest AV delay possible that will still allow for full ventricular activation by the pacemaker.[117–119] This is a challenging set of requirements. While the "optimal" AV delay can be easily set with the patient at rest, one cannot predict the degree of shortening of AV nodal conduction during physiological stress to ensure complete ventricular capture by the pacemaker. Hence, any arbitrary rate-responsive AV delay algorithm may be less than optimal. It may shorten the AV delay either too much or too little.

In negative AV delay hysteresis, the physician programs a hysteresis interval by which the pacemaker will shorten the paced or sensed AV delay if an R wave, presumably a conducted R wave, is sensed within the AV interval.[115] It will measure this interval and on the next cycle, automatically shorten the AV delay by a programmable

interval such that it is shorter than the measured AR interval (Figure 16). In a manner similar to positive AV delay hysteresis, after a set number of cycles, the system will automatically search for the intrinsic AV interval. If there is AV or PV pacing at the longer interval, the pacemaker's AV timing will return to that original programmed setting.

Capture

AutoCapture and AutoThreshold

Since the early days of cardiac pacing, it has been known that the capture threshold, the lowest output setting of the pacemaker that results in consistent stable capture, will wax and wane during the course of the day. The capture threshold is affected by a multiplicity of physiological and pharmacological factors.[120,121] Hence, in order to assure capture, the output of the conventional pacemakers has to be programmed at some level above the measured threshold.[122] The difference between the programmed output and the capture threshold is termed the safety margin.

The higher the programmed output, the greater the battery current drain with a resultant reduction in device longevity. Hence, it would be desirable to program the output as low as possible. Although acute and chronic capture thresholds are significantly lower at the present time as compared to the first generation of devices, assuring capture with the lowest output possible continues to be an important goal, but in a conventional pacemaker, programming a low output, even if there is a good safety margin, requires continued close follow-up.[123] Since Preston's early work about a threshold tracking pacemaker starting in 1973,[124,125] industry has been trying to develop a reliable technique by which capture can be automatically monitored on a beat-by-beat basis by the implanted pacemaker allowing the output to be automatically adjusted and maintaining it as low as possible, hence minimizing battery current drain but with the capability of providing a higher output back-up pulse in case of loss of capture. Various techniques have been used in an effort to recognize the capture[126–134] (charge balancing or use of low polarization leads) or hemodynamic consequences of capture (impedance measurements or T wave sensing) but all have been less than successful until the implementation of the **AutoCapture Pacing System**® incorporated in the St. Jude Medical Microny® and Regency® pacemakers which were commercially released in Europe in 1995 and approved by the FDA in 1998 in Regency SC + ®.

At this time, AutoCapture is available only in the single chamber ventricular pacing mode. An integral part of the algorithm requires sensing of the pacemaker evoked potential and at the moment, this requires a low polarization bipolar electrode utilizing unipolar stimulation via the tip electrode and sensing of the evoked response via the proximal electrode. Work is actively in progress to incorporate AutoCapture capability in single chamber atrial pacing[139] and on both channels of a dual chamber pacemaker[140] while eliminating the requirement for special leads.

In Microny® and Regency®, the pacemaker monitors capture by sensing the evoked potential. This requires a bipolar low-polarization lead. It also requires an evoked potential of >4 mV in amplitude and a low-polarization signal, both of which are measured by the pulse generator to determine if AutoCapture can be enabled. Stimulation is unipolar (tip to case) with sensing of the evoked potential via the ring electrode. At the present time, high polarization leads can cause a false positive response (diagnosis of capture in the presence of loss of capture) and should not be used with this system. Capture is monitored every beat. Each time loss of capture occurs, a 4.5 volt back-up pulse is delivered 64 ms after the initial ineffective output pulse (Figure 17). If loss of capture associated with the primary output pulse occurs in two consecutive cycles, the system automatically increases the amplitude of the initial pulse by 0.3 volts. The system continues to step up the amplitude of the primary pulse until capture is present on two consecutive primary outputs. At that point as well as every 8 hours, the system performs a capture threshold assessment (Figure 18). Once the capture threshold is identified, the system automatically programs the output to 0.3 volts above the capture threshold.

In ventricular AutoCapture, the system periodically performs a capture threshold search and logs the results in a special histogram (Figure 19). When the patient returns for routine follow-up, the sequential history of the capture threshold can be retrieved from the pulse generator and printed via the programmer for inclusion in the office or hospital record. Based on the clinical studies, there has been a superb correlation of the AutoCapture threshold reports with the capture threshold measured with Vario at the time of routine office evaluation. The ability of the system to automatically monitor and record its output behavior is essential to the documentation of the system performance between scheduled office or clinic follow-up sessions.

A limitation in the present algorithm involves fusion and pseudofusion beats (Figure 20). These may be interpreted as noncapture causing the pacemaker to automatically

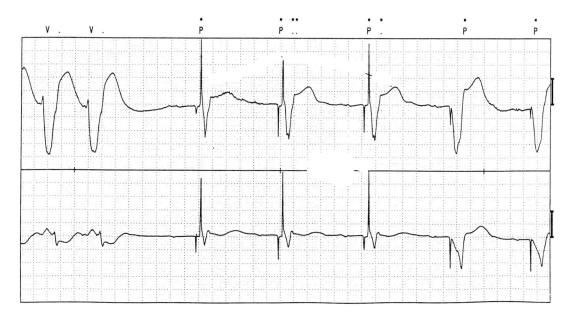

Figure 17. Recording from a 24-hour Holter monitor from a patient with a St. Jude Medical Regency® VVI pacemaker where AutoCapture was enabled. Following a ventricular couplet, there are a total of three cycles that demonstrated failure to capture associated with the primary output pulse. This was followed by a 4.5-V output pulse 64 ms after the ineffective pulse restoring capture with a subjectively nondetectable change in the pacing rate. The fourth and fifth paced complexes demonstrate capture associated with the primary pulse.

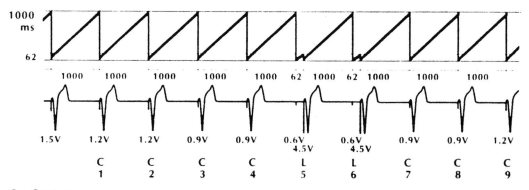

C = Capture
L = Loss of Capture

Figure 18. Schematic diagram of the periodic capture threshold assessment. The system steps down the output in 0.3-V steps until loss of capture occurs in two consecutive cycles. It then increases the output by 0.3 V and when capture is present on two consecutive cycles, labels this the capture threshold. The system then automatically sets the pacemaker to an output that is 0.3 V above threshold.

increase its output. This has been minimized by changing the rate ever so slightly when "noncapture" is diagnosed after the high-output back-up pulse is delivered. If the programmed output does increase due to fusion beats and a false interpretation of noncapture, the periodic capture thresholds that are performed will identify the correct threshold automatically resetting the pacemaker's output to a lower level thus minimizing any im-

pact on battery current drain and projected longevity.

The AutoCapture Pacing System allows the system to maximize longevity by providing as low an output as possible while absolutely assuring maintenance of capture on a beat-by-beat basis. Other systems are being introduced that automatically performs periodic capture threshold determinations by measuring changes in impedance, the T

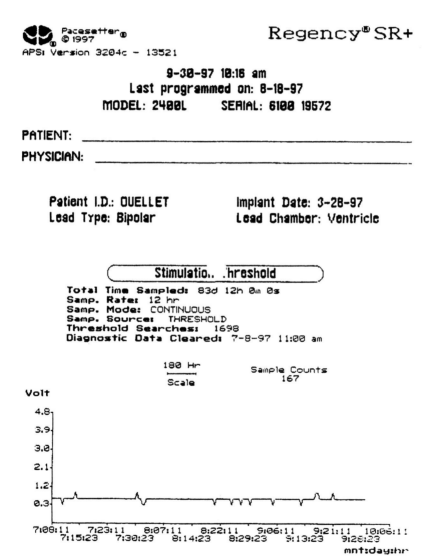

Figure 19. The pacemaker records the capture threshold results and displays this in graphic form retrievable at the time of a routine follow-up evaluation. This particular graph represents the behavior of the capture threshold over the preceding 83 days being monitored every 12 hours.

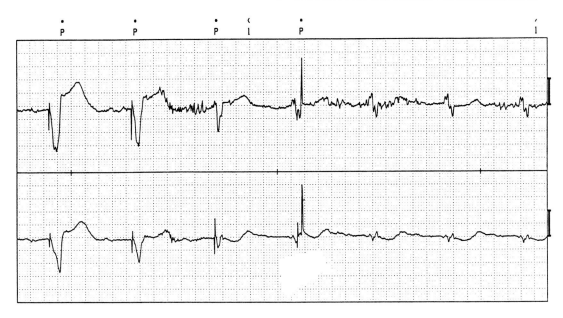

Figure 20. The first two complexes are fully paced. The third complex is a fusion beat but with a significant portion of the depolarization due to the pacemaker. The fourth complex is either a fusion or pseudofusion beat. The ventricular output coincides with a native QRS resulting in a cancellation of the amplitude of the evoked potential. As the pacemaker could not document capture, it delivered a high output back-up pulse.

wave or the evoked response associated with the primary output pulse with the physician defining the desired margin of safety. However, this does not assess capture on a beat-by-beat basis and cannot respond instantaneously to episodic loss of capture between the threshold assessments.

Sensing

ICDs have the challenge of recognizing both normal ventricular rhythms which are usually associated with relatively large endocardial potentials and ventricular fibrillation commonly associated with very small signals. Early systems programmed to a very sensitive setting combined with very short refractory periods in order to detect the rapid ventricular fibrillatory signals experienced oversensing of nonphysiologic signals and physiologically inappropriate signals such as T waves triggering multiple inappropriate responses with either a sequence of antitachycardia pacing and/or delivery of a shock. To minimize the episodes of oversensing while assuring the sensing of very low-amplitude signals, many ICDs incorporate a feature termed ***automatic gain control* (AGC).** Set appropriately to sense the normal ventricular depolarization, the system becomes progressively more sensitive as the timing interval progresses until there is release of therapy, either pacing or shock. In the period following a relatively large sensed complex, the system is relatively insensitive thereby minimizing T wave oversensing. As the interval between signals lengthen, the unit becomes progressively more sensitive so that small fibrillation or tachycardia signals are able to be recognized after a relatively short period of time for prompt diagnosis and delivery of therapy.

A similar **autosensitivity** capability has been incorporated in standard bradycardia pacemakers.[141, 142] This is not identical to the AGC in ICDs. The goal is to attain a sensitivity that provides consistent sensing while avoiding oversensing (Figure 21). This is more critical for the unipolar sensing configuration where oversensing is a potential

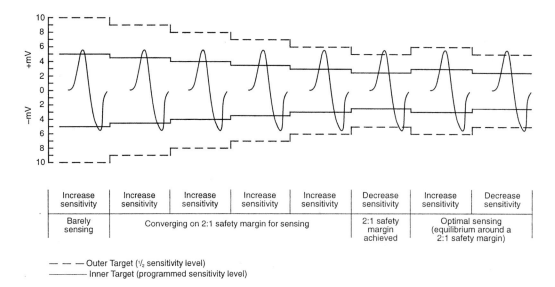

Increase sensitivity	Increase sensitivity	Increase sensitivity	Increase sensitivity	Increase sensitivity	Decrease sensitivity	Increase sensitivity	Decrease sensitivity
Barely sensing	Converging on 2:1 safety margin for sensing				2:1 safety margin achieved	Optimal sensing (equilibrium around a 2:1 safety margin)	

— — — Outer Target (½ sensitivity level)
———— Inner Target (programmed sensitivity level)

Figure 21. Diagrammatic representation of the autosensing function of the Intermedics DDDR pacemakers. The autosensing function maintains a 2:1 sensing safety margin automatically during sensing of atrial or ventricular activity by dynamically adjusting the gain of its sense amplifiers. The amplitude of the sensed signal is maintained at a level close to the outer target, thus helping to assure proper sensing in the presence of a varying electrogram. Sensing occurs at the inner target. The sensitivity level is not adjusted on every cycle and the time between adjustments depends on the amplitude and timing of sensed signals. The broken line represents the outer target sensitivity level and the unbroken line represents the inner target sensitivity test. Courtesy of Intermedics, Inc.

problem if the pacemaker is routinely programmed to a very sensitive setting. The ICD does not have to identify absolutely every complex for recognition of a tachyarrhythmia. Missing an occassional complex will not impair its function. However, a bradycardia support pacemaker must recognize every native complex. Even when there is a large endocardial signal associated with the sinus P wave or conducted R wave, an ectopic beat arising from either chamber may generate a relatively diminutive signal. A pacemaker with autosensitivity must be ready and able to sense the unexpected isolated premature beat. If it automatically reduces its sensitivity in the presence of a large intrinsic signal, it may miss the isolated smaller ectopic beat. Hence, if there is marked variation in signal amplitudes as with frequent ectopic beats, this feature is best disabled at the present time.

The alternative to autosensitivity is to program the pacemaker to a very sensitive setting. While this will predispose the system to an increased risk of oversensing, this has not been a serious clinical problem with the bipolar sensing configuration. The option of programming a high sensitivity (low number) in a unipolar system is associated with an increased incidence of oversensing.

Timing circuits that directly impact sensing are the various refractory periods. Originally incorporated in pacemakers to preclude the sensing of physiologically inappropriate signals such as the evoked potential or repolarization waves, filtering techniques have reduced but not eliminated the need for these blind periods. The longer the refractory period, the greater the chance that the system will not recognize or respond to an appropriate intrinsic event. In either the single chamber ventricular system or the dual chamber pacing systems, a long ventricular refractory period will preclude sensing early ectopic beats or native conducted beats in the presence of atrial fibrillation with a fast ventricular rate. With sensors driving the pacing system to higher rates, a long PVARP and a long VRP could result in functional undersensing and competition.

In dual chamber pacing systems, the PVARP is essential to minimize sensing of retrograde P waves and the propensity for PMT but limits the total atrial refractory period (TARP) thus limiting the MTR. While rate responsive AV delay mitigates the impact of a long PVARP to some degree, the automatic shortening of the PVARP with progressively higher rates would protect the patient from initiation of a PMT at the lower rates while allowing the system to track higher atrial rates. The advent of Automatic Mode Switch algorithms has allowed sensing within the PVARP for detection of pathologic atrial rates but this does

not impact the allowed MTR. Some systems also allow sensing within PVARP to minimize the misidentification of intrinsic conducted R waves as VEs. Sensing will be optimized by minimizing the duration of the refractory periods.

Special Circumstances

Lead Supervision

Lead supervision is the ability of the pacemaker to automatically monitor lead impedance. In the first iteration of this capability, an open circuit involving the proximal conductor of a bipolar lead resulted in the system automatically switching to the unipolar output and sensing configuration that utilized the distal conductor (Figure 22). While this would correct the acute prob-

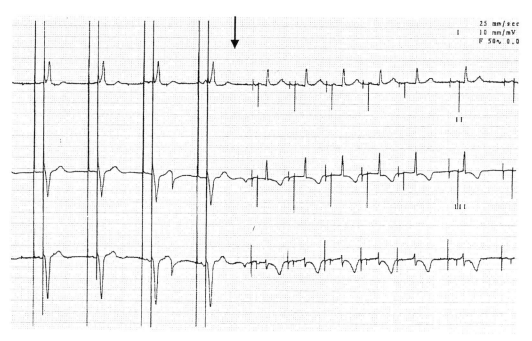

Figure 22. Intermedics Relay DDDR pacemaker showing automatic conversion of bipolar to unipolar pacing secondary to erroneous programming. The patient had a bipolar atrial lead and a *unipolar* ventricular lead. The pacemaker was unwittingly programmed to the bipolar mode by a junior member of the pacemaker team. At the next visit, the ECG showed large (unipolar) atrial and ventricular stimuli (left). Application of the magnet (arrow) restored the programmed bipolar mode with successful atrial capture but loss of ventricular capture. This illustrates how a high impedance in the outer coil of a bipolar ventricular lead (fracture or misprogramming) automatically converts bipolar DDD pacing to unipolar DOO pacing. This type of security is only temporary in the case of a fracture because the integrity of the other electrode is at risk. Used with permission from Gencel L, et al.[144]

lem and convert it from a potential emergency to a condition that could be managed electively, programming to unipolar is not a definitive cure for the lead problem. In addition, the first capability responded only to open circuit associated with a high-stimulation impedance and would not respond to a major insulation failure with a very low lead impedance.[143]

Future iterations of this algorithm will respond to either a very high impedance reflecting an open circuit or a very low impedance representative of a problem with the internal insulation in a bipolar coaxial lead. When either a very high or a very low impedance is recognized by the pacemaker, it automatically switches to the unipolar output and sensing configuration. This will restore pacing if the fracture involves the proximal conductor, which is likely in a coaxial bipolar lead or an internal insulation failure but as mentioned above, is a temporizing measure only converting a potential emergency into a condition that can be electively managed.

Summary

Increasing automaticity means that pacemakers can automatically adjust a variety of functional parameters based on a multiplicity of native and technological inputs to the system. This has the potential to improve the quality of pacing by virtually all physicians, not just the "pacemaker expert." In addition, it enables the pacemakers to intelligently respond to changes that might be required between scheduled office visits thus increasing both the safety and the physiological behavior of the implanted system for the benefit of the patient. Various automatic features include adjustment of various timing parameters including rate and AV delay. Automatic mode switch and unique PMT algorithms allow the system to respond to either endogenous pathological atrial tachyarrhythmias or pacemaker-mediated tachyarrhythmias. AutoCapture allows the system to maximize device longevity while maximizing safety with beat-to-beat monitoring of capture. The true role for autosensitivity remains to be determined with respect to the day-to-day automatic adjustment of the sensitivity setting. Although not required on a frequent basis, a variety of algorithms are being introduced to enhance the treatment of recurrent neurocardiogenic syncope when pacing is required. Histograms and other event counter diagnostics detailing the performance of these various algorithms and device behavior between scheduled visits facilitate the clinician's ability to fully evaluate the performance of the implanted pacing system. Although we are not yet at the "set it and forget it" stage with the system self-optimizing its own behavior, this is a goal that is on the horizon due to the enhanced sophistication and automaticity enabled by microprocessor technology incorporated in the modern pacemaker.

References

1. Preston TA. Future trends in pacing. Heart Lung 1978;7:781.
2. Auerbach AA, Furman S. The autodiagnostic pacemaker. PACE 1979;2:58–68.
3. Kruse I, Arnman K, Conradson TB, et al. A comparison of the acute and long-term hemodynamic effects of ventricular inhibited and atrial synchronous ventricular inhibited pacing. Circulation 1982;65: 846–855.
4. Davis MJE, Mundin HA, Mews GC, et al. Functional benefits of physiologic compared with ventricular pacing in complete heart block. Clin Prog Electrophysiol Pacing 1985;3:457–460.
5. Fananapazir L, Srinivar V, Bennett DH. Comparison of resting hemodynamic indices and exercise performance during atrial synchronous and asynchronous ventricular pacing. PACE 1983;6:202–209.
6. Faerestrand S, Breivik K, Ohm OJ. Assessment of the work capacity and relationship

between rate response and exercise tolerance associated with activity sensing rate responsive ventricular pacing. PACE 1987; 10:1277–1290.

7. Nordlander R, Hedman A, Pehrsson JK. Rate responsive pacing and exercise capacity (editorial). PACE 1989;12:749–751.

8. Alt E, Matula M, Theres H, et al. The basis for activity controlled rate variable cardiac pacemakers: an analysis of mechanical forces on human body induced by exercise and environment. PACE 1989;12:1667–1680.

9. Humen DP, Kostuk WJ, Klein GJ. Activity-sensing rate responsive pacing: improvement in myocardial performance with exercise. PACE 1985;8:52–59.

10. Benditt DG, Mianulli M, Fetter J, et al. Single-chamber cardiac pacing with activity-initiated chronotropic response: evaluation by cardiopulmonary testing. Circulation 1985;75:184–191.

11. Mond H, Strathmore N, Kertes P, et al. Rate responsive pacing using a minute ventilation sensor. PACE 1988;11:1866–1874.

12. Lau CP, Antoniou A, Ward DE, et al. Initial clinical experience with a minute ventilation sensing rate modulated pacemaker: improvements in exercise capacity and symptomatology. PACE 1988;11:1815–1822.

13. Alt E, Hirgstetter C, Heinz M, et al. Rate control of physiology pacemakers by central venous blood temperature. Circulation 1986;73:1206–1212.

14. Fearnot NE, Smith HJ, Sellers D, et al. Evaluation of the temperature response to exercise testing in patients with single chamber, rate adaptive pacemakers: a multicenter study. PACE 1989;12:1806–1815.

15. Rickards AF, Norman J. Relation between QT interval and heart rate: new design of physiologically adaptive cardiac pacemaker. Br Heart J 1981;45:56–61.

16. Mehta D, Lau CP, Ward DE, et al. Comparative evaluation of chronotropic response of activity sensing and QT sensing rate responsive pacemakers to different activities. PACE 1988;11:1405–1414.

17. Ovyshcher I, Guetta V, Bondy C, et al. First derivative of right ventricular pressure, dp/dt, as a sensor for a rate adaptive VVI pacemaker: initial experience, PACE 1992; 15:211–218.

18. Callaghan Fvollmann W, Livingston A, et al. The ventricular depolarization gradient: effects of exercise, pacing rate, epinephrine and intrinsic heart rate control on the right

ventricular evoked response. PACE 1990; 12:1115–1120.

19. Paul V, Garrett C, Ward DE, et al. Closed loop control of rate adaptive pacing, clinical assessment of a system analyzing the ventricular depolarization gradient. PACE 1989;12:1896–1992.

20. Ruiter JH, Heemels JP, Kee D, et al. Adaptive rate pacing controlled by the right ventricular pre-ejection interval: clinical experience with a physiologic pacing system. PACE 1992;15:886–894.

21. Shaldach M. Automatic adjustment of pacing parameters abased on intracardiac impedance measurements. PACE 1990;13: 1702–1710.

22. McGoon MD, Shapland JE, Salo R, et al. The feasibility of utilizing the systolic pre-ejection interval as a determinant of pacing rate. J Am Coll Cardiol 1989;14: 17534–17538.

23. Stangl K, Wirtzfeld A, Gobe G, et al. Rate control with an external SO₂ closed loop system. PACE 1986;9:992–996.

24. Stangl K, Wirtzfeld A, Henize R, et al. First clinical experience with an oxygen saturation controlled pacemaker in man. PACE 1988;11:1182–1887.

25. Soldati E, Bongiorni MG, Arena G, et al. Endocardial acceleration signals detected by a transvenous pacing lead: do they reflect local contractility? PACE 1996;19: 659A.

26. Witte J, Reibis R, Greco OT, et al. Influence of contractility changes on unipolar intracardiac impedance: clinical validation. Eur J Cardiol Pacing Electrophysiol 1996;6:178.

27. Hayes DL. Dual-sensor, rate-adaptive pacemakers: current status. Cardio 1994;11: S17–S25.

28. Griffith M. Advances in rate responsive pacing? Br Heart J 1994;72:405–406.

29. Sulke N, Tan K, Kamalvand K, et al. Dual sensor VVIR mode pacing: is it worth it? PACE 1996;19:1560–1567.

30. Lau CP, Leung SK, Lee ISF. Delayed exercise rate response kinetics due to sensor cross-checking in a dual sensor rate adaptive pacing system: the importance of individual sensor programming, PACE 1996;19: 1021–1025.

31. Benditt DG, Mianulli M, Lurie K, et al. Multiple-sensor systems for physiologic cardiac pacing. Ann Int Med 1994;121:960–968.

32. Gentzler R, Lucas EH, et al. Automatic sensor adjustment in a rate-modulated pacemaker. Eur J Cardiac Pacing Electrophysiol 1996;6:156.

33. Phillippon F, O'Hara G, Desaulniers D, et al. Rate response optimization: a new fully integrated dual sensor DDDR pacemaker. Circulation 1997;96:1–707.

34. Ritter P, Anselme F, Saoudi N, et al. Clinical evaluation of an automatic slope calibration function in a minute ventilation controlled DDDR pacemaker. Proceedings of Europace '97, 8th European Symposium on Cardiac Pacing, 1997, pp 507–511.

35. Clarke JM, Hammer J, Shelton JR, et al. The rhythm of the normal human heart, Lancet 1976;2:508–512.

36. Bjerregaard P. Mean 24 hour heart rate, minimal heart rate and pauses in healthy subjects 40–79 years of age. Eur Heart J 1983;5:44–51.

37. Kostis JB, Moreyra AE, Amendo MT, et al. The effect of age on heart rate in subjects free of heart disease, studies by ambulatory electrocardiography and maximal exercise stress test. Circulation 1982;65:141–145.

38. Chew PH, Bush DE, Engel BT, et al. Overnight heart rate and cardiac function in patients with dual chamber pacemakers. PACE 1996;19:822–828.

39. Lee MT, Baker R. Circadian rhythm variation in rate adaptive pacing systems, PACE 1990;13:1797–1801.

40. Adkins RA, Baker R. Implantable device with circadian rhythm adjustment. U.S. Patent number 5, 143, 065.

41. Bornzin GA, Arambula ER, Florio J, et al. Adjusting heart rate during sleep using activity variance. PACE 1994;17:1933–1938.

42. Wildiers A, de Vusser Ph. Sleep rate pacing based on activity variance. In Sethi KK, ed. Proceedings of VIth Asian Pacific Symposium on Cardiac Pacing and Electrophysiology. Monduzzi Editore Spa, Bologna, Italy, 1997, pp 159–163.

43. Candinas R, Duru F, Buckingham TA, et al. Pacemaker automaticity: automatic rate modulation, when and how to use it? Santini M, ed. Progress in Clinical Pacing, Futura Media Services, Armonk, NY, 1997, pp 321–330.

44. Djordjevic M, Kocovic D, Pavlovic S, et al. Circadian variations of heart rate and Stim-T interval: adaptation for nighttime pacing. PACE 1989;12:1757–1763.

45. Park E, Gibb W, Bornzin G, et al. Next generation of rate-adaptive algorithm using activity. In Vardas PE, ed. Proceedings of Europace '97, 8th European Symposium on Cardiac Pacing. Monduzzi 331i, Editore Spa, Bologna, Italy, 1997, pp 501–505.

46. Rea RF, Thames MD. Neural control mechanisms and vasovagal syncope. J Cardiovasc Electrophysiol 1993;4:587–595.

47. Kosinski D, Grubb BP, Temesy-Armos P. Pathophysiologic aspects of neurocardiogenic synocope: current concepts and new perspectives. PACE 1995;18:716–724.

48. Benditt DG, Petersen M, Lurie KG, et al. Cardiac pacing for prevention of recurrent vasovagal syncope. Ann Int Med 1995;122:204–209.

49. Fitzpatrick AP, Travill CM, Vardas PE, et al. Recurrent symptoms after ventricular pacing in unexplained syncope. PACE 1990;13:619–624.

50. Ahmed R, Guneri S, Ingram A, et al. Double blind comparison of DDI, DDI with rate hysteresis, VVI and VVI with rate hysteresis in symptom control in carotid sinus syndrome. PACE 1991;14:623A.

51. Petersen MEV, Chamberlain-Webber R, Fitzpatrick AP, et al. Permanent pacing for cardioinhibitory malignant vasovagal syndrome. Br Heart J 1994;71:274–281.

52. Gammage MD, Hess M, Markowitz T. Initial experience with a rate drop algorithm in malignant vasovagal syndrome. Eur J Cardiac Pacing Electrophysiol 1995;5:45–48.

53. Sheldon R, Koshman ML, Wilson W, et al. Effect of dual-chamber pacing with automatic rate-drop sensing on recurrent neurally mediated syncope. Am J Cardiol 1998;81:158–162.

54. Sheldon R, Connolly S, Benditt DG, et al. presentation at 1997 Annual Scientific Sessions of NASPE on the North American Vasovagal Pacing Study, May 1997.

55. Mabo P, Druelles P, Kermarrec A, et al. Haemodynamic mechanisms of arterial hypotension in carotid sinus syndrome and of prevention by dual chamber pacing. Eur J Cardiac Pacing Electrophysiol 1992;2:129–138.

56. Crilley JG, Herd B, Khurana CS, et al. Permanent cardiac pacing in elderly patients with recurrent falls, dizziness and syncope and a hypersensitive cardioinhibitory reflex. Postgrad Med J 1997;73:415–418.

57. McIntosh SJ, Lawson J, Bexton RS, et al. A study comparing VVI and DDI pacing in elderly patients with carotid sinus syndrome. Heart 1997;77:553–557.

58. Bana G, Locatelli V, Piatti L, et al. DDI pacing in the bradycardia-tachycardia syndrome. PACE 1990;13:264–270.

59. Markewitz A, Schad N, Hemmer W, et al. What is the most appropriate stimulation mode in patients with sinus node dysfunction. PACE 1986;9:1115–1120.

60. Zimerman L, Geiger M, Newby K, et al. Effects of AV node ablation and pacemaker implantation in patients with depressed

ejection fraction and chronic atrial fibrillation with "normal" ventricular response. Reblampa 1995;8:187–190.

61. Brignole M, Gianfranchi L, Menozzi C, et al. Assessment of atrioventricular junction ablation and DDDR mode switching pacemaker versus pharmacologic treatment of patients with severely symptomatic paroxysmal atrial fibrillation: a randomized controlled study. Circulation 1997;96:2617–2624.

62. Kim SG, Sompalli V, Rameneni A, et al. Symptomatic improvement after AV nodal ablation and pacemaker implantation for refractory atrial fibrillation and atrial flutter. Angiology 1997;48:933–938.

63. Geelen P, Goethals M, de Bruyne B, et al. A prospective hemodynamic evaluation of patients with chronic atrial fibrillation undergoing radiofrequency catheter ablation of the AV junction. Am J Cardiol 1997; 80:1606–1609.

64. Buys EM, van Hemel NM, Kelder JC, et al. Exercise capacity after His bundle ablation and rate response ventricular pacing for drug refractory atrial fibrillation. Heart 1997;77:238–241.

65. Mond HG, Barold SS. Dual chamber, rate adaptive pacing in patients with paroxysmal supraventricular tachyarrhythmias: protective measures for rate control. PACE 1993;16:2168–2185.

66. Ovsyshcher IE, Katz A, Bondy C. Initial experience with a new algorithm for automatic mode switching from DDDR to DDIR mode. PACE 1994;17:1908–1912.

67. Provenier F, Jordaens L, Verstraeten T, et al. The "automatic mode switch" function in successive generations of minute ventilation sensing dual chamber rate responsive pacemakers. PACE 1994;17:1913–1919.

68. den Dulk K, Dijkman B, Pierterse M, et al. Initial experience with mode switching in a dual sensor, dual chamber pacemaker in patients with paroxysmal atrial tachyarrhythmias. PACE 1994;17:1900–1907.

69. Levine PA, Bornzin GA, Barlow J, et al. A new automode switch algorithm for supraventricular tachycardias. PACE 1994;17: 1895–1899.

70. Delay M, Bruls A, Mounier C, et al. Evaluation of a new sensor-based algorithm to protect against atrial arrhythmias. PACE 1996;19:1704–1707.

71. Gencel L, Geroux L, Clementy J, et al. Ventricular protection against atrial arrhythmias in DDD pacing based on a statistical approach, clinical results. PACE 1996;19: 1729–1733.

72. Mayumi H, Matsuzaki K, Kohno H, et al. Effectiveness and limitations of the Fallback I algorithm for transient supraventricular tachyarrhythmias in DDD pacing. J Artif Organs 1996;20:810–814.

73. Bonnet JL, Brusseau E, Limousin M, et al. Mode switch despite undersensing of atrial fibrillation in DDD pacing. PACE 1996;19: 1724–1728.

74. Fahraeus T, Verboven Y, Bruls A. Evaluation of a new sensor-based protection algorithm in patients with paroxysmal atrial arrhythmias. Heartweb, 1996, 2: article number 96110018, http://www.webaxis.com/heartweb/1196/pacing0001.htm.

75. Kamalvand K, Kotsakis A, Tan K, et al. Evaluation of a new pacing algorithm to prevent rapid tracking of atrial tachyarrhythmias. PACE 1996;19:1714–1718.

76. Palma EC, Kedarnath V, Vankawalla V, et al. Effect of varying atrial sensitivity, AV interval and detection algorithm on automatic mode switching. PACE 1996;19: 1734–1739.

77. Kamalvand K, Tan K, Kotsakis A, et al. Is mode switching beneficial? A randomized study in patients with paroxysmal atrial tachyarrhythmias, J Amer Coll Cardiol 1997;30:496–504.

78. Ellenbogen KA, Mond HG, Wood MA, et al. Failure of automatic mode switching, recognition and management. PACE 1997; 20:268–275.

79. Levine PA, Florio J, Bornzin GA. Automatic mode switching in the Pacesetter Trilogy DR + and DC + pulse generators. In Sethi KK, ed. Proceedings of the VIth Asian Pacific Symposium of Cardiac Pacing and Electrophysiology, Monduzzi Editore S.p.A, Bologna, Italy, 1997, pp 167–174.

80. Mond HG, Sparks PB, Jayaprakash S. Dual chamber, rate adaptive pacing in patients with paroxysmal supraventricular tachyarrhythmias, the role of automatic mode conversion algorithms. In Sethi KK, ed. Proceedings of the VIth Asian Pacific Symposium of Cardiac Pacing and Electrophysiology, Monduzzi Editore S.p.A, Bologna, Italy, 1997, pp 153–157.

81. Akhtar M. Retrograde conduction in man. PACE 1981;4:548–562.

82. Narula OS. Retrograde pre-excitation, comparison of antegrade and retrograde conduction intervals in man. Circulation 1974; 50:1129–1143.

83. Goldreyer BN, Bigger JT. Ventriculo-atrial conduction in man. Circulation 1970;41: 935–946.

84. Westveer DC, Stewart JR, Goodfleish R, et al. Prevalence and significance of ventric-

ulo-atrial conduction. PACE 1984;7:784–789.

85. Klementowicz P, Ausubel K, Furman S. The dynamic nature of ventriculoatrial conduction. PACE 1986;9:1050–1054.

86. Hayes DL, Furman S. Atrio-ventricular and ventriculo-atrial conduction times in patients undergoing pacemaker implant. PACE 1983;6:38–46.

87. Rubin JW, Frank MJ, Boineau JP, et al. Current physiologic pacemakers: a serious problem with a new device. Am J Cardiol 1983;52:88–91.

88. Harthorne JW, Eisenhauer AC, Steinhaus DM. Pacemaker-mediated tachycardias: an unresolved problem. PACE 1984;7: 1140–1147.

89. den Dulk K, Lindemans FW, Bar FW, et al. Pacemaker related tachycardias. PACE 1982;5:476–485.

90. Furman S, Fisher JD. Endless loop tachycardia in an AV universal (DDD) pacemaker. PACE 1982;5:486–489.

91. Levine PA, Selznick L. Prospective management of the patient with retrograde ventriculoatrial conduction; prevention and management of pacemaker mediated endless loop tachycardias, Pacesetter Inc, 1990 (Sylmar, CA).

92. Levine PA. Postventricular atrial refractory periods and pacemaker mediated tachycardias. Clin Prog Pacing Electrophysiol 1983; 1:394–401.

93. Haffajee C, Murphy J, Gold R, et al. Automatic extension vs programmability of the atrial refractory period in the prevention of pacemaker mediated tachycardia. PACE 1985;8:A–56A.

94. den Dulk K, Hamersa M, Wellens HJJ. Role of adaptable atrial refractory period for DDD pacemakers. PACE 1987;10:425A.

95. Satler LF, Rackley CE, Pearle DL, et al. Inhibition of a physiologic pacing system due to its anti-pacemaker mediated tachycardia mode. PACE 1985;8:806–810.

96. Cranefield PF, Aronson RS. Torsade de pointes and other pause-induced ventricular tachycardias: the short-long-short sequence and early after depolarizations. PACE 1988;11:670–678.

97. Alt E, Coenen M, Baedeker W, et al. Ventricular tachycardia initiated solely by reduced pacing rate during routine pacemaker follow-up. Clin Cardiol 1996;19:668–671.

98. Karbenn U, Borggrefe M, Breithardt G. Pacemaker-induced ventricular tachycardia in normally functioning demand pacemakers. Am J Cardiol 1989;63:120–122.

99. Goldman DS, Levine PA. Pacemaker me-

diated polymorphic ventricular tachycardia, PACE 1998 (in press).

100. van Gelder LM, El Gamal MIH. Ventriculoatrial conduction: a cause of atrial malpacing in AV universal pacemakers: a report of two cases. PACE 1985;8:140–143.

101. Barold SS. Repetitive reentrant and nonreentrant ventriculoatrial synchrony in dual chamber pacing. Clin Cardiol 1991;14: 754–763.

102. van Gelder LM, El Gamal MIH, Baker R, et al. Tachycardia-termination algorithm: a valuable feature for interruption of pacemaker-mediated tachycardia, PACE 1984;7: 283–287.

103. Duncan JL, Clark MF. Prevention and termination of pacemaker-mediated tachycardia in a new DDD pacing system (Siemens Pacesetter model 2010T). PACE 1988;11: 1679–1683.

104. Limousin M, Bonnet JL, et al. A new algorithm to solve endless loop tachycardia in DDD pacing: a multicenter study of 91 patients. PACE 1990;13:867–874.

105. Cameron DA, Gentzler RD, Love CJ, et al. Initial clinical experience with a new automatic PMT detection and termination algorithm to discriminate between pacemaker mediated tachycardia due to ventriculoatrial conduction and normal sinus tachycardia. Heartweb 1996; 2: article 96110035, http://www.webaxis.com/1196/pacing 0018.htm.

106. Ritter P, Daubert C, Mabo P, et al. Hemodynamic benefit of a rate adapted AV delay in dual chamber pacing. Eur Heart J 1989; 10:637–646.

107. Ritter P, Vai F, Bonnet JL, et al. Rate adaptive atrioventricular delay improves cardiopulmonary performance in patients implanted with a dual chamber pacemaker for complete heart block. Eur J Cardiac Pacing Electrophysiol 1991;1:31–38.

108. Sulke AN, Chambers JB, Sowton E. The effect of atrioventricular delay programming in patients with DDDR pacemakers. Eur Heart J 1992;13:464–472.

109. Rosenqvist M, Isaaz K, Botvinick EH, et al. Relative importance of activation sequence compared to atrioventricular synchrony in left ventricular function. Am J Cardiol 1991; 67:148–156.

110. LeClercq C, Gras D, Le Helloco A, et al. Hemodynamic importance of preserving the normal sequence of ventricular activation in permanent cardiac pacing. Am Heart J 1995;129:1133–1141.

111. Harper GR, Pina IL, Kutalek SP. Intrinsic conduction maximizes cardiopulmonary

performance in patients with dual chamber pacemakers. PACE 1991;14:1787–1791.

112. Jutzy RV, Feenstra L, Pai R, et al. Comparison of intrinsic versus paced ventricular function. PACE 1992;15:1919–1922.

113. Pierterse MGC, den Dulk K, van Gelder BM, et al. Programming a long paced atrioventricular interval may be risky in DDDR pacing. PACE 1994;17:252–257.

114. Mayumi H, Kohno H, Yasui H, et al. Use of automatic mode change between DDD and AAI to facilitate native atrioventricular conduction in patients with sick sinus syndrome or transient atrioventricular block. PACE 1996;19:1740–1747.

115. Linde C. The clinical utility of positive and negative AV/PV hysteresis. In Santini M, ed. Progress in Clinical Pacing. Futura Media Services, Armonk, NY, 1997, pp 339–345.

116. Vardas PE, Simantirakis EN, Parthenakis FI, et al. AAIR versus DDDR pacing in patients with impaired sinus node chronotropy: an echocardiographic and cardiopulmonary study. PACE 1997;20:1762–1768.

117. Jeanrenaud X, Schlapfer J, Fromer M, et al. Beneficial effects of atrioventricular junction ablation for optimal left ventricular capture and filling. PACE 1997;20:293–300.

118. Kappenberger L, Linde C, Daubert JC, et al. Pacing in hypertrophic obstructive cardiomyopathy, a randomized cross-over study. Eur Heart J 1997;19:1249–1256.

119. Losi MA, Betocchi S, Briguori C, et al. Dual chamber pacing in hypertrophic cardiomyopathy: influence of atrioventricular delay on left ventricular outflow tract obstruction. Cardiology 1998;89:8–13.

120. Preston TA, Fletcher RD, Lucchesi BR, et al. Changes in myocardial threshold: physiologic and pharmacologic factors in patients with implanted pacemakers. Am Heart J 1967;74:235–242.

121. Dohrmann ML, Goldschlager NF. Myocardial stimulation threshold in patients with cardiac pacemakers: effect of physiologic variables, pharmacologic agents and lead electrodes. Cardiol Clin 1985;3:527–537.

122. Zarling J, Belott P, Sieckhaus J, et al. Is a high voltage output still needed in a new pacemaker. Eur J Cardiac Pacing Electrophysiol 1992;2:254.

123. Schwaab B, Schwerdt H, Heisel A, et al. Chronic ventricular pacing using an output amplitude of 1.0 V. PACE 1997;20:2171–2178.

124. Preston TA, Bowers DL. The automatic threshold tracking pacemaker. Med Inst 1974;8:322–355.

125. Preston TA, Bowers DL. Clinical applications of the threshold tracking pacemaker. Am J Cardiol 1975;36:322–326.

126. Thalen H, Rickards A, Wittkampf F, et al. Evoked response sensing as automatic control of pacemaker output. Cardiac Pacing, Piccin Medical Books, Padova, Italy, 1982, pp 1229–1234.

127. Bolz A, Hubmann M, Hardt R, et al. Low polarization pacing lead for detecting the ventricular evoked response. Med Prog Techno 1993;19:129–137.

128. Brouwer J, Nagelkerke D, de Jongste M, et al. Analysis of the morphology of the unipolar endocardial paced evoked response. PACE 1990;13:302–313.

129. Curtis A, Vance F, Miller K. Automatic reduction of stimulus polarization artifact for accurate evaluation of ventricular evoked responses. PACE 1991;14:529–537.

130. Kadhiresan V, Olive A, Hauck J, et al. Automatic capture verification by charge neutral sensing. PACE 1995;18:116A.

131. Schuller H, Fahraeus T, Thuesen L, et al. First clinical experience with an automatic output adaption pacemaker based on evoked response. PACE 1995;18:115A.

132. Baig MW, Walton C, Economides AP, et al. A comparison of two techniques for the elimination of post-stimulus polarization potentials. Eur J Cardiac Pacing Electrophysiol 1992;2:31–40.

133. Leung ZKC, Lau CP, Leung SK. Feasibility of an automatic atrial and ventricular threshold determination using transthoracic impedance. PACE 1996;19:631A.

134. Alt E, Kriegler C, Fotuhi P, et al. Feasibility of using intracardiac impedance measurement for capture detection. PACE 1992;15:1873–1879.

135. Schuller H, Lindgren A. Principles and utility of autocapture. In Sethi KK, ed. Proceedings of VIᵗʰ Asian Pacific Symposium on Cardiac Pacing and Electrophysiology, Monduzzi Editore S.p.A., Bologna, Italy, 1997, pp 187–192.

136. Ebner E, Hummer A. Autocapture: ein neuer algorithmus zur kontinuierlichen anpassung der stimulations-amplitude an die reizschwelle. Herzschrittmacher 1996;16:114–120.

137. Giovanzana P, Beretta R. Autocapture: benefici e principio di funzionamento. Cardiostimulazion 1995;13:284–289.

138. Sermasi S, Marconi M, Libero L, et al. Italian experience with AutoCapture in conjunction with a membrane lead. PACE 1996;19:1799–1804.

139. Livingston AR, Callaghan FJ, Byrd CL, et al. Atrial capture detection with endocardial electrodes. PACE 1988;11:1770–1776.

140. Bornzin GA, Florio J, Sloman L, et al. Dual-chamber autocapture system algorithm that saves pacing energy and avoids fusion in patients with intact conduction. HeartWeb 1996; 2: article 96110024, http://www.webaxis.com/heartweb/1196/pacing0007.htm.

141. Berg M, Frohlig G, Schwerdt H, et al. Reliability of an automatic sensing algorithm. PACE 1992;15:1880–1885.

142. Wilson JH, Love CJ, Wettenstein EH. Clinical evaluation of an automatic sensitivity adjustment feature in a dual chamber pacemaker. PACE 1990;13:1220–1227.

143. Mauser JF, Huang SKS, Risser T, et al. A unique pulse generator safety feature for bipolar lead fracture. PACE 1993;16: 1368–1372.

144. Gencel L, Clémenty J, Barold SS. Stimucoeur 1996;24:296–298.

Chapter 38

Treatment of Vasovagal Syncope:
Is There a Role for Cardiac Pacing?

David G. Benditt, Keith G. Lurie, Gerard Fahy, Demosthenes Iskos,
Scott Sakaguchi

Introduction

Vasovagal syncope is usually a solitary and relatively innocent event.[1-3] Consequently, prophylactic therapeutic interventions are, more often than not, unnecessary. Furthermore, many vasovagal episodes are clearly attributable to circumstances that can be either avoided or modified. Examples include syncope associated with venipuncture, hot stuffy environments, excessive dehydration, or vigorous physical exercise. In other instances, patients readily learn to anticipate certain common "triggers" such as anger, anxiety, or pain. As a result, they can take evasive action and thereby minimize risk of injury; often this can abort the event entirely.

Despite the generally "benign" nature of vasovagal syncope, there remains a small proportion of affected individuals in whom preventive treatment is important. For example, in certain individuals, recurrent or unusually severe syncopal episodes may cause substantial lifestyle difficulties, economic loss, or physical injury. In others, syncope may have occurred without warning, leading to an excessive risk of accident and physical injury. The latter scenario (i.e.,

absence of warning symptoms) is particularly prevalent in older patients with vasovagal spells.[4] Finally, even infrequent recurrences may be unacceptable in certain individuals such as airline pilots, machinery operators, and drivers of commercial vehicles.

At the present time, apart from education and reassurance, strategies for prevention of vasovagal symptoms largely focus on pharmacological interventions, despite controversy surrounding treatment efficacy. Nonpharmacological treatments, including support hose, exposure to graded periods of upright posture, and in some instances cardiac pacing, tend to be reserved for selected difficult to treat cases. With regard to cardiac pacing in vasovagal syncope, current practice is typically restricted to a relatively small subset of those individuals in whom there appears to be evidence favoring a predominantly cardioinhibitory process.

This chapter reviews the more common approaches to prevention of vasovagal syncope. Particular attention is directed toward the current role of cardiac pacing, findings of recent pacemaker therapy trials, and po-

From Singer I, Barold SS, Camm AJ (eds): Nonpharmacological Therapy of Arrhythmias for the 21st Century: The State of the Art. Futura Publishing Co, Inc., Armonk, NY, © 1998.

tential implantable device developments which may impact future therapy decisions.

Prevention of Recurrent Vasovagal Syncope

Pathophysiological Considerations

In vasovagal syncope, hypotension may be due to marked bradycardia (cardioinhibition), inappropriate peripheral vasodilatation (vasodepression) or, as is most often the case, both (mixed form). Consequently,

it would be of considerable value to understand the relative importance of "cardioinhibitory" and "vasodepressor" components in each patient in order to establish a rational treatment strategy. Thus, patients with severe bradycardia alone may be prime candidates for cardiac pacing therapy (Figure 1), and those individuals with an exclusive vasodepressor response may be better served by focusing on pharmacological and volume control management. Patients with a "mixed" picture may require a combination of techniques. Unfortunately, current diagnostic techniques do not allow

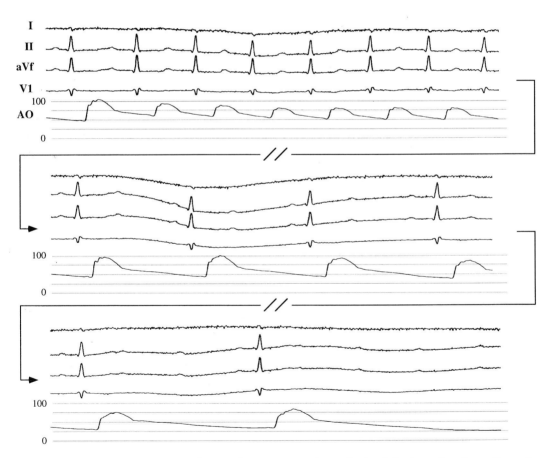

Figure 1. Electrocardiographic and arterial pressure tracings obtained during a head-up tilt study in a young woman with recurrent syncope in the absence of structural heart disease. The tracings are very nearly continuous. As the study progressed, the patient developed paroxysmal AV block of increasing severity. A moderate vasodepressor component is also evident (see lower panel). The latter is evident by the drop in systolic pressure from approximately 105 mm Hg (top panel) to 80–90 mm Hg in the lower panel. Since this patient appears to exhibit predominantly a cardioinhibitory response, cardiac pacing may be an effective treatment option.

adequate differentiation of cardioinhibitory, vasodepressor, and mixed events in most cases. In particular, it is not yet possible to conclude that tilt-table testing results correspond well with spontaneous syncope in terms of the relative magnitudes of cardioinhibitory and vasodepressor components. Further, it remains uncertain whether spontaneous vasovagal events always exhibit the same features in a given individual.

Pharmacological and Nonpharmacological Strategies

In recent years, prevention of vasovagal syncope recurrences has focused on pharmacological interventions, with the apparent efficacy of a wide variety of drugs having been examined.[2,5–17] In uncontrolled studies, beta-adrenergic blocking drugs, disopyramide, certain vasoconstrictor agents (e.g., etilephrine, midodrine), and serotonin re-uptake blockers have been reported to be helpful in preventing syncope recurrences. However, for any of these drugs only a small experience currently exists. The few small controlled studies that have been reported (atenolol, cafedrine, disopyramide, scopolamine, and etilephrine) all have methodological problems. Nonetheless, only one of these studies, using the beta-adrenergic blocker atenolol, has shown a drug benefit over a 1-month follow-up.[15] Outcomes for the remaining agents have tended to question their effectiveness. By way of example, an important international randomized trial examining the efficacy of etilephrine in vasovagal syncope (VASIS trial[18]) recently terminated the drug-testing arm due to an apparent greater frequency of syncope in the "active" medication group than among controls. A cardiac pacing arm of this study is ongoing.

Volume expanders (e.g., fludrocortisone, salt tablets) are also commonly utilized in the pharmacological management of vasovagal syncope. In general, although attempts at maintaining central volume seem

to make sense on theoretical grounds, the utility of these agents is even less well delineated than has been the case for the drugs listed above. Finally, belladonna alkaloids (e.g., scopolamine) and purinergic antagonists, such as theophylline, have received only very limited evaluation. They do, however, appear to be helpful in selected cases.

Nonpharmacological approaches to prevention of vasovagal syncope include stress and anxiety management, development of insight into recognition and avoidance of provoking events, and education regarding useful evasive actions (e.g., lying or sitting down as soon as premonitory symptoms appear). In some cases, exposure to a "controlled" faint using tilt-table technique can be beneficial by facilitating earlier and more accurate recognition of warning symptoms, and by reducing anxiety and apprehension. As an extension of the latter concept, Reybrouck et al.[19] have recently described the successful use of head-up tilt conditioning as a means of treatment to prevent vasovagal syncope recurrences. Anti-gravity clothing, such as support hose, also fall into the category of nonpharmacological treatments; unfortunately, this approach is often perceived by patients as being inconvenient and uncomfortable thereby leading to poor compliance.

Not infrequently, combination therapy is needed. Thus, education, volume expansion, drugs, and support hose may be necessary in a very difficult to treat patient. In some individuals, the addition of cardiac pacing to a pharmacological regimen may also be of value. In the not too distant future, more sophisticated implantable systems having both pacing and drug infusion capabilities may become available for the most difficult cases.

Role of Tilt-Table Testing in Treatment Selection

In the past decade, tilt-table testing has become widely used both to better understand the pathophysiology of vasovagal syncope and to assess the efficacy of proposed therapies. In regard to the latter, reproducibility of the test is an important issue. The reproducibility of tilt-table testing in terms of inducing syncope has been the subject of a number of studies. In general, there has been a relatively high concordance of outcomes within individuals (approximately 80%-85%) for two tests carried out either on the same day or many days apart.[20–23] However, the intrapatient reproducibility of cardioinhibitory versus vasodepressor characteristics during induced vasovagal spells has been less well characterized. In one of the earliest examinations of this issue, Chen et al.[20] reported outcomes of two sequential 80° head-up tilt tests (approximately 1 hour apart) in 23 patients (6.5–74 years) undergoing evaluation for recurrent syncope of unknown origin. Overall, 15 of the 23 (65%) individuals developed syncope in either the first or second tilt procedure, while eight patients remained asymptomatic. The findings in the two tests were concordant with respect to provocation of syncope (i.e., positive in both tests or negative in both tests) in 20 of 23 (87%) of cases. Furthermore, there was a strong concordance in terms of heart rate and hemodynamic findings in each of the tests suggesting that these characteristics of the induced episodes also tended to be reproducible within a given patient. On the other hand, Fish et al.[24] found that although syncope or presyncope was reproduced by tilt-table testing in the majority of cases, the pattern of physiological response (i.e., cardioinhibitory, vasodepressor, mixed) varied. Thus, despite a 67% reproducibility rate (with respect to symptoms), the utility of head-up tilt testing as a useful method for assessing therapeutic interventions was questioned. Additional studies providing even more careful evaluation of moment-to-moment heart rate and blood pressure changes are needed.

Clinical Endpoints for Evaluating Treatment Efficacy

The establishment of realistic endpoints for assessing treatment efficacy in vasova-gal syncope patients is crucial. In this regard, it is highly unlikely that any tolerable intervention will entirely eliminate all events. Furthermore, in the absence of a life-threatening condition (which is almost always the case for vasovagal syncope) a goal of total symptom elimination would almost certainly expose patients to an excessively high risk of adverse treatment effects, particularly drug toxicity. Therefore, endpoints comparable to those proposed for evaluation of drug treatment in supraventricular tachycardias are more appropriate for future clinical trials.[25–27] Specifically, the number of symptomatic episodes, the duration of symptom-free intervals, the presence or absence of a premonitory phase, and the occurrence of physical injury or accident should be reported.

In regard to the method of patient follow-up, it seems premature to assess effectiveness of a candidate treatment based solely on repeated tilt-table testing. Currently the value of such an approach for predicting long-term treatment benefit outside the laboratory is unknown. Consequently, randomized and appropriately controlled trials utilizing spontaneous "endpoints" such as those outlined above are essential. To date, with the possibility of one very recent exception, all reported clinical studies of treatment efficacy suffer from important endpoint assessment limitations, inadequate controls, or absence of randomization. Consequently, their interpretation must be undertaken with caution.

Status of Pacing for Vasovagal Syncope

Guidelines from several major professional societies (American Heart Association/American College of Cardiology,[28] British Pacing and Electrophysiology Working Group[29]) provide a class II indication for pacing in vasovagal syncope. Nevertheless, in contrast to a closely related condition, carotid sinus syndrome, where cardiac pacing is often the cornerstone of the treatment plan, pacing has been relatively infrequently utilized in vasovagal syncope.

Several factors may account for the marked difference in therapeutic approach to carotid sinus syncope and vasovagal syncope. First, physical injury is a greater concern in the usually older patients with carotid sinus syndrome. Second, there is a widespread clinical impression that the cardioinhibitory component is more consistent and important in carotid sinus syndrome than in vasovagal syncope. Third, a substantial percentage of vasovagal fainters are young otherwise healthy individuals who would be reluctant to accept pacemakers. Finally, unlike for carotid sinus syndrome,[30–36] there have been only a limited number of reports demonstrating benefits of pacing in vasovagal syncope, and most of these incorporate only a small number of patients followed for a brief period.

Clinical Studies of Cardiac Pacing in Vasovagal Syncope

The potential utility of cardiac pacing for treatment of patients with recurrent vasovagal syncope has only recently become a subject of substantial clinical interest. In an early study of this issue, Fitzpatrick et al.[37] reported findings in two patients who originally received single chamber ventricular pacemakers in an attempt to prevent syncope of unknown origin. However, symptoms later recurred in both cases. Subsequent tilt-table testing not only confirmed susceptibility to neurally mediated hypotension/bradycardia (i.e., vasovagal mechanism) in these individuals, but also suggested that symptomatic hypotension was probably aggravated by ventricular pacing (i.e., "pacemaker effect"). Following conversion of the pacing systems to dual chamber modes (DDI mode, with a basic rate of 50 bpm) and a bradycardia (<50 bpm) triggered hysteresis rate of 80 bpm, one of the two patients became asymptomatic and the other continued to experience symptoms.

In a later prospective evaluation of the effects of temporary dual chamber pacing in vasovagal syncope, Fitzpatrick et al.[38] examined hemodynamic and symptom status in seven patients with recurrent syncope and reproducible vasovagal reactions during tilt studies on 2 successive days. The pacing protocol in this study utilized a hysteresis feature in which the base rate was 50 bpm with an intervention pacing rate of 90 bpm. With these settings, pacing was associated with greater cardiac index (baseline, 1.0 ± 0.2 L/min/m^2 vs. paced 1.6 ± 0.3 L/min/m^2) and mean arterial blood pressure (baseline 30 ± 11 mm Hg vs. paced 48 ± 12 mm Hg), and longer head-up tilt tolerance during induced vasovagal reactions. Further, in five cases syncope was prevented despite evident onset of a vasovagal reaction. Two other patients exhibited no apparent symptomatic benefit.

Samoil et al.[39] have also examined the effects of temporary pacing during tilt-table study. Six patients were evaluated in the baseline unpaced state, during single chamber ventricular pacing, and again during dual chamber cardiac pacing. The pacing algorithm used rate hysteresis with an intervention pacing rate set to 20 bpm above resting rate. Findings indicated that with respect to endpoints such as time to onset of symptoms or total tolerated upright tilt time, ventricular pacing proved to be essentially ineffective. On the other hand, dual chamber pacing significantly improved upright tilt tolerance (dual chamber pacing, 25 ± 6 min vs. unpaced, 12 ± 6 min). In addition, dual chamber pacing prevented syncope during tilt-table testing in three of six patients. Finally, in a somewhat larger study, Sra et al.[40] examined the impact of temporary conventional cardiac pacing techniques for prevention of tilt-induced hypotension and bradycardia in 22 syncope patients in whom an initial tilt-test was associated with bradycardia of presumably sufficient magnitude (heart rate nadir <60 bpm) to trigger a pacing system. The pacing intervention rate was set at approximately 20% higher than the supine resting heart rate, and was initiated while the patient was supine, and was continued throughout the tilt. Twenty patients were evaluated during

AV sequential pacing, while two others with atrial fibrillation were tested in a single chamber ventricular pacing mode. Findings revealed that despite pacing, mean arterial pressure fell significantly during upright tilt. However, the magnitude of tilt-induced hypotension was less during pacing than during tilt-testing undertaken in the baseline untreated state (blood pressure decline, paced 41 ± 19 vs. unpaced $59 \pm \pm 16$). Furthermore, symptoms were much improved. One patient remained asymptomatic and one other complained of dizziness but was not hypotensive during pacing. Fifteen patients had only presyncopal symptoms while five developed syncope. In contrast, all had been syncopal in the baseline state. In essence, pacing proved to be remarkably effective in converting syncope to less severe manifestations of vasovagal reactions (i.e., presyncope) in a considerable percentage of patients in this study.

The strongest evidence supporting a potential long-term benefit of pacing in vasovagal syncope was the report by Petersen et al.[41] examining the effectiveness of pacing in 37 patients in whom vasovagal syncope appeared to exhibit a predominantly cardioinhibitory character as assessed by tilt-testing. The devices were programmed to the DDI mode to detect at heart rates in the 40–50 bpm range, and respond with pacing rates of 80–90 bpm. Patients were followed for 39 ± 19 months. Symptomatic improvement was noted in 84% of cases, with complete resolution of symptoms in 35%. The overall frequency of syncopal episodes (annual syncope burden) was reduced approximately tenfold.

To date, there has been only one completed prospective randomized controlled trial of pacing in vasovagal syncope, the North American Vasovagal Pacemaker Study.[42] An interim unpublished analysis of findings from this study was provided in the spring of 1997, after the study had been terminated due to having achieved a statistically significant result earlier than originally anticipated. The principal clinical endpoint was syncope recurrence.[42] Syncope

patients qualified for inclusion if they had both a positive head-up tilt test and either or both of (1) at least six syncopal episodes preceding the tilt test, or (2) at least one syncope recurrence within 6 months of a positive tilt test. Additionally, during the tilt test, patients had to exhibit degrees of bradycardia exceeding certain preestablished thresholds. In the interim analysis, 24 patients were randomized to pacing (22 of 24 received devices) and 22 were randomized to no pacemaker. Syncope recurrence occurred in 4 of 24 of the pacemaker group and 13 of 22 control patients, resulting in an actuarial 1-year rate of recurrent syncope of 18.5% for pacemaker patients and 59.7% for controls. A detailed assessment of these results cannot be provided until a complete report is published by the investigators. Nevertheless, the findings seem to further support the view that cardiac pacing does offer benefit to a select group of very symptomatic vasovagal fainters.

Optimal Pacing Modes for Vasovagal Syncope

Although much remains unknown regarding the efficacy of cardiac pacing in vasovagal syncope, experience to date has provided insight into both pacing mode selection and potentially useful stimulation algorithms. In general, the most important observation is that a dual chamber pacing mode is essential. Atrial pacing (AAI, AAIR modes) alone is contraindicated due to the potential for transient AV block during vasovagal events (a concern also well known in carotid sinus syndrome). Similarly, an atrial tracking mode alone (e.g., VDD or VDDR) is inadequate since the atrial rate is almost always inappropriately slow for the magnitude of hypotension.[43] A modified DDI or DDIR pacing mode appears to be the best option to turn to after detection of an event. At other times, the patient should be permitted to remain in a more physiological DDD or DDDR pacing mode.

The optimum pacing algorithm for use during an impending vasovagal episode is as yet unclear. Nevertheless, a form of rate hysteresis appears to be necessary. Essentially, after the pacing system detects what appears to be an imminent vasovagal event, the pulse generator responds by pacing at a rate rapid enough to overcome or at least stabilize the developing hypotension. Based on available clinical experience, the intervention rate probably needs to be in the range of 110–120 bpm. Periodically, the device will need to terminate pacing and assess native heart rate. If the latter has returned to normal, the pacing sequence will terminate. If not, a further period of pacing support will be offered. Unfortunately, it is not yet possible to monitor and respond to an even more crucial parameter, systemic pressure.

Possible Future Developments

Vasovagal Episode Detection and Implantable Device Therapy

At the present time, detection of vasovagal syncope relies solely on recognition of relatively abrupt heart rate slowing, a marker that we have learned may not be sufficiently sensitive, and lacks adequate specificity (e.g., detection of abrupt heart rate slowings during sleep have been an issue of concern). Consequently, it would be desirable for future pacing systems to collect additional information and correlate this information with the heart rate findings. For example, markers of change in systemic pressure, respiratory and heart rate variability, and PR or QT intervals could prove helpful. The goal is to provide more sensitive and specific recognition of vasovagal syndromes at an earlier stage in the progression of events. Furthermore, application of one or more of these alternative sensors would allow extension of implantable device therapy, perhaps through a drug delivery system, to those patients who never develop severe bradycardia during their faints.

Currently, pacing interventions are initiated only after onset of bradycardia. However, since vasodilatation tends to precede marked heart rate slowing, late onset pacing may not be able to compensate sufficiently. Conceivably, pacing at an earlier stage could enhance treatment effectiveness. In this regard, the findings from Sra et al.,[40] in which pacing was initiated in the supine posture prior to tilt, are supportive of this notion. On the other hand, Sutton.[44] had less success when pacing was manually triggered at what appeared to be an early stage of the vasovagal event. Further study of this concept is needed.

The combination of drug infusion systems with pacemaker therapy may be a necessary strategy in order to treat the most troublesome forms of vasovagal syncope. Agents such as midodrine, ephedrine, or perhaps even disopyramide could be candidates for parenteral delivery. However, before such an approach becomes feasible, considerable progress must be made both in the development of diagnostic algorithms and in our understanding of drug dosing and routes of delivery.

Conclusion

Several lines of evidence suggest that cardiac pacing may be a useful adjunctive therapy in selected patients with recurrent troublesome vasovagal syncope. However, maximum benefit may not be attainable until a number of important barriers are overcome, namely: (1) development of practicable techniques that permit implantable systems to recognize vasovagal syncope at an early stage; (2) a better understanding of the most effective pacing algorithms; and (3) combining pacing systems with as yet evolving physiological sensor technologies and drug infusion systems.

Acknowledgment: The authors would like to thank Barry L.S. Detloff for technical assistance and Wendy Markuson for preparation of the manuscript.

References

1. Benditt DG, Ferguson DW, Grubb BP, et al. Tilt-table testing for assessing syncope. An American College of Cardiology expert consensus document. J Am Coll Cardiol 1996; 28(1):263–275.

2. Benditt DG, Sakaguchi S, Schultz JJ, et al. Syncope: diagnostic considerations and the role of tilt table testing. Cardiol Rev 1993;1: 146–156.

3. Kapoor W. Evaluation and outcome of patients with syncope. Medicine 1990;69: 160–175.

4. Fitzpatrick A, Theodorakis G, Vardas P, et al. The incidence of malignant vasovagal syndrome in patients with recurrent syncope. Eur Heart J 1991;12:389–394.

5. Raviele A, Gasparini G, Di Pede F, et al. Usefulness of head-up tilt test in evaluating patients with syncope of unknown origin and negative electrophysiological study. Am J Cardiol 1990;65:1322–1327.

6. Kosinski DJ, Grubb BP. Neurally mediated syncope with an update on indications and usefulness of head-up tilt table testing and pharmacologic therapy. Curr Opin Cardiol 1994;9:53–64.

7. Milstein S, Buetikofer J, Dunnigan A, et al. Usefulness of disopyramide for prevention of upright tilt-induced hypotension-bradycardia. Am J Cardiol 1990;65:1339–1344.

8. Fitzpatrick AP, Ahmed R, Williams S, et al. A randomised trial of medical therapy in "malignant vasovagal syndrome" or "neurally-mediated bradycardia hypotension syndrome." Eur J Cardiac Pacing Electrophysiol 1991;2:99–102.

9. Nelson S, Stanley M, Love C, et al. Autonomic and hemodynamic effects of oral theophylline in patients with vasodepressor syncope. Arch Intern Med 1991;90:2425–2429.

10. Brignole M, Menozzi C, Gianfranchi L, et al. A controlled trial of acute and long-term medical therapy in tilt-induced neurally-mediated syncope. Am J Cardiol 1992;70: 339–342.

11. Sra JS, Murthy VS, Jazayeri MR, et al. Use of intravenous esmolol to predict efficacy of oral adrenergic blocker therapy in patients with neurocardiogenic syncope. J Am Coll Cardiol 1993;19:402–408.

12. Morillo C, Leitch JW, Yee R, et al. A placebo-controlled trial of intravenous and oral disopyramide for prevention of neurally mediated syncope induced by head-up tilt. J Am Coll Cardiol 1993;22:1843–1848.

13. Grubb BP, Wolfe D, Samoil D, et al. Useful-ness of fluoxetine hydrochloride for prevention of resistent upright tilt-induced syncope. PACE 1993;16:458–464.

14. Kosinski DJ, Grubb BP, Temesy-Armos PN. The use of serotonin re-uptake inhibitors in the treatment of neurally mediated cardiovascular disorders. J Serotonin Res 1994;1: 85–90.

15. Mahanonda N, Bhuripanyo K, Kangkagate C, et al. Randomized double-blind placebo-controlled trial of oral atenolol in patients with unexplained syncope and positive upright tilt table results. Am Heart J 1995;130: 1250–1253.

16. Moya A, Permanyer-Miralda G, Sagrista-Sauleda J, et al. Limitations of head-up tilt test for evaluating the efficacy of therapeutic interventions in patients with vasovagal syncope: results of a controlled study of etilephrine versus placebo. J Am Coll Cardiol 1995;25:65–69.

17. Jankovic J, Hiner BC, Brown DC, et al. Neurogenic orthostatic hypotension: a double-blind placebo-controlled study with midodrine. Am J Med 1993;95:38–48.

18. Sutton R, Petersen M, Brignole M, et al. Proposed classification for tilt-induced vasovagal syncope. Eur J Cardiac Pacing Electrophysiol 1992;2:180–183.

19. Reybrouck T, Ector H, Heidbuchel H, et al. Tilt training: a new treatment for recurrent neurocardiogenic syncope and severe orthostatic intolerance. PACE 1997;20(Pt 2):1441.

20. Chen XC, Chen MY, Remole S, et al. Reproducibility of head up tilt table testing for eliciting susceptibility to neurally mediated syncope in patients without structural heart disease. Am J Cardiol 1992;69:755–760.

21. Sheldon R, Splawinski J, Killam S. Reproducibility of upright tilt-table tests in patients with syncope. Am J Cardiol 1992;69: 1300–1305.

22. Grubb BP, Wolfe D, Temesy-Armos P, et al. Reproducibility of head upright tilt-table test results in patients with syncope. PACE 1992; 15:1477–1481.

23. Brooks R, Ruskin JN, Powell AC, et al. Prospective evaluation of day-to-day reproducibility of tilt-table testing in unexplained syncope. Am J Cardiol 1993;71:1289–1292.

24. Fish FA, Strasburger JF, Benson DW Jr. Reproducibility of a symptomatic response to upright tilt in young patients with unexplained syncope. Am J Cardiol 1992;70: 605–609.

25. Pritchett EL, Smith MS, McCarthy EA, et al. The spontaneous occurrence of paroxysmal

supraventricular tachycardia. Circulation 1984;70:1–6.

26. Greer GS, Wilkinson WE, McCarthy EA, et al. Random and nonrandom behavior of symptomatic paroxysmal atrial fibrillation. Am J Cardiol 1989;64:339–342.

27. Clair WK, Wilkinson WE, McCarthy EA, et al. Spontaneous occurrence of symptomatic paroxysmal atrial fibrillation and paroxysmal supraventricular tachycardia in untreated patients. Circulation 1993;87:1114–1122.

28. Dreifus LS, Fisch C, Griffin JC, et al. Guidelines for implantation of cardiac pacemakers and antiarrhythmia devices. American Heart Association/American College of Cardiology Task Force report. J Am Coll Cardiol 1991;18:1–13.

29. British Pacing and Electrophysiology Group Working Party. Recommendations for pacemaker prescription for symptomatic bradycardia. Br Heart J 1991;66:185–191.

30. Sugrue DD, Gersh BJ, Holmes DR, et al. Symptomatic "isolated" carotid sinus hypersensitivity: natural history and results of treatment with anticholinergic drugs or pacemaker. J Am Coll Cardiol 1986;7:158–162.

31. Morley CA, Perrins EJ, Grant P, et al. Carotid sinus syncope treated by pacing: analysis of persistent symptoms and role of atrioventricular sequential pacing. Br Heart J 1982;47:411–418.

32. Morley CA, Perrins EJ, Chan SL, et al. Long-term comparison of DVI and VVI pacing in carotid sinus syndrome. In Steinbach K, ed. Cardiac Pacing. Proceedings of the VIIth World Symposium on Cardiac Pacing. Steinkopff Verlag, Darmstadt, 1983, pp 929–935.

33. Madigan NP, Flaker GC, Curtis JJ, et al. Carotid sinus hypersensitivity: beneficial effects of dual-chamber pacing. Am J Cardiol 1984;53:1034–1040.

34. Brignole M, Sartore B, Barra M, et al. Is DDD superior to VVI pacing in mixed carotid sinus syndrome? An acute and medium-term study. PACE 1988;11:1902–1910.

35. Brignole M, Sartore B, Barra M, et al. Ventricular and dual chamber pacing for treatment of carotid sinus syndrome. PACE 1989;12:582–590.

36. Deschamps D, Richard A, Citron B, et al. Hypersensibilite sino-carotidienne. Evolution a moyen et a long terme des patients traites par stimulation ventriculaire. Arch Mal Coeur 1990;83:63–67.

37. Fitzpatrick AP, Travill CM, Vardas PE, et al. Recurrent symptoms after ventricular pacing in unexplained syncope. PACE 1990;13:619–624.

38. Fitzpatrick AP, Theodorakis G, Ahmed R, et al. Dual chamber pacing aborts vasovagal syncope induced by head-up 60 degree tilt. PACE 1991;14:13–19.

39. Samoil D, Grubb BP, Brewster P, et al. Comparison of single and dual chamber pacing techniques in prevention of upright tilt induced vasovagal syncope. Eur J Cardiac Pacing Electrophysiol 1993;1:36–41.

40. Sra J, Jazayeri MR, Avitall B, et al. Comparison of cardiac pacing with drug therapy in the treatment of neurocardiogenic (vasovagal) syncope with bradycardia or asystole. N Engl J Med 1993;328:1085–1090.

41. Petersen MEV, Chamberlain-Webber R, Fitzpatrick AP, et al. Permanent pacing for cardio-inhibitory malignant vasovagal syndrome. Br Heart J 1994;71:274–281.

42. Sheldon RS, Gent M, Roberts RS, et al, on behalf of the NAVPAC Investigators. North American Vasovagal Pacemaker Study: study design and organization. PACE 1997;20:844–848.

43. Petersen MEV, Price D, Williams T, et al. Short AV interval DDD pacing does not prevent tilt induced vasovagal syncope in patients with cardioinhibitory vasovagal syndrome. PACE 1994;17:882–891.

44. Sutton R. Personal communication.

Index